D1508418

Fundamentals of

COMPLEMENTARY AND INTEGRATIVE MEDICINE

THIRD EDITION

Fundamentals of

COMPLEMENTARY AND INTEGRATIVE MEDICINE

MARC S. MICOZZI, MD, PhD
Director
Informatics Institute for Complementary and Integrative Medicine
Bethesda, MD

Former Director
Center for Complementary and Integrative Medicine
Thomas Jefferson University
Philadelphia, PA

Senior Fellow
Health Studies Collegium
Sterling, VA
and
American Society for Integrative Medicine
Washington, DC

With forward by C. EVERETT KOOP, MD, ScD
Former Surgeon Genaral of the United States

THIRD EDITION

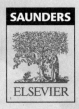

SAUNDERS

ELSEVIER

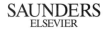

SAUNDERS
ELSEVIER

11830 Westline Industrial Drive
St. Louis, Missouri 63146

FUNDAMENTALS OF COMPLEMENTARY
AND INTEGRATIVE MEDICINE
Copyright © 2006, 2001, 1996 by Elsevier Inc.

ISBN-13: 978-1-4160-2583-2
ISBN-10: 1-4160-2583-9

All rights reserved. No part of this publication may be reproduced or transmitted in any form or by any means, electronic or mechanical, including photocopying, recording, or any information storage and retrieval system, without permission in writing from the publisher.
Permissions may be sought directly from Elsevier's Health Sciences Rights Department in Philadelphia, PA, USA: phone: (+1) 215 239 3804, fax: (+1) 215 239 3805, e-mail: healthpermissions@elsevier.com. You may also complete your request on-line via the Elsevier homepage (http://www.elsevier.com), by selecting 'Customer Support' and then 'Obtaining Permissions'.

Notice

Knowledge and best practice in this field are constantly changing. As new research and experience broaden our knowledge, changes in practice, treatment and drug therapy may become necessary or appropriate. Readers are advised to check the most current information provided (i) on procedures featured or (ii) by the manufacturer of each product to be administered, to verify the recommended dose or formula, the method and duration of administration, and contraindications. It is the responsibility of the practitioner, relying on their own experience and knowledge of the patient, to make diagnoses, to determine dosages and the best treatment for each individual patient, and to take all appropriate safety precautions. To the fullest extent of the law, neither the Publisher nor the Editors assumes any liability for any injury and/or damage to persons or property arising out or related to any use of the material contained in this book.

The Publisher

Third Edition

ISBN-13: 978-1-4160-2583-2
ISBN-10: 1-4160-2583-9

Publishing Director: Linda Duncan
Acquisitions Editor: Kellie White
Developmental Editor: Kim Fons
Publishing Services Manager: Melissa Lastarria
Project Manager: JoAnn Amore
Designer: Jyotika Shroff
Cover Art: Jyotika Shroff

Printed in the United States of America.

Last digit is the print number: 10 9 8 7 6 5 4 3 2

Working together to grow
libraries in developing countries

www.elsevier.com | www.bookaid.org | www.sabre.org

ELSEVIER   BOOK AID International   Sabre Foundation

Contributors

PATCH ADAMS, MD
Executive Director of
Gesundheit Institute
Arlington, Virginia

AMY L. AI, PhD
Associate Professor
Health Sciences
University of Washington
Seattle, Washington
and Cardiac Rehabilitation Affiliated Researcher
University of Michigan Health System
Ann Arbor, Michigan

HAKIMA AMRI, PhD
Assistant Professor
Director, Master's of Science Program in Physiology
with Complementary and Alternative Medicine Track
Department of Physiology and Biophysics
Georgetown University School of Medicine
Washington, D.C.

GERARD C. BODEKER, EdD
Adjunct Professor of Epidemiology,
Columbia University
Senior Clinical Lecturer in Public Health,
University of Oxford Medical School
Clinical Medicine
University of Oxford
Oxford, United Kingdom

MICHAEL CARLSTON, MD
Santa Rosa, California

CLAIRE MONOD CASSIDY, PhD, DIPL AC, LAC
Paradigms Found Consulting
Windpath Healing Works LLC
Bethesda, Maryland

PATRICK COUGHLIN, PhD
Professor
Department of Anatomy
Philadelphia College of Osteopathic Medicine
Philadelphia, Pennsylvania

ELLIOT DACHER, MD
Aquinnah, Massachusetts

VICTOR DOUVILLE
(Sicangu-Lakota)
Lakota Studies Department
Sinte Gleska University
Mission, South Dakota

E. DANIEL EDWARDS, DSW
Professor of Social Work
Director of American Indian Studies
University of Utah
Salt Lake City, Utah

KEVIN V. ERGIL, MA, MS, LAC
Director, Graduate Program in Oriental Medicine
Associate Professor, Graduate Program in Oriental Medicine
Touro College
New York, New York

SUSAN M. GERIK, MD
Associate Professor of Pediatrics and Family
Medicine
University of Texas Medical Branch at Galveston
Galveston, Texas

HOWARD HALL, PhD, PsyD
Department of Pediatrics
Case University and
Rainbow Babies and Children's Hospital
Cleveland, Ohio

MARIANA G. HEWSON, PhD
Professions Education Consultant
Madison, Wisconsin

CAROLINE HOFFMAN, BSW
Registered General Nurse
Complementary Therapies Practitioner
Therapies Director, Breast Cancer Haven
London, United Kingdom

TED J. KAPTCHUK, OMD
Assistant Professor, Harvard Medical School
Osher Institute
Boston, Massachusetts

RICHARD A. LIPPIN, MD
Founder, International Arts-Medicine Association
Southampton, Pennsylvania

LISA MESEROLE, MS, ND
Phytomedicine Research Advisor
Bastyr University and
Sage Healing Clinic
Seattle, Washington

MARC S. MICOZZI, MD, PhD
Director
Informatics Institute for Complementary
and Integrative Medicine
Bethesda, Maryland
and
Former Director
Center for Integrative Medicine
Thomas Jefferson University
Philadelphia, Pennsylvania

DANIEL E. MOERMAN, PhD
William E. Stirton Professor of Anthropology
University of Michigan-Dearborn
Editor-in-Chief: *Economic Botany*
Ypsilanti, Michigan

KERRY PALANJIAN, MBA, CMT
Nationally Certified Massage Therapist
Shiatsu Therapy & Owner, Shiatsu On-Site
Corporate and Private Practice
More than just Massage-in-a-Chair
Hatboro/Greater Philadelphia, Pennsylvania

JOSEPH E. PIZZORNO, Jr, ND
President, SaluGenecists, Inc.
President Emeritus, Bastyr University
Seattle, Washington

MAURIE D. PRESSMAN, MD
Emeritus Clinical Professor, Temple University,
Department of Psychiatry
Emeritus Chairman Pyschiatry, Albert Einstein
Medical Center
Philadelphia, Pennsylvania

DANIEL REDWOOD, DC
Redwood Chiropractic and Acupuncture
Virginia Beach, Virginia

DENISE RODGERS, MDiv, CHT
Executive Director
Association for the Development of Mind/Body
Potential, Inc.
Austin, Texas

HARI M. SHARMA, MD, FRCPC
Professor Emeritus
Former Director, Division of Cancer Prevention and
Natural Products Research
Department of Pathology, College of Medicine and
Public Health
The Ohio State University College of Medicine
Columbus, Ohio

VICTOR S. SIERPINA, MD
WD and Laura Nell Nicholson Family Professor in
Integrative Medicine
Associate Professor Family Medicine
Principal Investigator, CAM Education Project
University of Texas Medical Branch
Galveston, Texas

DEVNA SINGH, MD
Chief Resident
Family Practice
Underwood Memorial Hospital,
Woodbury, New Jersey

PAMELA SNIDER, ND
Adjunct Faculty
College of Naturopathic Medicine
Bastyr University
Vice President, Integrated Health Care Policy
Consortium Board of Directors
College of Naturopathic Medicine
Bastyr University
Seattle, Washington

ROBERT T. TROTTER, II, PhD
Arizona Regent's Professor
Department of Anthropology
Northern Arizona University
Flagstaff, Arizona

RICHARD W. VOSS, DPC, MSW, MTS
Associate Professor
Department of Social Work
West Chester University of Pennsylvania
West Chester, Pennsylvania

KENNETH G. ZYSK, PhD, DPhil
Associate Professor
Institute for Cross-Cultural and Regional Studies
Department of Asian Studies
University of Copenhagen
Copenhagen, Denmark

To my wife, Carole, and
my daughter, Alicia.

Preface to Third Edition

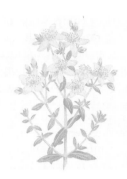

The use of complementary/alternative medicine (CAM) and integrative medicine (CIM) is widespread and increasing among all segments of US adults. This fact underlines the importance of communicating with your patients about CAM and integrative medicine. A recent survey showed that two-thirds of adults show lifetime use of CAM by age 33. Further, CAM use is currently highest among post-babyboomers (7 out of 10), with 5 out of 10 boomers, and 3 out of 10 preboomers. These trends may represent an interest in use of CIM that is primarily related to managing medical conditions. Such conditions are more prevalent among older Americans. Lifelong attitudes that are inclusive of "holistic" healing among younger Americans may lead them to CIM in even greater numbers when the need arises in older age.

In addition, two-thirds of HMOs offer at least one type of alternative/complementary therapy, with acupuncture, massage and nutritional therapy the most likely modalities to be added. The best predictor of CAM use is higher education perhaps reflecting disposable income as well as knowledge, awareness and attitudes.

Regional variations are quite consistent, with such diverse areas as South Carolina, Northern California, Florida and Oregon all registering in the range one-half to two-thirds of respondents using CIM. However, up to half of all clients do not tell their regular physicians about their use of CIM, indicating that much additional work on integration of CAM into the continuum of care is needed (Chapter 3).

A high proportion of adults with cancer utilize CAM. Several surveys found rates of 80% or higher. In one study, 40% of CAM users abandoned conventional care after adopting CAM. For breast cancer, despite the relative effectiveness of conventional care, CAM use was as high as 74%. CAM use is also marked in neurological diseases, psychiatric disorders, physical disabilities, psoriasis, diabetes and other chronic disorders. The range of CAM modalities utilized are well reflected in the topics covered in this book.

In addition to the management of medical conditions, CAM therapies have gained increasing attention in chronic disease prevention. Although CAM is often thought of as more related to healthy lifestyle and the prevention of disease, in fact, there has been more evidence about the effectiveness of CAM in treatment. Clinical treatment trials on CAM are increasing in number, while prevention trials are larger, longer, more costly, more complex and ultimately less commonly undertaken.

Constitutional factors such as body weight (long recognized in traditional health systems such as Chinese medicine and Ayur Veda) is now increasingly recognized by public health agencies as a major risk factor for chronic medical conditions, and a major source of morbidity and mortality. Efforts at weight loss and weight management represent an important means toward prevention of disease. In the realm of CAM, recent controversies over the use of ephedra for weight loss have clouded the issue of herbal remedies in general and have motivated efforts by the US Congress to attempt actions against all dietary supplements (Chapter 11).

Dietary supplements also have an increasingly recognized role in optimal health. The JAMA article on Vitamins for Chronic Disease Prevention in Adults by Fairfield and Fletcher in June 2002 documented the importance of nutrition and clearly provided substantiation for the role of dietary supplementation in light of the typical US diet and nutrient composition of foods. Dietary supplement use is already prevalent among many segments of the US population. Guidance in the appropriate uses and sources of dietary supplements is an increasingly important aspect of integrative medicine.

As the public investment in CIM increases, efforts are underway to match government resources to growing requirements for education and training, basic infrastructure and applied research and development, as well as basic research. Health care professionals remain the greatest resource for helping patients understand the appropriate use of alterna-tive, complementary and integrative medicine. As knowledge increases, what works best will not be seen as complementary, alternative or mainstream, but simply as "good medicine".

The third edition of Fundamentals of Complementary & Integrative Medicine marks ten years continuously in print for this edited volume, with many expert contributors and a growing number of topics. Our goal is that the chapters in this new edition will continue to provide a useful guide to our readers.

MARC S. MICOZZI, MD, PhD

Preface to Second Edition

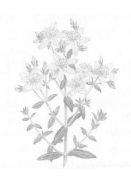

A NEW ECOLOGY OF HEALTH: A COMMON SENSE GUIDE TO COMPLEMENTARY AND ALTERNATIVE MEDICINE

The history of both medicine and physical science over the last 100 years has been the history of relentlessly breaking material reality into smaller and smaller parts.

In the effort to reduce reality to the smallest components physics encountered a point at which it is impossible to observe matter without influencing the reality of what one is trying to observe. It also became clear that all matter also has an energetic nature—and that the further one looks the more the matter-energy duality becomes impossible to separate.

We have also begun to perceive that not all physical phenomena may be explained by reducing matter to its smallest constituent parts and explanations at this end point become increasingly elusive.

THE NATURE OF MEDICINE

The central idea in medicine over the past 100 years, propagated as part of general science, is that health can also be broken down into its smallest component parts and studying the parts can be made relevant to the experience of the health of the whole. In its "reduced" state modern medicine has focused on cells, genes, and molecules—an understanding of which is central to the modern practice of biomedical science. While much of science is necessarily beginning to move beyond basing all understanding of reality on reductionist studies, modern Western medicine remains rooted in this central idea.

In the meantime contemporary studies in biology and ecology increasingly demonstrate that the behavior of biological systems, whether at the level of the whole organism, the whole community or population, or the whole planet, is not predicated, predicted, or perceivable on the basis of the isolated parts—but can be observed and understood only as phenomena at the level of the whole. Likewise, "health" is not a property that can be ascribed to or experienced by cells or molecules but only at the level of the whole person in the context of his or her physical and social environment.

Science has also attempted to produce laws to explain and predict observable behavior. The most obvious and successful examples have been in the physical sciences. In the biological sciences we have found scientific laws alone to be often insufficient in the interpretation of the natural reality that surrounds us. For in nature it has become clear that what we observe is based not only on scientific law but also on the history of everything that has ever happened before in nature. As stated by the natural scientist Stephen Jay Gould, "biology is a science with a history," and in this way biological phenomena can be made sense of only by a reading of the history of nature—a truly natural history. If one thinks of life on earth as part of a continuum connected to all other forms of life at every point in time and through time, it is not possible to think of human life or health as separate from nature. Certainly, the celebrated gene provides the mechanism by which life is linked to nature through individuals and communities through time, but it does not provide a new central idea in biomedical science.

Similarly, modern biomedicine is a science with a history and the modern practice of medicine and medical science is as influenced by social history as it is by scientific laws. The central idea of modern medicine has been to master the minutiae while missing the whole—and it is the whole that people are missing most in modern medicine. In the laudable effort to make medicine scientific, we have emphasized that knowledge about the world, including nature and human nature, must be pursued by the following criteria: (1) *objectivism*—the observer is separate from the observed, (2) *reductionism*—complex phenomena are explainable in terms of simpler, component phenomena, (3) *positivism*—all that can be known is derivable from physically measurable data, (4) *determinism*—phenomena can be predicted from a knowledge of scientific law and initial conditions. This is not the only way of knowing things, but it has become the modern test to determine whether such knowledge is "scientific" (see Chapter 1).

In fact, science requires only empiricism—making and testing models of reality by what can be observed, guided by certain values and based on certain metaphysical assumptions. Science itself is not reality but a system of human knowledge like any other human knowledge system. Often we cannot tell the difference between metaphysical reality and the scientific model that has been constructed through human intellectual activity to describe it. In this way new thoughts about the nature of medicine do not represent a "new science" so much as a new philosophy.

In the fundamental science of physics we already know that objectivism is ultimately not possible at the fundamental level because of the Heisenberg uncertainty principle—the act of observing phenomena necessarily influences the behavior of the observed. Modern biological and ecological science has produced a wealth of observations about how living organisms and communities interact with each other and their environment in transactional, multidirectional, and synergic ways that are ultimately not subject to reductionist explanations. For positivism and determinism to provide a complete explanation we must assume that science has all the physical and intellectual tools to ask the right questions, and knows the right questions to ask. However, the tools we have and the questions we ask are based on the history of science itself as part of the history of human intellectual enquiry.

Nature and Human Nature

The self-conscious experience of humans in their natural and social environments is a common and ancient topic of human enquiry. Virtually every human society around the world through time has had ways of describing and understanding the experience of the human condition—a broad and general way of describing "health." Without modern biomedical science, the ancients and the elders of human society came to understand the experience of the human condition at the level of the experience itself. And all human experience has a material nature and an energetic nature. The ancients and elders did not know that mind is separate from the body and did not know that experience could be reduced to cells and molecules, so their explanations were based on whole phenomena. The ancients and elders also did not know about the new physics, but they knew that the human body and living things have energy, as well as matter, whereas we now know that fundamental particles have a material nature and a wave (energy) nature. And despite the fact that the ancients and elders of human society did not always have sophisticated technology (although the appropriateness of many of their technologies is amazingly sophisticated) their central idea of medicine, their philosophy of health, was perhaps more sophisticated than ours has become.

Ancient and indigenous medical systems think of the human body as having energy, the balance of which is critical for health and the flow of which can be manipulated to maintain and restore health. In this way medicine is not about the putting of things into the body but using outer resources to help mobilize the inner resources of the body. The body heals itself and maintains its own health.

Modern Western medicine works on the material aspects of the body: sending in drug molecules to affect cell receptors, cutting out parts that do not work, replacing parts that fail. But the body is not a machine. Although these mechanistic approaches have clearly had great success in fixing problems, they do not always provide the best approaches to maintaining health.

Modern Western medicine knows the body has its own energy. We know the body can heal itself. Practitioners know that the "placebo" effect is real. They know that the "laying on of hands" can heal. But these things have not been in the realm of science for modern biomedicine, and even though we know they exist, they have not been studied until now. And although we know the body has energy, we have not until now used energy to heal. We measure the energy of the heart (ECG), and muscle (EMG) to help address the material aspects of the body. We know now that bones can heal by using energy. However, this has not changed the central idea of modern medicine.

Alternative Medicine Means Medical Choices

What today is called *complementary* and *alternative* medicine in the United States and Europe covers a broad range of health and medical systems often derived from ancient and indigenous societies and variously called in recent years unconventional, nontraditional, integral, holistic, and wholistic. Most have in common the idea that the body has energy, as well as material, reality. So what is really an old idea has become a new idea consistent with the frontiers of physics but not yet the frontier of modern medicine, which still operates with 100-year-old central ideas. Although alternatives are very diverse in terms of cosmology in the *causes* of disease, they generally share an idea about the cures of disease—that the body can heal itself (as modern medicine knows) and that healing comes only from the inner resources of the body, which can be mobilized by external manipulation.

When focusing on the energetic aspects of the body, the emphasis is on the flow of energy and the balance of energy, implying a dynamic interaction that is different from the static grasp of matter. Much of our modern knowledge of medicine comes from the historically important idea more than 100 years ago that diseases of the whole organism can be understood at the cell level and that observations at the cell level are directly related to diagnosis, prognosis, and therapy of the patient. Great advances have come from this approach to the material aspects of disease. When studying the dynamic energy of life processes, however, we may have reached our limits in what can be understood through the study of dead tissue cells. Many neuroscientists now believe that we will further advance our fundamental understanding of the brain only when we "remap" what we know about the brain from studying dead brain cells to studying living brain tissue.

Many believe that a new central idea, a new philosophy, is needed for medicine to maintain its relevance to a broadened definition of health. Today there are many approaches through different models and medical philosophies. It is not so much that there are many alternatives to modern Western (allopathic) medicine, but that allopathic medicine is one of many alternatives. How can we make sense of so many different modalities of health and healing? It makes sense only if we realize that the final common pathway for the way that all medical systems work is by their ability to influence the body to heal itself, to mobilize inner resources, and to address the energetic, as well as material, aspects of a living human organism.

Alternative medicine means having choices that people want and are willing to pay for. Americans are not primarily interested in propagating any particular model of medical practice or science. People want what works. Increasingly, medical practitioners who know and respect the power of the placebo effect, the laying on of hands, and other "nonscientific" medicine also are on a search for what works for their patients and what works for their own personal perceptions as healers.

Healing is not solely about a given medical system or tradition. It is about the human body, human biology, and human physiology—how the body works and how it heals. Formulary approaches to alternative medicine (e.g., acupuncture, herbalism, homeopathy) taken out of the complete context of their traditional practices still are observed to work because they draw on the body's biology in the same ways. These formulary approaches provide evidence that empirical traditions of alternative medicine have discovered certain truths about human physiology and encoded them into their medical practice and/or cultural knowledge systems.

Nonetheless, no medicine works as well if the patient (and practitioner) does not believe it. And any medicine works better if patient and practitioners share a belief in its efficacy. As stated in the foreword by Dr. C. Everett Koop, the health care practitioner operates within and between the realms of the art and the science of medicine. Integration of complementary and alternative therapies into medical practice affords the opportunity to expand our knowledge and utilization of both.

MARC S. MICOZZI, MD, PhD

Preface to First Edition

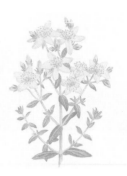

Fundamentals of Complementary and Alternative Medicine provides the reader with a basis of knowledge about systems of medical thought and practice referred to today in the United States as complementary and alternative medicine. The book's approach is to present medical, health, and science students and practitioners, as well as other interested individuals, with the intellectual foundations and tools to understand and make sense of these various fields that demonstrate great diversity and yet can be unified around certain themes. To provide a useful introduction to these topics, the book is carefully organized with subjects presented in the order in which they should be read for a progressive, comprehensive overview and understanding of the material.

Alternative and complementary medicine, natural medicine, and the use of natural products represent a classic consumer movement and a current social phenomenon of significant dimensions. Students, practitioners, patients, and consumers need a common language for understanding this movement.

Physicians and patients are becoming increasingly involved in alternatives driven by the perceived need for health care reform, the desire to move toward a wellness orientation in medical practice, and an intellectual interest and curiosity about the ability of what well-established ancient and historic medical systems continue to offer us today.

In sum, this book presents the contemporary complementary and alternative medical approaches that come from observations within, around, and beyond the current Western, biomedical paradigm. The approaches discussed expand our view of the possibilities for light, time, touch, sensation, energy, and mind to enter into health and medicine. The ultimate goal is a synthesis of mind-body medicine, its relation to the emerging field of psychoneuroimmunology, and a possible model for a final common pathway among complementary and alternative medical systems.

MARC S. MICOZZI, MD, PhD

Foreword

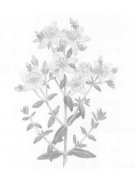

For more than 50 years I have tried to identify the mix of personal attributes and technical skills that make one an outstanding doctor. I am sure that most physicians in the United States have pondered the same question. Now, through the work of the C. Everett Koop Institute at Dartmouth I have an opportunity to influence the way medical students are trained. The Institute, working in partnership with the Dartmouth Medical School and the Dartmouth-Hitchcock Medical Center, is actively engaged in training physicians for the new century.

Because doctors must remain abreast of a growing volume of new information, our medical schools help both their graduates and society by producing physicians who are computer literate and comfortable with telemedicine. As a scientific pursuit, medicine should take advantage of the technologic innovations that allow us to better serve the lifetime learning needs of physicians as well as the health education needs of patients. Nonetheless, because medicine is also an art, doctors still need to listen to their patients. This aspect of medical practice has not changed.

As I travel across the country many of the people I meet are eager to share their ideas for improving the nation's health care system. The most common complaint I hear focuses on poor communication in the doctor-patient relationship. Too many patients feel that their physician does not really listen to them. When the patient attempts to explain his or her problem, the doctor interrupts. Subsequently, when the doctor tries to explain what conditions the patient has and attempts to outline a treatment regimen, the patient is confused because the physician does not communicate to the level of the patient's understanding.

From my perspective, medical students need to master the art of listening to and communicating with their patients just as much as they need to learn the fundamentals of human biology. We have found at the Koop Institute that a student's communication skills are greatly improved by having to explain the first principles of health promotion and disease prevention to second graders. Medical students who choose to participate in programs sponsored by the Koop Institute work in and with local communities from their very first year. Some choose to advise junior high and high school students on the risks associated with alcohol, tobacco, and sexually transmitted diseases; others help rural physicians take better advantage of the computer revolution.

Just as a physician should be sensitive to the feelings of a patient and the needs of the community, he or she must be conversant with major trends and developments in society. I would like to tell you about one current trend that is of interest to me. Studies conducted at Harvard Medical School and reported in the *New England Journal of Medicine* focused on attitudes toward complementary and alternative medicine in the United States. They indicate that one third of adult Americans regularly use some kind of complementary or alternative treatment even though it was not covered by insurance and they had to pay for it themselves. This is an opportune time for us to take a second look at such alternative treatment approaches as acupuncture, botanical medicine, homeopathy, and others; not to offer these treatment modalities blindly but to expose them to the scientific method. Physicians have to depend on facts—on empirical data—when they determine treatment strategy for a particular patient. Today we do not have enough data on the potential of alternative approaches to help or harm human health. It is time to discover the value of these treatment regimens. We can conduct the necessary studies and assemble the data that doctors and health policy makers need, a type of biomedical research that would be a prudent long-term investment.

In my lifetime we have achieved great successes in the fight against infectious diseases. We have more work to do in our effort to improve the quality of life and make people more comfortable as they endure chronic health problems such as cancer, heart disease, and arthritis. Drugs and surgery can be useful tools in the effort to treat these diseases, but when possible I would like to see us increase the range of approaches that can be used. My experience as a doctor has taught me that often a mix of different approaches is necessary to achieve success. We need to be flexible and adaptable because the diseases that challenge us certainly are not static.

A recent trend that concerns me is the growth of drug resistant bacteria. Today it is easy to forget that prior to the development of antibiotics in the 1940s a child's ear infection could be a frightening and fatal experience. I well remember patients with serious complications and death caused by the lack of antibiotics. If drugs we have depended on for decades are compromised, we may return to a time when even routine infections could be dangerous. As both a grandfather and a physician, I would hate to see that happen.

There is an element of good news in this picture. If some of the synthetic drugs we have developed are no longer as dependable as they once were, studies have shown that the botanical substances these drugs are based on are still effective in treating disease. I have never claimed to be an expert on botany or ecology, but current trends suggest that we need to do more. We need to conserve the plants that may contain the medicines of the future and more important, we need to learn what local experts seem to understand about the pharmacologic properties and uses of these medicines.

Reduced health care costs are an important by-product of the work we are doing at the Koop Institute. Our students know that the physician of the future must be a health educator first and foremost. Today, the challenge is to treat the patient once he or she has gone to the hospital. Tomorrow, the challenge will be to keep the patient out of the hospital in the beginning.

Preventive medicine means education, empowerment, and personal responsibility. Many patients want alternatives to invasive medical procedures and long stays in the hospital. Physicians can conserve time and resources by teaching patients how to reduce their risk of cancer, heart disease, and other life-threatening diseases. As our students know, the most inexpensive treatment is to keep the patient from becoming sick in the first place. Demand reduction in the health care system is the most immediate cost saving effort.

I think that alternative/complementary therapies may potentially be an important part of this overall educational process. One must have an open mind about complementary therapies and understand belief systems that emphasize the mind-body connection. At a time when many Americans complain of stress, make poor nutritional choices, and are increasingly concerned about environmentally induced illnesses these messages could not be more timely.

Many people are confused about alternative medicine, and I do not blame them. For many Americans alternative therapies represent a *new* discovery, but in truth, many of these traditions are hundreds or thousands of years old and have been used by millions of people worldwide. To ease the uncomfortableness of the word *alternative* one must realize that while treatments may look like alternatives to us, they have long been part of the medical mainstream in their cultures of origin.

When I worked in Washington as Surgeon General for eight years, President Reagan had an important credo in his approach to foreign policy: "Trust but verify!" So it is with complementary and alternative medicine. So many people have relied on these approaches for so long that they may have something of value to offer. Let us begin the necessary research so that we could have substantive answers in the near future.

One reason such research is worth doing is that eighty percent of the world's people depend on these alternative approaches as their primary medical care. For years, we have attempted to export Western medicine to the developing world. The sad truth is that the people we are attempting to help simply cannot afford it. I have doubts about how much longer we can afford some of it ourselves. It is possible that in this new millennium, we may be more ready to ask the peoples of the developing world to share their wisdom with us.

During the nineteenth century, American medicine was an eclectic pursuit where a number of competing ideas and approaches thrived. Doctors were able to draw on elements from different traditions in attempting to make people well. Perhaps there is more to this older model of American medicine than we in the twentieth century had been willing to examine. My experience with physicians has convinced me that they are healers first. As such, they are willing to use any ethical approach or treatment that has been proven to work. However, in the opinion of many doctors, there is not yet a definitive answer on the value of complementary and alternative medicine. I would like us to undertake the study and research that will provide definitive answers to prudent questions about the usefulness of complementary and alternative medicine for society at large.

C. EVERETT KOOP, MD, ScD
Former Surgeon General of the United States
Senior Scholar, The Koop Institute at Dartmouth,
Hanover, New Hampshire

About the Author

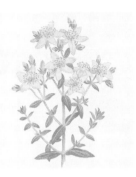

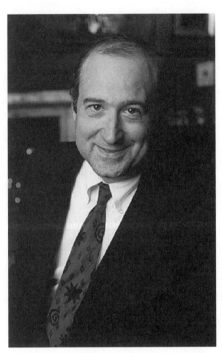

MARC S. MICOZZI, MD, PhD, is Former Director of the Center for Integrative Medicine, Thomas Jefferson University, Philadelphia, PA, and Director of the Informatics Institute for Complementary and Integrative Medicine (IICIM), Bethesda, MD. He was previously Executive Director of The College of Physicians of Philadelphia, Founding Director of the National Museum of Health and Medicine in Washington, DC, and a Senior Investigator at the National Cancer Institute, National Institutes of Health (NIH). He has published sixteen books and over 250 articles in medical and health topics. He was the founding editor-in-chief of the first medical journal on complementary and alternative medicine and is editor of this first textbook, *Fundamentals of Complementary and Alternative Medicine,* now in its third edition. He has served as consultant to the U.S. Federal Trade Commission and the Commonwealth of Pennsylvania Bureau of Professional and Occupational Affairs on complementary and alternative medicine and is Principle Investigator on a grant from the US Health Resources and Services Administration for developing an internet-based professional reference resource on integrative medicine. He has been a frequent speaker to medical and consumer audiences worldwide on integrative medicine. He frequently lectures to medical and graduate students for the Department of Physiology and Biophysics, Georgetown University School of Medicine, Washington, DC. e-mail: MarcMicozzi@aol.com

Contents

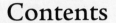

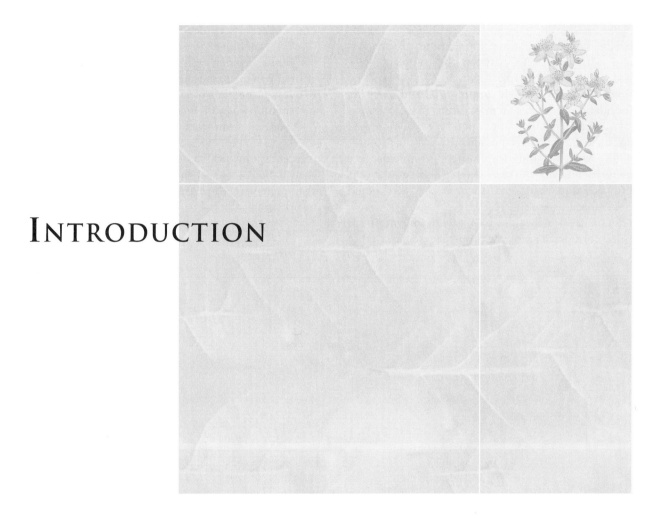

INTRODUCTION

The aim of this text is to provide clear and rational guides for health care professionals and students so they have current knowledge about:

- Therapeutic medical systems currently labeled as complementary medicine
- Complementary approaches to specific medical conditions
- Integration of complementary therapy into mainstream medical practice

Each chapter is written specifically with the needs and questions of a health care audience in mind. Where possible, basic applications in clinical practice are addressed.

Complementary medicine is being rapidly integrated into mainstream health care largely in response to consumer demand, as well as in recognition of new scientific findings that are expanding our view of health and healing—pushing against the limits of the current biomedical paradigm.

Health care professionals need to know what their patients are doing and what they believe about what has been called alternative medicine. In addition, a basic working knowledge of complementary medical therapies is a rapidly growing requirement for primary care, family practice, general internal medicine, many medical specialties, and throughout the allied health professions. These approaches also expand our view of the art and science of medicine and contribute importantly to the intellectual formation of health professions students.

This text provides a survey of the fundamentals and foundations of complementary medical systems currently available and practiced in North America and Europe. Each topic is presented in ways that are *understandable* and that provide an important *understanding* of the intellectual foundations of each system—with translation between the complementary and conventional medical systems. These explanations draw appropriately on the social and scientific foundations of each system of care.

Rapidly growing contemporary research results are included whenever possible. In addition to providing evidence indicating where complementary medicines may be of therapeutic benefit, guidance is provided as to when complementary therapies should not be used, as well.

This field of healthcare is rapidly moving from being considered *alternative* (implying exclusive use of

one medical system or another), to *complementary* (used as an adjunct to mainstream medical care), to *integrative medicine* (implying an active, conscious effort by mainstream medicine to incorporate alternatives on the basis of rational clinical and scientific information and judgment).

Likewise, healthcare professionals and students must move rapidly to learn the fundamentals of complementary medical systems in order to better serve their patients, protect the public health, and expand their scientific horizons and understandings of health and healing.

Fundamentals of
COMPLEMENTARY AND INTEGRATIVE MEDICINE

THIRD EDITION

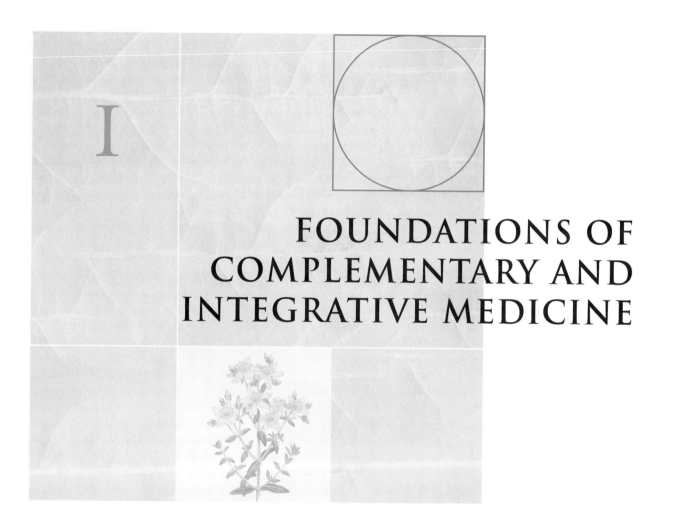

FOUNDATIONS OF COMPLEMENTARY AND INTEGRATIVE MEDICINE

This section and Section II provide an introduction to the whole topic of complementary and integrative medicine (CIM), its themes and terminology, and the various contexts relative to its proper interpretation. The chapters provide a social and cultural recontextualization of CIM, referred to as *complementary and alternative medicine* (CAM) in the first two edition of this book. The ubiquitous use of plants and natural products among alternatives is reviewed through underlying themes from both the social and the biological sciences. ❧

1

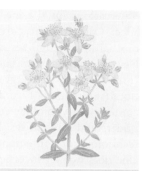

CHARACTERISTICS OF COMPLEMENTARY AND INTEGRATIVE MEDICINE

MARC S. MICOZZI

The different medical systems subsumed under the category *complementary and integrative,* previously called *complementary and alternative,* are many and diverse, but these systems have some common ground in their views of health and healing. This overall philosophy can be called *a new ecology of health,* sustainable medicine, or "medicine for a small planet."

ROLE OF SCIENCE

Allopathic medicine is considered the "scientific" healing art, whereas the alternatives have been considered "nonscientific." However, perhaps what is needed is not *less science* but *more sciences* in the study of complementary and integrative medicine (CIM). Some of the central ideas of biomedicine are very powerful but may be intellectually static. The study of dead tissue cells, components, and chemicals to understand life processes and the quest for "magic bullets" to combat disease are based on a reductionist, materialist view of health and healing. Tremendous advances have been made over the past 100 years by applying these concepts to medicine. However, the resulting biomedical system is not always able to account for and use many observations in the realms of clinical and personal experience, natural law, and human spirituality.

Contemporary biomedicine conceptually uses Newtonian physics and pre-evolutionary biology. Newtonian physics explains and can reproduce many observations on the mechanics of everyday experience. Contemporary quantum physics (quantum mechanics) recognizes aspects of reality beyond Newtonian mechanics, such as matter-energy duality, "unified fields" of energy and matter, and wave functions (see Chapters 17 and 18). Quantum physics and contemporary biology-ecology may be needed to understand alternatives. Nuclear medicine uses the technology of contemporary physics, but biomedicine does not yet incorporate the concepts of quantum physics in its fundamental approach to human health and healing. Contemporary biomedicine measures the body's energy using electrocardiography, electroencephalography, and electromyography for diagnostic purposes, but it does not explicitly enlist the body's energy for the purpose of healing.

The biomedical model relies on a projection of Newtonian mechanics into the microscopic and molecular realms.

As a model for everything, Newtonian mechanics has limitations. It works within the narrow limits of everyday experience. It does not always work at a *macro* (cosmic) level, as shown by Einstein's theory of relativity, or at a *micro* (fundamental) level, as illustrated by quantum physics. However useful Newton's physics has been in solving mechanical problems, it does not explain the vast preponderance of nature: the motion of currents; the growth of plants and animals; or the rise, functioning, and fall of civilizations. Per Bak once stated that mechanics could explain why the apple fell but not why the apple existed or why Newton was thinking about it in the first place.

Mechanics works in explaining machines. But no matter how popular this metaphor has become (with acknowledgment of *National Geographic*'s popular "incredible machine" imagery), the body is not a machine and it cannot be entirely explained by mechanics. It is becoming increasingly clear that an understanding of energetics is required. This duality between the mechanical and the energetic has been accepted in physics for most of the past century. This duality is famously illustrated by the fact that J.J. Thomson won the Nobel Prize for demonstrating that the electron is a particle. His son, George P. Thomson, won the Nobel Prize a generation later for demonstrating that the electron is a wave.

"Hard scientists," such as physicists and molecular biologists, accept the duality of the electron but sometimes have difficulty accepting the duality of the human body. The "soft sciences," which attempt to be inclusive in their study of the phenomena of life and nature, are often looked on with disdain according to the folklore of the self-styled real scientists. However, real science must account for all of what is observed in nature, not just the conveniently reductionistic part.

The biological science of contemporary medicine is essentially pre-evolutionary in that it emphasizes typology rather than individuality and variation. Each patient is defined as a clinical entity by a diagnosis, with treatment prescribed accordingly. The modern understanding of the human genome does not make this approach to biomedical science less pre-evolutionary. Both the fundamentals of inheritance (Mendel) and those of natural selection (Darwin and Alfred Russel Wallace) were explained long before the discovery of the structure of the gene itself. Although modern biology-ecology continues to explore the phenomena of how living systems interact at the level of the whole—which cannot be seen under a microscope or in a test tube—molecular genetics continues to dissect the human genome.

It may seem outrageously complex to construct a medical system based on the concepts of modern physics and biology-ecology while maintaining a unique diagnostic and therapeutic approach to each individual. This would indeed be complex if not for the fact that the body is its own entity, a part of nature, and each body has an innate ability to heal itself.

One way of studying and understanding alternative medicine is to view it in light of contemporary physics and biology-ecology and to focus not just on the subtle manipulations of alternative practitioners, but also on the physiological responses of the human body. When homeopathy or acupuncture is observed to result in a physiological or clinical response that cannot be explained by the biomedical model, it is not the role of the scientist to deny this reality, but rather to modify our explanatory models to account for it. In this way, science itself progresses. In the end there is only one reality. Integrative (or alternative) medical systems, which are relatively "old" in terms of human intellectual history, always have been trying to describe, understand, and work with the same reality of health and healing as biomedicine. While contemporary biomedicine uses new technologies in the service of relatively old ideas about health and healing, alternative methods use old technologies whose fundamental character may reflect new scientific ideas on physical and biological nature (Box 1-1).

> If biomedicine cannot explain scientific observations of alternatives, the biomedical paradigm will be revised.

Science must account for *all* of what is observed, not just part of it. That is why physics has moved beyond Newtonian mechanics—biology beyond typology. Is it possible for a biomedical model to be constructed for which its validity includes observations from CIM? Although it may be necessary to wait for new insights from physics and biology to understand CIM in terms of biomedicine, clinical pragmatism dictates that successful therapeutic methods should not be withheld while mechanisms are being explained—or debated. We live in a world filled with opportunities to observe the practice of integrative medicine; all that remains is to apply scientific standards to its study. In the meantime, patients are now waiting for mainstream physicians to understand the mechanisms of CIM. Also, we can come to understand the underlying intellectual content and history of alternatives as complete systems of thought and practice.

WELLNESS

The CIM systems generally emphasize what might be called "wellness" by the mainstream medical system. The goal of preventing disease is shared by integrative and mainstream medicine alike. In the mainstream medical model this involves using drugs and surgery to prevent disease in those who are only at risk, rather than reserving these powerful methods for the treatment of disease. I have called this trend the *medicalization* of prevention. In this approach, one can continue to engage in risky lifestyle behaviors while medicine provides "magic bullets" to prevent diseases that it cannot treat. Wellness in the context of complementary medicine is more than the prevention of disease. It is a focus on engaging the inner resources of each individual as an active and conscious participant in the maintenance of his or her own health. By the same token, the property of being healthy is not conferred on an individual solely by an outside agency or entity, but rather results from the balance of internal resources with the external natural and

---

BOX 1-1

A Note about Nomenclature

Although the term *complementary and integrative medicine* (CIM) is used in this third edition, "complementary and alternative medicine" was the title of the first two editions of this text. The word *alternative,* or the term *complementary and alternative medicine,* now seems to be culturally encoded in the English language. Workers at Harvard Medical School have provided a basis for a functional definition of the term:

> Alternative medicine refers to those practices explicitly used for the purpose of medical intervention, health promotion or disease prevention which are not routinely taught at U.S. medical schools nor routinely underwritten by third-party payers within the existing U.S. health care system.

The Harvard definition seems to be a diagnosis of exclusion, meaning that alternative medicine (or now CIM) is everything not being presently promoted in mainstream medicine. This definition may remind us of a popular song from the 1960s called "The Element Song," which offers a complete listing of the different elements of the periodic table (set to the tune of "I Am the Very Model of a Modern Major General" from Gilbert and Sullivan's *The Pirates of Penzance*). It ends with words to this effect: "These are the many elements we've heard about at Harvard. And if we haven't heard of them, they haven't been discovered." I have likened the recent "discovery" of alternative medicine to Columbus's discovery of the Americas. Although his voyage was a great feat that expanded the intellectual frontiers of Europe, Columbus could not really discover a world already known to millions of indigenous peoples who used complex systems of social organization and subsistence activities. Likewise, the definitional statement that alternatives are not "within the existing U.S. health care system" is a curious observation for the tens of millions of Americans who routinely use them today.

social environment. This latter point relates to the alternative approach that relies on the abilities of the individual to get well and stay healthy.

SELF-HEALING

The body heals itself. This might seem to be an obvious statement because we are well aware that wounds heal and cells routinely replace themselves. Nonetheless, this is a profound concept among CIM systems because self-healing is the basis of *all* healing. External manipulations simply mobilize the body's inner healing resources. Instead of wondering why the body's cells are sick, alternatives ask why the body is not replacing its sick cells with healthy cells. The body's ability to be well or ill is largely tied to inner resources, and the external environment—social and physical—has an impact on this ability.

What is the evidence for self-healing? The long and common history of clinical observations of the "placebo" effect," the "laying on of hands," or "spontaneous remissions" may be included in this category. To paraphrase Jung: Summoned or unsummoned, self-healing will be there. Self-healing is so powerful that biomedical methodology mainly designs double-blind, controlled clinical trials to see what percentage of benefit powerful drugs can add to the healing encounter.

BIOENERGY

A related concept is that the body has energy (see Chapters 17 and 18). Accordingly, as a living entity, the body is an energetic system. Disruptions in the balance and flow of energy cause illness, and the body's response to energetic imbalance leads to perceptible disease. Because the body heals itself, the body can also make itself sick. Restoring or facilitating the body to restore its own balance restores health. The symptoms of a cold, flu, or allergy are caused by the body's efforts to rid itself of the offending agent. For example, by raising the body's temperature, a fever reduces bacterial reproduction (like an antibiotic, fever is literally bacteriostatic), and sneezing physically expels offending agents (see Chapter 8).

Pathologists know that there are only so many ways that cells can look sick because cellular reactions have a defined repertoire for manifesting malfunction. We have also learned a great deal over the past 100 years by correlating the appearance of dead tissue cells under the microscope with clinical diagnosis and prognosis. However, studying dead tissue cells for clinical significance does not allow direct observation of the dynamic energy of living cells, systems, organisms, and communities. Although correlation of the appearance of stained tissue cells under a microscope to clinical conditions is a powerful concept in medicine, alternatives appear to provide a path to study the energy of living systems for health and healing, perhaps before the development of overt disease, as so often encountered among the many "functional complaints" in modern medicine (see Chapter 2).

NUTRITION AND NATURAL PRODUCTS

The reliance on nutrition and natural products is fundamental to CIM and does not play merely a supportive or adjunctive role. Nutrients and plant products are taken into the body and incorporated in the most literal sense. They provide the body with energy in the form of calories and with the material resources to stay healthy and get well.

Because the basic plan of the body, as a physical entity and as an energy system, evolves and exists in an ecological context, what the body needs it obtains from the environment in which it grew. Lao Tzu states that "what is deeply rooted in nature cannot be uprooted." The human organism is designed to obtain nutrients from natural food sources present in the natural environment, and the body is often best suited to obtain nutrients in their natural forms (see Chapter 11).

PLANTS

Plants are an important part of nature relative to health and a dominant part of the nature in which humans evolved. In addition to producing the oxygen that we breathe, plants are seen as sources of nutrients, medicines (e.g., phytochemicals), and essential oils (e.g., volatiles for inhalation and transdermal absorption); some systems also view plants as sources of vibrational energy. Many systems see the use of plants as sources of nutrients in continuity with their use as sources of medicine, paralleling contemporary biomedical guidelines for nutrition as disease prevention. As in Chinese medicine, foods exist in continuity with medicines among plant sources.

INDIVIDUALITY

The emphasis of CIM is on the whole person as a unique individual with his or her own inner resources. Therefore the concepts of normalization, standardization, and generalization may be more difficult to apply to research and clinical practice compared with the allopathic method. Some believe that alternatives restore the role of the individual patient and practitioner to the practice of medicine; the biomedical emphasis on standardization of training and practice to ensure quality may leave something lost in translation back to restoring the health of the individual (see Chapter 8).

> The focus on the whole person as a unique individual provides new challenges to the scientific measurement of the healing encounter. Mobilizing the resources of each individual to stay healthy and get well also provides new opportunities to move health care toward a model of wellness and toward new models for helping solve our current health care crisis, which is largely driven by costs.

If the body heals itself, has its own energy, and is uniquely individual, then the focus is not on the healer but on the healed. Although this concept is humbling to the role of practitioner as heroic healer, it is liberating to realize that in the end, each person heals himself or herself. If the healer is not the sole source of health and healing, there is room for humility and room for both patient and practitioner to participate in the interaction.

For the purposes of this book, a functional definition of complementary and integrative medicine is offered, limited here to what may be called *complementary medical systems*. Complementary medical systems are characterized by a developed body of intellectual work (1) that underlies the conceptualization of health and its precepts; (2) that has been sustained over many generations by many practitioners in many communities; (3) that represents an orderly, rational, conscious system of knowledge and thought about health and medicine; (4) that relates more broadly to a way of life (or lifestyle); and (5) that has been widely observed to have definable results as practiced.

Although the term *holistic* has been applied to the approach to the "body as person" among CIM systems, I apply holism to the medical system itself as a complete system of thought and practice (what I have called "health beliefs and behaviors," Chapter 2). This system of knowledge is therefore shared by patients and practitioners—the active, conscious engagement of "patients" is relative to the focus on *self-healing* and *individuality* that are among the common characteristics of these systems.

In this regard it might be considered that we are trying to document here the "classic" practice of CIM systems. In trying to build a bridge between a well-developed system of allopathic medicine and complementary medical systems, it is necessary to have strong foundations on both sides of this bridge. It is not possible to apply these criteria to the work of individual alternative practitioners who have unilaterally developed their own unique techniques over one or two generations (what might be called "unconventional"), just as it is not possible to build a bridge to nowhere. This definition is meant to apply to systems of *thought* and not just techniques of practice. Often an underlying philosophy of individual practitioners surrounds new techniques they have developed, or new techniques may be subsumed under existing systems of practice.

Eclecticism is itself a historical form of alternative medicine that drew from among different traditions and was popular in the United States in the nineteenth century. In such a system, treatment is determined by the needs of each individual patient, not limited to what one given system has to offer. At present a chiropractor may practice in an Ayurveda clinic; osteopaths may practice in allopathic clinics; and chiropractors, osteopaths or allopaths may use acupuncture. *Naturopathy,* in some ways the most recent of homegrown alternatives from the Euro-American tradition, consciously uses a variety of traditions ranging from acupuncture to herbal medicine. I have termed naturopathy as *neoeclecticism,* with the underlying philosophy that the body heals itself using resources found in nature (see Chapter 13).

In the end a given system develops in answer to human needs. Alternatives vary widely, but their characteristics cluster around the self-healing capabilities of the human organism and the ability (and reliance) of the human organism to use resources present in nature. What is constant and at the center of such CIM systems is the individual human. Therefore, if the focus is not on the medical system itself but on the person at the center, there is really only one system.

FUNDAMENTALS OF COMPLEMENTARY AND INTEGRATIVE MEDICINE

Contemporary biomedicine is a scientific paradigm with a particular history, as much influenced by social history as by scientific laws. In the laudable effort to make medicine scientific, we have emphasized that knowledge about the world, including nature and human nature, must be pursued by the following criteria: (1) *objectivism*—the observer is separate from the observed, (2) *reductionism*—complex phenomena are explainable in terms of simpler, component phenomena, (3) *positivism*—all information can be derived from physically measurable data, and (4) *determinism*—phenomena can be predicted from a knowledge of scientific law and initial conditions. We all know that this is not the only way of "knowing" things, but it became the twentieth-century test to determine whether such knowledge is "scientific."

In fact, science simply requires *empiricism*—making and testing models of reality by what can be observed, guided by certain values, and based on certain metaphysical assumptions. Science itself is a system of human knowledge. Scientists often detect differences between metaphysical reality and the scientific models constructed through human intellectual activity. These new thoughts about the nature of medicine do not represent a new science so much as they represent a new philosophy.

Therefore the four criteria just listed are not always applicable. In the science of physics, objectivism is ultimately not possible at the fundamental level because of the *Heisenberg uncertainty principle*, which states that the act of observing phenomena necessarily influences the behavior of the phenomena being observed. Contemporary biological and ecological science has produced a wealth of observations about interactions among living organisms and their environments in transactional, multidirectional, and synergic ways that are not ultimately subject to reductionist explanations. For positivism and determinism to provide a complete explanation, we must assume that science has all the physical and intellectual tools to ask the right questions. However, the questions we ask are based on the history of science itself as part of the history of human intellectual inquiry.

> A final point about alternatives: In a way, perhaps particular to the United States, CIM systems imply the importance of individuality and choice. In an era when the active engagement of the individual in his or her own health is a paramount goal, the importance of individuality and of choice could not be more salient.

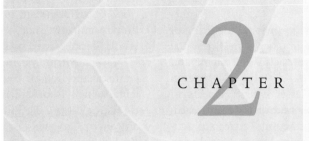
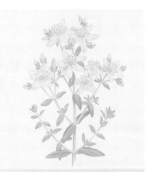

CHAPTER 2

TRANSLATION FROM CONVENTIONAL MEDICINE

MARC S. MICOZZI

What has been labeled "alternative medicine" in the United States is, first of all, a social phenomenon and consumer movement of significant dimensions. The term *complementary medicine,* or now *complementary and integrative medicine* (CIM), has been used interchangeably and is a more accurate functional description of this social phenomenon because patients in the United States generally use "alternative medicine" as an *adjunct* to (not a replacement for) conventional medical care. Much of what we call "complementary and alternative medicine" (CAM, or now CIM) in the United States, in fact, represents time-honored traditions of medical practice originating from other countries and other cultures or from the history of European and American society.

One of the most important distinctions we can make in studying and understanding CIM is to note the differences between two types of practices: (1) practices that are many years or centuries old and have a large body of practitioners and patients and a well-developed fund of clinical "wisdom" that is encoded into the belief system of a particular society or subgroup of people and (2) practices that have been developed recently by one or few practitioners in isolation from peers and without benefit of scientific testing and clinical studies (what may be called "unusual therapy"). Practices in this second category often fit conceptually within the biomedical model but simply have not been tested by use of the standards of biomedical research and practice.

For example, for the topics in this volume, CIM systems (alternatives) in the first category of time-tested traditions include the traditional medicine of China (with heterogeneous practice styles), manual therapies (osteopathy, chiropractic, massage), and homeopathy. Many time-tested traditions have in common, to a greater or lesser extent, aspects of mind-body medicine, a focus on nutrition and natural products, hands-on interaction between practitioner and patient, and an emphasis on listening to the patient. The five common characteristics of complementary and integrative (alternative) medicine described in this book are (1) a wellness orientation, (2) a reliance on self-healing, (3) an inference that bioenergetic mechanisms play a role, (4) the use of nutrition and natural products in a fundamental role, and (5) an emphasis on individuality.

Because homeopathy, for example, stresses the importance of eliciting detailed symptoms and symptom complexes from the patient (and is not a system for placing patients into disease-based diagnostic categories), the practitioner must spend a great deal of time listening to the patient. The therapeutic benefits (and diagnostic value) of listening to the patient continue to be actively used among the "talk therapies" of contemporary mainstream medical practice in psychiatry and psychology, as well as general clinical practice (Adler, 1997).

Because complementary and integrative therapies do not necessarily stress the assignment of patients to disease-based diagnostic categories, they are routinely prepared to deal with "functional" disorders and complaints (e.g., pain, gastrointestinal dysfunction, menstrual dysfunction, other "subjective" symptoms) that do not carry a pathological diagnosis. Many CIM systems see these functional disorders as precursors of disease (rather than, for example, results of disease) and approach the clinical intervention on that basis.

VITALISM AND HOLISM

Various CIM systems also refer to the importance of "energy" in the development of disorders and diseases and in their treatment and cure. Energy has a dynamic quality and is not measured in the usual ways that conventional medicine is accustomed to describing on the basis of materialist, reductionist biomedical mechanisms. The idea that whole, living systems and organisms have a "vital energy" that may

not be present in nonliving entities or in parts or portions of an organism is an ancient concept among human cultures that is also reflected in European and U.S. intellectual traditions (Figure 2-1).

CIM medical systems are sometimes considered vitalistic and holistic compared with allopathic medicine, which is considered materialistic and reductionistic (Table 2-1). Vitalism contends that there is an "energy" to living organisms that is nonmaterial. *Vitalism* is a nonecological concept historically and

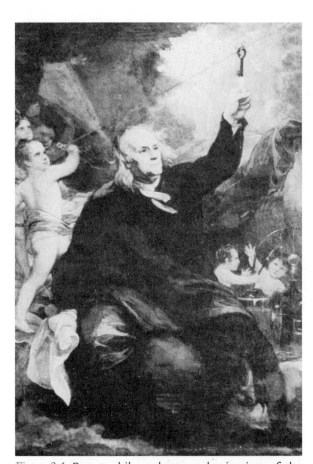

Figure 2-1 Poets, philosophers, and scientists of the late eighteenth and early nineteenth centuries were all interested in vitalism—the energy that animated life and the universe. Here Benjamin Franklin is shown in this heroic pose by Benjamin West figuratively "taming lightning." In fact, Franklin, like his contemporaries, was searching for insights into nature and human nature, not just exploring electricity in a contemporary utilitarian sense. Later, scientists thought that reductionist, materialist explanations substituted for the need for vitalist interpretations.

TABLE 2-1

Vitalism and Holism in Complementary Medicine

Biomedicine	Complementary medicine
Reductionist	Holistic
Materialist	Vitalist

posits nonnaturalistic explanations for life. *Holism* is an ecological concept that the totality of biological phenomena in a living organism or system cannot be reduced, observed, or measured at a level below that of the whole organism or system (Smuts, 1926). Holism as an ecological concept is not consistent with the vitalist idea that living systems are independent of nature. Holism was meant to be both antimechanistic and antivitalist.

However, it is generally interpreted that vitalism and holism go together in studying the characteristics of CIM. However, some interpretations of homeopathy, for example, rely on a vitalist mechanism while basing therapy on an essentially reductionist approach; that is, a whole organism's energetic mechanism is postulated for the effect elicited by minute doses of specific materia medica in pills. Likewise, in Chinese medicine the post-1949 traditional Chinese medicine (TCM) "style" of practice veers toward a reductionist model while maintaining an essentially vitalist mechanism. Since 1978 the World Health Organization (WHO) has referred to traditional (cultural) medical systems as holistic, meaning "viewing humans in totality within a wide ecological spectrum, and emphasizing the view that ill health or disease is brought about by imbalance or disequilibrium of humans in the total ecological system and not only by the causative agent and pathogenic mechanism" (WHO, 1998).

Historically, we might say that premodern medical systems could understand medicine only on the basis of observations of the whole organism, whose components were not well known or understood. Modern reductionist biomedical science has allowed knowledge to be built on the basis of studying dead parts and pieces of the whole organism (e.g., tissue cells, DNA). A postmodern medicine might permit translation of the biomedical model back to the realm of the whole, vital organism. For example, new imaging technologies that permit observation of

living cells for diagnostic and therapeutic purposes may provide one mechanism.

This view might consider that biomedicine has new technologies generally in the service of old ideas about health and healing, whereas CIM systems represent old technologies that may be interpreted in light of new ideas about health and healing.

Outcomes-based research has begun to be helpful in demonstrating the therapeutic benefit (or lack of benefit) of alternative (integrative) practices that are unexplainable on the basis of postulated mechanisms of action foreign to the biomedical model. In this way, some regard such ideas as nonsense, or perhaps more accurately, "unsense." However, some sense may be made of these ideas by considering a medical ecological or adaptational model.

MEDICAL ECOLOGICAL AND ADAPTATIONAL MODEL

With medical traditions that have been encoded and carried as knowledge in different cultures for many years, it is possible to study the adaptiveness and adaptive value of such practices. What benefits do these traditions confer on members of a society who follow certain health-related beliefs and practices?

Human physiology allows adaptation to occur in response to environmental pressures in the short term in the individual. Evolution allows adaptation to occur over the long term in the population. Human culture is learned behavior that also has adaptive value.

At the end of the nineteenth century, European interpretations regarded traditional medical practices as myth, superstition, or magic (and sometimes madness), as illustrated in Sir James Frazer's *The Golden Bough* (Frazer, 1890, 1959). During the twentieth century, social scientists searched for the functional meanings and purposes of medically related traditions. European and North American social scientists began describing the meanings of traditional medical practices in the 1920s. For example, if traditional societies, through plant domestication and agriculture, learn to obtain nutrients (foods) from the environment in which they live, they may also learn to obtain medicines from their environments and to develop therapeutic techniques to provide medical care.

As previously stated, many contemporary CIM paradigms and practices derive from complex and sophisticated ancient health systems and from indigenous cultures closely in touch with their natural and social environments. These health systems form part of the adaptation of these societies and cultures to their respective environments, representing integral components of traditional societies (Micozzi, 1983). Health-related beliefs and behaviors that are widespread and persistent merit study to determine their adaptive value (Table 2-2).

To accept the validity of the premise for scientific investigation of integrative (alternative) medical systems, one need only accept the possibility (or probability) of the adaptiveness of human belief and behavior systems that are persistent and widespread. The adaptiveness of human behavior is an important concept to both social and biological scientists. Whether human behavior is adaptive represents a persistent question in intellectual discourse. Some point to cultural practices that are widespread and that persist over generations as evidence of the adaptiveness of such practices.

Although many hold out the symbolic power of beliefs and the transcendental value of ideas regardless of "adaptive" value, belief and behavior systems can often be demonstrated in a scientific sense to have associated outcomes relative to human health and disease. The British anthropologist-physician W.H.R. Rivers showed that traditional health systems are not magic or superstition but represent rational, ordered systems of knowledge and useful ways of understanding and interacting with the environment (Rivers, 1924).

Bringing together social science and biomedical science in a more effective and integrated way must be rigorous in the application of the social sciences to the study of health and medicine. Social scientists often study health belief systems without adequately measuring health outcomes in a scientific sense, whereas biomedicine measures outcomes scientifically without being able to study the underlying belief systems. Social and cultural factors are amenable to study by techniques extrinsic to biomedical science. A conceptual paradigm may be considered to have reached the limits of explanation or inquiry when dependent variables can be measured but independent variables are unknown or immeasurable in the system of study (Kuhn, 1973). If health outcomes are considered *dependent* variables, the explanatory limits of biomedical science are exceeded because relevant *independent* variables are not made an explicit component of the explanatory model.

For example, there are different ways of explaining how manual therapies work. Although their clinical applications and associated health outcomes have been accepted on the basis of biomechanical mechanisms, many manual therapy traditions invoke the manipulation of bioenergy as the mechanism.

BIOENERGETIC EXPLANATIONS FOR MANUAL THERAPIES

First, all manual therapies imply that touching the patient in a particular manner is a primary means of therapy. The traditional view of the "laying on of hands" is to focus the attention of both practitioner and patient on the intention to heal and on the practitioner undertaking to treat the patient.

TABLE 2-2

Representation of Traditional Health Systems

Conceptual paradigm	Health system component	Methodology	Representation

"Social reality"	Health beliefs
	Health behaviors
	• Health practices, *wellness* maintenance
	• Care seeking, *illness* perceived
	  —Structural-functional access
	  —Cultural access
		Informant interview/survey
		Participant-observation
			Cognitive
			Observational

"Scientific reality"	Health outcomes, *disease* defined	Technical evaluation: health and nutrition status indicators	Analytical

Manual therapies as CIM combine several approaches to healing traditions. Manual therapies can be seen to include North American historic traditions such as osteopathy and chiropractic and more recently "body work" (e.g., massage therapy, rolfing, Trager method, applied kinesiology, Feldenkrais method). Asian manual systems include Chinese tui na and Japanese shiatsu. Techniques that are often seen as manual therapy but more explicitly relate to manipulation of bioenergy are the Asian systems of qi gong (Qigong) and reiki and the North American technique of therapeutic touch.

The founder of *chiropractic,* Daniel David Palmer, was originally an "energy healer" or "magnetic healer," as was the founder of traditional *osteopathy,* Andrew Taylor Still. Both traditions were established within a few years and a few hundred miles of each other in the American Midwest of the 1890s. In addition to embracing the concept of "vital energy," both Palmer and Still also rejected the use of drugs, which were especially toxic during that period of history (Palmer, 1910; Still, 1902). In this regard, Still and Palmer were joined by such mainstream medical figures as Sir William Osler and Oliver Wendell Holmes. In a famous statement, Holmes opined that if the entire materia medica of contemporary medicine were thrown to the bottom of the sea, it would be better for humankind and worse for the fishes. However, chiropractic and traditional osteopathy went further by specifically identifying themselves as "drugless healing," which found many adherents, in reaction to the therapeutic excesses in mainstream medicine. After World War II, osteopathy was largely mainstreamed into modern medicine, partially driven by the chronic shortage of medical personnel in the U.S. military (who recruited DOs to supplement MDs), as well as the desire of osteopaths to participate in the full benefits of medical mainstream training and practice.

Therapeutic touch and *healing touch* are more recent developments, largely promulgated initially by two nurses in the United States, Dolores Krieger and Dora Kunz. Healing "touch" is notable in that the patient is not actually physically touched. The technique therefore may be explained as a form of "energy healing" (perhaps the form most in practice in clinical settings in the United States) rather than manual therapy. The hands of the practitioner are thought to manipulate the flow of energy around the patient's body (Krieger, 1979; Kunz, 1991).

Other forms of hand-mediated healing modalities include polarity therapy, Tibetan-Japanese reiki, Japanese jin shin jyutsu, external qigong, touch for health, reflexology, acupressure, and shiatsu massage.

Bioenergetic mechanisms are invoked to explain clinical observations of the efficacy of therapeutic touch. These concepts are difficult to translate in clinical medicine, which at the same time recognizes that there is experimental reality beyond the realm of the contemporary biomedical paradigm.

AYURVEDA

Bioenergetic mechanisms have also been invoked in attempting to understand some aspects of Ayurveda, or the traditional medicine of India (see Chapters 25 to 27). Traditionally, Ayurveda is not only a medical system; rather, it is described as the science of *longevity* and relates more to what we would think of as a way of life or "lifestyle." A contemporary view of Ayurveda as provided by Maharishi Ayurveda represents a revival of Ayurvedic traditions lost through centuries of foreign rule (Moslem/Mogul and European/British) in India, blended with "bioenergetic" interpretations of mechanism.

Empirically, Ayurveda makes use of correspondences among five cosmic elements of earth, air, fire, water, and space (similar to ancient Greek concepts and "humoral" Western medical systems extending into the nineteenth century). There are three constitutional body types based on the balance of three *doshas,* which represent these five elements as they occur in the human body (Table 2-3). The three primary body types *(prakriti)* represent an empirical system for describing predisposition to illness, proscribing against unhealthy behavior, and prescribing for treatment of disease. The three primary body types of vata, pitta, and kapha may be roughly translated to the Sheldon somatotypes of twentieth-century Western science describing body constitution as ectomorph, mesomorph, and endomorph. Ayurveda also demonstrates systematic correspondences among a number of cosmic elements, seasons, constitutions, personalities, diseases, and treatments.

The idea that body constitution predisposes to certain diseases is an old one, and in biomedicine this idea now finds expression in the association of genetic factors with disease, a current preoccupation of contemporary biomedical science.

TABLE 2-3

Characteristics of Three Constitutional Types in Ayurveda

	Dosha		
	Vata	Pitta	Kapha
Somatotype (Sheldon)	*Ectomorph*	*Mesomorph*	*Endomorph*
Body type	Light, thin	Moderate	Solid, heavy
Skin type	Dry	Reddish	Oily, smooth
Personality	Anxious	Irritable	Tranquil, steady
Digestion	Irregular, constipation	Sharp	Slow
Activity	Quick	Medium	Slow, methodical
Season	Winter	Fall	Spring
Diseases	Hypertension	Inflammation	Sinusitis
	Arthritis	Inflammatory bowel disease	Respiratory diseases
	Rheumatism	Skin diseases	Asthma
	Cardiac arrhythmia	Heartburn	Obesity
	Insomnia	Peptic ulcer	Depression

CHINESE MEDICINE

As with Ayurveda, we can also think of Chinese medicine as an empirical tradition of systematic correspondences making reference to five cosmic elements ("five phases") that dates back to about 3000 BC (Table 2-4). Although for comparative purposes Chinese medicine is often treated as a homogeneous monolithic structure, this view neglects the changing interpretations of basic paradigms offered by Chinese medicine through the ages and the synchronic plurality of differing opinions and ideas over thousands of years (Unschuld, 1985).

Likewise, I prefer to use the term *China's traditional medicine* or *traditional medicine of China*. The popular term "traditional Chinese medicine" is a twentieth-century invention, concoction, or perhaps convention that blends certain aspects of Chinese medicine with a scientific underpinning put into place by the Communist government of Mao

TABLE 2-4

Correspondences of Five Phases in Chinese Medicine

Category	Wood	Fire	Earth	Metal	Water
Organ	Liver	Heart	Spleen	Lungs	Kidney
Bowel	Gallbladder	Small intestine	Stomach	Large intestine	Urinary bladder
Season	Spring	Summer	Late summer	Autumn	Winter
Time of day	Before sunrise	Forenoon	Afternoon	Late afternoon	Midnight
Climate	Wind	Heat	Damp	Dryness	Cold
Direction	East	South	Center	West	North
Development	Birth	Growth	Maturity	Withdrawal	Dormancy
Color	Cyan	Red	Yellow	White	Black
Taste	Sour	Bitter	Sweet	Pungent	Salty
Sense organ	Eyes	Tongue	Mouth	Nose	Ears
Odor	Goatish	Scorched	Fragrant	Raw fish	Putrid
Vocalization	Shouting	Laughing	Singing	Weeping	Sighing
Tissue	Sinews	Vessels	Flesh	Body hair	Bones

Tse-Tung to provide basic health care to the Chinese population.

Much of what the Chinese medical practitioner does is thought to influence the flow or balance of the body's energy called "qi." In my view, the Chinese concept of qi, which is translated as "energy," "bioenergy," or "vital energy," has a metabolic quality because the Chinese character for qi may be described as vapor or steam rising over rice (Figure 2-2). The term *rice* has a specific quality that we associate with a specific food, but it also has a generic meaning, "food" or "foodstuff." For example, the character "rice hall" is used to describe a restaurant in Chinese. The elusive meaning of qi may therefore be likened more to living metabolism than to the energy that we associate with electromagnetic radiation.

Energy or qi also has the dynamic qualities of "flow" and "balance." Because flow and balance are dynamic, they may be described in changing terms from one patient to the next or in the same patient from one day to the next (again, not using static, fixed pathological diagnostic categories). Such concepts present great challenges in translation to the biomedical model.

Acupuncture is a major modality for the manipulation of qi. Clinical observations of efficacy are increasing, and some biomedical explanations focus on the physiological effects of skin puncture and modulation of neurotransmitter substances. Some experiments indicate that the acupuncture needle has the same effect when it is merely held in place over the appropriate point (without puncturing the skin). If acupuncture needles operate by influencing the flow of energy, which is not limited by internal or external barriers, then puncturing the skin is not a necessary part of the mechanism of action. Perhaps practical Chinese acupuncturists simply found a way to hold the needles in place by puncturing the skin when they were trying to influence more than two acupuncture points simultaneously (and had only two hands to hold the needles in place).

HOMEOPATHY

Homeopathy challenges certain assumptions of allopathic medicine with the concept that "like cures like." A symptom may be seen as an attempt on the part of the body to correct itself, to fight disease, and to restore balance (homeostasis). For example, in the case of fever this may be seen as an adaptation to bacterial infection. Increased temperatures (above the normal body temperature) are seen to slow the rate of bacterial reproduction significantly. In this way, raising body temperature above normal is bacteriostatic and, as with many antibiotics, may slow bacterial growth, giving the immune system a chance to clear the infection.

Homeopathy originally gave the name "allopathic" medicine to the "regular" medical mainstream approaches of the time (early nineteenth century) because the medical focus is on the elimination or control of symptoms. In homeopathy, symptoms are everything, and describing them is the primary goal and guide to therapy. In classic homeopathy an empirical approach is taken by administering "provings" of substances (largely materia medica) in minute doses and observing whether the patient shows clinical improvement. This practice may also be considered reductionistic. Because many symptoms tend to improve over time, these "provings" cannot be considered controlled experiments, but the same observation may be applied to the administration of "cures" in other traditions as well.

NATUROPATHIC MEDICINE AND HERBALISM

Naturopathy is the most recent of alternative approaches to have developed as a complete system in North America (see Chapter 13). It emphasizes the

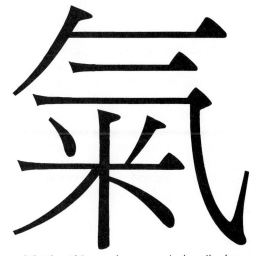

Figure 2-2 The Chinese character qi, described as vapor or steam rising over rice.

healing power of nature and can also be understood in terms of the adaptational model. In practice, contemporary naturopathy is eclectic, consciously drawing on a number of models and systems (e.g., Chinese, Ayurveda, homeopathy, manual therapies, Islamic healing) in an effort to fit the patient profile and the clinical problem with appropriate medical systems and techniques. Naturopathy is well organized in a few western states (notably Oregon, Washington, and Montana) and in Connecticut and northern New England but may be practiced in a less formal fashion in other parts of the United States.

The use of nutrition, herbs, natural remedies, and other natural products is an important component of naturopathic medicine. Medical traditions around the world, from the most basic shamanistic approaches to healing to the highly complex and sophisticated systems of Chinese and Ayurvedic medicine, make use of medicinal plants in light of their biological activity. Homeopathy (often included in the range of practice of naturopathic medicine) is also based largely on minute doses of materia medica.

From the standpoint of evolutionary biology, it is not surprising that plants develop biologically active constituents as an adaptation to compete in nature with each other and with animal species. Because plants form a primary feature of the terrestrial environment in which humans evolved, it is also not surprising that human physiology and metabolism are adapted to obtaining nutrients and medicines from plants in their environments. Societies learn over time which plants have value, and how to obtain, harvest, and prepare them and encode this knowledge and behavior into their cultures. In addition to the traditional medical settings for the use of medicinal plants, an eclectic system of herbal medicine has historically developed in the West, which can be referred to as "Western herbalism." Biologically active constituents of plants include carbohydrates, glycosides, tannins, lipids, volatile oils, resins, steroids, alkaloids, peptides, and enzymes.

Volatile oils form the primary basis of the practice of aromatherapy. The active constituents have various physiological effects throughout the body (Table 2-5). Because biologically active constituents are present in combination in medicinal plants, they are often observed to have synergistic effects. These synergistic effects have been useful, for example, in the application of crude extracts of medicinal plants to antibiotic-resistant bacterial infections and to

TABLE 2-5		
Medicinal Plant Constituent Actions		
Respiratory	Gastrointestinal	Neural
Expectorant	Emetic	Sedative
Antitussive	Antiemetic	Stimulant
Immuno- modulative	Laxative	Cardiotonic
	Spasmolytic	Antidepressant

chloroquine-resistant malaria. However, it is difficult to translate this approach to the active ingredient model of reductionist biomedical research, as described in the next section.

GLOBAL PERSPECTIVES

Understanding complementary medical systems described here as traditional or cultural medicine in an ecological model, we can compare and contrast how they "fit" in their indigenous settings with the interpretations made in the contemporary United States. In the U.S. health care system, we assume traditional herbal medicines are of value only when their active principal or ingredient is known and can be purified for mass production. However, this "active ingredient" approach to medicinal plants and traditional medicine reflects a particular conceptual paradigm rather than a particular truth about how natural medicines may work. On the basis of findings from U.S. biomedical plant-screening programs, therapeutic benefits are often observed to be limited. However, methodologies used in biomedicine often overlook the effects by which traditional medicines produce results because of a fixed and defined view of what constitutes therapeutic action. Although traditional health systems have acknowledged use in chronic, low-level conditions, they are assumed to be of no value in providing acute or emergency care. In some countries (China, Vietnam, Nicaragua), however, traditional medicine is mandated and used effectively for trauma and major acute diseases; historically, this resulted from political and economic exclusion from other health care technologies. Much research already exists in other countries (often in other languages besides English).

Traditional medicines are now seen as valuable because they serve as sources of leads for new pharmaceuticals (so-called biodiversity prospecting), and the potential medical value of tropical rainforest species provides a basis for support to preserve and conserve regional biodiversity. However, this "biodiversity prospecting" assumption overlooks the role of traditional medical systems in addressing the needs of the people from whence come the medicinal plants and the knowledge about their appropriate use. Whereas old views assume the marginalization of traditional medical systems, a new perspective looks to them to provide complementary therapies and, in some cases, new solutions to our contemporary "health care crisis" (Table 2-6).

Much of what is called complementary or integrative (alternative) medicine in the United States represents primary care for 80% of the world's people (WHO, 1998). In this way, CIM may be considered to represent appropriate technology and affordable, sustainable medicine both for indigenous people traditionally and now for industrialized societies as well, on a global basis.

References

Adler HM: The history of the present illness as treatment: who's listening, and why does it matter? *J Am Board Fam Med* 10:28-34, 1997.

Frazer JG: *The golden bough* (1890), new edition, New York, 1959, New American Library (Translated by TH Gaster).

Hahnemann S: *Organon of medicine* (1933), ed 6, New Delhi, 1980, B Jain Publishers (Translated by W Boericke).

Krieger D: *The therapeutic touch: how to use your hands to help or to heal,* New York, 1979, Prentice-Hall.

Kuhn T: *The structure of scientific revolutions,* New Haven, Conn, 1973, Yale University Press.

Kunz D: *The personal aura,* Wheaton, Ill, 1991, Quest.

Lust B: *Universal directory of naturopathy,* Butler, NJ, 1918, Lust Publisher.

Micozzi MS: Anthropological study of health beliefs, behaviors and outcomes, *Hum Org* 42:351-353, 1983.

Palmer DD: *Textbook of the science, art and philosophy of chiropractic,* Portland, Ore, 1910, Portland Printing House.

Rivers WHR: *Medicine, magic and religion,* New York, 1924, Harcourt & Brace.

Smuts JC: *Holism and evolution,* New York, 1926, Macmillan.

Still AT: *Philosophy and mechanical principles of osteopathy,* Kansas City, Mo, 1902, Hudson-Kimberly Publishing.

Unschuld P: *Medicine in China: a history of ideas,* Berkeley, 1985, University of California.

World Health Organization: *Traditional medicine,* Geneva, 1998, WHO Publications.

TABLE 2-6

Old Assumptions and New Perspectives on Complementary Medical Systems

Old assumptions	New perspectives
"Primitive"	Holistic
Ineffective	Cost-effective
Marginalized	Locally available
Extinct	Renewed
Should be regulated	Should be studied
Prospects for biomedicine	Valid in own right
Active ingredient model	Synergistic activity

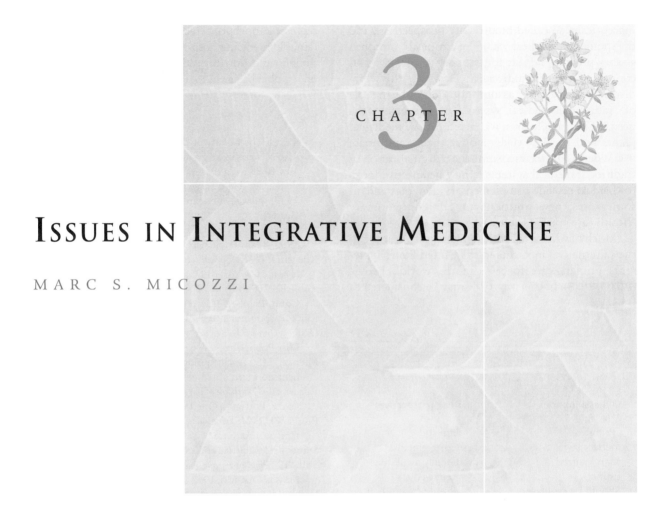

CHAPTER

3

ISSUES IN INTEGRATIVE MEDICINE

MARC S. MICOZZI

As discussed in Chapters 1 and 2, one of the major popular health movements of the twenty-first century is widespread interest in, and utilization of, what has been called alternative, complementary, or now, integrative medicine. Following recognition by the medical and scientific community during the 1990s, there has been a corresponding movement among medical practitioners, administrators, academicians, and scientists to incorporate these modalities into their existing spheres of research, practice, and teaching. These movements are now leading the private sector, through health systems and insurers, and the public sectors of state and federal governments to invest more deeply and broadly in integrative medicine from the standpoint of public health and health care practice.

In recent years, estimates indicated that the American public made more visits to alternative practitioners than to primary care physicians. Utilization of herbal remedies and dietary supplements is now supported by an estimated $30 billion industry in the United States. The 2004 report on CAM Utilization by the U.S. National Center for Health Statistics, the largest and most methodologically sophisticated survey to date, indicated that almost three quarters of Americans had experienced lifetime use of complementary and alternative medicine (CAM), and almost two thirds had experienced use sometime in the prior year. These statistics seem to indicate "once a user, always a user" (Barnes et al, 2004).

Significantly, American consumers have paid for most of these products and services as out-of-pocket costs, receiving only limited if any insurance or tax benefits until recently (see later discussion). It is also estimated that the out-of-pocket amount spent by consumers for alternative care exceeds the out-of-pocket co-payments and deductibles consumers make for health care covered by insurance. These observations are important when making assumptions or debating the roles of third-party payers in the provision of health care. A reality for health care professionals is that one last bastion of traditional fee-for-service medicine resides among alternative and many integrative practitioners. Furthermore, the workforce supplying alternative, complementary, and integrative care is strikingly small compared with the current workforce of approximately 600,000 practicing physicians (see Availability of Services).

NOMENCLATURE AND PHILOSOPHIES OF CARE

In trying to develop a nomenclature for these modalities for descriptive purposes in the 1990s, the medical and scientific professions advanced various labels, such as nontraditional, unconventional, unorthodox, holistic, and "wholistic" (a revival from the 1960s). In the midst of the call for greater scientific evidence and objectivity, these labels had the characteristic of betraying cultural values, prejudices, and judgments about the validity and appropriateness of such modalities. The more properly descriptive terminology of "alternative and complementary medicine" became generally accepted at the time. "Alternative" came to imply a mutual exclusivity by comparison to the regular practice of medicine, whereas "complementary" was more accurate in describing a compatibility between the utilization and acceptance of these modalities as an adjunct to, and not a replacement for, regular medicine. Institutions such as Thomas Jefferson University Hospital pioneered the utilization of the term (and the practice of) *integrative medicine* in 1997. In 2002 a national clinical network of seven integrative medical centers was established, with infrastructure support from the Philanthropic Collaborative for Medicine.

"Integrative medicine" implies an active, conscious effort by the health professions and medical science to seek and sort out the evidence and application of various complementary modalities for appropriate incorporation into the continuum of health care within the current parameters of the health care system. A potentially irresolvable philosophical question relates to the intangible costs and benefits of integration within one system versus the continued existence of pluralism among healing choices for consumers. "Integration" is interpreted to mean improved standards of evidence, quality, appropriateness, and availability of care within the mainstream health care system. "Alternatives" imply greater choices to consumers for those (perhaps relatively few) willing and able to create their own menu of healing modalities.

One view pivots on the present workforce situation, which may dictate that more appropriate care will be provided to more Americans through continued integration than with an uncoordinated landscape of different practices, each vying for primacy within as-yet incompletely defined, articulated, and accepted, evidence-based scopes of practice.

MODALITIES OF CARE

Many of the various physical modalities variously described as alternative, complementary, and integrative medicine can be seen to exist in a continuum with regular medicine and are believed and increasingly proved to have a measurable, physiological effect on the body. In this textbook, we have found it useful and instructive to arrange these techniques from "least invasive" to "most invasive" (see Chapter 4, Figure 4-4). Such an array also provides the beginnings of an approach to cost-effectiveness analyses in light of the general correlation between degree of invasiveness and costs, both the cost of providing the care and the cost of managing the known and accepted complications of that care.

One such array is provided by meditation, talk therapies, bioenergetic manipulation, massage, physical manipulation, insertion, ingestion, injection, and surgery. Alternative/complementary systems of practice are then organized around the utilization of one or more of these techniques. For example, Chinese medicine uses bioenergy ("qi"), manipulation (tui na, qi gong), insertion (acupuncture needles), and ingestion (herbs and foods) for medicinal purposes, approximating a more "complete" system of care. Chiropractic is traditionally limited to manipulative therapy, although many chiropractors incorporate acunpuncture, herbal medicine and nutrition into their individual practices.

Thus, individual practitioners within one system of care may incorporate other healing modalities that are traditionally outside that system of care (e.g., physician or chiropractor who incorporates acupuncture). Finally, individual techniques, when practiced in a manner that is removed from the traditional system of care (what may be called "formulary approaches"), are increasingly proved to be effective. For example, in the traditional practice of Chinese medicine (as may be found in China or in urban United States in Chinatown) the client generally seeks the services of a seventh-generation Chinese practitioner who may also want to incorporate herbs, manipulation, and other remedies for the treatment of a medical condition, despite historic debates among various Chinese practitioners over the use of herbs versus acupuncture. Meanwhile, in the United States, a licensed physician may attend a 6-week course in acupuncture in California and become a licensed acupuncturist. Research shows that acupuncture provided by the physician on a "formulary" basis is effective and may meet cultural expectations better for the average American when delivered by a practitioner in a white coat in an antiseptic clinic than with delivery of care in Chinatown.

AVAILABILITY OF SERVICES

The availability of these modalities is determined by (1) the existence, number, and location, of practitioners trained (and licensed, where applicable) to provide these services and (2) access to these practitioners through, in increasing order of complexity, clinics, hospitals, academic medical centers, health care systems, and networks. Individual practices have often thrived independent of the mainstream health care system. Given the dimensions of the movement, it is often striking how few "alternative" providers presently exist relative to the mainstream medical workforce. Manual and manipulative therapies are relatively well represented, with approximately 100,000 massage therapists and more than 50,000 licensed chiropractors. There is approximately half that number of osteopaths, with perhaps fewer than one quarter of them maintaining any practice in manipulative therapy. Manipulative therapy is also relatively well regulated, with licensure for chiropractic in all 50 states and the District of Columbia (D.C.) and accreditation of graduate schools of chiropractic,

while osteopathy has been fully subsumed under the credentialing processes of mainstream medicine.

In contrast, other fields of complementary medicine are sparsely represented.

There are approximately 10,000 licensed acupuncturists in the United States, with licensure available in most states and D.C. Approximately 3000 are MD-acupuncturists, and the remainder of this category include a number of traditional Chinese practitioners. There are approximately 3000 homeopaths, most of them licensed physicians. There are approximately 4000 naturopaths, with licensure available only in a dozen states, primarily in the northwestern United States and New England and five accredited graduate schools, primarily in the northwest and southwest. Naturopaths represent the practice of an eclectic style of medicine and "Western herbalism," drawing from the herbal traditions of other cultures worldwide. Hundreds of Ayurvedic practitioners may exist, many following highly individuated practices, with others ascribing to a tightly controlled Maharishi Ayur Veda school of practice in North America. In another tradition from India, thousands of yoga masters offer somewhat attenuated training in a variety of yoga, primarily designed as a meditative practice, intended to influence the physical body (Hatha-Yoga). Energy healers now come from several organized schools of energy healing nationwide. The practice of energy healing is widely incorporated among members of the U.S. nursing professions through healing touch and therapeutic touch and among a number of physical therapists, who may also include such modalities as craniosacral therapy.

MODELS OF INTEGRATION

To provide integrated care, the health care system requires access to licensed health care providers and training of existing providers in one or more modalities of complementary care. The health care system may provide credibility, appropriate practice environments, and access to new clients for practitioners. Often the health care system has opportunities to make capital investments in facilities required to provide care that are not available to individual practitioners. Sometimes the success of the integrated care clinic is based on attracting the individual practitioner's existing client base, while the individual practitioner comes to the health care system looking for new referrals. An important area for expansion of services is represented by appropriate referrals from within the health system hosts to their integrated clinics and inpatient services.

When complementary medical services are added onto existing services (instead of selectively replacing them), they become a cost center rather than a cost-effective source of savings. In response to consumer demand, some managed care systems have offered access to a network of complementary care providers who have agreed to accept reduced rates. For example, an innovative approach is available through the WellPower (Denville, NJ, www.wellpoweronline.com) network of licensed "holistic" health providers, which offers an insurance rider to employers, unions, and associations for access to members at negotiated rates.

Academic medical centers offer a further opportunity to develop the integration of clinical research and training with the practice of integrative medicine. Many academic medical centers adopted an "arms-length" relationship to CAM in the 1990s with internally isolated efforts at research or teaching or practice. The Jefferson–Myrna Brind Center for Integrative Medicine (www.JeffersonHospital.org/cim) was an early leader by developing a resource for academic, research, and clinical integration that has grown into a national model while serving increasing numbers of clients in the region.

Integrated care has been taken to imply the provision of various medical modalities under the supervision of a physician. To the extent that such physician-supervised centers function as full-service (or even fuller-service) primary care facilities, the concern is that if primary care "gatekeepers" refer patients for complementary care, they may never come back. Within a health care system, an integrative medical practice may be successfully managed as part of a primary care referral system for general hospital services. The national American Whole Health Network, based on a successful clinic in Chicago to provide integrated medical services under physician supervision, was unable to receive adequate physician patient referrals nationally and had to embark on costly direct-to-consumer marketing. One response to the concern about physician referrals, developed by the late William Fair, Sr., a leader in integrated care, was a facility for complementary care not supervised by a physician. This concept, initially developed as Synergy Health opened in New York City in the late 1990s under the name Health.

Another important implication of integrated medicine takes the provision of complementary care beyond the primary care provider and "gatekeeper" to the integration of appropriate complementary medical modalities into medical specialty practice for the management of chronic diseases. The initial primary care focus of integrated medicine is being supplemented by information on integrative medicine targeted to medical specialists such as the quarterly review journal *Seminars in Integrative Medicine* (www.elsevierhealth.com).

EFFECTIVENESS AND COST-EFFECTIVENESS

The establishment and expansion of the CAM research program at the National Institutes of Health (NIH) by leaders in the U.S. Congress has increasingly emphasized clinical trials research to create the research data base for evidence on the efficacy or lack of efficacy of available alternative medical modalities. Therefore the health care system has access to increasingly available, abundant, and credible data on effectiveness. Understanding appropriateness and cost-effectiveness of care requires health care utilization research to better understand (1) patient motivation and satisfaction, (2) willingness to pay for care, (3) preference of one effective modality of care for another, (4) willingness to substitute care, (5) multidisciplinary guidelines for best practices in disease management, and (6) related types of analyses that can better inform health care decision makers, whether policy makers, administrators, or consumers. The Agency for Health Care Quality has worked within a limited budget to provide important analyses on effectiveness and cost-effectiveness of various modalities for the management of low back pain, the most common cause of disability in working Americans; pharmaceuticals, surgery, spinal manual therapy, acupuncture, massage, and other therapies are all present at various levels of availability, cost, and effectiveness.

The U.S. Health Resources and Services Administration is currently sponsoring projects for development and dissemination of best practices for the treatment of lower back pain, for example, as well as an Internet-based, distance learning network for applied aspects for the management and administration of integrative medical practice. Under the new

Health Insurance Portability and Accountability Act (HIPAA, originally the Kennedy-Kassebaum bill, developed by the Congressional Energy and Commerce Committee), the Center for Medicare and Medicaid Services is mandated to develop CPT (current practice terminology) codes for every therapy "in commerce," implying that codes will exist for CAM therapies currently in practice and for which consumers are paying. These codes will provide a basis for expanded reimbursement of CAM by Medicare and Medicaid and as a precedent for other third-party payers. For improved effectiveness and cost savings to be realized by consumers, the health care system, and third-party payers, it is necessary to determine which therapeutic options can be appropriately and specifically provided to which patients in what order for cost-effective medical management.

PRODUCTS FOR THE PRACTICE OF INTEGRATIVE MEDICINE

Reliance on the appropriate use of nutrients and herbs is a critical and fundamental component of many integrative medical practices (see Figure 4-4). Presently in the United States, these natural products are widely available, classified, and regulated as dietary supplements. As such, they are regulated by the Food and Drug Administration (FDA) for identity, purity, and safety, but not for efficacy. However, unlike pharmaceuticals, information about the health effects may not be provided on the product label or with the product. Credible third-party research is increasingly available on the efficacy of herbal and nutritional ingredients. In addition, the medical profession is increasingly recognizing the importance of dietary supplementation for optimal health and for the prevention and management of many medical conditions (Fairfield et al., 2002). Practitioners of integrative medicine are able to maintain a medical standard of information and practice about herbal and nutritional ingredients. Part of this requirement is to develop and maintain an appropriate clinic- or hospital-based formulary of high-quality sources of herbs and nutrients, available in appropriate forms, doses, and combinations.

In addition to the chaotic regulatory environment, much of the natural products industry does not operate to medical and scientific standards, many irresponsible marketing claims are made, and many medical and scientific professionals are not knowledgeable about the science behind herbal and nutritional medicine. This volatile mix produces much confusion and misinformation on both sides, even promulgated periodically by such well-intentioned sources as the *New England Journal of Medicine*. Most medical professionals are presently on their own in trying to understand the proper indications, ingredients, and dosages for the appropriate scientific use of herbal and nutritional remedies. Consumers can only look to health professionals for guidance. New information technologies are being brought online to provide distributors, consumers, and practitioners fair and accurate information about the appropriate use of dietary supplements (see Chapter 11).

MEDICAL EDUCATION

The issues considered thus far point to the clear need for enhanced and improved education at the medical school, postgraduate medical training, and continuing medical education (CME) levels. CME programs are met with the challenge that current practitioners have generally had no exposure in medical school or in postgraduate medical training.

According to surveys conducted by the Center for Research in Medical Education at Thomas Jefferson University, the majority of today's medical students in all graduation years and among all classes desire more education in integrative medicine. The proportion is increasing with each graduating year. Among classes in medical school, the proportion is relatively high in the first year (when entering students carry the culture of the general population), declines somewhat in the second and third years (as students become professionalized and may observe little reinforcement for the teaching of integrative medicine), and rises again in the fourth year (after students have been exposed to the problems and questions of patients).

The literature of integrative medicine is in the process of creation, with the need for both "basic science" and clinical texts and journals in integrative medicine. Elsevier has developed many titles in complementary medicine, including a series on Medical Guides to Complementary and Alternative Medicine for which this text serves as the foundation (www.elsevierhealth.com). Much curriculum development and faculty development remains to be done in this area, and the traditional support of state and federal governments for medical education and training could be well utilized to help provide medical schools with the needed resources and incentives. In the interim, it is incumbent on health care providers to help stimulate appropriate CME and in-service training for health profession staffs so that practitioners may be knowledgeable and helpful to their patients in seeking guidance on the use of integrative medicine.

PUBLIC POLICY ISSUES

State governments have developed a traditional role in regulating medical practice and in supporting medical education. The federal government has developed a unique and critical role in stimulating and supporting medical research, regulating medical products and devices, protecting the public health, and helping build health care infrastructure, and it is now paying approximately one third of U.S. health care costs. Policy makers at the state and federal levels are becoming more knowledgeable about the needs and opportunities relative to integrative medicine. The bipartisan Congressional Caucus on Complementary & Alternative Medicine and Dietary Supplements was organized for this purpose and co-chaired in the Senate by Sen. Tom Harkin (D-Iowa) and Sen. Orrin Hatch (R-Utah) and in the House of Representatives by Rep. Dennis Kucinic (D-Ohio) and Rep. Dan Burton (R-Indiana), who also chaired the Subcommittee on Health and Human Rights of the Government Reform Committee. The Policy Institute for Integrative Medicine (www.piimed.org) and others are working with members of the Caucus and other elected representatives to broaden and deepen federal support for appropriate analyses and programs in integrative medicine. It is unlikely that the current regulatory legislation governing dietary supplements will be changed (Dietary Supplement Health and Education Act of 1994). Although funding for the National Center for Complementary and Alternative Medicine had increased each year commensurate with the multiyear doubling of the overall NIH budget, that rate of growth is no longer planned by NIH.

Other federal agencies charged with programs relative to health resources and services, primary care, health professions training and workforce development, consumer education, health services research, and other areas are being brought to bear on the important challenge and opportunity of integrative medicine. Public support together with private innovation has been the hallmark for medical advancement in the twentieth century and should continue to be the case for integrative medicine in the twenty-first century.

References

Barnes PM, Powell-Griner E, McFann K, Nahin RL: Complementary and alternative medicine use among adults: United States, 2002, *Semin Integr Med* 2:54-71, 2004.
Fairfield KM, Fletcher RH: Vitamins for chronic disease prevention in adults: Scientific evidence, JAMA 287: 3116-3126, 2002.

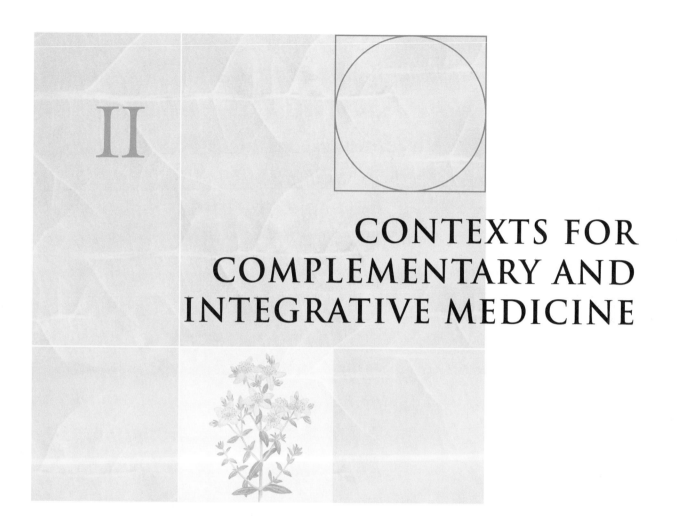

CONTEXTS FOR COMPLEMENTARY AND INTEGRATIVE MEDICINE

This section continues the introduction to complementary and integrative medicine (CIM) presented in the previous section. The following chapters discuss social and cultural factors, an integrated medical model, and global dimensions of CIM practice. Also, the social history of the use of CIM is provided through a review of the concept of "vitalism" in intellectual and medical discourse, which is important to understanding the common themes of bioenergy and self-healing among CIM systems. ∾

CHAPTER 4

SOCIAL AND CULTURAL FACTORS

CLAIRE MONOD CASSIDY

There are a great many health care systems in the world. All share the goals of alleviating the suffering of the sick, promoting health, and protecting the wider society from illness.

Despite this universality, systems differ profoundly. They differ in degree of expansion into the world, so that some systems are practiced only locally, as among a single rainforest tribe, whereas others have spread to every corner of the globe. They differ in degree of technology, from systems that require virtually none, to others that can barely function in the absence of electricity and perfect sanitation. Most importantly, these systems differ in their perceptions of the sick and well human body and in how they deliver health care.

These similarities and differences have been systematically studied for more than 100 years. As a result, we can now discuss both why so many systems exist and how differences among them matter. Basically, health care systems arise and persist because each one serves a need. Moreover, patients report satisfaction with care—no matter what kind—if that care is delivered in a manner that meshes with their cultural expectations. The form health care takes is first and fundamentally a matter of sociocultural interpretation. In other words, the "truth" that guides any health care system is relative and is learned.

This point, although implied by the very existence of numerous health care systems, surprises North Americans because, almost alone in the world, we have encouraged the belief that there is only one "best" health care approach. This belief is couched in language that argues for the primacy of scientific medicine, including the claim that only one medicine—biomedicine or allopathy—is scientific. As the voices of other types of practitioners gain strength, however, and as the world's cultural diversity increasingly bears in on Americans, it becomes clear that most of what we know, even scientific fact, is culturally modeled. We remain unaware of this situation most of the time because our cultural assumptions are learned at an early age and are embedded within us to the point that we take them for granted. Only when these assumptions are challenged, as they will be by the material in this book, do we become aware of them. Once aware, we can choose either to expand our thinking or to defend the status quo.

Biomedicine (or *allopathy*) is the formal name for the health care system in which the primary practitioners earn the degree of MD. These names emphasize aspects of this system's explanatory model. Other names are flavored by cultural politics and emphasize biomedicine's expanded or dominant position, such as Western, cosmopolitan, modern, orthodox, and conventional. All these names are inaccurate in various degrees, and it is best to refer to medical systems by their formal names. In this chapter, all health care practices, including biomedicine, are treated as alternatives, meaning that all are options available to users. They are complementary to the extent that they can be and are used together. Rarely are they integrated as yet, for sociopolitical reasons discussed below, but there is hope for the future.

This chapter offers an opportunity to expand thinking through a series of conceptual models that contextualize the variety of health care systems. It considers three questions:

1. What are the many health care realities?
2. How do they resemble each other?
3. What are the implications of the differences?

REALITY, INTERPRETATION, AND RELATIVITY

A psychiatrist told me about a Mormon woman who came to him deeply distressed because 20 years and four children into her second marriage, she realized that she would be spending eternity with her first husband, a man who had died 6 months after their wedding. Mormon couples can be married both for this life and for "eternity," and she and her first husband had chosen to be linked in both ways. Now her first husband was a stranger to her, and she desperately wanted to spend the afterlife with her present husband and children. To his credit the psychiatrist realized that he could not help this patient. He called a Mormon colleague who quickly linked the patient with a bishop of the Mormon Church. In a single visit the bishop helped the woman straighten out her fears about the afterlife.

Why could the first psychiatrist not help the patient himself? Because he did not share her reality model. He could have denied her suffering and told her "not to be so silly." Instead, he took a logical and compassionate step and linked the sick woman with health care workers who did share her reality model.

Consider another example. On a chilly wet day, a young woman laughingly pointed out her red tights and red boots to me, saying, "I always wear red on my feet on days like this, to keep me cooking from below up." Was this an amusing poesy shared on an elevator? A sign of psychosis? Certainly, this remark did not make sense from within the biomedical model. But an acupuncturist would understand that the cold element, water, is chased by the hot element, fire, and the symbolic color of fire is red. A similar behavior pattern would be recognized by practitioners of Ayurveda, the traditional medicine of India, or curanderismo, the folk medicine tradition of Mexico, Central America, and of many Hispanic people in the United States. It also survives in mainstream America when a mother boots up her kids on rainy days to keep them warm and to prevent colds.*

These stories provide small illustrations of the statement that the form health care takes is first and fundamentally a matter of interpretation. The wide variety of lifeways shows that humans have found many different ways to answer the same life questions. We can enjoy these differences much as we enjoy a good conversation, or we can grapple with their meanings and implications. Those involved in delivering health care must grapple with these differences.

---

*That the remark makes sense within the logic of humoral models does not mean that practitioners would say that red boots "work," that is, that the boots themselves, or their color specifically, prevented the young woman from being invaded by cold damp. To determine whether an action is instrumental requires an entirely different level of analysis.

Unfortunately, the same derisive tone that labels the interpretation of personal experience as merely superstition is also found in comparisons of medical belief systems. If one is modern then others are, by inference, outmoded; if one is based on fact then others must be laced with superstition. In this way, biomedicine is seen as somehow more true than any alternative system could possibly be.... Such a view ... fails to consider the internal logic of other explanatory models. But most health systems are logical and rational systems of thought if the underlying assumptions are known; this does not necessarily mean that these assumptions are correct, only that they can be viewed as having been reached by the coherent use of reason (Snow, 1993).

Grappling with issues of meaning can be difficult if we do not even know why we are reacting with laughter, anger, or defensiveness. The process of socialization—into our culture as children and into our profession as adults—provides us with truths and logical structures that answer life's questions well. We even learn to deal with the ambiguities and inconsistencies within what we have learned, and we may not notice that we believe two mutually incompatible things until someone with a different perspective points it out to us. Even then, why should we question our own truths or pay other truths heed? Strange answers make no sense and provide little guidance or comfort. It is tempting to think that others are irrational or ignorant. In the following quotation, a biomedical practitioner rejects user models of health care while insisting on the truth of his own reality, but would he be likely to convince mothers with this tonality?

> Mothers may not believe this, but colds are *not* caused by standing in drafts, going without a hat, or getting feet wet. They occur when one sneezing, coughing child shares germs with another (Sears, 1991).

That there are numerous cogent *models* of reality is often disturbing to people. In the West, battles have been fought and lives lost in defense of the ideal of a singular reality (Ames, 1993). Earlier in our history the search for this reality was mainly expressed in religious terms, but for more than 150 years, many have believed that science provides that singular reality. By this logic, health care practices that are not considered scientific are not trustworthy, and the path to acceptance demands "scientific research."

This situation helps explain why the preceding psychiatric example might be shrugged off. Lay-

people are known to have beliefs, and clinicians must deal with them. But the point of this discussion is that *everyone* has beliefs, and *all* realities are constructed; the facts of science are as culturally contextualized as those of law, theology, or social manners. Scientific fact is only as stable as the logic that produced it and the systems that apply it. Thus, science also experiences paradigm shifts. Plasma physics operates by a different logic and perceives reality differently from how Newtonian physics does; population biology is quite a different kettle of fish from Linnaean systematics; and an ecological or holistic approach to gathering scientific knowledge is very different from a reductionistic one.

The curious thing about modular reality is that you are likely to find exactly what you expect. The observer is not separate from the observed (see Heisenberg uncertainty principle, Chapter 1). Expectations are based on assumptions and the application of logic. When the assumptive base changes, so does the logic and, as a result, the appropriate response. Consider, for example, streptococcal pharyngitis. According to biomedicine the *Streptococcus* bacterium causes the sore throat. Logically, one could treat with antibiotics to destroy that bacterium. However, approximately 20% of the population carries this germ in their throat without developing an illness (Greenwood and Nunn, 1994). Only a minority of people who are exposed to the sore throat contract it. Thus, other factors must be involved; the presence of bacterium, although necessary, is not sufficient. Most "holistic" health care systems, such as homeopathy, Ayurveda, and Chinese medicine, understand this concept and focus more attention on the other factors—the reacting body, the person—than on infectious microorganisms. Care is aimed at strengthening the person rather than destroying bacteria.

But surely, you might ask, people use universal definitions for such material body parts as the heart or blood? Not necessarily. For example, although everyone might agree that the heart is a pulsating organ located in the center of the chest, its energetic and spiritual capabilities are debated. Biomedical thinkers describe the heart as a pump, using a material and mechanical metaphor. Even biomedical physicians, however, once thought of the heart as the "seat of the soul," a memory our society revisits in many romantic songs. This idea still is active in Chinese medical thought, in which the physical heart beats while the energetic "Heart" fills the role of sovereign ruler: "Sovereign of being and pivot of life, the heart is the guarantor of the unity of a person's existence" (Larre and de la Vallee, 1995, p. 174). In Chinese anatomy the heart even has a special "Protector," an organ unknown in biomedical anatomy.

Again, in biomedicine, blood is a living red substance that contains red and white cells and carries food, enzymes, hormones, and oxygen; it is complex and constantly renews itself. In popular Jamaican thought, however, blood does not renew itself. Its purity (a social rather than medical concept) determines one's success in life (Sobo, 1993). Following this logic, many Jamaicans are loath to give or receive blood for transfusions. Resistance to donating blood (e.g., Jehovah's Witnesses, www.religioustolerance.org) or to receiving organ transplants (O'Connor 1995) is common wherever people believe the soul imbues all body parts.

Cultural Relativity

In each of the preceding examples a reader might ask, "Who's right?" This is not a useful question, however, because answers are judged "right" from within the logic of the model in use. "Rightness" also is modular or relative.

A truly useful question is, "How does this model serve its users?" To be able to ask this question, one must stand back from one's own beliefs and models and recognize them as constructed and not exclusively correct. To ask this question is to practice *cultural relativity*.

Cultural relativity is a technique for dealing with the many ways in which people explain themselves. It tells practitioners and researchers to remain in a fairly neutral, nonjudgmental stance, *knowing the values of people without adopting or rejecting them* (Kaplan, 1984). From this position, clinicians, researchers, or students can observe their own perceptions and those of others and understand how these interpretations serve users' lives. They can avoid becoming mired in determining which method is true, because nothing is exclusively true when all realities are constructed.

On the other hand, ideas can be true in certain contexts or situations; that is, they make sense to their users. Therefore the observer must learn to synthesize his or her position with those of others, so as to design an effective response strategy. For example,

if people think of penicillin as a cooling drug and therefore hesitate to use it to treat a "cold" illness such as pneumonia, the practitioner can neutralize the cold of penicillin by suggesting that the patient take the medicine along with a food perceived as "hot" (Harwood, 1977). Alternately, as in the previous example of the Mormon woman, the clinician can refer a patient to a practitioner whose reality model more closely resembles that of the patient.

The practice of cultural relativity is pivotal to the study of medicine because each system of medicine provides a different set of ideas about the body, disease, and medical reality. Readers will find it much easier to absorb and use this material if they can willingly—even playfully—step aside from their current beliefs and appreciations to let in new ones.

THE BEHAVIORAL FIELD OF HEALTH CARE

What belongs under the rubric of health care? Once we know, we can examine which components are addressed by which particular health care system, because no single system addresses the whole.

Field of Health Care from Ego's Point of View

Imagine that each person is immersed in a potential field of health care that instructs how to prevent illness, treat illness, and, more positively, enhance wellness. Figure 4-1 depicts this idea as three triangles (shown as nonoverlapping, although in reality they do overlap, at least partially). The three triangles are embedded in a semicircle labeled historical, cultural, and social environment, which reminds us that all health care is delivered within a context of experience, belief, and expectation that is not always obvious to us.

The central triangle deals with health care as it is delivered to groups of people, and the right and left triangles deal with health care that is received primarily by individuals or families. The small circle in the center represents a person, Ego,* to whom all the con-

---

*"Ego" is used in the anthropological or geneological sense, that is, the person from whose point of view the figure is to be understood. It is not used in the common psychiatric sense, that is, the "I" that deals with reality.

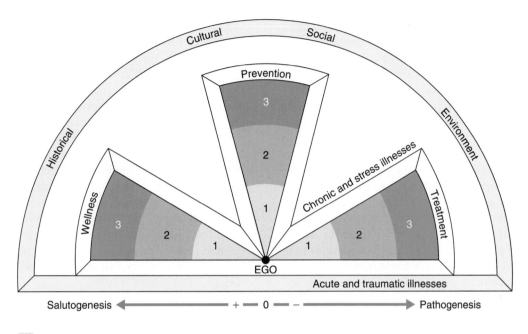

1 Self-care

2 Lower intensity specialist care

3 Higher intensity specialist care

Figure 4-1 The behavioral field of health care from the perspective of an individual.

tents of the field are available. Lines at the bottom of the drawing mark the health condition, from increasing health (left) to decreasing health (right). The central triangle covers prevention, that is, the avoidance of sickness without seeking high-level wellness.

Each triangle is divided into three sections. Section 1 represents the forms of health care that Ego can seek and deliver without the intervention of a specialist. Examples include praying, exercising, brushing teeth, bathing, eating fruit, cleaning house, paying utility bills for receipt of electricity and pure water, taking dietary supplements, washing and bandaging minor wounds, and taking an analgesic or sleeping to treat a headache.

Section 2 represents a degree of complexity or severity that requires specialist intervention. Most health care needs fall at this level, and most health care systems deliver most care at this level. At this level of wellness, we might find Ego seeking help with finding appropriate work, consulting a dietary specialist, taking a parenting class, or learning meditation techniques. Under treatment, we would find Ego seeking help for traumas, discomforts, or mal-

functions that have not responded to home remedies or that Ego believes requires the attention of a specialist. This section also includes ongoing care and control of chronic conditions and handicaps. Prevention at this level involves preventive dental care, screening tests, vaccinations, and community prevention activities, such as pure food and drug controls and pollution prevention—activities of which Ego is generally unaware and over which he or she has little control.

Section 3 represents a high degree of complexity and intensity that few specialists emphasize and that Ego calls on rarely. This level of treatment deals with extreme illnesses, malformations, and trauma, including care that is delivered in emergency departments, operating rooms, and intensive care units. This level in the prevention triangle deals with responses to major catastrophes such as epidemics and earthquakes. In the wellness triangle this level deals with an issue that is not easily expressed in English and is generally described in terms with psychological and spiritual overtones, such as *self-actualization, enlightenment,* or *awakening.*

Note that the cost of health care rises from level 1 to 3, attaining the highest cost in the prevention and treatment triangles at level 3 but, paradoxically, potentially the lowest cost at wellness level 3.

Now having drawn and laid out this concept in a linear form, I must critique it. The alert reader already will be asking such questions as, What if Ego has diabetes and is taking all kinds of proactive steps to increase wellness despite his or her condition? What about healing communities that increase wellness for terminally ill patients? Where do healthy pregnant women belong on this figure? These are appropriate criticisms: distinctions between the sections are not as precise in real life. A healthy woman who seeks a midwife's care during delivery might belong in wellness section 2, whereas one who delivers in a hospital with medical intervention belongs in treatment section 2—not because she is sick, but because her pregnancy is being treated as if it were an illness, as it has been for most North American women since the middle of the twentieth century.

Field of Health Care from Point of View of Variant Practices or Systems

Activities included in the wellness triangle in Figure 4-1 range from those that are widely accepted in our society, such as diet and exercise, to behaviors such as praying that many do not classify as health related (but see Dossey, 1997). Why include them here?

The dominant biomedical system's materialist effort to segregate medicine from religion grew out of the secularist urge to embrace science late in the nineteenth century; this concept is artificial and is not shared by most of the world's health care systems. Indeed, most systems argue that the nonmaterial aspects of the body-person are as real and cogent as the material aspects, and further, that there is no true separation of these aspects.

> Sister Erma Allen once told me of having healed a small boy who had cut his head; she had silently said the [bloodstopping] verse over and over while at the same time applying ice to the wound. I asked how she knew that it was not the *ice* that had stopped the bleeding. After a pause she reprimanded me gently, "God sewed it with *His* needle, darlin'" (Snow, 1993).

The fact that biomedicine prefers materialist explanations also implies that it does not deliver care in all parts of the triangles. This is equally true for other systems. Each emphasizes a distinctive viewpoint (explanatory model) and develops expertise in only some of the potential areas of health care. For example, biomedicine has had great success in treating acute illness and trauma. Its control of technology allows for remarkable success in extending life and in producing pharmaceuticals and technology to address the physical and physiological components of disease. Simultaneously, however, biomedicine is criticized for its relatively ineffective care of many chronic conditions and for repeated inefficiencies in human kindness and humane care, areas that easily escape its materialist model.

Other systems, notably the so-called holistic systems, *integrate* human development into their usual care patterns. These systems also control technologies and techniques that address physical and physiological functioning. Patients praise these systems for their care of chronic conditions and for their efforts to enhance wellness, which include weaning patients from excessive dependence on pharmaceuticals and even on health care specialists.

Figure 4-2 portrays these different approaches. Note that neither the biomedical system nor the Chinese medical system deals much with prevention on a mass scale. That is the prerogative of different specialists, especially of public health specialists.

Two vital points emerge from the field discussion and recur throughout this chapter, as follows:

1. No one health care system addresses the whole field.
2. All health care systems address a considerable part of the field.

The logical corollaries are (1) no one system is best for everything, and (2) existing systems overlap considerably in what they offer. There is a temptation to argue that societies ought to achieve economies of scale by making sure that only the best survive. However, considering our discussion of cultural relativity, it is impossible to define "best" in a manner that satisfies everyone. Logic demands that we determine who will be served well by which system and why. We will return to this issue after discussing some of the important ways in which health care systems differ.

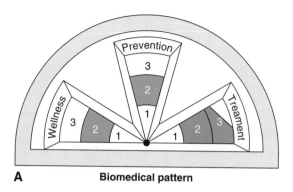
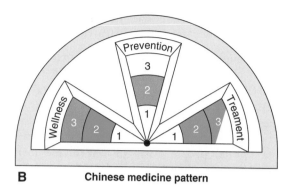

A   Biomedical pattern

B   Chinese medicine pattern

■ Strong emphasis
■ Moderate emphasis

Figure 4-2 The behavioral field of health care, highlighting the components addressed by two particular health care systems. **A,** Biomedicine. **B,** Chinese medicine.

CULTURAL CONCEPT OF THE HEALTH CARE SYSTEM

A cultural medical system is a complex of beliefs, models, and linked activities that providers and users consider useful in bettering health or well-being and in relieving stress and disease (Box 4-1).

This definition makes it clear that a health care *system* is complex and multilayered. Even simple systems, such as those limited in scope to one ethnic group, are difficult for one person to master or describe. Larger systems are correspondingly more complex, encompassing a wide range of viewpoints, numerous subspecialties, and distinctive styles of practice. Biomedicine includes specialties ranging from the intensely material practice of surgery to the much more relational specialties of family medicine and psychiatry. Biomedical complexity is compounded by the fact that it is practiced rather differently in different countries.

> Even the best simultaneous translator is going to have trouble dealing with the fact that *peptic ulcer* and *bronchitis* do not mean the same things in Britain that they do in the United States; that the U.S. *appendectomy* becomes the British *appendicectomy;* that the French tendency to exaggerate means there are never headaches in France, only migraines, and that the French often refer to real migraines as "liver crises"; that the German language has no word for chest pain, forcing the German patient to talk of heart pain, and that

BOX 4-1

Components of a Health Care System

1. A developed theory of the body-person, known as the explanatory model (Kleinman, 1980). This theory includes the causes of malfunction, as well as appropriate ways to address this malfunction.
2. Plans to educate and train new practitioners through apprenticeship, schooling, or both.
3. A health care subsystem that delivers care to needy persons.
4. Associated means of producing substances or technologies necessary to delivery systems and educational subsystems.
5. Professional organizations of practitioners who monitor each other's practices and promote the system to potential users.
6. A legal mandate that provides for the official recognition of practitioners and maintains a minimum standard of quality.
7. A social mandate that informally reveals levels of community acceptance, as by frequency of use, willingness to pay, and stereotypes about practitioners, among other markers.

> when a German doctor says "cardiac insufficiency" he may simply mean that the patient is tired. . . . How can [bio]medicine, which is commonly supposed to be a science, . . . be so different in four countries whose peoples are so similar genetically? The answer is that while [bio]medicine benefits

from a certain amount of scientific input, culture intervenes at every step of the way (Payer, 1988).

This complexity is equally true of Chinese medicine, which embraces many *styles*, including traditional Chinese medicine (TCM), Worsley Five Element style, French Energetic, and numerous Japanese, Korean, and other styles. Even community-based or folk systems may have different specialties. Lakota (Sioux) people distinguish medicine men and women who emphasize herbal treatment from holy men and women who practice shamanically (Hultkrantz, 1985). The Dineh (Navajo) recognize three types of diagnosticians and singers who work with ritual, herbs, and the psychosocial body to deliver health care (Morgan, 1977). Biomedicine is famous for its numerous *specialties*, and other health care systems also offer specializations.

On a much smaller scale than the system or the style is the *technique* (Figure 4-3). A technique is comparatively simple; it might be single therapy and often can be practiced without being linked to an explanatory model, detailed training, or professional oversight. Some practitioners specialize in offering single therapies, such as bee-sting injections, colonic irrigations, biofeedback, specific dietary supplements, or Swedish massage.

Single-therapy practitioners can provide *symptomatic relief* to their patients, but they cannot provide *systematic care,* that is, care guided by a well-developed model of how the body-person works, how the malfunction arose, and how intervention can help. The expansive power and persistence of health care systems correlate with the effectiveness of their explanatory models and linked therapeutic modalities.

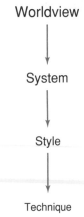

Figure 4-3 Scale of complexity in understanding health care.

Systems Embedded in Larger Constructs

But where do explanatory models come from? As noted earlier, health care systems are embedded in the sociocultural system surrounding them. This provides not only access to natural resources but also ideas, assumptions, and patterns of logic. All these are reflected in explanatory models and health care delivery formats. In formal terms, health care systems are guided by the worldview principles of their society. The larger and more heterogeneous the surrounding society, the wider the range of health care ideas that society can encompass.

Nevertheless, certain worldviews tend to predominate. In the United States and Europe the *hierarchical* or *reductionistic* worldview dominates. This worldview model emphasizes hierarchies of value, a tendency to be judgmental, and appreciation for competition, forcefulness, "modernity," and materialism (Cassidy, 1994; Kenner 2002). Biomedicine reflects these patterns in (1) its concern for the expertise of the practitioner over that of the layperson or patient; (2) its tendency to magnify the importance of some specialties or diseases over others (cardiology over pediatrics, cancer over asthma); (3) its preference for specialist-delievered technological treatment modalities that cause obvious reactions in the physical body (surgery, pharmaceuticals); and (4) its focus on end-stage physical malfunction while generally ignoring less-developed conditions and rejecting nonmaterial explanations of cause.

> [Cartesian] assumptions permeate Western society and form the modus operandi of conventional medicine. They have led to our belief in rationalism, causality, objectivity, and the separation of [bio]medicine and psychiatry. The assumptions work very well in acute emergency situations, but are limited when illness becomes chronic. . . . Cartesian thinking can be classified broadly as yang, and its inferred opposite as yin. Chinese philosophic thought can therefore be seen to be inclusive of Western thought, while Western thought has no way of incorporating Chinese holistic thinking (Greenwood and Nunn, 1994).

Other Western health care systems literally originated in reaction to biomedicine (allopathy), including homeopathy, osteopathy, naturopathy, chiropractic, and Christian Science. Others have been imported from Asia, such as Chinese medicine and Ayurveda. All argue (not always convincingly) that their approaches to care are more egalitarian, less judgmental, and gentler than biomedicine. Several offer nonmaterialist explanations of cause and care. In making such arguments, these systems are calling on another worldview currently held in the United States, namely, the *relational* (ecological or holistic) worldview. This worldview sees all things as connected in a network of relationships and deals with how people, things, and energy interact and how these interactions can better the whole. Reflected into health care, this idea means that practitioners model health in terms of achieving balance, and patients are seen to have expertise different from that of the practitioner but expertise nonetheless. Thus, practitioner and patient form a partnership, and patients take some responsibility for their own care and development.

Professionalized and Community-Based Systems

The terms *professionalized* and *community-based* systems distinguish between systems that serve large, heterogeneous patient populations and those smaller, more localized systems that serve culturally homogeneous populations.

A professionalized system tends to be found in urban settings, is taught in schools with the aid of written texts, and demands formal, usually legal, criteria for practice (Foster and Anderson, 1978; Shahjahan, 2004). Students enter the system by choice and are approved by entrance examinations. They become practitioners on completing a designated plan of study, passing more examinations, and often being licensed by the state or nation. Health care typically is delivered on a one practitioner–to–one patient basis in locales that have been set aside for this purpose, such as offices, clinics, and hospitals. Practitioners form membership organizations dedicated to policing their respective specialties and presenting them in a positive light to outsiders. The dominant health care systems of modern nations always are professionalized systems. Examples include Ayurveda, biomedicine, Chinese medicine, chiropractic, homeopathy, osteopathy, and Unani (the traditional system of Pakistan and neighboring Muslim nations).

Community-based systems, also known as *folk* or *tribal* systems, are less expanded than professionalized systems, although they may have equally complex explanatory models and equally lengthy histories. These systems are found in both urban and rural settings, and training is often by apprenticeship. People enter training sometimes by inheritance but most often by receiving a call from the unseen world, indicating that he or she has the special capacity necessary to become a healer. Training ends when the teacher considers the student ready to practice. Rather than written examinations, students are tested by practicing medicine under guidance; essentially the community itself determines whether a student is "good enough." Care is often offered in people's homes, and community-based healers often practice on a part-time basis. Some folk healers form professional associations, with the same goals as professionalized doctors. Examples of community-based systems include Alcoholics Anonymous and similar urban self-help groups, curanderismo (among the most expanded of folk systems), rootwork (an African-derived system used by some African-Americans), and traditional health care in Native American and Euro-American rural groups.

Box 4-2 provides sources for details about community-based systems in North America.

A third type of system is often called "popular" health care. Popular health care is not organized systematically; rather, it consists of simple techniques associated with the care of particular conditions. Examples include using cranberry juice for bladder infections, chicken soup for colds, and hot toddies for sore throats. Much of what is published in general-reader magazines or discussed on talk shows is popular medicine. It is typically presented using biomedical terminology and is often simplified biomedicine.

Distinctions of complexity among health care systems are not absolute. For example, most professionalized systems continue to insist on considerable hands-on training, similar to apprenticeships. Some folk systems, especially urbanized ones, train practitioners in schools and do not expect students to have received a call to practice; these practitioners often earn their living through full-time health care work.

Language Issues

Distinctions made in this section deal with differences of *scale*. A *system* is remarkably more complex than a *technique* or a single *therapy;* a professionalized

BOX 4-2

Sources Describing Community-Based Systems in North America

American Folk Medicine (Hand, 1976)

Black Elk: the Sacred Ways of a Lakota (Black Elk and Lyon, 1990)

Cry of the Eagle: Encounters with a Cree Healer (Young et al., 1989)

Curanderismo: Mexican-American Folk Healing (Trotter & Chavira 1997)

Ethnic Medicine in the Southwest (Spicer, 1979)

Feeling the Qi: Emergent Bodies and Disclosive Fields in American Appropriations of Acupuncture (Emad, 1998 [Dissertation])

Healing by Hand: a Cross-Cultural Primer for Manual Therapies (Oths, 2004)

Healing Traditions, Alternative Medicine and the Health Professions (O'Conner, 1995)

Herbal and Magical Medicine: Traditional Healing Today (Kirkland et al., 1992)

Masters of the Ordinary: Integrating Personal Experience and Vernacular Knowledge in Alcoholic Anonymous (Scott, 1993 [Dissertation])

Powwowing in Union Country: a Study of Pennsylvania German Folk Medicine in Context (Reimansnyder, 1989)

Ritual Healing in Suburban America (McGuire, 1994)

Susto: a Folk Illness (Rubel et al., 1984)

The Hands Feel It: Healing and Spiritual Presence among a Northern Alaskan People (Turner, 1996)

This Other Kind of Doctors: Traditional Medical Systems in Black Neighborhoods in Austin, TX (Terrell, 1990)

Walkin' over Medicine (Snow, 1993)

comparing a baseball bat to the entire Olympics, or an orange to a grocery chain.

This problem is common in commentary about alternative and complementary medicine, because one system (biomedicine) has been set up as "standard" while everything else, of whatever scale of complexity, has been set aside into the "other" category. This "contrast habit," itself, is invalid, and it is hoped that a wider view of medical care will soon result in *all* medical systems being seen as alternatives to one another. Meanwhile, one must be careful of terms that lend themselves to scalar confusion. The single term *acupuncture* can refer to a system, a modality, or simply a needling technique. Which does a given writer or speaker mean? Massage can mean a single technique, or it can refer to a rapidly professionalizing and systematizing practice. Some people use the term *medicine* to refer exclusively to biomedicine; for most, however, medicine is a term that encompasses all the ways in which people deliver health care.

Another confusing term is *traditional* (a good one not to use). Biomedical publications often refer to their own practice as "traditional medicine," categorizing all other practices by a term such as "alternative." However, when biomedicine is referred to as "modern" medicine, its worldwide nature is being contrasted with the indigenous systems of non-Western societies, which are then called "traditional." Systems other than biomedicine are used worldwide, so the expanded systems are sometimes classified as the "Great Tradition" systems and others, in contrast, as "little tradition" or "folk" systems.

In summary, it is most effective to refer to health care systems by their specific names and to distinguish clearly the scale at which one wants to speak or write.

MODALITIES OF HEALTH CARE

Whatever the other aspects of their character, all health care practices care for people. To do so, these practices use a variety of interventions, such as surgery, injection or ingestion of pharmaceuticals, use of delete biologicals or botanicals, needling, dietary management, manipulation, bodywork, meditative exercises, dancing, music therapy, art therapy, water and heat treatments, bioenergetic manipulation, talk therapy, shamanic journeying, sitting meditation, and prayer.

system is expanded further than a community-based system. Failing to understand this point can lead to confusion and can also result in invalid "data." For example, researchers attempting to describe attitudes to those in nonbiomedical practices often offer respondents lists of "alternative therapies" of completely different scale, from garlic supplementation (a small-scale, single therapy a layperson can select from reading a popular magazine) to Ayurvedic medical care (a large-scale, professionalized urban health care system). Creating a list of such wildly different scalars cannot yield meaningful data; it is as pointless as

Figure 4-4 sorts selected modalities along a line from intensely to lightly physically invasive. This correlates roughly with a movement from materialist to nonmaterialist views of the body-person. The more invasive modalities enter the physical body by cutting, pricking, insertion or ingestion. Less invasive techniques involve touching the surface of the body; even softer modalities access energetic or spiritual levels of the body without touching the skin. Even techniques that break into the body have differing degrees of intensity: Replacing a hip is more intrusive than removing a cataract. Pharmaceutical drugs generally are more toxic than phytomedicines (semipurified plant medicines), which are in turn more forceful than herbs. However, forcefulness does not connote effectiveness: Mild and gentle modalities can be as effective as intrusive ones.

Actual health care systems employ several of these modalities and can be roughly mapped with regions of the line in the figure, providing further evidence that each system emphasizes certain parts of, but not the entire spectrum of, health care options.

For example, a community-based system such as curanderismo uses bodywork, dietary manipulation, herbs, first-aid techniques, and shamanic techniques to treat a wide range of physical, psychosocial, and spiritual malfunctions (Rubel et al., 1984; Spicer, 1979; Trotter and Chavira, 1997). Ayurveda offers surgery, a variety of water treatments from purges to baths, numerous biological and herbal remedies, bodywork, dietary management, and both sitting and moving forms of meditation (Krishan, 2003; Morrison, 1995). Biomedicine is unusual in focusing at the left of the line in Figure 4-4, the most invasive region, but associated practitioners such as physical therapists, nurses, and psychotherapists use modalities farther to the right along the line.

EXPLANATORY MODELS

We have discussed intervention modalities, but we have yet to understand the "madness" behind each method. Each system has its own explanatory model that summarizes the perceptions, assumptions, beliefs, theories, and facts that guide the logic of health care delivery. To develop the idea of the explanatory model, we explore how different systems perceive the body-person and sickness and disease, their preferred causal explanations, and the preferred relationship between patients and practitioner.

Concepts of the Body-Person

There is not one human body, not one anatomy, not one physiology, but many. To understand any system, we must understand its concept of the body. Figure 4-5 depicts the body-person as four intersecting circles. The figure is simplified, because even within each of the circles, there are many ways in which systems can phrase their material, energetic, spiritual, or social perceptions of the body-person.

The biomedical model of the body-person focuses on the physical body, specifically the structure of its tissues and the movement and transformation of chemicals within cells. Classic chiropractic and osteopathic* models of the body are also materialistic, emphasizing connections and communications between bones, nerves, and muscles and the rest of the physical body, although newer versions increasingly employ an "energy" model to help explain changes. Note that such primarily materialist systems "enter" the body through the physical route and view this aspect as the goal of treatment, only hesitantly accepting that the psychosocial being may also be affected.

Other medical systems focus initial care on other aspects of the body-person and characteristically assume care will redound on all parts. Several systems begin with "energy," and much current research aims to develop this concept (Jobst, 2004; Oschman, 2003; Stux and Hammerschlag 2001). Existing systems use traditional language; for example, homeopathy views the physical body as having three significant layers and the body-person as having three distinct aspects (Vithoulkas, 1980), each imbued with *vital spirit* or *vital energy*. Acupuncture analyzes the physical body in terms of the flow of energy through pathways, or *meridians*, that do not directly correlate with known anatomical entities. The energy that flows through and animates the material body is called *qi (ch'i, ki)* and closely resembles the homeopathic concept of vital spirit or the Ayurvedic concept of *prana*.

Biofield or bioenergetic therapies intervene in aspects sometimes referred to as energy "whorls," "emanations," or "auras," and specialists identify them somewhat differently. Wirkus (1993), using

---

*Osteopathy originated as a manipulative system. Currently, only a minority of practitioners maintain this tradition; the remainder practice biomedicine (allopathy) or a combination.

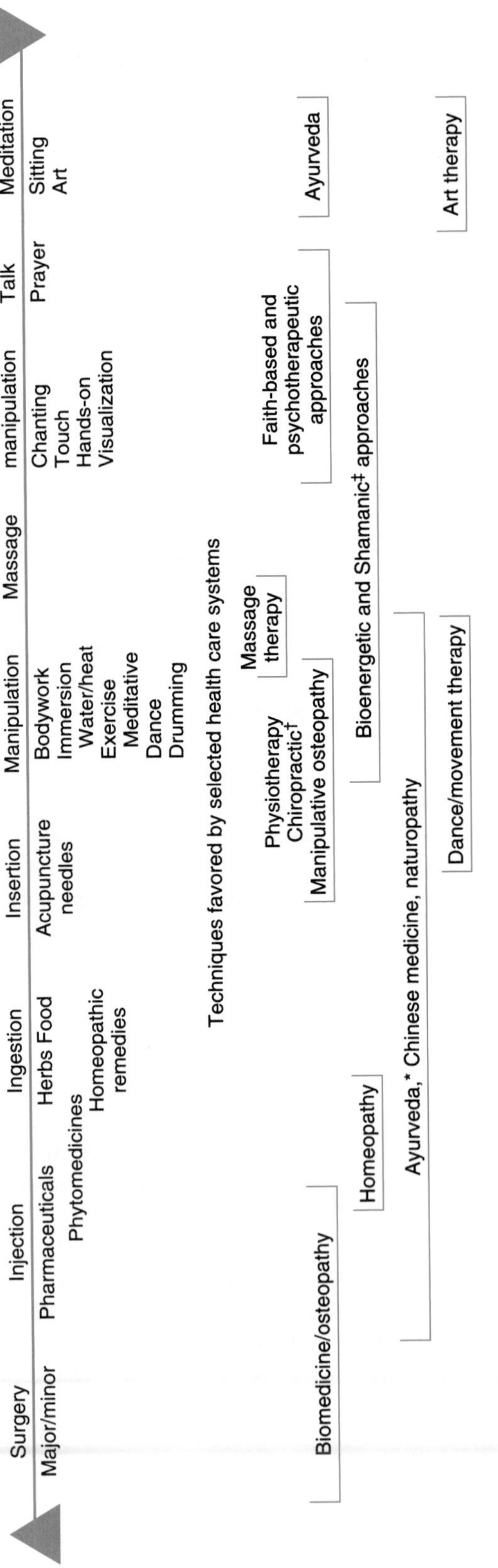

Figure 4-4 Relative physical invasiveness of selected therapeutic techniques, from most invasive (*left*) to least invasive (*right*).

* Ayurveda also provides minor surgery.
† Some chiropractors offer dietary management, acupuncture needling, etc.
‡ Many Shamanic practitioners also provide herbs.

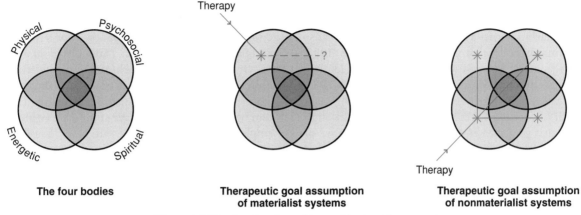

Figure 4-5 The four bodies addressed by health care.

bioscience terminology, refers to the thermal, electromagnetic, and acoustic fields. Brennan (1988), using esoteric science terminology, labels these three as the etheric, astral, and mental bodies. Bruyere (1989) focuses on chakras.

Spiritual and shamanic healers also work with nonmaterial and normally invisible bodies. Most believe that these spiritual forces imbue the physical body, although some say they extend beyond it, and some say that parts can travel (as during sleep), be removed (exorcism), or get lost (Eliade, 1964; Ingerman, 1991, 1994; Targ and Katra, 1999).

Psychotherapists typically begin work with the psychosocial body, that is, the "person" who lives within the other bodies and interacts with the world outside. Terms for this aspect include *mind* and *emotions,* as well as technical terms that each subspecialty uses to showcase its particular explanatory model.

The several bodies are not separate: only one body-person stands before the practitioner seeking help. But who can say where the physical body, with its ongoing chemical and electrical changes, merges into the energetic body and where the latter extends into the spiritual body? All are immersed in the psychosocial body; what a person believes greatly affects how he or she will respond to illness and to treatment or what he or she will deliver in the way of health care.

With the exception of heavily materialist models that perceive themselves as treating the physical body and only reluctantly acknowledge the psychosocial body, all health care systems argue that there are both material and nonmaterial aspects to the body (Figure 4-5), and that intervention in one area will affect all others. Thus, when a professional acupuncturist nee-

dles a patient who is having an asthma attack, he or she enters the energetic body and moves energy. The acupuncturist expects the physical, psychosocial, and spiritual bodies to respond as well: the bronchial tubes will dilate, and pain, anxiety, and fear will dissipate. These changes are not thought to be coincidental; according to this system's explanatory model, all the aspects of the body can work at ease when energy flows smoothly. Similarly, a shamanic practitioner offers healing first through the spiritual body, but assumes harmoniousness will result in improved function in all bodily aspects. Gathering scientific evidence for bodily interrelatedness is the subject of the field of psychoneuroimmunology (Martin, 1999; Moss et al., 2002).

CONCEPTS OF SICKNESS, DISEASE, AND IMBALANCE

Although often used generically, the terms *sickness* and *illness* formally refer to an experience of discomfort or malfunction. Disease and imbalance, however, are abstracted concepts. Thus a person has an illness or sickness, and a practitioner assigns meaning to this experience by diagnosing and explaining what has happened. The answers provided by the practitioner are guided by the explanatory model of his or her health care system. Cultural learning also guides the expression of the patient's illness and the practitioner's diagnostic values, so much so that even the pain people feel and report is related to such learned aspects of being as gender and ethnicity (Bachiocco et al., 2002; Bates et al 1995; Bates 1996; Emad, 1994).

A system's preferred malfunction concept is closely linked to its perception of the body-person, particularly whether a system tends to perceive cause as primarily *external* or *internal* (Cassidy, 1982, 1995; Fabrega, 1974; Foster and Anderson, 1978; Helman, 2000; Kleinman, 1980; Lindenbaum and Lock 1993; Mattingly and Garro 2000; Murdock, 1980). Most health care systems accept that both occur, although most also prefer to emphasize either the invader or the responding organism. External models argue that malfunctions attack from outside the body-person, invading and destroying. Internal models argue that something must first go wrong internally, allowing outer influences to penetrate where they previously could not. These conceptual differences affect each system's view of patient and practitioner. External theorists see the patient as passive and the practitioner as authority, whereas internal ideology interprets the patient as responsible and the practitioner as partner to that responsibility.

Disease

The concept of *disease* is preferred by external models. In this view the body-person is relatively passive, whereas the surrounding environment teams with danger. Body-persons are thought to respond similarly to invaders; that is, one person with mumps, leukemia, or pneumonia experiences it much as others do. If people are similar and the environment is dangerous, it is logical to emphasize the actions of the invader, and to find that every different type of invader creates a different disease. These assumptive patterns lead to the naming of many different diseases, and a major function of practitioners is to distinguish among them (diagnose *disease*). Their second job is to remove, destroy, or immobilize invaders, thereby curing the patient.

This model has long been preferred by biomedicine and has yielded familiar metaphors (Sontag, 1977). Tumor cells and microorganisms that have been awaiting their chance in "reservoirs" invade human "victims." The body "wages war," and surgeons and physicians are "warriors in white," battling the invaders.* Diseases that fit this classic model have

distinctive symptoms and signs, single causes, and respond to specific therapies. Treatment results in cure. To emphasize the separation between ailments and patients, the former often are called *disease entities*.

Only a minority of the disease entities defined by biomedicine fit the invasion model. Chronic, degenerative, and stress-related disorders frustrate the system because they do not have specifiable boundaries, single causes, or predictable outcomes. These disorders force biomedicine to consider explanations that fall outside the usual framework: (1) the body-person is not passive but plays some part in the genesis of disease; (2) many (often unspecifiable) factors must interact before disease arises; (3) some of these factors might be psychosocial; and (4) the practitioner's role is less to prescribe than to educate. The area of biomedicine that best reflects this opening state of mind is that of "lifestyle" diseases, or conditions that arise from and can be ameliorated by changes in how people behave and believe. Interestingly, even this door has not opened too widely; most lifestyle discussions still focus on ameliorative factors that address the physical body, such as diet and exercise. Biomedical practitioners who recommend visualization or meditation are likely to consider themselves "avant-garde."

As noted, chiropractic and osteopathy share biomedicine's primarily material and mechanistic view of disease, although these systems focus on the spine and nerves rather than cells and chemicals. Patient instructions also tend to take a physical form, such as a change in diet or more exercise.

Imbalance

Many health care systems emphasize internal models of disorder and emphasize *imbalance* rather than disease. Their therapeutic goal is to return the person to a state of balance. These systems often name conditions according to their process within the person. For example, in Chinese medicine, *rising Liver fire* describes a person's condition momentarily or repeatedly, but it is not a freestanding and categorical concept such as the biomedical disease entity *hepatitis*.

Balance can be perturbed by external invaders or by interruptions in the smooth working of the internal milieu. External causes, however, rarely harm a body-person who is in balance. Health care therefore tends to the self-protective abilities of the body-person, maintaining and strengthening them. This is not

---

*Similar metaphors are used to describe the need for exorcism: Invasion by an evil entity demands a spiritual battle to defeat it. Faith-based systems that use exorcism therapeutically also use external models of disease causation.

curing but healing; the practitioner's goal is not to battle the invader or fix the patient but rather to prune, weed, and plant within the patient, enabling the person to grow a vibrant internal garden in which all aspects of his or her body-person function harmoniously despite the vagaries of the external environment.

Treatment within internal-cause systems is individualistic because the logic of this model is such that each person has a unique history and constitution that affect how he or she will respond to the myriad circumstances of life. The practitioner examines the current condition of the patient, relates it to the patient's social and medical history, and then selects therapy on the basis of the entire assessment.

Although diet, exercise, rest, and other physical interventions are prescribed, these are usually offered in formats that also address the spiritual and energetic bodies. For example, exercises such as yoga, t'ai chi, or Qigong offer movement, energy balancing and storage, and meditation simultaneously. A patient might be advised to develop his or her spiritual and emotional body through creative skills, such as art, dance, and chanting, or may be encouraged to minimize vulnerability to psychic attack by meditation, shamanic journeying, or prayer. Diet counseling may include attention not only to nutrient content but also to seasonal, constitutional, and essential (as opposed to literal) temperature appropriateness.

Constitutional Types

The disease entity and imbalance models represent ideals. Practitioners know that neither model works all the time. Thus, biomedicine recognizes as *syndromes* those conditions with multiple linked causes, not all of which can be specified. Similarly, internal-cause systems know that individuality is not absolute because people do present commonalities or patterned responses to similar challenges.

Many health care systems have developed sophisticated models to link certain constitutional types with the probability of their developing particular illnesses. In the European and Middle Eastern system that preceded biomedicine, persons were categorized as melancholic, phlegmatic, sanguine, or choleric. Although current biomedical practitioners may view these concepts with an indulgent smile, the underlying idea is by no means absent in modern biomedicine:

In the mid-twentieth century, bioscientists attempted to link physical and psychosocial diseases with the endomorphic, mesomorphic, and ectomorphic types (Sheldon et al., 1949). At present there is much interest in type A personalities, which are said to be prone to heart disease, and type C, prone to cancer. A popular diet links blood type to diet (Adamo, 1996). Constitutional typologies are well developed in the Ayurvedic system (the *doshas* of pitta, vata, and kapha) and in some styles of Chinese medicine (the five elements of wood, fire, earth, metal, water). The old European categories survive in the hot-cold systems of Latin America and the Philippines.

Figure 4-6 summarizes the data of this section on a linear model. The "categorical disease entities" model forms one extreme on a continuum, with the "process-related imbalance" model at the other end. At the midpoint are patterned responses, including constitutional types. At the end featuring diseases, the individual person essentially has been deleted from the argument ("one person suffers much like others, so focus on identifying the disease"), whereas at the other extreme the person is the final focus and arbiter of interpretation ("in this individual these symptoms mean x, which I know from experience of him/her . . . they may mean y in another individual"). In the middle are positions that share both interpretive energies: "Certain characteristics make it more likely that he or she will experience these symptoms, so perhaps I can reduce my diagnostic chore."

Language Issues

Biomedical disease entity names have become standard vocabulary, but these diseases (not the symptoms) are "real" only to people who use the biomedical model. Practitioners of other systems may use these terms out of familiarity to communicate with patients or granting agencies or to complete insurance claim forms, but within their own system of health care, these labels have little cogency. Acupuncturists, for example, treat what their patients and referring physicians call "depression," but the concept does not exist in Chinese medicine. Research has shown that in samples of people with the biomedical diagnosis of depression, Chinese medical practitioners can recognize at least five distinct energetic imbalance conditions (Schnyer, 2002; Schnyer and Allen, 2001). The significant point is that two

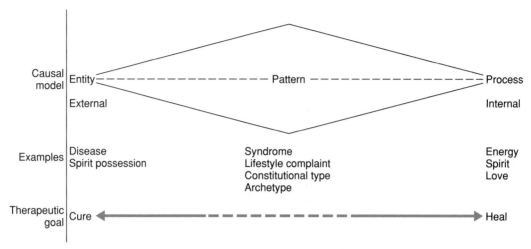

Figure 4-6 Three major approaches to interpreting symptoms.

patients with the same biomedical diagnosis might appropriately receive different herbal or needle therapies from a Chinese medicine practitioner.

Practitioners and scientists therefore must be careful in their use of biomedical terminology, not assuming it is sufficient to describe what is understood by other systems. Specialists should describe the symptoms and then, if they wish, affix a biomedical label while clearly stating that the biomedical label may not reflect the way of knowing of another system. This can serve its purpose because symptoms are recognized everywhere; it is the interpretations that differ. By focusing on symptoms, the malfunction labels of the other systems would begin to take on the kind of reality that now is owned only by the biomedical labels. The medical conversation would become more accurate and broader.

Concepts of Deep Cause

External and internal causative factors mentioned so far can be understood as proximate causes of malfunction. With the issue of deep cause, we contemplate why *this* person at *this* time or in *this* place has become ill in *this* way. We want to consider sociocultural answers, not epidemiological ones. We explore the issue by first, returning to our discussion of the body-person and considering the developmental nature of sickness, and second, considering the intentional component of sickness.

Developmental Nature of Sickness

An ancient chicken-and-egg philosophical argument questions whether the physical body comes first, giving rise to nonmaterial constructs such as emotions and mind, or whether mind (spirit, soul) comes first and animates the physical body. Materialist models prefer the first argument, whereas nonmaterialist models favor the second.

This choice affects both the theory and the politics of health care. If one accepts as real only what one can see, hear, or measure with machines, delivering care to the nonmaterial bodies is, at the least, puzzling, but more likely, ridiculous. Efforts to test nonmaterialist systems include designing machinery to "prove" that the claimed bodies exist, such as using electrical point locators to find acupuncture points and meridians or Kirlian photography to find auras. Materialists suspect nonmaterialist practitioners of misleading their patients or achieving effects primarily by activating the placebo response. Cynics also argue that nonmaterialist practitioners have their greatest successes in the care of functional, or psychosomatic, diseases. Such diseases are disvalued in materialist systems precisely because they lack specific material signs such as germs, malfunctioning genes, tumor cells, abnormal metabolic values, or broken bones. Materialists suspect that those who have functional conditions are not really sick.

Nonmaterialist thinkers consider malfunction in the nonmaterial aspects of the body to be as real as physical malfunction. All patient complaints signal true distress; the diagnostic concern is not with triaging between the real and the imaginary, but with identifying what aspect of the person will respond most efficaciously to treatment.

Many such systems use a developmental model of malfunction, in which sickness starts in the nonmaterial bodies and is expressed in the physical body only later. They fault materialist systems for paying attention only to end-stage (i.e., physical) malfunction and failing to treat conditions before they become entrenched. They further argue that a focus on the material level alone provides only symptomatic relief and ignores deep cause, allowing underlying malfunctions to remain unaddressed. Nonmaterialist systems assume that care can modify all parts of the body-person. Some also claim that as persons heal, they cycle backward through layers of long-buried symptoms until finally they express the oldest symptoms, release them, and are well. This pattern is called the "law of cure."

For example, a child might experience a spiritual trauma such as loss of intimacy (Jarrett, 1998). Afterward this child has eczema. Later still the child has allergies and asthma. Untreated, the original spiritual wound or deep cause has been magnified and becomes overt and disabling. Appropriate treatment of the asthma not only will relieve wheezing but also might instigate a recrudescence of eczema and grief until the spiritual wound is healed.

Thus, by the logic of internal-cause systems, it is advantageous to treat complaints before malfunction is manifested physically. Nonmaterial complaints are real because any suffering affects the whole body-person.

Systems that use only nonmaterial therapies, such as bioenergetic healing, psychotherapy, and shamanism, focus care on the nonmaterial aspects of the person but expect that the physical body will respond. However, many systems use a combination of material and nonmaterial therapeutic modalities. The techniques themselves often have a layered character. For example, acupuncture points have multiple functions and in combination have predictable and specific physical, spiritual, and emotional effects (Ross, 1995). The same is true of herbal remedies and some forms of bodywork. Nonmaterialist models also view the person as having an active role in creating and treating his or her own condition. The role of practitioner is reformulated from authority to facilitator, from the one who does the curing to the one who

helps persons heal themselves. As treatment is administered, such practitioners encourage patients to consider what attitudes of mind or spirit may have played a part in their illness and to explore new, life-enhancing ways of believing and behaving—wellness training. The goals of nonmaterialist health care are to care for the nonsomatic aspects of the patient so completely that the somatic aspect rarely suffers.

Unfortunately, in the hands of some practitioners the focus on patient responsibility becomes excessive, and patients feel guilt about their sickness. The materialist emphasis on the patient as the victim of disease can be equally harmful, resulting in patients who feel helpless to change themselves or learn health-enhancing behaviors.

Intentional Component of Sickness

While practitioners discuss proximate and deep causes of sickness, medical social scientists recognize another cross-cutting domain of causality and contrast, called the naturalistic and personalistic explanatory approaches. According to the *naturalistic* approach, the causes of sickness are found in the natural world and lack intention; they cause malfunction by unintentionally ending up in the wrong place or by causing damage as they go about their own lifeways. Sickness is considered a normal experience of life, natural and inevitable. The *personalistic* approach, in contrast, maintains that some form of intention is present, and sickness is an unnatural result of one's own misbehavior, or of attracting the attention of the wrong entities (Foster and Anderson, 1978).

When a person says he or she has lung cancer and attributes it to 30 years of smoking, the person speaks in a naturalistic mode. However, if the person complains of having been inveigled into smoking or that this habit is an expression of weak character, the person is moving in a personalistic direction. If people attribute their cancer to the corrective or punitive actions of a spiritual entity such as God, they speak fully in the personalistic mode.

These tendencies coexist in most health care systems, although one or the other usually is emphasized. Professionalized health care systems generally prefer such naturalistic explanations as microorganisms, malformations, toxins, age-related degeneration, winds, hot and cold, or damp and dry. Within these systems, however, some practitioners recognize, even specialize in, the personalistic approach. In biomedicine, psychiatry and psychology emphasize this structure, usually attributing malfunction to troubles in the psychosocial body rather than in the spiritual or energetic bodies. In other major systems, practitioners deal with expressions of self-distrust or the results of psychic attacks in much the same way as they deal with physical conditions.

Faith-based systems are primarily personalistic in approach. They ask patients to confess ways in which they have angered God, who may have retaliated by sending disease. Some also recognize invasion by evil spiritual entities and offer exorcism as a treatment. Prayer is offered to alleviate pain and prevent sickness. Some faith-based systems also practice the "laying on of hands."

> "But she seems to be an intelligent woman," one family practitioner kept repeating as he told me of the woman who had refused the surgical removal of uterine fibroids. What he viewed as a completely medical (and secular) situation his patient took to be a tangible sign of divine displeasure . . . God would heal her if it would be his will; no scalpels necessary (Snow, 1993).

Shamanic systems combine naturalistic and personalistic approaches. Natural events, such as experiencing a severe emotional or physical shock, may cause parts of the soul to be lost. The shaman recognizes the situation from the symptoms and takes a spiritual journey to retrieve the soul parts. Again, a person with an insufficient degree of psychic protection may be psychically attacked by someone else, either purposefully, during an argument, or even by being looked at with envious eyes. The shaman's task is to heal the psychospiritual wound and then help the patient to develop stronger personal protective skills. Shamans also serve communities by mediating arguments, changing weather, and treating physical illness with herbs and psychospiritual support.

Notice that the naturalistic-personalistic frame cuts across the materialist-nonmaterialist frame. Naturalistic explanations often deal with causes that are nonmaterial, such as temperature changes or wind invasions. Similarly, personalistic explanations can be materialist; some people see, hear, or feel entities such as ghosts and spirits, and material objects such as hair and fingernails store aspects of soul and thus can be used to heal or harm. Most importantly, however, even when the system and practitioner prefer naturalistic explanations, patients regularly demand to know, "Why me, Lord?" and offer answers couched in the personalistic framework.

CONCEPTS OF THE PRACTITIONER-PATIENT RELATIONSHIP

Systems that prefer external causative models characteristically view the body-person as passive, a victim, and, logically enough, interpret the practitioner as active, the one who cures. By contrast, systems that prefer internal causative models view the body-person as active and as already capable of healing. The practitioner's task is to facilitate the discovery of this capacity and develop it. The patient in this model has life expertise, and the practitioner must use medical expertise in partnership with the patient.

Some patients are passive regardless of what is asked of them, and others always demand a say in their care. The biomedical literature discusses this issue under the rubrics of external locus and internal locus of control. However, this chapter makes the point that not only practitioners or patients, but entire systems are modeled to emphasize one style of caregiving. Systems that want patients to be passive find active patients frustrating, irritating, and intrusive. Systems that want patients to be active find passive patients unresponsive, helpless, and in denial.

A lucid practitioner might be able to match his or her style to the patient's needs, providing either authoritarian or relational (patient-centered) care to fit the situation. However, practitioners also have preferences and personal styles that cannot be modified easily. Students are likely to select health care practices that fit their personal styles.

MAKING SENSE OF ALL THE VARIABILITY

The chapter began with the claim that health care systems vary in many ways and that the variety can be analyzed with the help of conceptual models. Now we must ask, "How can this information be applied in a world in which patients use many health care modalities and practitioners are advised to understand and sympathize?"

This section explores this question by discussing an example that compares biomedicine and Chinese medicine. I have developed a conceptual map that allows any system to be rapidly compared with another (Figure 4-7). I end by summarizing what makes biomedicine unusual, yet convinced that it is normative.

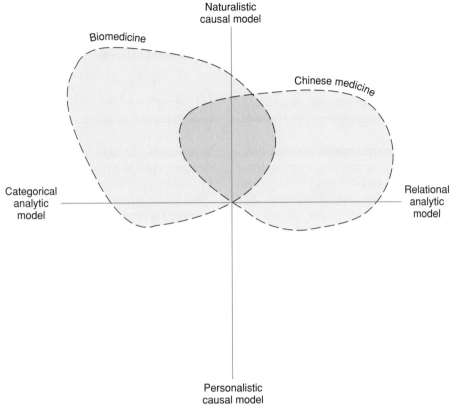

Figure 4-7 A cognitive map for health care systems.

Comparison of Care in Two Medical Systems

As discussed, biomedicine prefers reductionistic, categorical explanatory models, whereas Chinese medicine prefers relational, process-related explanatory models (Beinfield and Korngold, 1991; Cassidy 2002; Kaptchuk, 1983; Lock and Gordon, 1988; Stein, 1990). Both are heterogeneous systems, so relational tendencies can be found in biomedicine, and categorical tendencies exist in Chinese medicine. How different do these preferences really make these two systems?

Similarities Between Biomedicine and Chinese Medicine

1. Both aim to provide comprehensive health care, which includes health-enhancing, preventive, reproductive, acute and chronic illness, and trauma care.
2. Both prefer to deliver care in specific locales such as clinics or hospitals and in practitioner-to-patient dyads; group-based and home- or community-based practices are viewed as possible but nonmodal.
3. Both prefer naturalistic explanations of malfunction, arguing that impersonal forces are the main sources of ill health. However, if sometimes reluctantly, both also recognize that personalistic explanations sometimes make sense.
4. Both subsume a wide range of practices or specialties. Although specialties within internal medicine represent the intensively reductionistic naturalistic components of biomedicine, psychiatry veers toward personalistic explanatory models, and immunotherapy, clinical ecology, and approaches emphasizing lifestyle intervention use a relational flavor. Again, although some styles of acupuncture practice aim to be primarily relational and holistic in outlook, the post-1949 TCM style veers toward the reductionistic model and borrows many ideas from biomedicine.

Differences Between Biomedicine and Chinese Medicine

1. Biomedicine focuses on trauma, acute illness, and end-stage chronic disease intervention. Although prevention is discussed as part of biomedical care, wellness is not a core concept. Chinese medicine emphasizes wellness and preventive care, treats chronic and acute illness conditions, but avoids surgery (see Figure 4-2).

2. Biomedicine emphasizes materialist explanations, whereas Chinese medicine emphasizes nonmaterialist explanations based on a distinctive concept of qi (ch'i, vital energy). Their views of anatomy and physiology and their favored bodily metaphors (machinery and warring vs. gardening) are distinctly different.

3. Biomedicine emphasizes the physical body as the locus for intervention, recognizes but remains uncomfortable with the concept of the psychosocial body, and largely denies the existence of the energetic and spiritual bodies. By contrast, Chinese medicine uses the energetic body as the locus for intervention and assumes that interventions at that level will redound on all the other bodies.

4. Biomedicine sees humans as biologically similar; therefore, diseases will present similarly and can be treated similarly. Chinese medicine sees each human as unique and assumes that even if symptoms appear to be similar, the deep cause might be dissimilar; thus, care should be delivered individualistically.

5. Biomedicine has defined an immense universe of distinct disease entities, assumes they will present similarly in most people, focuses much energy on disease diagnosis, and defines success as cure. Controlling or palliating symptoms is considered a lesser success, and death is commonly thought of as a failure. Chinese medicine focuses on the flow of energy within the body and between the patient and the cosmos. Ill health arises when this flow is disrupted or impeded or when there is insufficient energy. Because this can happen in many ways, the practitioner also spends much time diagnosing by assessing the character of the flow, hearing the patient's story, and listening in to the energetic body (e.g., by taking the pulses). Imbalance is viewed as commonplace and natural, and there is little to cure; instead the practitioner hopes to maintain or improve the coherence of the

body-person, that is, heal the person. Death is also deemed natural; the dying patient can use acupuncture to ease pain and to achieve a final energetic balance.

Conceptual Mapping of Health Care Systems

It is possible to map differences among health care systems to allow these similarities and differences to be rapidly grasped and applied. Figure 4-2 maps the systems in terms of individual needs; Figure 4-7 redraws Figure 4-2 in terms of the conceptual models explored in this chapter.

Figure 4-7 shows a matrix with the categorical (reductionistic) versus relational (process-related) worldview represented on the horizontal axis and the naturalistic to personalistic causal model on the vertical axis. Using this map, we can—hypothetically—locate virtually any system of health care in such a way as to compare it rapidly with any other system. Knowing more about the terrain of systematic health care differences makes it easier to understand and use the insights from other systems of health care. Practitioners can use such information to design research, to make themselves and their patients aware of their own prejudices, and to listen more openly to the users of different health care systems.

Figure 4-7 maps only the two systems cited in our example; readers are encouraged to map others as they learn about them in this text. Note that each of the two systems mapped, however, covers a wide area. Biomedicine, although clearly within the realm of categorical naturalistic thinking, spills over the horizontal line into personalistic models (psychology, psychiatry) and over the vertical line into relational territory (family practice, psychoneuroimmunology, lifestyle arguments). In fact, biomedical practice overlaps the Chinese medicine outline at the center of the figure.

The map also shows that in terms of preferred worldview, Chinese medicine is opposite that of biomedicine. On the other hand, it is similar to biomedicine in its general preference for naturalistic causal explanations. These twin characteristics map Chinese medicine into the upper right quadrant. Note again, however, the wide range of practice under the umbrella of Chinese medicine. The more symptomatic and categorical styles of practice map left toward the reductionistic quadrant, and the traditional shamanistic components of Chinese medicine map below the horizontal line.

This map reminds us that no single health care system serves the whole field, and that systems differ but also share similarities.

Why Biomedicine Finds Other Systems Unconventional

Although not drawn onto the map, the other health care systems tend to cluster more centrally or to the right of the center on both sides of the horizontal axis. Thus the mapping exercise also provides a visual clue as to why biomedicine, from its perch in the upper left quadrant, might find the other systems unconventional. They are nonmodal when judged from biomedicine's position. Biomedicine is equally unconventional when viewed from the position of most systems. From a worldwide viewpoint, biomedicine is unusual in the following ways:

1. Its intense attachment to materialist interpretive models
2. Its focus on the physical body, almost to the exclusion of other possibilities
3. Its focus on the disease, often to the virtual exclusion of the person
4. Its vast development of disease types
5. Its highly technological delivery system
6. The invasiveness of its care modalities
7. Its emphasis on acute disease, trauma, and end-stage malfunction, with relatively little focus on prevention or wellness
8. Its high cost

Despite these oddities, biomedicine considers itself conventional and other systems "alternative." How did this situation come about, and why is it not surprising to most Western urban people? Furthermore, why is it difficult for people to consider biomedicine as just one more alternative?

Health care is not free of culture or politics. In the United States, we are accustomed to thinking of biomedicine as the best system because it is the most expanded, being practiced in every country in the world, although Chinese medicine and homeopathy are close seconds. Biomedicine also has the largest educational, legal, and economic mandate. Finally, its explanatory model closely fits the dominant European and North American worldview paradigm: categorical or reductionistic.

As part of the expression of this worldview, many state that biomedicine is the most scientific system. This argument is controversial and must be examined carefully.

Science is a particular method for gathering information and constructing knowledge. In contrast to other systems, such as theology, which allows for revelation, and law, which allows for precedence, science demands that information be sought in the natural world and that interpretations be tested for accuracy. This is extremely unusual; it means that a person's opinion or mere observation and consequent certitude are not enough to make the person's position acceptable to scientists. Instead, the person must show that he or she has gathered data systematically and accounted for potential biases, then must submit his or her interpretations to others for examination and retesting. Furthermore, the researcher is enjoined to be a relativist; that is, not to become enamored with his or her interpretations but to hold them always as models of reality or approximations. This provides remarkable training in humbleness, and to be frank, not many researchers achieve it.

ROLE OF SCIENCE

Euro-American society in particular has developed science to be *the* believable knowledge method, the knowledge orthodoxy since the late nineteenth century. The determination with which Westerners cling to their cultural preference concerning the power of science approaches a religious fervor. Biomedicine gradually took on the cloak of scientism with the rise of clinical medicine in the early nineteenth century, moving toward a laboratory-based experimental model by the late nineteenth century. Although the experiment is only one way to gather valid data by use of the scientific method, this became accepted as the "scientific" approach. By the early twentieth century, American biomedicine already contrasted itself to other systems by claiming to be experimental and thus uniquely scientific. Given that the other major systems are generally not experimental—they depend on well-developed clinical observation skills and experience guided by their explanatory models—it becomes clear why a system that perceives itself as scientific can consider nonscientific systems as inferior *in our cultural milieu.*

The biomedical model assumes diseases to be fully accounted for by deviations from the norm of measurable biologic (somatic) variables. It leaves no room within its framework for the social, psychological, and behavioral dimensions of illness. . . . The biomedical model has thus become a cultural imperative, its limitations easily overlooked. In brief, it has now acquired the status of dogma. In science, a model is revised or abandoned when it fails to account adequately for all the data. A dogma, on the other hand, requires that discrepant data be forced to fit the model or be excluded (Engel, 1977).

But is biomedicine really scientific if judged from the perspective of science rather than cultural preference? Recent studies suggest that only 30% of what biomedicine achieves has been tested adequately (Altman, 1994; American Iatrogenic Association; Andersen, 1990). A full 70% of practice uses the same well-developed clinical observation skills and experience guided by the explanatory model that powers the other health care systems.

Those who can stand back dispassionately—that is, those who really do think like scientists—understand that a great deal of the argument over which systems are modal or alternative is really an argument over cultural turf. As such, victory in this argument serves the usual political purpose of maintaining power by insisting on the virtue of one's own values, often by attacking the perceptions of one's rivals, but these are political, not scientific, acts.

IMPORTANCE OF VIEWING HEALTH CARE AS A MATTER OF CULTURAL MODELING

That health care is a matter of cultural modeling rather than scientific truth is important to practitioners whose goals are to relieve suffering. It also is important to those who want to be scientific in their thoughts and choices. Differences must be addressed. So, pragmatically, we end by asking, "Who do the differences serve?" and "How do the differences serve?"

Users of Alternative Medicine

Demand for nonbiomedical health care in Europe and North America is at a peak that has not been seen for about 150 years. Surveys of users of alternative or integrative medicine tell similar stories. People want to feel cared for, and biomedicine's emphasis on laboratory medicine, factoring the person out of the diagnostic and treatment equation, invasive treatments including high levels of painful side effects,* rushed delivery of care, and immensely high cost, all connote an uncaring system and are making biomedicine unattractive to increasing numbers of people.

Who are these people? Surveys indicate that the users of the major non-biomedical systems are mainly urban, female, well educated, with middle to high incomes (Cassidy, 1998a; Cassileth et al., 1984; Eisenberg et al., 1993, 1998; McGuire, 1994). These people are in excellent positions to judge the quality of the care they receive from the variety of practitioners that they consult. This point matters because mainstream practitioners and researchers often attack nonbiomedical health care by saying that the users are being misled, either purposefully by the practitioners or by their own desires, distress, and ignorance.

Such defensive, politically motivated arguments are increasingly weakened by the following:

1. Studies show that where health care is obviously pluralistic, laypeople are astute at matching systems with complaints (Cassidy 1998a; Young, 1981).
2. On the whole, patients report satisfaction with alternative health care (Cassidy, 1998b; Eisenberg et al., 1998; Emad, 1994; O'Connor, 1995; Workshop on Alternative Medicine, 1994).
3. Rapidly accumulating results of scientific research on alternative treatments show that they are often as effective or more effective, or safer, than biomedical treatments of identical conditions, or that they provide valuable complementary effects when biomedicine is in use (Benor, 1993; Byrd, 1988; Carlson, 2003; Cassidy, 2002; Edzard et al., 2001; Jacobs et al., 1994; Jobst, 1995; O'Connor, 1995; Reilly et al., 1994; see also articles in *Journal of Alternative and Complementary Medicine, Alternative Therapies,* and other journals; access Medline; and see reports of NIH Center for Complementary and Alternative Medicine).
4. Methodological skills for analyzing systems that differ deeply from biomedicine are developing

---

*Approximately 20% of illnesses that lead to hospitalization are *iatrogenic,* that is, caused by the biomedical care itself (Greenwood and Nunn, 1994).

rapidly (Cassidy, 1995; Edzard et al., 2001; Grimes, 2003; Jonas and Crawford, 2003, Wisnesky and Anderson 2005).

The Constituency for Alternative Medicine

Current biomedical discussion on the best use of nonbiomedical alternatives focuses either on annexing particular techniques (in the process, jettisoning the systemic embedding of the techniques in their native explanatory models) or on using the alternatives adjunctively (e.g., recommending acupuncture as adjunctive therapy to minimize the side effects of chemotherapy). Readers are now prepared to interpret these proposals as expressions of a biomedical perspective that claims its health care reality is superior to all others.

Of course, the situation looks a little different from the viewpoints of alternative practitioners, as well as from the perspective of potential patients, many of whom are glad that modern health care provides a menu of alternatives from which to choose. At times, for example, Chinese medical practitioners might want to use biomedicine adjunctively, and some biomedical diagnostic techniques are well integrated into nonbiomedical systems of health care.

Many would benefit if the U.S. health care system were organized such that several alternatives were widely available and people learned about them from childhood (Box 4-3).

Note that this discussion assumes that there is space for all forms of health care. This should be true in a democratic society, and it is true in the sense that all the systems already exist and serve people. The drive behind current research is to discover what services each system can provide and to compare their effectiveness in providing these services. Interestingly, this drive will fail if it is expressed solely in terms of conditions or complaints, which is only half the equation. The other half consists of the people who are to receive the care. There always will be a range of desires and needs; some patients will always prefer care that is technological and has rapid overt effects, whereas others will always prefer care that is relational, gentle, and virtually contemplative.

It is hoped that the world's people will become more skilled at using all our health care resources and options, to make it possible for everyone—practitioners

BOX 4-3

Beneficiaries of Widely Available Alternative (or Integrative) Health Care Systems in the United States

- Those who have a high need for affiliation and who therefore want a relational style of health care
- Those who want to alleviate symptoms gently or with fewer side effects
- Those who will not take "hopeless" for an answer
- Those who want to prevent disease or enhance wellness
- Those who interpret the body-person as having more than a physical aspect and who want to be able to address the energetic, psychosocial, and spiritual bodies when receiving or delivering health care
- Those who are concerned with the end-stage focus and invasiveness of typical biomedical care

and patients—to know enough about their options to triage care successfully in a manner that maximizes patient satisfaction and health while minimizing suffering, iatrogenic disease, and cost.

It remains for you to consider your own goals for practice. Where do you fall on the various continua discussed in this chapter? Are you satisfied with the care that you deliver, or would you like to modify some rough spots? How can the existing range of medical options help you do so? How can developing your skill and referral base in complementary and integrative medicine (CIM) aid your current or future patients?

CONCLUSION

This chapter introduces concepts that are fundamental to understanding values and issues in the practice of health care and provides a sociocultural context and models that will be useful in understanding the practices described in subsequent chapters.

Health care is fundamentally a matter of sociocultural interpretation. It should now be clear that health care systems differ in important ways and that no one system provides all the answers, or even the best answers, for all users or circumstances. Differences among systems are not random but are driven and logically organized by underlying assumptive patterns that are revealed in explanatory models, therapeutic modalities, and styles of practice.

These differences are *not* unbridgeable; the concepts developed in this chapter should allow most practitioners and researchers to approach even strange ideas with new appreciation, as well as provide them with tools that allow for better communication and understanding. After all, the deepest and most common goal of all health care systems is to relieve pain and prevent suffering.

Acknowledgments

Special thanks to Haig Ignatius, MD, MAc, and Marc Micozzi, MD, PhD, for their generous reading of the original chapter in its draft stages. More thanks to Jean Edelen for bibliographic help with the newer version. Continuing thanks to many colleagues whose deep thinking about medical philosophical and practice issues guides and sustains my own explorations. And to my husband and daughter, always, your love and support are most precious.

References

Adamo PJ: *Eat right for your type,* New York, 1996, Putnam.

Altman D: The scandal of poor medical research, *BMJ* 308:283-284, 1994.

Ames R: *Sun-Tzu: the art of warfare,* New York, 1993, Ballantine.

Andersen B: *Methodological errors in medical research,* Oxford, 1990, Blackwell.

Bachiocco V, Tiengo M, Credico C: The pain locus of control orientation in a health sample of the Italian population: sociodemographic modulating factors, *J Cultur Divers,* 9(2):55-62, Summer 2002.

Bates MS: *Biocultural dimensions of chronic pain: implications for treatment of multi-ethnic populations,* Plattsburgh, NY, 1996, State University of New York Press.

Bates MS, Rankin-Hill L, Sanchez-Ayendez M, Mendez-Bryan R: A cross-cultural comparison of adaptation to chronic pain among Anglo-Americans and native Puerto Ricans, *Med Anthropol* 16(2):141-173, 1995.

Beinfield H, Korngold E: *Between heaven and earth: a guide to Chinese medicine,* New York, 1991, Ballantine.

Benor D: *Healing research: holistic energy medicine and spirituality,* Munich, 1993, Helix Verlag.

Black Elk W, Lyon WS: *Black Elk: the sacred ways of a Lakota,* San Francisco, 1990, Harper & Row.

Brennan B: *Hands of light: a guide to healing through the human energy field,* Toronto, 1988, Bantam.

Bruyere R: *Wheels of light: Chakras, Auras and the Healing Energy of the Body.* Fireside Publications (Simon & Schuster Inc), New York, 1994.

Byrd RC: Positive therapeutic effects of intercessory prayer in a coronary care unit population, *South Med J* 81:826-829, 1988.

Carlston M: *Classical homeopathy,* Edinburgh, 2003, Churchill Livingstone.

Cassidy CM. Protein-energy malnutrition as a culture-bound syndrome, *Cult Med Psychiatry* 6:325-345, 1982.

Cassidy CM: Unraveling the ball of string: reality, paradigms, and the study of alternative medicine, *Adv J Mind-Body Health* 10:3-31, 1994.

Cassidy CM: Social science theory and methods in the study of alternative and complementary medicine, *J Altern Complement Med* 1:19-40, 1995.

Cassidy CM: Chinese medicine users in the United States. I. Utilization, satisfaction, medical plurality, *J Altern Complement Med* 4:17-28, 1998a.

Cassidy CM: Chinese medicine users in the United States. II. Preferred aspects of care, *J Altern Complement Med* 4:17-28, 1998b.

Cassidy CM, editor: *Contemporary Chinese medicine and acupuncture,* Edinburgh, 2002, Churchill Livingstone.

Cassileth B, Lusk E, Strouse R, Bodenheimer B: Contemporary unorthodox treatments in cancer medicine: a study of patients, treatments and practitioners, *Ann Intern Med* 101:105-112, 1984.

Dossey L: *Prayer is good medicine: how to reap the healing benefits of prayer,* San Francisco, 1997, Harper San Francisco.

Edzard M, Ernst D, Pittler M, et al: *Desktop guide to complementary and alternative medicine: an evidence-based approach,* St Louis, 2001, Mosby.

Eisenberg D, Davis RB, Ettner S, et al: Trends in alternative medicine use in the United States, 1990-1997: results of a follow-up survey, *JAMA* 280:1569-1575, 1998.

Eisenberg D, Kessler R, Foster C, et al: Unconventional medicine in the United States, *N Engl J Med* 328:246-252, 1993.

Eliade M: *Shamanism: archaic techniques of ecstasy,* Princeton, NJ, 1964, Princeton University Press.

Emad M: Does acupuncture hurt? Ethnographic evidence of shifts in psychobiological experiences of pain, *Proc Soc Acupunct Res* 2:129-140, 1994.

Emad M: Feeling the qi: emergent bodies and disclosive fields in American appropriations of acupuncture, Houston, 1998, Rice University (Dissertation).

Engel G: The need for a new medical model challenge for biomedicine, *Science* 196(4286):129-136, 1977.

Fabrega H: *Disease and social behavior: an interdisciplinary perspective,* Cambridge, Mass, 1974, MIT Press.

Foster G, Anderson B: *Medical anthropology,* New York, 1978, Wiley & Sons.

Greenwood M, Nunn P: *Paradox and healing: medicine, mythology and transformation,* ed 3, Victoria, British Columbia, 1994, Paradox.

Grimes D: Identifying worthy medical research, *Network* 23(1), 2003.

Hand WD, editor: *American folk medicine: a symposium,* Berkeley, 1976, University of California Press.

Harwood A: The hot-cold theory of disease: implications for treatment of Puerto Rican patients, *JAMA* 216:1153-1158, 1977.

Helman CG: *Culture, health and illness,* ed 4, London, 2000, Arnold Publishers.

Hultkrantz A: The shaman and the medicine man, *Soc Sci Med* 20:511-515, 1985.

Ingerman S: *Soul retrieval: mending the fragmented self,* San Francisco, 1991, HarperCollins.

Ingerman S: *Welcome home: following your soul's journey home,* San Francisco, 1994, Harper San Francisco.

Jacobs J, Jimenez LM, Gloyd SS, et al: Treatment of acute childhood diarrhea with homeopathic medicine: a randomized clinical trial in Nicaragua, *Pediatrics* 93(5):719-725, 1994.

Jarrett L: *Nourishing destiny: the inner tradition of Chinese medicine,* Stockbridge, Mass, 1998, Spirit Path Press.

Jobst KA:. A critical analysis of acupuncture in pulmonary disease: efficacy and safety of the acupuncture needle, *J Altern Complement Med* 1:57-85, 1995.

Jobst KA, editor: Energy medicine: science and healing from bioelectromagnetics to the medicine of light, *J Altern Complement Med* 10(1) 1-5), 2004.

Jonas W, Crawford C, editors: *Healing, intention and energy medicine: science, research methods, and clinical implications,* Edinburgh, 2003, Churchill Livingstone.

Kaplan A: Philosophy of science in anthropology, *Annu Rev Anthropol* 13:25-39, 1984.

Kaptchuk T: *The web that has no weaver: understanding Chinese medicine,* New York, 1983, Congdon & Weed.

Kenner D: Putting it all together: practicing Oriental medicine. In Cassidy CM, editor: *Contemporary Chinese medicine and acupuncture,* Edinburgh, 2002, Churchill Livingstone.

Kirkland J, Mathews HF, Sullivan CW III, Baldwin K, editors: *Herbal and magical medicine: traditional healing today,* Durham, NC, 1992, Duke University Press.

Kleinman A: *Patients and healers in the context of culture,* Berkeley, 1980, University of California Press.

Krishan S: *Essential Ayurveda: what it is and what it can do for you,* Novato, Calif, 2003, New World Library.

Larre C, de la Vallee ER: *Rooted in spirit, the heart of Chinese medicine,* Barrytown, NY, 1995, Station Hill Press.

Lindenbaum S, Lock M: *Knowledge, power and practice: the anthropology of medicine and everyday life,* Berkeley, 1993, University of California Press.

Lock M, Gordon DR, editors: *Biomedicine examined,* Dordrecht, The Netherlands, 1988, Kluwer.

Martin P: *The healing mind: the vital links between brain and behavior, immunity and disease,* New York, 1999, St Martin's Griffin.

Mattingly C, Garro L: *Narrative and the cultural construction of illness and healing,* Berkeley, 2000, University of California Press.

McGuire MB: *Ritual healing in suburban America,* New Brunswick, NJ, 1994, Rutgers University Press.

Morgan W: Navajo treatment of sickness; Diagnosticians. In Landy D, editor: *Culture, disease and healing: studies in medical anthropology,* New York, 1977 (1931), Macmillan, pp 163-168.

Morrison J: *Book of Ayurveda: a holistic approach to health and longevity,* New York, 1995, Fireside.

Moss D, McGrady A, Davies T, Wickramasekera I: *Handbook of mind-body medicine for primary care,* Thousand Oaks, Calif, 2002, Sage.

Murdock GP: *Theories of illness: a world survey,* Pittsburgh, 1980, University of Pittsburg Press.

O'Connor BB: Hmong cultural values, biomedicine and chronic liver disease. In *Healing traditions, alternative medicine and the health professions,* Philadelphia, 1995, University of Pennsylvania Press.

Oschman J: *Energy medicine in therapeutics and human performance,* Philadelphia, 2003, Butterworth-Heinemann.

Oths K: *Healing by hand: a cross-cultural primer for manual therapies,* Walnut Creek, Calif, 2004, Alta Mira Press.

Payer L: *Medicine and culture: varieties of treatment in the United States, England, West Germany, and France,* New York, 1988, Penguin.

Reilly D, Taylor MA, Bettie N, et al: Is evidence for homeopathy reproducible? *Lancet* 344(8937):1601-1606, 1994.

Reimansnyder BL: *Powwowing in Union County: a study of Pennsylvania German folk medicine in context,* New York, 1989, AMS Press.

Ross J: *Acupuncture point combinations: the key to clinical success,* Edinburgh, 1995, Churchill Livingstone.

Rubel A, O'Nell CW, Ardon RC: *Susto: a folk illness,* Berkeley, 1984, University of California Press.

Schnyer R: Acupuncture in depression and mental illness. In Cassidy CM, editor: *Contemporary Chinese medicine and acupuncture,* Edinburgh, 2002, Churchill Livingstone.

Schnyer R, Allen J: *Acupuncture in the treatment of depression: a manual for practice and research,* Edinburgh, 2001, Churchill Livingstone.

Scott AW: Masters of the ordinary: integrating personal experience and vernacular knowledge in Alcoholics Anonymous, Ann Arbor, 1993, Michigan Microfilms (Dissertation).

Sears: Sick Enough to Stay Home? *Redbook,* September, 1991.

Shahjahan R: Standards of education, regulation, and market control: perspectives on complementary and alternative medicine in Ontario, Canada, *J Altern Complement Med* 10:409-412, 2004.

Sheldon WH, Hartl EM, McDermott E: *Varieties of delinquent youth: an introduction to constitutional psychiatry,* New York, 1949, Harper & Brothers.

Snow LF: *Walkin' over medicine,* Boulder, Colo, 1993, Westview Press.

Sobo EJ: *One blood: the Jamaican body,* Albany, 1993, State University of New York Press.

Sontag S: *Illness as metaphor,* New York, 1977, Farrar, Straus, & Giroux.

Spicer EH, editor: *Ethnic medicine in the Southwest,* Tucson, 1979, University of Arizona Press.

Stein HF: *American medicine as culture,* Boulder, Colo, 1990, Westview Press.

Stux G, Hammerschlag R, editors: *Clinical acupuncture: scientific basis,* Berlin, 2001, Springer.

Targ R, Katra J: *Miracles of mind: exploring nonlocal consciousness and spiritual healing,* Novato, Calif, 1999, New World Library.

Terrell SJ: *This other kind of doctors: traditional medical systems in black neighborhoods in Austin TX,* New York, 1990, AMS Press.

Trotter R, Chavira JA: *Curanderismo: Mexican-American folk healing,* Atlanta, 1997, University of Georgia Press.

Turner E: *The hands feel it: healing and spirit presence among a northern Alaskan people,* DeKalb, 1996, University of Northern Illinois Press.

Vithoulkas G: *The science of homeopathy,* New York, 1980, Grove Press.

Wirkus M: School of bioenergy, the healing art, *Newslett Int Soc Study Subtle Energies Energy Balance* 4(2):8-10, 1993.

Workshop on Alternative Medicine: *Alternative medicine: expanding medical horizons,* Chantilly, Va. Report to the National Institutes of Health on Alternative Medical Systems and Practices in the United States, NIH Pub No 94-066, Washington, DC, 1994, US Government Printing Office.

Young JC: *Medical choice in a Mexican village,* New Brunswick, NJ, 1981, Rutgers University Press.

Young D, Ingram G, Swartz L: *Cry of the eagle: encounters with a Cree healer,* Toronto, 1989, University of Toronto Press.

Wisnesky L, Anderson L: *The Scientific Basis of Integrative Medicine.* Boca Raton, 2005, CRC Press.

Websites

American Iatrogenic Association: www.iatrogenic.org

Ontario Consultants on Religious Tolerance: Jehovah's Witnesses, www.religioustolerance.org

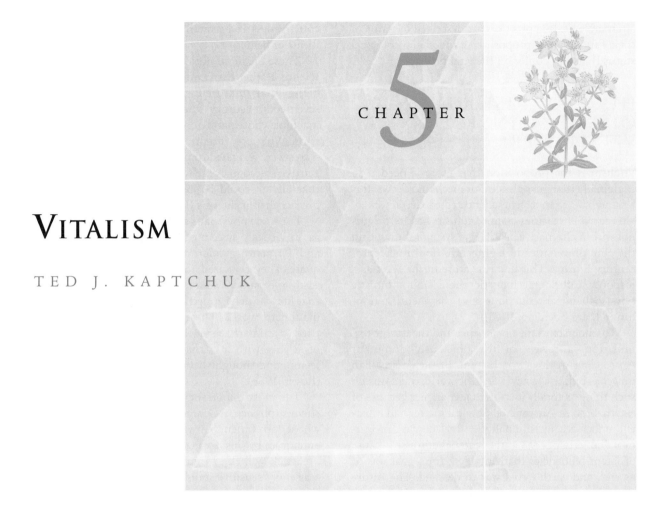

CHAPTER

5

VITALISM

TED J. KAPTCHUK

Practitioners of most alternative healing believe that one source of their intervention is a type of "vital energy" used by their system and still not appreciated by conventional biomedical science. Subtle health-promoting influences pervade the alternative (or now integrative) healing world. Health is accessible through gentle technologies that activate, evoke, or redirect universal beneficent healing influences. The universe is thought to provide an endless influx of forces that can help to "put things right." Health is harmony in the cosmic energy; illness is cured by reordering the protective forces. A person threatened by disorder and disease is guaranteed a response from fundamentally benign, lawful, coherent, potent, and even meaningful powers. One can almost speak of a faucet that pours out healing juice.

Homeopathy connects with the "spiritual vital force" (Hahnemann, 1980); chiropractic calls it "innate" or "universal intelligence" (Palmer, 1910); psychic healing manipulates "araruic," "psi," or psionic powers (Moore, 1977; Reyner, 1982); believers in New Thought are restored by correct "mind" (Braden, 1987); acupuncture uses "qi" (Eisenberg, 1985); Ayurvedic medicine and yoga teachers are in touch with "prana" (Lad, 1984); and naturopaths invoke the "vis medicatrix naturae" (Turner, 1990). Unseen powers are said to permeate the universe and have a profound effect on humans that is undetectable by scientific instruments.

This chapter delineates this concept of alternative and integrative medicine by tracing the historical development of the idea of vital energy. Individual alternative healing practices are described in terms of their fundamental propositions and the ontological status that they confer on the vital principle.

HISTORY: RISE AND FALL OF THE MAINSTREAM VITALIST PRINCIPLE

Vitalism is the proposition that more is needed to explain life than just physical or mechanical laws. It is less archaic than recent advocates or detractors of alternative medicines claim. Vitalism has its origins not within alternative health care systems, but within the elite universities of eighteenth- and nineteenth-century Europe. This doctrine arose in the West as a response to the mechanistic thesis and atomistic physicochemical reductionism of the scientific revolution (Lain Entralgo, 1948).

To understand the new science and the vitalist formulation, a review of the previously dominant Aristotelian worldview is helpful. In the Aristotelian universe, unlike the new scientific world, there was no such thing as totally inert matter changing because of external forces. Aristotelian physical matter had inherent tendencies, intentionality, and teleological properties. Things happened in the material universe because of latent tendencies that unfolded; fire's goal was to ascend, and earth's goal was to descend. The future exerted a compulsion on the present. The organic universe was the model for the inorganic universe; the acorn both embodied and obeyed its future potential as an oak tree. The material realm was a continuum of the organic realm but at a reduced level of complexity.

In terms of humans, this sense of continuation persists. Medieval biology could not conceive of an extreme dichotomy of *soma* (body) and *psyche* (mind), much less their separate existence (Gilson, 1940; Hartman, 1977). This would have conflicted with theology (Kemp, 1990). Psyche had no reality apart from soma. A human's material body overlapped and interpenetrated and was given actuality and form by a subtle substratum of souls. Each soul organized the soma into a distinct hierarchy of function and awareness. Somehow, *pneuma,* a mediator of the same eternal essence as the celestial bodies, allowed for both an embodied and mindful integrity of psyche and soma (Hall, 1975). Pneuma served as a common denominator of all phenomena and allowed all forms of being—from human to minerals—to maintain their cohesiveness and growth and to transform into other forms of being.

These medieval notions were replaced by the new science. Rather than conceiving nature as an organic being that matured through self-development, seventeenth-century scientists viewed nature as a machine whose parts only moved in response to other parts. Volition, intentions, cognition, and mental states were relegated to peripheral or epiphenomenal status in biology. Some scientists even came to believe that all life could be explained in mechanical and physicochemical terms (Ledermann, 1989).

For some physicians and scientists, explaining life as an intricate system of levers, pulleys, or bubbling and fermenting microchemical flasks was inadequate. They criticized the new philosophy as excessively mechanical, material, and simple and argued that life was determined by more than the laws of the inanimate world. These physicians and biologists tried to animate the newly constituted passive matter of science with a vitalist hypothesis to explain the feeling and thought behind organic and human life (Roger, 1986).

The most important figure in this effort was the chemist-physician George Ernest Stahl (1659-1734), whose prominent university status at Halle was enhanced by his former position as physician to Frederick Wilhelm I (Rather, 1961). He proposed the *anima,* or "sensitive soul," to fill the perceived void in the new science. Anima was the agency that made life distinct from lifeless matter. Stahlian animism was undoubtedly influenced by the earlier "archeus" of Paracelsus (1493-1541) and van Helmont (1577-1644), two pre-Cartesian chemist-physician-mystics of the Nordic renaissance who were involved in an entirely different dialogue (Lain Entralgo, 1948). Francois Boissier de Sauvages (1706-1767) introduced the anima into the teaching of Montpellier, one of Europe's oldest and most important medical schools, but he preferred using the word "soul" for this animating life force. His student, Paul Joseph Barthez (1734-1806), whose credentials included having been Napoleon's physician, believed that both words were too occult and old-fashioned and in 1778 introduced the phrase *principe vitale,* or *vital principle* (Haight, 1975; Wheeler, 1939).

The vitalist hypothesis could not totally obliterate the newly created Cartesian chasm of an inert matter *(res extensa)* and a mind *(res cognitans)*—it conceded too much to the new physics. However, the power relationship had been reversed; in life, primary agency was no longer physicochemical or mechanical, but rather a benevolent power with a self-directive healing power.

Unbound by the precise and quantifiable laws of physics and chemistry, the vitalism argument, by its nature, quickly fractured into many interpretations. Some physicians took a phenomenal position and saw the vital principle to be a regulative principle (Lipman, 1967). Others took a realist position and postulated that a constitutive part animated matter; this approach is much more important to alternative healing (Benton, 1975). Realist theories took various forms: from various shades of incorporeal and spirit agency; to diverse mental powers; to different types of distinctive forces analogous and on the same plane of reality as conventional electromagnetism but still not scientifically measurable (Larson, 1979; Toulmin and Goodfield, 1962).

In the nineteenth century the mechanistic physicochemical view gained complete ascendancy in biology and medicine. From Wohler's synthesis of organic material in 1828 to Atwater and Rosa's demonstration in 1897 that the laws of thermodynamics apply to life, as well as inorganic matter, there was a gradual elimination of any need to believe in a vital principle or life force to explain perceived inadequacies of physicochemical explanations (Needham, 1955). Vitalism's main argument was the opponent's weakness; vitalism had to retreat before each new scientific discovery. This weakened vitalism migrated to the alternative medical worldview that was being created in the nineteenth century, where it was welcomed and eventually merged with other important forms of vitalism.

MESMERIC VITAL ENERGY

At the time that vitalism was being developed in elite academia and just before it received an official name, the Viennese physician Anton Mesmer (1734-1815) uncovered what he believed to be the real vital energy. In 1775, Mesmer discovered that the source of a popular religious exorcist's powers was not divine intervention but rather a vital force. The cures were caused by "animal magnetism," a subtle fluid that pervades the universe and is analogous to gravitation (Ellenberger, 1970). Mesmer declared that the scientific evidence of the new vital force is the healing influx; harmony with the cosmic fluid is health. All disease was caused by an unequal distribution or blockage of this fluid. Healing is the restoration of equilibrium, and healers can manipulate this fluid to cure patients (Mesmer/Bloch, 1980). An influx of subtle fluids from the celestial bodies is the substantive basis of all life and health, and later even mortality (Darton, 1968).

Mesmer relocated to Paris, and his popularity quickly generated controversy. In 1784, King Louis XVI, through the Royal French Academy of Science, appointed a prestigious investigatory commission that included ambassador Benjamin Franklin, chemist Antoine Lavoisier, and physician-inventor J.I. Guillotin. Mesmer demanded clinical outcome comparisons. Instead, the blue ribbon panel wanted to investigate mechanism. In a series of some of medicine's earliest controlled, blinded trials, the panel discovered that healing occurred whenever subjects believed they were being mesmerized, and no effect occurred if subjects were ignorant of magnetic passes. The commission sentenced mesmerism to the medical fringe, where it became a critical component of alternative medical thought (Fuller, 1982).

Mesmer's followers quickly split into denominations. Mesmerists divided between those who understood the force as a physical agency and those who detected a more incorporeal power. A lower mesmeric interpretation made the force analogous to a physical electromagnetic vibration that resembled more-recognized scientific energies. A higher mesmeric interpretation that quickly fused with earlier mystical and occult traditions saw the force as ethereal and reduced the physical agency to an epiphenomenon of no consequence. In addition to healing, the force had abilities for clairvoyant medical diagnosis and telepathy and became a scientific vehicle to contact spiritual forces or spiritual beings (Darton, 1968). Between the poles of lower and higher mesmerism were various intermediate versions, each spawning complex lineage; all shared the distinctive mesmeric view that life's agency and healing potential can be found in a vital energy or presence distinct from the ordinary mechanical forces. Mesmerism became the inspiration for many unconventional therapies.

Lower Mesmerism and Psychic Healing

Tracing the history of mesmerism can be difficult because many of Mesmer's descendants often changed their names, like other new arrivals on Ellis Island, to avoid the stigma associated with the term *mesmerism* since its excommunication from official science. New designations, however, could be helpful. If an earlier vital energy was discredited, new forces could be discovered to take its place. For example, Robert Hare (1781-1858), a chemist at the University of Pennsylvania and the inventor of the oxyhydrogen blowpipe, was an early convert to mesmerism. In 1856 he developed a "spirit-scope" to measure mesmeric and spiritual presences and also coined the scientific-sounding term *psychic force* in 1856 (McClenon, 1984; Moore, 1977). In 1935, Joseph Bank Rhine (1885-1980), who spent most of his career at Duke University trying to shift psychical research from the seance room to the laboratory, adopted the more respectable "parapsychology" from German (McVaugh and Mauskupf, 1976; Moore, 1977). In 1947, Robert Thouless (1894-1984), a British psychologist and parapsychologist at Cambridge, thought psi phenomena or psionic energy was a noncommittal label for paranormal energetics (Moore, 1977). Historically, theosophists preferred the word *auric* or *astral* force (Campbell, 1980; Coddington, 1990), whereas modern researchers have recently chosen the phrase *subtle energy*. These name substitutions indicate the lower mesmeric concern for keeping vital energy on a par with other more physically established forces as the primary agency for life.

> Lower mesmeric forms of healing energy are easily recognized in the contemporary alternative therapies that speak of an electromagnetic dimension which can become depleted or unbalanced . . . [causing] the blockage of energy flow, requiring physical or spiritual cleaning in order for healing to occur (Glick, 1988).

Alternative therapies—therapeutic touch (Krieger et al., 1979), laying on of hands (Vlamis, 1978), polarity (Vlamis, 1978), and paranormal healing (Rose, 1954)—as well as the countless individual psychic, auric, and psionic healers, although often unaware of their heritage, all bear the characteristic mesmeric style of manipulating unseen and refined forces that evade biomedical detection. The proof of the force is healing, and secondary evidence can be sensations of heat, tingling, or vibratory motions (Fuller, 1989). Curiously, despite the suspicions and even hostility of colleagues, some conventional researchers hover on the edge of this type of healing and continue to investigate the phenomenon scientifically (Benor, 1990; Beutler et al., 1988).

Higher Mesmerism and Channeling

The trance states of higher mesmeric traditions were used to contact noncorporeal realities. Healing dispensations, medical diagnosis, and medical advice were common products of "tuning-in," as were clairvoyance, spirit sightings, levitations, ectoplasmic emissions, table turning, spirit tapping, and spirit photographs. This higher trance phenomenon quickly merged with earlier occult and theurgic movements (e.g., neo-Platonism, Renaissance occult and kabbala, pre-Christian religions, theurgical traditions, and Swedenborgianism [Galbreath, 1971]), creating a mass phenomenon in the nineteenth century (Braude, 1989; Oppenheim, 1988). This spiritualist movement was later reincarnated in various theosophical and occult movements in today's New Age scene (Beckford, 1984; Melton, 1988). Such contemporary phenomena as "experiencing the healing powers of interplanetary Brotherhoods and curing their medical ailments by soul travel to different planes of reality" (Levin and Coreil, 1986) are all direct descendants of higher mesmerism. Alternative healing methods and associations, such as Spiritual Frontiers Fellowship, Edgar Cayce's Association for Research and Enlightenment (Carter, 1972), and Great White Brotherhood, and modalities such as past lives therapy (Netherton and Shiffrin, 1978) are involved with a panoply of spiritual beings that are detectable by mesmeric trances, currently referred to as altered states of consciousness, channeling, higher states of awareness, or transmissions from spiritually evolved beings. These are rarely organized as healing professions and routinely exceed the limits of healing practices, becoming instead alternative or emergent religions.

ELECTRICAL DEVICES AND CRYSTALS

Electrical devices and crystals that emit or harmonize energies for healing are important first cousins of mesmerism. The experiments of Luigi Galvani (1737-1798), which caused the severed legs of frogs to jump as if alive, coincided with Mesmer's own research. This discovery of animal electricity, or electrical body fluid, was considered to be analogous or identical with animal magnetism and all mysterious vital forces (Sutton, 1981). Electrical machines and gadgets with healing properties were ubiquitous in the nineteenth century (Marvin, 1988) and continued into the twentieth century. Contemporary radionic machines, magnetic beds, transcranial electrostimulators, neuromagnetic vibrators, and electromagnetic chairs all bear the imprint of their preceding mesmeric electrical cousins (Easthope, 1986; Schaller and Caroll, 1976). Important scientific research has been generated by scientists interested in low-frequency electromagnetic devices despite the stigma of an association with charlatanism (Macklin, 1993).

Crystal healing, a form of *lithotherapeutics,* has ancient roots distinct from mesmerism (Forbes, 1972). In the last 200 years, however, it has repositioned itself to become part of the vital energy family. In the 1840s and 1850s, Baron Charles von Reichenbach (1788-1869), the discoverer of kerosene, also managed to detect a refined and definitive mesmeric energy in crystals. He gave it the scientifically oriented name *odic force.* Modern crystal healers continue this merged tradition and speak of crystals as "able to tap the energies of the universe" and being an especially potent "focus of healing energy" (Fuller, 1989).

MIND CURE

Mind Cure, or the healing systems that consider thoughts or deep feeling to be the primary arbitrator of health, is an important offshoot of mesmerism. The discovery of the mind as the ultimate unseen force of healing is related directly to Phineas P. Quimby (1802-1866). Quimby first worked as a magnetizer or magnetic healer (reconstituted names for a mesmerist) in Portland, Maine. He decided that healing was not so much animal magnetism or an esoteric energy, but rather that it resulted from changes in the mind. The force was not a physical force, but a mental state. Mesmer's fluid was really "Mind," and everything was controlled by Mind. Disease is what follows the disturbance of the mind or spiritual matter (Dresser, 1969).

Quimby began the New Thought movement that believes disease is "wrong thinking." Change the thought, and you have health (Judah, 1967). Divine Mind, Divine Truth, and Love are primary agency, not the physical world. Physical reality is clay in the hands of the Mind. New Thought and positive thinking all derive from Mind Cure, as do such metaphysical

groups as Unity Church of Christianity, United Church of Religious Science, and International Divine Science (Braden, 1987). New and more contemporary forms of this approach to healing are constantly being offered. For example, "a course on miracles" (Perry, 1987), "prosperity consciousness" (Chopra, 1993; Cole-Whittaker, 1983), and "living love" (cornucopia) (Keyes, 1989) are all based on the same premise. Beyond any organization, this notion of "what you think is what is real" infuses important sectors of the modern alternative health community, resonating through history in uncanny ways. For example, the words Quimby wrote in 1859 could easily have been taken from Bernie Siegel's best-selling alternative healing book *Love, Medicine and Miracles* (1986): "Love is the true answer to our desire . . . it contains nothing but true knowledge and love, no sorrow, nor pain, nor grief, nor shame nor fear (Dresser, 1969). Love or True Mind heals all."

Mind Cure often advocated "entering the silence" to make mind impressions, self-love, or autosuggestion imprint more effectively (Fuller, 1982; Meyers, 1965). Almost 100 years ago, William James (1842-1910) described a phenomenon that still is current when he said that the "mind-cure principles are beginning to so pervade. . . . One hears of the Gospel of Relaxation of the Don't Worry Movement or people who repeat to themselves Youth, Health, Vigor" (James, 1961). Mind Cure's meditation, relaxation, and breathing techniques (which partially derive from somnambulistic or mesmeric trance states [Davis, 1885]) were some of the indigenous Western practices that prepared the way for Asian-style meditations that are so influential in the alternative health movement (see later discussion).

CHRISTIAN SCIENCE

Quimby's most famous legacy to unconventional healing is through his student and patient who later became known under the name Mary Baker Eddy (1821-1919). She went on to establish Christian Science, radically declaring that all disease, pain, misfortune, and evil are illusion. Knowing Divine Truth and Divine Science allows perception of the underlying perfection. Divine Mind is the only reality. Rigid, doctrinaire, exclusive, and sectarian, Mrs. Eddy denied any relationship with Mind Cure, mesmerism, or alternative healing, but her venomous denunciations of Quimby and malicious animal magnetism revealed her origins only too clearly and assured Christian Science a place in the history of vital energy (Feldman, 1963; Fox, 1984; Schoepflin, 1988).

CHIROPRACTIC, OSTEOPATHY, AND MASSAGE

Mesmeric vital energy took a somatic and even mechanical twist in the creation of *chiropractic*, the largest contemporary alternative health care profession in North America, licensed in 50 states (Wardwell, 1992). Discovered in 1895 by D.D. Palmer (1845-1913), chiropractic's origin is a unique marriage of the indigenous healing craft of bonesetting (Cooter, 1987; Schiotz and Cyriax, 1975) and the American tradition of mesmeric healing (Beck, 1991). For 10 years before his discovery of chiropractic, Palmer worked as a magnetic healer. Like Quimby, he occasionally used hand passes and magnetic rubbings of the spine (Fuller, 1982). In an intuitive flash (or, some say, clairvoyant communication [Beck, 1982]), Palmer realized that "putting down your hands" worked better than an esoteric "laying on of hands." Mechanical adjustment was more precise than magnetic activity administered from a distance. Yet even 20 years after abandoning his magnetic clinical work, Palmer's mesmeric heritage is readily evident in his writings: "Disease is a manifestation of too much or not enough energy. Energy is liberated force; in the living being it is known as vital force. . . . It is an intelligent force, which I saw fit to name Innate, usually known as spirit" (Beck, 1991).

Disease is disruption in what Palmer calls *innate intelligence.* The nervous system is the conduit for this force. By aligning the spine, one frees the nerves so that this force can move without interference and produce healing. The vital energy is guided and shaped by the structure of the body. The noncorporeal agency of life is housed in the nerves and guarded by the spinal vertebrae. Chiropractic and spinal manipulation, despite its alternative associations, recently has generated considerable interest from researchers, in terms of basic science (Goldstein 1975), controlled clinical trials (Anderson et al., 1992; Shekelle et al., 1992), and comparative health care outcome trials (Meade et al., 1990). Official government reports, such as the Manga Report in Canada

(Manga et al., 1993) and a recommendation from the Agency for Health Care Policy and Research (Bigos et al., 1994) on chiropractic for acute low back pain, have blurred the demarcation between alternative and mainstream medicine and encouraged wider acceptance of chiropractic.

Osteopathy, chiropractic's older cousin, was developed by Andrew Still (1828-1917), who was also a magnetic healer for many years. In 1874 he discovered that misaligned bones impeded the flow of fluids and blood, and he developed the system of osteopathy. In addition to having episodes of clairvoyance and channeling, Still also had connections to metaphysical, Mind Cure, and spiritualist groups (Gevitz, 1988; Terrett, 1991). Obviously, osteopathy has taken a different trajectory from chiropractic. By breeding out its mesmeric influence, it has become practically indistinguishable from mainstream medicine (Baer, 1987; Gevitz, 1982).

Massage is one of the earliest and most pervasive forms of healing (Sigerist, 1961). In the last 100 years, however, many unconventional massage therapies have increasingly found their rationale in vital energy theory. Many styles of massage therapies exist (Knapp and Antonucci, 1990) with different theories and therapeutic goals, including Rolfing (Rolf, 1977), reflexology (Carter 1969), Aston-Patterning (Low, 1988), Hellerwork, and shiatsu (Namikoshi, 1969). The multiplicity of forms, the fact that anyone can give a massage, and constant introduction of new methods have hampered the regulation, licensing, and professional development that is analogous to chiropractic. Nonetheless, "bodywork" provides an extensive and important network of much energy work (Good and Good, 1981).

HOMEOPATHY

Although mesmerism dominated the vital energy tradition, the mainstream vitalist hypothesis also continued to survive and remained operational in the alternative medical world. Often this survival was made possible by an explicit or implicit strategic union with mesmerism. Homeopathy is the most important system of medicine to derive from this tradition.

For a considerable period during the last century, homeopathy was the most serious challenge to conventional medicine (Rothstein, 1985) and currently is enjoying a serious revival (Kaufman, 1988). Discovered by Samuel Hahnemann (1755-1843), homeopathy espouses the belief that whatever symptom-complex a substance can cause in a healthy person, infinitesimally small amounts of the same substance can cure diseases with the same symptom configuration. The small dosage has the capacity to evoke the spiritual, self-acting (automatic) vital force, which is present throughout the organism (Hahnemann, 1980). *Sililia similibus curentur*—"like cures like." The tiny dosage enhances the spiritual essence of the bodily response to disease. The alchemical homeopathic remedy was to rescue the insufficient self-help mechanisms of the physical body and supply a corrective to nature (Neuburger, 1933). Hahnemann's idea of vital energy derived from early German romantic sources (from Paracelsus and van Helmont) and the later academic tradition of G.E. Stahl (Coulter, 1977). Even from its inception, however, an alliance with mesmerism was discernible. Hahnemann himself ascribed mesmeric healing as a marvelous, priceless gift of God to humankind (Hahnemann, 1980). At present it is virtually impossible to distinguish homeopathy's vital force from other conceptions rooted in mesmerism. Despite its alternative status, homeopathy has generated considerable conventional biomedical research and debate (Hill and Doyon, 1990; Kliejnen et al., 1991a; Linde et al., 1994).

HERBALISM AND THE "VIS MATECATRIX NATURAE"

Another energy in alternative medicine is the healing force of nature, which has a long history independent of mesmerism or the vitalist hypothesis (Neuburger, 1933). In 1772, William Cullen (1710-1790), a professor at the University of Edinburgh—himself no friend of this approach in medicine—proposed the term *vis matecatrix naturae* to describe this power (Neuburger, 1933). Again, as with the academic vitalist hypothesis, the natural force became more important in the alternative world and eventually was indistinguishable from the whole concept of vital energy.

The rise of the market economy and industrialization allowed for nostalgia and a romantic view of nature, which made possible the natural healing movements that date from the early nineteenth century. Alternative healing movements "irregulars" launched crusades to overthrow the orthodox medi-

cine "regulars," who used "contaminated unnatural poisonous" drugs and bleeding (Warner, 1987). The earliest American natural healing movement was Thomsonian herbalism. The history of herbal medicaments lies deep in antiquity (Wheelwright, 1974), but Samuel Thomson (1769-1843), a native of New Hampshire, initiated the first herbal social reform movement in the 1820s and 1830s. Borrowing from indigenous colonial and Indian treatments, Thomsonians substituted herbal purges and soporifics for mainstream minerals, chemicals, and bloodletting. This movement developed into the profession of eclectic medicine, which mounted a challenge to conventional medicine with a systematic herbal approach, its own medical schools (Berman, 1951), and eventually a strong following in Europe (Griggs, 1981). Somewhere in this history, herbalism formed an alliance with mesmerism. The two languages fused. Herbalists insisted that treatment must be in harmony with nature and the vital force and must assist the vital force instead of destroying it (Brown, 1985). The last eclectic medical school closed in Ohio in 1939 (Rothstein, 1988), and herbalism as a professional system of healing had practically disappeared in the United States, although it survived in Great Britain (Sharma, 1992).

In the United States, vestiges of the herbal movement remain in popular self-help manuals, and the concept of medicinal herbs remains an important symbol for alternative medicine. Some scientific research continues into popular herbal remedies (Ernst, 1995; Johnson et al., 1985; Melchart et al., 1994), but much of the conventional biomedical discussion is in terms of potential adverse effects (Huxtable, 1992).

HYDROPATHY AND NATUROPATHY

Water cure, or hydropathy, is another healing movement that relied on a natural force. As with herbalism, hydrotherapy has early roots but became a health reform movement only in the nineteenth century (Donegan, 1986). It has practically disappeared, except for spas and in physical therapy. Nevertheless, its legacy has important ramifications for contemporary alternative healing.

Originally, hydropathy was imported to the United States from Germany in the 1840s as the

Priessnitz method and later reimported in the 1890s as the Kneipp method. In these systems, water was the pure force of healing. Often combined with massage, exercise, and health food, water could purify the body of "morbid matter" (toxins), stimulate nervous energy, and promote natural healing (Cayleff, 1988). Quickly, the water cure movement became a catchall for other methods; by 1850 it was associated with dietary regimens, dress reform, home doctor, and finally with all-natural methods, including herbs, mesmeric energies, electropathy, and manipulation. This natural healing movement took on many forms and names, such as drugless healing, sanipractic, vita-o-pathy, sagliftopathy, panpathy, and physculopathy (Fishbein, 1932; Whorton, 1986), but the most enduring one is the name associated with Benedict Lust (1872-1945), a water cure therapist who trained under the Bavarian hydropath Father Kneipp.

In 1895, Lust purchased the term *naturopathy* to describe his eclectic water cure system, and the term was used publicly for the first time in 1902 in association with Lust's New York–based American School of Naturopathy (Baer, 1992; Cody, 1985). His naturopathy was a nature cure system, defined as "the art of natural healing and the science of physical and mental regeneration on the basis of self-reform, natural life, clean and normal diet, hydropathy (Priessnitz, Kneipp, Lehmann, and Just systems), osteopathy, chiropractic, naturopathy [sic], electrotherapy, sun and air cult, diet, physiotherapy, physical and mental culture to the exclusion of poisonous drugs and non-adjustable surgery" (Fishbein, 1932). Naturopathy, whose eclecticism resembles the current holistic movement, was common practice in many states during the 1920s and 1930s under the name "drugless practitioner" (Gort and Coburn, 1988; Whorton, 1986) but now functions legally only in eight states, the stronghold being the Pacific Northwest (Baer, 1992). Legal constraint prevents its widespread adoption as a unifying ideology for all natural therapies. Nevertheless, naturopathy is a potent concept in the alternative health movement and sometimes is used as a synonym for alternative health.

ACUPUNCTURE AND ASIAN MEDICAL SYSTEMS

The vital energy of alternative medicine received a dramatic infusion of credibility and possibility with the introduction of acupuncture and other Asian medicines into the United States in the 1960s after several unsuccessful introductions (Haller, 1973).

The Chinese notion of *qi* (as well as the Indian and Tibetan equivalents) obviously developed before any Western Cartesian detachment of mind from matter. Qi was not so much an entity added to lifeless matter, but the state of being—either animate or inanimate (Chiu, 1986; Kuriyama, 1986; Sivin, 1987). Qi was more akin to pneuma than any other Western idea (Needham, 1956). Asian medical systems, similar to archaic Western systems, relied on hierarchies and gradations of organizations to explain differences between organic and inorganic forms of being. Qi was characteristic of rocks, plants, and even human rationality. It was the common thread that allowed for "ladders of the soul" that extended from minerals to human life (Yoke, 1985).

The qi of acupuncture or the *prana* of India have been swept in the undertow of Western vitalistic ideas. Contemporary Western literature generally translates qi as "vital energy." Ancient Chinese notions, which defy severing of mind-body, have been discarded from modern Asian medical dialogue (in both Asia and the West) in favor of vital energy. Nonphysician acupuncturists have gained licensing, registration, or certification in 27 states plus the District of Columbia between 1977 and 1993 (Lytle, 1993; McRae, 1982). Although still small, acupuncture is one of the most rapidly growing health care professions, and its success provides an important ideological boost to alternative health care. The excitement of acupuncture has generated basic scientific investigations (Pomeranz and Stux, 1988) and more than 200 controlled clinical biomedical research studies (Eisenberg, 1995; Kleijnen et al., 1991b; ter Riet et al., 1990).

The Eastern opening also brought new massage (shiatsu, anmo, tui na, acupressure, jin shin jyutsu), new esoteric psychic energies (reiki johrei, qi gong), and countless new forms of meditation to supplement and supplant indigenous American forms. Again, they usually are formulated in nineteenth-century vitalist terms (Miura, 1989).

PSYCHOLOGICAL INTERVENTIONS

Of all the mesmeric forces, the most complex, prolific, and hidden ones lie concealed in psychology, which deals with "mind." Significant aspects of clinical psychology's origins are connected with attempts to legitimize, mainstream, or find the real source of mesmerism and vital energy. In 1843, James Braid (1795-1860), an English physician, sought to clean up mesmerism's tainted reputation by postulating that its effects were caused by a mental force, not a mysterious fluid. He changed its name to *hypnosis,* after the Greek god for sleep, Hypnos (Kaplan, 1974). Hypnosis became a major concern in psychology—and depending on the perspective, even a legitimate mesmerism—and retains its importance in some areas of conventional medicine (Hall and Crasilneck, 1978). Hypnosis was taken seriously by such figures as Jean Martin Charcot (1825-1893) and Hippolyte Bernheim (1840-1919) and is a crucial ingredient in the early development of the psychodynamic psychiatry of Sigmund Freud (1856-1939) (Ellenberger, 1970). Hypnosis became less critical after Freud, becoming simply a porthole to the unconscious. Vital energy transforms into various forms of dynamic tensions that are thought to have potent psychological and physiological consequences. A clinical research agenda has also become a companion for psychotherapies (Strupp and Howard, 1992).

Hypnosis and such forms of passive volitional intention as *autogenic training* and *guided imagery* also later interact with the academic behavioral psychology developed by I.P. Pavlov (1849-1936), the rigorous investigations of classic conditioning by J.B. Watson's (1878-1958), and the work of E.L. Thorndike (1874-1949) in operant conditioning (Thorndike, 1931). This cross-fertilization of disciplines and ideas eventually contributed to the formation of such modern cognitive-behavioral mind-body interventions as *biofeedback* (Basmajian, 1981), modern autogenic training (Linden, 1990), visualization and guided imagery (Sheikh, 1983), the relaxation response (Benson, 1975), and the reexamination of older self-control practices such as meditation (West, 1991).

These cognitive-behavioral interventions, along with the psychosomatic movement, began as academic pursuits but have become valuable intellectual and clinical resources for alternative and integrative medicine. The vital force now can be conceptualized in psychosomatic terms or in the current mind-body framework. These mind-body techniques shift between conventional and nonconventional. They are less on the fringe, almost accepted, and are often wholly accepted aspects of vitalist ideology. They are

the lowest, most scientific aspects of the mesmeric legacy, a kind of legitimate mesmerism. Because of university connections, these mind-body interventions have generated much research (Eisenberg et al., 1993; Holroyd and Penzien, 1990; Turner and Chapman, 1982).

The vital energy has gone psychological. This has lent significant credibility to alternative medicine. Psychology has been a rich source of new interventions and theory for both conventional and integrative medicine. Occasionally, however, these efforts have been used to support more outlandish alternative healing ideas, to the discomfort of more scientifically inclined researchers. In either case, the mesmeric force has become a hyphenated mind-body connection between the invisible mind and the visible body. In the last 50 years, more new psychological interventions and names probably have been developed—between 250 (Herink, 1980) and 400 (Karasu, 1986) types, depending on who counts and when—than in the entire history of mesmeric forces.

HOLISTIC MEDICINE

Vital energy and vitalism underwent regrouping and reorganization during the post-1960s renaissance. *Holism,* or holistic medicine, has become the new family name, coined to avoid the tarnished image of older, discredited medical ideas. The term originates within conventional medical debates of the early twentieth century over vitalism and reductionism.

Reductionism has been the corollary of the ascendancy of physicochemical mechanistic viewpoint. The trajectory of reductionism is basically described by Morgagni's situation of life-activity and pathology in organs (1761), followed by Bichat's focus on tissue (1800), leading to Broussais' attention to lesions in tissues (1830s), to Virchow's localization in cells (1848), to Koch's germ theory (1882), and all the way to modern dissection of genes. This process is complex and nonlinear (Mendelsohn, 1965). Emphasis on a mechanical physicochemical agency leads to progressively smaller analytical pieces. Again, however, academic medicine has provided important antidotes to reductionism, with organismic tendencies attempting to counterbalance or prevail over excessive reductionism. Antireductionist tendencies within conventional medicine emphasize homeostasis, predisposition, susceptibility, and psychosocial factors, as opposed to tendencies that emphasize an idea of disease that Tauber calls ontological, autonomous, well-circumscribed states (Tauber, 1994). A few of the many names associated with nonreductionism within biomedicine include Claude Bernard, Walter Cannon, L.J. Henderson, George Draper, Charles Sherrington, Hans Selye, Helen Dunbar, George Engels, and Arthur Kleinman (Tracy, 1992).

One antireductionist position developed in the philosophy of biology was by J.C. Smuts, the Cambridge-educated, South African statesman who in 1926 coined the word *holism* (Smuts, 1926). Holism was meant to be both antivitalist and antimechanistic and argued that the entirety of an organism necessarily implied a teleological purpose that could not be exhaustively explained by the laws governing component parts. The idea and word were appropriated by a few conventional scientists (Needham, 1955) and were later used positively by conventional medicine to imply humanistic, psychosocial, or systemic approaches in health care. For example, a December 1948 editorial in the *Journal of the American Medical Association* referred to the holistic concept as being "an integrated approach to the sick person as a being in a state of mental, moral, and physiological imbalance with his environment." In the 1970s, holistic partially changed its association. A 1979 *New England Journal of Medicine* editorial criticized holistic medicine, as follows:

> Patients must be dealt with as whole people. But this worthwhile philosophy is ill served by those who seek quick solutions to all the ills of mankind through the abandonment of science and rationality in favor of mystic cults (Relman, 1979).

The word *holism* is adopted by many unconventional health practitioners, most of whom are seemingly unaware of Smuts or his philosophy (Whorton, 1989), causing confusion. Holism has become an amorphous label often glibly used or made trivial (Kopelman and Moskop, 1981) for any perspective that sees biomedicine as too reductionist or materialist. It also has become a generic name for any therapy that does not consider its clinical perspective to be reductionist. Also, holism has become the new family name for any intervention, regardless of how reductionist (e.g., chiropractic, crystals), that is informed, knowingly or unknowingly, by some nineteenth-century vitalist perspective. The term *complementary*, introduced first in the United Kingdom in the 1980s and then in the United States in the 1990s, now often replaces "holistic."

VITALISM'S ATTRACTION

Vitalism can be attractive. Life is more than chemicals and mechanism. Agency is more than chemistry and physics. Mind, ideas, volition, intentions, spiritual entities, beliefs, innate intelligence, feelings, and mysterious vital forces can all become critical phenomena. The multivalent possibilities of vital energy—its lower, higher, natural, psychological, or supernatural forms—allow practitioners and patients to customize explanations and treatment options. Its very imprecision allows for enormous flexibility and adaptibility.

In conventional medicine it is sometimes too easy for a person to become an irrelevant spectator, overwhelmed by a mechanical world of technology, tests, and surgery. The vitalist perspective, on the other hand, aligns itself with coherent, life-affirming principles. The vitalist universe is not random, detached, or mindless; it is benign, coherent, and extremely hospitable for people. Instead of a medicine whose central issues can seem coldly mechanical and buried in inaccessible physiology, vitalism instinctively invites a person to experience a unifying, transcendent, and reassuring ontological presence.

Whatever the outcome of the recent scientific investigations of vitalist medical traditions, vitalism's attractiveness for practitioners and patients is likely to remain a growing presence in health care.

References

Anderson R, Meeker WC, Wirick BE, et al: A meta-analysis of clinical trials of spinal manipulation, *J Manipulative Physiol Ther* 15, 1992.

Baer HA: Divergence and convergence in two systems of manual medicine: osteopathy and chiropractic in the United States, *Med Anthropol Q* 1:2176-2193, 1987.

Baer HA: The potential rejuvenation of American naturopathy as a consequence of the holistic health movement, *Med Anthropol* 13:369-383, 1992.

Basmajian JV, editor: *Biofeedback: principles and practice for clinicians,* New York, 1981, Institute for Psychosomatic Research.

Beck BL: Magnetic healing, spiritualism and chiropractic: Palmer's union of methodologies, 1886-1895, *Chiro Hist* 11(2):11-16, 1991.

Beckford JA: Holistic imagery and ethics in new religious and healing movements, *Soc Compass* 21(2/3):259-272, 1984.

Benor DJ: Survey of spiritual healing research, *Comp Med Res* 4(3):9-33, 1990.

Benson H: *The relaxation response,* New York, 1975, Morrow.

Benton E: Vitalism in nineteenth-century scientific thought: a typology and reassessment, *Stud Hist Philos Sci* 5:1, 1975.

Berman A: The Thomsonian movement and its relation to American pharmacy and medicine, *Bull Hist Med* 25:5, 1951.

Beutler JJ, Attenvelt JT, Schooten SA, et al: Paranormal healing and hypertension, *BMJ* 296:1491-1494, 1988.

Bigos SJ, Bowyer OR, Braen GR, et al: Acute low back problems in adults, Clinical Practice Guideline No 14, PHS Agency for Health Care Policy and Research, Rockville, Md, 1994, US Department of Health and Human Services.

Braden CS: *Spirits in rebellion: the rise and development of new thought,* Dallas, 1987, Southern Methodist University Press.

Braude A: *Radical spirits,* Boston, 1989, Beacon Press.

Brown PS: The vicissitudes of herbalism in late nineteenth- and early twentieth-century Britain, *Med Hist* 29:71-92, 1985.

Campbell BF: *Ancient wisdom revived: a history of the theosophical movement,* Berkeley, 1980, University of California Press.

Carter M: *Helping yourself with reflexology,* West Nyack, NY, 1969, Parker.

Carter ME: *My years with Edgar Cayce,* New York, 1972, Harper & Row.

Cayleff SE: Gender, ideology and the water-cure movement. In *Other healers: unorthodox medicine in America,* Baltimore, 1988, The Johns Hopkins University Press.

Chiu ML: Mind, body and illness in Chinese medical tradition, Cambridge, Mass, 1986, Harvard University (Unpublished PhD thesis).

Chopra D: *Creating affluence,* New York, 1993, New World Press.

Coddington M: *Seekers of the healing energy,* Rochester, Vt, 1990, Healing Arts Press.

Cody G: History of naturopathic medicine. In Pizzorno JE, Murray MJ, editors: *A textbook of natural medicine,* Seattle, 1985, John Bastyr College Publications.

Cole-Whittaker T: *How to have more in a have-not world,* New York, 1983, Fawcett Crest.

Cooter R: Bones of contention? Orthodox medicine and the mystery of the bone-setter's craft. In Bynum WF, Porter R, editors: *Medical fringe & medical orthodoxy, 1750-1859,* London, 1987, Croom Helm, pp 158-173.

Coulter HL: *Divided legacy: a history of the schism in medical thought.* Vol II, Washington, DC, 1977, Wehawaken Books.

Darton R: *Mesmerism and the end of the Enlightenment in France,* Cambridge, Mass, 1968, Harvard University Press.

Davis AJ: *The harbinger of health,* Boston, 1885, Colby & Rich, Banner Publishing.

Donegan JB: *Hydropathic highway to health,* Westport, Conn, 1986, Greenwood Press.

Dresser HW, editor: *The Quimby manuscripts,* Secaucus, NJ, 1969, Citadel Press.

Easthope G: *Healers and alternative medicine,* Aldershot, England, 1986, Gover.

Editorial: Holistic medicine, *JAMA,* Dec 18, 1948.

Eisenberg D: *Encounters with qi: exploring Chinese medicine,* New York, 1985, Norton.

Eisenberg D: Traditional Chinese medicine. In *Alternative medicine: implications for clinical practice,* Boston, 1995, Harvard Medical School, Department of Continuing Education.

Eisenberg D, Delbanco TL, Berkey CS, et al: Cognitive behavioral techniques for hypertension: are they effective? *Ann Intern Med* 118:964-972, 1993.

Ellenberger HF: *The discovery of the unconscious,* New York, 1970, Basic Books, pp 53-60.

Ernst E: St. John's wort, an anti-depressant? A systematic, criteria-based review, *Phytomedicine* 2(1):67-71, 1995.

Feldman AB: Animal magnetism and the mother of Christian Science, *Psychoanal Rev* 50:153-160, 1963.

Fishbein M: *Fads and quackery in healing,* New York, 1932, Blue Ribbon.

Forber TR: Lapis Bufonis: the growth and decline of a medical superstition, *Yale J Biol Med* 45:139-149, 1972.

Fox M: Conflict to coexistence: Christian Science and medicine, *Med Anthropol,* Fall 1984, pp 292-300.

Fuller R: *Mesmerism and the American cure of souls,* Philadelphia, 1982, University of Pennsylvania Press.

Fuller R: *Alternative medicine and American religious life,* New York, 1989, Oxford University Press, p 104.

Galbreath R: The history of modern occultism: a bibliographical survey, *J Pop Cult* 5:726-754, 1971.

Gevitz N: *The D.O.'s: osteopathic medicine in America,* Baltimore, 1982, The Johns Hopkins University Press.

Gevitz N: Andrew Taylor Still and the social origins of osteopathy. In *Studies in the history of alternative medicine,* New York, 1988, St Martin's Press.

Gilson E: *The spirit of medieval philosophy,* New York, 1940, Charles Scribner's Sons.

Glick DC: Symbolic, ritual and social dynamics of spiritual healing, *Soc Sci Med* 27(11):1197-1206, 1988.

Goldstein M: *The research status of spinal manipulative therapy,* Bethesda, Md, 1975, Public Health Service, National Institutes of Health, US Department of Health, Education and Welfare.

Good BJ, Good MJ: Alternative health care in one California community, Sacramento, 1981, Public Regulation of Health Care Occupations in California.

Gort EH, Coburn D: Naturopathy in Canada: changing relationships to medicine, chiropractic and the state, *Soc Sci Med* 26(10):1061-1072, 1986.

Griggs B: *Green pharmacy: a history of herbal medicine,* London, 1981, Jill Norman & Hobhouse.

Hahnemann S: *Organon of medicine,* ed 6, New Delhi, 1980, B Jain Publishers, p 97 (Translated by W Boericke).

Haight E: The roots of the vitalism of Xavier Bichet, *Bull Hist Med* 49:72-86, 1975.

Hall JA, Crasilneck HB: Hypnosis, *JAMA* 239(8):760-761, 1978.

Hall TS: *History of general physiology.* Vol 1, Chicago, 1975, University of Chicago Press.

Haller JS: Acupuncture in nineteenth century western medicine, *NY State J Med,* May 1973, pp 1213-1221.

Hartman E: *Substance, body and soul: Aristotelian investigations,* Princeton, NJ, 1977, Princeton University Press.

Herink R, editor: *The psychotherapy handbook,* New York, 1980, New American Library.

Hill C, Doyon F: Review of randomized trials of homeopathy, *Rev Epidemiol Sante Publique* 38:139-147, 1990.

Holroyd KA, Penzien DB: Pharmacological versus non-pharmacological prophylaxis of recurrent migraine headache: a meta-analytic review of clinical trials, *Pain* 42:1-13, 1990.

Huxtable RJ: The myth of beneficent nature: the risks of herbal preparations, *Ann Intern Med* 117(2):165-166, 1992.

James W: *The varieties of religious experience,* New York, 1961, Collier.

Johnson ES et al: Efficacy of feverfew as prophylactic treatment of migraine, *BMJ* 291:569-573, 1985.

Judah JS: *The history and philosophy of the metaphysical movements in America,* Philadelphia, 1967, Westminster Press.

Kaplan F: "The Mesmeric Mania": the early Victorians and animal magnetism, *J Hist Ideas* 35:4, 1974.

Karasu TB: The specificity vs. non-specificity dilemma: towards identifying therapeutic change agents, *Am J Psychiatry* 14:3-6, 1986.

Kaufman M: *Homeopathy in America: the rise and fall and persistence of a medical heresy,* Baltimore, 1988, The Johns Hopkins University Press.

Kemp S: *Medieval psychology,* New York, 1990, Greenwood Press.

Keyes K: *Discovering the secrets of happiness,* Coos Bay, Ore, 1989, Love Line Books.

Kleijnen J, Knipschild P, ter Riet G: Clinical trials of homeopathy, *BMJ* 302:316-323, 1991a.

Kleijnen J, ter Riet G, Knipschild P: Acupuncture and asthma: a review of controlled trials, *Thorax* 46:799-802, 1991b.

Knapp JE, Antonucci EJ: *A national study of the profession of massage therapy/bodywork,* Princeton, NJ, 1990, Knapp & Associates.

Kopelman L, Moskop J: The holistic health movement: a survey and critique, *J Med Philos,* May 1981, pp 209-235.

Krieger D, Peper E, Ancoli S: Therapeutic touch: searching for evidence of physiological change, *Am J Nurs,* April 1979, pp 660-662.

Kuriyama S: Varieties of haptic experience: a comparative study of Greek and Chinese pulse diagnosis, Cambridge, Mass, 1986, Harvard University (Unpublished PhD thesis).

Lad V: *Ayurveda,* Sante Fe, NM, 1984, Lotus Press.

Lain Entralgo P: Sensualism and vitalism in Bichat's "Anotomie Generale," *J Hist Med* 3, 1948.

Larson JL: Vital forces: regulative principles or constitutive agents? *Isis* 70, 1979.

Ledermann EK: *Philosophy and medicine,* Aldershot, England, 1989, Gower.

Levin JS, Coreil J: "New Age" healing in the U.S., *Soc Sci Med* 23:9, 1986.

Linde K, Jonas WB, Melchart D, et al: Critical review and meta-analysis of serial agitated dilutions in experimental toxicology, *Hum Exp Toxicol* 13:481-492, 1994.

Linden W: *Autogenic training: a clinical guide,* New York, 1990, Guilford Press.

Lipman TO: Vitalism and reductionism in Liebig's physiological thought, *Isis* 58:167-185, 1967.

Low J: The modern body therapies: Aston-Patterning, *Massage Magazine* 16:48-55, 1988.

Lytle CD: *An overview of acupuncture,* Washington, DC, 1993, US Department of Health and Human Services, Public Health Service, Food and Drug Administration.

Macklin RM: Magnetic healing, quackery and the debate about the health effects of electromagnetic fields, *Ann Intern Med* 118(5):376-383, 1993.

Manga P, Angus DE, Papadopoulos C, et al: A study to examine the effectiveness and cost-effectiveness of chiropractic management of low-back pain, Ottawa, 1993, Pran Managa.

Marvin C: *When old technologies were new: thinking about electric communication in the late nineteenth century,* New York, 1988, Oxford University Press.

McClenon J: *Deviant science: the case of parapsychology,* Philadelphia, 1984, University of Pennsylvania Press.

McRae G: A critical overview of U.S. acupuncture regulation, *J Health Polit Policy Law* 1:163-196, 1982.

McVaugh M, Mauskupf JD: Rhine's extra-sensory perception and its background in psychical research, *Isis* 67:161-189, 1976.

Meade TW, Dyer S, Browne W, et al: Low back pain of mechanical origin: randomized comparison of chiropractic and hospital outpatient treatment, *BMJ* 300, 1990.

Melchart D et al: Immunodulation with *Echinacea*—a systematic review of controlled clinical trials, *Phytomedicine* 1:245-254, 1994.

Melton JG: A history of the New Age movement. In Basil B, editor: *Not necessarily the New Age: critical essays,* Buffalo, NY, 1988, Prometheus Books.

Mendelsohn E: Physical models of physiological concepts: explanation in nineteenth-century biology, *Br J Hist Sci* 2:7, 1965.

Mesmer FA: Dissertation on the discovery of animal magnetism. In Bloch GJ, editor: *Mesmerism: a translation of the original medical and scientific writings of F.A. Mesmer, M.D.,* Los Altos, Calif, 1980, William Kaufmann.

Meyers D: *The positive thinkers: a study of the American quest for health, wealth, and personal power from Mary Baker Eddy to Norman Vincent Peale,* Garden City, NJ, 1965, Doubleday.

Miura K: The revival of qi gong in contemporary China. In *Taoist meditation and longevity techniques,* Ann Arbor, 1989, Center for Chinese Studies, University of Michigan.

Moore RL: *In search of white crows: spiritualism, parapsychology, and American cult,* New York, 1977, Oxford University Press.

Namikoshi T: *Shiatsu,* New York, 1969, Japan Publications.

Needham J: *Mechanistic biology and the religious consciousness in science, religion & reality,* New York, 1955, George Brazziler.

Needham J: *Science and civilization in China.* Vol 2, Cambridge, Mass, 1956, Cambridge University Press.

Netherton M, Shiffrin N: *Past lives therapy,* New York, 1978, William Morrow.

Neuburger M: *The doctrine of the healing power of nature,* New York, 1933, New York Homeopathic College.

Oppenheim J: *The other world: spiritualism and psychical research in England, 1850-1914,* Cambridge, 1988, Cambridge University Press.

Palmer DD: *Chiropractic,* Portland, Ore, 1910, Portland Printing House, p 691.

Perry R: *An introduction to a course in miracles,* Fullerton, Calif, 1987, Miracle Distribution Center.

Pomeranz B, Stux G, editors: *Scientific basis of acupuncture,* Berlin, 1988, Springer-Verlag.

Rather LJ: G.E. Stahl's psychological physiology, *Bull Hist Med* 35:27-49, 1961.

Relman AS: Holistic medicine, *N Engl J Med* 300(6):312-313, 1979.

Reyner JH: *Psionic medicine,* London, 1982, Routledge & Kegan Paul.

Roger J: The mechanistic conception of life. In *God and nature,* Berkeley, 1986, University of California Press.

Rolf IP: *Rolfing: the integration of human structure,* New York, 1977, Harper & Row.

Rose L: Some aspects of paranormal healing, *BMJ* 4:1329-1332, December 1954.

Rothstein WG: *American physicians in the 19th century,* Baltimore, 1985, The Johns Hopkins University Press.

Rothstein WG: The botanical movements and orthodox medicine. In *Other healers: unorthodox medicine in America,* Baltimore, 1988, The Johns Hopkins University Press.

Schaller WE, Caroll CR: *Health, quackery and the consumer,* Philadelphia, 1976, Saunders.

Schiotz EH, Cyriax J: *Manipulation: past and present,* London, 1975, Heinemann.

Schoepflin RB: Christian Science healing in America. In *Other healers: unorthodox medicine in America,* Baltimore, 1988, The Johns Hopkins University Press.

Sharma U: *Complementary medicine today: practitioners and patients,* London, 1992, Tavistock/Routledge.

Sheikh AA: *Imagery: current theory, research and application,* New York, 1983, Wiley.

Shekelle P, Adams AH, Chassin MR, et al: Spinal manipulation for low-back pain, *Ann Intern Med* 117:7, 1992.

Siegel BS: *Love, medicine and miracles,* New York, 1986, Harper & Row.

Sigerist HE: *A history of medicine,* New York, 1961, Oxford University Press.

Sivin N: Traditional medicine in contemporary China, Ann Arbor, 1987, Center of Chinese Studies, University of Michigan.

Smuts JC: *Holism and evolution,* New York, 1926, Macmillan.

Strupp HH, Howard KI: A brief history of psychotherapy research. In Frehen DK, editor: *History of psychotherapy,* Washington, DC, 1992, American Psychological Association.

Sutton G: Electric medicine and mesmerism, *Isis* 72(253): 375-392, 1981.

Tauber AT: Darwinian aftershocks: repercussions in late twentieth century medicine, *J R Soc Med* 87:27-31, 1994.

ter Riet G, Kleijnen, Knipschild P, et al: Acupuncture and chronic pain: a criteria-based meta-analysis, *J Clin Epidemiol* 43:1191-1199, 1990.

Terrett AJ: The genius of D.D. Palmer: an exploration of the origin of chiropractic in his time, *Chir Hist* 11:1 1991.

Thorndike EL: *Human learning,* New York, 1931, Century.

Toulmin S, Goodfield J: *The architecture of matter,* New York, 1962, Harper & Row, pp 322-330.

Tracy SW: George Draper and the American constitutional medicine, 1916-1946: reinventing the sick man, *Bull Hist Med* 66:53-89, 1992.

Turner JA, Chapman CR: Psychological interventions for chronic pain: a critical review. I. Relaxation training and biofeedback, *Pain* 12:1-21, 1982.

Turner RW: *Naturopathic medicine,* Northamptonshire, England, 1990, Wellingborought, p 21.

Vlamis G: Polarity therapy, *Alternatives* 2(4):23-26, 1978.

Wardwell WI: *Chiropractic: history and evolution of a new profession,* St Louis, 1992, Mosby–Year Book.

Warner JH: Medical sectarianism, therapeutic conflict, and the shaping of orthodox professional identity in antebellum American medicine. In Bynum WF, Porter R, editors: *Medical fringe & medical orthodoxy, 1750-1850,* London, 1987, Croom Helm.

West AM, editor: *The psychology of meditation,* Oxford, NY, 1991, Clarendon Press.

Wheeler R: *Vitalism,* London, 1939, HF & G Witherby.

Wheelwright EG: *Medicinal plants and their history,* New York, 1974, Dover.

Whorton JC: Drugless healing in the 1920's: the therapeutic cult of sanipractic, *Pharm Hist* 28:14-24, 1986.

Whorton JC: The first holistic revolution: alternative medicine in the nineteenth century. In Stalker D, Glymour C, editors: *Examining holistic medicine,* Buffalo, NY, 1989, Prometheus Books.

Yoke HP: *Li, qi, and shu: an introduction to science and civilization in China,* Hong Kong, 1985, Hong Kong University Press.

Suggested Readings

Carlson CJ: Holism and reductionism as perspectives in medicine and patient care, *West J Med* 131(6):466-470, 1979.

Gardner M: Isness is her business: Shirley MacLaine. In Basil R, editor: *Not necessarily the new age: critical essays,* Buffalo, NY, 1988, Prometheus Books, p 193.

Kaufman M: *Homeopathy in America: the rise and fall of a medical heresy,* Baltimore, 1971, The Johns Hopkins University Press.

Pavlov IP: *Lectures on conditioned reflexes,* New York, 1928, International Publishers.

Zefron LJ: The history of the laying-on of hands in nursing, *Nurs Forum* XIV(4):350-363, 1975.

CHAPTER 6

INTEGRATED MEDICAL MODEL

ELLIOTT DACHER

Today we find ourselves living in an extraordinary in-between time—a gap in history between two sets of values. This gap has been created by the decline of our previously unquestioned optimism and faith in modernism, its values and institutions, and the slow and as-yet uncertain emergence of a new postmodern worldview. Disillusionment with the limitations and excesses of biomedicine and efforts to revitalize our approach to health and healing emerge from this historical moment. To understand this circumstance is to understand that the changes that we now envision are fundamental rather than cosmetic and as much compelled as chosen. Because of the highly personal nature of health, this shift in worldview is most publicly and passionately played out in the arena of health and healing.

DEVELOPMENT OF THE BIOMEDICAL MODEL

The practice of American medicine has been slowly maturing for the past 150 years of the modern era. We can readily identify four distinct phases in its development: (1) its inception as a frontier medicine in the eighteenth and early nineteenth centuries; (2) the rise of the institutions of scientific medicine in the late nineteenth and early twentieth centuries (Figure 6-1); (3) the recognition of the high costs of scientific medicine and the resulting cost sharing and cost containment initiatives of the past 60 years; and (4) the current emergence of a postmodern medicine based on an expanded set of assumptions and values. To understand the maturation of American medicine accurately,

67

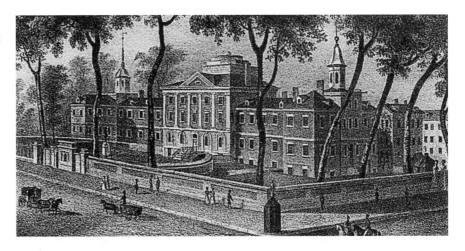

Figure 6-1 Pennsylvania Hospital, circa 1800, America's first hospital. (Courtesy The Pennsylvania Hospital, Philadelphia.)

we must begin by examining the forces that have shaped our current approach to health and healing.

Scientific medicine as it is presently known was nonexistent before the late nineteenth century. With a few notable exceptions, medical schools were free-standing commercial ventures unaffiliated with universities and lacking the bare essentials of an educational curriculum. For a moderate fee any individual, regardless of previous educational achievement, could attend a 3- to 6-month course of study conducted by local physicians, who shared the tuition as personal income. Written examinations were not possible because of the lack of writing skills; licensing procedures were minimal; clinical training with actual patients was nonexistent; and the general status of physicians was fairly low. In 1869, Harvard Medical School, one of the best in the United States, had 300 students, of whom no more than 20% had a college degree and fewer than 50% were reportedly able to write English (Harrington, 1905).

This situation began to change toward the end of the nineteenth century as universities slowly improved their undergraduate programs and then focused their attention on professional training. The changes were initiated at Harvard in 1870 by the new and dynamic president Charles Eliot, who strongly supported the German university model that emphasized the scientific and laboratory-based teaching methods that had proved highly successful in identifying the microbial causes of the infectious diseases that had devastated Europe for millennia. The new medical program at Harvard created more stringent admission criteria, a longer course of study, written examinations, a full-time faculty, a complete integra-

tion of the medical school into the university, and a laboratory-based teaching method. In summary, as the study of disease shifted from the context of the individual within the family and community to the laboratory, the patient's disease became the physician's disease, and the unique human story line gave way to generic diagnostic coding.

Over the decades an increasing number of medical schools embraced these ideas, a movement that culminated in the opening of the Johns Hopkins Medical School in 1893 (Gilman, 1969 [1906]). As a result of the philanthropy of Johns Hopkins, the medical faculty, under the guidance of Daniel Coit Gilman, William Welch, John Shaw Billings, Sir William Osler, Howard Kelly, and William Halsted, were able to develop fully the new model of medical education unencumbered by the traditions and politics of an existing institution. Despite these new approaches, however, most of the more than 100 existing commercial medical schools had failed to undertake these changes by the turn of the century.

As a result, in 1907, Andrew Carnegie, through his newly formed Carnegie Foundation, funded a study of medical education by Abraham Flexner (Figure 6-2), an aggressive and highly capable educator. The study was designed to document the poor state of medical education that continued in most medical schools (Flexner, 1910). In this famous report, Flexner insisted that all medical schools comply with the Hopkins approach or shut down. He, as the medical reformers preceding him, promoted a university-based, scientifically trained practitioner.

These efforts were readily accepted by a general public immersed in the spirit of progressivism and, by

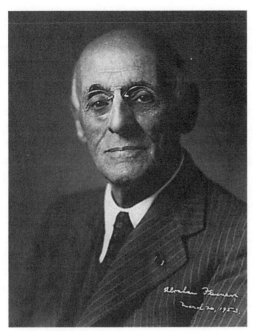

Figure 6-2 Abraham Flexner. (Courtesy National Library of Medicine, Bethesda, Md.)

the 1900s, increasingly aware of the practical results of medical science (identification of bacterial causes of specific disease; use of antisepsis and asepsis; use of the x-ray; development of vaccines against rabies, typhoid, and bubonic plague; discovery of Salvarsan, the first effective antibacterial drug). The general public sought an educated, skillful, modern-day medical practitioner. Flexner, subsequently serving as general secretary of the General Education Board, a Rockefeller philanthropy, directed extensive funds (estimated at more than $1.7 billion in current dollars) toward the promotion of his report (Ludmerer, 1985). The result of these efforts, as well as those of others, led to the complete transformation of medical education and practice into a disciplined, highly structured applied science, what is now called *biomedicine.*

As faith in the possibilities of scientific medicine expanded, research blossomed, medical centers emerged, new technologies evolved, and by the 1930s the high costs of scientific medicine became evident. Slowly, over decades, third parties began to take over the funding of medical services with the goal of distributing their cost among large groups of the sick and well populations. A lengthy process took place that would determine the ultimate third party, the

federal government or private industry. At the beginning of the twenty-first century, it appears that private industry has won this competition, although not completely free from federal regulatory efforts. Health care has become a commodity subject to market forces and values. The changes promoted by Eliot, Gilman, Welsh, Flexner, and others had unexpectedly resulted in a cascade of changes, many of which would have been unimaginable and unacceptable to these great innovators.

A considered analysis of the development of biomedicine from 1870 to 1920 demonstrates that it was an appropriate and highly successful response to the *circumstances and needs of that era.* At present, our circumstances and needs are different because of (1) the success of the biomedical model, (2) changing social conditions accompanied by a shift in the burden of disease from acute to chronic, and (3) the rapid expansion over the past century of our understanding of the relations among consciousness, health, and disease. Our task must be to facilitate the further evolution of medicine in a manner that responds to the imperatives of the new millennium.

NEW INITIATIVES

Much as the escalating costs of scientific medicine became apparent by the 1930s, by the 1960s its effectiveness, given the needs and temperament of our time, and its more covert iatrogenic effects became further causes for concern. Rene Dubos in *Mirage of Health* (1961) and Thomas McKeown in *The Role of Medicine: Dream, Mirage, or Nemesis* (1976) expressed an emerging skepticism about the ability of scientific medicine to resolve contemporary medical problems. Ivan Illich in *Medical Nemesis* (1976) articulated a growing concern for the clinical and social iatrogenic consequences of scientific medicine. A recognition of the shift in the burden of disease from infectious diseases to stress-related illness, chronic disease, emotional disorders, and lifestyle and environmentally related disorders further highlighted the limitations of biomedicine when confronted with the complexities of modern existence.

Simultaneously, other developments were occurring in the field of psychology and consciousness research. These included an expanded understanding of the interactions of mind and body (Dacher, 1996; Locke, 1986), the impact of personal relationships

(Berkman and Syme, 1979) and socioeconomic status (Adler et al., 1993; Hause et al., 1982) on health and disease, and a renewed interest in the healing powers of the spirit (Benor, 1992). The turn outward in biomedicine to science, manipulative interventions, and technology led to the constellation of a complementary force—the turn inward toward self-care, mind-body resources, holism, and psychological and spiritual development as counterpoints to the limitations and excesses of scientific medicine.

Emerging social and personal forces have given rise to four major new initiatives in the arena of health and healing: the wellness, holistic, mind-body, and alternative therapies movements. Beginning in the 1970s, these initiatives began to confront the dominant medical model with a new set of values and perspectives, perspectives that at their core were inconsistent with those of biomedicine. They heralded the potential for a revitalization of health and healing, and the infusion of these new ideas was well received by a culture that no longer held an unquestioned faith in the values and practices of biomedicine.

Shedding further light on these developments, Paul Ray in *The Integral Culture Survey* (1996) identified the recent emergence of three coexisting subcultures: traditional, modern, and cultural creatives. Each had its unique value system, perspectives, and language. The *traditionalists* were most clearly identified by their religious and traditional values; the *modernists* by their focus on materialism; and the most recent group, the *cultural creatives,* by their emphasis on community, ecology, and self-actualization. This third group, which Ray suggests may comprise as many as 44 million Americans, is the subculture that most challenges the values and perspectives of contemporary medicine.

However, an existing perspective invariably tends to sustain itself. Thomas Kuhn suggests in *The Structure of Scientific Revolutions* (1970) that, when challenged from without, those invested in the dominant perspective, both individuals and institutions, first deny the significance of new initiatives, then characterize them as "fringe," and finally attempt to co-opt them by incorporating these initiatives into the mainstream of existing culture, reshaping them in a way that conforms to the old rather than supporting the new. This is largely the fate of each of the movements previously mentioned. The "wellness movement," a rich blend of psychological, social, and spiritual perspectives, was reduced to its most physical elements:

nutrition, exercise, smoking cessation, and relaxation training. The rich philosophical vision of "holism," often mistaken for humanism and a multiplicity of practices, became a commodity to be labeled, bottled, and sold. The "mind-body movement" has failed to be significantly integrated into the biomedical model. Also, in their urgency for licensure, social legitimization, and reimbursement, the alternative (or integrative) and complementary movements are in danger of losing the essential uniqueness of their traditions as they become mainstreamed and increasingly perceived as merely one more set of therapeutic tools (Duggan, 1995).

These initiatives may expand our therapeutic options and open up the dominant medical system, but once exposed to the system and its unchanged worldview and core values, they cannot prosper. A school that trains students in Oriental medicine and instills within them a broader set of values must then release these students into the world of contemporary practice and managed care. A well-designed clinical research program that is inclusive of a broader set of values is unlikely to have its research accepted by the dominant medical model, and well-meaning practitioners may change the character of their practice but not the cultural context within which it is embedded. Much the same can be said for any effort that does not address in a more global sense the fundamental issue of values, particularly the values that are emerging in our current time as a counterforce to the limits and excesses of biomedicine. As a result, what seems hopeful in the beginning turns out to be much less innovative than originally imagined. Although these movements have managed to shake up the system and to catalyze the dissolution of the existing worldview, they have not served to transform it. This failure can be directly attributed to the absence of a guiding dialogue focused on values and vision.

VALUE-CENTERED DECISION MAKING

Values are not addressed in the modern worldview. They are considered "soft" issues, subjective ones that cannot be seen, touched, or measured through our senses. The objectivistic worldview maps, categorizes, and models the surface of reality. It neither legitimizes nor allows for any discussion about the *context* in which physical reality is embedded: the human and cultural experience. When new initiatives arise, they are seen only in terms of their physical and external aspects: nutrition, exercise, smoking cessation, objectified models of holism, techniques, and therapies. The underside is simply not seen; human meaning, significance, and values are excluded from discussion—the map maker is lost from view. Where there appears to be change, there is none.

Although value-centered decision making is an ongoing and natural part of the human experience, we are generally unaware of its occurrence. The choices we make and the actions that we take are too often unconsciously compelled by our personal and collective value systems. For example, in a culture that values objectivism (i.e., sensory-based knowledge) our actions are exclusively based on factual information and data, and intuitive, nonrational knowledge is treated with skepticism and disregard. Our values and actions are predetermined by hidden cultural assumptions. They are not freely chosen. They are neither conscious nor intentional.

Lawrence Kohlberg enhanced our understanding of this issue with his theory of moral development and its three stages: (1) preconventional, the undeveloped perspective of the child; (2) conventional, the unconscious assimilation of enculturated values; and (3) postconventional, the evolution of an authentic individual value system (Kohlberg, 1984). Only in the postconventional level of development is the individual capable of participating in conscious and intentional, value-centered decision making.

At any one moment in time, individuals are spread throughout each of these three stages of development, but with the maturing of a culture and the expansion of consciousness, an increasing number of individuals develop a postconventional capacity to consciously choose and assert their unique value system. The term *value-centered decision making* refers to a manner of decision making that occurs when an individual, community, and culture are capable of consciously reflecting on their values within a context of moral development and then freely choosing the values consistent with the needs of the individual within the framework of the imperatives of the historical age.

Consider the following situation. When caring for the severely ill individual, physicians and families are called on to make critical decisions. In the usual scenario the underlying yet covert conventional assumption is that a goal of rational medicine is "the

prolongation of life, the effort to eradicate or deter disease, aging, and death." Our medical expertise and technology are used to promote the value we attribute to this assumption. But what would happen if we made this value explicit to the individuals involved and offered a competing value? For example, the goal of medicine and medical science is "to support the individual in living through the natural cycles of life." Now we have two values to consider and choose from, and when we choose the one that we value most, it will serve as a compass that guides our actions. This is an example of conscious and intentional value-centered decision making.

Thus it is apparent that value-centered decision making is an ongoing process. The issue is whether it is conscious or unconscious. In the latter case, we are automatically chained to the past; in the former case, we are free to consider the imperatives of our present lives and to choose with a fully informed and aware mind. *Consciousness* and *intention* are the two qualities that distinguish conscious decision making from conditioned decision making. These qualities can allow us to engage each other in the communal effort of choosing what is *good* for us as individuals and as a culture. Existing assumptions can be made explicit so that we may choose to continue to value them or not, and the full range of alternative assumptions can become available for us to examine. In this process we become involved in consciously envisioning the future, and as a result of this process the power over our lives that has been inexorably compelled by covert assumptions is brought to an end.

To bring the process of conscious and intentional value-centered decision making into the arena of health and healing, we must become familiar with the underlying assumptions of the existing medical model (biomedicine) and of an alternative set of assumptions. With these choices in mind, we can attribute value in the direction that seems most appropriate to our current needs and to our vision of the future.

To address this issue, in a study for the Institute of Noetic Sciences, we examined, from a value-centered perspective, the full range of issues involved in an expanded, comprehensive, and fully integrated approach to health and disease. We undertook a series of targeted interviews with individuals who are working toward a postmodern approach to health care, convened a series of focused group meetings, and completed a qualitative analysis of the patterns that emerged from these discussions.

This dialogue included representatives from diverse groups who share a common interest in the outcome of the health care debate: health care providers of various types of practices, consumer groups, policy makers, and key leaders in the reconceptualization of health care. This study considered a variety of issues, including the influence of social and cultural perspectives on health care; the epistemological assumptions of various health care systems; the impact of the expanding accessibility of health information; the role of consciousness, intentionality, and spiritual dimensions in health and healing; the changing role of the practitioner and patient; the education of the health care practitioner; the scope and character of related health care research; and the role of public policy and health care financing.

In individual interviews and small group discussions there was a remarkable similarity in the articulation of values on which a postmodern medicine can be formulated. In analyzing this research, we identified a specific set of values that could form the basis of a postmodern medicine and the recurrence of several general themes related to the enculturation of these values.

From Encounter to Relationship

Our study participants uniformly focused on the importance of renewing and revitalizing the relationship between physician and patient. The content and character of this relationship continue to hold value and meaning to them. There is general agreement that the proper relationship should emphasize mutuality, empathy, compassion, caring, authenticity, integrity, and trust. Stated briefly, the practitioner-patient relationship, which currently focuses on efficiently "doing" the standardized activities of diagnosis and therapy, should reconfigure itself toward "being," the process of sharing a relationship, a process that some characterize as a "partnership." This is a shift in emphasis from data collection to human interaction. Both the practitioners and the lay individuals interviewed were aware that the character and quality of the "healer-healee" relationship can itself become a potent healing force.

The Pew-Fetzer Task Force report on *Advancing Psychosocial Health Education* focused on "relationship-centered care" (Tresolini and Pew-Fetzer Task Force, 1994). To work effectively in the patient-practitioner relationship, the report defined the essential knowledge, skills, and values that practitioners must develop in four areas: (1) self-awareness and continuing self-growth; (2) the patient's experience of health and illness; (3) developing and maintaining a relationship with patients; and (4) communicating clearly and effectively. Self-awareness is seen as serving as the foundation for an empathic understanding of another's circumstance, and a sustained healing relationship is based on honest, open, and trusting communication. These views were mirrored in our participant comments.

From Disease Centered to Person Centered

Our study participants went beyond their emphasis on the importance of the quality of the physician-patient relationship to speak about the focal point of the interaction. They expressed a dissatisfaction with the disease-centered orientation of the medical encounter, preferring it to be person centered and individualized. A disease-centered perspective collapses the uniqueness and intactness of an individual and the context in which his or her life is embedded, substituting instead the generic search for data, normative or nonnormative, with the sole intent to define the presence or absence of disease categories. Individuals appear to want to be seen, particularly by their healers, as the unique and complex individuals that they are, and similarly, healers express the desire for the time, opportunity, and support that is necessary to hold their patients in this manner. As stated by one participant, ". . . there should be a radical emphasis on the individuality of each person."

The shift from a focus on disease categories to a focus on the individual addresses two further values raised by our participants: *wholeness* (the appreciation of context) and *integrity*. To be seen and known as an individual whose experiences constitute a dynamic unity requires the practitioner to expand his or her worldview so as to be large enough to contain both a reductionistic and integrated view of the individual, a perspective that is both analytic and synthetic at the same time. To be seen in a reductionistic manner confirms the observation that for specific purposes, the body may be seen as a closed mechanical system. To be seen from an integrative perspective affirms an individual's wholeness, integrity, uniqueness, complexity, and sense of coherence, allowing for empathic understanding. One cannot have empathy for a body part. To be seen as a whole acknowledges the centrality of the individual in the healing process.

From Practitioner and Corporate Empowerment to Personal Empowerment

The power relationships in contemporary medicine derive from the conditions of their historical development. The shift to a science-centered medicine resulted from (1) the simultaneous choice of and extraordinary financial investment in the expansion of medical science and its research facilities, (2) the reinvention of the medical school curriculum by basing it in the laboratory sciences, and (3) the integration of medical education into the emerging academic centers. The consequent development of the profession of medicine as an autonomous and authoritative profession granted to it the exclusive rights to practice medicine and to define and manage its domain, a right that was increasingly formalized by state licensing boards in the early part of the twentieth century. The power over the healing process shifted from household family members to an eclectic group of healers and then to physicians and their institutions.

The second shift in power occurred as the financial costs of a scientific-centered medicine became apparent in the 1930s. The high costs of health care, which rapidly became unaffordable to most families, resulted in the development of the third-party payer system and the subsequent decades-long drama that was to decide the central third-party payer—government or private industry—a drama that has been resolved in one direction or another nation-by-nation. This process has resulted in a shift of power, and the accompanying capacity to define the character of health care, from the professional domain of physicians to governmental institution or the board room of the corporation. This can be seen as the shift in health care from a *service* to a *product*.

However, these shifts in power occurred in an era of expanding social and political citizen activism that has created another potentially powerful center of interest: the *consumer* of health care. The wellness, holistic, mind-body–self-regulation, and complementary and integrative (alternative) care movements are each a demonstration of this new and growing force. Individuals are discovering their central role in the healing process, their capacities for self-healing, their ability to access scientific and other health-related information rapidly and effectively through the Internet, and their right to question the actions of physicians, corporations, and government.

From Illness to Wellness

In the 1970s, John Travis, MD, opened the first wellness center in Mill Valley, California. Influenced by Halbert Dunn's book *High Level Wellness,* Travis sought to expand our ideas about health beyond the customary focus on preventing and curing disease to include a concern for the promotion of well-being. Health and healing were seen in a broader context as a psychological-social-spiritual process of education, lifestyle change, and personal growth and development. This concept was rapidly accepted by an increasingly health-conscious self-help culture, resulting in a proliferation of exercise facilities and fitness programs, health food stores, self-help books, corporate employee wellness programs, and wellness workshops and seminars conducted by individuals and institutions. Prevention, usually considered to reside within the domain of public health and population-based interventions, expanded into a social and private activity as it extended its vision toward health promotion.

The shift from an exclusive focus on illness to an emphasis on wellness, even in the context of illness, is related to the values we have already discussed: the emphasis on the practitioner-patient relationship, person-centered care, and personal empowerment. Although the interest in wellness and health promotion, an interest that should be seen as a radical expansion of all previous conceptualizations of health, has been apparent in our culture for 25 years, it has yet to be fully enculturated into our health care system or our popular culture.

GENERAL THEMES

Absence of a Bridging Language

The language of government and corporate health and market forces is increasingly becoming the dominant language that defines the character of health care. Words and terms like *consumer, provider, payer, capitation, market share, per member per month costs, stream of revenue, managed care, delivery of services, utilization, encounters, purchasers of care,* and *lives covered* reflect a specific set of values applied by the corporate culture to the process of health care. This language relates to a specific view of medicine that emphasizes the economics of disease and curative therapeutics.

In contrast, participants in the our study previously discussed have been working to develop a very different set of words and terms, ones that define the human dimensions of health care rather than its commodification. Such a language may include words and terms such as *holism, integrity, caring, listening, mind-body, spirituality, consciousness,* and *soul.* This reflects a view of medicine that emphasizes the relational aspects of healing and focuses on health as a broader experience of mind, body, and spirit, an experience that is ongoing and multidimensional.

Absence of Enculturation

When values have failed to become enculturated, they are neither *collectively* held nor acknowledged, affirmed, or supported by the culture at large. External social structures that bring tangibility and affirmation through acknowledged social roles, community rituals, and institutional structures are absent. As a result, the emerging values can only be personally embodied (in contrast to enculturated), individually expressed by those who nurture them, and supported by islands of like-minded individuals or institutions.

If one considers the three subcultures defined by Ray—traditionalists, modernists, and cultural creatives—it becomes apparent that the first two subcultures have clear social contexts (enculturation) within which to live out and affirm their core values. Traditionalists can look toward their fundamentalist religious affiliations and institutions for ongoing support and validation. Modernists need only to turn to the dominant institutions of contemporary culture that readily offer the roles and rituals to support their value system. For both these groups, interior values are reflected in external social structures that bring tangibility in the form of community, roles, and institutional structures to what otherwise would remain a set of values that can only be experienced

and validated internally or interpersonally. Cultural creatives, the prime proponents of the emerging postmodern values, lack the built-in external social contexts within which they can readily live and experience their new value system (Ray, 1996).

The absence of normalized social contexts (enculturation) within which to "talk and walk" postmodern values appears to impose both a burden and a responsibility on those who hold these values. The burden is the inability to easily and routinely live and affirm these values within the existing cultural roles and models. This will continue until these values become enculturated. The responsibility appears to be a personal sense of importance attributed to finding a way to infuse these values successfully into the normative life of our culture. In the arena of health and healing, this effort is to instill the emerging postmodern values discussed previously into a scientifically and technologically based medicine (education, research, and clinical practice).

AN INTEGRAL MODEL OF HEALING

The following model draws on the values research discussed earlier and uses *systems theory,* a theory that first developed as a modern response to the accumulation of expanding volumes of information and data and an increasing emphasis on microspecialization (Dacher, 1996). Systems, or *organizational,* theory is an attempt to integrate, to create wholes out of parts. It is in essence a science of wholeness. Its concepts and principles are based on the observation that nature is organized in patterns of increasing complexity and comprehensiveness and that these larger "wholes," or units, have characteristics and qualities unique to the whole and cannot be identified or accessed through an analysis of their component parts (van Bertalanffy, 1968; Weiss, 1977). For example, the human organism, composed of cells, tissues, and organ systems, contains qualities and characteristics that cannot be exclusively accounted for through the linear summation of its parts. These include the capacity for self-organization, integrated action and adaptability, will, intention, and creativity.

Each of the subsystems of this model is a complete and distinct whole in itself, yet at the same time it is part of a more comprehensive healing system. As an intact system, each of these component systems has its own frame of reference, operating principles, internal stability, characteristics, and research methodology. As we ascend the hierarchy of healing systems, we expand our conceptualization of healing, adding both complexity and comprehensiveness at each new level. Each component of the systems can be studied separately, and the entire system can be studied in terms of both its system-wide characteristics and the interrelations of its component parts. For the scientific researcher, it is appropriate to study a particular system selectively, applying the research methodology appropriate to the system under study. The practitioner, however, whose focus is always the whole person, must have the dual concern of attending to the individual components of the healing system while considering these components within the context of a more inclusive and comprehensive multisystem approach to healing.

The model is composed of four healing systems: homeostasis, treatment, mind-body, and spiritual. Figure 6-3 illustrates the relation of the component parts to the whole.

Homeostatic Healing System

Walter Cannon described the most primary and basic healing system available to the human organism, the homeostatic system (Figure 6-4). This built-in instinctual system of internal physiological checks and balances evolved over the millennia of human development, providing the human organism with the potential to respond automatically to internal states of disequilibrium with immediate, reflexlike physiological corrections. This system ensures the maintenance of a steady physiological state, which in turn ensures survival.

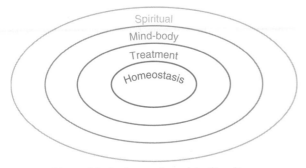

Figure 6-3 An integral model of healing.

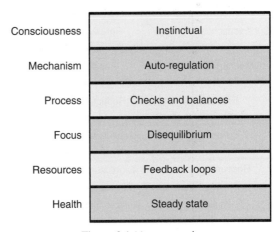

Figure 6-4 Homeostasis.

However, our homeostatic system is much more suited to the life of early humans than it is to the more recent and dramatic changes in lifestyle and environment that characterize and accompany "civilized" urban life (Weiss, 1977). As a consequence, the homeostatic system is often maladapted to the changing lifestyles, practices, and environments of modern humans: our nutritional choices, exercise patterns, physical environments, and stress levels. This mismatch between primitive adaptive mechanisms and the realities of modern life has resulted in significant limitations and deficiencies in the natural protective mechanisms designed into this system. For example, the maintenance of normal glucose levels and the integrity of the vasculature are undermined by our modern diets and sedentary lifestyles, and the on-and-off mechanism of the stress response and the maintenance of normal levels of blood pressure are distorted by the presence of unrelenting mental stress. To remedy the results of the mismatch between the built-in mechanisms of the homeostatic healing system and the realities of urban life, civilized humans have developed "treatment" models with the purpose of "stepping in" when homeostasis has failed to restore normal function.

Treatment Healing System

The treatment system is activated when the patient seeks assistance from a health care practitioner as a reaction to the appearance of a symptom or the presence of overt disease, an indication of the breakdown of the natural homeostatic system. This step is

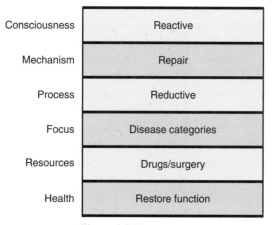

Figure 6-5 Treatment.

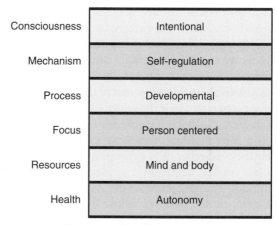

Figure 6-6 Mind-body healing.

routinely followed by the requisite testing, establishment of a diagnosis, and the prescription of therapy, usually, in the biomedical treatment system, in the form of external agents such as drugs, surgery, or physical therapy. Biomedicine, the dominant form of treatment in Western society, seeks to establish and explain causation by reducing the field of study to a single-body system and its associated biochemistry. Its aim is to repair the biophysiological abnormality and reestablish health, which in the biomedical system is defined as the "restoration of normal function" (Figure 6-5).

The success of biomedicine has resulted in a shift in the burden of illness from acute infectious disease to chronic, often stress-related, degenerative disease, the causes of which are largely a result of personal attitudes and lifestyles. Although biomedicine is well equipped to diagnose and treat these diseases, which are currently the major source of premature death and morbidity, its therapies rarely result in cure. The characteristics that have been responsible for biomedicine's many accomplishments by necessity also define its limits.

Mind-Body Healing System

The mind-body healing system relies on the assumption of personal responsibility and the self-motivated effort to develop and use the personal skills and capacities (psychological, psychosocial, and physical) that are available to assist in the process of self-regulation and healing (Figure 6-6). Mind-body healing is inten-

tional and preferably proactive. Its focus is on personal attitudes and lifestyle, the central factors in the development of stress-related degenerative disorders. The concern here is with psychological development, individuation, personal transformation, and mastery, to the extent possible, over the activities of the mind and body.

This aspect of healing finds its scientific legitimacy in the emerging research in the field of psychoneuroimmunology (Ader et al., 1991). The discovery of the interconnectedness of psychic and physiological functions mediated by the mobile neuropeptide messenger system has assisted in establishing the biochemical pathways that account for the long-accepted relations between mind and body. Furthermore, we are now able to demonstrate the specific psychological qualities and psychosocial influences that appear to provide enhanced resistance to the detrimental effects of physiological stress (Antonovsky, 1988, 1991; Kobassa, 1979).

The shift in focus from diagnostic categories to issues of personal attitudes, lifestyle, and psychological development alters the relationship of the health practitioner to the patient. The relationship is more of a *partnership* than the hierarchical relationship that characterizes biomedical healing. The focus is long term, and the treatment modalities, which can more accurately be termed *health promotion practices,* are more internal than external. Examples include meditation, exercise, nutritional practices, psychosocial education, biofeedback, and yoga. The intent is more educational than therapeutic, and the health practitioner serves more as an educator and coach.

As with each of the preceding systems, the defining focus of the mind-body healing system—self-regulation, psychological development, and individuation—also accounts for its deficiencies and defines its limits. This system fails to consider the spiritual aspects of the human experience, which transcend and extend the boundaries of personal development, conveying to the individual a more comprehensive and sustaining understanding of the living experience.

Spiritual Healing System

Spirituality has many definitions. For the purposes of this model, I define spirituality as "an individual's capacity to view the living experience in the context of an organized and unifying perspective that transcends day-to-day experience and provides meaning and purpose to essential human concerns about life and death." A spiritual perspective can have a profound effect on personal attitudes, values, and behaviors and consequently on biochemistry and physiology. These effects on the mind and the body are termed *spiritual healing* (Figure 6-7).

CHARACTERISTICS OF THE FOUR SYSTEMS AS A WHOLE

When these four healing systems are considered as an integrated comprehensive system, certain characteristics appear that are not evident when each is taken

Consciousness	Intuitive
Mechanism	Integration
Process	Unifying
Focus	Myth/symbol
Resources	Consciousness
Health	Wholeness

Figure 6-7 Spiritual healing.

separately. We are able to see the evolving characteristics of healing as we approach Figure 6-8 in a horizontal direction; for example, the expansion of consciousness from instinctual to reactive, intentional, and intuitive and the shift in resources from built-in automatic feedback loops to drugs and surgery, mind and body, and expanded consciousness. Similarly, we can see an increasingly inclusive and comprehensive vision of health as we shift from the goal of maintaining a physiological steady state to restoring function, to individuation, and finally to the attainment of wholeness. Taken as a whole, the movement through each healing system reflects the natural developmental sequence of a human life. We discover that much like this model, we are both parts and wholes—mechanical, interactive, and integrated all at the same time.

	Homeostasis	Treatment	Mind-body	Spiritual
Consciousness	Instinctual	Reactive	Intentional	Intuitive
Mechanism	Auto-regulation	Repair	Self-regulation	Integration
Process	Checks and balances	Reductive	Developmental	Unifying
Focus	Disequilibrium	Disease categories	Person centered	Myth/symbol
Resources	Feedback loops	Drugs/surgery	Mind/body	Consciousness
Health	Steady state	Restore function	Autonomy	Wholeness

Figure 6-8 Integrative model.

The adversarial distinction between the conventional and the complementary and integrative (or alternative) therapies disappears as we consider the intent, usefulness, and mechanism involved in each form of therapy and properly assign it to one of the four healing systems: homeostasis, treatment, mind-body, and spiritual. This is a more functional way to categorize a therapeutic practice than the current arbitrary and capricious view of its status as "conventional" or "complementary and integrative." To the extent that a practice, whether conventional or complementary and integrative, fits within a specific system, it then by necessity must attain its legitimacy and credibility through the disciplined exploration of its efficacy by means of the research methodology appropriate to that specific system.

This model is inclusive rather than exclusive, honoring and respecting the contributions, independence, and interdependence of each of these healing systems and the integrity and professionalism of the many and varied practitioners whose practices, when proved efficacious through a rigorous system-based research methodology, serve as accepted and valuable resources for one or more of the healing systems. Reductionistic and holistic thinking and conventional and alternative practices are each seen as essential components of a comprehensive intellectual process and a unified approach to health and healing. Of the healing systems discussed in this chapter, the spiritual healing system is the most difficult to define and presents the most significant challenge to our current research methodologies. However, it conveys an essential completeness and wholeness to this comprehensive healing model by encouraging an existential exploration of the meaning and purpose of primal human issues of pain and suffering, disease, aging, and death.

In the biomedical system, practitioners-in-training and the active clinician can incorporate these perspectives into the daily practice of healing. In this system we are accustomed to using a symptom as the "ticket of admission" to the clinical setting and as the basis for the ensuing interview, which begins with a general review of the body systems and progresses, in a reductionistic manner, toward a subsequent focus on the particular single system most directly related to the presenting symptom. This process can be directly applied to the expanded approach proposed here by adding an initial level of *triage*, which precedes the more detailed interview process. This initial triage decision determines which one or more of the healing systems—homeostatic, treatment, mind-body, or spiritual—is to be applied to the presenting problem. For example, a minor acute illness is not the basis for a multisystem interview. In contrast, a myocardial infarction requires full attention to the homeostatic, treatment, mind-body, and spiritual healing systems. An individual's age further assists in determining the applicability and usefulness of the mind-body and spiritual healing systems. Mind-body healing cannot be introduced until the attainment of a certain level of maturity, and similarly, a spiritual approach is generally inappropriate for the adolescent or young adult. Mind-set is the final indication of which direction to proceed. Mind-body and spiritual healing systems require a certain openness, interest, and intellect because they call on the direct and enthusiastic participation of the patient.

Once made, this triage decision defines the next level of inquiry, which consists of an *interview* related to the particular healing system(s) that has been selected. If the problem seems most appropriately resolved through the biomedical approach, the traditional review of systems ensues. If an alternative (or integrative) approach is selected, the specific approach-based interview is conducted. If the problem calls for the mind-body or the spiritual system, the inquiry appropriate to one of these systems is inserted. The homeostatic system is concerned with the circumstances (environmental, dietary, and physical) that support the normal autoregulatory functions of the mind and body; the treatment system focuses on the traditional issues of diagnosis and therapy; the mind-body system is concerned with personal attitudes and lifestyle; and the spiritual system considers issues of meaning and purpose. As with the traditional review of systems, an inquiry into each of these aspects of healing proceeds with a series of questions and responses between practitioner and patient.

With the preceding considerations and the appropriate inquiry into the nature of the presenting problem, a comprehensive *plan* can be agreed on in partnership with the patient. This plan will apply the appropriate range of resources from each of the selected healing systems. In its most complete form, such a plan would aim to support the normal operations of the homeostatic system, restore function where dysfunction has developed (the treatment system), expand personal resources and capacities (the mind-body healing system), and assist the individual in the attainment of a more whole and balanced life (the spiritual healing system). As with any plan, a continuing reiterative process occurs throughout the life cycle.

To illustrate this process better, let us consider the case of an individual who presents for the first time with the symptoms of atherosclerotic heart disease. The initial triage would suggest that the age at which this disease presents itself and the intensity and severity of this particular illness indicate the need to consider, at a minimum, the homeostatic, treatment, and mind-body healing systems (Figure 6-9). Further inquiry, which may continue over weeks, will clarify whether this specific individual is amenable to viewing the implications of this disease within the framework of a spiritual perspective. Initially, the appropriate steps related to treatment, diagnosis, and therapy are pursued. Concurrently, an inquiry into personal attitudes and lifestyle is initiated. Finally, if appropriate, a dialogue can be initiated, seeking an understanding of the meaning, purpose, significance, and implications of this disease for the individual's life.

In the patient with atherosclerotic disease, development of a comprehensive plan would include a mixture of approaches: (1) the use of appropriate diagnostic and therapeutic interventions (treatment system); (2) the introduction of attitudinal and lifestyle changes in the areas of stress management, nutrition, exercise, and insight-based psychological counseling (mind-body system); and (3) an ongoing consideration of the impact of this illness on previously held values, beliefs, and priorities (spiritual system). The goal for

the practitioner is to begin to perceive disease and the individual in a larger context. The goal for the individual is to use disease as a doorway into a more considered and expanded life that serves to remedy the problem at hand, reverse the personal factors that contributed to the development of the illness, and enhance the overall quality of life.

This proposed model has definite implications for practitioners and their patients. If primary care practitioners are to perform the role of triage officers as proposed here, they must be provided with the elements of a comprehensive approach to health and healing. Such a practitioner must be knowledgeable in the dynamics of each of the four healing systems, but the distinctive aspect of his or her education will be an understanding of the principles, concepts, and structural issues that underlie a comprehensive approach to healing. We are not seeking experts in specific domains; the level of data and information available makes that task impossible. Rather, we are seeking practitioners, conventional and "alternative," whose training is expanded to include an understanding of each of the essential aspects of healing complemented by a strong emphasis on integrative studies. The latter is not merely an emphasis on structure and organization but contains a value system that emphasizes synthesis and wholeness, a perspective that is largely absent from current educational programs.

However, it must be remembered that *technique,* whether conventional or alternative, is only one of two important healing forces. Although this force has been the central focus of biomedicine, a second

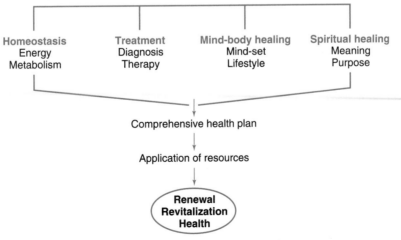

Figure 6-9 Comprehensive health plan.

healing force complements technique. The force of *personal presence* is marked by active empathic listening, caring, ongoing support, and by the special type of love that passes through the healing relationship. This traditional aspect of healing is much subtler than the development and use of technique, and although the source of its healing power is largely unknown in a mechanistic sense, most of us know it through personal and direct experience. The personal presence is partly acknowledged and is termed the *placebo effect* by modern science. The development of this healing capacity requires the shift from an emphasis on disease categories toward the following:

1. Consideration of the unique contextual elements of the individual story line.
2. Rediscovery of the art of tending to the patient as a corrective balance to the current overemphasis on treatment.
3. An understanding, appreciation, and patience with suffering, disease, aging, and death, which in part characterize and mature human life.
4. A commitment by the practitioner to a lifetime process of personal development that parallels the process of professional development.

Patients must also review their monotheistic and fragmented approach to health care and their incessant conditioned demand for professionals and treatments. It will be increasingly necessary to view health as an artistic creative act that is engaged for the duration of the life cycle. The expansion of consciousness, self-knowledge, capacities, resources, and skills is the very process of health itself. In these terms, *health* becomes more a verb than a noun, an intentional and proactive orientation to life that values personal growth and development. Health is then viewed as a lifetime journey rather than as a response to illness. In this context, a consciously lived life cycle will engage an individual in exploring each of the healing systems, maximizing its contributions toward enhancing the quality and duration of life while compressing morbidity into the final years of life.

CONCLUSION

The development of a postmodern integral medicine can be best accomplished by a full discussion of the values and perspectives that can appropriately underlie an expanded approach to health and healing. On the basis of these values and perspectives, it is then possible to create one or more comprehensive healing models that reflect the needs of our time and provide a framework for practitioner education, clinical practice, and research.

References

Ader R, Felten DL, Cohen N: *Psychoneuroimmunology,* ed 2, New York, 1991, Academic Press.

Adler NE, Boyce WT, et al: Socioeconomic inequalities in health, *JAMA* 269:3140-3145, 1993.

Antonovsky A: *Unraveling the mystery of health,* San Francisco, 1988, Jossey-Bass.

Antonovsky A: *Health, stress, and coping,* San Francisco, 1991, Jossey-Bass.

Benor DJ: *Healing research: holistic energy medicine and spirituality.* Vol 1. Research in healing, Munich, 1992, Helix.

Berkman LF, Syme SL: Social networks, host resistance, and mortality: a nine year follow up study of Alameda County residents, *Am J Epidemiol* 109:186-204, 1979.

Dacher ES: *Intentional healing,* New York, 1996, Marlowe.

Dacher ES: *Whole healing,* New York, 1996, Dutton.

Dubos R: *Mirage of health,* Garden City, NY, 1961, Doubleday.

Duggan RM: Complementary medicine: transforming influence or footnote to history? *Altern Ther* 1(2):28-31, 1995.

Flexner A: Medical education in the United States and Canada, Bulletin #4, New York, 1910, Carnegie Foundation.

Gilman DC: *The launching of a university,* New York, 1969 (1906), Garrett Press.

Harrington TF: *The Harvard Medical School: a history, narrative, and documentary.* Vol III, New York, 1905, Lewis Publishing.

Hause JS, Robbins C, Metzner HL: The association of social relationships with mortality: prospective evidence from the Tecumseh Community Health Study, *Am J Epidemiol* 116:123-140, 1982.

Illich I: *Medical nemesis,* New York, 1976, Pantheon Books.

Kobassa SC: Stressful life events, personality, and health: an inquiry into hardiness, *J Pers Soc Psychol* 37:1-11, 1979.

Kohlberg L: *The psychology of moral development,* San Francisco, 1984, Harper & Row.

Kuhn TS: *The structure of scientific revolutions,* Chicago, 1970, University of Chicago Press.

Locke S: *The healer within,* New York, 1986, Dutton.

Ludmerer KM: *Learning to heal,* Baltimore, 1985, Johns Hopkins University Press.

McKeown T: *The role of medicine: dream, mirage, nemesis,* London, 1976, Neuffeld Provincial Hospitals Trust.

Ray PH: The Integral Culture Survey, Research Report 96-A, Sausalito, Calif, 1996, Institute of Noetic Sciences.

Tresolini CP, Pew-Fetzer Task Force: *Health professions education and relationship-centered care,* San Francisco, 1994, Pew Health Professions Commission.

Von Bertalanffy L: *General systems theory,* New York, 1968, Braziller.

Weiss P: The system of nature and the nature of systems: empirical holism and practical reductionism harmonized. In Schaeffer KE, Hensel H. Brody R, editors: *Toward a man-centered medical science,* Mount Kisco, NY, 1977, Futura.

Williams GC, Neese RM: The dawn of Darwinian medicine, *Q Rev Biol* 66:1-22, 1991.

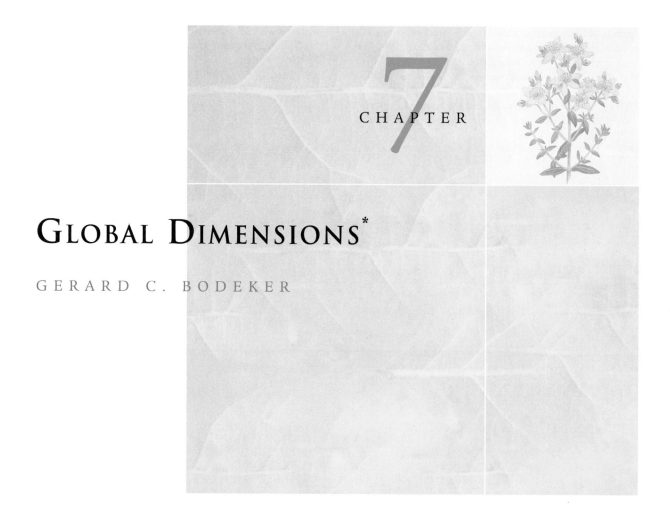

CHAPTER

7

GLOBAL DIMENSIONS*

GERARD C. BODEKER

At the basis of the global concern about the ever-increasing cost of health care lies the issue of *sustainability*. Developing countries recognize that their health care systems are based on expensive, imported medicines and technologies, and that continued reliance on these systems will result in health care costs consuming national finances and stifling national economic growth.

Basic questions are now being asked about priorities in health expenditures and national economic development: How can countries address the health needs of their people without continuing to rely on expensive, imported medicines? Furthermore, how can local, existing systems of health care be utilized to provide basic health services to rural and poor communities? Increased attention is being paid to the potential of locally available medicinal plants and inexpensive herbal medicines in providing effective primary health care. This in turn has raised concerns about the sustainable use of wild sources of medicinal plants, the conservation of biodiversity, appropriate forms of local cultivation and production, the safety and effectiveness of natural medicines, and the regulatory environment that should accompany the incorporation of traditional systems of health into national health care.

This chapter discusses some of these recent trends with experiences from countries and communities in

*This chapter is modified and updated from the original article "Traditional health knowledge and public policy," in *Nature & Resources* 30(2), 1994, UNESCO.

Africa, the Americas, and Asia. The primary focus is the economic, cultural, environmental, and other factors that have led to the resurgence of interest in traditional systems of health. The chapter concludes with a discussion of policy options for incorporating traditional ecological and medicinal knowledge into national and international environmental, health, and economic policy and planning.

BACKGROUND

The terms *traditional medicine* and *traditional systems of health* refer to the long-standing indigenous systems of health care found in developing countries and among the indigenous populations of industrialized countries. The paradigms of these traditional medical systems view humanity as being linked intimately with the wider dimensions of nature (Bodeker, 2000). Long relegated to marginal status in the health care plans of developing countries, traditional medicine—or more appropriately, traditional systems of health care, since they provide comprehensive approaches to prevention and treatment that are beyond the scope of medicine alone—has undergone a major renewal in the past 15 or more years.

The World Health Organization (WHO) has referred to these systems as *holistic,* meaning, "that of viewing man in his totality within a wide ecological spectrum, and of emphasizing the view that ill health or disease is brought about by an imbalance, or disequilibrium, of man in his total ecological system and not only by the causative agent and pathogenic evolution" (WHO, 1978). Traditional medicine has been described as "one of the surest means to achieve total health care coverage of the world population, using acceptable, safe, and economically feasible methods."

The treatment strategies utilized by traditional systems of health include the use of herbal medicines; mind-body approaches such as meditation; physical therapies such as massage, acupuncture, and exercise programs; and approaches that address both physical and spiritual well-being. These methods incur limited costs, are available locally, and, according to WHO, are utilized as the primary source of health care by 80% of the world's population.

An essential feature of traditional systems of health is that they are based in cosmologies or paradigms that take into account mental, spiritual, physical, and ecological dimensions in the conceptu-

alization and evaluation of health and well-being. Assumptions of causality frequently differ from those of Western medicine, and treatments are designed to reflect those underlying theories of causality. Indeed, classification of diseases, medicinal plants, and ecosystems in traditional knowledge systems may vary substantially from those of Western taxonomies.

A fundamental concept found in many systems is that of *balance:* the balance between mind and body; between different dimensions of individual bodily functioning and need; between the individual and community; among the individual, community, and environment; and between the individual and the universe. Disease is understood to arise from a breakdown in the state of balance in one or more of these areas. Treatments are designed not only to address the locus of the disease, but also to restore a state of systemic balance to the individual and the inner and outer environment.

Historically, the paradigms of traditional knowledge systems have been considered "primitive" by modern or Western science. However, recent advances in environmental sciences, immunology, medical botany, and pharmacognosy have led to a new appreciation for the precise descriptive nature and efficacy of many traditional taxonomies, as well as for the efficacy of the treatments employed. There is an emerging awareness that any meaningful appraisal of a traditional system of health and its contribution to health care must take into account the paradigm or cosmology that underlies diagnosis and treatment.

ORGANIZATIONAL RELATIONSHIPS BETWEEN MODERN AND TRADITIONAL MEDICINE

Under colonial influence, traditional medical systems were frequently outlawed by authorities. In the postcolonial era the attitudes of Western medical practitioners and health officials have maintained the marginal status of traditional health care providers, despite the role that these practitioners play in providing basic health care to the rural majority, to developing countries, and within indigenous communities.

Traditional medicine and modern medicine have interfaced with each other in the following four broad ways:

1. *Monopolistic:* Modern medical doctors have the sole right to practice medicine.
2. *Tolerant:* Traditional medical practitioners are not officially recognized, but they are free to practice on the condition that they do not claim to be registered medical doctors.
3. *Parallel:* Practitioners of both modern and traditional systems are officially recognized. They serve their patients through separate but equal systems, such as in India.
4. *Integrated:* Modern and traditional medicine merged in medical education and jointly practiced within a unique health service, such as in China and Vietnam.

FACTORS INFLUENCING POLICY DEVELOPMENT

Despite the historical suppression of traditional medicine by modern medical interests, an increasing number of developing countries are displaying policy interest in traditional approaches to health care. This has led to a resurgence of interest in research, investment, and program development in this field (Bodeker and Kronenberg, 2002). Economic factors, cultural factors, and national crises (e.g., war, epidemics) underlie this new interest.

Economic Factors

The majority of the rural populations of developing countries cannot afford Western medical health care. In Vietnamese peasant communities, there is a common saying that traditional medicine costs one chicken, modern medicine costs one cow, and modern hospital treatment costs many cows. Rural people may have to travel for a day or more to reach a modern medical clinic or pharmacy. This results in lost wages, which is compounded by the cost of transport and the relatively high cost of medicines.

Typically, more than 80% of health budgets in developing countries are directed to services that reach approximately 20% of the population. Of this, 30% of the total health budget is spent on the national pharmaceutical bill.

In Asia, traditional systems of health have been incorporated as formal components of national health care for approximately 35 years. The Indian

Medicine Central Council Act of 1970 gave an official place in national health programs to the Ayurvedic and Unani medical systems of India. India now has more than 200,000 registered traditional medical practitioners, the majority of whom have received their training in government colleges of Ayurvedic or Unani medicine. China has had a policy of integrating traditional medicine into national health care for more than three decades, and it has an extensive national program in which modern and traditional medicine are combined as formal components of health care provision. In both India and China the traditional health sector provides the majority of health care to the poor and rural communities.

In recent years, other countries have begun to provide increased support for their long-standing traditional medical systems, recognizing that they cannot afford Western medicine. In Thailand, for example, the Ministry of Health promotes the use of 66 traditional medicinal plants in primary health care, based on scientific evidence of the efficacy of these plants, as well as on traditional patterns of utilization. The Fourth Public Health Development Plan of Thailand (1977-1981) stated the country's general policy to promote the use of traditional medicinal plants in primary health care. The Seventh Plan (1992-1996) promoted the integration of traditional Thai medicine into community health care and prioritized research on medicinal plants. The Thai Ministry of Public Health also promotes the use of medicinal plants in state-run hospitals and health service centers (Koysooko and Chuthaputti, 1993). A study by the Royal Tropical Institute of the Netherlands found that traditional herbal medicines were used most effectively in primary health care in Thailand when self-administered. Since most rural people treat themselves before seeking help from either modern or traditional medical practitioners, herbal medicines offer a low-cost intervention in the early treatment of disease and provide a safe alternative to the growing problem of self-medication with inappropriate doses and harmful combinations of over-the-counter drugs (Le Grand and Wondergem, 1990).

In Korea, 15% to 20% of the national health budget is directed to traditional medical services, and government reports indicate that traditional medicine is favored equally by all levels of society. Health insurance coverage is available for Oriental medical treatments. In Japan, where physicians have been authorized to prescribe and dispense medications, more than two thirds of all physicians reportedly prescribe herbal medications (Norbeck and Lock, 1987).

Cultural Factors

Cultural factors play a significant role in the continued reliance on traditional medicine. Often, villagers seek symptomatic relief with modern medicine but turn to traditional medicine for treatment of what may be perceived as the "true cause of the condition" (Kleinman, 1980). Traditional medical knowledge typically is coded into household cooking practices, home remedies, and health prevention and health maintenance beliefs and routines. The advice of family members or other significant members of a community has a strong influence on health behavior, including the type of treatment that is sought (Nichter, 1978).

Decolonization and increased self-determination for indigenous groups have led some countries to reevaluate and promote their traditional medical systems. At a 1993 Pan American Health Organization conference on indigenous peoples and health, representatives from South America reported increasing activity and interest in traditional medicine in their countries (Zoll, 1993). Several Latin American countries have departments or divisions of traditional medicine within their health ministries.

Mexico has undertaken an extensive program of revitalizing its indigenous medical traditions. More than 1000 traditional medicines have been identified as a result of a program of ethnomedical and pharmacognostic research; training centers have been established by the government to pass traditional medical knowledge on to new generations of health care workers; and hospitals of traditional medicine have been established in a number of rural areas. The Mexican Constitution was revised to include traditional medicine in the provision to national health care (Argueta, 1993). Nongovernment organizations (NGOs) have played a strong role in revitalizing traditional health in Mexico, organizing national and international meetings on traditional approaches to health care. More than 50 different traditional medicine associations were represented at a 1992 meeting of the Instituto Nacional Indigenista.

Native North American communities have been incorporating traditional forms of treatment into health programs for some years. In the United States,

Indian Health Service (IHS) alcohol rehabilitation programs include traditional approaches to the treatment of alcoholism. An analysis of 190 IHS contract programs revealed that 50% of these programs offered a traditional "sweat lodge" at their site or encouraged the use of sweat lodges (Hall, 1986). Treatment outcomes improved when a sweat lodge was available. Often these sweat lodges include the presence of medicine men or healers, and the presence of a traditional healer greatly improved the outcome when used in combination with the sweat lodge. In northern Canada the Inuit Women's Association developed a program to revitalize traditional birth practices (Flaherty, 1993). Women who were midwives in their own communities for many years were interviewed and recorded on videotape, and these tapes are being used to train young midwives in the use of traditional methods.

National Crises

In addition to economic and cultural factors, national crises have spurred governments to evaluate their indigenous medical traditions as a means of providing affordable and available health care to their citizens. War and national epidemics (e.g., AIDS, malaria) are two common crises faced by these nations.

War

During the war in Nicaragua, there was an acute shortage of pharmaceutical supplies. In 1985, out of necessity, the country turned to its herbal traditions as a means of fulfilling the country's medical needs. A department was established within the health ministry to develop "popular and traditional medicine as a strategy in the search for a self-determined response to a difficult economic, military and political situation" (Castellon, 1992). This department for traditional medicine initiated a program of ethnobotanical research in the midst of war. More than 20,000 people nationwide were interviewed regarding their use of traditional and popular remedies, the methods of preparing these remedies, and the sources of plant ingredients. Previously, nurses and health workers in rural areas frequently manned outposts without medical supplies. They often were surrounded by medicinal herbs about which they knew nothing.

Based on this extensive survey, a national toxicology program in Nicaragua was begun. Over 6 to 7 years, pharmacognostic studies attempted to determine the chemistry and medicinal properties of commonly used plants. As a result of this effort, inexpensive medicines were produced locally and sustainably in rural areas to treat a wide range of conditions, including respiratory ailments, skin problems, nervous disorders, diarrhea, and diabetes.

After Vietnam's war of independence from France, an official policy was articulated by President Ho Chi Minh in 1954, asserting the importance of preserving and developing traditional medicine as a basic component of health care throughout the country, because a significant proportion of the population could not afford modern medicine. A national heritage program in traditional medicine was established to ensure that the medical knowledge of experienced practitioners was gathered, recorded, and passed on to future generations through formal training programs. Simultaneously, a policy was developed to promote the modernization of traditional medicine and to incorporate it into health service provision integrated with modern medicine. This policy was expanded and strengthened during the 1960s and 1970s, during the war between North and South Vietnam. Emergency medical strategies were generated, including the development of a traditional medical program for the treatment of burns.

After several decades of pharmacognostic and toxicological research, the National Institute of Materia Medica in Hanoi developed a list of 1863 plants of known safety and efficacy in the treatment of common medical conditions. Traditional medicine now accounts for one third of all medical treatments provided in Vietnam (Institute of Materia Medica, 1990).

Forced migration resulting from war or persecution of political dissidents can remove people from mainstream medical care and force an increased reliance on medical practices from their cultural traditions, even in the face of unfamiliar biodiversity. In one study of Burmese refugees at the Thai-Burma border, high use of traditional medicine was found despite the views of health officials that there was little or no traditional medicine use among these displaced groups (Bodeker et al., 2005).

Surveys of outpatients at a refugee-run clinic at the Thai-Burma border revealed that 59 refugee respondents listed 271 traditional remedies used for common health conditions. Research on psychoso-cial health found that separation from ancestral spiritual practices and shrines in the home country may exacerbate and even prolong mental health conditions.

Refugee aid agencies set the global agenda for refugees and ultimately determine the fate of refugees' health and well-being. By not looking at traditional systems of health care, these agencies may be overlooking a valuable, sustainable resource and may be contributing to a loss of important cultural knowledge. In contrast, by harnessing this knowledge and its practices, agencies could help facilitate new global strategies for coping and new prospects for development.

Acquired Immunodeficiency Syndrome

African governments face huge drug bills for the growing AIDS crisis and are looking to their indigenous medical traditions and medicinal plants for inexpensive and effective methods of at least alleviating the suffering of AIDS victims. The Health Ministry of Uganda has been active in generating research into the role of traditional medical practitioners in treating people with AIDS. The Uganda AIDS Commission and the Joint Clinical Research Centre in Kampala have worked with traditional healers' associations to evaluate several traditional treatments for opportunistic infections associated with human immunodeficiency virus and acquired immunodeficiency syndrome (HIV/AIDS). Commenting on research findings, a Uganda AIDS Commission official stated that traditional medicine is better suited to the treatment of some AIDS symptoms, such as herpes zoster, chronic diarrhea, shingles, and weight loss (Kogozi, 1994).

As the AIDS crisis leads an increasing number of countries to question their priorities in health expenditures, there is a new awareness that *traditional health practitioners* (THPs) can play an important role in delivering an AIDS prevention message. It is increasingly recognized that some THPs may be able to offer treatment for opportunistic infections. At the same time, there are concerns about unsafe practices and growing claims of traditional cures for AIDS. Partnerships between modern and traditional health sectors are a cornerstone for building a comprehensive strategy to manage the AIDS crisis.

In Uganda, where there is only one physician for every 20,000 people, there is one THP per 200 to 400 people (Green, 1994). In such settings, partnerships may be the only way that effective health care coverage can be achieved in managing the twin epidemics of AIDS and malaria. Clearly, such partnerships not only make good public health sense but, based on a growing body of pharmacological evidence, may also yield important preventive and treatment modalities.

In light of the widespread availability of traditional health care services and the reliance of the population on these services, it is inevitable that people with AIDS will turn to THPs for treatment. Collaborative AIDS programs have been established in many African countries, including Malawi, Mozambique, Uganda, Senegal, South Africa, Swaziland, Zambia, Zimbabwe.

Information sharing and educational programs in South Africa have resulted in THPs providing accurate HIV/AIDS advice as well as demonstration of condom use. One such program trained 1510 THPs, and during the first 10 months of the program, an estimated 845,600 clients were potentially reached with messages on AIDS and sexually transmitted disease (STD) prevention. In similar programs in Mozambique, traditional healers learned that AIDS is transmitted by sexual contact, blood, and nonsterile razor blades used in traditional practice. In a follow-up evaluation, 81% of those trained reported that they had promoted condom use with at least their STD patients (Green, 1997).

One of the challenges in such workshop situations is to move beyond "training" to genuine information sharing. It is difficult to modify health professionals' teaching approach to AIDS, which tends toward didactics and use of scientific jargon. Removing such communication barriers is a necessary first step in ensuring that training is an effective tool in mobilizing THPs as partners in AIDS control.

In Brazil, for example, face-to-face educational intervention by healersblended traditional healing, using its language, codes, symbols, and images, with scientific medicine and simultaneously addressed social injustices and discrimination. New information about HIV/AIDS transmission was conveyed using languages and concepts intimately familiar to THPs. A controlled evaluation found significant increases in AIDS awareness, knowledge about risky HIV behavior, information about correct condom use, and acceptance of lower-risk, alternative ritual blood practices among the 126 members of the trainee group compared with 100 untrained controls. There were significant decreases in prejudicial atti-tudes related to HIV transmission among the trainee group compared with controls (Nations and de Souza, 1997).

The Ugandan NGO called Traditional and Modern Health Practitioners Together Against AIDS (THETA) was established in 1992 to conduct research on potentially useful traditional medicines with HIV-related illness and to promote a mutually respectful collaboration between traditional and modern health workers in the fight against AIDS. THETA has conducted workshops to share knowledge on AIDS prevention as well as treatment of opportunistic infections using local herbal remedies.

Traditional healers participating in clinical observational studies of their herbal medicines have subsequently sought training in prevention, education, and counseling issues as well as in basic clinical diagnostic skills. A 1998 UNAIDS-sponsored evaluation of THETA found that it had reached 125 THPs (44 women and 81 men) in five districts of Uganda. Over 2 years an estimated 50,000 people benefited from the improved services offered by THPs (Kabatesi, 1998).

Malaria

The emergence of multidrug-resistant strains of malaria that has accompanied each new class of antimalarial drug is one of most significant threats to the health of people in tropical countries. Although there is widespread agreement that a fresh approach to the prevention and treatment of malaria is urgently needed, solutions have tended to focus on the development of new classes of drugs. More recently, practitioners have emphasized combination therapy with existing drugs to prevent resistance.

Historically, however, local communities in tropical regions have used local flora as a means of preventing and treating malaria (Kirby, 1997). It can be argued that these traditional medicines, based on the use of whole plants with multiple ingredients or of complex mixtures of plant materials, constitute combination therapies that may well combat the development of resistance to antimalarial therapy.

Resistance, Synergism, and Traditional Medicines

Combination therapy for malaria, cancer, and AIDS is based on the principle of synergistic action among multiple drugs. However, little significance has yet been attributed to (1) all the major antimalarials being derived from plants and (2) combinations existing in the traditional formulations before the process of extraction. For example, flavinoids in *Artemisia annua,* which are structurally unrelated to the antimalarial drug *artemisinin,* enhance the in vitro antiplasmodial activity of artemisinin (Phillipson et al., cited in Kirby, 1997).

Elsewhere, synergism has been observed between the alkaloids of the antimalarial plant *Ancistrocladus peltatum.* A total alkaloid extract of this plant had much greater antiparasitic activity than any of the six alkaloids isolated subsequently. In studies on antimalarial plants from Madagascar, the bisbenzylisoquinoline alkaloids and novel pavine and benzyl tetrahydroisoquinoline alkaloids all were found to potentiate the antiparasitic activity of chloroquine in vitro and in some cases in vivo. Preparations of these plants are currently being tested as adjuvants to chloroquine therapy in Madagascar (Kirby, 1997). In Uganda, clinical case reports and a cohort study suggest that a traditional Ugandan herbal remedy is effective against malaria (Bitawha et al., 1997; Willcox, 1999).

As with other conditions, people with malaria often combine conventional drugs and traditional medicines, sometimes simultaneously or as first-line or second-line treatments (Agyepong and Manderson, 1994; Bugmann, 2000; Gessler et al., 1995; Jayawardene, 1993; Lipowsky et al., 1992; McCombie, 1996; Pagnoni et al., 1997). Herbalists then report their view that this combination provides an additional therapeutic effect (Rasoanaivo et al., 1994). Perceived efficacy is an important reason for people using traditional antimalarial medicines. Affordability is another reason. However, when patients were asked why they choose traditional medicine over conventional drugs, a study in Burkina Faso found that the cost of medicines accounted for only 50% of responses. Lack of faith in doctors was the reason for the other 50% using traditional medicine (Abyan and Osman, 1993). Elsewhere it has been reported that medical staff at Burkina Faso hospitals are less trusted because they are frequently young, do not speak the local languages, and are not courteous or welcoming to patients (Bugmann, 2000).

Several cohort studies have been conducted to evaluate the outcomes of traditional herbal treatments used by herbalists in managing malaria. A few studies have shown complete parasite clearance by day 7 (Makinde et al., unpublished; Mueller et al., 2000; both cited in Willcox et al., 2004). Makinde et al. showed 100% parasite clearance in adults by a leaf extract of *Morinda lucida.* However, there was not full parasite clearance from infected children. Further preclinical and clinical studies on the antimalarial effects of plants have been reviewed in the book *Traditional Medicinal Plants and Malaria* (Willcox et al., 2004).

POLICY OF WORLD HEALTH ORGANIZATION

In response to rising demand for traditional medicines globally and the call from health ministries for formal regulation of this sector, WHO developed a Traditional Medicines Strategy (2002-2005) that focuses on four areas identified as requiring action to maximize the potential role of traditional medicine in public health. These areas are (1) policy; (2) safety, efficacy, and quality; (3) access; and (4) rational use. Within these areas, WHO identifies respective challenges for action, as listed next.

National Policy and Regulation

- Lack of official recognition of traditional, complementary, and alternative medicine (TCAM) and TCAM providers.
- Lack of regulatory and legal mechanisms.
- TCAM not integrated into national health care systems.
- Equitable distribution of benefits in indigenous medical knowledge and products.
- Inadequate allocation of resources for TCAM development and capacity building.

Safety, Efficacy, and Quality

- Inadequate evidence base for TCAM therapies and products.
- Lack of international and national standards for ensuring safety, efficacy, and quality control.
- Lack of adequate regulation of herbal medicines.
- Lack of registration of TCAM providers.
- Inadequate support of research.
- Lack of research methodology.

Access

- Lack of data measuring access levels and affordability.
- Lack of official recognition of role of TCAM providers.
- Need to identify safe and effective practices.
- Lack of cooperation between TCAM providers and allopathic practitioners.
- Unsustainable use of medicinal plant resources.

Rational Use

- Lack of training for TCAM providers.
- Lack of training for allopathic practitioners in TCAM.
- Lack of communication between TCAM and allopathic practitioners and between allopathic practitioners and consumers.
- Lack of information for the public on rational use of TCAM.

The WHO Center for Health Development in Kobe, Japan, has developed a global atlas on TCAM to provide policy makers with a frame of reference on global utilization and policy trends and examples of policy development in this field (WHO, 2005).

INTERNATIONAL PRESSURE TO CONSERVE BIODIVERSITY

Traditional health systems intersect with areas of the national economy other than health care. These systems interface with environmental concerns as well.

Environmental factors such as land degradation through erosion or development have contributed to the loss of natural habitats. Loss of natural habitats can affect the availability of medicinal plants and therefore local health standards. In countries where this has occurred, herb gatherers must walk increasingly longer distances to find herbs that previously grew nearby. This contributes to increasing the cost, availability, and sustainability of naturally occurring sources of medicines that traditionally provided basic health care to rural communities.

National economic development may be linked to the cultivation and use of traditional medicines. Wild harvesting of medicinal plants can provide an additional source of family income and also saves expenditure on other forms of medicine. However, overharvesting constitutes a serious threat to biodiversity. Overharvesting of medicinal plants occurs in China, where approximately 80% of the raw materials (animal and plant) for traditional medicines come from wild sources, increasing the need for new policies to integrate health, environmental, and economic perspectives. Investments are needed to develop appropriate cultivation and harvesting strategies that will meet the demand for inexpensive and accessible medicines while ensuring the conservation of diverse biological resources.

Most developing countries lack the information and resources to apply the contemporary methods of studying the inventory of flora and fauna. It has not been possible to track resource depletion systematically in medicinal plants or in animal species that are used in traditional formulae. International collaboration in developing taxonomic capabilities of environmental and forestry departments is one means by which donor agencies can protect diverse medicinal plant species, thus influencing the long-term health of local populations in developing countries.

Although local health needs have constituted the primary beneficiary of the world's medicinal plant resources, traditional medicine has also interested the international pharmaceutical industry. However, pharmaceutical interest has declined in the past decade as challenges to intellectual property rights (Bodeker, 2003) and low yield from high-throughput screening programs have led to more interest in genetic and marine sources of drugs. Another source interested in traditional medicine is the natural products industry in Europe and the United States. In Europe, where there is a large industry in phytomedicines, extracts of medicinal plants are sold in purified form to treat and prevent a wide variety of conditions.

The trends just reviewed have led to a situation where traditional medicine is viewed as a source for the production of other medicines, rather than viewed in terms of its intrinsic value. The traditional medicine community has expressed such concerns. A prevailing view is that this trend does not contribute to the development of traditional medicine as a health care system for poor or rural communities, the main constituency of traditional medical care. Rather, the international drug development initiative is seen to take medicinal knowledge from these communities to serve the demand for new drugs in industrial countries. The drugs that are being developed are for the treatment of cancer and heart disease, which are the major killers in industrialized societies, rather than for the treatment of malaria and other endemic diseases that decimate the populations of the developing countries from where the knowledge derives.

There has been no attempt, to date, to develop a scientific understanding of the efficacy of medicinal plants in addressing the primary health care needs of the populations in the areas from where the plants derive. Some projects, however, have recognized this imbalance, such as the New York Botanical Garden's ethnobotany program in Belize, and are addressing the situation through community-based projects to produce natural medicines for local consumption (Balick, 1995). They also are working to include knowledge of medicinal plants in school curricula as a means of conserving endangered traditional medical knowledge, as well as to conserve medicinal plants and rain forest areas. The National Institutes of Health (NIH) is supporting research and policy evaluation on the role of traditional medicine in the provision of cost-effective primary health care in developing countries (www. nccam.nih.gov).

A broader economic perspective would recognize that the health status of developing countries is central to the economic health of those countries and thus to the world economy. Traditional medicine and medicinal plants play an important role in meeting the basic health needs of the majority of the world's population.

CONCLUSION

Currently, wide variability exists in health planners' consideration of traditional health systems. In some countries, traditional medicine is incorporated routinely into health planning. However, this occurs in only a minority of cases, primarily in Asia. In most cases, the revival has come from nongovernment organizations. National and international funding currently is directed to the provision of Western-style health services in developing countries and indigenous communities. Research consistently links reductions in morbidity and morality rates to economic conditions, educational levels (particularly years of female education), and large-scale public health measures (e.g., sanitation, water supply). Although these factors—rather than the availability of Western medicines—have been found to lead to improved levels of health, health planners continue to operate under the view that Western medicine provides the primary means of improving health in these communities. This belief is not based in a scientific appraisal of the world's natural systems of health. Some traditional treatments are still more effective than modern treatments.

Old and limited views of traditional systems of health continue to exist, but an emerging intellectual and policy climate is giving expression to a fresh perspective. Whereas the old view favors the marginalization of traditional systems of health, the new view looks to these systems to provide complementary therapy, and in some cases, new solutions to major health crises. This new view is consonant with the

BOX 7-1

Myths Contributing to Marginalization of Traditional Health Care

Myth 1: Traditional medicines are of value only when their active ingredient is known and they are purified for mass production.

Myth 2: Based on findings from the plant screening programs of the pharmaceutical industry and national drug development programs, the therapeutic benefit of traditional medicines is limited.

Myth 3: Traditional health systems may have some use in the provision of care for chronic, low-level conditions, but they are of no value in providing acute or emergency care.

Myth 4: Little scientific knowledge is available on the safety and efficacy of traditional medicine, and all international efforts regarding traditional medicine should be directed to toxicity and efficacy research.

Myth 5: The global value of traditional medical knowledge is twofold: it serves as a source of leads for the development of new Western drugs, and the potential medicinal value of tropical rain forest species provides a basis for generating international support to preserve the world's rain forest areas and to conserve regional biodiversity.

ancient or traditional concepts of health and human potential that underlie many of the world's traditional systems of health. Table 2-6 presents an outline of how this shift affects perspectives of traditional health care systems. Box 7-1 lists the myths that contribute to the marginalization of traditional health care.

References

Abyan IM, Osman AA: Social and behavioural factors affecting malaria in Somalia, TDR/SER/PRS/11, 1993, World Health Organization.

Agyepong IA, Manderson L: The diagnosis and management of fever at household level in the Greater Accra Region, Ghana, *Acta Trop* 58:317-330, 1994.

Argueta A: Presentation to World Bank Conference on Indigenous Knowledge and Sustainable Development, Washington, DC, 1993.

Balick M: Conservation in today's world. In *Proceedings of WHO Symposium on the Utilization of Medicinal Plants* (Philadelphia, April 1993), Philadelphia, 1995, University of Pennsylvania Press.

Bitawha N, Tumwesigye O, Kabariime P, Tayebwa AK, Tumwesigye S, Ogwal-Okeng JW: Herbal treatment of malaria—four case reports from the Rukararwe Partnership Workshop for Rural Development (Uganda). *Trop Doct* 1997;27 Suppl 1:17-9.

Bodeker G: Traditional health systems: valuing biodiversity for human health and well being. In Posey D, editor: *Cultural and spiritual values in biodiversity,* Nairobi, 2000, United Nations Environment Programme, pp 261-284.

Bodeker G: Traditional medical knowledge, intellectual property rights and benefit sharing, *Cardozo J Int Compar Law* 11(2):785-814, 2003.

Bodeker G, Kronenberg F: A public health agenda for complementary, alternative and traditional (indigenous) medicine, *Am J Public Health* 92(10):1582-1591, 2002.

Bodeker G, Neumann C, Lall P, Oo ZM: Traditional medicine use and healthworker training in a refugee setting at the Thai-Burma border, *J Refugee Studies,* 18, 1, 76-99, 2005.

Bugmann N: Le concept du paludisme, l'usage et l'efficacité in vivo de trois traitements traditionnels antipalustres dans la région de Dori, Burkina Faso, Basel, 2000, Faculty of Medicine, University of Basel (Inaugural dissertation).

Castellon U: Report of the Fundacion Centro Nacional de Medicina Popular Tradicional, Nicaragua, 1992, Alejandro Davila Bolanos, MD.

Flaherty M: *Proceedings of Conference on Indigenous Peoples and Health,* Winnipeg, Canada, April 1993, pp 1-72.

Gessler MC, Msuya DE, Nkunya MH, et al: Traditional healers in Tanzania: sociocultural profile and three short portraits, *J Ethnopharmacol* 48(3), 145-160, 1995.

Green EC: *AIDS and STDs in Africa: Bridging the Gap Between Traditional Healers and Modern Medicine.* Boulder, Co., and Oxford, U.K.: Westview Press. (South African edition published by University of Natal Press, 1994).

Green EC: The participation of African traditional healers in AIDS/STD prevention programmes. *Tropical Doctor* 27: Supplement 1, 56-59, 1997.

Hall RL: Alcohol treatment in American Indian communities: an indigenous treatment modality compared with traditional approaches, *Ann NY Acad Sci* 472:168-178, 1986.

Institute of Materia Medica: *Medicinal plants in Viet Nam,* Western Pacific Series No 3, Hanoi, Manila, 1990, WHO Regional Publications.

Jayawardene R: Illness perception: social cost and coping strategies of malaria cases, *Soc Sci Med* 37:1169-1176, 1993.

Kabatesi D: Use of traditional treatments for AIDS-associated diseases in resource-constrained settings. In: *Health in the Commonwealth: challenges and solutions 1998/99* (eds. L. Robertson, K. Bell, L. Laypang & B. Blake), 1998, London: Kensington Publications.

Kirby GC: Plants as a source of antimalarial drugs. *Trop Doct* 1997;27 Suppl 1:7-11.

Kleinman A: *Patients and healers in the context of cultures,* Berkeley, 1980, University of California Press.

Kogozi J: Herbalists open hospital, Kampala, *The New Vision,* Feb 4, 1994, p 14.

Koysooko R, Chuthaputti A: Promising practices in the use of medicinal plants in Thailand. Presented at WHO Symposium on the Utilization of Medicinal Plants, Philadelphia, April 1993.

Le Grand A, Wondergem P: *Herbal medicine and promotion,* Amsterdam, 1990, Royal Tropical Institute, KIT Press.

Lei SH, Bodeker G: Changshan: ancient febrifuge and modern antimalarial—lessons for research from a forgotten tale. In Willcox M, Bodeker G, Rasaoanaivo P, editors: *Traditional medicinal plants and malaria,* London, 2004, CRC Press, Taylor & Francis.

Lipowsky R, Kroeger A, Vazquez ML: Sociomedical aspects of malaria control in Colombia, *Soc Sci Med* 34:625-637, 1992.

McCombie SC: Treatment seeking for malaria: a review of recent research, *Soc Sci Med* 43:933-945, 1996.

Nations MK, de Souza MA: *Umbanda* healers as effective AIDS educators: case-control study in Brazilian urban slums (*favelas*). *Tropical Doctor* 27: 1997, Supplement 1, 60-66.

Nichter M: Patterns of curative resort and their significance for health planning in south Asia, *Med Anthropol* 2:29-58, 1978.

Norbeck E, Lock M: *Health, illness and medical care in Japan,* Honolulu, 1987, University of Hawaii Press.

Pagnoni F, Convelbo N, Tiendrebeogo J, et al: A community-based programme to provide prompt and adequate treatment of presumptive malaria in children, *Trans R Soc Trop Med Hyg* 91:512-517, 1997.

Rasoanaivo P, Ratsimamanga-Urverg S, Milijaona R: In vitro and in vivo chloroquine-potentiating action of *Strychnos myrtoides* alkaloids against chloroquine-resistant strains of *Plasmodium* malaria, *Planta Med* 60:13-16, 1994.

Willcox ML: A clinical trial of "AM," a Ugandan herbal remedy for malaria, *J Public Health Med* 21(3):318-324, 1999.

Willcox M, Bodeker G, Rasaoanaivo P, editors: *Traditional medicinal plants and malaria,* London, 2004, CRC Press, Taylor & Francis.

World Bank: *World development report on health,* Washington, DC, 1993, World Bank.

World Health Organization: *Traditional medicine,* Geneva, 1978, WHO Publications.

World Health Organization Global Atlas on Traditional, Complementry and Alternative Meddicine (G Bodeker, C-K Ong, G Burford & C Grundy) (eds), Kobe, Japan, 2004, WHO Center for Health Development.

Zoll AC: *Proceedings of Conference on Indigenous Peoples and Health,* Winnipeg, Canada, April 1993.

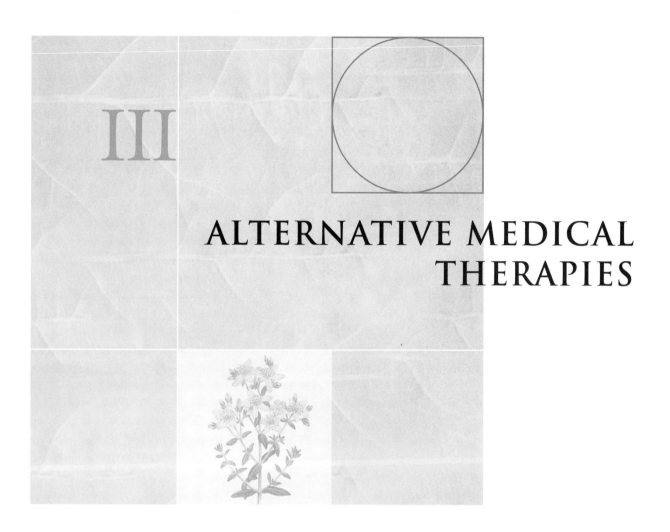

III

ALTERNATIVE MEDICAL THERAPIES

his section describes the background, context, and clinical approaches of select alternative therapeutic systems as these have developed throughout European and American history. Chapters 8 to 14 also describe individual approaches as suggested from contemporary Western research, both within and beyond the biomedical paradigm. Where these systems and approaches can be understood in light of the contemporary biomedical paradigm, this view is examined; where they cannot be understood in these terms, this paradox is acknowledged. When and how medical systems are embedded in the natural environment is clarified, as well as when and how they are embedded in technology. In each case, these medical practices are presented as products of history that make sense in terms of that history. ∽

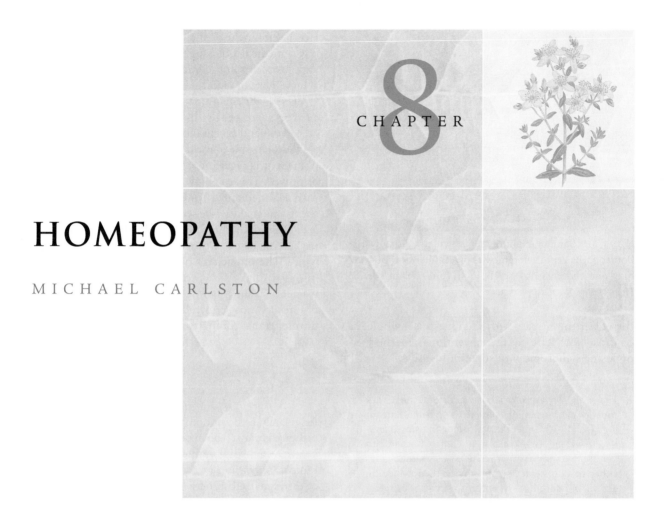

CHAPTER 8

HOMEOPATHY

MICHAEL CARLSTON

Homeopathy is a highly systematized method of healing that utilizes the principle of "use likes to treat likes" practiced by licensed physicians and other health care professionals throughout the world. In the United States, homeopathic medicines are protected by federal law, and most are available over the counter. The greatest challenge that homeopathy may pose to conventional medicine and science is the common use of extremely diluted medicinal substances.

HISTORY

The homeopathic method was developed by Samuel Hahnemann, MD (1755-1843), a German physician, chemist, and author of a well-known textbook on the preparation and use of contemporary medicines (Figure 8-1). In a series of experiments from 1790 to 1810, Hahnemann demonstrated (1) that medicinal substances elicit a standard array of signs and symptoms in healthy people and (2) that the medicine whose symptom-picture most closely resembles the illness being treated is the one most likely to initiate a curative response for that patient (Hahnemann, 1833).

Hahnemann understood these experiments to mean that the outward manifestations of illness represent the concerted attempt of an organism to heal itself and that the corresponding remedy reinforces that attempt in some way. He coined the term *homeopathy* to describe his method of using remedies with

95

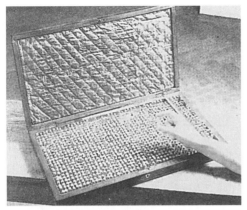

Figure 8-1 Samuel Hahnemann's remedy box. Many homeopaths kept their remedies in a similar box, but few had one that was so splendid. (From Richardson S: *Homeopathy: the illustrated guide.*)

the power to resonate with the illness as a whole, in contrast with the more conventional method of opposing symptoms with superior force.

> The word *homeopathy* is derived from the Greek roots *omoios,* meaning "similar," and *pathos,* meaning "feeling." Hahnemann also began using *allopathy,* from the Greek *alloios,* meaning "other," to denote the standard practice of using medicines either to counteract symptoms or to produce an action unrelated to symptoms, such as purging, bloodletting, or blistering of the skin.

Hippocrates, Celsus, Paracelsus, and others advocated treatment with "similars" for some patients. Hahnemann credited his teacher, Quarin, as the source of his own medical capabilities. Quarin's teacher, Stoereck, advocated testing drugs for their "like" effects: "If stramonium makes the healthy mentally sick through a confusion of the mind, why should one not determine whether it gives mental health in that it disturbs and alters the thoughts and sense in mental disease, and that if it gives health to those with spasms, to try and see if, on the other hand, they get spasms" (Stoerck, 1762).

Hahnemann was the first to base his entire therapeutic approach on the "likes cure likes" methodology. He believed that the detailed correspondence between the clinical symptoms of patients and the experimental pathogenesis of remedies indicated a universal law of healing with medicinal substances.

His development of such a rigorous system integrating a medical philosophy, formalized drug testing, and protocols for clinical application is a unique achievement in medical history.

The Hahnemannian law of similars—*similia similibus curentur,* or "Let likes be cured by likes"—never gained general acceptance in medicine and is considered implausible to most physicians. Even committed homeopaths regard it as a mystery not yet explained or proved. This tolerance of uncertainty is consistent with Hahnemann's commitment to the belief that theory must always be secondary to the patient's clinical benefit. In the founding document of homeopathic medicine, *Organon of Medicine,* Hahnemann wrote: The physician's highest calling, his **only** calling, is to make sick people healthy—to heal as it is termed" (Hahnemann, 1982). He then noted that physicians must remember medical philosophies are unimportant compared with the recovery of the patient.

THEORETICAL BASIS

Essentially a methodology for treating sick patients rather than a set of hypotheses about the nature of health and disease, homeopathy begins and ends as a radical innovation in the experimental investigation of medicinal substances. Its cardinal principles follow logically from the law of similars and the conceptual transformations required to accommodate this law.

Provings

In 1790, while experimenting with cinchona (Peruvian bark), Hahnemann decided to ingest a therapeutic dose because he was frustrated by the conventional explanation of its medicinal action. He soon felt cold, numb, drowsy, thirsty, and anxious and experienced palpitations, prostration, and aching bones. He recognized these symptoms as those of *ague,* or intermittent fever, the syndrome that was then being treated with cinchona (Bradford, 1895). He allowed the dose to wear off before taking a second and a third dose that confirmed his original results.

Hahnemann recognized this response as a confirmation of principles taught in Hippocratic writings and by Paracelsus. Excited by the possibilities of a fuller application of the approach, Hahnemann devoted the rest of his life to ascertaining the therapeutic properties of medicinal substances by administering them to healthy people: himself, his colleagues, and his students. His *Materia Medica Pura* records the detailed symptoms of more than 90 medicines, a monumental achievement that represents 20 years of painstaking labor (Hahnemann, 1833, 1880).

In these *provings,* as he called them, Hahnemann administered the substance in question to a group of reasonably healthy people in doses sufficient to elicit symptoms without provoking irreversible toxicity, anatomical changes, or organic damage. These experiments developed a unique composite portrait, or "symptom picture," for each substance. Therefore a homeopathic remedy is a shorthand sum of the responses of all people who have taken that remedy, a distinctive totality that must be studied as a whole and for its own sake, rather than simply as a weapon against a particular disease or a group of symptoms.

THE HOMEOPATHIC MATERIA MEDICA

The Hahnemannian concept of medicinal action remains the most distinctive contribution of homeopathy to medical science, with implications for pharmacology, ethnobotany, and industrial medicine and toxicology. Without recourse to pathological models or unconsenting animal subjects, provings offer a purely experimental technique for investigating the medicinal action of any substance.

The homeopathic pharmacopeia currently recognizes more than 2000 remedies, with more added all the time. Most are of plant origin, including flowers, leaves, roots, barks, fruits, and resins. Although many are poisonous in their crude state (e.g., aconite, belladonna, digitalis, ergot, hellebore, nux vomica), others are common medicinal herbs (comfrey, eyebright, mullein, yellow dock); foods and spices (cayenne, garlic, mustard, onion); fragrances, resins, and residues (amber, petroleum, charcoal, kreosote); and mushrooms, lichens, and mosses.

Mineral remedies include metals (copper, gold, lead, tin, zinc), metalloids (antimony, arsenic, selenium), salts (calcium sulfate, potassium carbonate, sodium chloride), alkalis, acids (hydrochloric, nitric, phosphoric, sulfuric), elemental substances (carbon, hydrogen, iodine, phosphorus, sulfur), and constituents of the earth's crust (silica, aluminum oxide, ores, rocks, lavas, mineral waters).

Remedies from the animal kingdom include venoms (jellyfish, insects, spiders, molluscs, crustaceans, fish, amphibians, snakes); secretions (ambergris, cuttlefish ink, musk); milks, hormones, and glandular or tissue extracts (sarcodes); entire creatures (*Apis mellifera,* or honeybee; tarentula); and nosodes, or disease products (tuberculosis, gonorrhea, syphilis, abscesses, vaccines).

The investigative method of provings is equally applicable to the study of conventional drugs, unproven folk remedies, toxic or laboratory chemicals, pollutants, and commercial or industrial products (dyes, insecticides, paints, solvents). The homeopathic materia medica is as boundless as the creation of the earth and as inexhaustible as its transformation by human or environmental forces.

Finally, the richness and diversity of the materia medica database increases the likelihood that some degree of medicinal help can be found for most people. At the same time, its basic principles are simple enough that even a novice can achieve some results with a small number of remedies. As long as a few commonsense guidelines are observed, the method is perfectly safe for laypeople of average intelligence to learn at their own pace and to use for first aid and for the treatment of common domestic ailments. Considerable study and experience are required, however, to take full advantage of this enormous tool.

The Vital Force

Like acupuncture, herbalism, and other natural methods, homeopathy belongs to the vitalist tradition in medicine, based on the old *vis medicatrix naturae,* the natural healing capacity, and summarized in the aphorisms of Paracelsus, as follows:

> The art of healing comes from Nature, not the physician. . . . Every illness has its own remedy within itself. . . . A man could not be born alive and healthy were there not already a Physician hidden in him (Jacobi, 1958).

Underlying these approaches is the coherent philosophy of ancient lineage (traced elsewhere in this book), the precepts of which still ring true despite modern efforts to ignore or surpass them (Box 8-1).

BOX 8-1

Precepts of Healing

- Healing is a concerted effort of the entire organism and cannot be achieved by any part in isolation from the whole.
- All healing is essentially self-healing, which is a basic property of all living beings.
- Healing applies only to individuals and therefore is inherently problematic, even risky, and never reducible to any technique or formula, however scientific its foundation.

Within homeopathy, curative remedies imitate and therefore resonate with manifested signs and symptoms. Illness is viewed as the organisms attempt to heal itself. Hahnemann identified the life energy itself (the vital force) as the ultimate source of health and illness alike, ending only with the death of the organism. Whatever we choose to call it, some version of the vital force is required to refer to the bioenergetic integrity of living beings.

The Totality of Symptoms

Just as provings include the full range of symptoms elicited by each remedy, homeopathy teaches that illness is primarily a disturbance of the vital force and manifests itself as a totality of physical, mental, and emotional responses that is unique to each patient and cannot be adequately understood as a mere specimen of any disease process. Hahnemannian totality of symptoms simply describes the principal signs and symptoms as they appear in the patient and is complete as soon as a reasonable sense of the illness as a whole is discernible.

To the practicing homeopath, this composite totality or psychophysical style—much more than any abstract disease category or printout of laboratory abnormalities—furnishes the truest picture of the health and illness of the patient as a whole, as well as of the particular condition for which treatment is being sought.

In practice the totality of the symptoms demands that the remedy selection take into account the living experience of the patient, including the full range of thoughts and feelings. This determination by no means rejects or ignores the technical expertise of the physician and does not hesitate to make use of pathological diagnosis or of conventional drugs or surgery. Homeopathy uses the technical language of abnormalities to educate the patient, allowing the patient to retain control and to participate at every step. The conventional diagnosis also is important in predicting patient response to homeopathic treatment.

The totality of symptoms also explains why mental and emotional symptoms sometimes weigh heavily in choosing the remedy. Whereas most physical symptoms refer to a certain part of the body (e.g., arm, nose, back, stomach), psychological states describe how patients feel as a whole (e.g., afraid, depressed, happy, confused). The totality of symptoms gives special importance to describing the condition of the patient as a whole.

Other aspects of the patient's symptoms are also evaluated by the homeopath. Symptoms that are strange, rare, or peculiar help the homeopath understand that patient's unique response to the illness. Symptoms affecting the person's emotions and mental abilities are more important because they most deeply impact the person's well-being. Similarly, symptoms reflecting more serious disease must be given more attention because a remedy without power to influence these problems cannot be the correct choice for a patient with such a condition.

The Single Remedy

Based on the materia medica, the Hahnemannian method uses one remedy at a time for the whole patient, comparing the totality of symptoms of the individual with those of various remedies until the closest possible match is found. The reason is that the homeopathic material medica has been compiled testing individual substances. Although almost all homeopathic remedies are made from a complex mix of substances (e.g., plants, insects), they have been tested in toto, and the homeopathic material medica establishes that even slight differences (e.g., mineral *calcarea phosphorica* vs. *calcarea corbonica*) produce distinctly different symptom patterns.

The encyclopedic scale of the homeopathic materia medica ensures that it can never be grasped in its entirety. As a result, some have tried to abbreviate and simplify it, and competent and reputable physicians use two, three, or more remedies simultaneously.

Over-the-counter (OTC) combination remedies also are available in many pharmacies and health food stores and are safe and effective if used properly.

Administering different remedies to affect each part of a patient makes it difficult to know which remedy has acted. As such, remedies would have to be selected according to the rough indications of folk medicine or the technical language of abnormalities, much as in conventional drug treatment. Under these conditions, what is learned will not yield an experience that can build on itself or a method that can be taught.

Studying the totality of symptoms enables the serious student to accumulate detailed personal experience with remedies and generates much of the excitement about learning how to use them. The revival of American homeopathy in recent years has been achieved largely on the strength of the single-remedy concept. Only the totality of symptoms can display remedies, and patients are unique individuals worthy of study for their own sake.

The Minimum Dose

Because homeopathic remedies stimulate an ailing self-healing mechanism rather than correcting a specific abnormality, large or prolonged doses are seldom required and might even have harmful effects. Homeopaths use the smallest possible doses and only repeat them if necessary, allowing remedies to complete their action without further interference. The remedy will not work unless it fits the illness so closely as to render the patient uniquely susceptible to its action. The minuteness of the dose makes it unlikely that any untoward or dangerous adverse effects will occur.

Hahnemann's advocacy of infinitesimal doses remains one of the most controversial aspects of his work. No one has explained satisfactorily how medicines diluted beyond the molecular threshold of Avogadro's number could possibly have any effect, let alone a curative one. However, the standard argument that "the remedies are simply placebos" cuts both ways. People do heal themselves of serious illnesses without drugs or surgery. With a variety of basic scientific investigations ongoing and many showing evidence of physical change in homeopathic dilutions, homeopathy envisions a new bioenergetic science that is still in its infancy.

The Laws of Cure

The totality of symptoms also makes clear why drugs that successfully lower the blood pressure, kill bacteria, or correct physiological abnormality may leave the patient feeling as bad or worse than before. Judgments about improvement, worsening, and the effectiveness of treatment are difficult to interpret apart from the totality of symptoms, from how patients feel as a whole, and from how they function according to their own individual standards. Perhaps the greatest shortcoming of the biomedical model is its failure to comprehend patients as integrated energy systems and to follow them throughout their lifetime.

Since the era of Hahnemann, classical homeopathy has addressed this critical issue by attempting to track the order in which symptoms and illnesses appear, the grouping of symptoms that appear and disappear together, and the relation of each group to the overall health and functioning of the patient. Constantine Hering (1865, 1875) proposed four general directions in which symptoms tend to move or redistribute themselves during the recovery process (Box 8-2).

Although the fourth principle has proved most reliable for case management, and the relative importance of organs and tissues often is difficult to assess, some approximation of the totality of symptoms over time remains indispensable to the general assessment of the patient as a whole, for clinician and researcher alike.

These "laws of cure" provide clear standards by which to evaluate the actions of all therapies, including homeopathic medicine. When the intervention is

---

BOX 8-2

Hering's Directions of Symptom Movement in the Cure and Recovery Process

1. From above downward, from the head toward the feet.
2. From inside outward, from interior to peripheral parts.
3. From more vital to less vital organs, from more visceral to less essential structures.
4. From the most recent to the oldest, in the reverse order of their appearance in the life history of the patient.

(Hering, 1865, 1875)

followed by a lasting decline in the patient's condition as defined in this manner, the intervention was an ill choice. This pertains to homeopathy as well as conventional medicine or other healing approaches.

METHODOLOGY

Pharmacy

The Homeopathic Pharmacopoeia of the United States (American Institute of Homeopathy, 1989) is the official standard for the preparation of homeopathic medicines. Crude medicinal substances are made into remedies by serial dilution and succussion in a liquid or solid medium. First crushed and dissolved in a specified volume of 95% grain alcohol, crude plant materials are shaken and stored, and the supernatant liquid is kept as the "mother tincture." The same procedure is used for animal products, nosodes, and any other substances that are soluble in alcohol. Metals, ores, and other insoluble remedies are pulverized with mortar and pestle and diluted with lactose, succussing until they become soluble.

Tinctures are further diluted with alcohol or lactose, either 1:10 (the decimal scale, written "X") or 1:100 (the centesimal, written "C") and succussed vigorously, yielding the 1X or 1C dilution. The process is repeated for the 2X, 3X, 4X (or 2C, 3C, 4C), and on up as desired.

In clinical practice any dilution may be used, but the most popular for self-care are the 6th, 12th, and 30th (X or C). Higher dilutions for professional work are in the centesimal scale, namely, the 200th, 1000th, 10,000th, and 50,000th, written 200C, 1M, 10M, and 50M, and representing dilutions of 10^{-400}, 10^{-2000}, $10^{-20,000}$, and $10^{-100,000}$, respectively.

The general skepticism about diluted remedies, as expressed by Oliver Wendell Holmes and modern critics, is readily understandable because even the 12C and 30C are well beyond the apparent limits imposed by Avogadro's number and therefore out of the realm of conventional chemistry entirely (Holmes, 1842).

CASE TAKING

As in general medicine, seeing patients requires more than simply taking down information or selecting remedies. Allowing patients to tell their story, in its entirety, relieves their burden of pain and suffering, making the homeopathic interview a powerful healing experience in its own right. It even might suggest a path of recovery, allowing remedies to continue the process.

Patients are invited to speak and allowed to continue for as long as possible without interruption, while homeopaths ask, "What else?" as often as necessary to elicit more symptoms and to remind the patient that no one disease is being sought but rather the totality of symptoms. Symptoms are written down verbatim whenever possible, supplemented by the homeopath's own observations about the patient's temperament, behavioral patterns, and personality style.

After the patient finishes his or her story and the principal symptoms have been noted, the homeopath must investigate further to characterize symptoms in detail. Conventional diagnosis is based on common symptoms such as fever, pain, cough, and bleeding, whereas homeopaths look for unusual or idiosyncratic features that tend to be ignored or discarded by conventional physicians (Box 8-3). Medical school faculty who learn about the process of homeopathic interviewing often comment that the careful attention to the patient's descriptions and nonjudgmental respect for the patient's experience would be useful skills for all medical students to learn.

The interview also includes physical examination and laboratory work as needed to establish a diagnosis.

BOX 8-3

Fully Characterized Symptoms Described in a Homeopathic Interview

- Subjective sensations such as pain, vertigo, fatigue, and anger
- Localization of symptoms (one-sided, wandering, radiating, circumscribed, or diffuse)
- Modalities, that is, factors by which symptoms are modified (intensified or relieved) according to changes in the time of day, the weather, diet, or emotional state
- Concomitants, or symptoms that appear simultaneously or in sequence (nausea with headache, fever after chill)

Selecting the Remedy

Remedy selection, homeopathic "diagnosis" in a sense, is the product of the homeopath's understanding of the patient. Homeopathic prescribing is the clinical implementation of the correspondence between the database of the materia medica and the details of each patient's case record.

Because of the mass of information contained in the homeopathic material medica, an encyclopedic memory or a computer with a similar capacity would be required to fully grasp the treatment options for each patient. Even experienced homeopathic specialists must use reference materials.

For professional homeopaths to gain access to as many remedies as possible, they need help in proceeding from the clinical totality to a menu of possible remedies that they can study and choose from. This is the purpose of the *repertory*. Patients complain of problems and symptoms, but homeopathic material medicas are organized by the name of the medicinal substance. The repertory overcomes this problem by indexing the symptoms and the remedies that have either elicited them in provings or cured them clinically. By finding the remedies that match the leading symptoms in a case, the search for a cure can be narrowed, and the homeopathic specialist can study most effectively.

Whether in the form of a book or computer software, the largest, most comprehensive repertories (Archibel, 2004; Kent Homeopathic Associates, 2003; van Zandvoort, 1996) include all types of symptoms from every anatomical region and physiological system, as well as mental and emotional symptoms, "generalities" (physical symptoms or modalities attributable to the patient as a whole), and rare symptoms, the oddity of which may point directly to the remedy. The repertory is only a tool for locating remedies; these remedies must then be studied in the materia medica. The final selection is based on a total or qualitative fit more than on any narrow, technical calculation.

Regimen and Precautions

Although they remain stable in the cold and across a wide range of temperatures, dilute remedies are inactivated by direct sunlight and should be stored in a dark, dry place and shielded from heat and radiation.

Patients are instructed to put nothing in the mouth for at least 30 minutes before and after each dose because competing tastes can interfere with the remedy action. Coffee and camphorated products might reverse the effects of the remedy, so patients should avoid them throughout the treatment period, even when no remedies are actually being taken. The use of medicinal herbs and exposure to mothballs and other aromatic substances also should be curtailed. Homeopaths may differ on how compulsive patients need to be about avoiding possible interferences.

Although conventional drugs often interfere and should be avoided when possible, severely ill patients should not stop taking medications. Because of their potentially synergistic effect, some homeopaths believe that acupuncture and chiropractic should not be started concurrently with homeopathic remedies. Relapse might also follow dental work that includes drilling and local anesthesia.

Administration and Dosage

Remedies are dispensed in the form of tablets or pellets of sucrose or lactose that are taken dry on the tongue or dissolved in water. Lower dilutions are preferred in acute situations because they can be repeated as often as necessary and will be somewhat effective even if only broadly similar to the totality of the case. Higher dilutions are used mainly by professionals for chronic treatment. More care must be taken in the selection of higher dilutions, which and they should not be repeated while their action is in progress.

In homeopathy the term *dosage* refers primarily to the number and frequency of repetitions, which must be tailored to fit the patient, similar to the choice of the remedy. In both acute and chronic cases, the rule is to stop the remedy once the reaction is apparent, repeating only when the reaction has subsided.

Pros and Cons

There are few, if any, absolute contraindications to homeopathic treatment. Although patients with severely disabling illnesses or chronic drug dependence are difficult to help—by any method—homeopathy at least might be considered before resorting to more drastic measures or after conventional methods have failed. Homeopathic remedies are relatively safe, economical, simple to administer, and gentle in their action, with very few serious or prolonged adverse effects. Although subtle at first, the effects of treatment are prompt, thorough, and long lasting. Simple acute illnesses and injuries are easy for even untrained laypeople to treat homeopathically because the amount of information required is minimal.

On the other hand, homeopathy is far from a panacea for all ills. It is a difficult and exacting art. Even after years of study and practice, a skilled prescriber might need to try several remedies before any benefit is obtained. Some patients might show little or no improvement, despite the most conscientious efforts. Remedies are rather delicate and easily inactivated, so certain precautions must be observed. Finally, we do not understand how dilute remedies act, and we cannot predict with absolute certainty how a patient will respond or which symptoms will change and in what order. As with all medicine, homeopathy is an art dependent on the living energy and variability of individual humans.

HISTORICAL DEVELOPMENT

Early Controversies

Although his successful treatment and prophylaxis of a scarlet fever epidemic brought fame to homeopathy widely throughout Europe, Hahnemann was ridiculed and persecuted for his heresies until 1822, when he was awarded a stipend to publish his writings (Bradford, 1895). He fueled the controversy by his unflagging convictions and determination to speak out. Famously, he upset the local medical community when he published a letter in the paper decrying the care other physicians provided to the newly deceased Emperor of Austria, claiming that instead of helping the patient, they hastened his demise.

In addition to his *Organon of Medicine* and *Materia Medica Pura,* he wrote many technical and expository works, maintained a busy correspondence, and continued to practice and conduct experimental research. Hahnemann died secure in the knowledge that his students were practicing homeopathy throughout Europe and America. Fired by ambition and gifted with intellect, Hahnemann left a body of work and a method that have stood the test of time.

HOMEOPATHY IN AMERICA

In the latter half of the nineteenth century, the United States became the center of the homeopathy movement and produced some of its greatest masters, whose works still enjoy international use. Three major factors contributed to the rapid growth and development of American homeopathy.

The first was the absence of laws or bureaucracy to license the practice of medicine, a tolerant attitude born of the hope to break free from the oppressive social and economic constraints of Europe. When the first school of homeopathy opened in Pennsylvania during the 1830s, American physicians were organized on a voluntary basis, and state legislatures were reluctant to prevent uneducated or lay healers from helping anyone who wanted to use their services (Starr, 1982).

The second factor was the great migration of those seeking land and fortune in the west, where doctors were scarce and people were forced to heal themselves and their families. Homeopathy was well suited for self-care, and popular manuals on first aid and the treatment of common domestic ailments began to appear during this period (Hering, 1844).

Third, the concept of the materia medica itself was easily adapted to Native American medicine. Introducing dozens of Native American herbs into the pharmacopeia, American homeopathy was enriched by the botanical lore of midwives, medicine men, eclectics, and other herbalists whose recipes are still in use today (Hale, 1867).

Under these conditions, homeopathy flourished in the United States, inspiring the creation of hospitals, medical schools, and "insane asylums" that scored notable triumphs and attracted public attention (Coulter, 1973). During epidemics of cholera, typhus, and scarlet fever, published accounts indicate that homeopathy proved its superiority over the often toxic conventional treatments then in vogue (Bradford, 1900).

Physicians practicing this new method quickly rose to social prominence, treating such rich and famous patients as members of President Lincoln's cabinet (Coulter, 1973). By the turn of the nineteenth century, 10% of all physicians used homeopathy in their practices (Ullman, 1991).

During and after the Civil War, however, the tremendous expansion of American industry transformed the nature of medicine. American homeopathy—

with its use of minimal doses at rare intervals—never created a large or profitable industrial base capable of financing large educational or research institutions. Experimental medicine, based on rigorous physicochemical causality, generated such unprecedented technical achievements as anesthesia, antisepsis, surgery, microbiology, vaccines, and antibiotics (Bernard, 1957).

The American Medical Association (AMA) and its state societies forbade its members to consult or fraternize with homeopaths (Coulter, 1973). Such persecution had little effect until state legislatures began to license physicians and accredit medical schools, and the pharmaceutical industry won control of the process (Starr, 1982). Thereafter the AMA invited homeopaths and physicians of all schools to become members in exchange for licensing, creating a monopoly against lay healers, midwives, and herbalists. The Flexner Report, published in 1914, proposed a uniform standard of medical education for all physicians and used the power of accreditation to phase out homeopathic colleges that fell short of these standards (Starr, 1982). Philosophical disputes within the homeopathic community precluded unified action to maintain homeopathy's foothold in American medicine (Coulter, 1973).

The AMA strategy succeeded. By the 1920s, the homeopathic schools had closed or conformed to the new model, and homeopathy was reduced to a postgraduate specialty for the few physicians who were prepared to swim against the tide. Although some fine homeopathic physicians continued to practice, the movement declined rapidly over the next 40 years. By 1970, homeopathy appeared to be moribund, its teachers aged or dead (Kaufman, 1971).

American homeopathy has begun to flourish once more, largely because of the rebirth of the self-care movement, the health care crisis, and the technological overemphasis that provoked these events (Illich, 1976; Lown, 1996). By eliminating lay healers and aspiring to control every abnormality by purely technical means, American medicine has become a colossus that thrives on great cost and great risk (Moskowitz, 1988), generating more iatrogenic illness (Steel, 1981) and consuming a greater share of the gross national product than anywhere else in the world. Facing crises in health insurance, malpractice litigation, and the physician-patient relationship (Moskowitz, 1988), the public—and now the medical profession itself—have turned to alternatives such as those described in this text.

Safe, effective, and inexpensive enough to sustain busy practices even without third-party reimbursement, homeopathy has become increasingly popular with young family physicians, whose instant waiting lists approximate the virtually limitless demand for their services. As in frontier days, the renaissance of American homeopathy would not be occurring were it not for the devotion of laypeople—not only for self-care, but also for organizing study groups in their communities and teaching these methods to their friends and neighbors.

RESEARCH

Hahnemann's system of provings—using individuals to determine the symptoms that a medicine could produce—was the first research in homeopathy. Indeed, the whole field is based on this experimental work, which was unprecedented both in method and in scope. Provings are still conducted on many herbal medicines that have been used by traditional healers for centuries, particularly in Asia and in South America. The proving method also is being modernized; statistical methods are used to determine the significance of various symptoms. Some historians of medicine credit Hahnemann with conducting the first Phase I drug trials (Kaptchuk, 1998). Following Hahnemann's scientific bent, homeopaths have been conducting all types of research investigating the method since its inception. The Samueli Institute recently published a very good overview of the field of homeopathic research (Walach et al., 2002).

Basic Science Research

Basic scientific research in homeopathy primarily has investigated the chemical and biological activity of highly diluted substances. As discussed previously, Hahnemann found that if the homeopathic remedies were highly diluted to concentrations as low as 10^{-30} to $10^{-20,000}$, medicinal effect could be preserved while simultaneously minimizing adverse effects. Most scientists reject homeopathic theory because of this extreme dilution of the medicine beyond Avogadro's number of 1×10^{-23}, beyond which point no molecules of the original material should remain.

Although some believe that conventional scientific knowledge already encompass the most unlikely homeopathic principles (Eskinazi, 1999), the general belief is that the purest scientific research is necessary to overcome entrenched intellectual resistance to this theory.

Toxicology

The model most often used for investigating biological effects of homeopathic dilution is toxicological research. Generally these studies have used rats subjected to lethal doses of toxic metals (arsenic, mercury, lead). In a meta-analysis and critical review of published and unpublished work on this topic (Linde et al., 1994), the quality of the studies overall was poor. Although this problem significantly impaired definitive conclusions, interestingly the best studies used post-Avogadran dilutions, and more than 70% of these studies reached findings in support of the homeopathic dilutions.

Immunology

A number of studies on the effects of high dilutions have been conducted in the fields of immunology (Bastide, 1994; Belon, 1987), including one of the most notorious controversies in recent scientific literature. This study of the effects of high dilutions showed degranulation of human basophils by immunoglobulin E (IgE) antibodies diluted as much as 10^{-120} (Davenas et al., 1988). This article was highly criticized not only because it challenged the basic tenets of biomedicine, but also for its handling by the *Nature* editors (Anderson, 1991; Benveniste, 1988; Coles, 1989; When to believe, 1988), who published it conditional upon a subsequent investigation by a team that included a professional magician, but no immunologist (Maddox et al., 1988). The controversy over this study continues, with attempts to repeat the experiment reporting both success and failure (Belon et al., 2004; Benveniste et al., 1991; Hirst et al., 1993).

Miscellaneous Life Sciences

There have been a great number of research studies have used utilizing animal, organ, tissue, plant, and cellular studies to evaluate ing aspects of homeopathic principles published in scientific journals. In fact, this line of inquiry has been followed for nearly 80 years; in 1927, investigators first published a study investigating the effects of a homeopathic dilution on developing tadpoles (Konig, 1927). To explore the foundations of these areas of homeopathic research further, refer to Bellavite and Signorini (1995 and 2002) and Endler and Schulte (1994).

Fundamental Science

The two crucial aspects of homeopathic theory have often been investigated independently of each other. The *similia* principle ("likes cure likes") is often linked to well-established paradoxical effects of nearly all conventional medicines. Systematic study of the *similia* principle has mostly appeared under the guise of "hormesis" (Calabrese and Baldwin, 2001). However, others have extended investigations of this concept as a general physiological principle (van Vijk and Wiegant, 1994).

Investigations searching for evidence of physical changes created by the potentization process have a long and creative history. In the 1960s, researchers first assayed homeopathic dilutions using nuclear magnetic resonance (NMR) imaging (Smith and Boericke, 1966 and 1968). As might be expected when attempting to apply new technology to an unconventional subject, these studies have generally been of very poor quality and demand both cautious interpretation and data of better quality (Aabel et al., 2001; Demangeat and Poitevin, 2001). More recently, as technology advances with finer instruments capable of measuring more subtle phenomena, scientists have begun to apply these tools to study homeopathic principles (Becker-Witt et al., 2003; Bellavite and Signorini, 2002; Berezin, 1994; Lo and Bonavida, 1998; Poitevin and Demangeat, 2000).

Clinical Research

Before the mid-1980s, little clinical research in homeopathy was published outside of homeopathic journals. The first double-blind experiment published in a peer-review medical journal showed statistically significant results in treating rheumatoid arthritis with individualized prescribing of remedies (Gibson et al., 1980). A later study on arthritis, comparing response to a single homeopathic remedy with that to a conventional drug, showed the homeopathic treatment was inferior on almost nearly every outcome measure (Shipley et al., 1983). This study is an excellent example of the difficulties adapting classical homeopathic practice to double-blind, randomized controlled trial (RCT) protocols. Unlike the standard individualized remedy selection and dosing scheme, as well as long-term frame for treatment of chronic conditions, the Shipley study design violated all these essential components and led one of the experimenters later to recant the negative finding, as follows:

> One cannot logically extrapolate from this any conclusions about other potencies of Rhus tox., other homeopathic remedies, or homeopathic medicine in general. The most important lesson that we have learned from this study is that a double-blind crossover trial of short duration using a single potency of a remedy prescribed on local features is unlikely to be a fruitful method of seriously studying homeopathic medicine (Lancet, 1983).

A study of recurrent respiratory illnesses in a pediatric population (de Lange de Klerk et al., 1995) recalls the Shipley study because of the problems interpreting the data. Superficially, the pediatric study found no significant benefits. However, good reasons exist to contest this conclusion. As one of the confounding factors, the "placebo" intervention included all the components (homeopathic interview, dietary and lifestyle advice, clinical management avoiding overuse of medication) typical of homeopathic clinical consultations. Other studies have shown that these interventions appear to be effective in themselves, and the investigators found that both groups improved dramatically. Although the group who received the remedy improved even more, the difference between the groups was not statistically significant. Was the placebo group improvement in this case simply the course of natural history, or was it the effect of the homeopathic approach minus the remedy?

Other notable studies include work on pediatric diarrheal disease (Jacobs et al., 1993, 1994, 2000, 2003), fibrositis (Fisher et al., 1989), hay fever/pollinosis (Ludtke and Wiesenauer, 1997), vertigo (Weiser et al., 1998), otitis media (Jacobs et al., 2001) and the homeopathic standard arnica in surgery, trauma, and physical overexertion (Campbell, 1976; Hart et al., 1997; Ramelet et al., 2000; Stevinson et al., 2003; Tveiten and Bruset, 2003; Tveiten et al., 1991, 1998; Vickers et al., 1998; Wolf et al., 2003).

Ferley's early positive findings for a homeopathic treatment for influenza (Ferley et al., 1989) have received equivocal support best summarized by a recent meta-analysis (Vickers and Smith, 2004).

Probably the most impressive series of trials were conducted by Reilly's group investigating allergic rhinitis and asthma (Reilly et al., 1986, 1994; Taylor et al., 2000). For 15 years this group conducted research in these allergic diseases using homeopathically prepared allergens as an intervention in sensitive patients. They repeatedly achieved positive findings of such a degree that the pooled patient subjective data (visual analog scale) resulted in a p value of 0.0007. This highly impressive finding was tarnished by a failed but admittedly imperfect attempt at replication (Lewith et al., 2002).

Systematic Reviews

In homeopathy, as in all areas of medicine, systematic reviews and meta-analyses have been in vogue as a means of refining our understanding of the research data. Some studies, as discussed earlier, were disease specific. Others were meta-analyses of general research, a few studies specifically looked at study quality, and one review even considered the quality of the meta-analyses (Cucherat et al., 2000; Jonas et al., 2001; Ernst, 2002; Linde and Melchart, 1998; Linde et al., 1997, 1999). Among the conclusions, every review commented on the poor quality of most of the studies. Each found results favoring homeopathy, which became more ambiguous as the quality of the studies improved.

The *British Medical Journal* published the first meta-analysis of homeopathic clinical trials (Kleijnen et al., 1991). The authors' comments still sum up not only homeopathic research but also the intellectual and emotional milieu of the discussion, as follows:

> The amount of published evidence even among the best trials came as a surprise to us. Based on this evidence we would be ready to accept that homeopathy can be efficacious, if only the mechanism of publication were more plausible. . . . The evidence presented in this review would probably be sufficient for establishing homeopathy as a regular treatment for certain indications. There is no reason to believe that the influence of publication bias, data massage, bad methodology, and so on is much less in conventional medicine and the financial interests for regular pharmaceutical companies are many times greater. Are the results of randomized double-blind trials convincing only if there is a plausible explanation? Are review articles of the clinical evidence only convincing if there is a plausible mechanism of action? Or is this a special case because the mechanisms are unknown or implausible?

Global Measures of Homeopathy: Cost-Effectiveness and Outcomes

Another relevant area of research in homeopathy is cost-effectiveness and outcomes. Many believe that outcomes research will prove to be the most important area of homeopathic research (Jacobs et al., 1994; Carlston, 2003). As with many forms of complementary and integrative alternative medicine, homeopathic treatment is directed toward the patient's global well-being, not specific disease features. Therefore, outcomes measures such as overall health status (using widely accepted scales), patient satisfaction, days missed from school or work, and the cost of treatment are most suitable for evaluating homeopathic treatment. Also, patients do not care if their treatment is merely statistically superior to placebo. They only want to get better, and thus many conventional medical researchers argue that measuring patient satisfaction is crucial. As Ian Chalmers, the founder of the Cochrane Collaboration, states, "The patient's opinion is the ultimate outcome measure."

> In France the annual cost to the Social Security System for a homeopathic physician is 15% less than that of a conventional physician, and the price of the average homeopathic medicine is one-third that of standard drugs (CNAM, 1991). Fisher found that expenditures for patients of the London Homeopathic Hospital were significantly reduced compared with matched, conventionally treated patients. The reduction in expensive services documented in other studies also suggests a potential for cost-effectiveness (Jacobs et al, 1998; Swayne, 1992).

HOMEOPATHY TODAY

The use of homeopathy is increasing rapidly throughout the world, particularly in Europe, Latin America, and Asia. In many European countries, homeopathy is the most popular form of alternative and integrative medicine. Other developing countries have turned to homeopathy as the cost of conventional, Western medicine becomes too costly to afford. In both Argentina and Brazil, several thousand physicians use homeopathy, and Mexico has five medical colleges that provide homeopathic training. South Africa has homeopathic medical colleges in several major cities, and the health ministry in Israel recently approved the importation of homeopathic preparations for sale in pharmacies (Kayne, 2003).

The use of homeopathy by the United States has increased tremendously in the last 20 years. A survey showed that 1% of the American population used homeopathy in 1989 (Eisenberg et al., 1993). Sales of homeopathic remedies increased by 1000% during the 1980s (Food and Drug Administration, 1985) and were reported to be $200 million in 1992, climbing at the rate of 25% per year (Swander, 1994). A 1999 survey found that 17% of Americans were using homeopathy for self-care (Roper Starch Worldwide, 1999).

Physician interest parallels patient enthusiasm. In Germany, 25% of all physicians use homeopathy (Ullman, 1991a, 1991b): in France, 32% of general-practice physicians use it (Bouchayer, 1990); and in Great Britain, 42% of physicians refer patients to homeopaths (Wharton and Lewith, 1986). In India, homeopathy is practiced in the national health service, at several hundred homeopathic medical schools, and by more than 100,000 homeopaths (Kishore, 1983). In 1995, about 10% of conventional U.S. medical offered elective instruction about homeopathy (Carlston et al., 1997). By 1998, almost 15% of U.S. medical school required that students study homeopathy (Barzansky et al., 1998).

Because education in complementary, alternative, and integrative medicine (CIM) has expanded dramatically, even more recent numbers for homeopathy would likely be much higher. Recent data show that almost nearly 50% of American schools of osteopathic medicine include homeopathy in the required coursework (Saxon et al., 2004).

Appropriate Use

Homeopathic remedies are most likely to be successful and to optimize overall health for several types of conditions (Box 8-4).

Homeopathy is not appropriate (1) for the treatment of chronic diseases involving advanced tissue damage, such as cirrhosis of the liver or severe cardiovascular disease; (2) for people with prolonged dependence on conventional medication such as corticosteroids, anticonvulsants, and antipsychotics; or (3) as a substitute for appropriate conventional treatments such as emergency surgery or reduction of fractures. Homeopathy is often used by homeopathic specialists as a treatment complementing conventional

BOX 8-4

Uses of Homeopathic Remedies

- Functional complaints with little or no tissue damage, such as headache, insomnia, chronic fatigue, and premenstrual syndrome
- Conditions for which conventional medicine has little to offer, such as viral illnesses, traumatic injuries, surgical wounds, and multiple sclerosis
- Chronic health conditions, such as allergies, recurring infections, arthritis, skin conditions, and digestive problems
- Conditions that have not been cured by conventional treatments because of the inappropriateness of the medication, determined nature of the disease, or noncompliance of the patient

medicine in these circumstance or as a palliative measure when no other effective treatment exists.

PRACTICE PATTERNS

Surveys of American physicians document interesting differences between those using homeopathic medicines in their practices and those using more conventional remedies (Jacobs et al., 1998; Schappert, 1992). Physicians using homeopathy saw fewer patients and spent more than twice as much time with each patient as conventional physicians: averaging 30 minutes per visit versus 12.5 minutes. In addition, homeopathic physicians ordered half as many diagnostic procedures and laboratory tests as conventional physicians and prescribed fewer standard medications.

Asthma, headaches, depression, allergies, psychological problems, and skin problems were among the top 10 conditions treated most frequently by homeopathic physicians (Jacobs et al., 1998). Schappert's contemporaneous survey found that conventional physicians, on the other hand, saw more patients with hypertension, upper respiratory tract infections, diabetes, sore throats, bronchitis, back disorders, and acute sprains and strains. These practice patterns suggest that patients were seeking homeopathic care mostly for chronic conditions not managed adequately by conventional medicine. The low number of acute problems seen by homeopaths may be the result of patients treating these conditions on their own.

CONCLUSION

Homeopathic medicine has persisted both in spite of and because of its dissident voice. Its theories usually contradict conventional medicine, and the intensive clinical interaction between patient and practitioner stands in opposition to the time pressures of managed care. Although its controversial aspects would seem to weaken homeopathic practice severely, in fact this distinction attracts interest, and in many ways this controversy serves to invigorate conventional and homeopathic thought.

References

Aabel S, Fossheim S, Rise F: Nuclear magnetic resonance (NMR) studies of homeopathic solutions, *Br Homeopath J* 90(1):14-20, 2001.

American Institute of Homeopathy: *The homeopathic pharmacopoeia of the United States,* Falls Church, Va, 1989, The Institute.

Anderson C: Robocops: Stewart and Feder's mechanized misconduct search, *Nature* 350(6318):454-455, 1991.

Archibel, Inc: Synthesis/RADAR version 9.0, Namur, Belgium, 2004, Archibel.

Barzansky B, Jonas HS, Etzel, SI: Educational programs in U.S. medical schools, 1997-98, *JAMA* 280(9):803-808, 827-835, 1998.

Bastide M: Immunological examples of UHD research. In Endler PC, Schulte J, editors: *Ultra high dilution: physiology and physics,* Dordrecht, The Netherlands, 1994, Kluwer Academic.

Becker-Witt C, Weisshuhn TE, Ludtke R, Willich SN: Quality assessment of physical research in homeopathy, *J Altern Complement Med* 9(1):113-132, 2003 (review).

Bellavite P, Signorini A: *Homeopathy: a frontier in medical science,* Berkeley, Calif, 1995, North Atlantic Books.

Bellavite P, Signorini A: *The emerging science of homeopathy: complexity, biodynamics and nanopharmacology,* Berkeley, Calif, 2002, North Atlantic Books.

Belon P: Homeopathy and immunology. In *Proceedings of the 42nd Congress of the LMHI,* Arlington, Va, 1987, pp 265-270.

Belon P et al: Histamine dilutions modulate basophil activation, *Inflamm Res* 53(5):181-188, 2004.

Benveniste J, Davenas E, Ducot B, et al: L'agitation de solutions hautement diluees n'induit pas d'activite specifique, *Comptes Rendus Acad Sci Paris* 312(II):461-466, 1991.

Benveniste J: Dr. Jacques Benveniste replies, *Nature* 334(6180): 291, 1988.

Berezin AA: Ultra high dilution effect and isotopic self-organization. In Endler PC, Schulte J, editors: *Ultra high dilution: physiology and physics,* Dordrecht, The Netherlands, 1994, Kluwer Academic, pp 137-169.

Bernard C: *An introduction to the study of experimental medicine,* New York, 1957, Dover, pp 65-67 (Translated by HC Greene).

Bouchayer F: Alternative medicines: a general approach to the French situation, *Complement Med Res* 4:4-8, 1990.

Bradford TL: *The life and letters of Samuel Hahnemann,* Philadelphia, 1895, Boericke and Tafel, pp 37, 124-126.

Bradford TL: *The logic of figures, or comparative results of homeopathic and other treatments,* Philadelphia, 1900, Boericke and Tafel, pp 141-145.

Calabrese EJ, Baldwin LA: U-shaped dose-responses in biology, toxicology, and public health, *Annu Rev Public Health* 22:15-33, 2001.

Campbell A: Two pilot controlled trials of *Arnica montana, Br Homeopath J* 65:154-158, 1976.

Carlston M, Stuart MR, Jonas W: Alternative medicine education in U.S. medical schools and family practice residency programs, *Fam Med* 29:559-562, 1997.

Carlston M, editor: *Classical homeopathy,* Philadelphia, 2003, Churchill Livingstone, pp 97, 143.

Cazin J, Cazin M, Gaborit JL, et al: A study of the effect of decimal and centesimal dilutions of arsenic on the retention and mobilization of arsenic in the rat, *Hum Toxicol* 6:315-320, 1987.

CNAM: Healthcare professionals in private practice in 1990, CNAM Pub No 61, Paris, 1991, Social Security Statistics.

Coles P: Benveniste controversy: INSERM closes the file, *Nature* 340(6230):178, 1989.

Coulter H: *Divided legacy,* Washington, DC 1973, McGrath, pp 140-238, 285-316.

Cucherat M, Haugh MC, Gooch M, Boissel JP: Evidence of clinical efficacy of homeopathy: a meta-analysis of clinical trials, Homeopathic Medicines Research Advisory Group (HMRAG), *Eur J Clin Pharmacol* 56(1):27-33, 2000.

Davenas E, Beauvais F, Amara J: Human basophil degranulation triggered by very dilute antiserum against IgE, *Nature* 333:816-818, 1988.

Davenas E, Poitevan B, Benveniste J: Effect on mouse peritoneal macrophages of orally administered very high dilutions of silica, *Eur J Pharmacol* 135:313-319, 1987.

de Lange de Klerk ESM, Blommers J, Kuik DJ, et al: Effect of homeopathic medicines on daily burden of symptoms in children with recurrent upper respiratory tract infections, *BMJ* 309:1329-1332, 1995.

Demangeat PL, Poitevin P: Nuclear magnetic resonance: let's consolidate the ground before getting excited! *Br Homeopath J* 90:2-4, 2001.

Eisenberg DM, Kessler RC, Foster C, et al: Unconventional medicine in the United States, *N Engl J Med* 328:246-252, 1993.

Endler PC, Schulte J, editors: *Ultra high dilution: physiology and physics,* Dordrecht, The Netherlands, 1994, Kluwer Academic.

Endler PC, Pongratz W, Kastberger G, et al: The effect of highly diluted thyroxine on the climbing activity of frogs, *Vet Hum Toxicol* 36:56-59, 1994.

Ernst E: A systematic review of systematic reviews of homeopathy, *Br J Clin Pharmacol* 54(6):577-582, 2002.

Eskinazi D: Homeopathy re-revisited: is homeopathy compatible with biomedical observations? *Arch Intern Med* 159(17):1981-1987, 1999.

Ferley JP, Smirou D, D'Adhemar D, Balducci F: A controlled evaluation of a homeopathic preparation in the treatment of influenza-like syndromes, *Br J Clin Pharmacol* 27:329-335, 1989.

Fisher P: The influence of the homeopathic remedy Plumbum Metallicum on the excretion kinetics of lead in rats, *Hum Toxicol* 6:321-324, 1987.

Fisher P, Greenwood A, Huskisson EC, et al: Effect of homeopathic treatment on fibrositis (primary fibromyalgia), *BMJ* 299:365-366, 1989.

Food and Drug Administration: Riding the coattails of homeopathy, *Food and Drug Administration Consumer,* 1985, p 31.

Gibson RG, Gibson SL, MacNeill AD, Buchanan WW: Homoeopathic therapy in rheumatoid arthritis: evaluation by double-blind clinical therapeutic trial, *Br J Clin Pharmacol* 9:453-459, 1980.

Hahnemann S: *Organon of medicine,* ed 5, Calcutta, 1833, Roy, pp 45, 53-70, 269-270 (Translated by W Boericke and E Dudgeon).

Hahnemann S: *Materia medica pura,* Liverpool, 1880, Hahnemann Publishing Society (Translated by E Dudgeon).

Hahnemann S: *Organon of medicine,* Los Angeles, 1982, Tarcher.

Hale EM: *Homeopathic materia medica of the new remedies,* Detroit, 1867, Lodge.

Hart O, Mullee MA, Lewith G, Miller J: Double-blind, placebo-controlled, randomized clinical trial of homoeopathic arnica C30 for pain and infection after total abdominal hysterectomy, *J R Soc Med* 90(2):73-78, 1997.

Hering C: *The homeopathist or domestic physician,* New Delhi, 1984, India Jain Publishing.

Hering C: Hahnemann's three rules concerning the rank of symptoms, *Hahnemannian Monthly* 1:5-12 1865.

Hering C: *Analytical therapeutics,* Philadelphia, 1875, Boericke and Tafel, p 24.

Hirst SJ et al: Human basophil degranulation is not triggered by very dilute antiserum against human IgE, *Nature* 366(6455):525-527, 1993.

Holmes OW Sr: *Homeopathy and its kindred delusions,* Boston, 1842, Ticknor.

Homoeopathy, *Lancet* 1(8322):482, 1983.

Illich I: *Medical nemesis,* New York, 1976, Pantheon.

Jacobi J, editor: *Paracelsus: selected writings,* New York, 1958, Pantheon, pp 50, 76 (Translated by N Guterman).

Jacobs J: Future directions in homeopathic research, *J Am Inst Homeopath* 87:155-159, 1994.

Jacobs J, Chapman EH, Crothers D: Patient characteristics and practice patterns of physicians using homeopathy, *Arch Fam Med* 7(6):537-540, 1998.

Jacobs J, Springer DA, Crothers D: Homeopathic treatment of acute otitis media in children: a preliminary randomized placebo-controlled trial, *Pediatr Infect Dis J* 20(2):177-183, 2001.

Jacobs J, Jonas W, Jiménez-Pérez M, Crothers D: Homeopathy for childhood diarrhea: combined results and metaanalysis from three randomized, controlled clinical trials, *Pediatr Infect Dis J* 22:229-234, 2003.

Jacobs J, Jiménez LM, Gloyd SS, et al: Treatment of acute childhood diarrhea with homeopathic medicine: a randomized clinical trial in Nicaragua, *Pediatrics* 93:719-725, 1994.

Jacobs J et al: Homeopathic treatment of acute childhood diarrhea, *Br Homeopath J* 82(5):83-86, 1993.

Jacobs J et al: Homeopathic treatment of acute childhood diarrhea: results from a clinical trial in Nepal, *J Altern Complement Med* 6(2):131-139, 2000.

Jonas WB, Anderson RL, Crawford CC, Lyons JS: A systematic review of the quality of homeopathic clinical trials, *BMC Complement Altern Med* 1(1):12, 2001 (Epub).

Kaptchuk TJ: Intentional ignorance: a history of blind assessment and placebo controls in medicine, *Bull Hist Med* 72(3):389-433, 1998.

Kayne S. In Carlston M, editor: *Classical homeopathy,* Philadelphia, Churchill Livingstone, 2003, pp 49-52, 58-60.

Kaufman M: *Homeopathy in America: the rise and fall of a medical heresy,* Baltimore, 1971, Johns Hopkins University Press.

Kent Homeopathic Associates: *MacRepertory,* San Anselmo, Calif, 2003, Kent.

Kishore J: Homeopathy: the Indian experience, *World Health Forum* 4:105-107, 1983.

Kleijnen J, Knipschild P, ter Riet G: Clinical trials of homeopath, *BMJ* 302:316-323, 1991.

Konig K: On the effect of extremely diluted ("homeopathic") metal salt solutions on the development and growth of tadpoles, *Z Gesamte Exp Med* 56:581-593, 1927.

Lewith GT et al: Use of ultramolecular potencies of allergen to treat asthmatic people allergic to house dust mite: double blind randomised controlled clinical trial, *BMJ* 324(7336):520, 2002.

Linde K, Melchart D: Randomized controlled trials of individualized homeopathy: a state-of-the-art review, *J Altern Complement Med* 4(4):371-388, 1998.

Linde K et al: Critical review and meta-analysis of serial agitated dilutions in experimental toxicology, *Hum Exp Toxicol* 13:481-492, 1994.

Linde K, Clausius N, Ramirez G, et al: Are the clinical effects of homeopathy placebo effects? A meta-analysis of placebo-controlled trials, *Lancet* 350(9081):834-843, 1997.

Linde K, Scholz M, Ramirez G, et al: Impact of study quality on outcome in placebo-controlled trials of homeopathy, *J Clin Epidemiol* 52(7):631-666, 1999.

Lo SY, Bonavida B, editors: *Physical, chemical and biological properties of stable water (IE) clusters,* Singapore, 1998, World Scientific Publications.

Lown B: *The lost art of healing,* Boston, 1996, Houghton Mifflin.

Ludtke R, Wiesenauer M: [A meta-analysis of homeopathic treatment of pollinosis with Galphimia glauca], *Wien Med Wochenschr* 147(14):323-327, 1997.

Maddox J, Randi J, Stewart J: "High-dilution" experiments a delusion, *Lancet* 334:287-290, 1988.

Moskowitz R: Some thoughts on the malpractice crisis, *Br Homeopath J* 77:17, 1988.

Poitevin B, Davenas E, Benveniste J: In vitro immunological degranulation of human basophils is modulated by lung histamine and apis mellifica, *Br J Clin Pharmacol* 25:439-444, 1988.

Poitevin B, Demangeat JL: Effects of potentization, *Br Homeopath J* 89:155-156, 2000.

Ramelet AA, Buchheim G, Lorenz P, Imfeld M: Homeopathic *Arnica* in postoperative haematomas: a double-blind study, *Dermatology* 201(4):347-348, 2000.

Reilly DT, Taylor MA, McSharry C, Aitchison T: Is homoeopathy a placebo response? Controlled trial of homoeopathic potency, with pollen in hayfever as model, *Lancet* ii:881-885, 1986.

Reilly DT, Taylor MA, Beattie NGM, et al: Is evidence of homeopathy reproducible? *Lancet* 344:1601-1606, 1994.

Roper Starch Worldwide: The growing self-care movement, Washington, DC, 1999, Food Marketing Institute.

Saxon DW, Tunnicliff G, Brokaw JJ, Raess BU: Status of complementary and alternative medicine in the osteopathic medical school curriculum, *J Am Osteopath Assoc* 104(3):121-126, 2004.

Schappert SM: National Ambulatory Medical Care Survey: 1990 summary. Advance data from *Vital and Health Statistics,* No 213, Hyattsville, Md, 1992, National Center for Health Statistics.

Shipley M, Berry H, Broster G, et al: Controlled trial of homeopathic treatment of osteoarthritis, *Lancet* i:97-98, 1983.

Smith RB, Boericke GW: Modern instrumentation for the evaluation of homeopathic drug structure, *J Am Inst Homeopath* 59:263-280, 1966.

Smith RB, Boericke GW: Changes caused by succussion on NMR patterns and bioassays of BKTA succussions and dilutions, *J Am Inst Homeopath* 61:197-212, 1968.

Starr P: *The social transformation of American medicine,* New York, 1982, Basic Books, pp 30-59, 99-123.

Steel K: Iatrogenic illness on a general medical service at a university hospital, *N Engl J Med* 304:638, 1981.

Stephenson J: A review of investigations in the action of substances in dilutions greater than 1×10^{-24} (microdilutions), *J Am Inst Homeopath* 48:327-335, 1955.

Stevinson C, Devaraj VS, Fountain-Barber A, et al: Homeopathic arnica for prevention of pain and bruising: randomized placebo-controlled trial in hand surgery, *J R Soc Med* 96(2):60-65, 2003.

Stoerck: Libellus quo demonstratur stramonium, hyoscyamus, aconitum..., Vindebonnae, 1762, p 19 (Translated by Boyd).

Swander H: Homeopathy: medical enigma attracts renewed attention, *Am Acad Fam Pract Rep* XXI(6):1-2, 1994.

Swayne J: The cost and effectiveness of homeopathy, *Br Homeopath J* 81:148-150, 1992.

Taylor MA et al: Randomised controlled trial of homeopathy versus placebo in perennial allergic rhinitis with overview of four trial series, *BMJ* 321:471-476, 2000.

Tveiten D, Bruset S: Effect of *Arnica* D30 in marathon runners: pooled results from two double-blind placebo controlled studies, *Homeopathy* 92(4):187-189, 2003.

Tveiten D, Bruseth S, Borchgrevink CF, Lohne K: [Effect of *Arnica* D30 during hard physical exertion: a double-blind randomized trial during the Oslo Marathon 1990], *Tidsskr Nor Laegeforen* 111(30):3630-3631, 1991.

Tveiten D, Bruseth S, Borchgrevink CF, Norseth J: Effects of the homeopathic remedy *Arnica* D30 on marathon runners: a randomized double-blind study during the 1995 Oslo Marathon, *Complement Ther Med* 6:71-74, 1998.

Ullman D: *Discovering homeopathy,* Berkeley, Calif, 1991, North Atlantic Books.

Ullman D: The international homeopathic renaissance, *Berl J Homeopath* 1(2):118-120, 1991.

Van Wijk R, Wiegant FA: *Cultured mammalian cells in homeopathy research: the similia principle in self-recovery,* Utrecht, The Netherlands, 1994, Utrecht University Press.

Van Zandvoort R, editor: *The complete repertory,* Leidschendam, The Netherlands, 1996, Institute for Research in Homeopathic Information and Symptomatology.

Vickers AJ, Fisher P, Smith C, et al: Homeopathic *Arnica* 30x is ineffective for muscle soreness after long-distance running: a randomized, double-blind, placebo-controlled trial, *Clin J Pain* 14(3):227-231, 1998.

Vickers AJ, Smith C: Homoeopathic Oscillococcinum for preventing and treating influenza and influenza-like syndromes, *Cochrane Database Syst Rev* (1):CD001957, 2004.

Walach H, Schneider R, Chez R: *Proceedings: Future directions and current issues of research in homeopathy,* Corona del Mar, Calif, 2002, Samueli Institute for Information Biology.

Weiser M, Strosser W, Klein P: Homeopathic vs conventional treatment of vertigo: a randomized double-blind controlled clinical study, *Arch Otolaryngol Head Neck Surg* 124(8):879-885, 1998.

Wharton R, Lewith G: Complementary medicine and the general practitioner, *BMJ* 292:1498-1500, 1986.

When to believe the unbelievable, *Nature* 333:787, 1988.

Wolf M, Tamaschke C, Mayer W, Heger M: [Efficacy of *Arnica* in varicose vein surgery: results of a randomized, double-blind, placebo-controlled pilot study], *Forsch Komplementarmed Klass Naturheilkd* 10(5):242-247, 2003.

Suggested Readings

Carlston M, editor: *Classical homeopathy,* Philadelphia, 2003, Churchill Livingstone.

Clarke JH: *Dictionary of practical materia medica,* Rustington, UK, 1962, Health Science Press.

Hering C: *Guiding symptoms,* Philadelphia, 1891, Hering Estate.

Resch G, Gutmann V: *Scientific foundations of homeopathy,* Germany, 1987, Barthel & Barthel.

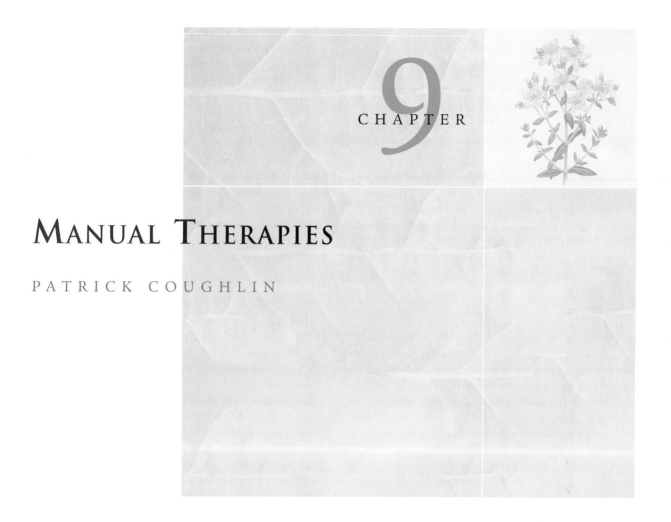

CHAPTER 9

MANUAL THERAPIES

PATRICK COUGHLIN

Manipulation as a therapeutic practice has existed for thousands of years. Although the date of origin of the earliest forms of manipulative therapy is unknown, it has been recorded that Hippocrates was skilled in the use of manipulation and taught it in his school of medicine, more than 2000 years ago. In China the history of manual therapy (tui na) predates the development of the technology necessary to produce the needles used for acupuncture, 3000 to 5000 years ago. Actually, all the world's cultures can demonstrate the use of manipulation as a form of therapy. However, much of this information has been passed on as an oral rather than a written tradition, so documentation is difficult or impossible to obtain in many cases. Consequently,

the styles of manipulation presented here are those for which information is readily available. In addition, this chapter discusses the basic principles and theories of manipulative practice.

As with other complementary or integrative therapies, manipulation espouses a holistic philosophy that has the following outstanding tenets:

1. The body is a unit.
2. Structure and function are interrelated.
3. The body has an inherent ability to heal itself.
4. When normal adaptability is disrupted, disease may ensue.

Based on these defining principles, manipulation seeks to correct structural imbalances in order to optimize the body's ability to self-correct or repair itself, which includes the defense against invasion from foreign substances or organisms.

CONCEPTS APPLICABLE TO ALL MANIPULATION PRACTICES

A number of concepts based on physical laws and anatomical principles universally apply to manipulative practices. These concepts are briefly described here so that they can be associated with the various forms (styles) of manipulative therapy, providing the reader with a greater understanding of the reasons for applying or seeking this type of treatment.

Concept 1: Bilateral Symmetry

The musculoskeletal system is usually described as being bilaterally symmetrical. That is, if the body is divided in half by a slice made from top to bottom and front to back along the midline (midsagittal), the right side should be a mirror image of the left side. This is an idealized assumption, of course, because few if any human bodies are really symmetrical. Certain behaviors that we engage in, both consciously and unconsciously, are specifically designed to compensate for a lack of bilateral symmetry.

Concept 2: Gravity

The human organism is similar to all other organisms in that we are subject to the laws of physics. As such, the way we interact with planet earth is governed by the pull of the earth on our bodies: the force of gravity. Because of this constant force and because our bodies have mass, we are given the weight that we must carry as we go about our activities.

Concept 3: Tensegrity

Tensegrity was developed as a concept in the late 1940s by the renowned architect Buckminster Fuller and the sculptor Kenneth Snelson. The basic premise of *tensegrity* ("tensional integrity") is that in many systems a balance exists between compression and ten-

sion. Tensegrity is "an architectural system in which structures stabilize themselves by balancing the counteracting forces of compression and tension which gives shape and strength to both natural and artificial forms." (http://www.bfi.org/tensegrity.htm, 2004). Architectural systems such as suspension bridges employ this concept, but it also is seen in biological systems, including the musculoskeletal system. The muscles and other soft tissues (e.g., joint capsules, tendons, ligaments) act as tensional elements while the bones resist the compression of weight bearing. By maximizing the ratio of tensional elements to compression elements, such a system enables the organism to maintain balance and move with a minimum amount of energy expenditure.

Concept 4: Postural Maintenance and Coordinated Movement

As we evolved from a quadrupedal (four-legged) to a bipedal (two-legged) stance, we became able to "manipulate" our environment by freeing up our hands, but we also became more unstable (visualize the result of removing two legs of a four-legged table). From an architectural point of view, we became a buttressed arch system (the feet, legs, and pelvic girdle) supporting an elongated tower (the spine and head), with two cantilevered upper appendages (the arms) that can assist with balance. However, we are designed for movement (being necessary for survival) and are rarely stationary, even when seated. Consider the act of walking, when for about 40% of the time allotted to the normal gait cycle (the period of two strides), we are moving with only one foot on the ground. Because we engage in considerable movement, we are constantly adapting to our position relative to the earth, which exerts its gravitational pull. As such, we have programmed into our neuromusculoskeletal system a device that lets us know what that position is at all times, as well as directing the constant physical adjustments that we make. This is commonly referred to as the "equilibrial triad," which consists of the proprioceptive system, vestibular system, and visual system.

The *proprioceptive* system gives us positional information based on the state of contraction of each muscle in the body, as well as the position of each joint. The *vestibular* system is our "gyroscope," which gives us information on the position of the head and how it and the rest of the body are rotating or accelerating in space. The *visual* system allows us to be well aware of our surroundings and position because we can see where we are. In fact, since the visual system is so important in our normal range of activity, the other two parts of the triad act to support it. The proprioceptive and vestibular systems sense the position of the head relative to the body and adjust the posture so that the head is situated with the eyes aligned parallel to the horizon. Together, these three systems act with the motor system to produce coordinated movement, balanced posture, and a properly aligned head.

Concept 5: Connective Tissue (Fascia)

Connective tissue can be highly organized, as in the case of joint capsules, ligaments, tendons, the meninges of the central nervous system (CNS), intervertebral discs, and articular cartilage, or it can be more diffuse and seemingly less organized. *Fascia* is another name for the connective tissue that surrounds and gives architectural form to the tissues and organs of the body.

Fascia can be divided into two major components: superficial fascia and deep fascia. The *superficial* fascia resides just under the skin (the hypodermis) and serves as a staging center for the immune system (large quantities of antigens from the skin are presented to immune cells in this layer) and as a fat storage depot (the cause of significant attention). The *deep* fascia is much more extensive than the superficial fascia and exists throughout the body, serving to "connect" virtually all the tissues and organs. Skeletal muscles are surrounded by capsules of deep fascia, as are nerves and blood vessels (e.g., neurovascular bundles are wrapped in deep fascia). In this sense the deep fascia forms compartments that separate these tissues, but it also forms a structural continuum, where, if physical stress is applied to one area of fascia, this continuity will result in effects being "felt" in other areas or fascial layers as well. The compartmentalization of tissues by the deep fascia also results in specific pathways for, and limits to, the spread of infection (i.e., along fascial planes), as well as for the accumulation of fluid. Both superficial fascia and deep fascia are richly supplied by blood and lymphatic vessels and by nerves (especially pain fibers) (Figure 9-1).

On the molecular level, fascia is composed of a fibrous component (primarily the macromolecular proteins collagen and elastin) and a soluble, gel-like

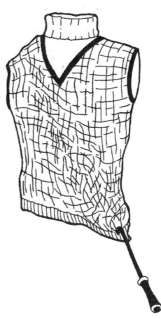

Figure 9-1 A force applied to one part of the fascial continuum affects the entire system.

component, mostly water. The combination of fibrous and soluble components of the fascia creates, in effect, a molecular sieve through which chemical compounds diffuse to and from the cells of the body. Therefore the fascia has a great impact on the function of the organs it surrounds and infiltrates. Cells also reside in the fascia, including the fat and immune cells in the superficial fascia. *Fibroblasts,* a major population of connective tissue cells, are responsible for the secretion of fibrous proteins that make up the scaffold of the fascia. Immune cells constantly patrol the fascia, seeking out foreign antigens as well as ingesting and destroying extracellular debris, including used constituents of the fibrous matrix. This creates a significant turnover in the components of the fascia and contributes to its innate adaptability to changing body conditions. The cellular component of the fascia can be significantly altered by a state of inflammation, where large numbers of immune cells migrate into the area in response to tissue damage or antigenic challenge. Inflammation also stimulates fibroblasts to secrete larger amounts of collagen to reseal any breaches in the continuum, which results in scar formation or fibrosis.

Not only is the fascia very adaptable to the ever-changing internal environment, but it is also significantly affected by the aging process. As the human body ages, the chemical bonds that bind collagen molecules together, known as *cross-links,* become more prevalent. As this occurs, less space is available in the fascia for water and the other soluble components. The end result is a loss of tissue water and an increase in the fibrous component, which in turn decreases the relative elasticity and physical adaptability of the tissue. In other words, the tissues dry up and become more brittle. This leaves the musculoskeletal system in particular significantly more susceptible to microtrauma and macrotrauma.

The physical properties of fascia have stimulated manual therapy practitioners to devise specific techniques to address these properties and the relationship between the fascia and the tissue it surrounds. Just as the fascial matrix can become distorted from the forces brought to bear on it, it also can be restored to its original structural relationships by manual means. In addition, because of the continuity of the fascia throughout the body, local fascial distortions can produce distant effects. This is especially true in the case of muscle-associated deep fascia, which, if distorted, can alter the vector and function of that muscle.

The gel-like consistency of the soluble component of the fascia enables it to behave as a colloid, which resists force in direct proportion to its velocity. Conversely, due to this property, fascia, like a colloid, will respond much more readily if force is applied slowly and gently. In addition, gentle application of force results in gradual yet sustained realignment of the fibrous component of the fascia, which can be palpated in the form of a "release." This is the rationale behind the development of myofascial, craniosacral, and other low-velocity techniques.

Concept 6: Segmentation (Functional Spinal Unit)

Anatomically, the human body is arranged lengthwise as a series of building blocks or segments. This can be observed most directly by the looking at the individual vertebrae that make up the spinal column, which extends from the base of the skull to the coccyx ("tailbone"). Just above the coccyx is the sacrum, a single bone resulting from the fusion of five vertebrae. This fusion is significant because the sacrum articulates with the pelvic bones, which in turn articulate with the femurs. This relationship produces an arch that has the sacrum as its keystone.

Passing between the vertebrae and going from the spinal cord to the periphery are 31 pairs of spinal nerves (one for each side, with the exception of the coccygeal nerve, which is fused at the midline of the body). Each of these spinal nerves contains sensory and motor nerve fibers that are distributed around the body (Figure 9-2).

Most nerves are accompanied by arteries that supply blood to the same region supplied by the spinal nerve. In addition, the *neurovascular bundle* contains veins and lymphatic vessels, which serve to drain away waste products from the same territory. Thus, each segment of the body receives information (and is sending information back to the CNS) as well as nourishment, and each is being drained of waste products. It might appear that each segment functions as a separate entity, but this is not the case. Because of significant overlap both inside and outside the CNS, each segment is "aware" of what is transpiring in the segments adjacent to it.

The individual spinal nerve and all the tissues that it innervates, called the *segment* or the *spinal segment,* is also referred to as the *functional spinal unit* (FSU). The FSU thus includes two adjacent vertebrae and the spinal nerves, skeletal muscles, and fascia between them; other bones, muscles, and fascia associated with the segment (e.g., ribs, intercostal muscles); the blood and lymphatic vessels that supply these tissues; and visceral structures within the body cavities that receive innervation from the autonomic portion of the spinal nerves.

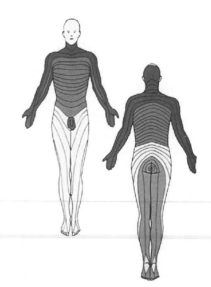

Figure 9-2 Spinal nerves and dermatomes.

Concept 7: Reflexes and Autonomic Nervous System

The CNS, consisting of the brain and spinal cord, can be compared to a computer in that it is designed to integrate and process information. This information basically takes two forms: sensory (input) and motor (output). The most fundamental unit of information processing is the *reflex*. Information enters the CNS through a sensory neuron and is processed in the spinal cord or brain stem through an interaction between the sensory neuron and the motor neuron, known as a *synapse*. Motor information then leaves the CNS directly through a motor neuron to effect a response in a skeletal muscle. The most common example of this type of reflex (called *somatic* for the type of tissue involved) is the withdrawal response when a painful stimulus is encountered (e.g., hand on a hot burner). The painful information is relayed through the spinal cord and out to the muscles that affect the removal before the sensation reaches the cerebral cortex and is perceived.

Although much of the sensory information coming into the CNS reaches consciousness (is perceived), much does not, and we go about our business neither knowing nor feeling what is happening. The same is true of motor activity, which can be voluntary or involuntary (see ANS below). An example of this involuntary phenomenon is the digestive system, which, under normal circumstances, functions without our knowledge (with an important daily exception). With respect to postural maintenance, if we are asked to attend to our position, we are usually able to do so (a test of this system [conscious proprioception] is to ask the subject to close the eyes and state the location and position of different parts, such as the hands and feet). However, we usually are not particularly attentive to our position (unless we lose our balance), and there is an entire division of the proprioceptive system (unconscious proprioception) that is never perceived. In short, we are constantly adjusting ourselves to adapt to the gravitational pull of the earth and our position relative to it, and most of this activity takes place at the level of the reflex.

The autonomic nervous system (ANS) is responsible for the unconscious control of visceral structures. These structures include smooth muscle (e.g., surrounding blood vessels and the bronchial tubes), cardiac (heart) muscle, glands, and lymphoid (immune) tissue. There are two divisions that act opposite one another: the *sympathetic* (thoracolumbar) division, responsible for arousal, or the "fight or flight" reaction, and the *parasympathetic* (craniosacral) division, responsible (among other functions) for stimulating the activity of the digestive system, or the "rest and digest" function. Although each division predominates in certain situations, the two divisions normally coexist in balance with one another to maintain a state of homeostasis, which is a form of internal equilibrium. The names "thoracolumbar" and craniosacral" indicate the origin of the motor nerves of each division. Therefore the spinal nerves of the thoracolumbar region contain both somatic and sympathetic nerve fibers, whereas some of the cranial nerves and sacral nerves contain both somatic and parasympathetic nerve fibers.

Within the CNS, interactions between sensory and motor nerves are constantly taking place through reflexes. Although it has been long known that somatic and visceral reflexes occur, it has only recently been discovered that the two types of reflex loops overlap with one another. That is, stimulation of a visceral structure can produce a somatic response, and stimulation of a somatic structure can elicit a visceral response. This discovery is of extreme importance to the practitioners of manipulation, because it essentially validates the claim that manipulation has global effects on the body, especially with the maintenance or reestablishment of proper blood and lymphatic flow. In fact, it is quite arguable that manipulation of somatic structures (the musculoskeletal system) is entirely capable of restoring proper blood flow to visceral structures through reflexes mediated through the CNS.

Concept 8: Pain and Guarding, Muscle Spasm, and Facilitation

> Patient: "Doc, it hurts when I do this."
> Doctor: "Then don't do that!"

Pain is the result of a noxious stimulus that produces tissue damage. This stimulus can come from outside the body, such as a thermal or chemical burn, which is perceived at the skin, producing a classic withdrawal response. The stimulus can also come from inside the body, such as a sprained ankle, where the damage is perceived at a muscle, joint, or ligament.

If pain results from damage to a bone, joint, or ligament, a natural response is for the surrounding muscles to contract reflexively, producing a natural splint of the area. This is also known as *guarding*. Another result of this type of damage is an altered gait pattern (a limp), which is merely an attempt to "get off" the affected joint, if weight bearing causes additional pain. This can also happen when a paravertebral muscle is overstretched from a bending or lifting maneuver. Proprioceptors in that muscle would report the stretch, causing a reflex contraction of that muscle. If the amount of damage is sufficient, the reflex contraction becomes stronger, and other muscles in the area are recruited to "guard" against further stretching and damage. The involved muscles are now considered to be in *spasm*. This reaction can spread (through reflex spread within the CNS) until much of the back musculature is involved. This is what happens when the back "goes out" and the person suffers back spasms. Because of the altered position of the body away from the norm and the prolonged spastic contraction, the involved muscles are required to do much more work than normal, which results in fatigue. When this occurs, muscle contraction results in the compression of local blood vessels, which in turn affects the nutrition of local tissue, thereby exacerbating the problem by causing more pain. A downward spiral of pain → spasm → more pain → spasm can result.

Over time, as more and more sensory input is being fed to the CNS, the nerves that are reporting this information, as well as the nerves that are reacting (the motor neurons), become more sensitive. That is, their threshold for activity becomes significantly reduced. This situation is known as *facilitation* and is responsible to a large extent for the downward spiral just mentioned.

Presumably, muscle spasm lasts until the injury is healed and the surrounding muscles are allowed to release their grip on the area. This is why most allopathic physicians prescribe bed rest for back pain (and tell patients, "Don't do that"). Sooner or later the spasm will resolve on its own. However, this is not always the case, and the spasm can persist on a reduced level. This can cause the vertebrae normally moved by that muscle to become fixed in a certain position. The vertebrae may remain in that fixed position even when the muscle spasm is completely resolved. This also creates a need for a compensatory

reaction or altered behavior to avoid the generation of more pain, as with a limp (see following discussion). In many patients it is possible to break the cycle of pain → spasm → more pain by the application of manipulative therapy.

Concept 9: Compensation and Decompensation

As mentioned, the proprioceptive system is constantly reporting sensory information to the CNS regarding body position so that postural adjustments can be made, primarily to maintain the eyes parallel to the horizon (horizontal gaze). However, such compensatory behavior becomes more prolonged in certain situations. For example, in a person with one leg longer than the other (asymmetry), the pelvis on the "longer" side would be elevated relative to the other side. Since the sacrum is strongly connected to the pelvic bones, the base on which the fifth lumbar vertebra (L5) rests would be tilted toward the short side. This information would be reported by the proprioceptive system, and the FSU above the L4-5 level would begin a compensatory reaction (through muscular contraction) to move the spine back into vertical alignment, creating a scoliotic curve. These compensatory reactions can occur all the way up the spine, as long as the result is a level head. This creates an overall increased load on the system as a whole and significantly increases the amount of work needed to maintain proper alignment.

In most cases, these responses work well, and no pain or damage is produced. This is especially true in younger people. As persons age, however, changes in body tissues, most notably loss of water and reduced elasticity, alter the mechanical properties of the body as a whole. Eventually the system fails and begins to decompensate. This results in an increase in the amount and number of compensatory reactions as the system becomes further decompensated, eventually leading to tissue damage (usually on the microscopic level), which ultimately leads to pain, which may be chronic. This scenario explains in part the preponderance of complaints of low back and neck pain in the general population. In fact, musculoskeletal complaints cause about one third of all the office visits to physicians in the United States. On a holistic or preventive level, intervention to correct a musculoskeletal problem or dysfunction before it becomes chronic or debilitating would be sensible and cost-effective in the long run. This is where manipulative therapy is indicated and most effective.

Concept 10: Range of Motion and Barrier Concept

Each joint of the body has a normal direction and amount of motion associated with it. This is referred to as *range of motion* (ROM). When motion is outside of this normal range (a statistical norm that can very considerably), that joint is said to be "hypermobile" or "hypomobile." In addition, joints with a greater ROM are generally less stable than those with less ROM (e.g., hip and shoulder joints). In the spine the lumbar and cervical areas have the greatest ROM, which establishes an increased probability of instability and injury, especially in the lumbar spine, where significantly greater weight is being borne. This is the principal reason for the relative frequency of lumbar and cervical problems in the general population.

Typically, if there is pain around a joint for any reason, ROM will be decreased or limited. In this case, motion is said to be "restricted." The restriction of motion in a particular direction or plane of space produces a "barrier" to normal motion. However, motion barriers may not necessarily be accompanied by or be the result of pain. In fact, barriers exist to motion under normal circumstances as "anatomical" barriers or "physiological" barriers. A good example of an anatomical barrier is the elbow joint, where the olecranon process of the ulna locks into the olecranon fossa of the humerus, thus preventing overextension of the joint. Therefore the bones themselves present a motion barrier. Joint capsules and ligaments also create anatomical barriers. Physiological barriers are produced by the normal tone of the muscles around a joint, which also act in balance with one another, so that no individual muscle becomes too taut or stretched, producing damage. The proprioceptive system plays an important role in maintaining physiological barriers. If a guarding reaction is present, or if a muscle is in spasm, a temporary physiological motion barrier can be established, in this case referred to as a *restrictive barrier*. In this situation, as previously noted, manipulation can be effective in reducing or eliminating musculoskeletal dysfunction and restoring normal motion.

Concept 11: Active vs. Passive and Direct vs. Indirect

In treating musculoskeletal disorders with manipulation, two approaches can be used through a variety of techniques. *Active* versus *passive* refers to the activity level of the patient: is the patient actively participating in the treatment, or is the practitioner doing the mechanical work?

Direct versus *indirect* refers to the motion barrier and the practitioner's approach to it. As discussed, a motion barrier is a decrease in normal ROM caused by an increase in the normal physiological motion barrier. The practitioner seeks to remove or release this barrier and restore normal motion. The technique employed can move the affected joint either toward the motion barrier (direct) or away from the barrier (indirect). As a simple example, consider that the flexors of the elbow joint are in spasm, thus holding the elbow in flexion (bent) and creating a barrier to extension (straightening). A direct technique would be an attempt to move the joint into extension, that is, into or toward the motion barrier. An indirect technique would move the elbow joint further into flexion, producing a change in the position of the joint, which would be reported by the muscle and joint proprioceptors. Over a short time, this causes a reflex release of the spastic contraction of the flexor muscles, thereby eliminating the motion barrier.

In summary, the practitioner of manual therapy seeks to restore proper anatomical and physiological balance in the patient. At least three types of balance are potential targets of the various styles and techniques employed, as follows:

1. The restoration of proper joint range of motion and body symmetry.
2. The restoration of balance of nervous activity:
   a. Between sensory and motor systems.
   b. Between somatic and autonomic nerves.
   c. Between sympathetic and parasympathetic divisions of autonomic nervous system.
3. The restoration of proper arterial flow and venous and lymphatic drainage for proper nutrition of all tissues of the body.

OSTEOPATHIC MEDICINE

Osteopathy was founded by Andrew Taylor Still (1828-1917), son of a practicing physician and ordained Methodist minister. Trained in medicine by his father and during a short stint at a medical school in Kansas City, Still ministered principally to the settlers and Indian tribes then living in the state of Missouri and the Kansas territory. He received additional "training" as a surgeon for the Union army during the Civil War.

In 1864 an outbreak of meningitis claimed the lives of three of Still's children. This tragic event and his helplessness to affect its outcome, coupled with his critical awareness of the methods of medicine practiced at the time (e.g., application of leeches, bleeding, purging, treatments with such toxic elements as mercury and arsenic), sowed the seeds of his discontent with his profession. During this period, Oliver Wendell Holmes, Sr., the renowned physician, declared, "If the whole *materia medica* as now used could be sunk to the bottom of the sea, it would be better for mankind—and all the worse for the fishes." Still began to search for a better way.

His search led him to a prolonged and detailed study of human anatomy, particularly the bones. He ultimately concluded that if the bones of the body were not in the proper relationship to one another and could not move properly, other systems of the body would become affected, and disease could develop. He apparently became acquainted with the principles of "bonesetting," a tradition of adjustment practiced primarily in Europe. With modifications, especially the emphasis on spinal mobilization, the style evolved into what he called "osteopathy."

Still strongly espoused the theory of holism, where all body systems are considered both structurally and functionally interrelated. Still was also a strong advocate of the importance of balance (homeostasis) within the body, with a specific emphasis on the unimpeded arterial flow and venous/lymphatic drainage to and from the organs (the "rule of the artery"). He also believed in the inherent ability of the body to defend and repair itself. Bearing in mind that these observations were made before the discovery of the immune and endocrine systems by Western science, Still's ideas were considered quite radical at the time.

In 1892, Still founded the American School of Osteopathy (ASO) in Kirksville, Missouri, where he remained until his death. Between the time he "dis-

covered" osteopathy and the establishment of the ASO, Still was developing his osteopathic technique and billed himself as a "Lightning Bonesetter." The ASO has evolved into the A.T. Still University of Health Sciences (formerly the Kirksville College of Osteopathic Medicine). The success of the ASO was such that the founding of osteopathic colleges in De Moines, Chicago, Philadelphia, and Kansas City followed within the next 15 years. After Still's death, osteopathy sought to gain legal if not philosophical equality with the allopathic profession, which had established itself as the gold standard of medical practice. Through the American Medical Association (AMA), the doctors of medicine (MDs), or allopathic physicians, were making a concerted effort to eradicate perceived competition (see later discussion on chiropractic).

The first step toward parity for the osteopaths was to provide equivalent education for their students, which was based on the Flexner model of medical education adopted by the medical profession (2 years of basic science, followed by 2 years of clinical rotations, internship, and residency). The unity engendered by persecution from the AMA and the loyalty of its patients led to the slow but steady growth of the osteopathic profession until after World War II. Hospitals were built, legal battles for practice rights were fought on a state-by-state basis, and the profession developed on a "separate but equal" basis; doctors of osteopathy (DOs) now prescribe drugs, perform surgery, offer obstetrical and gynecological services, and practice emergency medicine.

The post–Word War II period brought accelerated growth to osteopathy, largely because of the commissioning of DOs into the U.S. armed services. New colleges were established, and full practice rights were finally granted in all 50 states in the 1960s (osteopathic physicians are still not fully licensed in Canada). The struggle for equality was won, but not without a price. The push for equivalence with the MDs created a desire to shed what originally made osteopathy unique. As a result, the DOs began to deemphasize manipulation as the benchmark of their clinical practice, and many today view it as archaic and an embarrassment. Most DOs in the United States, although they learned manipulative theory and technique as students, do not use manipulation or use it only sparingly, especially since the advent of managed care. Manipulation is not cost-effective for physicians because reimbursements by insurance companies are insufficient. This is the rationale for using the term *osteopathic medicine* as the title of this section rather than the more traditional "osteopathy." As a result, manipulation may become the lost art of osteopathic practice. Also, there are currently about 50,000 DOs in the United States, compared with more than 600,000 MDs. These trends seem to indicate that osteopathic medicine's days as a distinct profession are numbered, at least in the United States. The growth of the osteopathic profession in Europe and Asia, however, appears to indicate that the profession is alive and well. These practitioners are not licensed as physicians, however, and only practice manipulation (and perhaps other forms of complementary and integrative medicine for which they are certified).

Despite these developments, the American Academy of Osteopathy (AAO), a component society of the American Osteopathic Association (AOA), has dedicated itself to the preservation and nurturing of osteopathic manipulation and philosophy. Through the efforts of this association, as well as the paradigm shift in medicine brought on by the complementary medicine movement, osteopathic manipulation may yet surge again within the profession. In addition, osteopathic movements are growing in Europe and Asia, although issues of licensing and scope of practice must be resolved separately in each country.

Osteopathic manipulative treatment (OMT) is based on the diagnosis of somatic dysfunction. This term was coined by Ira Rumney, DO, when the *International Classification of Diseases* (ICD) coding system was developed for insurance reimbursement. Until then, the more provincial term "osteopathic lesion" was used. The following criteria must be met for a diagnosis:

1. *Asymmetry*. Asymmetry can be observed while the patient is standing (uneven shoulder height, pelvic tilt, scoliosis, kyphosis, genu valgum [knock knees], foot pronation), walking (limp, pelvic tilt, uneven arm swing), lying supine (pelvic rotation, leg-length discrepancy), prone (scoliosis, abnormal bony prominence), or in other positions or during other movements.
2. *Restriction*. Motion restriction is diagnosed with ROM testing, usually passive ROM, by attempting to move the affected joint through normal ROM and observing any restrictions, changes in motion characteristics, and discomfort. In the spine, ROM can be analyzed regionally (e.g., thoracic spine) or intersegementally (e.g., T4-5). ROM testing also extends to the fascial system, which is assessed by a variety of techniques.
3. *Tissue texture changes*. Tissue changes include excessive dryness or oiliness, redness or pallor, a feeling of "ropiness," and excessive hardness or softness compared with the surrounding tissues. The tissues involved can be skin, fascia, muscles, joint capsules, or visceral structures.
4. *Tenderness*. Pain can be elicited with active or passive ROM and by palpation with light to deep pressure. Occasionally the patient does not notice tenderness until the operator points it out.

Diagnosis is usually made on the basis of combining observation and palpation, with palpation by far the more important of the two elements (see later discussion on cranial osteopathy).

As with other forms of manual therapy, the discretion of the practitioner is operative when selecting specific techniques to be used with individual patients. Different combinations and sequences are observed, depending on the physician's preference and observations of the patient's tolerance level. Since DOs are fully licensed, drugs and injections may also accompany manipulative treatment, when considered necessary or beneficial. The following sections discuss some of the more common osteopathic techniques.

Muscle Energy Technique

Muscle energy technique can be applied directly or indirectly. When applied *directly* (i.e., toward the motion barrier, or in an attempt to lengthen a shortened or spastic muscle), this technique is based on the principle of *reciprocal inhibition,* which states that as a muscle (e.g., flexor) contracts, its antagonist (the associated extensor) reflexively relaxes. If a muscle in spasm is contracted against resistance and then relaxed, the effect is to break the reflex spasm cycle, resulting in increased ROM (reduction of the motion barrier). When applied *indirectly,* muscle energy technique is based on the principle of *postisometric relaxation* (also known as *postcontraction relaxation*). This technique is one of the few "active" techniques in manual therapy, that is, where the patient does the work. Individual muscles can be treated as well as muscle groups.

A distinction of muscle energy technique is the amount of effort exerted by the patient. Usually, less than 20% of the total strength of the muscle is brought to bear during the interval of contraction. Another way of showing this is through the "one-finger rule," where the amount of force necessary is that force needed to move a single finger of the therapist, lightly resisting the contraction. This is in contradistinction to the proprioceptive neuromuscular facilitation (PNF) technique used by physical therapists, which employs a maximum muscle contraction (exposing the patient to the risk of injury). A thorough knowledge of muscle attachments and their motion vectors is necessary to apply muscle energy effectively and efficiently.

High-Velocity Low-Amplitude Technique

The high-velocity low-amplitude (HVLA) technique is probably the most publicly recognized technique of the osteopath or chiropractor. This is a thrust-oriented technique designed to break through a motion barrier aggressively. More often than not, an audible pop is heard, the result of a brief cavitation of the involved joint. The HVLA technique can be applied directly (toward the barrier) of indirectly (away from the barrier), using short or long levers. Although often associated with manipulation of the spine, the HVLA technique can also be performed on the extremities. This technique is *not* indicated in patients with osteoporosis, bone tumors, or severe atherosclerosis. Recently, much discussion has focused on the safety of HVLA when performed in the high cervical (neck) region; however, research indicates that this technique is relatively safe.

Strain and Counterstrain

The strain and counterstrain technique is a very gentle, passive technique developed by Lawrence Jones, DO. The therapist palpates a muscle in spasm, and the patient is brought into a position that shortens the muscle *(counterstrain)*, thereby exaggerating the motion restriction. This position is held usually for 90 to 120 seconds, and the patient is slowly returned to the original position. The technique is designed to interrupt the reflex spasm loop by changing and holding altered proprioceptive input into the CNS. This technique can also be done directly *(strain)*, that is, gently stretching the involved muscle, with the same result. Tender points are also treated in this manner, where the patient is brought to a position of ease, held in the position until a "softening" or change in tissue texture is felt, then slowly returned to the original position.

Myofascial Release

Myofascial release is a gentle technique that uses knowledge of the physical properties of the fascia as it relates to muscles. A high level of palpation skill is necessary to apply this technique effectively. The operator uses light or deep pressure to palpate motion restriction and moves toward or away from the restriction. The position is held until a "release," or softening, is felt; the tissues are then slowly returned to their original position. The release can be the relaxation of muscle, the slow breaking of fascial adhesions, or the realignment of the fascia to its correct orientation.

Myofascial–Soft Tissue Technique

The myofascial–soft tissue technique is a combination direct/indirect massage technique for reducing muscle spasm and fascial tension. It is similar to petrissage (see later discussion), except that more parts of the hand are typically employed. This technique can be used as a prelude to the HVLA technique.

Lymphatic Drainage Techniques (Pumps)

Lymphatic drainage techniques are similar to effleurage (see later discussion) in that light pressure is applied to the skin and superficial fascia in the direction of the heart to increase the venous and lymphatic drainage of the involved structure(s). Lymphatic pumps are rhythmic techniques applied over organs such as the liver and spleen to increase drainage. The thoracic diaphragm is also sometimes used as a lymphatic pump.

Cranial Osteopathy

Cranial osteopathy (or osteopathy in the cranial field) was developed by W.G. Sutherland. His work was based on the observation that the joints between the skull bones are meant to permit motion just as joints do in other areas of the body. While palpating these bones and joints, he discovered the existence of a very subtle rhythm in the body unrelated to respiration or cardiovascular rhythms. Sutherland named this rhythm the *cranial rhythmic impulse* (CRI). This impulse, he learned, was capable of moving the cranial bones through a very small ROM, but still palpable to well-trained hands. Cranial theory posits that there is inherent motility of the CNS, resulting in fluctuations of the cerebrospinal fluid, which bathes the brain and spinal cord. This fluctuation in turn moves the cranial bones through their small yet palpable ROM, primarily at the sutural joints. However, motion is not restricted to the cranial bones by this rhythm. Through the dural membranes, which cover the CNS, the sacrum is linked to the cranium, and motion is palpable there as well. In addition, through the fascial/fluid system of the body, the CRI has effects all over the body. Motion restrictions in this system can be palpated and corrected (either directly or indirectly) through very gentle manipulation, also with global effects (see previous discussion on fascia). As releases are produced in this fascial system and throughout the body, and perhaps because of its proximity to the brain, memories (sometimes painful) can be reawakened, producing the "somatoemotional release," a form of mind-body connection.

Evidence of the effectiveness of cranial osteopathy comes almost exclusively in the form of clinical case reports and testimonials. Successes have been reported for a variety of conditions. Cranial osteopathy has been reported to improve such conditions as chronic headache, cerebral palsy, autism, and behavioral disturbances.

Cranial osteopathy has been controversial from its inception because of the lack of definitive experimental evidence (although workers in the field would dispute this). However, data are being gathered and outcome-based studies conducted, which lends credence to its effectiveness. Because of the time and effort necessary to develop this skill, relatively few osteopaths practice cranial osteopathy. However, training in cranial osteopathy (or "craniosacral therapy") is now being offered to other practitioners of manual therapies by the Upledger Institute (Palm Beach, Florida).

Visceral Manipulation

Visceral manipulation generally involves gentle massage of the accessible internal organs (abdominopelvic organs). Although not indicated in patients with tumors or inflammatory disease, visceral manipulation can be useful in stabilizing and balancing blood flow and autonomic innervation and can even dislodge certain obstructions of the gastrointestinal system. Visceral manipulation, along with cranial osteopathy, is practiced extensively by European osteopaths.

Articulatory Technique

In the articulatory technique the operator moves the affected joint through its ROM in all planes, gently encountering motion barriers and gradually moving through them to establish normal motion. This would be considered a passive, direct/indirect, oscillatory technique.

Functional Technique (Facilitated Positional Release)

In the functional technique the patient is positioned so as to produce a "position of ease" or comfort. Typically the operator places a hand or finger over a tender area and positions the patient until the discomfort is significantly reduced, and the patient holds this position for a certain period. The patient is then brought slowly back to the original position. The position of ease reduces nociceptive and aberrant proprioceptive input to the CNS, thus breaking the cycle of pain and spasm. Realignment of fascia is also a result of the functional technique.

CHIROPRACTIC

During the mid-1890s, D.D. Palmer, a practicing magnetic healer, relieved a man of his long-standing deafness by administering an adjustment to his thoracic vertebrae. This was his first experience with what he began to call "chiropractic." Within 2 years he had established the Palmer School of Chiropractic in Davenport, Iowa. Interestingly, at approximately the same time and within 200 miles of one another, the professions of chiropractic and osteopathy grew up together. It has been rumored (by the osteopaths) that Palmer was a patient of Still's at Kirksville and carefully observed his technique and its results. Although this has not been confirmed, it does reflect the atmosphere of intellectual freedom during that period and in that part of the United States.

Palmer was a devotee of vitalism, which states that the universe and its inhabitants are imbued with an innate intelligence. He believed that this intelligence accounted for the self-healing capacity of the body. Using vitalism as a foundation, he developed the "one cause, one cure" theory, which posits that all disease can be traced to subluxations of the vertebral column. Therefore, he stated, all disease can be cured by chiropractic adjustment. Vertebral subluxation was explained by the "bone out of place," or static, model. This model stated that the malpositioned vertebra entrapped the spinal nerve at the neural foramen, thereby affecting normal body tonus and causing disease. The treatment involved a thrusting technique to put the bone back in its proper alignment. Palmer took great effort to explain the technique, which used the spinous and transverse processes of the vertebra as short levers; this distinguished Palmer from Still and the osteopaths, who taught both short-lever and long-lever techniques.

In 1906, Palmer spent 3 months in the Scott County (Iowa) jail for practicing medicine without a license. This event marked the beginning of a long period of conflict between the chiropractic and medical professions. It has been estimated that by 1930, chiropractors had served more than 30,000 jail terms.

Over the next few years, several additional chiropractic schools were established. In contrast to the early growth in the number of osteopathic colleges (to expand and promote the profession), the outgrowth of chiropractic colleges primarily resulted from intractable philosophical conflicts between their founders and Palmer. One of these, S.M. Langworthy, established the American School of Chiropractic and Nature Cure (1903). Langworthy, along with O. Smith and M. Paxson, published a textbook that delineated what would later become the dynamic model of spinal subluxation, proposing that vertebral subluxation is a result of motion restriction or "fixation." Palmer also had serious differences of opinion with his son, B.J., who took over the administration of the Palmer School after his father's death. (Palmer was struck by a car driven by his son; chiropractors continue to speculate on whether the incident was really an accident.)

B.J. believed that the upper cervical vertebrae were the seat of all spinal subluxations and treated his patients accordingly. Treating all patients with the same technique gave rise to the term "hole in one" to describe the procedure.

As a defender of the profession, B.J. was tireless. In 1907, he retained lawyers in the defense of S. Morikobu, another chiropractor accused of practicing medicine without a license. Using the Langworthy textbook, the defense pointed out that chiropractic was not medicine and that the profession was separate and distinct from the allopathic profession. Therefore, Dr. Morikobu was not in fact practicing "medicine" without a license, but rather was practicing chiropractic. The case was won, and the "separate and distinct" concept was publicly established.

B.J. Palmer was also enamored of technology. He purchased and extensively used the first available x-ray equipment, advocating its use in documenting subluxations. As a means of earning additional money to support the college, he became involved in the wireless communication business, eventually starting WOC (World of Chiropractic) radio in Davenport, Iowa. One of WOC's more famous alumni was Ronald Reagan, known during his radio days as "Dutch."

By the 1930s the rift between the Palmer philosophy (one cause–one cure, bone out of place, hole in one) and the rationalists came to a critical point when Gillet, a Belgian chiropractor, put forth the dynamic model, based in part on Langworthy's earlier work. Gillet stated that subluxations were caused by vertebral fixations, which could be muscular, articular, ligamentous, or bony. The fixation in turn caused a nerve entrapment, causing symptoms associated with that segment. This theory is by far the most widely espoused today, and it is the origin of the common terms *vertebral subluxation complex* (VSC) and *segmental dysfunction* (SDF). By the 1940s the chiropractors falling on the side of the Langworthy-Gillet theory, disavowing the one cause–one cure theory of Palmer, became known as the "Mixers," whereas those adhering to the Palmer theory were referred to as "Straights."

In conjunction with the split in the chiropractic profession, the persecution by the allopaths continued. In the 1960s and 1970s, MDs were forbidden by the AMA to have any professional association with doctors of chiropractic (DCs). This led to an antitrust suit brought against the AMA *(Wilk v AMA)*. That lawsuit was won early in the early 1990s, a major victory for the profession.

At the time of the original schism, the National Chiropractic Association (NCA) had been established for more than 10 years. C.O. Watkins, the NCA's chairman, strongly advocated embracing the scientific method and establishing educational standards. He believed that the greatest hope for the profession was through the validation of chiropractic theory by research. The NCA eventually became the American Chiropractic Association (ACA), from which grew the Foundation for Chiropractic Research and Council on Chiropractic Education (CCE). The CCE now accredits all chiropractic colleges in the United States, including those who continue to profess the one cause–one cure philosophy (the "Straights"). The research effort in the profession has been somewhat centralized in the form of the Consortial Center for Chiropractic Research (CCCR) at the Palmer College. The center was one of the first recipients of large-scale National Institutes of Health (NIH) funding for research in complementary medicine.

Currently, most chiropractors primarily treat musculoskeletal complaints and restrict their manipulation ("adjustment") to the spine and pelvis, although treatment occasionally may be given to the cranium and extremities. Because of research conducted by Korr, Patterson, Sato, and others on the effects of somatovisceral reflexes and the continuing research on many questions related to manual therapy in general, the impact of spinal adjustment on other ailments may yet be more clearly elucidated.

The hallmarks of the VSC or SDF are similar (if not identical) to the osteopathic somatic dysfunction. Motion restriction in the form of a fixation is present; that is, something is restricting movement of the vertebra in one of the three planes of space. Possibilities include a joint (articulatory), usually a facet joint; a ligament; a muscle (in spasm); or a bone (as a result of arthritis or other pathology). Tenderness is also present, along with texture changes in the surrounding tissues.

The disorders treated by chiropractors are commonly classified into the following three groups:

1. *Type M (musculoskeletal).* This group includes, but is not limited to, such complaints as facet syndrome, sacroiliac joint dysfunction, tension headache, myositis, fibromyalgia, trigger points, strain and sprain injuries, torticollis (wryneck), some forms of sciatica, and undifferentiated low back and neck pain. Successes have been reported in cases of herniated disc, but treating this ailment with high-velocity technique is somewhat controversial.
2. *Type N (neurogenic).* Some successes have been reported in cases of nystagmus, migraine, Bell's palsy, Tourette's syndrome, and other neurogenic complaints, but these reports are anecdotal, and no controlled studies have yet been conducted to confirm the results.
3. *Type O (organic, stress related).* These disorders would include, but again are not be limited to, hypertension, headache, bowel and bladder dysfunction, dysmenorrhea, infantile colic, gastritis, angina, and asthma. As noted, reports of success using chiropractic manipulative therapy (CMT) are anecdotal, and research is needed to confirm these claims.

As mentioned earlier, chiropractic adjustment technique is primarily thrust (HVLA) oriented, using a short-lever approach. The classic joint "pop" or "crack" is a hallmark of chiropractic treatment. Four types of thrusts are presented here, although variations on each exist. These thrusts are used to increase joint mobility and decrease or eliminate muscle spasm, as follows:

1. *Impulse.* In this thrust the motion barrier is engaged with the hands, and a quick, short thrust is applied.
2. *Recoil.* The thrust is delivered with force generated from the operator's chest, arms, and hands. After it is delivered, the hands recoil from the spinous process of the vertebra.
3. *Body drop.* This thrust is performed with the operator's arms fully extended and the elbows locked in. The operator's weight is quickly brought to bear on the vertebra to be manipulated.
4. *Leverage.* This thrust is performed with counterstabilization applied to prevent the loss of force during the thrust.

Thrusts can be applied singly or in groups (multiple thrust) with gradually increasing force. The direction of the thrust and selection of fulcrum depend on the type of fixation and direction of motion restriction.

Over the years, many different models for the analysis and treatment of the VSC/SDF have been developed. Almost all are HVLA oriented, and all are passive (i.e., the patient does no work), as follows:

- *Diversified.* This is by far the most common of the chiropractic approaches. The HVLA technique is delivered to individual segments or groups of segments, as determined by motion analysis and palpation diagnosis.
- *Gonstead.* This approach uses direct HVLA (thrust). X-ray analysis is typically employed, with lines drawn on the films to aid in the diagnosis.
- *Cox/flexion-distraction.* This approach uses a traction-mobilization technique. It is used primarily in cases of intervertebral disc pathology and is one of the few non-HVLA techniques in the chiropractic armamentarium.
- *Activator.* This technique is applied with a device that delivers a very-high-velocity impulse. It is used with muscles and other soft tissues, as well as joints.
- *Thompson.* In this approach, HVLA is applied primarily to the pelvis to correct dysfunction there and dysfunction as a result of leg-length discrepancy. The legs and pelvis are regarded as a supportive arch system for the body and the seat of dysfunction.
- *Sacro-occipital technique* (SOT). Modeled after cranial osteopathy, SOT attempts to balance the cerebrospinal fluid system through gentle, direct technique.
- *Nimmo/tonus receptor.* This technique is designed to treat trigger points with direct pressure for about 7 to 8 seconds. When one trigger point releases, the next is treated in the same manner (see later discussion on neuromuscular therapy).
- *Applied kinesiology* (AK). AK is one of the most controversial of the chiropractic techniques. Promulgated by G. Goodheart, AK theory states that the VSC creates weakness in specific muscle groups. Therefore, if a muscle group is found to be weak when pressure is applied to a particular segment, that segment is expressing a spinal dysfunction. This system is also applied to various points on the body that, when pressure is applied, will induce weakness in specific muscle groups. When the point is treated with pressure, the weakness subsides and the dysfunction is corrected. The points identified

in AK are similar to acupuncture points and correspond to visceral as well as somatic dysfunction.
- *Logan basic.* The sacrum is the center of this theory, with the focus on the sacrotuberous ligament. Sacral dysfunctions are relieved by a fascial release–oriented treatment.
- *Palmer upper cervical* ("hole in one," HIO). As described earlier, B.J. Palmer proposed that all vertebral subluxations were secondary to the first two cervical vertebrae (C1-2). He therefore devised the HIO technique, in which a lateral thrust is applied to C1-2.
- *Meric.* In this system it is believed that the third thoracic vertebra (T3) is the primary center of subluxation. HVLA technique is applied.
- *Pierce-Stillwagon.* This approach targets the cervical spine and pelvis with HVLA thrusts.

Along with adjustment, chiropractors also use treatment modalities typically associated with physical therapy. Hot packs, ultrasound, transcutaneous electric nerve stimulation (TENS), and other treatments can be found in the modern chiropractors office.

Despite the philosophical departure from the original theories of the Palmers, the chiropractic profession has never, in contrast to the osteopathic profession, attempted to attain equivalency with allopathic medicine, a fact that would please B.J. Palmer. Even though intramural disagreements still exist, the chiropractors have remained essentially true to their roots as a separate and distinct health care profession.

See Chapter 10 for further information on chiropractic.

MASSAGE

Massage, as with other manipulative forms of therapy, predates written history. The Greek physician Aesciclipides became perhaps the first practitioner of the "one cause, one cure" approach when he abandoned the other forms of contemporary medical treatment in favor of massage to restore the free movement of body fluids and return the patient to a state of health. During the Renaissance the physician Ambroise Paré, author of a widely used surgery text, espoused the application of massage and manipulation and was reportedly the first to use the term "subluxation." In 1813, Pehr Henrik Ling, a gymnastics instructor, founded the Central Royal Institute of Gymnastics, where his theory of massage as passive gymnastics was developed. This work was the genesis of what is now referred to as "Swedish massage," and Ling is considered the father of massage.

The basic classification of massage techniques was completed by Johann Georg Metzger, a Dutch physician and student of Ling. Although Metzger's work was never published, his students von Mosengeil and Helleday wrote and published descriptions of the techniques. In the late nineteenth century the prominent French physician Marie Marcellin Lucas-Champonnière advocated the use of massage therapy in the treatment of fractures, arguing the case for consideration of soft tissue union in the healing process. His students, the English physicians William Bennett and Robert Jones, effectively brought massage to England. Bennett incorporated the use of massage at St. George's Hospital in London around 1899, and Jones used massage therapy at the Southern Hospital in Liverpool. Jones taught both James Mennell, author of the text *Physical Treatment by Movement, Manipulation, and Massage* (1917) and a tireless advocate of massage, and Mary McMillan, who was very influential in the introduction and promotion of massage in the United States.

As awareness of this form of treatment grew, so did the science of physiology, and the two entities became intertwined with the growth of the scientific basis of medicine. Some authors attribute the development of the physical therapy profession as an outgrowth of massage and its incorporation into the Euro-American therapeutic armamentarium. Many other forms of so-called bodywork are also outgrowths of massage and its various techniques and styles.

The essential theory of massage therapy is based on the principle that the tissues of the body will function at optimal levels when arterial supply and venous and lymphatic drainage are unimpeded ("rule of the artery"; see earlier discussion on osteopathic medicine). When this flow becomes unbalanced for any reason, muscle tightness and changes in the nearby skin and fascia will ensue, which may produce pain. The basic techniques of massage are designed to reestablish proper fluid dynamics and are directed at the skin, muscles, and fascia, although nerve pathways occasionally are included. In general, articulations are not directly addressed in this form of therapy. Contraindications to massage or areas to avoid during the application of massage include skin infections or melanoma, bleeding (especially within 48 hours of a traumatic event causing bleeding into tissues), acute inflammation (e.g., rheumatoid arthritis, appendicitis), thrombophlebitis, atherosclerosis, varicose veins, and immunocompromised state (to avoid transmission of infection from massage therapist to patient).

The techniques of massage are generally applied in the direction of the heart to stimulate increased venous and lymphatic drainage from the involved tissues. Muscles are treated in groups, with one group being treated before advancing to the next. Different combinations of techniques are used depending on the objectives of treatment. Treatment typically begins with more gentle techniques before progressing to deeper, more aggressive applications. Massage is usually performed with a powder, oil, or other type of lubricant applied to the skin of the patient (or client), who lies prone, supine, or laterally on a table, or who may be seated in a massage chair. Verbal communication between the operator and patient is important because the operator will use the cues given by the patient as a guide to treatment.

The visceral effects of massage include the general vasoactivity in somatic tissues as regulated by the ANS. Also, effects on blood pressure and/or heart rate (usually decreases in both) can be observed as the client relaxes into the treatment.

There are five basic techniques of massage, and all are of the passive variety (i.e., operator does the work). These techniques are effleurage, petrissage, friction, tapotement, and vibration.

Effleurage

The most frequently used massage technique, effleurage typically is used to begin a treatment session and introduce the patient to the process of touching. Effleurage is a stroking technique applied with light to moderate pressure (superficial or deep), serving to modulate the arterial supply and venous/lymphatic drainage of the tissues contacted. The amount of pressure applied determines the layer of the body contacted; very light pressure would only affect the skin, deeper pressure the superficial fascia, even deeper pressure the deep fascia, and so on. The entire palmar surface of the hand is used, or a "knuckling" technique may be employed (after Hoffa, see below). When used during the initial stages of treatment, effleurage is also used as a palpation diagnostic tool, as the operator "looks" for areas of altered texture, asymmetry, or tenderness. Specific long strokes are also used at the conclusion of treatment, especially if sleep induction is desired.

Petrissage

Petrissage is somewhat more aggressive than effleurage, with the thumb and fingers working together to lift and "milk" the underlying fascia and muscles in a kneading motion. Care is taken not to pinch or produce bruising. The effect of petrissage is to increase venous and lymphatic drainage of the muscles and to break up adhesions (small areas of local fibrosis), which may be present in the fascia. Depending on the direction of application and vector of motion restriction (if any), this technique can be considered direct or indirect.

Friction

Friction can be the most deeply applied massage technique. The tips of the fingers or thumb are used in a circular or back-and-forth movement. If deeper pressure is desired, or if the operator is easily fatigued, the heel of the hand can be used, or sometimes even the elbow. Friction can be used in cases of tenosynovitis, where adhesions are present, or where the target tissue is too deep for petrissage. Cyriax developed the technique of transverse friction massage, which is widely used by physical therapists. As with petrissage, the direction of the applied technique, relative to any motion restriction, will determine whether the application is direct or indirect.

Tapotement

Often seen in classic fight films, tapotement involves rapid, repeated blows of varying strength done with the sides or palms of the hands, with the hands cupped, or with the fists. Occasionally, rapid pinching of the skin is done. The purpose of tapotement is to stimulate arterial circulation to the area. Again, the technique should not produce bruising and is not applied over the area of the kidneys or on the chest, or over any recent incisions or areas of inflammation or contusion.

Vibration

Usually considered to be one of the more difficult of the massage techniques to master or to perform without becoming fatigued, the application of vibration typically employs a mechanical vibrator of some type. When the hands are used, a light, rhythmic, quivering effect is achieved.

Other Styles of Massage

Albert Hoffa

The techniques described in Hoffa's text, *Technik der Massage*, published in 1900, are still in use today. Hoffa advocated the limitation of massage to 15-minute treatments, with no pain experienced by the patient. Like Ling, Hoffa stated that massage should be applied from distal to proximal, with the point of reference being the heart. His adaptations included knuckling and circular effleurage, two-finger petrissage, and other forms.

Mary McMillan

McMillan is credited with the categorization of massage into its five basic techniques. In each of those categories, she introduced innovative variations. She advocated the use of olive oil as a lubricant for its nutritional value when absorbed through the skin. Her influence in the development of massage is universally recognized, and her techniques have been widely adopted by massage therapists in the United States.

Bindgewebmassage (Dicke)

Elisabeth Dicke was a student of Hoffa who described massage based on the connective tissue system of the body. She described areas of referred pain on the back that indicate internal pathology but do not necessarily correspond to segmental distribution. Areas of tenderness do correspond to certain acupuncture points. Treatment is given with the middle finger in a series of sequenced strokes without lubricant.

James Cyriax

Cyriax was a strong advocate of friction as the most effective technique in massage. He developed the "transverse friction massage" technique, which is widely used by manual therapists. Deep friction massage is used to stimulate increased circulation to the affected area. It can be applied to muscles, tendons, ligaments, and bones. Cyriax' methods are described in detail in his book, *Textbook of Orthopedic Medicine, Volume II.*

Current Massage Therapies

Massage is used in a variety of clinical scenarios. The expertise of the masseur/massuese is essential in determining which techniques may or may not be indicated and how the massage may be delivered. Application may be based on the motion restrictions that may be present in the patient or in the environment, such as in a hospital. Massage is routinely applied to pediatric and geriatric patients (infant massage is a burgeoning field). Frequently, massages therapists expand their therapeutic horizons by taking postgraduate study in other forms of bodywork (see following discussion). It is not uncommon to find a therapist who not only does Swedish massage, but who also employs Trager work, Feldenkrais, and craniosacral therapy.

OTHER FORMS OF BODYWORK

Neuromuscular Therapy

Neuromuscular therapy (NMT) was pioneered by Lief and Leon Chaitow (DO) in Europe and Nimmo in the United States, and its development continues today through Judith Delany, Paul St. John, and others. As with osteopaths, neuromuscular therapists use the term *somatic dysfunction* when describing the former "neuromuscular lesion" (Chaitow being an osteopath). Somatic dysfunction is characterized by an area of tenderness and limited motion. Causes of these lesions include, but are not limited to, connective tissue changes, ischemia, nerve compression, and postural disturbances. Causes can include trauma, stress, and repetitive microtrauma (stress due to work and recreationally related activities).

The concept of reflex points (Chapman's points, Jones' Tender points, Bennett's points), especially trigger points, is also emphasized and treated in NMT. *Trigger points,* as named by Janet Travell, MD, are areas of tenderness within a muscle that radiate in a defined zone when pressure is applied. Reflex and

trigger points (like the connective tissue zones described by Dicke) may or may not correspond to the distribution of a segmental nerve (i.e., common referred pain patterns) and appear to have some association with acupuncture points.

NMT is generally applied with a combination of effleurage or gliding, petrissage (for specific muscles) or grasping, friction (especially transverse friction), muscle energy, and strain/counterstrain techniques. Lubricants may be used, depending on the technique employed, and the therapist may use the fingers, thumbs, forearms, elbows, or pressure bars to apply force. When deep muscles or muscle groups are treated, some discomfort may be felt, followed by pain relief.

Trager Work (Psychophysical Integration and Mentastics)

Milton Trager, MD, was originally a boxer and gymnast and developed (almost by accident) his technique of psychophysical integration more than 50 years ago. To obtain the credentials he believed were necessary to bring his technique to the medical community, he obtained a medical degree from the University of Guadalajara in 1955. While there, he was able to demonstrate his technique and treat polio patients, with a relatively high degree of success. After developing the technique over many years in his medical practice, he began to teach the method in 1975. The Trager Institute (Mill Valley, California) was founded shortly thereafter and is responsible for dissemination of information and certification programs.

Trager work is a two-tiered approach, along the lines of Feldenkrais (see following discussion). The psychophysical integration phase, also known as "table work," consists of a single treatment or a series of treatments. Mentastics, as described later, is an exercise taught to patients so that they may continue the work on their own.

Psychophysical integration is essentially an indirect/functional technique. The patient lies on a table, and the practitioner applies a very gentle rocking motion to explore the body for areas of tissue tension and motion restriction. No force, stroking, or thrust is used in this technique, merely a light, rhythmic contact. The purpose is to produce a specific sensory experience for the patient, one that is positive and pleasurable. Any discomfort serves to break the continuum of "teaching" and "learning."

The focus of the treatment, however, is not on any specific anatomical structure or physiological process, but rather on the *psyche* of the patient. An attempt is made to bring the patient into a position (or motion) of ease, where a sensation of lightness or freedom is experienced. This sensation is "learned" by the patient during the process of sensorimotor repatterning. In the words of Dr. Trager, the patient learns "how the tissue should feel when everything is right." This mind-body interaction is the core of the treatment, where the patient's psyche is brought to bear on the CNS in order to break the feedback loop of pain → guarding → muscle spasm and induce a change. The result is deep relaxation and increased ROM (i.e., the sense of lightness).

Patterns of behavior and posture are learned during a person's lifetime in part as reactions to trauma or withdrawal from pain, either physical or emotional (see following discussion on structural integration). Initially, the body may be able to compensate for such reactions, but it will eventually decompensate, resulting in various somatic or visceral symptoms. The Trager treatment "allows" the patient to reexperience the norm through this exploratory process.

The practitioner seeks to integrate with the patient by entering a quasimeditative state of awareness referred to as the "hookup." This allows the operator to attend acutely to the work at hand and feel very subtle changes in tissue texture and movement, not unlike the level of attention necessary to practice cranial osteopathy (see earlier discussion). Without any specific anatomical protocol, the work is very intuitive, and "letting go" is necessary by both parties. The practitioner maintains a position of "neutrality" and makes no attempt to "make anything happen," since it is actually the patient who is sensing and learning. The practitioner's role is one of a facilitator, where he or she seeks to provide a safe and nurturing environment for the patient to explore new and pain-free patterns of motion.

Mentastics, the continuing phase of Trager work, is short for "mental gymnastics" and follows table work. A basic exercise set is taught, and patients are instructed to practice on their own. These exercises consist of repetitive and sequential movements of all the joints, designed to relieve tension from the body. They are to be performed in an effortless, relaxed state of awareness, where the individual "hooks up" with the self. The basic principles of Hatha-Yoga and t'ai chi are used in these exercises. Once the set is learned, individuals can then continue to explore independently, creating their own custom-designed series.

Practitioners of Trager work have reported success (not necessarily cures) in patients with multiple sclerosis, muscular dystrophy, and other debilitating diseases. Athletes have also reported significant improvements in performance as a result of applying Trager techniques.

Feldenkrais (Awareness through Movement, Functional Integration)

Moshe Feldenkrais (1904-1985) was an Israeli physicist who developed a system of movement and manipulation over several decades. The Feldenkrais method is divided into two "educational" processes. The first, *awareness through movement,* is a sensorimotor balancing technique that is taught to "students" as active participants in the process. The students are verbally guided through a series of very slow movements designed to create a heightened awareness of motion patterns and to reeducate the CNS as to new patterns, approaches, and possibilities (as in learning t'ai chi).

The second process is referred to as *functional integration*. This is a passive technique using a didactic approach, not at all unlike Trager table work. The operator acts as "teacher" and the patient as "student." The teacher brings the student through a series of manipulons to reestablish proper neuromotor patterning and balance. *Manipulons* are a manipulative sequence of information, action (as initiated by the operator), and response. They are gentle and are treated as exploratory, with the therapist introducing new motion patterns to the patient. Manipulons are referred to as "positioning," "confining," "single," or "repetitive." They can also be oscillating. In all cases the teacher plays a supportive and guiding role while creating a nonthreatening environment for change. Functional integration could be considered a combination of passive, articulatory, or functional techniques.

Structural Integration (Rolfing)

Structural integration was developed by Ida Rolf. A PhD in biochemistry, Rolf was treated for pneumonia by an osteopath whom she had sought out after being dissatisfied with conventional medical treatment. After this experience, Dr. Rolf embarked on a lengthy period of study, including yoga, which resulted in the manipulative system that now bears her name. In 1971, she founded the Rolf Institute in Boulder, Colorado, which now trains and certifies practitioners of this style.

The theory of *rolfing* (or Rolfing) is based primarily on physical consideration of the interaction of the human body with the gravitational field of the earth. As a dynamic entity, the human body moves around and through this field in a state of equilibrium, storing potential energy and releasing kinetic energy. In this system, form (potential energy) is in direct proportion to function (kinetic energy), and the balance between the two is equivalent to the amount of energy available to the body. In simple terms, the worse the posture, the more energy we consume on a baseline level, and thus the less we have available for normal activity. Furthermore, the physical energy of the body is in direct proportion to the "vital energy" of the person. Ideally, the body is always in a position of "equipoise," as shown below, but this is seldom if ever the case.

$$\text{Balance} \leftrightarrow \text{Energy}$$
$$\text{Form} \leftrightarrow \text{Function}$$

Rolfing traditionally involves a 10-session treatment protocol designed to integrate the entire myofascial system of the body. Photographs are taken of each patient before and after each session to evaluate progress.

The body is treated as a system of integrated segments consolidated by the myofascial system (see earlier discussion on segmentation). Attempts are made through "processing," as the treatment is called, to lengthen and center through the connective tissue system by a series of direct myofascial release techniques. As distortions in the system are released, the patient may experience pain. The pain experienced, however, is not merely structural. It is thought that emotions are expressed through the musculoskeletal system as behavior, which is reflected in various postures and movement patterns, (i.e., the widely accepted psychological concepts of Pavlovian conditioning and body language). In other words, the musculoskeletal system is viewed as a link between the body and mind. Emotional or physical traumas are stored in the body as postures, which mirror a with-

drawal response from the offending or painful agent. Over time, compensatory reactions occur, but the body ultimately decompensates, resulting in somatic or visceral dysfunction (see previous discussion on compensation). The direct technique seeks to put the energy of the operator into the system of the patient in an attempt to overcome the resistance to change affected in the withdrawal response. As releases are affected through the treatment, the emotional component may also be expressed (i.e. the somatoemotional release; see earlier discussion on cranial osteopathy).

The result of the treatment is a feeling of balance and "lightness" experienced by the patient. In addition, the patient should experience a heightened sense of well-being because the treatment releases the effects of emotional trauma. Thus the feeling of "lightness" is greater than simply an increase in the basal physical energy in the body; it is an increase in the body's vital energy as well.

Acupressure and Jin Shin Do

Acupressure is the application of the fingers to acupuncture points on the body, or "acupuncture without needles." It is based on the meridian or channel system, which permeates Asian medical arts and philosophy. According to this system, there are 12 major channels through which the body's energy, or *chi* (or *qi*), flows. Although most of the channels are named for specific organs, they do not necessarily correspond to the anatomical body part, but rather are more functional in nature. Interruptions in the flow of chi (prana, ki, vital energy, as described in other cultures) cause functional aberrations associated with that particular channel. These interruptions can be released by the application of needles or fingers.

Jin Shin Do, or the "way of compassionate spirit," was developed by psychotherapist Iona Teeguarden. It is a form of acupressure in which the fingers are used to apply deep pressure to hypersensitive acupuncture points. Jin Shin Do represents a synthesis of Taoist philosophy, psychology, breathing, and acupressure techniques. In accordance with this philosophy, the body is linked to the mind and spirit, and tender points found in the body can represent expressions of emotional trauma or locked memories (i.e., the somatoemotional component).

The theory of Jin Shin Do states that various stimuli cause energy to accumulate in acupuncture points. Repeated stress in turn causes a layering of tension at the point, known as *armoring*. The most painful point is termed the *local point* as a frame of reference. Other related tender points are referred to as *distal points*. Deep pressure applied to the point ultimately causes a release, and the tension dissipates. The overall effect is to reestablish flow in the channel and balance body energy.

During the treatment session the operator identifies a local point and asks permission nonverbally to treat it. A finger is placed on the local point while another finger is applied to a distal point. Gradually increasing pressure is applied to the local point. After 1 or 2 minutes the operator feels the muscle relaxing, followed by a pulsation (practitioners of craniosacral therapy refer to this phenomenon as the "therapeutic pulse"). When the pulsing stops, the patient usually reports a decreased sensitivity at the point, indicating a successful treatment.

Myofascial releases are sometimes accompanied by emotional releases as painful memories are brought to consciousness. The context of the Jin Shin Do treatment is as much psychological as physical and reiterates the importance of the body-mind-spirit philosophy of this treatment form.

Shiatsu (Zen Shiatsu)

Shiatsu means "finger pressure" in Japanese. It originally developed as a synthesis of acupuncture and Anma, traditional Japanese massage. During the eighteenth and nineteenth centuries, Anma became more associated with carnal pleasure and subsequently lost its place as a therapeutic practice. Shiatsu further diverged and became systematized in the twentieth century, with the Nippon Shiatsu School opening in the 1940s.

As with other Asian-derived systems, shiatsu employs the meridian or channel concept of the human body. The points along the channels are referred to as *tsubos* (Japanese for "vase"). Shiatsu theory states that when a channel becomes blocked, the tsubos along it can express a "kyo" state (weak energy, low vibration, cold, open) or a "jitsu" state (strong energy, high vibration, heat, closed). The hands are used for three purposes: to diagnose, to treat, and for maintenance (to strengthen the newly attained balance).

During a shiatsu treatment the practitioner (or "giver") uses acupressure to open or close jitsu or kyo tsubos, respectively. The technique is applied with the thumb, elbow, or knee, perpendicular to the skin of the "receiver." The body part used by the practitioner and the duration of application depend on the state of the tsubo. Acupressure is combined systematically with passive stretching and rotation of the joints to stimulate flow of *ki* through the channels. Treatments are described for the whole body (basic) and for each of the 12 major meridians.

Several issues are raised in observing the Asian styles of manual therapy. The intertwining of body-mind-spirit becomes evident as a holistic method of treatment born of an ancient philosophy. The practitioner-patient (giver-receiver) relationship is one of partnership because each is a participant in the healing process. This is born of the yin-yang principle (giver = yang, receiver = yin). The intention of the practitioner plays a major role in the effectiveness of the treatment; the giver is a nonjudgmental observer or plays an empathetic role. As opposed to the more neutral "do no harm" principle of Western caregivers, there appears to be more of a natural expression of love as a defined part of these systems (see later discussion on reiki). Intuition is also an important part of the treatment because each session is an exploration of the process of healing and of the individuals involved.

Reflexology

In the Asian meridian system of the body, all the major meridians or channels are represented in the hands and feet. Since acupuncture is usually not done on the feet because of their sensitivity, a system of foot massage was developed in China. This system was brought to the United States in 1913 by Fitzgerald, who called it "zone therapy." Now referred to as *reflexology*, the technique involves deep pressure on various points on the hands and feet (the feet receive the preponderance of attention in this method), applied with the thumbs and fingers of the operator. The various identified points not only correspond to the energy channels of the body, but also to specific organs and systems. When treatment is given, areas of tenderness or texture change are identified and pressure is applied. When treatment is given, areas of tenderness or texture change are identified and pressure is applied. This has the effect of opening that channel and allowing body energy to flow unimpeded through its entirety. When all points are successfully treated, the energy system is flowing and balanced.

TUI NA

Tui na is the manipulative practice within traditional Chinese medicine (TCM). The literal translation is "pushing and grasping." Tui na is more than 4000 years old and predates the manufacture of acupuncture needles. It was the forerunner of shiatsu in Japan. Tui na may be practiced by TCM physicians as part of their general practice, or they may specialize in it, as do members of the osteopathic profession.

As with the other Chinese medical arts, tui na is based on the meridian or channel view of the human body, the yin-yang principle, and the five elements theory. The organs of the body exist not only as anatomical structures, but also in a functional context (e.g., the "triple burner"), as well as in relation to one another. Yin and yang, as opposite forces, coexist in equilibrium with one another. Of the 12 major meridians of the body that correspond to the organs, six are yin, the others yang.

Chi, or vital energy, is a universal force that permeates everything. It is manifest as five separate elements: fire, wood, metal, water, and earth; the organs of the body are categorized accordingly. Chi (or qi) flows through all the meridians once each day in 2-hour cycles. Therefore each meridian, and thus its associated organ, has its daily strong and weak periods. When the flow of chi is impeded in any channel, that organ/function may become dysfunctional, resulting in disease.

Tui na can be applied to virtually anyone and has few contraindications. The existing contraindications are similar to those for massage, including skin lesions or infection, skin or lymphatic cancer, and osteoporosis. In addition, it is recommended that the low back and abdomen be avoided during pregnancy.

Anatomically, tui na is applied to the musculoskeletal system and viscera, with attention being paid to the meridians and flow of chi (as specific meridians flow through specific joints, muscle groups, and visceral structures). As with other forms of manipulative treatment, tui na seeks to produce a feeling of well-being and health in the patient. In addition, as the emotional and spiritual components of the patient are addressed, emotional release can also be produced.

The techniques of tui na combine soft tissue, visceral, and joint manipulation. Typically, the patient is lying on a table or is seated. Soft tissue techniques, which are applied to the limbs, trunk and head, precede joint mobilization to prepare the joint for movement and to relax the surrounding musculature. The techniques are designed to stimulate local blood flow, venous and lymphatic drainage, and the flow of chi (see previous discussion on shiatsu). These soft tissue techniques include the following:

- *Pressing,* using the thumbs elbows or palms
- *Squeezing,* using the whole hand, or finger-thumb combination
- *Kneading,* a circular pressing technique, using the thumbs, heel of the hand, elbow, or forearm
- *Rubbing,* a high frequency technique, using the palms, heels of the hands (chafing) or forearms
- *Stroking* (see effleurage), moving the hand over the skin in a long stroke, in one direction only
- *Vibration,* similar to that used in massage
- *Thumb rocking,* for deep penetration of acupuncture points
- *Plucking,* a transverse friction type of technique (see Cyriax) applying deep pressure with the palm of the hand to the thumb of the opposite hand and moving across individual muscles or muscle groups
- *Rolling,* using the back of the hand to roll over the skin and underlying tissue
- *Percussion* (see tapotement), which includes pummeling with the fists, hacking with the heels of the hands, and cupping the hands

Included in the joint manipulative techniques are the following:

- *Shaking,* where traction is applied to the limb and it is shaken with low amplitude movements (HVLA) from 10 to 20 times
- *Flexion/extension,* primarily applied to the elbow and knee joints (i.e., the hinge joints). These are both high and low velocity techniques designed to engage a motion barrier but not to challenge it. In addition, in some of these techniques a thumb is simultaneously applied to an acupuncture point to open a meridian.
- *Rotation,* an articulatory technique used for the ankles, wrists, hips, and shoulders. Practitioners of tui na do not apply this technique to the neck.

- *Pushing and pulling*, a low velocity technique designed to directly engage a motion barrier. A counterforce is applied by the opposing hand in the opposite direction.
- *Stretching*, a general, low velocity flexion-extension technique used to loosen the joints of the spine.
- *Thrust*, used in a similar manner as with osteopathic and chiropractic methods on the spinal joints.

AYURVEDIC MANIPULATION

In Sanskrit, *Ayurveda* means "the study of life." As a healing art, Ayurveda is one of the world's oldest and, like the Indian culture, probably predates TCM. As with TCM, Ayurveda has many concepts and components, as discussed in Chapters 25 to 27. However, several principles pervade Ayurveda (as does TCM) and apply to the manual component of Ayurvedic treatment.

Both Ayurvedic and Chinese theory present five basic elements. In contrast to those of Chinese theory (fire, water, earth, wood, metal), however, Ayurveda defines space (ether), air, fire, water, and earth as the five basic elements. These elements flow through the body with one or more predominating in certain areas, corresponding to specific organs, emotions, and other categories. *Prana*, or the life force (qi, ki), also flows through the body, permeating the organs and tissues, and is especially concentrated at various points along the midline of the body, known as *chakras*.

The unity and balance of body, mind, and spirit have deep cultural roots in Ayurveda. Body structure and a person's actions, feelings, and beliefs all reflect his or her constitution. The human constitution is based on the relative proportions and strengths of these three constituents (mind, body, spirit) and the five elements. Three basic types of constitutions (*doshas*) are recognized, which are based on different combinations of the five elements. The first, *vata*, is a combination of air and space and is reflected in kinetic energy. The second, *pitta*, combines fire and water and reflects a balance between kinetic and potential (stored) energy, which is expressed in the third constitution, *kapha*, a combination of earth and water.

The manipulative treatment developed within the Ayurvedic tradition offers three types of touch. *Tamasic* is strong and solid, firmly rooted in the earth (and might be well suited for a kapha constitution). The application is fast, and time is needed for the mind and spirit to "catch up." Tamasic might correspond to HVLA technique (osteopathy, chiropractic), tapotement (massage), or rubbing and thumb rocking (TCM). The second type of touch, *rajasic*, is slower and is used to expand and integrate initial manual explorations and findings. It is more in resonance with the mind and spirit. As mentioned earlier, greater depth can be achieved with less tissue resistance due to the makeup of the body fascia. Effleurage (massage) and myofascial release (osteopathy) might correspond with this type of touch, which in turn might be more suited to a pitta constitution. The vata constitution might benefit from the third type of touch, *satvic*, where the application is very slow and gentle and can follow the intention of the mind and spirit. This might correspond to cranial osteopathy, SOT (chiropractic), counterstrain (osteopathy), Trager work, Feldenkrais, or healing/therapeutic touch.

In a massage-oriented treatment, different oils are used as lubricants according to the constitution of the individual and the problem to be treated. The patient is prone or supine, lying on either side, or sitting up, with the positions arranged in a specific sequence. Strokes are applied either toward or away from the heart, also in a specific sequence. Another technique, which is rarely encountered, uses the feet to perform the manipulation. The operator stands above the patient, who is lying prone on a reed mat, and applies the technique with his feet. Oils again are used as lubricants, and to maintain balance, the operator holds onto a cord strung lengthwise above the patient. The strokes go from the sacrum up the spine and out to the fingers, then back down to the feet. One side is done, then the other. The patient then lies supine, and the process is repeated.

Techniques can be direct or indirect relative to motion barriers. They can also be active or passive. Both the patient and the practitioner act as partners during treatment, exploring tissue and motion in an attempt to unlock the body and restore the unimpeded flow of prana and constitutional balance. Visualization, nonverbal communication, and mind intent are elements of treatment, regardless of the technique employed.

ENERGY WORK

Energy work refers to the techniques that have developed either as part of ancient traditions (e.g., qi gong,

QiGong), or as recently "discovered" methods in which the operator manipulates the bioenergy of the patient. The theory of bioenergy basically states that a life force, or vital energy, permeates the entire universe. This energy flows through all living things in distinct patterns. These patterns of flow are reflected in the meridian system (where *qi*, or *chi*, is the name of the life force) originally conceived by the Chinese and the chakra system of Hindu tradition (where the word *prana* is used to indicate this force). Various forms of exercise have been developed for the cultivation of bioenergy, including yoga, internal QiGong, and t'ai chi.

Three basic concepts are important in understanding energy work: intent, cooperation, and the tripartite nature of the human. *Intent* is important in that the practitioner projects his or her mind intent to heal into the patient. As such, that intent must go one step further than the "do no harm" doctrine of Western therapeutics to an attitude of love and concern. Intent also assumes a high level of visualization. *Cooperation* implies the partnership between the practitioner and patient as participants in the healing process, with neither being exclusively active or passive. The *tripartite concept* refers to the acceptance of three parts of the human: body, mind, and spirit. This concept is imbued in the much older Asian cultures as to go beyond religion, whereas Western cultures rely on belief systems driven by faith. In addition, the "scientific," reductionist approach to conventional Western medicine is rather dismissive of spiritual aspects and has only recently acknowledged the mind-body connection.

QiGong (China)

The term *qi gong* (or qigong, Qigong, QiGong) refers to the manipulation of bioenergy and loosely translated means "chi work." QiGong can be internal, where an individual can strengthen and balance the flow of chi within the self, or external, where a trained practitioner can project his or her chi into a patient to induce a therapeutic effect.

Although the vast majority of the vital energy of an organism is contained within the body, some of it radiates off the skin, the "aura," which has been visualized using Kirlian photography. The qigong practitioner is able to palpate the meridian system through this aura, locate points of blockage, and free these blockages by projecting his or her qi into the patient,

using intent and visualization. As in Trager work, Feldenkrais, and yoga, specific "external QiGong" exercises have been developed, which, when performed by an individual, serve to cultivate qi within the self. QiGong is also a natural result of long-term "internal" martial arts training, in which practitioners are capable of seemingly superhuman feats of strength and balance.

Reiki

Reiki (literally "universal energy") was "rediscovered" by Dr. Mikao Usui in the mid-nineteenth century. Usui was interested in determining the nature of spiritually oriented healing power, as expressed through such individuals as Jesus Christ and the Gautama Buddha. After much study, including a doctorate from the University of Chicago, he began an extended period of fasting and meditation. At the end of this period, he reportedly received a vision and the ability to channel "reiki" through his body to effect healing in others. From that point, he continued healing, eventually training others in his method. Usui handed the title of Grand Master to Dr. Hiyashi Chugiro, who in turn passed it to Hawayo Takata, a Hawaiian woman of Japanese descent. In this way, reiki was exported from Japan to the West.

For practitioners, reiki must be "received" from a master or teacher. Only then is an individual able to effect healing. There are three degrees of reiki training. The first-degree practitioner is capable of giving a basic treatment with the hands on the patient, or about 1 inch away from the skin if touching is not possible. The second-degree practitioner can effect healing with the hands removed from the body (see QiGong), and treatments can be given at a faster rate. The third-degree practitioner is referred to as a "master" and is qualified to teach reiki.

The five principles of reiki are as follows:

1. Today I give thanks for my many blessings.
2. Just for today, I will not worry.
3. Today I will not be angry.
4. Today I will do my work honestly.
5. Today I will be kind to my neighbor and to every living thing.

The objective of reiki treatment is to restore internal harmony to the body and to release any blockages, which may be physical or emotional.

During a reiki treatment the hands of the practitioner are placed with the fingers together on the patient. As energy is transferred from giver to receiver, the hands and the area treated become warm, indicating a release of tension in the area and an increase in the blood flow. The head of the patient is treated first (four locations or positions), followed by the front (five positions) and back of the body (five positions). Each position is held for 8 to 10 minutes (or less, if the practitioner is above first degree). Problem areas may be "held" longer until a result is sensed. The hand positions correspond to the energy points or chakras, identified in Hindu tradition, as well as other points. The treatment is completed with a series of general myofascial techniques, including kneading, counterforce, and stroking (effleurage), to close the energy channels.

As with other energy-oriented manipulative techniques, reiki requires significant verbal and nonverbal communication between the giver and receiver, who act in partnership. Permission must be granted both consciously and subconsciously for healing to be successful. Somatoemotional release is quite possible in this treatment.

From a historical and practical standpoint, the reiki method likely was originally derived from QiGong as practiced by the Chinese Taoists and Buddhists. It probably disappeared from practice in Japan at some point, only to be rediscovered by Usui, hundreds of years later.

Therapeutic Touch and Healing Touch

Therapeutic touch was developed by Dr. Dolores Krieger and Dora Kunz in the late 1960s and early 1970s. In this style of bodywork, energy is directed through the hands (either on or off the body, usually off) of the "giver" to activate the healing process of the "receiver." The therapist essentially acts as a support system to facilitate the process. Therapeutic touch treatments typically last 20 to 25 minutes and are accompanied by a relaxation response and a decrease in perceived pain. Although skeptics have claimed that this technique merely elicits a placebo effect (an interesting concept in itself), successes have been reported with comatose patients, patients under anesthesia, and premature infants.

Therapeutic touch posits that humans are open energy systems, that we are bilaterally symmetrical (see earlier discussion), and that illness is the result of an imbalance in the patient's energy field. The healer places himself or herself between the patient's illness and the patient's energy field to affect the healing process. The receiver must accept the energy of the healer and the necessity of change for the healing to occur. This should happen both consciously and subconsciously.

There are two phases of the treatment: assessment and balancing. Before balancing the practitioner "centers" himself or herself, entering a state of relaxation and awareness. The hands are moved around the patient's body at a distance of 2 to 3 inches. The patient's energy field is encountered and assessed by feeling for changes in temperature, pressure, rhythm, or a tingling sensation. Simultaneously, the practitioner nonverbally requests the permission of the patient to enter the patient's field and effect a change. During the balancing phase the healer (sometimes referred to as the "sender") then attempts to bring the two energy fields into a harmonic resonance through intent and visualization.

The attitude of the sender is one of empathy and compassion. The intent of the treatment is to facilitate the flow of vital energy, to stimulate it, to dissipate areas of congestion, and to dampen any areas of increased activity. In addition, the concept of rhythm and vibration is used, with color observed as a product of different frequencies within the field. At the beginning of the treatment, at the end of the treatment, or at both times, the practitioner "smoothes" out the patient's energy field by running the hands from head to toe. This sometimes has a cooling effect and is referred to as *unruffling*.

Healing touch, as developed by Barbara Brennan, is similar to therapeutic touch in that the healer seeks to balance the energy field of the patient. A specific sequence of techniques is used in which the healer encounters, assesses, and treats different layers of the patient's visible "aura," correcting any imbalances and smoothing out the field. Healing touch is somewhat more spiritually oriented that therapeutic touch, using techniques such as channeling, and uses colors and crystals to assist in the process.

The successful application of these "energy-based" techniques (in addition to many of the other styles mentioned) underscores the importance of psychoemotional cooperation and participation by the patient (i.e., the mind-body connection). In addition, the mind intent of the manipulator comes into play as the director of his or her internal energy outward and into the patient. This concept is quite controversial by Western standards of scientific analysis.

Although critics refer to these and other manipulative techniques as "pseudoscience" because of a lack of supportive evidence, clinical outcomes studies have indicated that the intent of both the patient and the clinician has a demonstrable effect in determining treatment outcome. This evidence sheds new and interesting light on the placebo effect as a real phenomenon (especially in light of the fact that placebos are "effective" in randomized drug trials about 30% of the time). It also indicates that treatment of the somatic component of disease can be approached effectively through acknowledgment of the "three-legged stool" model of the human: body, mind, and spirit.

CONCLUSION

In closing, it is important to note the preventive aspect of manipulation as a holistic practice. Manipulative treatment can be used for proactive general maintenance as well as for reactive treatment of dysfunction. I like to use the automobile analogy in describing how we as Americans think nothing of periodically getting our cars tuned up and paying considerable sums for the privilege. Why don't we do the same for our own bodies? In addition, the concept of manual treatment for young persons cannot be overstated. Structural corrections can be made before fascial distortions become relatively locked in or before continuous aberrant sensory input results in facilitated sensorimotor patterning. Corrections can be made before compensatory reactions in muscles, fascia, and behavior can create unbalanced anatomy and physiology that function poorly and eventually lead to a decreased resistance to disease (pathology). As Alexander Pope once proclaimed, "Just as the twig is bent, the tree's inclined."

Suggested Readings and Resources
Osteopathic Medicine

Books

Fulford RC, Stone, G: *Dr. Fuller's touch of life: the healing power of the natural life force,* New York, 1997, Simon & Schuster. (Appropriate for general reading.)

Gevitz N: *The D.O.s: osteopathic medicine in America,* ed 2, Baltimore, 2004, Johns Hopkins University Press. (Appropriate for general reading.)

Associations

American Osteopathic Association
142 East Ontario St
Chicago, IL 60611
Phone: 800-621 1773
www.DO-Online.org (for health industry professionals)
www.Osteopathic.org (for patients, consumers, and media)

American Association of Colleges of Osteopathic Medicine
5550 Friendship Blvd, Suite 310
Chevy Chase MD 20815-7231
http://www.aacom.org

American Academy of Osteopathy
3500 DePauw Blvd, Suite 1080
Indianapolis, IN 46268
http://www.academyofosteopathy.org

Chiropractic

Books and Journal

McGill L: *The chiropractor's health book: simple, natural exercises for relieving headaches, tension, and back pain,* New York, 1997, Crown Publishing Group. (Appropriate for general and professional reading.)

Redwood D, Cleveland C: *Fundamentals of chiropractic,* St. Louis 2003, Mosby. (Appropriate for general and professional reading.)

Rondberg TA: *Chiropractic first: the fastest growing healthcare choice . . . before drugs or surgery,* 1996, World Chiropractic Alliance. (Appropriate for general reading.)

Journal of Manipulative and Physiologic Therapeutics
www.mosby.com/jmpt/

Associations
American Chiropractic Association
1701 Clarendon Blvd
Arlington, VA 22209
Phone: 800-986-4636
http://www.amerchiro.org
E-mail: memberinfo@amerchiro.org

World Federation of Chiropractic
1246 Yonge St, Suite 202/203
Toronto, Ontario, Canada, M4T 1W5
http://www.wfc.org
E-mail: info@wfc.org

International Chiropractors Association
1110 North Glebe Rd, Suite 1000
Arlington, VA 22201
Phone: 800-423 4690
Fax: 703-528 5023
http://www.chiropractic.org
E-mail: chiro@chiropractic.org

Canadian Chiropractic Association
1396 Eglinton Ave, West
Toronto, Ontario, Canada, M6C 2E4
http://www.ccachiro.org
Email: ccachiro@ccachiro.org

The Foundation for Chiropractic Education and Research
PO Box 400
Norwalk, IA 50211-0400
Phone: 800-622-6309
http://www.fcer.org
E-mail: FCER@fcer.org

Massage
Books and Journal
Fritz S: *Mosby's fundamentals of therapeutic massage,* ed 3, St Louis, 2005, Mosby. (Appropriate for therapeutic massage students and practitioners.)
Tappan FM, Benjamin PJ: *Tappan's handbook of healing massage techniques: classic, holistic, and emerging methods,* Norwalk, Conn, 1997, Appleton & Lange. (Appropriate for general and professional reading.)
Journal of Bodywork and Movement Therapies
Elsevier Journals Customer Service
6277 Sea Harbor Dr
Orlando, FL 32887
Phone: 877-839-7126
http://www.harcourt-international.com/journals/jbmt
E-mail: usjcs@elsevier.com

Associations
American Massage Therapy Association
820 Davis St
Evanston, IL 60201
Phone: 847-864-0123
http://www.amtamassage.org
E-mail: info@amtamassage.org

Touch Research Institutes
University of Miami School of Medicine
PO Box 016820
Miami FL 33101
http://www.miami.edu/touch-research/
This is the premiere center for massage research in the world. It is directed by Tiffany Field, LMT, PhD, who has been featured in many publications and media.

Neuromsuscular Therapy
Book
Chaitow L: *Modern neuromuscular techniques,* ed 2, New York, 2002, Churchill Livingstone.

Association
American Version NMT
NMT Center
Judith Delany, Director
900 14th Ave North
St Petersburg, FL 33705
E-mail: nmtcenter@aol.com

Shiatsu
Books
Liechti E: *The complete illustrated guide to shiatsu: the Japanese healing art of touch for health and fitness,* Rockport, Mass, 1998, Element Books. (Appropriate for general and professional reading.)
Lundberg P, Dorelli F (photographer): *The book of shiatsu,* New York, 1992, Simon & Schuster. (Appropriate for general reading.)

Association
American Association for Bodywork Therapies of Asia
1010 Haddonfield-Berlin Rd, Suite 408
Voorhees, NJ 08043-3514
http://www.aobta.org
E-mail: office@aobta.org

Trager Work
Books
Liskin J: *Moving medicine: the life work of Milton Trager, M.D.,* Barrytown, NY, 1995, Station Hill Press. (Appropriate for general reading.)
Trager M, Hammond C: *Movement as a way to agelessness: a guide to Trager mentastics,* Barrytown, NY, 1994, Station Hill Press. (Appropriate for general reading.)

Associations
United States Trager Association (USTA)
http://www.trager-us.org

Trager International
21 Locust Ave
Mill Valley, CA 94941
www.trager.com
E-mail: trager@trager.com
This is the official designation and website of the Trager Institute.

Feldenkrais
Books
Feldenkrais M: *Awareness through movement: easy-to-do health exercises to improve your posture, vision, imagination, and personal growth,* San Francisco, 1991, Harper San Francisco. (Appropriate for general and professional reading.)
Rywerant Y, Mohor D (illustrator): *The Feldenkrais method,* New Canaan, Conn, 1991, Keats Publishing (foreword by Moshe Feldenkrais, preface by Thomas Hanna). (Appropriate for general and professional reading.)

Associations

Feldenkrais Guild of North America
3611 SW Hood Ave, Suite 100
Portland, OR 97239
Phone: 800-775-2118
http://www.feldenkraisguild. com/trainings/index.lasso

The International Feldenkrais Federation (IFF)
http://www.peak.org/~iff
E-mail: info@feldenkrais-method.org

Structural Integration (Rolfing)

Books
Rolf IP: *What in the world is rolfing?* 1975, Dennis-Landman Publishers. (Appropriate for general reading.)
Rolf IP: *The integration of human structures,* 1997, Dennis-Landman Publishers. (Appropriate for general reading.)
Rolf IP, Thompson R: *Rolfing: reestablishing the natural alignment & structural integration of the human body for vitality and well-being,* Rochester, Vt, 1989, Inner Traditions International. (Appropriate for general and professional reading.)

Associations
The Rolf Institute of Structural Integration
5055 Chaparral St
Boulder, CO 80301
Phone: 800-530-8875
www.rolf.org
This is the principal Rolf educational institution in the United States, responsible for the education and certification of practitioners of Rolfing. The web site is also an excellent information source for structural integration.

Acupressure and Jin Shin Do

Book
Teeguard I: *Acupressure way of health: Jin Shin Do,* 1978, Japan Publications (USA). (Appropriate for general and professional reading.)

Association
Jin Shin Do Foundation of Bodymind Acupressure
PO Box 416
Idyllwild, CA 92549
Phone/Fax: 951-659-5707
www.jinshindo.org
Good clearinghouse site for information and referrals.

Reflexology

Books
Dougan I, Townley A (editor), Allen P (illustrator), Ryecart G (photographer): *The complete illustrated guide to reflexology: therapeutic foot massage for health and well-being,* Lanham, Md, 1999, Barnes & Noble Books. (Appropriate for general reading.)

Wills P, Atkinson S (photographer): *The reflexology manual: an easy-to-use illustrated guide to healing zones of the hands & feet,* Rochester, Vt, 1995, Inner Traditions International. (Appropriate for general and professional reading.)

Association
Association of Reflexologists
27 Old Gloucester St
London, WC1N 3XX, England
E-mail: info@aor.org.uk
http://www.aor.org.uk
http://www.reflexology.org
Information site linked to the Association of Reflexologists (above)

Tui Na

Book
Pritchard SM: *Chinese massage manual: the healing art of tui na,* Bulverde, Tx, 1999, Omni Publishers (Sterling Publishing) (foreword by Wang Jianmin). (Appropriate for general and professional reading.)

Resource
http://www.acupuncture. com/TuiNa/TuinaInd.htm
Good links to general references on Chinese medicine.

Ayurvedic Manipulation

Books
Dash VB, Dash B: *Massage therapy in AyurVeda,* 1992, Concept Publishing. (Appropriate for general and professional reading.)
Govindan SV: *Massage for health and healing: AyurVedic and spiritual energy approach,* 1996, South Asia Books. (Appropriate for general reading.)
Johari H: *Ayurvedic massage: traditional Indian techniques for balancing body and mind,* Rochester, Vt, 1995, Inner Traditions International. (Appropriate for general and professional reading.)

Association
National Institute of Ayurvedic Medicine
584 Milltown Rd
Brewster, NY 10509
http://niam.com/corp-web/index.htm
An organization headed by Scott Gerson, MD, PhD. The site contains good information on Ayurvedic medicine in general and refers to manipulation as part of holistic treatment.

Qigong

Books
Liu H, Perry P: *Mastering miracles: the healing art of qi gong as taught by a master,* 1996, Brilliance Corporation. (Appropriate for general reading.)
Wang S, Liu JL: *Qi gong for health and longevity: the ancient Chinese art of relaxation, meditation, physical fitness,* 1999,

East Health Development Group. (Appropriate for general and professional reading.)

Associations
QiGong Association of America
http://www.qi.org/
Good site for general information on QiGong

QiGong Research Society
3201 Route 38, Suite 201
Mount Laurel, NJ 08054
http://www.qigongresearchsociety.com/
This site of QiGong Master Hou Faxiang contains general information on the practice of QiGong.

Reiki

Books
Lubeck W: *The complete reiki handbook: basic introduction and methods of natural application,* Twin Lakes, Wis, 1998, Lotus Light Publications. (Appropriate for professional reading.)
Rand WL, Martin SA (editor), Matsko SM (illustrator): *Reiki: the healing touch,* 1996, Vision Publications. (Appropriate for general reading.)
Stein D: *Essential reiki: a complete guide to an ancient healing art,* Freedom, Calif, 1995, Crossing Press. (Appropriate for general and professional reading.)

Associations and Resources
The International Center for Reiki Training
21421 Hilltop St, Unit #28
Southfield, MI 48034
E-mail: center@reiki.org
http://www.reiki.org

Reiki the World
http://shell.world-net. co.nz/~jimgould/rtw/
Clearinghouse site with discussion forums and general information.

The Reiki Alliance
PO Box 41
Cataldo, ID 83810
http://www.reikialliance.com/
This site contains general information as well as a reiki master locator.

Therapeutic Touch and Healing Touch

Books
Brennan BA, Smith JA (illustrator): *Hands of light: a guide to healing through the human energy field,* New York, 1988, Bantam Doubleday Dell Publishing Group. (Appropriate for general and professional reading.)
Juhan D: *Job's body: a handbook for bodywork,* 1998, Barrytown, Ltd (foreword by Ken Dychtwald). (Appropriate for general and professional reading.)
Krieger DK: *The therapeutic touch: how to use your hands to help or to heal,* New York, 1992, Simon & Schuster. (Appropriate for general and professional reading.)

Association and Resource
Healing Touch International
12477 West Cedar Dr, Suite 202
Lakewood, CO 80288
http://www.healingtouch.net
This organization offers a certificate program, and the site contains a referral directory of certified practitioners.

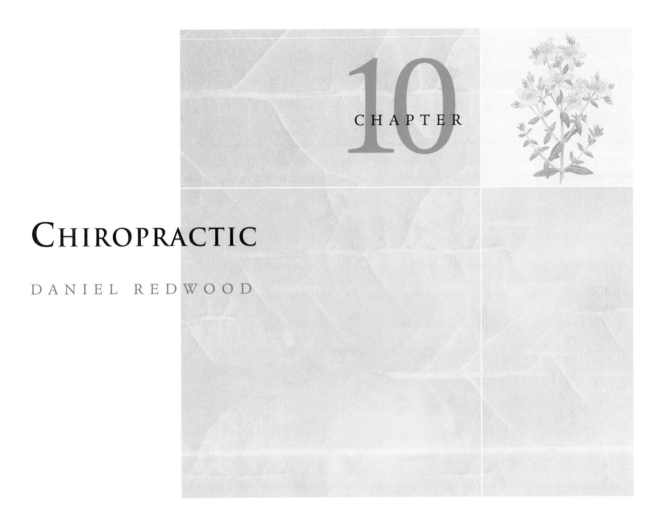

CHAPTER 10

CHIROPRACTIC

DANIEL REDWOOD

orn in the American Midwest in the late nineteenth century, chiropractic has evolved and matured toward mainstream status while largely preserving its essential principles. The contemporary chiropractic profession is in the unique position of having scaled many walls of the health care establishment (with licensure, an increasingly strong scientific research base, widespread insurance coverage, and approximately 30 million patients per year in the United States), while at the same time maintaining strong roots in the complementary and integrative medicine (CIM) community, with a philosophy that emphasizes healing without drugs.

Chiropractic is the third largest independent health profession in the Western world, following conventional (allopathic) medicine and dentistry. Its

practitioners are "portal of entry" providers, licensed for both diagnosis and treatment. Unlike dentistry, podiatry, and optometry, chiropractic practice is limited not by anatomical region but by procedure. The chiropractor's scope of practice excludes surgery and the prescription of pharmaceuticals; its centerpiece is the manual adjustment or manipulation of the spine.

The United States is home to approximately 65,000 of the world's 90,000 chiropractors (Chapman-Smith, 2000). Chiropractors are licensed throughout the English-speaking world and in an increasing number of other nations (Box 10-1). Rigorous educational standards are supervised by government-recognized accrediting agencies, including the Council on Chiropractic Education (CCE) in the United States. After fulfilling college science prerequisites analogous to

BOX 10-1

*Countries Where Chiropractors Are Recognized by National Health Authorities**

African Region	Guam[a]	Colombia[b]	Portugal[c]
Botswana[a]	New Caledonia[b]	Costa Rica[b]	Russian Federation[b]
Ethiopia[b]	New Zealand[a]	Ecuador[b]	Slovakia[b]
Kenya[b]	Papua New Guinea[b]	Guatemala[b]	Sweden[a]
Lesotho[a]		Honduras[b]	Switzerland[a]
Mauritius[b]	*Eastern Mediterranean*	Mexico[a]	
Namibia[a]	*Region*	Panama[a]	*North American Region*
Nigeria[a]	Cyprus[a]	Peru[b]	Bahamas[b]
South Africa[a]	Egypt[b]	Venezuela[b]	Barbados[a]
Swaziland[a]	Greece[b]		Belize[b]
Zimbabwe[a]	Israel[b]	*European Region*	Bermuda[b]
	Jordan[b]	Belgium[a]	British Virgin Islands[b]
Asian Region	Lebanon[b]	Croatia[b]	Canada[a]
China/Hong Kong[a]	Libya[b]	Denmark[a]	Cayman Islands[b]
Japan[b]	Morocco[b]	England[a]	Jamaica[b]
Malaysia[b]	Qatar[b]	Finland[a]	Leeward Islands[a]
Philippines[a]	Saudi Arabia[a]	Germany[b]	Puerto Rico[a]
Singapore[b]	Turkey[b]	Hungary[b]	Trinidad and Tobago[b]
Taiwan[b]	United Arab Emirates[b]	Iceland[a]	United States[a]
Thailand[c]		Ireland[b]	US Virgin Islands[b]
	Latin American Region	Italy[c]	
Pacific Region	Argentina[b]	Liechtenstein[a]	
Australia[a]	Brazil[b]	Netherlands[b]	
Fiji[b]	Chile[b]	Norway[a]	

From Chapman-Smith DA: *The chiropractic profession,* West Des Moines, Iowa, 2000, NCMIC Group, p 25.
*Listed according to the seven world regions adopted by the World Federation of Chiropractic. In most other countries, there are no chiropractors in practice, and national health authorities have not considered recognition or lack of recognition.
[a]Recognized pursuant to legislation.
[b]Recognized pursuant to general law.
[c]De facto recognition.

those required to enter medical or osteopathic schools, chiropractic students must complete a 4-year chiropractic school program, which includes a wide range of courses in anatomy, physiology, pathology, and diagnosis, as well as spinal adjusting, physical therapy, rehabilitation, and nutrition.

As noted by Meeker and Haldeman (2002), utilization of chiropractic in the United States has tripled, from about 3.6% (von Kuster, 1980) to an estimated 11%, according to a 1997 national random telephone survey (Eisenberg et al., 1998). American chiropractors log approximately 190 million patient visits per year, or about 30% of visits to all CIM practitioners. Almost 90% of chiropractic patients present as neuromusculoskeletal cases (Plamondon, 1995), principally back pain, neck pain, and headaches, the conditions for which spinal adjustment (also known

as spinal manipulation) is most effective. As described later, current chiropractic research seeks to define further the role of adjustment/manipulation in the management of various musculoskeletal conditions, as well as to evaluate its effectiveness for visceral organ disorders, including infantile colic, otitis media, dysmenorrhea, hypertension, and asthma.

In 1998 the National Institutes of Health (NIH) founded the Consortial Center for Chiropractic Research (CCCR) under the auspices of the National Center for Complementary and Alternative Medicine and the National Institute of Arthritis and Musculoskeletal and Skin Diseases. Based at the Palmer Center for Chiropractic Research in Davenport, Iowa, by 2003 CCCR had involved 13 chiropractic institutions and universities in 20 basic and clinical science projects and other efforts. CCCR's mission is to support a multidisciplinary group of researchers and clinicians to perform basic, preclinical, clinical, epidemiological, and health services research on chiropractic. It also aims to develop an environment for training future scientists and to encourage collaboration between basic and clinical scientists, as well as between the chiropractic and conventional medical communities. (For further information, see the CCCR website at www.c3r.org.)

HISTORICAL ROOTS, EVOLUTIONARY PROCESS

Precursors in Western Traditions

Spinal manipulation has been practiced for millennia in cultures throughout the world. Chiropractic's forebears have included prominent figures in the history of medicine.

Hippocrates was an early practitioner of spinal manipulation (Withington, 1959), and according to some scholars, he used manipulation "not only to reposition vertebrae, but also thereby to cure a wide variety of dysfunctions" (Leach, 1994). Galen, a Greek-born Roman physician who lived in the second century AD, and whose approach to healing set the officially recognized standard in Western medicine for 1500 years after his death, also used spinal manipulation and reported the successful resolution of a patient's hand weakness and numbness through manipulation of the seventh cervical vertebra (Lomax, 1975).

As Europe endured the Dark Ages, these healing traditions were preserved in the learning centers of the Middle East by the ascendant Arabic civilization. Later, this body of knowledge returned to Europe, and the works of Hippocrates and Galen helped form the foundations of Renaissance medicine. Ambroise Paré, sometimes called the "father of surgery," used manipulation to treat French vineyard workers in the sixteenth century (Lomax, 1975; Paré, 1968).

In the centuries that followed, up to the dawn of the modern era, manipulative techniques were passed down from generation to generation within families. These "bonesetting" methods, transmitted not only from father to son but often from mother to daughter, played an important role in the history of nonmedical healing in Great Britain, and similar methods are common in the folk medicine of many nations (Bennett, 1981).

In the second half of the nineteenth century, the United States was a vibrant center of natural healing theory and practice. Two manipulation-based healing arts, osteopathy and chiropractic, trace their origins to that era. Both began in the American Midwest.

Beginnings of a New Profession

Daniel David Palmer, a self-educated healer in the Mississippi River town of Davenport, Iowa, founded the chiropractic profession in 1895 with two fundamental premises: (1) the vertebral subluxation* (spinal misalignment causing abnormal nerve transmission) is the primary cause of virtually all disease, and (2) chiropractic adjustment (manual manipulation of the subluxated vertebra) is its cure (Palmer, 1910). This "one cause–one cure" philosophy played a central role in chiropractic history, first as a guiding principle, then later as a historical remnant, providing a target for the slings and arrows of organized medicine (Figure 10-1).

Although few if any contemporary chiropractors would endorse such a simplistic and all-encompassing formulation, it nonetheless remains true that the *raison d'être* of the chiropractic profession is the detection and correction of spinal subluxations. Chiropractors may do much more, but it is their ability to do this one thing well that has allowed the chiropractic art to survive for a century under a barrage of medical opposition, some of it justified, most of it not.

The one cause–one cure adherents among the early chiropractors had two major political effects on the development of the profession. First, their deep faith in the truth of their message, combined with the positive results of chiropractic adjustments, created a strong and steadily growing activist constituency of chiropractic patients and supporters. In their zeal, they generated a grassroots movement that ensured the survival of the profession through stormy years in the first half of the twentieth century. Civil disobedience was an integral part of the early development of the chiropractic profession, as it would later become in the American civil rights movement. Hundreds, including the founder himself, went to jail, charged with practicing medicine without a license.

That chiropractic would prove controversial was evident from its inception. In the first chiropractic adjustment the patient sought relief from back pain and attained results that greatly exceeded his

---

*This differs from the medical definition of subluxation, which is an incomplete or partial dislocation according to *Dorland's Illustrated Medical Dictionary*. Palmer's use of the term refers to more subtle malposition with neural involvement.

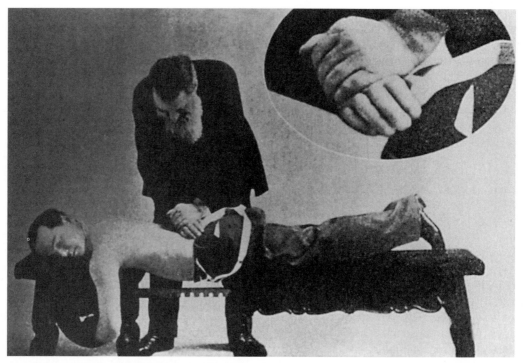

Figure 10-1 Daniel David Palmer, the founder of chiropractic, adjusting a patient (circa 1906). (Courtesy Palmer College of Chiropractic.)

expectations. Harvey Lillard, a deaf janitor in the building where Palmer had an office, came to him bent over with acute back pain. Noting an apparent spinal misalignment in the patient's upper back, Palmer administered the first chiropractic adjustment, after which Lillard is reported to have stood up straight, free of back pain, and able to hear for the first time in many years. This singular event illustrates the two chief symptomatic benefits ascribed to the chiropractic art of healing: (1) relief of musculoskeletal pain and disability, which is now well accepted, and (2) restoration of internal organ function, which remains unresolved.

At first there was hope that Palmer had discovered a cure for deafness, but similar results were not forthcoming when other deaf people sought his assistance. There have been other reports through the years of hearing restored through spinal manipulation, including one by a Canadian orthopedist (Bourdillion, 1982), but these have been rare. The story of Lillard's dramatic recovery has been used to disparage chiropractic, with charges that such an event is impossible, because no spinal nerves supply the ear.

Current knowledge of neurophysiology provides a credible theoretical basis for this and other apparent visceral organ responses to chiropractic adjustments.

The underlying physiological mechanism is the *somatoautonomic* (or *somatovisceral*) *reflex*. Chiropractors and osteopaths assert that signals initiated by spinal adjustment/manipulation are transmitted through autonomic pathways to internal organs. In the case of Palmer's first adjustment, the relevant nerve pathway begins in the thoracic region, coursing up through the neck and into the cranium along sympathetic nerves that eventually lead to the blood vessels of the inner ear. Normal function of the hearing apparatus depends on an adequate blood supply, which in turn depends on a properly functioning sympathetic nerve supply.

A key question is unresolved: why are there sometimes dramatic positive somatovisceral responses to chiropractic adjustments, while most such cases appear to be nonresponsive?

Legacy of Contention: Chiropractic and Allopathic Medicine in the United States

All nascent healing arts face serious challenges, particularly the need to maintain the enthusiasm generated by positive therapeutic results while clearly and consistently distinguishing among the proven, the probable, and the speculative findings. Some of the harshest criticism of chiropractic has been in reaction to the tendency of some chiropractors to "globalize" (Gellert, 1994), making broad, overarching claims on the basis of limited though powerful anecdotal evidence.

Whatever the validity of these medical critiques (some of which mirror intensive self-criticism within the chiropractic profession), the American medical establishment's policy on chiropractic has never been that of a disinterested group solely seeking to serve the public good. Its century-long campaign against chiropractic impeded chiropractic's advancement and at times posed a severe threat to its survival. Until very recently, allopathic medical students were taught that chiropractic is harmful, or at best worthless, and they in turn inculcated these prejudices in their patients.

That such a fiercely antichiropractic policy was pursued by the American Medical Association (AMA) is no longer in dispute. In 1990, the U.S. Supreme Court affirmed a lower court ruling in which the AMA was found liable for antitrust violations for having engaged in a conspiracy to "contain and eliminate" (the AMA's own words) the chiropractic profession (*Wilk v AMA*, 1990). The process that culminated in this landmark decision began in 1974 when a large packet of confidential AMA documents was left anonymously on the doorstep of the International Chiropractors Association's headquarters. As a result of the ensuing *Wilk v AMA* case, the AMA reversed its long-standing ban on interprofessional cooperation between medical doctors and chiropractors, agreed to publish the full findings of the court in the *Journal of the American Medical Association*, and paid an undisclosed sum, most of which was earmarked for chiropractic research.

This has not completely undone the effects of organized medicine's antichiropractic boycott, but it is nonetheless a laudable milestone on the long road toward reconciliation. Although the swords of contention have not yet been beaten into plowshares of amity, the pace of progress has accelerated substantially in the years after the *Wilk* decision, as men and women of goodwill in both professions strive to inaugurate a new era in which their patients are the beneficiaries of their mutual cooperation (Figures 10-2 and 10-3).

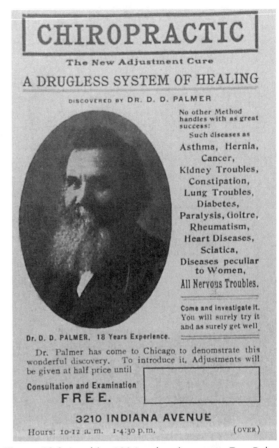

Figure 10-2 In this 1904 advertisement, Dr. Palmer touted chiropractic as a cure for virtually all human ailments. Such claims engendered great controversy. (Courtesy Palmer College of Chiropractic.)

Interprofessional Cooperation

Relations between the medical and chiropractic professions outside the United States have historically also been less than cordial. In certain instances, however, these relations have been sufficiently productive to permit closer collaboration between chiropractors and allopathic physicians. This has had particularly salutary effects in the research arena. Many of the key clinical trials that first established chiropractic's scientific credibility were conducted in Europe and Canada. Gradually, the tide turned in the United States as well. Research projects funded by the federal government have encouraged an atmosphere of growing medical-chiropractic cooperation, and multidisciplinary organizations such as the American Back Society also reflect

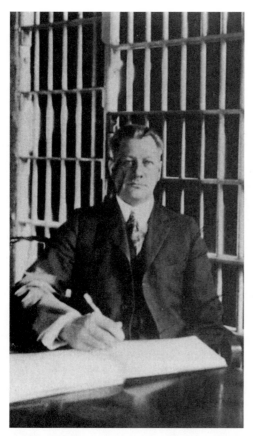

Figure 10-3 **Dr. D.S. Tracy behind bars in Los Angeles. Hundreds of chiropractors served time in jail to secure the right to practice their healing art freely. (Courtesy Palmer College of Chiropractic.)**

a newfound common ground. The recent incorporation of chiropractic into the health care system serving the U.S. military has provided an exceptional opportunity for interprofessional cooperation.

AHCPR Guidelines: Historical Breakthrough

The 1994 Guidelines for Acute Lower Back Pain, developed for the Agency for Health Care Policy and Research (AHCPR) of the U.S. Department of Health and Human Services by a blue-ribbon panel composed primarily of medical physicians and chaired by an orthopedic surgeon (2 of the 23 members were chiropractors), included a powerful endorsement of spinal manipulation (Bigos et al., 1994).

Based on an extensive literature review and consensus process, the AHCPR Guidelines concluded that spinal manipulation "hastens recovery" from acute low back pain (LBP) and recommended it either in combination with or as a replacement for nonsteroidal antiinflammatory drugs (NSAIDs). At the same time, the panel rejected as unsubstantiated numerous methods (including bed rest, traction, and various other physical therapy and pharmaceutical modalities) that for many years constituted the foundation of conventional medicine's approach to acute LBP, while endorsing the use of such self-care measures as exercise, ergonomic seating, and wearing low-heeled shoes. In addition, the panel cautioned against lumbar surgery except in the most severe cases.

Perhaps most significantly, the AHCPR Guidelines stated that spinal manipulation offers both "symptomatic relief" and "functional improvement." Because none of the other recommended nonsurgical interventions offers both, one might reasonably infer that for patients with acute LBP who show none of the guidelines' diagnostic "red flags" (e.g., fractures, tumors, infections, cauda equina syndrome), manipulation is now the treatment of choice.

The release of the AHCPR Guidelines was a landmark event in chiropractic history. Federal standards for the treatment of LBP, the most prevalent musculoskeletal ailment in the United States and the most frequent cause of disability for persons under age 45, now assign a pivotal role to spinal manipulation, of which 94% is provided by chiropractors (Shekelle and Adams, 1991). This may be the quintessential contemporary example of an "alternative" health care method achieving entry into the health care mainstream.

Assessment by government agencies in Canada (Manga et al., 1993), Great Britain (Rosen, 1994), Sweden (Commission on Alternative Medicine, 1987), Denmark (Danish Institute for Health Technology Assessment, 1999), Australia (Thompson, 1986), and New Zealand (Hasselberg, 1979) has brought similar approval of spinal manipulation for LBP.

INTELLECTUAL FOUNDATIONS

The history of chiropractic, as with all healing arts, is largely one in which empirical process has preceded theoretical formulation. From the earliest days, practitioners have applied new treatment methods on an intuitive, empirical basis, noted that some appeared to be more effective than others, and then theorized on the basis of these findings as to the underlying physiological mechanisms. The resultant body of chiropractic theory, philosophy, and practice draws from principles in the common domain shared by all natural healing arts. In addition, it contains unique chiropractic contributions to the cumulative sum and substance of health knowledge.

Common Domain Principles

Fundamental principles of natural healing, which have been part of chiropractic from the beginning and are incorporated into the curricula at chiropractic training institutions, include the following:

1. Humans possess an innate healing potential, an "inner wisdom of the body."
2. Maximally accessing this healing system is the goal of the healing arts.
3. Addressing the cause of an illness should take precedence over suppressing its surface manifestations in most cases.
4. Pharmaceutical suppression of symptoms can sometimes compromise and diminish the body's ability to heal itself.
5. Natural, nonpharmaceutical measures (including chiropractic spinal adjustments) should generally be an approach of first resort, not last.
6. A balanced, natural diet is crucial to good health.
7. Regular exercise is essential to proper bodily function.

These principles, endorsed and elucidated by chiropractors for more than a century, are currently recognizable as the foundation of the emerging holistic health or wellness paradigm.

Core Chiropractic Principles

In addition to precepts shared with other natural healing arts such as homeopathy and naturopathy, core theoretical constructs that form the underpinning of chiropractic are as follows:

1. Structure and function exist in intimate relation with one another.

2. Structural distortions can cause functional abnormalities.
3. Vertebral subluxation is a significant form of structural distortion and dysfunction and leads to a variety of functional abnormalities.
4. The nervous system occupies a preeminent role in the restoration and maintenance of proper bodily function.
5. Subluxation influences bodily function primarily through neurological means.
6. The chiropractic adjustment is a specific and definitive method for the correction of the vertebral subluxation.

These chiropractic principles reveal something unexpected: although chiropractic is best known for its success in the relief of musculoskeletal pain, its basic axioms do not directly address the question of pain relief. Instead, they focus on the correction of structural and functional imbalances, which in some cases cause pain. This fundamental paradox—that a profession renowned for the relief of musculoskeletal pain does not define its basic purpose in those terms—has been a persistent and sometimes discordant theme in chiropractic history.

Divergent Interpretations: Traditionalists and Modernists

Historically, a dichotomy has existed within the chiropractic profession between what have sometimes been called "straights" and "mixers," although most chiropractors are part of a broad middle ground between the extremes. Central to this controversy is the degree to which chiropractic practice should focus on symptom relief. Traditionalist, "straight" chiropractors see their approach as being subluxation based rather than symptom driven; they largely confine their role to analyzing the spine for subluxations, then manually adjusting the subluxated vertebrae. A minority within the profession, they generally reject the use of symptom-oriented ancillary therapies such as heat, electrical stimulation, and dietary supplementation. A few jurisdictions limit chiropractors to this circumscribed scope of practice.

Both groups agree that spinal adjusting is the paramount feature of chiropractic practice, and that advising patients on exercise and natural diet is appropriately within the chiropractor's scope. The chief philosophical difference between them is that whereas traditionalists seek to treat the cause and not the symptom (some even reject the term "treat" as excessively allopathic), broad-scope modernists seek to treat both the cause and the symptom. Although broad-scope chiropractors share their traditionalist colleagues' appreciation of spinal adjusting, they contend that patient care is sometimes enhanced by such adjuncts as electrical physical therapy modalities, hands-on muscle therapies, acupuncture, and nutritional regimens, including supplementation with vitamins, minerals, and herbs.

THEORETICAL CONSTRUCTS AND PRACTICAL APPLICATIONS

Bone-out-of-Place Theory

Pioneer-era chiropractors, following Palmer's lead, assumed that their adjustments worked by moving misaligned vertebrae back into line, thereby relieving pressure caused by direct bony impingement on spinal nerves. The standard explanation given to patients was the analogy of stepping on a garden hose: if you step on the hose, the water cannot get through, and then if you lift your foot off the hose, the free flow of water is restored. Similarly, the chiropractic adjustment removes the pressure of bone on nerve, thus allowing free flow of nerve impulses.

Based on the information available at the time, such nineteenth-century concepts were plausible. Chiropractors were able to feel interruptions in the symmetry of the spinal column with their well-trained hands, and in many cases they could verify this on x-ray examination. More often than not, when they adjusted the subluxated vertebra with manual pressure, patients reported significant functional improvements and healing effects.

Problems exist with this theory, however, as best illustrated by noting that, after an adjustment resulting in dramatic relief from headaches or sciatica, an x-ray study rarely shows any immediate, discernible change in spinal alignment. (The American Chiropractic Association Council on Diagnostic Imaging now considers such comparative x-ray films inappropriate because of the unnecessary radiation exposure.) Positive health changes have not been convincingly correlated with vertebral alignment.

Motion Theory and Segmental Dysfunction

Alternative hypotheses have been proposed to replace the bone-out-of-place concept. Chief among these is the theory of *intervertebral motion* and *segmental dysfunction* (SDF), the dominant chiropractic model of this era. Advocated by a small minority of chiropractors for many decades, this model first achieved profession-wide attention among chiropractors in the 1980s and now has broad acceptance in chiropractic college curricula throughout the world. This theory also allows a coherent explanation of chiropractic and the *vertebral subluxation complex* (VSC) to be communicated in familiar terms to medical practitioners and researchers.

Motion theory contends that loss of proper spinal joint mobility, rather than positional misalignment, is the key factor in the VSC. It posits that the subluxation always involves more than a single vertebra and that subluxation mechanics involve SDF, an interruption in the normal dynamic relationship between two articulating joint surfaces (Schafer and Faye, 1989).

Anatomically, the vertebral motor unit (or motion segment) consists of an *anterior segment,* with two vertebral bodies separated by an intervertebral disc, and a *posterior segment,* consisting of two adjacent articular facets, along with muscles, ligaments, blood vessels, and nerves, interfacing with one another. Restriction of joint motion, a common feature of the manipulable lesion or subluxation, is termed a *fixation.* Fixation-subluxations are the clinical entity most amenable to spinal manipulation.

Former Palmer College of Chiropractic president and national spokesperson for the American Chiropractic Association J.F. McAndrews, DC, an early advocate of motion theory and practice, offers a visual model of spinal motion principles (Figure 10-4), as follows:

> View it as a mobile hanging from the ceiling, with many strings on which ornaments are suspended. As the mobile hangs there, it is in a state of dynamic equilibrium. Then, if you cut one of the strings, the whole mobile starts moving, because its balance has been upset. Eventually, it slows down and reaches a new state of dynamic equilibrium. But things have changed. It doesn't look the same. All those ornaments have shifted, in relation to the central axis and also in relation to each other.
>
> The body's musculoskeletal system works in much the same way. If its normal balance is disrupted,

it must compensate. Structural patterns will be altered to a greater or lesser degree, depending on the nature and intensity of the forces that threw off the old pattern of balance.

Leach (1994) describes a triad of signs classically accepted as evidence for the existence of SDF: (1) point tenderness or altered pain threshold to pressure in the adjacent paraspinal musculature or over the spinous process, (2) abnormal contraction or tension within the adjacent paraspinal musculature, and (3) loss of normal motion in one or more planes. Chiropractic education includes extensive training in the development of the psychomotor skills necessary to diagnose the VSC or SDF and to perform the manipulative maneuvers best suited to its correction.

Much more problematic than fixations are subluxations involving joint hypermobility, characterized by ligamentous laxity, frequently of traumatic etiology. Hypermobility may be clinically diagnosed by eliciting a repeated click when a joint is moved through its normal range of motion. Hypermobile joints should not be forcibly manipulated because this can further increase the degree of hypermobility. However, nearby articulations that have become fixated to compensate for the hypermobile joint should be manipulated, and muscles in the area should be strengthened and toned to minimize the workload of the overstressed hypermobile joint.

The motion segment is the initial focus of chiropractic therapeutic intervention and is the site where the most direct and immediate effects of adjustment/manipulation are likely to be noted. More far-reaching effects are possible, however, through neural facilitation.

Segmental Facilitation

Segmental facilitation has been defined as a lowered threshold for firing in a spinal cord segment, caused by afferent bombardment of the dorsal horn associated with spinal lesions (Korr, 1976).

Once a segment has become facilitated, the effects can include local somatic pain or visceral organ dysfunction. Segmental facilitation is the dominant hypothesis proposed as the neurophysiological basis by which the VSC or SDF influences autonomic function.

Some models for the specific mechanisms of facilitation postulate that inflammation is a key factor (Dvorak, 1985; Gatterman and Goe, 1990; Mense, 1991), whereas others have proposed neurological models through which such facilitation could occur even in the absence of inflammation (Korr, 1975; Patterson and Steinmetz, 1986). When present, inflammation alters the local milieu of the nerve, causing chemical, thermal, and mechanical changes; inflammation surrounding a nerve is likely to compromise its function. Such aberrant nerve activity, researchers theorize, can disrupt the homeostatic mechanisms essential to normal somatic or visceral organ function.

A facilitated segment may result in either parasympathetic vagal dominance or excessive sympathetic output. As Leach (1994) concludes, "It appears that SDF is capable of initiating segmental facilitation and that certainly this is the most logical explanation for the use of [chiropractic] adjustment . . . for other than pain syndromes; certainly the

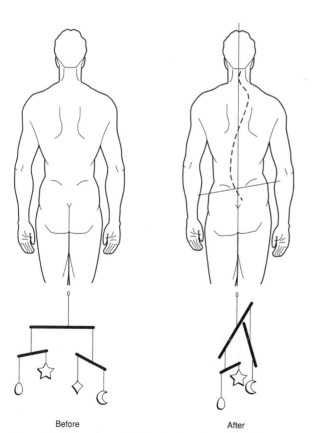

Figure 10-4 Visual model of spinal motion principles comparing mobile hanging from ceiling to body's musculoskeletal system before and after imbalance is introduced.

segmental facilitation hypothesis is gaining greater acceptance and is based upon a large body of acceptable scientific research."

RATIONALE FOR CHIROPRACTIC ADJUSTMENT

Indications and Contraindications

The central focus of chiropractic practice is the analytical process for determining (1) when and where spinal manipulative therapy (SMT) is appropriate and (2) the type of adjustment most appropriate in a given situation.

Proposed algorithms for this process detail procedures whereby the chiropractor, after arriving at an overall diagnostic impression (not limited to the spine) and methodically ruling out pathologies that contraindicate SMT, proceeds to evaluate SDF in order to arrive at a specific chiropractic diagnosis (Leach, 1994). This diagnostic process takes into account subluxations that are present, along with other clinical entities (e.g., degeneration, disc involvement, carpal tunnel syndrome), which in certain cases require additional treatment besides SMT or affect the style of SMT that is appropriate.

For example, the presence of advanced degenerative joint disease would not render SMT inappropriate but would rule out all forms of SMT that introduce substantial amounts of force into the arthritic joint. According to the *Guidelines for Chiropractic Quality Assurance and Practice Parameters* (Haldeman et al., 1993), the high-velocity low-amplitude (HVLA) thrust adjustment, the most common form of chiropractic SMT, is "absolutely contraindicated" in anatomical areas where the following occur:

- Malignancies
- Bone and joint infections
- Acute myelopathy or acute cauda equina syndrome
- Acute fractures and dislocations, or healed fractures and dislocations with signs of ligamentous rupture or instability
- Acute rheumatoid, rheumatoid-like, or nonspecific arthropathies, including ankylosing spondylitis characterized by episodes of acute

inflammation, demineralization, and ligamentous laxity with anatomical subluxation or dislocation
- Active juvenile avascular necrosis
- Unstable os odontoideum

These guidelines also rate, in descending order of severity, conditions in the following categories: "relative to absolute contraindication," "relative contraindication," and "not a contraindication." Listing all conditions in each category is beyond the scope of this chapter. The key point is that chiropractic diagnosis is geared toward evaluating where each case falls on this spectrum, then proceeding with appropriate medical referral, chiropractic treatment, or concurrent care.

Types of Manual Interventions Used by Chiropractors

The HVLA technique, also known as *osseous adjustment,* is performed by manually moving a joint to the end point of its normal range of motion (ROM), isolating it by local pressure on bony prominences, and then imparting a swift, specific, low-amplitude thrust. This thrust is frequently accompanied by a clicking sound indicating joint cavitation, as the joint moves into the "paraphysiological space" between normal ROM and the limits of its anatomical integrity. Properly applied, the adjustment usually involves little or no discomfort.

Other adjusting methods with wide application in the chiropractic profession include the following:

- High-velocity thrust with recoil
- Low-velocity thrust
- Flexion-distraction (originally an osteopathic technique for lumbar disc syndrome)
- Adjustment with mechanically assisted drop-piece tables
- Adjustment with compression-wave instruments
- Various specific light-touch techniques

Some of these procedures are "low-force" methods, developed to assist chiropractors in managing cases where standard HVLA adjustment is either contraindicated or otherwise undesirable. Nonadjustive manual measures are also employed by chiropractors, generally to supplement rather than replace SMT, and include trigger-point therapy, joint mobilization, and massage (Figure 10-5).

CLINICAL SETTINGS AND METHODOLOGIES

Independence Born of Necessity

Chiropractic's long-time role as a dissenting wing of the Euro-American healing arts has meant that its practitioners have functioned almost entirely within the context of freestanding private practice. Similarly, chiropractic educational facilities have been private institutions, functioning almost entirely without public funding.

This outsider status is changing. Chiropractors now serve on the staffs of a small but growing number of hospitals, and universities in Quebec, Australia, Denmark, Wales, and the United States now include chiropractic departments. Chiropractors serve in official capacities at the Olympic Games and play an increasingly prominent role in the treatment of sports and workplace injuries. In 1993, J.R. Cassidy became the first chiropractor to be named research director of a university hospital orthopedics department, at the University of Saskatchewan in Canada. In 1994, John Triano became the first member of the profession to join the staff of the Texas Back Institute, where he has worked in the dual role of staff chiropractic physician and clinical research scientist.

Among the most promising developments in the mainstreaming of chiropractic is the recent (post-2000) inclusion of chiropractic in the health care systems serving veterans and the active-duty military personnel in the United States.

Such developments bode well for the future but are still more the exception than the rule. Evolving outside the mainstream has been a struggle, although it has strengthened many practitioners committed to chiropractic. By far the most serious negative effect of chiropractic's peripheral status has been that the majority of patients who could benefit from chiropractic care have not received it, since referrals from allopathic physicians to chiropractors remain much rarer than referrals to other medical practitioners or physical therapists.

The most salient positive aspect of operating outside the establishment for so many years is that the cre-

ative impulses and capacities of individual chiropractors were encouraged rather than quashed. One of the greatest challenges currently facing the profession is developing uniform practice standards—the *Guidelines for Chiropractic Quality Assurance and Practice Parameters* (Haldeman et al., 1993), or "Mercy Guidelines," is an initial effort—while simultaneously maintaining the innovative atmosphere that has characterized the profession since its inception.

Diagnostic Logic

In the clinical setting the chiropractic model demonstrates both similarities and differences compared with the standard medical approach. Foremost, chiropractors seek to evaluate individual symptoms in a broad context of health and body balance, not as isolated aberrations to be suppressed. This holistic viewpoint shares much with both ancient and emerging models elsewhere in the healing arts.

Chiropractors recognize the need for thorough evaluation of symptoms, and they are trained to take histories and perform physical examinations in a similar manner as done at the typical medical office. However, the chiropractic paradigm does not hold the elimination of symptoms to be the sole or ultimate goal of treatment. Health is more than the absence of disease symptoms. The true goal is sustainable balance, a fact recognized by chiropractors and other holistically oriented health practitioners.

Chiropractors are trained in state-of-the-art diagnostic techniques, and chiropractic examination procedures overlap significantly with those used by orthodox medical physicians. However, chiropractors evaluate the information gleaned from these methods from a perspective that places greater emphasis on the intricate structural and functional interplay between different parts of the body.

Chiropractic and Medical Approaches to Pain

In my experience, conventional medical physicians engage in symptom suppression much more than chiropractors and also more frequently assume that the site of a pain is the site of its cause. Thus, knee pain is generally assumed to be a knee problem, shoulder pain is assumed to be a shoulder problem, and so

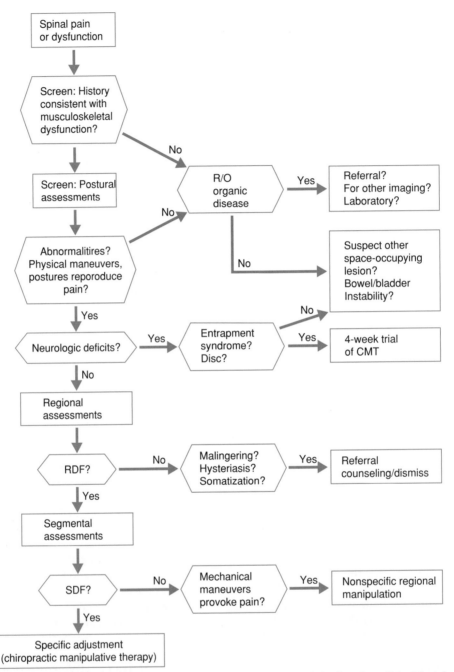

Figure 10-5 Proposed algorithm for the assessment of regional and segmental dysfunction. (Modified from Leach RA: An algorithm for chiropractic management of spinal dysfunction. In *The chiropractic theories: principles and clinical applications,* ed 3, Baltimore, 1994, Williams & Wilkins.)

forth. This pain-centered diagnostic logic frequently leads to increasingly sophisticated and invasive diagnostic and therapeutic procedures. For example, if physical examination of the knee fails to define the problem clearly, the knee is radiographed. If the x-ray film fails to offer adequate clarification, magnetic resonance imaging (MRI) of the knee is performed, and in some cases a surgical procedure follows.

As with their allopathic colleagues, chiropractors use diagnostic tools such as radiography and MRI

(Figure 10-6). The point here is not to criticize these useful technologies but to present an alternative diagnostic model. Chiropractors are familiar with patients in whom this entire high-tech diagnostic scenario, as in the previous knee example, is played out, after which the knee problem is discovered to be a compensation for a mechanical disorder in the lower back, a common condition that too often remains outside the medical diagnostic loop.

If the lower back is mechanically dysfunctional and in need of spinal adjustment/manipulation, this can often place unusual stress on one or both knees. In these patients, medical physicians can and often do spend months or years medicating the knee symptoms or performing surgery, never addressing the source of the problem.

Regional and Whole-Body Context: Neurology and Biomechanics

The chiropractic approach to musculoskeletal pain involves evaluating the site of pain in a regional and whole-body context. Although shoulder, elbow, and wrist problems can be caused by injuries or pathologies in these areas, pain in and around each of the shoulder, elbow, and wrist joints can also have as its

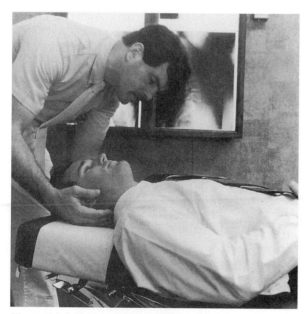

Figure 10-6 Contemporary chiropractors use state-of-the-art diagnostic and therapeutic methods.

source segmental dysfunction in the cervical spine. Similarly, symptoms in the hip, knee, and ankle can also originate at the site of the pain, but in many cases the source lies in the lumbar spine or sacroiliac joints. Besides pain, other neurologically mediated symptoms (e.g., paresthesia) can have a similar etiology. The need to consider this chain of causation is built into the core of chiropractic training.

Chiropractors since Palmer have intentionally refrained from assuming that the site of a symptom is the site of its cause. They assume instead that *the source of the pain should be sought along the path of the nerves leading to and from the site of the symptoms.* Thus, pain in the knee might come from the knee itself, but tracing the nerve pathways between the knee and the spine reveals possible areas of causation in and around the hip, in the deep muscles of the buttocks or pelvis, in the sacroiliac joints, or in the lumbar spine.

Furthermore, if joint dysfunction does exist, for example, at the fourth and fifth lumbar levels, it might have its primary source at L4-5, or it might represent a compensation for another subluxation elsewhere in the spine, perhaps in the lower or middle thoracic vertebrae or in a mechanical dysfunction of the muscles and joints of the feet. Such an integrative, whole-body approach to structure and function is of great value.

For patients whose presentation includes visceral organ symptoms, chiropractic diagnostic logic includes (once contraindications to adjustment/manipulation have been ruled out) evaluation of the spine, with particular attention to spinal levels providing autonomic nerve supply to the involved area, as well as consideration of possible nutritional, environmental, and psychological factors.

Criteria for Referral to Allopathic Physicians

Chiropractic practice standards mandate timely referral to an allopathic physician for diagnosis and treatment for conditions beyond the chiropractor's domain, or when a reasonable trial of chiropractic care (current standards in most cases limit this to about one month) fails to bring satisfactory results (Haldeman et al., 1993).

In addition, chiropractors frequently seek second opinions in less dramatic cases if chiropractic treatment, though helpful, fails to bring full resolution. Referrals from chiropractors to neurologists, neurosurgeons, orthopedic surgeons, internists, and other medical specialists are common. Referrals to complementary practitioners such as acupuncturists, massage therapists, homeopaths, and naturopaths also occur when appropriate, in areas where such practitioners are available.

Ethics of Referral

The medical profession has long had a clearly defined set of ethics for *intraprofessional* referral: a report is sent to the referring physician, and the patient remains the patient of the referring physician. In the era when the medical establishment prohibited collegial relations with chiropractors, physicians receiving referrals from chiropractors frequently failed to extend such professional courtesies to them. This still occurs, although in a decreasing number of cases.

The most insidious effect of this remnant of the old antichiropractic boycott is that it exerts a subliminal, if not overt, pressure on chiropractors *not* to refer. Ethical chiropractors resist the pressure, but such a vestige of the old order has no place in the modern health care arena and must be eliminated. At a time when many chiropractic patients still elect not to inform their allopathic physicians that they are seeing a chiropractor (Eisenberg et al., 1998), the need for breaking down all such barriers should be readily apparent.

RESEARCH

For years, chiropractors were attacked for offering only anecdotal evidence in support of their methods. Since the early 1990s, only those ignorant of the scientific literature can still make such claims. As summarized by Meeker and Haldeman (2002), 43 randomized trials of spinal manipulation for treatment of acute, subacute, and chronic LBP have been published. Thirty favored manipulation over the comparison treatments in at least a subgroup of patients, and the other 13 found no significant differences. None of these low back pain studies has shown SMT to be less effective than the comparison approaches or a control group. Eleven randomized, controlled trials of spinal manipulation for neck pain have been conducted; four

had positive findings, and seven were equivocal. Seven of nine randomized trials of manipulation for various forms of headache were positive.

University of Colorado Project

Contemporary chiropractic research began at the University of Colorado in the 1970s. First with grants from the International Chiropractors Association and later with added financial support from the American Chiropractic Association and the U.S. government, Chung Ha Suh and colleagues at the Biomechanics Department undertook a series of studies that provided an extensive body of chiropractic-related, basic science research.

Suh, the first American college professor willing to defy the AMA boycott to pursue chiropractic research, was a native of Korea, where he was not subjected to the same antichiropractic bias as the American health care academics of his era. In launching this research, he had to withstand intense pressure from powerful political forces within the American medical and academic establishments, which condemned chiropractic for lack of scientific underpinning while striving to prevent chiropractors from obtaining the funding and university connections necessary for the development of such a research base (*Wilk v AMA*, 1990).

The University of Colorado team pursued research in two major areas. First, Suh (1974) developed a computer model of the cervical spine that allowed a deeper understanding of spinal joint mechanics and their relationship to the chiropractic adjustment. The second area involved a range of studies on nerve compression and various aspects of neuron function (Kelly and Luttges, 1975; Luttges et al., 1976; MacGregor and Oliver, 1973; MacGregor et al., 1975; Sharpless, 1975; Simske and Schmeister, 1994; Triano and Luttges, 1982). Sharpless, for example, demonstrated that minuscule amounts of pressure (10 mm Hg) on a nerve root resulted in up to a 50% decrease in electrical transmission down the course of the nerve supplied by that root.

Manual Adjustment for Low Back Pain

A substantial body of research has addressed the efficacy of SMT in the treatment of LBP. As referenced earlier, consensus panels evaluating the data have consistently placed spinal manipulation on the short list of recommended procedures for acute, uncomplicated LBP.

In an influential trial with more than 700 patients, British orthopedic surgeon T.W. Meade compared chiropractic manipulation with standard hospital outpatient treatment for LBP, which consisted of physical therapy and wearing a corset (Meade et al., 1990, 1995). He concluded, "For patients with low-back pain in whom manipulation is not contraindicated, chiropractic almost certainly confers worthwhile, long-term benefit in comparison to hospital outpatient management." He described the applicability of these findings for primary care physicians as follows:

> Our trial showed that chiropractic is a very effective treatment, more effective than conventional hospital out-patient treatment for low-back pain, particularly in patients who had back pain in the past and who [developed] severe problems. So, in other words, it is most effective in precisely the group of patients that you would like to be able to treat. . . . One of the unexpected findings was that the treatment difference—the benefit of chiropractic over hospital treatment—actually persists for the whole of that three-year period [of the study]. . . . the treatment that the chiropractors give does something that results in a very long-term benefit (Meade, 1992).

Meade's study was the first large randomized clinical trial to demonstrate substantial short-term and long-term benefits from chiropractic care. Because it dealt with both acute LBP patients and chronic LBP patients, Meade's data support the use of SMT for both populations.

Acute vs. Chronic Low Back Pain

Consensus panels and meta-analyses have not fully resolved the question of whether the literature supports recommending spinal manipulation for both chronic and acute LBP patients. In general, strong agreement exists that the literature supports the appropriateness of SMT for many acute LBP cases, but debate still surrounds chronic LBP. The perceived current insufficiency of data favoring SMT for chronic LBP has led some analysts to rate it as "inappropriate" for chronic LBP.

When Shekelle and colleagues (1998) rated the "appropriateness" of decisions to initiate manipulative therapy, they deemed manipulation "inappropriate" for all cases of chronic lower back pain. Although

this lowered the percentage of cases in which chiropractic was considered appropriate, both Shekelle's group and Micozzi (1998) aptly noted that the study offered solid justification for primary care physicians to refer many more of their LBP patients to chiropractors.

Evidence for Manual Methods in Chronic Cases

Seeing that manipulation may be considered "inappropriate" for chronic LBP, physicians and other health practitioners might logically conclude that until further convincing evidence emerges, they should not refer patients with chronic LBP to chiropractors. However, physicians frequently refer chronic LBP patients to physical therapists, based on perceptions that its effectiveness and appropriateness significantly exceed its research documentation (Cherkin et al., 1995). Because a primary care physician's decision about whether and where to refer LBP patients hinges on which treatments are expected to yield the most satisfactory outcomes, a summary of studies on spinal manipulation for chronic LBP may aid the decision-making process.

Besides Meade's work (1990, 1995), an impressive prospective study of LBP was performed at the University of Saskatchewan hospital orthopedics department by Kirkaldy-Willis, a world-renowned orthopedic surgeon, and Cassidy, the chiropractor who later became the department's research director (1985). The approximately 300 subjects in this study were "totally disabled" by LBP, with pain present for an average of 7 years. All had gone through extensive, unsuccessful medical treatment before participating as research subjects. After 2 to 3 weeks of daily chiropractic adjustments, more than 80% of the patients without spinal stenosis had good to excellent results, reporting substantially decreased pain and increased mobility. After chiropractic treatment, more than 70% were improved to the point of having no work restrictions. Follow-up a year later demonstrated that the changes were long-lasting. Even those with a narrowed spinal canal, a particularly difficult subset, showed a notable response. More than half the patients improved, and about one in five were pain free and on the job 7 months after treatment.

In a randomized trial of 209 patients, Triano and colleagues (1995) compared SMT to education programs for chronic LBP, which they defined as pain lasting 7 weeks or longer, or more than six episodes in 12 months. These investigators found greater improvement in pain and activity tolerance in the SMT group, noting that "immediate benefit from pain relief continued to accrue after manipulation, even for the last encounter at the end of the 2-week treatment interval." They concluded, "There appears to be clinical value to treatment according to a defined plan using manipulation even in low back pain exceeding 7 weeks duration."

Koes and colleagues (1992) compared manipulation to physiotherapy (PT) and treatment by a general practitioner (GP) in a randomized trial of 256 chronic cases that included back and neck pain. Physiotherapy included exercises, massage, heat, electrotherapy, ultrasound, and short-wave diathermy. GP care included medication (analgesics, NSAIDs) and advice about posture, rest, and activity. Data indicated that both manipulation and PT were much more effective than GP treatment, with SMT marginally surpassing PT. This advantage was sustained at 12-month follow-up.

Another randomized trial compared the effects of SMT and NSAID treatments, each combined with supervised trunk exercise for 174 chronic LBP patients (Bronfort et al., 1996). Both regimens were found to produce similar and clinically important improvement over time that was considered superior to the expected natural history of long-standing chronic LBP. The SMT/trunk-strengthening exercise group showed a sustained reduction in medication use at 12-month follow-up. Also, continuation of exercise during the follow-up year was associated with better outcomes for both groups.

In a study of 115 patients with chronic spinal pain, Giles and Muller (2003) compared the effects of medication (NSAID or analgesic not previously ineffective for the individual patient), spinal manipulation, and acupuncture. Treating practitioners were told to follow their normal office procedures to determine whether manipulation or acupuncture was appropriate, as well as which adjustive/manipulative procedures or acupuncture points should be used. Electrical stimulation was not applied to the acupuncture needles. The highest proportion of early recovery (asymptomatic status) was found for manipulation (27.3%), followed by acupuncture (9.4%) and medication (5%). Manipulation also outperformed the other interventions on a variety of other measures, with one notable exception: acupuncture achieved the best results on the visual analog scale measurement for neck pain improvement (50% for acupuncture vs. 42% for manipulation).

Preventing Acute Cases from Becoming Chronic

Because the prognosis for patients with acute LBP is better than for those with chronic pain, high priority must be accorded to preventing acute cases from becoming chronic. However, a key factor leads physicians to minimize this concern: conventional wisdom that 90% of LBP resolves on its own within a short time. Findings published in the *British Medical Journal* call for urgent reassessment of the assumption that most LBP patients seen by primary care physicians attain resolution of their complaints. Contrary to prevailing assumptions, Croft and colleagues (1998) found that *at 3-month and 12-month follow-up, only 21% and 25%, respectively, had completely recovered in terms of pain and disability*. However, only 8% continued to consult their physician for longer than 3 months. In other words, the oft-quoted 90% figure actually applied to the number of patients who stopped seeing their physicians, not the number who recovered from their back pain. Their dissatisfaction with conventional medical care was also reminiscent of Cherkin's earlier work (Cherkin and MacCornack, 1989; Cherkin et al., 1991). Croft stated the following:

> We should stop characterizing low-back pain in terms of a multiplicity of acute problems, most of which get better, and a small number of chronic long-term problems. Low back pain should be viewed as a chronic problem with an untidy pattern of grumbling symptoms and periods of relative freedom from pain and disability interspersed with acute episodes, exacerbations and recurrences. This takes account of two consistent observations about low-back pain: firstly, a previous episode of low-back pain is the strongest risk factor for a new episode, and, secondly, by the age of 30 years almost half the population will have experienced a substantial episode of low-back pain. These figures simply do not fit with claims that 90 percent of episodes of low-back pain end in complete recovery (Croft et al., 1998).

The patients in Croft's study were not referred for manual manipulation, and most developed chronic LBP. Based on the AHCPR Guidelines, which emphasize the functionally restorative qualities of SMT, it seems reasonable to expect that early chiropractic adjustments could have prevented this progression in many patients. Recall that follow-up in both the Meade (1 year and 3 year) and the Kirkaldy-Willis (1 year) studies showed that the beneficial effect of manipulation was sustained for extended periods (Kirkaldy-Willis and Cassidy, 1985; Meade et al., 1990, 1995). The decision not to refer patients to chiropractors may mean that many LBP patients will develop long-standing problems that could have been avoided.

Low Back Pain Patients with Leg Pain

Differential diagnosis is crucial for cases in which LBP radiates into the leg. Specifically, motor, sensory, and reflex testing should be used to screen for signs of radicular syndromes and cauda equina syndrome. However, a British study of primary care practitioners found that a majority of these physicians do not routinely examine for muscle weakness or sensation, and 27% do not regularly check reflexes (Little et al., 1996). Such factors play a central role in determining which patients should be referred directly for surgical consultation and which should be referred for manual manipulation.

The AHCPR Guidelines state that manipulation is appropriate for acute LBP cases that include non-radicular pain radiating into the lower extremity (Bigos et al., 1994). In cases where radicular signs such as muscle weakness or decreased reflex response are present, however, preliminary evidence now suggests that chiropractic can yield beneficial results. In a series of 424 consecutive cases, Cox and Feller (1994) reported that 83% of 331 lumbar disc syndrome patients completing care (13% of whom had previous low back surgeries) had good to excellent results. ("Excellent" was defined as >90% relief of pain and return to work with no further care required, and "good" as 75% relief of pain, return to work, with periodic manipulation or analgesia required.) There was a median of 11 treatments and 27 days to attain maximal improvement.

BenEliyahu (1996) followed 27 patients receiving chiropractic care for cervical and lumbar disc herniations, the majority being lumbar cases. Pretreatment and posttreatment MRI studies were performed; 80% of the patients had a good clinical outcome, and 63% of the post-MRI studies showed herniations either reduced in size or completely resorbed.

In a study of 14 patients with lumbar disc herniation, Cassidy and colleagues (1993) reported that all but one obtained significant clinical improvement and relief of pain after a 2- to 3-week regimen of daily side-posture manipulation of the lumbar spine,

directed toward improving spinal mobility. All patients received computed tomography (CT) scans before and 3 months after treatment. In most patients the CT appearance of the disc herniation remained unchanged after successful treatment, although five showed a small decrease in the size of the herniation, and one patient showed a large decrease.

Headaches: Chiropractic Compared with Conventional Medicine

Probably the most noteworthy chiropractic research to emerge from the United States is the work on headaches conducted at Northwestern College of Chiropractic in Minnesota (Boline et al., 1995), in which chiropractic was shown to be more effective than the tricyclic antidepressant amitriptyline for long-term relief of headache pain.

During the treatment phase of the trial, pain relief among those treated with medication was comparable to the SMT group. Revealingly, however, the chiropractic patients maintained their levels of improvement after treatment was discontinued, whereas those taking medication returned to pretreatment status in an average of 4 weeks after its discontinuation. This strongly implies that although medication suppressed the symptoms, chiropractic addressed the problem at a more causal level.

A subsequent trial by this group of investigators employing a similar protocol for patients with migraine headaches demonstrated that migraines were similarly responsive to chiropractic, and that adding amitriptyline to chiropractic treatment conferred no additional benefit (Nelson et al., 1998).

Neck Pain

Chiropractors have treated acute and chronic neck pain and related upper extremity symptoms since the profession's beginnings, but research on this subject is not extensive, which is also the case for nonmanual methods of treating neck pain (e.g., medications). As noted earlier, Meeker and Haldeman (2002) found that of the 11 randomized controlled trials of spinal manipulation for neck pain conducted, four demonstrated positive findings, seven equivocal findings, and none negative. Rosner (2003) notes that "the RAND literature review (Coulter et al., 1995) suggested that short-term pain relief and enhancement of range of motion might be accomplished by manipulation or mobilization in the treatment of subacute or chronic neck pain; literature describing acute neck pain was regarded as extremely scanty, and remains so."

Somatovisceral Disorders

Although the bulk of recent and current chiropractic research still focuses on musculoskeletal disorders, research on somatovisceral disorders is also underway.

Infantile Colic

In late 1999 a breakthrough study in visceral disorders was published in *Journal of Manipulative and Physiological Therapeutics*. This randomized controlled trial by chiropractic and medical investigators at Odense University in Denmark showed chiropractic spinal manipulation to be effective for treating infantile colic (Wiberg et al., 1999). An estimated 22.5% of newborns suffer from colic, a condition marked by prolonged, intense, high-pitched crying. Numerous studies have explored a possible gastrointestinal (GI) etiology, but the cause of colic has long remained a mystery.

Health visitor nurses from the National Health Service recruited 50 participants for this study, whose parents consented to a 2-week trial of either dimethicone or spinal manipulation by a chiropractor. Dimethicone, which decreases foam in the GI tract, is prescribed for colic, even though several controlled studies have shown it to be no better than placebo (Illingworth, 1985; Lucassen et al., 1998).

The infants in the Wiberg study were 2 to 10 weeks of age and had no symptoms of diseases other than colic. Inclusion criteria included at least 1 violent crying spell lasting 3 hours or more for at least 5 of the previous 7 days. Mothers of infants in both groups also received counseling and advice on breastfeeding technique, mother's diet, air swallowing, feeding by bottle, burp technique, and other advice normally given to parents by health visitor nurses. The main outcome measure was the percentage of change in the number of hours of infantile colic behavior per day as registered in the parental diary, an instrument with validated reliability.

The 25 infants randomized to the chiropractic group were given a routine case history and a physical examination that included motion palpation of the spinal vertebrae and pelvis. The articulations

restricted in movement were manipulated (mobilized) with specific light pressure with the fingertips for up to 2 weeks (three to five sessions) "until normal mobility was found in the involved segments" (Wiberg et al., 1999). The areas treated were primarily in the upper and middle thoracic regions, the source of sympathetic nerve input to the digestive tract.

All 25 infants in the chiropractic group completed the 13 days of treatment, whereas the dimethicone group had nine dropouts. Those who dropped out before submission of the parental diary at the end of week 1 were omitted from the study's statistical analysis. Because some of these were reported by their mothers to have dropped out due to a significant worsening of symptoms, the relative benefit of spinal manipulation vis-à-vis dimethicone is understated in the final statistical analysis.

Nonetheless, the mean daily hours of colic in the chiropractic group were reduced by 66% on day 12, which is virtually identical to the 67% reduction in a previous prospective trial. In contrast, the dimethicone group showed a 38% reduction.

The Danish study on infantile colic is the first randomized controlled trial to demonstrate effectiveness of chiropractic manipulation for a disorder generally considered nonmusculoskeletal. Addressing this issue, the authors conclude that their data lead to two possible interpretations: "Either spinal manipulation is effective in the treatment of the visceral disorder infantile colic or infantile colic is, in fact, a musculoskeletal disorder" (Wiberg et al., 1999).

A contrasting view is provided by a study performed under the auspices of a university pediatrics department in Norway (Olafsdottir et al., 2001). In this study, 86 infants were randomly assigned to chiropractic care or placebo (held for 10 minutes by nurse, rather than given 10-minute visit with chiropractor). In the chiropractic group, adjustments were administered by light fingertip pressure. The methods used to identify involved segments were not described, and no mention was made of which regions were most frequently involved. Both groups experienced substantial decreases in crying, the primary outcome measure; 70% of the chiropractic group improved versus 60% of those held by nurses. However, no statistically significant differences were found between the two groups in terms of the number of hours of crying, or as measured on a five-point improvement scale (from "getting worse" to "completely well"). The researchers concluded that "chiropractic spinal manipulation is no more effective than placebo in the treatment of infantile colic." This conclusion raises a significant methodological issue regarding the role of control or placebo interventions in chiropractic research, described in detail later.

Other Visceral Disorders

A pilot study by Fallon, a New York pediatric chiropractor, evaluating chiropractic treatment for children with otitis media demonstrated improved outcomes compared to the natural course of the illness. Using both parental reports and tympanography with a cohort of more than 400 patients, data suggest a positive role for spinal and cranial manipulation in the management of this challenging condition (Fallon, 1997; Fallon and Edelman, 1998).

Two small controlled clinical trials evaluating the effects of chiropractic adjustment/manipulation for primary dysmenorrhea showed encouraging results, with both pain relief and changes in certain prostaglandin levels noted (Kokjohn et al., 1992; Thomasen et al., 1979). However, a larger random controlled trial failed to demonstrate significant benefits from adjustment/manipulation (Hondras et al., 1999).

A small random controlled study demonstrated that diastolic and systolic blood pressure decreased significantly immediately after chiropractic adjustments of the thoracic spine (T1-T5), while placebo and control groups showed no such change (Yates et al., 1988). This showed short-term effects of SMT on blood pressure and indicated a need for research on longer-term effects. No larger trials have been published.

A study at the National College of Chiropractic showed a marked increase in the activity levels of certain immune system cells (PMNs, monocytes) immediately after thoracic spine manipulation (Brennan et al., 1991). These increases were significantly higher than in control groups, who were given either sham manipulation or soft tissue manipulation. To date, no large trials on possible effects of adjustment/manipulation on the immune system have been published.

METHODOLOGICAL CHALLENGES IN CHIROPRACTIC RESEARCH

The most challenging methodological issues in chiropractic research are as follows:

1. What constitutes a genuine control or placebo intervention?
2. How can CIM practitioners properly interpret data collected in trials that compare active and control treatments?

These questions apply not only to chiropractic but to a broad range of procedures, particularly non-pharmaceutical modalities such as massage, acupuncture, physical therapy, and therapeutic touch. Depending on how one defines the placebo, the same set of research data can be interpreted as supporting or refuting the value of the therapeutic method under study (Redwood, 1999).

What Constitutes an Appropriate Placebo?

Two widely publicized studies illustrate the potential difficulties of defining the placebo or control too broadly. In their research on children with mild to moderate asthma, Balon and colleagues (1998) randomly assigned individuals to either active manipulation or simulated manipulation groups. Both groups experienced substantial improvement in symptoms and quality of life, reduction in the use of β-agonist medication, and statistically insignificant increases in peak expiratory flow. Because these two groups did not differ significantly in regard to these improvements, however, the researchers concluded that "chiropractic spinal manipulation provided no benefit."

If the simulated manipulation had no therapeutic effect, this is a reasonable conclusion, but a closer reading of the article's text reveals the following:

> For simulated treatment, the subject lay prone while soft-tissue massage and gentle palpation were applied to the spine, paraspinal muscles and shoulders. A distraction maneuver was performed by turning the patient's head from one side to the other while alternately palpating the ankles and feet. The subject was positioned on one side, a nondirectional push, or impulse, was applied to the gluteal region, and the procedure was repeated with the patient positioned on the other side; then the subject was placed in the prone position, and a similar procedure was applied bilaterally to the scapulae. The subject was then placed supine, with the head rotated slightly to each side, and an impulse applied to the external occipital protuberance. Low-amplitude,

low-velocity impulses were applied in all these non-therapeutic contacts, with adequate joint slack so that no joint opening or cavitation occurred. Hence, the comparison of treatments was between active spinal manipulation as routinely applied by chiropractors and hands-on procedures without adjustments or manipulation (Balon et al., 1998).

The validity of this study's conclusion hinges entirely on the assumption that these procedures are therapeutically inert. The following questions may be helpful in evaluating this claim:

1. Would massage therapists view these hands-on procedures as "nontherapeutic"?
2. Would acupuncturists or practitioners of Shiatsu concur that direct manual pressure on multiple areas rich in acupuncture points is so inconsequential as to allow its use as a "placebo"?
3. Perhaps most significantly for this study on chiropractic, would the average chiropractor agree that these pressures, impulses, and stretches are an appropriate placebo, particularly in light of the fact that they overlap with certain "low-force" chiropractic adjustments and mobilization procedures?

The authors of the study dismiss these concerns as follows: "We are unaware of published evidence that suggests that positioning, palpation, gentle soft-tissue therapy, or impulses to the musculature adjacent to the spine influence the course of asthma" (Balon et al., 1998). A reasonable alternative interpretation of this study's results, however, is that various forms of hands-on therapy, including joint manipulation and various forms of movement, mobilization, and soft tissue massage, appear to have a mildly beneficial effect for asthmatic patients (Redwood, 1999).

Active Controls

Another study that raises similar questions involves Bove and Nilsson's work (1998) on manipulation for episodic tension-type headache (ETTH). Patients were randomized into two groups; one received soft tissue therapy (deep friction massage) plus spinal manipulation, and the other (the "active control" group) received soft tissue therapy plus application of a low-power laser to the neck. All treatments were applied by

one chiropractor. Both groups had significantly fewer headaches and decreased their use of analgesic medications. As in the asthma study, differences between the two groups did not reach statistical significance. Thus the authors concluded that "as an isolated intervention, spinal manipulation does not seem to have a positive effect on tension-type headache."

Unlike the asthma study (Balon et al., 1998), Bove and Nilsson's carefully worded conclusion *is* justified by their data. But would it not have been more informative to affirm an equally accurate conclusion— that hands-on therapy, whether massage or manipulation, plus massage demonstrated significant benefits? Shortly after his paper's publication, Bove noted in a message to an Internet discussion group, "Our study asked one question [whether manipulation as an isolated intervention is effective for ETTH] and delivered one answer, a hallmark of good science. . . . We stressed that chiropractors do more than manipulation, and that chiropractic treatment has been shown to be somewhat beneficial for ETTH and *very* beneficial for cervicogenic headache. The message was that people should go to chiropractors with their headaches, for diagnosis and management."

The mass media's reporting on Bove and Nilsson's headache study provides a telling illustration of why defining the placebo or control correctly is more than an academic curiosity. Media reports on this study put forth a message quite different than Bove's nuanced analysis, with headlines concluding that chiropractic does not help headaches. Reports on the asthma study were similar. Moreover, future Medline searches will include the authors' tersely stated negative conclusions, with no mention of any controversy surrounding their interpretation.

The best way to avoid such confusion in the future is to emphasize increased usage of other valid methodologies, particularly direct comparisons of CIM procedures and standard medical care. Some comparative studies have shown adjustment/manipulation equal or superior to conventional medical procedures, with fewer side effects (Boline et al., 1995; Meade et al., 1990, 1995; Nelson et al., 1998; Wiberg et al., 1999; Winters et al., 1997). If fairly constructed, such studies will yield data that allow health practitioners and the general public to place CIM procedures in proper context. Comparing chiropractic and other nonpharmaceutical procedures to highly questionable placebos confuses the issue and delays the advent of a "level playing field."

SAFETY OF ADJUSTMENT/ MANIPULATION

All health care interventions entail risk, which is best evaluated in relation to other common treatments for similar conditions (i.e., adjustment/manipulation vs. antiinflammatory medications for neck pain). Medications with a safety profile comparable to that of spinal manipulation are considered quite safe. Although minor, temporary soreness after a chiropractic treatment is not unusual, major adverse events resulting from chiropractic treatment are few and infrequent. As a result, chiropractic malpractice insurance premiums are substantially lower than those for medical and osteopathic physicians.

The potential reaction to chiropractic treatment that has raised the greatest concern is cerebrovascular accident, or stroke, following cervical spine adjustment/manipulation. This occurs so rarely that it is virtually impossible study other than on a retrospective basis, because the cohort necessary for a prospective study would involve hundreds of thousands of patients, at a minimum.

Lauretti (2003) provides an excellent summary of chiropractic safety issues and makes the following key points:

- Every reliable published study estimating the incidence of stroke from cervical adjustment/manipulation agrees that the risk is less than 1 to 3 incidents per 1 million treatments and approximately 1 incident per 100,000 patients.
- Haldeman and colleagues (2001) found the rate of stroke to be 1 in 8.06 million office visits, 1 in 5.85 million cervical adjustment/manipulations, 1 in 1430 chiropractic practice years, and 1 in 48 chiropractic practice careers.
- NSAIDs, which are also widely used for neck pain and headaches, have a much less desirable safety record than adjustment/manipulation.

CHIROPRACTIC IN THE HEALTH CARE SYSTEM OF THE FUTURE

The greatest issue facing chiropractic in its first century was survival: whether it would remain a separate and distinct healing art, succumb to the substantial forces against it, or be subsumed into allopathic medicine. The question of survival has been resolved. Chiropractic has survived.

The key question for the new century, or at least the next generation, is: How can chiropractic best be integrated into the mainstream health care delivery system so that chiropractic services are readily available to all who can benefit from their application? A corollary follows as well: How can such integration be achieved without diluting chiropractic principles and practice to the point where chiropractic becomes a weak shadow of its former self?

It appears that an overwhelming majority of chiropractors do not want to pursue the path toward becoming full-scope allopathic physicians. Moreover, they will not willingly opt for any system in which chiropractic services are only available on medical referral. Chiropractors will function as contributing members of the health care team, but they will voluntarily surrender neither their political independence nor the holistic, wisdom-of-the-body worldview that has always been the core of their concept. How then can the desired integration be achieved, for the benefit of many millions of current and future patients?

To answer this question in a manner satisfactory to chiropractors, conventional physicians, and the general public, a mutually agreed-on framework based on common goals is essential. Fortunately, a common purpose does exist: all parties seek to create the most effective, efficient health care system possible for the greatest number of people. A framework for implementation also exists, at least in theory: based on the "level playing field" concept, which embodies a synthesis of two principles, democracy and hierarchy, coexisting in dynamic harmony.

The *democracy* of science is one in which equal opportunity is enjoyed by all, and all hypotheses are "innocent until proven guilty." Blind prejudice on the part of allopathic physicians, chiropractors, or anyone else, has no place in this environment. All methods, whether presently considered conventional or alternative (integrative), must prove themselves effective and cost-effective, and they must also demonstrate minimal iatrogenic effects. Approaches presently enjoying the imprimatur of the mainstream medical establishment should not be exempt from this scrutiny.

Hierarchy also has a place on the level playing field, as long as it is based on demonstrable skills and proven methods. In areas where conventional Western medicine has clearly established its superior quality (e.g., trauma care, certain surgeries, treatment of life-threatening infections), this expertise should be honored and deferred to, but this is a two-way street. Where a complementary method such as chiropractic is proved superior (low back pain is the first sphere where this has occurred), chiropractors must be accorded a similar role. Hierarchy in this sense does not imply a "control and domination" model. This is a lateral conception of hierarchy rather than a vertical one, a relationship among equals where precedence is based on quality, which in turn is determined through adherence to agreed-on standards.

To facilitate the integration of chiropractic into the mainstream, there is an immediate and pressing need to broaden lines of communication between the chiropractic and medical professions, on a one-to-one basis and in small and large groups, with the goal of offering to all patients the gift of their physicians' cooperation. Each side must learn to recognize their own strengths and weaknesses, as well as the strengths and weaknesses of the other side. No one has all the answers, and humility befits our common role as seekers after truth.

At present, even though chiropractors have clear guidelines for when to refer to medical doctors, neither the medical profession as a whole nor its various specialty groups have developed formal guidelines as to when to refer patients for chiropractic care. Given the legacy of contention surrounding chiropractic, this is not surprising. In the post–AHCPR Guidelines era, however, such criteria are essential for informed decision making. The time for creating these criteria is now. At a bare minimum, these guidelines should recommend referral to chiropractors of LBP patients who do not meet the AHCPR's tightly circumscribed criteria for surgical referral.

The future need not mirror the worst aspects of the past. It is incumbent on all health care providers, as well as wholly consonant with their role as healers, that practitioners heal not only sickness but old rifts among themselves. They now have an unprecedented opportunity to do so.

References

Balon J, Aker PD, Crowther ER, et al: A comparison of active and simulated chiropractic manipulation as adjunctive treatment for childhood asthma, *N Engl J Med* 339(15):1013-1020, 1998.

BenEliyahu DJ: Magnetic resonance imaging and clinical follow-up: study of 27 patients receiving chiropractic care for cervical and lumbar disc herniations, *J Manipulative Physiol Ther* 19(9):597-606, 1996.

Bennett GM: *The art of the bonesetter,* Isleworth, 1981, Tamor Pierston.

Bigos S, Bowyer O, Braen G: Acute lower back pain in adults. Clinical Practice Guideline, Quick Reference Guide No 14, AHCPR Pub No 95-0643, Rockville, Md, 1994, US Department of Health and Human Services, Public Health Service, Agency for Health Care Policy and Research.

Boline PD, Kassak K, Bronfort G, et al: Spinal manipulation vs. amitriptyline for the treatment of chronic tension-type headaches: a randomized clinical trial, *J Manipulative Physiol Ther* 18(3):148-154, 1995.

Bourdillion JF: *Spinal manipulation,* ed 3, East Norwalk, Conn, 1982, Appleton-Century-Crofts.

Bove G, Nilsson N: Spinal manipulation in the treatment of episodic tension-type headache: a randomized controlled trial, *JAMA* 280(18):1576-1579, 1998.

Brennan PC, Kokjohn K, Kaltinger CJ, et al: Enhanced phagocytic cell respiratory burst induced by spinal manipulation: potential role of substance P, *J Manipulative Physiol Ther* 14(7):399-408, 1991.

Bronfort G, Goldsmith CH, Nelson CF: Trunk exercise combined with spinal manipulative or NSAID therapy for chronic low back pain: a randomized, observer-blinded clinical trial, *J Manipulative Physiol Ther* 19(9):570-582, 1996.

Cassidy JD, Thiel HW, Kirkaldy-Willis WH: Side posture manipulation for lumbar intervertebral disk herniation, *J Manipulative Physiol Ther* 16(2):96-103, 1993.

Chapman-Smith DA: *The chiropractic profession,* West Des Moines, Iowa, 2000, NCMIC Group.

Cherkin D, Deyo RA, Berg AO: Evaluation of a physician education intervention to improve primary care for low back pain. I. Impact on physicians, *Spine* 16(10):1168-1172, 1991.

Cherkin DC, Deyo RA, Wheeler K, Ciol MA: Physician views about treating low back pain: the results of a national survey, *Spine* 20(1):1-9, 1995.

Cherkin DC, MacCornack FA: Patient evaluations of low back pain care from family physicians and chiropractors, *West J Med* 150(3):351-355, 1989.

Commission on Alternative Medicine, Social Departementete: *Legitimization for vissa kiropraktorer,* Stockholm, 1987, 12:13-16.

Coulter I et al.: The appropriateness of spinal manipulation and mobilization of the cervical spine: literature review, indications and ratings by a multidisciplinary expert panel. Monograph No DRU-982-1-CCR, Santa Monica, Calif, 1995, RAND.

Cox JM, Feller JA: Chiropractic treatment of low back pain: a multicenter descriptive analysis of presentation and outcome in 424 consecutive cases, *JNMS J Neuromusculoskel Syst* 2:178-190, 1994.

Croft PR, Macfarlane GJ, Papageorgiou AC, et al: Outcome of low back pain in general practice: a prospective study, *BMJ* 316(7141):1356-1359, 1998.

Danish Institute for Health Technology Assessment: Low-back pain: frequency, management, and prevention from an HTA perspective, *Danish Health Tech Assess* 1(1), 1999.

Dvorak J: Neurological and biomechanical aspects of pain. In Buerger AA, Greenman PE, editors: *Approaches to the validation of spinal manipulation,* Springfield, Ill, 1985, Charles C Thomas, pp 241-266.

Eisenberg DM, Davis RB, Ettner SL, et al: Trends in alternative medicine use in the United States, 1990-1997: results of a follow-up national survey, *JAMA* 280: 1569-75, 1998.

Fallon J: The role of the chiropractic adjustment in the care and treatment of 332 children with otitis media, *J Clin Chiropr Pediatr* 2(2):167-183, 1997.

Fallon J, Edelman MJ: Chiropractic care of 401 children with otitis media: a pilot study, *Altern Ther Health Med* 4(2):93, 1998.

Gatterman MI, Goe DR: Muscle and myofascial pain syndromes. In Gatterman MI, editor: *Chiropractic management of spine related disorders,* Baltimore, 1990, Williams & Wilkins, pp 285-329.

Gellert G: Global explanations and the credibility problem of alternative medicine, *Adv Mind Body Med* 10(4):60-67, 1994.

Giles LGF, Muller R: Chronic spinal pain: a randomized clinical trial comparing medication, acupuncture, and spinal manipulation, *Spine* 28(14):1490-1503, 2003.

Haldeman S et al: Arterial dissections following cervical manipulation: the chiropractic experience, *Can Med Assoc J* 165:905, 2001.

Haldeman S, Chapman-Smith D, Peterson DM, editors. Guidelines for chiropractic quality assurance and practice parameters. In *Proceedings of the Mercy Center Consensus Conference,* Gaithersburg, Md, 1993, Aspen.

Hasselberg PD: Chiropractic in New Zealand: report of a commission of inquiry, Wellington, NZ, 1979, Government Printer.

Hondras MA, Long CR, Brennan PC: Spinal manipulative therapy versus a low force mimic maneuver for women with primary dysmenorrhea: a randomized, observer-blinded, clinical trial, *Pain* 81(1-2):105-114, 1999.

Illingworth RS: Infantile colic revisited, *Arch Dis Child* 60:981-985, 1985.

Kelly PT, Luttges MW: Electrophoretic separation of nervous system proteins on exponential gradient polyacrylamide gels, *J Neurochem* 24:1077-1079, 1975.

Kirkaldy-Willis W, Cassidy J: Spinal manipulation in the treatment of low back pain, *Can Fam Physician* 31: 535-540, 1985.

Koes BW, Bouter LM, van Mameren H, et al: A blinded randomized clinical trial of manual therapy and physiotherapy for chronic back and neck complaints: physical outcome measures, *J Manipulative Physiol Ther* 15(1): 16-23, 1992.

Kokjohn K, Schmid DM, Triano JJ, Brennan PC: The effect of spinal manipulation on pain and prostaglandin levels in women with primary dysmenorrhea, *J Manipulative Physiol Ther* 15(5):279-285, 1992.

Korr IM: Proprioceptors and the behavior of lesioned segments. In Stark EH, editor: *Osteopathic medicine,* Acton, Mass, 1975, Publication Sciences Group, pp 183-199.

Korr IM: The spinal cord as organizer of disease processes: some preliminary perspectives, *J Am Osteopath Assoc* 76:89-99, 1976.

Lauretti WJ: Comparative safety of chiropractic. In Redwood D, Cleveland CS III, editors: *Fundamentals of chiropractic,* St Louis, 2003, Mosby, p 561.

Leach RA: *The chiropractic theories: principles and clinical applications,* ed 3, Baltimore, 1994, Williams & Wilkins.

Little P, Smith L, Cantrell T, et al: General practitioners' management of acute back pain: a survey of reported practice compared with clinical guidelines, *BMJ* 312:485-488, 1996.

Lomax E: Manipulative therapy: a historical perspective from ancient times to the modern era. In Goldstein M, editor: *The research status of spinal manipulation: 1975,* Washington, DC, 1975, US Government Printing Office, pp 11-17.

Lucassen PL, Assendelft WJ, Gubbels JW, et al: Effectiveness of treatments for infantile colic: a systematic review, *BMJ* 316:1563-1569, 1998.

Luttges MW, Kelly PT, Gerren RA: Degenerative changes in mouse sciatic nerves: electrophoretic and electrophysiological characterizations, *Exp Neurol* 50:706-733, 1976.

MacGregor RJ, Oliver RM: A general-purpose electronic model for arbitrary configurations of neurons, *J Theor Biol* 38:527-538, 1973.

MacGregor RJ, Sharpless SK, Luttges MW: A pressure vessel model for nerve compression, *J Neurol Sci* 24:299-304, 1975.

Manga P et al: *The effectiveness and cost-effectiveness of chiropractic management of low-back pain,* Richmond Hill, Va, 1993, Kenilworth.

Meade TW: Interview on Canadian Broadcast Corporation. In *Chiropractic: a review of current research,* Arlington, Va, 1992, Foundation for Chiropractic Education and Research.

Meade TW, Dyer S, Browne W, Frank AO: Randomised comparison of chiropractic and hospital outpatient management for low back pain: results from extended follow up, *BMJ* 311(7001):349-351, 1995.

Meade TW, Dyer S, Browne W, et al: Low back pain of mechanical origin: randomised comparison of chiropractic and hospital outpatient treatment, *BMJ* 300(6737):1431-1437, 1990.

Meeker WC, Haldeman S: Chiropractic: a profession at the crossroads of mainstream and alternative medicine, *Ann Intern Med* 136(3):216-227, 2002.

Mense S: Considerations concerning the neurobiological basis of muscle pain, *Can J Physiol Pharmacol* 69:610-616, 1991.

Micozzi MS: Complementary care: when is it appropriate? Who will provide it? *Ann Intern Med* 129:65-66, 1998.

Nelson CF, Bronfort G, Evans R, et al: The efficacy of spinal manipulation, amitriptyline and the combination of both therapies for the prophylaxis of migraine headache, *J Manipulative Physiol Ther* 21(8):511-519, 1998.

Olafsdottir E et al: Randomised controlled trial of infantile colic treated with chiropractic spinal manipulation, *Arch Dis Child* 84:138, 2001.

Palmer DD. *Textbook of the science, art, and philosophy of chiropractic,* Portland, Ore, 1910, Portland Printing House.

Paré A: *The collected works of Ambroise Paré,* New York, 1968, Milford House.

Patterson MM, Steinmetz JE: Long-lasting alterations of spinal reflexes: a potential basis for somatic dysfunction, *Man Med* 2:38-42, 1986.

Plamondon RL. Summary of 1994 ACA annual statistical study, *J Am Chiropr Assoc* 32(1):57-63, 1995.

Redwood D: Same data, different interpretation, *J Altern Complement Med* 5(1):89-91, 1999.

Rosen M: *Back pain: report of a clinical standards advisory group committee on back pain,* London, 1994, HMSO.

Rosner AL: Musculoskeletal disorders research. In Redwood D, Cleveland CS III, editors: *Fundamentals of chiropractic,* St Louis, 2003, Mosby, p 465.

Schafer RC, Faye LJ: *Motion palpation and chiropractic technique,* Huntington Beach, Calif, 1989, Motion Palpation Institute.

Sharpless S: Susceptibility of spinal roots to compression block. In Goldstein M, editor: *The research status of spinal manipulation: 1975,* Washington, DC, 1975, US Government Printing Office, pp 155-161.

Shekelle PG, Adams AH, et al: The appropriateness of spinal manipulation for low-back pain: project overview and literature review. Report No R-4025/1-CCR/FCER, Santa Monica, Calif, 1991, RAND.

Shekelle PG, Coulter I, Hurwitz EL, et al: Congruence between decisions to initiate chiropractic spinal manipulation for low back pain and appropriateness criteria in North America, *Ann Intern Med* 129(1):9-17, 1998.

Simske SJ, Schmeister TA: An experimental model for combined neural, muscular, and skeletal degeneration, *JNMS J Neuromusculoskel Syst* 2:116-123, 1994.

Suh CH: The fundamentals of computer aided x-ray analysis of the spine, *J Biomech* 7:161-169, 1974.

Thomasen PR, Fisher BL, Carpenter PA, Fike GL: Effectiveness of spinal manipulative therapy in treatment of primary dysmenorrhea: a pilot study, *J Manipulative Physiol Ther* 2:140-145, 1979.

Thompson CJ: *Second report: Medicare Benefits Review Committee,* Canberra, Canada, 1986, Commonwealth Government Printer.

Triano JJ, Luttges MW: Nerve irritation: a possible model of sciatic neuritis, *Spine* 7:129-136, 1982.

Triano JJ, McGregor M, Hondras MA, Brennan PC: Manipulative therapy versus education programs in chronic low back pain, *Spine* 20:948-955, 1995.

Van Tulder MW, Koes BW, Bouter LM: Conservative treatment of acute and chronic nonspecific low back pain: a systematic review of randomized controlled trials of the most common interventions, *Spine* 22:2128-2156, 1997.

Von Kuster T: *Chiropractic health care: a national study of cost of education, service, utilization, number of practicing doctors of chiropractic and other key policy issues,* Washington, DC, 1980, Foundation for the Advancement of Chiropractic Tenets and Science.

Wiberg JM, Nordsteen J, Nilsson N: The short-term effect of spinal manipulation in the treatment of infantile colic: a randomized controlled clinical trial with a blinded observer, *J Manipulative Physiol Ther* 22(8):517-522, 1999.

Wilk v AMA, 895 F2D 352 Cert den, 112.2 ED 2D 524, 1990.

Winters JC, Sobel JS, Groenier KH, et al: Comparison of physiotherapy, manipulation, and corticosteroid injection for treating shoulder complaints in general practice: randomised, single blind study, *BMJ* 314(7090):1320-1325, 1997.

Withington ET: *Hippocrates.* Vol 3, Cambridge, Mass, 1959, Harvard University Press.

Yates RG, Lamping DL, Abram NL, Wright C: Effects of chiropractic treatment on blood pressure and anxiety: a randomized, controlled trial, *J Manipulative Physiol Ther* 11(6):484-488, 1988.

Resources

Associations

American Chiropractic Association
1701 Clarendon Blvd
Arlington, VA 22209
Phone: 703-276-8800
E-mail: AmerChiro@aol.com
Website: www.amerchiro.org

World Federation of Chiropractic
3080 Yonge St, Suite 5065
Toronto, Ontario, M4N3N1, Canada
Phone: 416-484-9978
E-mail: worldfed@sympatico.ca
Website: www.wfc.org

International Chiropractors Association
1110 North Glebe Rd, Suite 1000
Arlington, VA 22201
Phone: 703-528-5000
E-mail: chiro@erols.com
Website: www.chiropractic.org

Canadian Chiropractic Association
1396 Eglinton Ave West
Toronto, Ontario, M6C2E4, Canada
Phone: 416-781-5656
E-mail: www.inforamp.net/~ccachiro
Website: www.ccachiro.org

Consortial Center for Chiropractic Research
Palmer Center for Chiropractic Research
741 Brady St
Davenport, IA 52803
Phone: 563-884-5150
Website: www.*c3r.org*

Foundation for Chiropractic Education and Research
704 East Fourth St
Des Moines, Iowa 50309
Phone: 515-282-7118
E-mail: fcernow@aol.com
Website: www.fcer.org

National Board of Chiropractic Examiners
901 54th Ave
Greeley, CO 80634
Phone: 970-356-9100
E-mail: nbce@nbce.org
Website: www.nbce.org

Council on Chiropractic Education
8049 N. 85th Way
Scottsdale, AZ 85258
Phone: 480-443-8877
E-mail: cce@cce-usa.org
Website: www.cce-usa.org

Council on Chiropractic Education International
8049 North 85th Way
Scottsdale, AZ 85282-4321
Phone: 480-922-8763
Fax: 480-922-8767
E-mail: ccei@cceintl.org
Website: www.cceintl.org

Other Informative Websites

Dynamic chiropractic:
www.chiroweb.com

The Chiropractic Resource Organization:
www.chiro.org

11

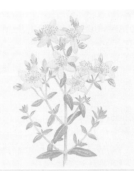

HERBAL MEDICINE

MARC S. MICOZZI
LISA MESEROLE

Plants have been used by humans for food, medicine, clothing, and tools, as well as in religious rites, since before recorded history, more than 60,000 years ago (Solecki, 1975). No continent, island, climate, or geography that is home to human culture lacks a formal tradition of incorporating local flora into daily and ceremonial life as a means of enhancing health and well-being. Prehistoric plant life prepared the earth to be a viable and hospitable habitat for *Homo sapiens,* and plant ecology continues to help maintain the oceans, continents, and atmosphere today.

DEFINITIONS

Herbalism is the study and practice of using plant material for food, medicine, and health promotion.

This includes not only treatment of disease but also enhancement of quality of life, physically and spiritually. A fundamental principle of herbalism is to promote preventive care and guided, simple treatment among the general population. An *herbalist,* or *herbal practitioner,* is someone who has undertaken specific study and supervised practical training to achieve competence in treating patients. Herbal medicines are recommended by physicians in the practice of integrative medicine and by other practitioners within the pharmacopeia of their traditions.

There is also an eclectic practice of herbal medicine in Europe and North America that draws on herbs from many healing traditions and has been called *Western herbalism.*

An herb can be an angiosperm (i.e., a flowering plant), shrub, or tree, or a moss, lichen, fern, algae, seaweed, or fungus. The herbalist may use the entire plant or just the flowers, fruits, leaves, twigs, bark, roots, rhizomes, seeds, or exudates (e.g., tapped and purified maple syrup), or a combination of parts. Botany defines an *herb* as a nonwoody, low-growing plant, but herbalists use the entire plant kingdom. In many herbal traditions, nonplants are used as healing agents, including animal parts (organs, bone, tissue), insects, animal and insect secretions, worm castings, shells, rocks, metals, minerals, and gemstones. These examples are recorded in ancient and contemporary materia medicae and formal manuscripts of healing agents with their indications and uses. Egyptian, Chinese, Tibetan, European, American, and other worldwide material medicae are important references for herbal practitioners. This chapter addresses only plant herbal agents.

Herbalism may be a misleading term because it implies that a single hidden "root" gives rise to the diverse ways in which all human cultures across the millennia have used plants for food, medicine, and ritual. The use of herbs by the peoples of the Americas, Europe, Africa, the Middle and Far East, the Pacific Islands, and other regions is specific to each society and paradigm. For example, contemporary Western scientists have been restricted until recently by the Western mechanistic premises of biology and physics (see Chapter 1).

Although there is no single, worldwide system of herbalism, all herbal traditions share certain themes.

 ### *"Herb" and Other Words*

*H*erb as a word has an ancient pedigree, originating with the Latin word *herba*, which refers to green crops and grasses and could also mean the same as we mean by *herb* today (*OED*). The word entered English through Old French. The English use of "herb" in the sense of a plant whose stem does not become woody and persistent, but which remains more or less soft and succulent, dying down to the ground (or entirely) after flowering, can be traced to the thirteenth century. In the thirteenth century it was also understood that "herb" (with variant spellings, e.g., "erbe") is a plant whose leaves and stems (and sometimes roots) could be used as food or medicine or for scent or flavor.

Herbarium, in the sense of a collection of dried plants, has its origins in the eighteenth century. A source that associates "herbarium" with the medicinal properties of plants is that the idea for drying plants for study originated with a professor in sixteenth-century Italy who also held a chair in "simples," where he studied medicinal and other plants.

"Herbalist" has shifted meaning. Originally (in the sixteenth century) an "herbalist" was one versed in the knowledge of herbs and plants—a collector of and writer about plants, more what we mean by "botanist" today. Usually, however, *herbalist* is now used to refer to early writers about plants, as well as a person who uses alternative medical therapy, although the *OED* does not mention this.

"Herbal," meaning a book containing names and descriptions of herbs (or other plants in general) that provides properties and virtues, came into use in the early sixteenth century. *Herbal*, meaning belonging to, consisting of, or made from herbs, has its origins in the early seventeenth century.

Early botanic gardens started in Renaissance Italy. These should properly be called "physic gardens" because they were used to help educated medical students, that is, to teach people—in this case medical students—about medicinal plants. Physic gardens appeared in England in the sixteenth century, in private hands. The Oxford Physic Garden began in 1621. (Chelsea Physic Garden was begun in 1673 by the Society of Apothecaries.) The Oxford Physic Garden became the Botanic Garden in 1840, an important and representative change. There was no real difference between a "physic garden" and a "botanic garden" because botany and the study of the medicinal properties of plants were not distinct fields. William Turner (1510-1568) was a physician, author of an herbal, and is considered the father of English botany. Taxonomy was not separate from pharmacology in the study of plants for Turner.

Although the process was gradual, by the nineteenth century the study of plants for their own sake—botany—was a clearly separate field. Pharmacopoeias and botanical atlases grew in importance as the need for herbals waned.

There are clear ways to classify types of gardens. In the 1790s, Dr. Benjamin Rush called for the establishment of a "botanic garden" at the College of Physicians of Philadelphia. In Rush's time this would have meant a garden to study the properties of plants, in this case, medicinal properties. Rush

(Continued)

"Herb" and Other Words—cont'd

suggests, however, that the garden could also be a *source* of medical preparations, as well as a place to grow plants that might be lost as Europeans settled North America. Although it was not the only purpose of Rush's garden, study was a component, and research lies at the heart of any botanical garden's purpose. (Botanical gardens are not limited strictly to taxonomy.)

Medical botany would be the study of the medicinal properties of plants, for example, chemical analysis to find new medically important compounds. A *medical botanical garden* would be the source of plants for studying their medical properties.

A *medicinal herb garden* would, in a technical sense, be a place that has examples of plants, from which samples could be taken to make medicinal preparations. Also, the garden would contain only herbaceous plants, not plants with woody stems and branches ∾

Common Themes of Herbalism

- *Optimization of health and wellness.* Most traditions include specific systems of food, spice, and herb taboos and recommended inclusions; adherence to these protects practitioners and users from undesirable consequences. A pregnant woman in Mexico avoids eggs because they could push her into a state of excess cold that could weaken her (curanderismo; see Chapter 30). During winter flu season, extra ginger and hot peppers are added to curries in Indian cuisine to protect against infection. Similarly, shitake mushrooms (powerful immunomodulators) are used in winter soups in traditional Japanese cooking.
- *Emphasis on the whole person.* This includes body, mind, and soul; past, present, and future; and community.
- *Emphasis on the individual.* In Chinese herbal medicine, 10 patients with high blood pressure might receive 10 different herbal formulas. Furthermore, the same patient might take different hypertension formulas at age 45 and at age 65, and each formula might be adjusted repeatedly according to pulse, tongue, and other readings.
- *Emphasis on the community.* The illness or recovery of a member might influence the community itself, beyond emotional group empathy.

- *Attention to finding and treating the root cause of a problem,* not only the manifestations and symptoms. However, as with most healers and medicine suppliers, if the cause remains unidentified or untreatable, symptomatic treatment is offered.
- *Application of the principle of duality* between both the healing and the life-threatening forces of nature. The fundamental assumption of this principle is that natural law is greater than the will of the individual or community, and that healing requires the healer, the patient, and the community be in alignment with natural forces.
- *Belief in the reality of the unmeasurable and abstract.* Although dual, the abstract and physical worlds are inseparable. An herbalist as healer devotes himself or herself to maintaining balance and communication between the visible and invisible. This goal might be accomplished through connecting with spirituality or by adjusting activities to natural cycles (e.g., in Tibetan medicine, blending a formula during a specific season, moon phase, or auspicious date).
- *Premise of recycling.* Nature is inherently circular and repetitive; generally sequential, but not predominantly linear; and predictable, but seldom certain. This leads to the common traditional practice of offering an object or prayer in return for healing plants and for addressing requests for healing to both the physical and the spiritual world.
- *Openness to exchange of knowledge.* Most traditions incorporate new medicinal plants and new herbal uses and preparations that have been learned about through trade or travel.
- *Regulation of the herbalist's practice* through local accountability to his or her community. Success and prestige arise primarily from professional reputation that grows by word of mouth, not from image, business acumen, or material wealth (see Chapter 4).
- *Humility* generated from the healer's recognition of his or her own limits and skills. Because reputation generally depends on treatment efficacy and community standing, an herbalist would be reluctant to take on a case without reasonable confidence that he or she could succeed. Complex or incurable cases would be referred to another kind of practitioner, or the patient would be advised that no treatment was available other than palliation of suffering.

CLASSIFICATIONS OF HERBALISTS

Each cultural or medical system has different types of herbal practitioners, all consistent with its paradigm. However, most paradigms identify professional herbalists, lay herbalists, plant gatherers, and medicine makers. (Professional or lay herbalists often collect their own plants and prepare their own medicines.)

Professional Herbalist

A professional herbalist undertakes formalized training or a long apprenticeship in plant and medical studies or alternatively in plant and spiritual or healing studies. This knowledge includes extensive familiarity—often a relationship—with specific plants, which involves their identification, habitat, harvesting criteria, preparation, storage, therapeutic indications, contraindications, and dosing. A professional herbalist is not necessarily the primary healer (Iwu, 1993). A professional herbalist might follow a family tradition or might be selected at a young age as being endowed with potential mastery of using plants as healing aids. In Europe and the United States, this group includes officially trained medical herbalists, clinical herbalists, licensed naturopathic doctors specializing in botanical medicine, licensed acupuncturists with training in Chinese herbal medicine, licensed Ayurvedic doctors, Native American herbalists and shamans, Latin American curanderos, and other lineage-recognized or culturally recognized professional herbalists. The shaman from Madagascar who—although never acknowledged or compensated for his contribution—revealed the usefulness of *Caranthas roseus,* the periwinkle plant developed in the West as vinblastine and vincristine against certain cancers, exemplifies the spirit and expertise of a professional healer and herbalist.

Many herbalists consider the patient's direct involvement in his or her own healing and the summoning of the patient's intellectual, emotional, physical, and spiritual attention to the process as critical. Partly for this reason and because of traditional herbalism's emphasis on "right relationship," social context, and self-responsibility, many herbal practitioners deliberately prescribe elaborate rather than convenient herbal therapies. For example, on returning home to Ghana, a merchant developed an infected leg ulcer. Instead of being supplied an herbal medicine by the herbalist, he was directed to the nearby live plant source (a local tree bark). He collected and prepared the antimicrobial and vulnery poultice and applied it daily until his wound healed. Although self-collection and medicine preparation is generally impractical in the United States, self-involvement in the healing process is possible in many ways and parallels the complex lifestyle changes now routinely recommended to patients with chronic ailments such as cardiovascular disease.

Lay Herbalist

A lay herbalist has a broad knowledge of plants useful for health problems but does not have extensive training in medical and spiritual diagnosis and management. He or she may be an herb vendor with a sensitivity to the needs and desires of the marketplace, whose livelihood has been passed down as a family business. Evaluation of medicinal plant quality, strength, uses, and dose is included in the lay herbalist's domain. The Irish herbalist who uses specific herbal treatments for certain skin or stomach symptoms is an example.

Plant Gatherer, Plant Grower, and Medicine Maker

Plant gatherers, plant growers, and medicine makers might consider themselves herbalists; actually, they are to the practicing herbalist what the contemporary pharmacist is to the clinical physician. In Chinese medicine, there is one specialist who produces and collects plants, one who processes and stores plants, and a clinical herbalist/doctor who prescribes the medicines. In some systems, preparing and handling medicines is considered a spiritual privilege and responsibility. Therefore, certain herbal medicines are prepared only by the herbalist or healer or by a designated assistant.

HERBS AND MEDICINAL PLANTS

Physicians in the United States studied and relied on plant drugs as primary medicines through the 1930s.

Until then, medical schools taught basic plant taxonomy and pharmacognosy and medicinal plant therapeutics. The term *drug* derives from an ancient word for *root,* and the roots and rhizomes of many medicinal plants continue to provide alkaloids, steroidal saponins, and many active constituents that are clinically useful at present. The *United States Pharmacopeia* listed 636 herbal entries in 1870; only 58 were listed in the 1990 edition (Boyle, 1991). Although some plants were dropped because they were found to be weak or unsafe, the majority of clinically useful plants were replaced with pharmaceuticals, which generated profits from patented drugs and contributed to the standardization and industrialization of medicine.

Characteristics and Composition

In many traditional systems the characteristics of a medicinal plant are emphasized without attention to its composition, because techniques and equipment for plant analysis are relatively new.

Preanalytical, chemical knowledge of medicinal and food plants is derived from direct perception through the five senses; from the herbalist's attentive, empirical observation of plants' effects on animals and humans; and in some traditions, from sacred teachings and "sixth sense" intuition. Plants' healing uses and properties are paradigm specific. In Chinese and Tibetan medicine the "five tastes" are sweet, sour, salty, pungent, and bitter. Each flavor is associated with certain qualities and corresponding physiological actions. For example, cinnamon *(Cinnamomum cassia)* bark is warm, sweet, and pungent and is used to warm the channels and disperse cold. It is prescribed for certain infections, correlating with more recent pharmacological and clinical research, which demonstrated that aqueous decoctions strongly inhibit *Staphylococcus aureus* and *Salmonella typhi* (Bensky and Gamble, 1986).

Knowledge of the chemical composition of food and medicinal plants is growing worldwide as access to analytical technology improves. Perhaps the only disadvantage to identifying, categorizing, and researching molecular constituents from plants is the risk of equating the plant's therapeutic efficacy to its composition. Analysis is reductionist in paradigm, and data cannot exist beyond the limits of the technology (and available funding to apply it) or the paradigm from which it arises.

Food, medicinal, and healing plants contain digestible fiber (carbohydrates and hemicellulose) and indigestible fiber (cellulose and lignins), nutritives (calories, vitamins, minerals, trace elements, amino acids, essential fatty acids, and water), and inert and active constituents.

Adhering to a Western paradigm, plant constituents can be classified according to their morphology, source plant taxonomy, therapeutic (pharmacological) applications, or chemical constituents (Tyler et al., 1988). A classic organization of the active chemical constituents includes the following:

1. *Carbohydrates:* sugars, starches, aldehydes, gums, and pectins
2. *Glycosides:* cardiac glycosides in *Digitalis purpurea* leaf, anthraquinone glycosides in *Aloe* species latex and rhubarb *(Rheum officinale)* root and rhizome, flavinol glycosides (rutin and hesperidin, used to reduce capillary bleeding), and other glycoside types
3. *Tannins:* present in coffee and tea
4. *Lipids:* fixed oils and waxes
5. *Volatile oils:* essential oils such as peppermint and eucalyptus
6. *Resins*
7. *Steroids:* including the steroidal saponins from Mexican yam *(Diocorea* species), the original source of early oral contraceptives
8. *Alkaloids:* atropine from *Atropa belladona,* quinine from chinchona, morphine from *Papaver somniferum*
9. *Peptide hormones*
10. *Enzymes:* bromelain from pineapple

Physiological Activities

Activities and correspondent indications for the use of plants are, again, paradigm specific (Box 11-1). In the United States alone, opinions vary regarding a particular plant's full spectrum of physiological action because of the complex nature of plants and their uses.

The many influences on plant activities and their therapeutic properties might threaten the confidence of the researcher, herbalist, or patient that the desired effect will be produced. However, every factor listed is present in the human food supply, which has supported human life since prehistory. Scientists might agree that there is no way to control all variables,

BOX 11-1

Influences on Plant Activities and Their Therapeutic Properties

- Specific plant species, variety, and sometimes individual plant itself.
- Habitat, including latitude, longitude, exposure, humidity, rainfall, sun, shade, wind, temperature and daily and seasonal variation, soil, soil microorganisms, insects, birds, animals, companion plants, pests, plant diseases, and interaction with humans (damage, cultivation, harvesting, and pollution).
- Composition and constituents (presence of active and inert ingredients).
- How and when the plant is collected, stored, processed; how the herb is dispensed and dosed.
- Presence of adulterants, pests, or disease.
- The prescriber; many traditional systems in Africa and Asia ascribe the ability to potentiate the plant's healing properties only to initiated healers or shamans.
- The patient's health status, disease, age, and receptivity to healing.
- The symbolic or cultural significance of the plant.
- The placebo effect.

although identifying, controlling, or tracking those most suspected of producing specific outcomes is a shared responsibility of healers and researchers. Plant actions are recorded in the pharamacopeia through the first half of the twentieth century in archaic terminology. Many terms are similarly used to describe the actions of contemporary pharmaceuticals.

A sample of some classic plant actions—often associated with identifiable nutritives or active constituents—are as follows:

- *Respiratory system:* stimulating expectorant (*Marrubrium vulgaris,* hoarhound), relaxing expectorant (*Prunus serotina,* black cherry bark), antitussive (*P. serotina),* and immunomodulator for upper respiratory tract infection (*Echinacea purpurea* and other species)
- *Gastrointestinal system:* emetic (*Cephaelis ipeca-cuanha),* antiemetic (*Zingiber officinale,* ginger), laxative (*Plantago ovata,* psyllium seed), and spasmolytic (*Papaver somniferum,* opium poppy)
- *Nervous system:* sedative (*Valeriana officinalis),* stimulant (*Piper methysticum,* kava kava), cardiotonic (*Crataegus oxycantha* or *C. monogyna,* hawthorn), and antidepressant (*Hypericum perforatum,* St. John's wort)

These examples illustrate a few of the many actions ascribed to classic Western-paradigm herbs. Often, contemporary research explains the constituents, mechanisms of action, and clinical responses that justify traditional uses. Occasionally, some plants are found to be inactive or ineffective or to contain potential toxins, resulting in their discontinuance or requiring special methods of preparation

and dosing. As with most current prescription medications, some strong herbs must be dosed carefully to render them safe and effective. However, to provide a realistic perspective, casava root—one of the leading sources of calories and carbohydrates for people worldwide—contains cyanide-like compounds that may produce permanent neurotoxicity, paralysis, and death if improperly prepared; traditional preparation involves cooking, which renders the toxins inert. Various cultural traditions of plant preparation have empirically developed to facilitate the extraction of nutritive and medicinal properties while eliminating toxic components.

There are other limitations to the direct association of active constituents to in vivo and clinical medicinal actions. Many times the active compounds remain unidentified, or the physiological response to the medicinal part of the whole plant is distinct from the actions of the individual active constituents (e.g., *Valeriana, Echinacea).* In addition, ingredients that appear inert are sometimes later found to be active when a more accurate mechanism of action or bioassay associated with the plant's effects is discovered. This occurred in the National Cancer Institute's screening program, when "inactive" plants were rescreened decades later with advanced methods and found to contain biologically active compounds.

From a nonreductionist paradigm, plant composition alone offers an incomplete explanation of the full scope of the properties and actions of food and healing plants. Traditional herbalists, turn-of-the-century vitalists (see Chapter 5), naturopathic doctors, and many contemporary medical doctors and practitioners share a belief in a "life force" that is yet to be fully understood. Many herbalists hold that healing energy is inherent to plants; it is this energy, in addition to nutritive or chemical constituents, that promotes healing. Shamans, traditional healers, and alchemists use their skills, knowledge, and power to instill certain plants with special healing properties in this view.

Herbal Therapeutics

Different cultural paradigms use plants for healing in a manner founded on each paradigm's premises. Herbal practitioners in the United States may rely primarily on one of the following, or a combination:

1. *The plant's pharmacological actions:* in some cases enhanced by specific processing and extractive solvents and techniques or formulating plant medicines into standardized extract products to concentrate and guarantee unit doses of active constituents.
2. *Individual plant pharmacokinetics*: best preserved by using single, whole plants or their extracts.
3. *Synergistic formulating:* blending a number of medicinal plants together to achieve specific therapeutic effects unachievable by using a single herb alone.
4. *Nutritive value*: as when *Urtica repens,* or nettles, is recommended as a tea rich in absorbable iron.
5. Energetics

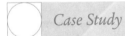

Case Study

A 35-year-old patient in the United States consults with a Western naturopathic doctor or medical herbalist about experiencing mild anxiety. The patient's family history and personal and psychological health history are medically "unremarkable."

A health screening and physical examination within the last 6 months identified no health problems. The patient is evaluated for a "constitutional" physiological profile, a personal and social profile, and a lifestyle profile (stress, diet, exercise, recreation, and spiritual values). Treatment for her simple, circumstantial, stress-induced anxiety is to increase exercise and gardening (time outdoors), make some minor adjustments to her diet and lifestyle, soak her feet each evening in a lavender (*Lavandula officionalus*) foot bath (mildly relaxing) for 10 days, use *Passiflora incarnata* tincture (specifically dosed) twice daily for 2 weeks, and then consult with the practitioner on her progress and symptoms.

P. incarnata is listed in Martindale's *Extra Pharmacopeia* (1994) and in the pharmacopeias of Egypt, France, Germany, Switzerland, and Brazil, although it is not listed in the *United States Pharmacopeia*. It acts as a mild sedative and antispasmodic. Among its constituents are a volatile oil (sedating on inhalation but of unknown composition), cyanogenic flavinoids 5-7-dihydroxyflavone ("chrysin," a monflavinoid shown to act as a partial agonist, displacing flunitrazepam from central benzodiazepine receptors from mice), and passiflorine (a hormone alkaloid).

Food and medicinal plants have multiple actions, caused at least in part by their multiple constituents. This is in relative contrast to many pharmaceuticals, which typically have a single or a few specific therapeutic actions. However, pharmaceutical side effects demonstrate how uncommon a true single action is physiologically—whether because of minor but concurrent nontherapeutic pharmacological actions or because a single action provokes the desired therapeutic physiological response along with unintended, nontherapeutic responses.

The multiple actions of plants, although a challenge to the isolation of single active constituents or primary single pharmacological or physiological actions, are only a problem if plants are classified as highly potent, synthetic pharmaceuticals. However, because most medicinal plants are much less potent than pharmaceuticals and because humans have evolved on plant-based diets (each individual plant or animal food a complex chemical soup of unknown formula), it seems appropriate to assume that humans are probably better adapted to plants as food and medicine (Chapters 1 and 2) than to strong pharmaceutical drugs that have 50 years or less of use in the population worldwide.

Herbal medicines can be delivered in many forms. Some plants are best used fresh but are seldom marketed fresh because they are highly perishable. Dried, whole, or chopped herbs can be prepared as *infusions* (steeped as tea) or *decoctions* (simmered over low heat). Flowers, leaves, and powdered herbs are infused (chamomile or peppermint), whereas fruits, seeds, barks, and roots require decocting (rose hips, cinnamon bark, licorice root). Many fresh and dried herbs can be tinctured as preserved medicines in alcohol; some plants are suited to acetracts (vinegar extracts), whereas others are active and well preserved as syrups, glycerites (in vegetable glycerine), or miels (in honey).

Powered or freeze-dried herbs are available in bulk, tablets, troches, pastes, and capsules. Fluid and solid extracts—strong concentrates (four to six times the crude herb strength)—and fresh plant juices preserved in approximately 25% alcohol (as in the fresh plant *Echinacea succus*) are other forms.

Nonoral delivery forms include herbal pessaries, suppositories, creams, ointments, gels, liniments, oils, distilled waters, washes, enemas, baths, poultices, compresses, moxa, snuffs, steams, and inhaled smokes and aromatics (volatile oils). The predominant plant delivery forms vary among different herbal traditions. Tinctures are widely used in Britain and the United States; tablets of standardized extracts of certain herbs (e.g., *Ginkgo biloba*) are popular in Germany and the United States; decoctions are common in Tibetan, Chinese, and African traditions; therapeutic oils are used topically and internally in Ayurvedic treatments; and teas, smokes, and compresses are used in the Native American tradition.

Another point must be made regarding herbal therapeutics as distinct from contemporary over-the-counter (OTC) and prescription pharmaceuticals. Herbal therapies have not always been used as traditionally intended, nor do they show highest efficacy when used as pharmaceutical substitutes. Crude or processed plant foods and medicines tend to work best preventively or therapeutically as slow-acting, gradual, healing agents. They must be taken consistently in the correct form and dose (although some medicinal plants may work rapidly). In addition, the herbal practitioner's familiarity with each medicinal plant or herbal formula usually may be greater than the medical familiarity with each individual pharmaceutical. This permits the herbalist to select precisely a particular plant or formula for each individual patient. Three different patients with a chief complaint of headache would likely each receive a different herbal prescription. The approach that an herbalist uses to arrive at which herbs to prescribe is distinct from how a conventional Western physician prescribes a pharmaceutical.

HERBS IN PREVENTIVE HEALTH AND SELF-CARE

As observed by the World Health Organization (WHO), herbs are essentially "people's medicine." In many parts of the world, traditional systems of herbalism generally make little distinction between food and medicinal plants, and local accessibility to food, spice, and therapeutic herbs generally is assumed in traditional agrarian, nonindustrialized societies.

Before the twentieth century, most people everywhere generally had closer personal contact with food and medicinal plants. The modern era has brought many advantages to human health and sanitation, but one potential disadvantage of economic and occupational specialization is the loss of this contact with the source of plant medicines. The marketplace has become multileveled, so the consumer usually has no direct or personal relationship with the herb producer. Sometimes, because of costs of production, taxes, and marketing, the packaged herbal product costs 20 times the price of the crude herb. There are undeniable advantages to certain prepackaged or concentrated herbal products, but two disadvantages are accountability and economic access. If fresh or bulk crude herbs are abandoned in the marketplace for less perishable and higher-return products, the patient has access to only highly processed products, and the cash-poor patient loses access altogether. This is particularly ironic in the case of medicinal plants; most traditional systems considered healing plants a gift of nature and access to them a basic human right.

A partial solution regarding access to high-quality herbs is renewed national interest in home gardens and urban "pea patches," thus embracing herbalism's unwritten dictum of self-responsibility and direct individual contact in the cycles of nature. Many culinary herbs such as thyme, oregano, and rosemary contain antioxidants and antimicrobial volatile oils and are digestive stimulants and antiseptics. Although specific herbs may vary depending on climate and region, such kitchen gardens could serve as preventive and therapeutic medicines for minor ailments.

In contemporary American culture, the context for using medicinal plants for preventive and therapeutic purposes already has been lost, except for subcultures in which it has been preserved, such as among the Amish and Native Americans. A restoration of the personal and symbolic relationship to food and medicine plants could be linked with contemporary scientific knowledge of herbal applications. Appropriate self-care could be encouraged with public education, access to consultation with professional herbalists and physicians, and access to fresh herbs and high-quality, processed herbal medicines when needed. This improved patient involvement in the self-care of the body and its signals might then improve the use of professional medical care.

RESEARCH IN FOOD AND MEDICINAL PLANTS

Although there is a relatively extensive contemporary literature on medicinal and healing plants, much of it exists outside the United States and often in languages other than English. In addition, there is little consistency in standard research designs and protocols among various countries.

The need for more research on food, spice, and medicinal plants is great, especially for their potential use in syndromes and conditions not well recognized or treated by conventional Western medicine. The challenge is to conduct the research in a holistic context. This requires creative funding of research that is unlikely to provide high-profit returns to a single source. Fortunately, research on crude or extracted traditional plant remedies is relatively inexpensive compared with the astronomical costs of new drug development by pharmaceutical companies. Many medicinal plants eliminated from the *United States Pharmacopeia* over the years were dropped because they lacked contemporary research documentation of efficacy, not because they were proved to be ineffective (although some plants proved less useful clinically than newly developed drugs).

Retaining a holistic context in medicinal plant research also involves addressing differences in paradigm. Involving traditional herbalists as research design consultants would protect against inadvertently eliminating a critical element of the paradigm in which the herb is used. In the past, plant collection for research has sometimes proved an environmental threat (habitats, species, or traditional knowledge were lost or threatened). A holistic approach to contemporary plant collection and research must be conducted in a way to conserve the traditional knowledge and ecology of the source plant and to avoid transgression of intellectual property rights, destruction of the plant habitat, or an imbalance of economic or intellectual returns to the source habitat and community.

Simple, well-documented analysis and outcomes-based research of crude and whole plant medicines are needed to determine their greatest potential applications and benefit to human health. British sailors were cured of scurvy with limes, subsequently presumed to be therapeutic against the disease solely because of their vitamin C content. However, limes and citrus proved more effective against scurvy than vitamin C supplementation alone. This observation was largely explained by the presence of bioflavonoids, later isolated and discovered to be prevalent in citrus pulp. It is desirable to perform bioassays and clinical efficacy studies on whole herbs and herbal formulas, as well as on identified active constituents within the plants.

Increasing contemporary research on medicinal plants is critical, but the importance of documenting and incorporating the empirical knowledge of healing plants cannot be overemphasized. One of the greatest disadvantages of modern research is its highly select study cohort (often a single gender/age group, ethnicity, or locality), its relatively brief treatment and monitoring intervals, and its failure to fully document subclinical or seemingly irrelevant symptoms of the participating individuals. Sample populations are relatively small compared with the worldwide population. However, if information gleaned from research is linked with empirical knowledge (usually derived from hundreds of years of human use across many generations and ethnic groups), along with contemporary clinical reporting from patients and practitioners on tolerance and efficacy, then herbal therapeutics and preventive protocols can be better targeted to enhance the health of future generations.

CHALLENGES AND OPPORTUNITIES FOR CONTEMPORARY HERBALISM

The greatest opportunity for human benefit from food, spice, and healing plants will be afforded only if at least some elements of the traditional contexts and paradigms in which herbs have been used are preserved. The special relationship of humans to the plant world is one of these traditions.

Challenges for the future include the following:

1. Ensuring preservation of germ plasm.
2. Maintaining conservation of biodiversity and plant habitat.
3. Training professional and other herbalists.
4. Exchanging information with traditional healers.
5. Providing physicians and other health care professionals with the resources to become familiar with plant medicines (Box 11-2).
6. Educating the public in the appropriate use of herbs for self-care.

BOX 11-2

General Guidelines for Use of Herbal Medicines

1. The clinician should take a careful history of the patient's use of herbs and other supplements.
2. An accurate medical diagnosis must be made before using herbs for symptomatic treatment.
3. *Natural* is not necessarily *safe;* attention should be paid to quality of product, dosage, and potential adverse effects, including interactions.
4. Herbal treatments should, for the most part, be avoided in pregnancy (and contemplated pregnancy) and lactation.
5. Herbal use in children should be done with care, using the appropriate dosage based on weight.
6. Adverse effects should be recorded, and dosage reduced, or the product discontinued. It can be carefully restarted to ascertain whether or not it is the source of the problem.

BOX 11-3

Legislative and Regulatory Environment for Herbal Medicines

Under the U.S. Dietary Supplement Health and Education Act (DSHEA) of 1994, as amended 1998, the FDA presently has power to regulate herbal remedies and dietary supplements in the following ways:
1. Institute "good manufacturing practices" (GMPs), including identity, potency, cleanliness, and stability (although FDA still has not promulgated GMPs 7 years after passage of DSHEA).
2. Refer for criminal action the sale of toxic or unsanitary products.
3. Obtain injunction against the sale of products making false claims.
4. Seize products that pose an unreasonable risk of illness and injury.
5. Sue any company making a claim that a product "cures" or "treats" disease.
6. Stop sale of an entire class of products if they pose imminent health hazard.
7. Stop products from being marketed if FDA does not receive sufficient safety data in advance (under "generally recognized as safe" [GRAS] provisions).

7. Ensuring funding of medicinal plant research that focuses on public health, clinical therapeutics, and wellness, not only drug development.
8. Preserving public access to inexpensive, tonic, and therapeutic herbs through economic, environmental, market, legislative, and health policy (Box 11-3).

The most trusted professional chosen by the American public is often the pharmacist. Many people value and need a personal, face-to-face relationship with the person who prepares and provides them with medicine. Traditionally, this was the role of the herbalist and healer, as well as the turn-of-the-century medical doctor. Currently, many pharmacists are becoming interested in learning about herbal medicines (see Box 11-2). Students in herbal training and naturopathic medical schools are becoming more interested in natural products chemistry. Physicians who practice integrative medicine actively incorporate herbal medicines and

dietary supplements into treatment of a variety of medical conditions. These developments appear to provide timely examples of nature's principle of reciprocity.

The reemergence of herbalism in the West might have been predicted by traditional herbalists and healers centuries ago, who believed in the recycling patterns of nature. All herbal traditions rely predominantly on an ecological relationship between the natural environment, the community, the herbal practitioner, and the individual. Self-sufficiency and personal responsibility are emphasized amid the irrevocable interdependence of human society with nature. The role of "herbalism" in contemporary Western society is not to serve as a substitute for the pharmaceutical advances of the last decades but to serve as an ancient paradigm that was less mechanistic and more holistic and humane in scope and that, if responsibly reclaimed

(Continued)

and integrated, could greatly benefit future health care worldwide. This is illustrated in the following quote by Paiakan, a contemporary Kayapo Indian leader. "I am trying to save the knowledge that the forest and this planet are alive, to give it back to you who have lost the understanding" (Odum, 1971).

GENERAL CONSIDERATIONS FOR USE OF HERBS IN INTEGRATIVE MEDICINE

Changes in the practice of medicine are causing a shift to increasing self-care with more benign, less invasive treatments. As such, it is critical that practicing clinicians (and, in turn, patients) be made aware of the indications, actions, and drug interactions of herbal remedies.

The WHO estimates that 80% of the world's population relies on herbal medicine. Meanwhile, the use of herbs in the United States is expanding rapidly; herbal products are readily found in most pharmacies and supermarkets. From 1990 to 1997, as the use of complementary and alternative (integrative) medicine rose from 34% to 42%, herbal use quadrupled from 3% to 12% (Eisenberg et al., 1998).

Importantly, these rapid changes have occurred because of popular demand. The public has discovered that natural medicines often provide a safe, effective, and economical alternative, and research is increasingly validating this finding. Many of those who use herbal and high-dose vitamin products fail to tell their physicians. Either they assume "natural" products are harmless and not worth mentioning, or they fear telling health professionals who may be skeptical about their use. Health professionals, however, are beginning to familiarize themselves with the subject. Aside from some advantages of natural products, herb-drug interactions are a growing concern: almost one in five prescription drug users are also using supplements (Eisenberg et al., 1998).

In Europe there is a less of a problem because herbs are classified with other pharmaceutical products and routinely prescribed by physicians. In Germany, prescriptions of St. John's wort outnumber those for all other antidepressants. Most of the research to date is European, since industry has had financial incentive to do the necessary research. The United States has recently joined in these efforts, and the National Institutes of Health (NIH) National Center for Complementary and Alternative Medicine (NCCAM) and the National Institute of Mental Health (NIMH) completed a $4.3 million joint clinical trial to determine the efficacy of St. John's wort (SJW) in major depression. Herbal studies are now in progress at a number of America's major medical universities.

Herbal Medicines in Health Care

In the Eisenberg survey (1998), two of the top five conditions for which consumers sought alternative treatment were anxiety and depression. Besides SJW, other herbs were often chosen for these and related problems, including kava for relief of stress and anxiety (until recent concerns about potential effects on the liver), ginkgo for senile dementia or benign forgetfulness, and valerian for sleep. A $20 million NIH trial comparing ginkgo to placebo in the development of dementia in older Americans began in 2000.

Many current drugs are derived from plants. Common examples are morphine, derived from the opium poppy; digitalis, from foxglove; and reserpine, from rauwolfia (Indian snakeroot). In many cases, pharmaceuticals remain the treatment of choice. When appropriate, however, herbs may be preferred for the following reasons:

1. Herbs generally are less likely to cause side effects. When they do occur, side effects are generally milder. In the absence of side effects, patients often fail to notice the subtle improvements that occur as these natural medicines begin to take effect. This contrasting lack of side of effects may also confound double-blind studies. A partial explanation for the milder side effects may be that the original plant constituents are more compatible with metabolism and body chemistry.
2. Although the isolated active ingredient has been assumed to be most effective, there are advantages to using the whole plant. Whereas Western biomedicine seeks to isolate a single active ingredient, herbal medicine relies on the synergistic action of a plant's many constituents.

3. These combinations may also yield a variety of effects. For example, by its action on the brain, kava acts as an anxiety reliever, while its relaxant effects result from its direct action on both smooth and striated muscle.
4. Herbs are working physiologically to restore balance rather than simply targeting a symptom. As a result, herbs often tend to take effect more gradually than pharmaceuticals.

Safety

Side effects of drugs can be serious or fatal; the worst is death by overdose. According to one report, overdoses yielded an annual rate of 30.1 deaths per 1 million prescriptions of antidepressant. On the other hand, to quote Norman Farnsworth, PhD, Professor of Pharmacognosy at the University of Illinois, Chicago: "Based on published reports, side effects or toxic reactions associated with herbal medicines in any form are rare. . . . In fact, of all classes of substances . . . to cause toxicities of sufficient magnitude to be reported in the United States, plants are the least problematic."

It is important to caution patients that if they feel any ill effects from an herbal product, they should inform the prescribing physician. Then, depending on the severity, the patient should either reduce the dose or stop taking the herb. Unlike with pharmaceuticals, withdrawal reactions are rarely an issue.

It is essential to obtain a complete drug and herbal history from the patient. Contraindicated combinations exist, and these should be covered individually. On the other hand, many combinations work well together. For example, individuals taking a drug that is metabolized by the liver can be protected by the liver-supporting herb "milk thistle" (*Silybum marianum*).

Pregnancy, Breastfeeding, and Children

Many herbs have not been approved for use by pregnant and nursing women in the guidelines of the German Commission E, a regulatory agency in some ways comparable to the U.S. Food and Drug Administration (FDA). Now available in English translation, the German Commission E has published a collection of reports based on safety and efficacy data on more than 200 herbs (Blumenthal et al., 2000).

Herbs may often be a treatment of choice for children. Despite lack of modern research, centuries of use have shown many products to be safe when dosed appropriately according to children's weight.

Aging

Considering the phenomenon of polypharmacy in elderly persons and problems of impaired metabolism and clearance, herbs may offer an alternative to drugs. On the other hand, the practitioner also must be aware of herb-drug interactions. SJW can be very useful for depression in the elderly patient, ginkgo for cognitive decline, and kava for sedation (see earlier), without the adverse effects of the benzodiazepines. These herbs can be used in combination with each other as well.

Selection and Use of Herbs

Standardized Extracts

For practitioners new to the medicinal use of herbs, dose selection can be confusing. As discussed, unlike synthetic drugs containing a single compound, herbs often have a number of different active ingredients. Even these will vary in proportion based on many factors, including where the plant was grown and when (season or even time of day) it was harvested. Manufacturers may adjust the mixture to help account for these variations.

To *standardize* the product, that is, to have a consistent, measured amount of product per unit dose, one ingredient is selected as the *marker,* usually the presumed active ingredient. Although research may reveal different or additional active ingredients, for convenience the designated constituent will usually remain the accepted marker. This situation is demonstrated in the example of St. John's wort.

SJW is standardized to hypericin, the long-accepted active antidepressant ingredient. Further research has found hyperforin to be a likely active ingredient. Some SJW products are actually standardized for both. In any case, all compounds (even as-yet-undiscovered contributors) remain distributed throughout the plant, alongside the hypericin. As a result, the standardization of hypericin serves as a useful guidepost for the strength of *all* the (active) ingredients.

Hypericin content is listed on the label, with most products using a 0.3% concentration, so that a 300-mg capsule contains 0.9 mg (0.3 × 300 mg) of hypericin.

In kava the marker is kavalactones, and in ginkgo, flavone glycosides.

Herbal Preparations and Dosing

Herbs can be purchased as teas, tinctures, tablets, and capsules. Teas and tinctures, being liquid, are absorbed more rapidly, with a shorter duration of action. *Tinctures* are made by soaking 1 part herbal material with 5 or 10 parts by weight of alcohol, making a 1:5 or 1:10 concentration. To remove the alcohol taste, the tincture can be placed in warm water or tea for a few minutes to let the alcohol evaporate. Glycerin may also be used instead of alcohol, but the resulting extract is weaker.

Capsules and tablets are the most common delivery system. Gelatin or vegetable-based *capsules* are filled with powdered dried herbs. *Tablets* are powdered herbs compressed into a solid pill, often with a variety of inert ingredients as fillers.

Herbs are supplied in a variety of sizes and strengths, so it is important to read the label carefully. The label also usually gives an average suggested dose as a guideline, based on research and clinical use. It is recommend to start at the low end; watch for a response, including unwanted effects; and adjust the dose accordingly.

For example, patients may do well on 300 mg of SJW once a day, whereas others need four times that dose. Most will fall in the middle range, with the recommended 300 mg three times daily. Some herbs take effect immediately (e.g., kava); others take days, weeks (e.g., SJW, ginkgo), or even months to do so, with individual variation.

Labeling and Patient Information

Most herbal products are regulated as "dietary supplements." In 1994 the U.S. Dietary Supplement Health and Education Act (DSHEA) set new guidelines with regard to quality, labeling, packaging, and marketing of supplements. It also sparked a surge of interest in herbal products. DSHEA allows manufacturers to make "statements of nutritional support for conventional vitamins and minerals." Because herbs are not nutritional in the conventional sense, DSHEA allows manufacturers to make only what they call "structure and function claims," but no therapeutic or prevention claims (see Box 11-3). Thus a label can claim that SJW "optimizes mood," but it cannot list "natural antidepressant," which would be a therapeutic claim.

Because the labels (by law) give insufficient information, it is particularly important for the health practitioner to be well educated in this area. Ideally, supplements would be labeled so that the purchaser would know exact indications and possible side effects, as with OTC medicines.

Quality control is essential, with assurance that the product contains the ingredients and quantities as labeled, and without such contaminants as bacteria, molds, or pesticides. Trade and professional organizations such as the American Herbal Products Association (AHPA) are setting standards called "good manufacturing practices" (GMPs) for the herbal industry. In general, we recommend buying herbal products from a recognized manufacturer.

CONSIDERATIONS FOR HERBAL MEDICINES IN PHARMACY

FDA regulatory authority over herbs is frequently misrepresented as "absent," including by the FDA Commissioner, according to hearings by the U.S. House of Representatives Committee on Government Reform in 2001. Nonetheless, the health care system must rely on vigilance by the medical profession and voluntary compliance by industry in safeguarding patients against adverse reactions. Although legislative efforts are periodically made to alter the regulatory environment, changes are not anticipated in DSHEA, which regulates herbs as dietary supplements, not as drugs. Sen. Orrin Hatch (R-Utah), Co-Chair of the Congressional Caucus on Complementary & Alternative Medicine and Dietary Supplements, documents the unprecedented involvement of a coalition of citizens and commercial groups in the passage of this bill (Hatch, 2002). It is likely that better information and education of consumers and health professionals will help to achieve what more regulation cannot achieve (see Box 11-3).

It is also important to interact with an active and growing natural products and dietary supplements industry in the United States. Some responsible natural products suppliers, manufacturers, and distributors are beginning to recognize that the integration of herbal and nutritional medicine into medical practice mandates higher standards of product ingredients and information about their efficacy.

Gingko biloba, kava kava, and St. John's wort have all come under attack in recent years, and ephedra has been removed from the market because of abuse (abuse may occur with herbs just as with prescription medicine). The case of each of these herbs illustrates a different aspect of problems in the study and regulation of herbal medicines, as information, and in some cases misinformation, comes to light.

Gingko is well established as an effective treatment for mild dementia and is documented to improve memory in those with memory impairment. However, it has been marketed irresponsibly as a "memory enhancer," leading to a misguided study of gingko using standard tests of memory in those without cognitive impairment. The subsequent promotion of this study's findings has led to great confusion.

Kava kava, after experience with approximately 70 million users, was claimed in a few cases to exhibit certain liver toxicity, as with many prescription and OTC drugs. A subsequent review examined each case and rejected the finding of liver toxicity (Gruenwald and Skrabal, 2003). Although an effective treatment for anxiety, kava is being voluntarily removed from the marketplace. A responsible approach to the risk-benefit ratio, as with other treatments manifesting side effects, could be developed in the case of real or claimed controversy.

St John's wort, although historically used only in ambulatory patients with mild to moderate depression, was used in a clinical trial of hospitalized patients with major depression and found to be no more effective than placebo (as has also been found in some studies with pharmaceutical antidepressants). As with the German Commission E, historical use may be wisely taken as a guide to the clinical use of herbs.

Ephedra has been used by millions for weight loss and was inappropriately used as a "performance enhancer." It was listed on autopsy reports as contributory to several fatalities among otherwise healthy individuals. This finding helped lead to its removal by the FDA. Obesity is a risk factor for many diseases, and effective weight loss regimens elude many overweight individuals. Is it possible to have safe, medically supervised regimens of appropriate ephedra formulations for weight loss, or does ephedra have no place in contemporary use?

Further abuses of herbal products adulterated with therapeutic drugs and contaminants (especially a problem with imports from overseas, particularly China) are a serious safety issue. Consumers, health professionals, and responsible elements of the U.S. natural products industry all suffer when irresponsibly adulterated products are imported from abroad. The NIH clinical trial on the Chinese herbal formulation PC-SPES for prostate cancer was undermined by the unwitting use of adulterated herbs. Some natural products from China have even been contaminated with chloramphenicol.

Improvements in manufacturing and marketing standards in the natural products industry will be required for effective integrative medical practice.

Integrative Medical Practice

Reliance on the appropriate use of nutrients and herbs is a critical and fundamental component of many integrative medical practices. Presently in the United States, these natural products are widely available. Unlike pharmaceuticals, information about the health effects cannot be provided on the product label or with the product as a product insert. Because of the increasing availability of credible third-party research on the efficacy of herbal and nutritional ingredients, as well as the increasing recognition by the medical profession of the importance of dietary supplementation for optimal health and for the prevention and management of many medical conditions (see *Journal of the American Medical Association,* July 2002), it is incumbent on practitioners of integrative medicine to maintain a medical standard of information and practice about herbal and nutritional ingredients. One approach to this requirement is to develop and maintain capability for clinic-based or hospital-based formularies of appropriate, effective, and high-quality sources of herbs and nutrients.

The current regulatory environment is coupled with the reality that much of the natural products industry does not operate to medical and scientific standards, that many irresponsible marketing claims are made, and that many medical and scientific professionals are not knowledgeable about the science behind herbal and nutritional medicine. This volatile mix produces much confusion and misinformation on both sides, documented periodically by such sources as the *New England Journal of Medicine*. Medical professionals presently are largely on their own in trying to understand the proper indications, ingredients, and dosages for the appropriate scientific use of herbal and nutritional remedies, and consumers can only look to practitioners for guidance.

New information technologies are being brought online to provide distributors, consumers, and practitioners fair and accurate information about the appropriate use of dietary supplements (see listing of websites after Suggested Readings and with Appendix 11).

PUBLIC POLICY ISSUES

State governments have developed a traditional role in regulating medical practice and in supporting medical education. The federal government maintains a unique and critical role in stimulating and supporting medical research, regulating medical products and devices, protecting the public health, and helping build health care infrastructure, and it is now paying approximately one-third the costs of health care in America.

Policy makers at the state and federal levels should become more knowledgeable about the needs and opportunities relative to integrative medicine. The bipartisan Congressional Caucus on Complementary & Alternative Medicine and Dietary Supplements was organized for this purpose. The Integrative Healthcare Policy Consortium, Policy Institute for Integrative Medicine, and other groups are working with members of the caucus and other elected representatives to broaden and deepen federal support for appropriate analyses and programs in integrative medicine. It is unlikely that the current regulatory legislation governing dietary supplements will be changed (Dietary Supplement Health and Education Act of 1994, as amended 1998). Although funding for The National Center for Complementary and Alternative Medicine has increased commensurate with the multiyear doubling of the overall NIH budget, it is critical that other federal agencies charged with programs relative to health resources and services, primary care, health professions training and workforce development, consumer education, health services research, and other areas be brought to bear on the important challenge and opportunity of integrative medicine. Integrative medicine has an important role that requires further articulation in current congressional actions on medical liability insurance reform and the national patient safety and quality assurance initiative.

Public support together with private innovation has been the hallmark for medical advancement in the twentieth century and should continue to be the case for integrative medicine in the twenty-first century.

References

Bensky D, Gamble A: *Chinese herbal medicine materia medica,* Seattle, 1986, Eastland Press, pp 34-35

Blumenthal M, Goldberg A, Brinckmann J: *Herbal medicine: expanded Commission E monographs,* Newton, Mass, 2000, Integrative Medicine Communications.

Boyle W: *Official herbs in the United States Pharmacopoeias: 1820-1990,* East Palestine, OH 1991, Buckeye Naturopathic Press.

Eisenberg DM, Davis RB, Ettner SL, et al: Trends in alternative medicine use in the United States, 1990-1997: results of a follow-up national survey, *JAMA* 280(18): 1569-1575, 1998.

Gruenwald J, Skrabal J: Kava ban highly questionable: A brief summary of the main scientific findings presented in the "In depth investigation on European Union member states market restrictions on kava products," *Sem Integrative Med* 1(4):199-210, 2003.

Hatch O: *Square peg: confessions of a citizen senator,* New York, 2002, Basic Books, pp 81-95.

Iwu MM: *Handbook of African medicinal plants,* Boca Raton, Fla, 1993, CRC Press, pp 343-349.

Odum H: *Environment, power and society,* New York, 1971, John Wiley & Sons, p 8.

Solecki RS, Shanidar IV: a neanderthal flower burial in northern Iraq, *Science* 190:880-889, 1975.

Tyler VE, Brady LR, Robbers JE: *Pharmacognosy,* Philadelphia, 1988, Lea & Febiger.

Suggested Readings

Astin JA: Why patients use alternative medicine: results of a national study, *JAMA* 279(19):1548-1553, 1998.

Bausell RB, Lee WL, Berman BM: Demographic and health-related correlates to visits to complementary and alternative medical providers, *Med Care* 39(2):190-196, 2001.

Berman BM: The Cochrane Collaboration and evidence-based complementary medicine, *J Altern Complement Med* 3(2):191-194, 1997.

Bisset NG, Wichtl M, editors: *Herbal drugs and phytopharmaceuticals: a handbook for practice on a scientific basis,* Boca Raton, Fla, 1994, CRC Press, pp 273-275.

Bourin M, Bougerol T, Guitton B, Broutin E: *Fundam Clin Pharmacol* 11(2):127-132, 1997.

Cott JM: In vitro receptor binding and enzyme inhibition by *Hypericum perforatum* extract, *Pharmacopsychiatry* 30(suppl. II):108-112, 1997.

Davies LP, Drew CA, Duffield P, et al: Kava pyrones and resin: studies on GABAA, GABAB and benzodiazepine binding sites in rodent brain, *Pharmacol Toxicol* 71(2):120-126, 1992.

DeFeudis FV: *Ginkgo biloba extract (Egb 761): parmacological activities and clinical applications,* Paris, 1991, Elsevier.

DeSmet, PA: Herbal remedies, *N Engl J Med* 347:2046-2056, 2002.

Donden Y: *Health through balance: an introduction to Tibetan medicine,* Ithaca, NY, 1986, Snow Lion Publications.

Dorn M. [Efficacy and tolerability of Baldrian versus oxazepam in non-organic and non-psychiatric insomniacs: a randomised, double-blind, clinical, comparative study], *Forsch Komplementarmed Klass Naturheilkd* 7(2):79-84, 2000.

Druss BG, Rosenheck RA: Association between use of unconventional therapies and conventional medical services, *JAMA* 282(7):651-656, 1999.

Eisenberg DM, Kessler RC, Foster C, et al: Unconventional medicine in the United States: prevalence, costs, and patterns of use, *N Engl J Med* 328(4):246-252, 1993.

Fairfield KM, Fletcher RH: Vitamins for chronic disease prevention in adults: scientific evidence, *JAMA* 287: 3116-3126, 2002.

Fletcher RH, Fairfield KM Vitamins for chronic disease prevention in adults: clinical applications, *JAMA* 287:3127-3129, 2002.

European Scientific Cooperative on Phytotherapy: *Monographs on the medicinal use of plants,* Exeter, UK, 1997, ESCOP.

Farnsworth NR, Bunyapraphatsara N: *Thai medicinal plants recommended for primary health care systems,* Bangkok, 1992, Medicinal Plant Information Center.

Fontana RJ, Lown KS, Paine MF, et al: Effects of a char-grilled meat diet on expression of CYP3A, CYP1A, and P-glycoprotein levels in healthy volunteers, *Gastroenterology* 117(1):89-98, 1999.

Fugh-Berman A, Cott JM: Dietary supplements and natural products as psychotherapeutic agents, *Psychosom Med* 61:712-728, 1999.

Garrett BJ, Cheeke PR, Miranda CL, et al: Consumption of poisonous plants by rats, *Toxicol Lett* 10:183-188, 1982.

Harkin T (D-Iowa), U.S. Senate: Personal communication, 2004.

Hoffmann DL: *The herb user's guide: the basic skills of medical herbalism,* Wellingborough, UK, 1987, Thorsons Publishing Group.

Johne A, Brockmoller J, Bauer S, et al: Pharmacokinetic interaction of digoxin with an herbal extract from St John's wort *(Hypericum perforatum)*, *Clin Pharmacol Ther* 66(4):338-345, 1999.

Junius MM: *The practical handbook of plant alchemy,* Rochester, New York, 1993, Healing Arts Press.

Kessler RC, Davis RB, Foster DF, et al: Long-term trends in the use of complementary and alternative medical therapies in the United States, *Ann Intern Med* 135(4): 262-268, 2001.

Kinzler E, Kromer J, Lehmann E: Wirksamkeit eines Kava-Spezial-Extraktes bei Patienten mit Angst: Spannungs-und Erregungszustanden nicht-psychotischer Genese, *Arzneim Forsch/Drug Res* 41:584-588, 1991.

Landes P: Market report, *HerbalGram* 42:64-65, 1998.

Landmark Healthcare: I. The Landmark Report II on HMOs and Alternative Care. II. 1999, Landmark Healthcare.

Linde K, Ramirez G, Mulrow CD, et al: St. John's wort for depression: an overview and meta-analysis of randomized clinical trials, *BMJ* 313:253-258, 1996.

Maurer A, Johne A, Bauer S, et al: Interaction of St. John's wort extract with phenprocoumon, *Eur J Clin Pharmacol* 55(3):A22, 1999.

McGuffin M, Hobbs C, Upton R, Goldberg A: *Botanical safety handbook,* Boca Raton, Fla, 1997, CRC Press, p 105.

Micozzi, M.S: Complementary medicine: what is appropriate? Who will provide it? *Ann Intern Med* 129:65-66, 1998.

Micozzi, MS: Culture, society and the return of complementary medicine, *Medical Anthropology Quarterly,* 2002.

Müller WE, Rolli M, Schäfer C, Hafner U: Effects of Hypericum extract (LI 160) in biochemical models of antidepressant activity, *Pharmacopsychiatry* 30(suppl. II):102-107, 1997.

Newall CA, Anderson LA, Phillipson JD: *Herbal Medicines: a guide for health-care professionals,* London, 1996, Pharmaceutical Press, pp 239-240.

Ohnishi A, Matsuo H, Yamada S, et al: Effect of furanocoumarin derivatives in grapefruit juice on the uptake of vinblastine by Caco-2 cells and on the activity of cytochrome P450 3A4, *Br J Pharmacol* 130(6): 1369-1371, 2000.

Piscitelli SC, Burstein AH, Chaitt D, et al: Indinavir concentrations and St John's wort, *Lancet* 355(9203):547-548, 2000.

Ruschitzka F, Meier PJ, Turina M, et al: Acute heart transplant rejection due to Saint John's wort, *Lancet* 355(9203):548-549, 2000.

Santos MS, Ferreira F, Faro C, et al: The amount of GABA present in aqueous extracts of valerian is sufficient to account for [3H]GABA release in synaptosomes, *Planta Med* 60(5):475-476, 1994.

Schelosky L, Raffauf C, Jendroska K, Poewe W (Neurology Department, Rudolf Virehote University, Berlin): Letter to the editor, *J Neurol Neurosurg Psychiatry* 45:639-640, 1995.

Scudder JM: *Specific diagnosis: a study of disease with special reference to the administration of remedies,* Cincinnati, 1874, Wilstach, Baldwin.

Shelton RC, Keller MB, Gelenberg A, et al: Effectiveness of St John's wort in major depression: a randomized controlled trial, *JAMA* 285(15):1978-1986, 2001.

Stetter C: *The secret medicine of the pharaohs: ancient Egyptian healing,* Chicago, 1993, Edition Q.

Suzuki D, Knudtson P: *Wisdom of the elders: sacred native stories of nature,* New York, 1992, Bantam Books.

Upton R, Graff A, Williamson E, et al: American herbal pharmacopoeia and therapeutic compendium on St. John's wort *(Hypericum perforatum)*: quality control, analytical and therapeutic monograph, *Herbal Gram* 40(suppl):1-32, 1997.

Upton R, Graff A, Williamson E, et al: American herbal pharmacopoeia and therapeutic compendium on valerian root: analytical, quality control, and therapeutic monograph, Santa Cruz, Calif, 1999, AHP.

Vorbach EU. Efficacy and tolerability of St. John's wort extract LI 160 vs. imipramine in patients with severe depressive episodes according to ICD-10, *Pharmacopsychiatry* 30(suppl 2):81-85, 1997.

Woelk H, Kapoula O, Lehrl S, et al: Behandlung von Angst-Patienten. *Z Allg Med* 69:271-277, 1993.

Wolfman C, Viola H, Paladini A, et al: Possible anxiolytic effects of chrysin, a central benzodiazepine receptor ligand isolated from *Passiflora coerulea, Pharmacol Biochem Behav* 47(1):1-4, 1994.

Wood M: Seven Herbs: *Plants as teachers,* Berkeley, Calif, 1986, North Atlantic Books.

Wooton, J, Sparber, A.: Surveys of complementary and alternative medicine usage: review of general population trends and specific populations, *Semin Integrat Med* 1(1), 2003.

Yue Q-Y, Bergquist C, Gerdén B: Safety of St John's wort *(Hypericum perforatum)*, *Lancet* 355: 576-577, 2000.

Websites

Alternative Medicine Foundation, Inc: HerbMed.org
American Botanical Council: www.herbalgram.org
Herb Research Foundation: www.herbs.org
Natural Product Research Consultants (NPRC): www.nprc.com
The Natural Pharmacist: www.TNP.com

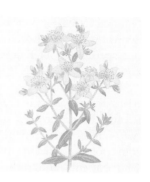

APPENDIX 11

Common Herbs for Integrative Care

VICTOR S. SIERPINA, SUSIE GERIK

Among the most popular and accessible alternative and integrative therapies are botanical or herbal medicines. These are readily available at drugstores and even grocery and convenience stores as well as the health food stores, are heavily marketed in print and electronic media, and are generally inexpensive compared with the cost of pharmaceuticals. As a result, patients frequently use these herbal medicines.

At the same time, practicing physicians are often uncomfortable with these products. Their concerns about product safety, reliability, bioavailability, and purity are real concerns in the United States, where little control is exercised by the Food and Drug Administration (FDA) or other government bodies over the manufacturing process. Although unsafe products can be recalled from the market, no standardized method exists to verify product quality. Independent laboratories such as Consumer Reports issue evaluations of individual products, and reputable manufacturers increasingly hold their own quality control program to a high standard of excellence and good manufacturing practices (GMPs). At this point, knowing the manufacturer by reputation and also the products that have actually been tested in clinical trials is useful (Blumenthal 2003; Blumenthal et al., 2000).

In addition to the heavy self-prescribed use of products by the public and the health care professionals' concerns about safety, a number of other issues must be addressed in the use of "botanicals."

First, instruction and reliable information must be available to physicians and other health professionals when patients inquire about botanicals. The physician can no longer be dismissive about a patient's honest request for reliable information on the safety and efficacy of over-the-counter (OTC) herbs and other supplements. Indeed, many reliable databases provide this information, including Natural Medicines Comprehensive Data Base, Natural Standard, HealthNotes Online, the federal Office of Dietary Supplements, and Longwood Herbal Project. Many texts and references are available, including the *Physicians' Desk Reference for Herbal Supplements*. Online databases often make personal digital assistant (PDA) applications of these materials available at low or no cost. In other words, ignorance about herbal products is no longer caused by "lack of good data," but rather the physician's reluctance to seek out sources of information for inquiring patients. Patients understand that physicians cannot possibly know everything about herbs, supplements, and other similar products and will accept an honest "I don't know" as an answer, at least at first. If this answer is repeated at subsequent visits, however, the patient may translate it as "I don't care." They may look to the Internet, advertisements, friends, and other, less reliable sources for information.

Second, identifying the potential for drug-herb interaction is a necessity in this era of self-medication and polypharmacy. Many of the references just noted and listed later (readings, websites) have up-to-date details on known or theoretically possible drug-herb interactions. This is a critical public health and public safety aspect to modern medical practice.

Third, it is not necessary to know every herbal product in use in the United States or in every culture. Certain herbs are widely used, for example, among Hispanic patients (Davidow, 1999), but not so much among non-Hispanic whites, Asians, or African Americans. The traditional Chinese medicine pharmacopeia is so extensive that years of study are required to master it. Those with practices that heavily involve such culturally defined groups must seek out specialized references to address their learning and patient care needs (Chen and Chen, 2004).

We have found that a short listing of common herbs in general use in the United States is most helpful for the majority of practicing physicians. These herbs are summarized briefly here in a table form. At some point, physicians should be able not only to ask your patients about their herbs and answer their questions, but also to feel comfortable in prescribing them. Tables 11-1 and 11-2 (at end of this appendix) can help physicians progress in their practice to actually using herbs as part of their treatment plans.

Online continuing medical education (CME) is also available (http://northwestahec.wfubmc.edu/learn/herbs/index.asp).

A "journey of a thousand plants" must begin with something useful. So we have distilled the number of plants down to the most common ones.

ALOE

Aloe vera is a common succulent houseplant (Figure 11-1 p. 194). Long kept in the kitchen for soothing burns, it is now available in commercial preparations for such indications as sunburn and the treatment of **stomach ulcers.** The solidified gel from the leaves, which extrudes when they are broken, can be used directly on the affected area of the skin and is useful in many **skin conditions** as a *vulnerary* (promotes wound healing). For internal use, aloe comes in a diluted liquid form.

Aloe can be a powerful *cathartic* and an *emmenagogue* (increases menstrual flow), and it should be avoided during pregnancy and lactation because of its *purgative* effects.

Dosage is simply putting some of the juice from the plants on the affected area, and the internal use is 0.1 to 0.3 gram (g). Commercial preparations of the juice are also available for internal use.

BLACK COHOSH

Cimicifuga racemosa is best thought of as a female herb (Figure 11-2 p. 194). Its traditional uses include the relief of **menstrual cramps, premenstrual syndrome (PMS),** and **menopausal symptoms.** It has

TABLE 11-1

Common Uses for Top 20 Herbs

Herb	Common Use
1. Aloe	Skin, gastritis
2. Black cohosh	Menstrual symptoms, menopause
3. Dong quai	Menstrual symptoms, menopause
4. Echinacea	Colds, immunity
5. Ephedra (ma huang)	Asthma, energy, weight loss
6. Evening primrose oil	Eczema, psoriasis, premenstrual syndrome, breast pain
7. Feverfew	Migraine
8. Garlic	Cholesterol, hypertension
9. Ginger	Nausea, arthritis
10. Ginkgo biloba	Cerebrovascular insufficiency, memory
11. Ginseng	Energy, immunity, mentation, libido
12. Goldenseal	Immunity, colds
13. Hawthorn	Cardiac function
14. Kava kava	Anxiety
15. Milk thistle	Liver disease
16. Peppermint	Dyspepsia, irritable bowel syndrome
17. Saw palmetto	Prostate problems
18. St. John's wort	Depression, anxiety, insomnia
19. Tea tree oil	Skin infections
20. Valerian	Anxiety, insomnia

been found to be useful in treating symptoms associated with menopause, such as hot flashes, mood and sleep disturbance, and vaginal atrophy. The American Indians used it for these indications and dysmenorrhea. Its active ingredients are triterpenes and flavonoids, some of which act on the pituitary gland to suppress luteinizing hormone. Black cohosh does not alter the production of follicle-stimulating hormone and prolactin. Stomach upset is the only reported side effect, and no other contraindications or drug interactions are reported. Some experts recommend limiting treatment to 3 to 6 months because long-term safety has not been evaluated.

A contemporary preparation of black cohosh is *Remifemin,* which is provided in a convenient tablet form for both dysmenorrhea (once or twice daily) and

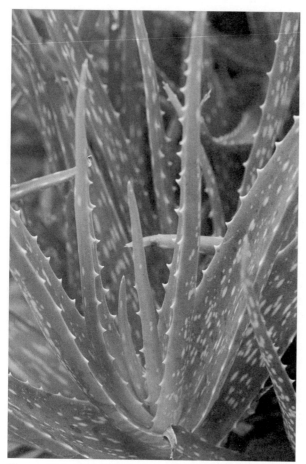

Figure 11-1 Aloe *(Aloe vera)*. (Courtesy Martin Wall, Botanical Services.)

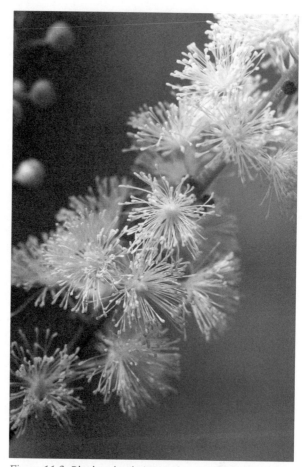

Figure 11-2 Black cohosh (*Cimicifuga racemosa* and *Actaea racemosa*). (Courtesy Martin Wall, Botanical Services.)

menopause (two tablets twice daily). Forty milligrams (mg) daily is a therapeutic dose. It can also be taken as a tea made of ½ to 1 tsp of the dried root. This tea is taken three times daily, or 2 to 4 milliliters (ml) of tincture is used three times daily.

DONG QUAI

Angelica sinensis is an Asian herb widely respected as a "women's remedy" (Figure 11-3). It has been widely used for **dysmenorrhea, menopause,** and **metrorrhagia.** It is useful in stabilizing the estrogenic activity and relieving hot flashes. Its imputed mechanism of action is through phytoestrogens, and it also contains ferulic acid, ligustilide, vitamin B$_{12}$, and vitamin E. Dong quai has been shown to have both a relaxing and stimulating effect on the uterus.

Some patients may experience hypersensitivity, which can cause excess bleeding and fever. Dong quai can also be photosensitizing. It should not be used during pregnancy and lactation, although various sources disagree on this point. There is a potential drug interaction with coumarin.

For PMS the three-times-daily dose is 1 to 2 g of powdered root or as tea, 1 tsp of tincture, or ¼ tsp of fluid extract starting on day 14 of the menstrual cycle. It is also available in teas.

ECHINACEA

Echinacea angustifolia is best known as an **immune stimulant** (Figure 11-4). Long favored by the American Indians, it is considered an antibiotic, useful against both bacterial and viral infections. It is

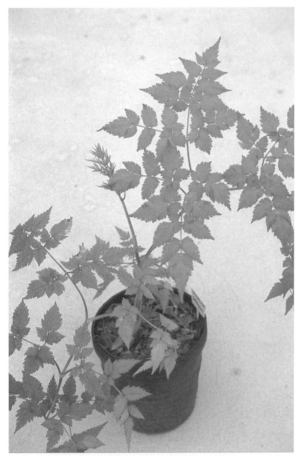

Figure 11-3 Dong quai *(Angelica sinensis)*. (Courtesy Martin Wall, Botanical Services.)

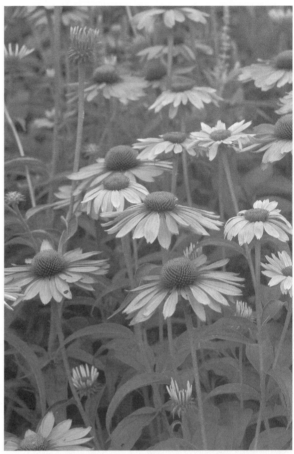

Figure 11-4 Echinacea (*Echinacea angustifolia* and *E. purpurea*). (Courtesy Martin Wall, Botanical Services.)

one of the best-selling herbs in U.S. health food stores.

Its imputed actions are encouraging the swarming of white blood cells to the site of an infection, stimulating phagocytosis, improving lymphocyte production, and increasing interferon production. Some sources discourage its use in autoimmune disease or tuberculosis. Echinacea is not recommended during pregnancy. Side effects are not reported.

The dosage is 3 to 4 cups of tea a day or 1 to 4 ml of tincture three times a day during an infectious episode, such as the **common cold** and **chronic respiratory tract infections.** Although sources vary on treatment dosing, a cycle of 5 days "on" and 2 days "off" during an infection is widely recommended. Taking it all the time is not considered to be as useful, and in any case, echinacea should not be taken for longer than 8 weeks.

EPHEDRA

Ephedra sinica or *ma huang* contains alkaloids, ephedrine, and pseudoephedrine (Figure 11-5). It is widely used for **asthma, allergy, low blood pressure,** and **cerebral insufficiency;** as a **stimulant;** and for **weight loss.** It has marked sympathomimetic effects and can be overused or even abused. Its effects on the central nervous system have been characterized as stronger than caffeine but less than amphetamines. Ephedra is best avoided in patients who are hypertensive or anxious and in those with glaucoma or diabetes.

The dosage is 1 to 2 tsp of dried herb steeped as a tea for 10 to 15 minutes taken three times a day, or 1 to 4 ml of the tincture three times a day. It is also found mixed in a number of other preparations.

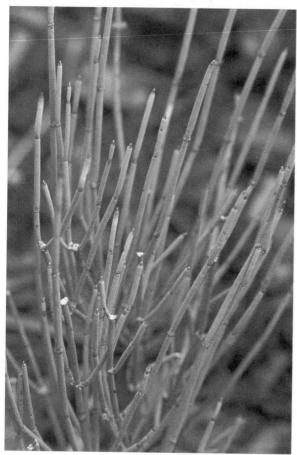

Figure 11-5 Ephedra (*Ephedra sinica* or *ma huang*). (Courtesy Martin Wall, Botanical Services.)

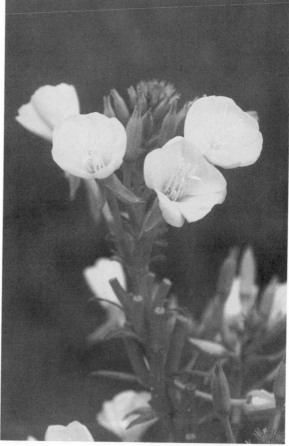

Figure 11-6 Evening primrose oil *(Oenothera biennis)*. (Courtesy Martin Wall, Botanical Services.)

EVENING PRIMROSE OIL

Oenothera biennis produces seeds that are a source of omega-6 essential fatty acids (Figure 11-6). It has a fairly long list of indications, but it is most often used for **atopic eczema, premenstrual syndrome, psoriasis, cyclical** and **noncyclical mastalgia.** Some trials have used it without benefit in multiple sclerosis. Its actions are thought to be related to antioxidant effects and the replacement of deficiency of the essential fatty acids linoleic acid and gamma-linolenic acid (GLA). Evening primrose oil should not be used with phenothiazines because it may precipitate seizures. Side effects are mild gastrointestinal effects and headache.

Based on a standardized GLA content of 8%, dosages are 2 to 4 g a day for children and 6 to 8 g for adults for atopic eczema, 3 to 4 g for mastalgia, and 3 g for PMS.

FEVERFEW

Tanacetum parthenium is a primary remedy in the treatment of **migraine headaches** and associated nausea and vomiting (Figure 11-7). It may also be useful for dizziness, tinnitus, and dysmenorrhea. It should not be used during pregnancy because of the stimulant action on the uterus or during lactation. It may cause mouth ulcers in some people, particularly those chewing the leaves. Feverfew treats and prevents migraine by inhibiting the release of blood vessel–dilating substances from platelets, inhibiting inflammatory mediators, and regulating vascular tone. The active

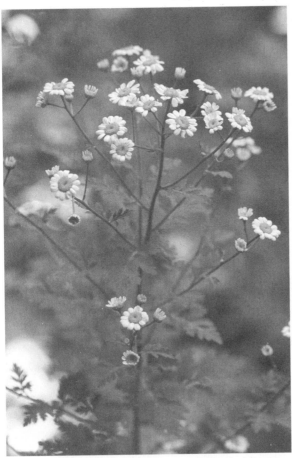

Figure 11-7 Feverfew *(Tanacetum parthenium).* (Courtesy Martin Wall, Botanical Services.)

ingredient is parthenolide, which should be present in at least a 0.2% concentration in preparations.

The dosage is one fresh leaf one to three times a day, fresh or frozen. The drug equivalent is 0.2 to 0.6 mg of parthenolide, which is equivalent to 50 to 200 mg of dried aerial parts in tablets or capsule. It also is available in a tincture of 1:5 in 25% ethanol with a dose of 5 to 20 drops. Continuous use for at least 4 to 6 weeks is recommended for prophylaxis at a dose of not less than 125 mg of dried feverfew containing a minimum of 0.2% parthenolide.

GARLIC

Allium sativum is a favorite kitchen herb in many cultures that has many health effects, including its antiplatelet activity (at about 1 clove a day), use as an antibiotic, and immune-enhancing effects (Figure 11-8). The volatile oil is largely excreted by the lungs and is useful in respiratory infections. Studies have shown its benefit in **reducing blood pressure and cholesterol** levels. The active ingredient is allicin. Fresh garlic has compounds such as S-allylcysteines and gamma-glutamylpeptides, which exert beneficial effects as well. Some gastrointestinal side effects, such as nausea, diarrhea, and vomiting or a burning sensation, may occur. It may potentiate the antithrombotic effects of antiinflammatory drugs or coumadin.

Dosages of up to three cloves a day (or in the form of garlic oil capsules) are recommended. The capsules should deliver at least 10 mg of allicin or a total allicin potential of 4000 µg. The German Commission E that reviewed herbal products recommended that commercial preparations contain no less than the equivalent of 4000 mg of fresh garlic. The bottom

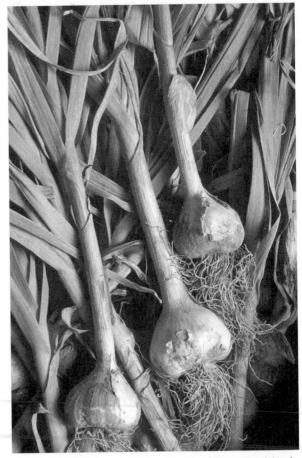

Figure 11-8 Garlic *(Allium sativum).* (Courtesy Martin Wall, Botanical Services.)

line is to take fresh garlic or standardized preparations. Cooking removes some of the benefits of garlic.

Preparations of garlic oil, 2 to 5 mg/day, or tincture, 1:5 in 45% alcohol 2 to 4 ml three times a day, are also available.

GINGER

Zingiber officinale is another favorite among Asians and cooks worldwide (Figure 11-9). It is useful in a variety of conditions, including use as an **antiinflammatory,** a **digestive aid,** a gargle for sore throats, and a compress for abdominal and gynecological problems. A recently marketed preparation claims effectiveness as a **rheumatological agent** through inhibition of leukotrienes and prostaglandins. It has been widely used as an **antinauseant,** particularly in pregnancy, in which a tea made from fresh grated ginger root, ginger ale, lemon, and honey or sugar is sipped in the morning. Its antiinflammatory and antiplatelet functions may account for its imputed effectiveness in some types of migraine.

The dosage is a standardized capsule three times a day. An infusion is prepared by pouring boiling water over the sliced root or a decoction from using 1½ tsp of dried root powder or finely chopped root. Ginger also is available in a tincture, 1.5 to 3 ml three times a day (a stronger tincture is available, taken as 0.25 to 0.5 ml three times daily). The tea or decoction can be sipped as needed. A compress made from fresh grated root in cheesecloth soaked in hot water and applied to the abdomen has long been favored as a stimulant for digestive and gynecological functions.

GINKGO

Ginkgo biloba is the most widely sold herb in Europe, where it is used for **cerebral insufficiency, circulatory disorders,** and **memory problems, vertigo,** and **tinnitus** (Figure 11-10). Studies have recently indicated its effectiveness in slowing the progression

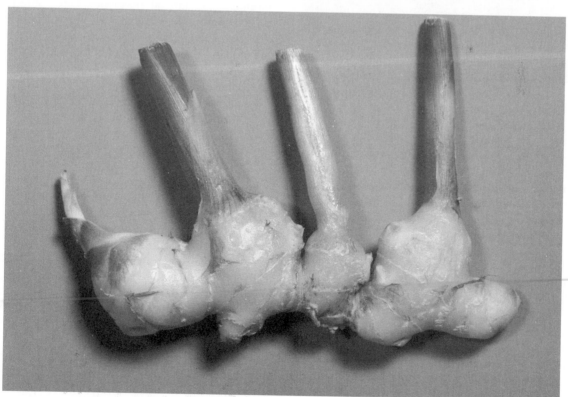

Figure 11-9 Ginger *(Zingiber officinale).* (Courtesy Martin Wall, Botanical Services.)

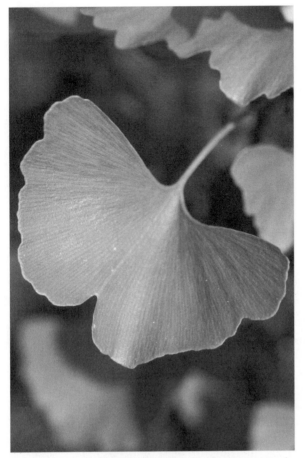

Figure 11-10 Ginkgo *(Ginkgo biloba)*. (Courtesy Martin Wall, Botanical Services.)

of Alzheimer's disease and multiinfarct dementia. Its mechanism of action is thought to be from its function as an antioxidant, a free radical scavenger, a membrane stabilizer, and from its inhibition of platelet-activating factor. This later effect makes its use in conjunction with coumarin potentially a problem, as does its use with aspirin. Clotting studies need to be followed carefully in this situation. Rarely, stomach or intestinal upsets, headaches, or skin rashes can occur.

Standardized extracts contain 24% mixed flavonoid glycosides and 6% terpene lactones. Dosage is 120 to 240 mg/day taken in two to three doses for memory problems and dementia. A lower dosage of 120 to 160 mg/day in two or three doses is used for vertigo, tinnitus, and peripheral arterial occlusive dis-

ease. An initial period of 6 to 8 weeks is recommended to assess the effectiveness of ginkgo.

GINSENG

Panax ginseng, Panax quinquifolius, Panax pseudoginseng, and *Eleutherococcus senticosus* (Oriental, American, Sanchi, and Siberian species) are widely reputed as tonics for **stress** and **fatigue** (Figure 11-11). A favorite among Orientals for centuries, it is considered an *adaptogen*—a substance that helps restore homeostasis during periods of physiological or psychological stress. Probably the simplest statement about ginseng is that the claims for its effectiveness are contradictory and difficult to verify. Nonetheless, it remains one of the top three best-selling herbs.

Improved athletic performance, sexual potency, memory, immune function, circulation, longevity, and treatment of cancer are all imputed to this panacea (the name *Panax* is derived from the Greek word meaning "all-healing"). Evidence of its effects on the endocrine system has been shown with increases in pituitary and adrenal hormones. Direct effects on potency have not been proved. Ginseng may reduce cholesterol levels. Many of the studies are in animal models, and the problems of source, standardization of dosing, and the opposing effects of the active ginsenosides account for the difficulty in studying this herb and proving its wide range of imputed effects.

The ginsenosides belong to a chemical group called *saponins,* which are similar in composition and structure to steroids such as testosterone, estrogen, and adrenocorticotropic hormone. Korean ginseng may raise blood pressure. Caution should be exercised when using ginseng in certain conditions, such as cardiac problems, diabetes, psychosis, and agitation; with steroid therapy or monoamine oxidase inhibitors; and possibly during pregnancy.

A standardized dose is 4% ginsenosides. Daily dosages vary from 0.5 to 1.0 g of root or equivalent preparations for healthy young persons for short-term use. Older and unhealthy people should take about half that amount. Doses can be taken in chronic states continuously. My conclusion on ginseng is that it is a mild stimulant tonic and probably best for older people rather than for young and healthy persons, although it is generally safe in both groups.

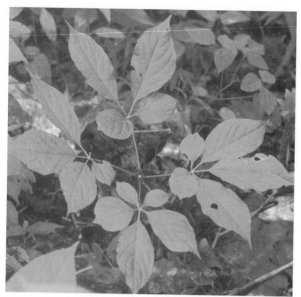

Figure 11-11 Ginseng (*Panax ginseng, P. quinquifolius, P. pseudoginseng,* and *Eleutherococcus senticosus*). (Courtesy Martin Wall, Botanical Services.)

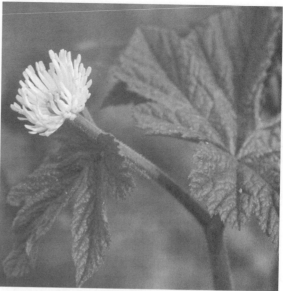

Figure 11-12 Goldenseal *(Hydrastis canadensis)*. (Courtesy Martin Wall, Botanical Services.)

GOLDENSEAL

Hydrastis canadensis is a widely used **immune stimulant** and **natural antibiotic** (Figure 11-12). It has an astringent effect, and its most common use is for **sore throats.** The berberine alkaloid of goldenseal exerts antibiotic effects and has been shown to inhibit the attachment of group A streptococci to the endothelial lining of the throat. It has effects against other microorganisms such as *Staphylococcus, Candida, Giardia, Escherichia coli, Trichomonas vaginalis,* and *Entamoeba histolytica.* The alkaloid berberine also has been shown to activate phagocytosis. As an external agent, goldenseal is used for eczema, ringworm, pruritus, earache, and conjunctivitis. It is also used for infectious diarrhea, gastritis, infection and inflammation of mucous membranes, and digestive disorders. Because of its stimulant effect on the uterus, it should not be used during pregnancy.

The dosage is dried root and rhizome ,0.5 to 1 g three times daily; tincture (1:10, 60% ethanol), 2 to 4 ml; liquid extract (1:1, 60% ethanol), 0.3 to 1 ml; or the extract standardized to contain 5% hydrastine, 250 to 500 mg, also three times daily.

HAWTHORN

Crataegus laeviagata is best known as a **cardiac tonic** (Figure 11-13). The hawthorn berries have been used for centuries in the Orient and Europe for their beneficial effects on the cardiovascular system. It is a traditional heart tonic, often used in conjunction with digoxin. Testing has shown that it increases myocardial contractility and coronary blood flow while decreasing heart rate and oxygen consumption. Its active constituents are proanthocyanidins and cardiotonic amines. It also contains antioxidant flavonoids that are produced in highest quantity from the young floral buds and leaves. It also inhibits angiotensin-converting enzyme and acts as a vasodilator and mild diuretic. Hawthorn is used clinically in angina, congestive heart failure, and hypertension, although it is best used as an adjunctive therapy in severe cases. The extracts are well tolerated, show no drug interaction, and have a wide therapeutic index.

The dosage is 2 tsp of berries and leaves infused for 20 minutes and sipped three times a day over a long period. The tincture is taken 2 to 4 ml three

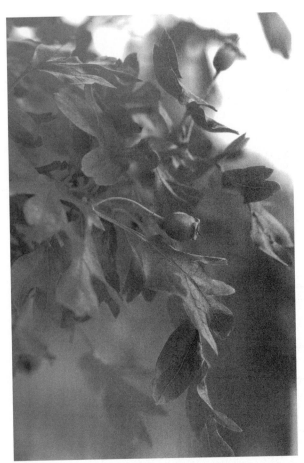

Figure 11-13 Hawthorn (*Crataegus laeviagata* and *C. monogyna*). (Courtesy Martin Wall, Botanical Services.)

times a day. The capsule dosage is 150 to 300 mg three times daily and should contain 1.8% vitexin-4'-rhamnoside or 10% procyanidins.

KAVA KAVA

Piper methysticum is a Polynesian euphoriant used primarily for **anxiety, depression,** and **insomnia** (Figure 11-14). The active ingredients are kavalactones, which are potentiated in the crude form and seem to have a gamma-aminobutyric acid (GABA) receptor augmentation effect compared with the pure extract. It is a member of the pepper family. Small doses improve mental function; for example, the chiefs of Polynesian tribes, when in council, often drank kava (originally prepared by chewing on the root and then expectorating the extract into a large pot for brewing) before serious negotiations.

Kava should not be used in patients with Parkinson's disease or in those currently taking benzodiazepines because the combination may cause disorientation. According to some sources, it may push limbic system impressions forward. It is safe and non-addictive according to clinical studies, mainly from Germany. It also has some benefit as a skeletal muscle relaxant, such as for nervous tension and stress headaches. High dosages of 400 mg/day or more over long periods may cause a scaly rash that resolves with discontinuance of the herb.

The dosage is 60 to 70 mg three times daily for anxiety or depression. For insomnia, 180 to 210 mg is taken 45 to 60 minutes before retiring. The dosage is based on the kavalactone content in the standardized preparation. The dried rhizome dosage is 1.5 to 3 g/day, and the alcoholic 1:2 extract is taken at a dosage of 3 to 6 ml/day. Kava's effects are potentiated by alcohol, and the standard bowl drunk by a group in its traditional social context has about 250 mg of

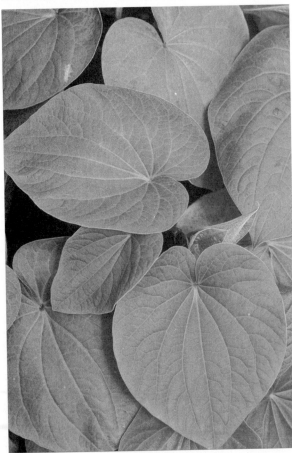

Figure 11-14 Kava kava *(Piper methysticum)*. (Courtesy Martin Wall, Botanical Services.)

kavalactones. Several bowls are often consumed at a sitting.

MILK THISTLE

Silybum marianum contains the active constituent silymarin (Figure 11-15). This herb acts as an antioxidant, inhibits leukotriene formation, stabilizes membranes, and is a choleretic and lipotropic. It has a decongesting effect on the liver and is most well known for preventing fibrosis and **cirrhosis** in toxic or chemical-induced **liver damage,** including **viral hepatitis.** No toxicity in animals or humans has been found. Patients with hepatitis C have shown a 30% reduction in abnormal liver enzymes in 2 to 3 months. It is also useful for psoriasis. Milk thistle promotes milk secretion and is safe during lactation.

It may also stimulate bile production and may have a cathartic effect as a result.

The standard dosage based on silymarin content is 70 to 120 mg three times daily. A phosphatidylcholine-bound form is available at 100 mg three times daily. The tea is prepared from 1 tsp of the dried herb and leaves infused for 10 to 15 minutes in a cup of boiling water. This is taken three times a day. A tincture of 1 to 2 ml can also be taken three times daily.

PEPPERMINT

Mentha piperita is considered a candy and breath mint, but it has significant medicinal value (Figure 11-16). Its presence at the checkout counter of most restaurants has to do not only with its breath-enhancing benefits but also its effects on the lower esophageal sphincter. Peppermint reduces the lower esophageal

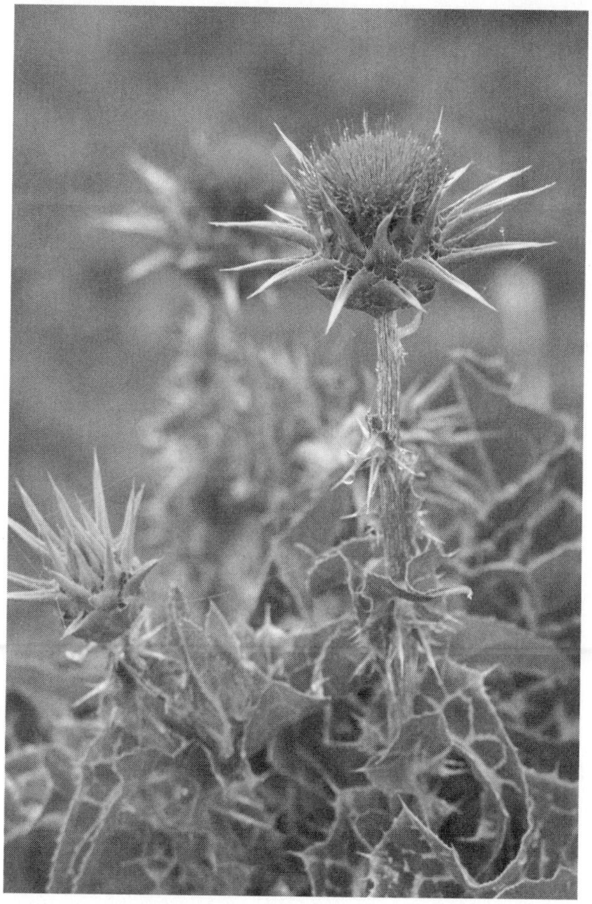

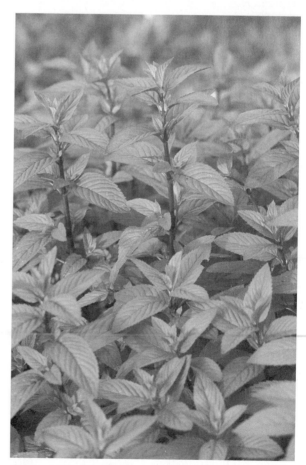

Figure 11-15 Milk thistle *(Silybum marianum)*. (Courtesy Martin Wall, Botanical Services.)

Figure 11-16 Peppermint *(Mentha piperita)*. (Courtesy Martin Wall, Botanical Services.)

sphincter tone, allowing for comfortable belching. Herbalists refer to it as a *carminative,* a digestive aid that stimulates peristalsis, relaxes the stomach, and prevents gas. Its volatile oils have been found to be useful for **irritable bowel syndrome** (IBS) in the form of enteric-coated peppermint oil (ECPO), which allows it to reach the small and large intestines. It acts as a smooth muscle relaxant by means of its calcium channel–blocking effects. It is an antispasmodic and reduces bile output. A study published in *Gastroenterology* showed peppermint had significant effects in reducing abdominal pain, distention, stool frequency, borborygmi (loud bowel sounds), and flatulence in patients with IBS.

The dosage is 0.2 to 0.4 ml of ECPO three times daily half an hour before meals. A tincture of 1 to 2 ml three times daily is also helpful. The preferred method of taking peppermint for **dyspepsia** is a teaspoon of the herb infused as a tea taken as often as desired. However, gastroesophageal reflux disease (GERD) may be worsened by peppermint because it can increase heartburn; it relaxes the lower esophageal sphincter tone, especially in those with a hiatal hernia, thereby encouraging acid reflux.

SAW PALMETTO

Serenoa repens is obtained from the berries of the saw palmetto plant, which contain fatty acids, sterols, and carotenes (Figure 11-17). These inhibit steroids essential to prostate metabolism such as 5α-reductase and also have a mild α_1-receptor antagonism. These effects result in a clinically beneficial effect on **benign prostatic hypertrophy** (BPH). It can also be used for **prostatitis** along with zinc, echinacea, and bearberry. It has been shown to be more effective than placebo in treating BPH. Some sources claim it does not reduce prostate-specific antigen levels, although others disagree with this point. In any case, saw palmetto is a safe product with a reduced side effect profile compared with the prescription α_1-receptor antagonists, particularly those with the side effect of low blood pressure.

An examination must be performed to rule out more serious problems of the prostate, especially prostate cancer in men older than 50. Saw palmetto is also considered a tonifier of the male reproductive system that boosts male sex hormones. Quality-of-life indicators show marked improvement with saw pal-

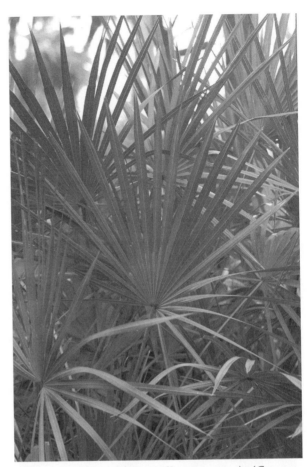

Figure 11-17 Saw palmetto *(Serenoa repens).* (Courtesy Martin Wall, Botanical Services.)

metto use. It is thought that the value of a good night's sleep caused by a reduction in nocturia contributes significantly to this improvement.

The dosage is 160 mg twice daily of the extract containing 85% to 95% fatty acids and sterols. Teas are primarily water soluble and have no benefit in prostate conditions. Most patients taking saw palmetto receive relief with a month of treatment.

ST. JOHN'S WORT

Hypericum perforatum is a well-researched herbal product used primarily for mild to moderate **depression** (Figure 11-18). It has active ingredients in the anthraquinone class such as hypericin and flavonoids. It acts primarily as an antidepressant and is a selective serotonin reuptake inhibitor

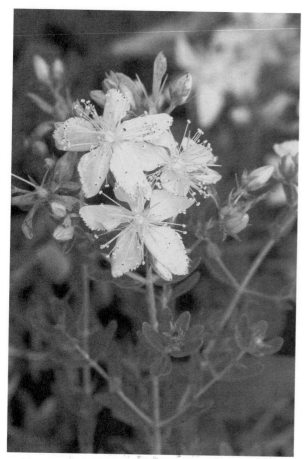

Figure 11-18 St. John's Wort *(Hypericum perforatum).* (Courtesy Martin Wall, Botanical Services.)

(SSRI). It has additional effects on the monoamine oxidase inhibitor (MAOI) pathway and on catecholamine methyl transferase (COMT). Although much has been made of its potential with MAOI-type drugs, no clinical evidence has been found verifying this concern. Its use with SSRIs, however, is of some concern. The potential of a serotonin syndrome with the use of such common antidepressants as paroxetine (Paxil), fluoxetine (Prozac), and sertraline (Zoloft) requires caution in concomitant use. Experts in this area recommend tapering of the SSRI drug while starting St. John's wort to reduce risk of serotonin syndrome. No other drug interactions are known.

Photosensitivity is a potential concern, especially in fair-skinned individuals, although the sunburn reported with St. John's wort has primarily been in range animals eating large amounts of the raw herb. Other side effects are mild but include hypersensitivity. It is not recommended during pregnancy or lactation because of lack of toxicity data.

St. John's wort is the most prescribed agent for depression in Germany, greatly exceeding fluoxetine sales. It has been tested against tricylic antidepressants and found to have improved depression scales with a significantly reduced side effect profile. It is also considered to be useful for anxiety, sleep disturbances, acquired immunodeficiency syndrome, and chronic fatigue syndrome.

The dosage is based on the standardized hypericin content of 0.3%. The usual dosage is 300 mg three times daily in capsules. For insomnia, 900 mg should be taken an hour before sleep. Tea is prepared by pouring boiling water over 2 to 4 g of the herb and steeping for 5 to 10 minutes; the infusion is also taken three times a day. There is a liquid extract (1:1 in 25% alcohol) taken 2 to 4 ml three times daily. The tincture (1:10 in 45% alcohol) is taken three times daily in a dose of 2 to 4 ml. Perhaps the greatest advantage of St. John's wort is patient compliance because of lack of side effects. It is also much less expensive than the leading SSRI antidepressants.

TEA TREE OIL

Melaleuca alternifolia is an Australian plant from which an essential oil is extracted (Figure 11-19). It is considered a useful **dermatological with antibacterial, antiviral, and antifungal properties.** It is used topically in full strength on boils, wound infections, and acne. At least one study showed it improved the healing of boils and reduced scar formation, presumably by its effect on *Staphylococcus aureus*. Another study showed it to be as effective as clotrimazole for treatment of tinea pedis.

Tea tree oil has a minimal tendency to irritate skin despite its penetrating qualities. Occasionally, it can cause contact dermatitis and irritation and will need to be diluted, or even discontinued, for a time.

VALERIAN

Valeriana officinalis yields valerenic acids, flavonoids, and valepotriates from its root; these are used for **nervousness, anxiety,** and **insomnia** (Figure 11-20).

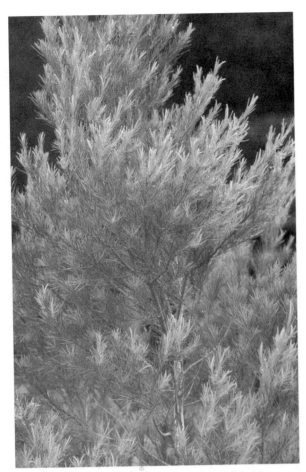

Figure 11-19 Tea tree oil *(Melaleuca alternifolia)*. (Courtesy Martin Wall, Botanical Services.)

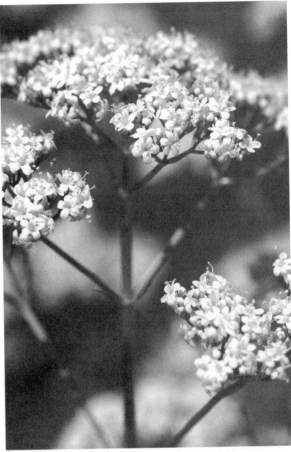

Figure 11-20 Valerian *(Valeriana officinalis)*. (Courtesy Martin Wall, Botanical Services.)

Valerian has been shown to improve the quality of sleep by improving slow waves in those with low baseline values. It is nonaddictive, unlike many of the sleep aids and anxiolytics, particularly those of the benzodiazepine class. It stimulates release of GABA and inhibits its reuptake. Its components bind directly to GABA receptors.

Because of its mechanism of action, valerian theoretically may potentiate the action of medications that have depressant effects on the central nervous system. Thus, if taking it with antidepressants or sedatives, it may be prudent to do so under medical supervision. Several studies showed that valerian did not cause daytime drowsiness, reduced concentration, or reduction in physical performance. Also, it does not have a synergy with alcohol, unlike many prescription sedatives. Although no evidence shows it to be harmful in pregnancy or lactation, like most herbs, it probably should be avoided during these times. There are no known side effects except occasional mild stomach upset, and there are no known interactions with other drugs.

The dosage of 0.8% valerenic extract for insomnia is 150 to 300 mg before sleep; for anxiety, 150 to 300 mg three times daily. The tea can be taken as needed three times a day or at bedtime and is made from steeping 1 to 2 tsp of the root in boiling water for 10 to 15 minutes. This yields 2 to 3 g of drug per cup. A tincture is available, and 2 to 4 ml is recommended three times daily. Valerian's odorous character has been likened to dirty socks.

TABLE 11-2

Common Herbs in Integrative Medicine

Herb	Common Uses*	Activity	Adverse Effects and Contraindications	Doses†	Drug Interactions‡
Aloe (*Aloe vera, Aloe barbadensis*)	**Burns and wound healing** **Constipation** Gastritis Ulcers Psoriasis	Antiinflammatory Antiseptic	Dermatitis GI upset (PO) Diarrhea Avoid in children and pregnancy. Avoid latex with inflammatory intestinal disease.	Liberal application of gel topically No more than 1 qt of juice per day	Cardiac glycoside containing herbs and drugs Licorice Stimulant laxatives
Bilberry (*Vaccinium myrtillus*)	**Eye disorder** **Antidiarrheal** Circulatory disorders Diabetes	Antioxidant Collagen stabilizer Vasoprotective Astringent ↓ Platelet aggregation	May alter insulin requirements	Anthocyanosides (calculated as anthocyanidin): 20-40 mg tid *V. myrtillus* (25% extract): 80-160 mg tid Fresh berries: 55-115 g tid	Warfarin (at high doses of bilberry)
Black cohosh (*Cimicifuga racemosa*)	**Menopause symptoms** **Menstrual problems** Rattlesnake bites	Probable SSRI-like effects Possible estrogenic activity Possible luteinizing hormone suppression	GI upset ↑ BP Avoid in pregnancy and lactation. Vertigo Rash Liver disease	27-Deoxyacteine: 2 mg bid Powdered rhizome: 1-2 g Tincture (1:5): 4-6 ml Fluid extract (1:1): 3-4 ml (1 tsp) Solid (dry powder) extract: (4:1): 250-500 mg	Hepatotoxic herbs and drugs
Cat's claw (*Uncaria tomentosa*)	**Arthritis** Cancer HIV Diverticulitis Herpes simplex and zoster	Immune stimulant Antiinflammatory Antimutagenic	Avoid in pregnancy and lactation, autoimmune illness, MS, TB, and leukemia (awaiting bone marrow transplant). Avoid in children <3 years old. Headaches	Tea (1 g/250 ml): 1 cup tid Tincture: 1-2 ml tid Standardized dry extract: 20-60 mg qd	Avoid combining with hormone drugs, insulin, vaccines, iron, NSAIDs, and salicylates. Antihypertensives Cytochrome P450 substrates

(Continued)

TABLE 11-2

Common Herbs in Integrative Medicine—cont'd

Herb	Common Uses*	Activity	Adverse Effects and Contraindications	Doses†	Drug Interactions‡
			Dizziness Vomiting		Chemotherapy Hyperimmune globulin IV thymic preparations
Cayenne (*Capsicum annum*)	**Arthritis** **Muscle pain** **Neuralgia** Postmastectomy pain Psoriasis Diabetes Antiflatulant Diarrhea	Blocks substance P (pain peptide) ↓ Lipids ↓ Platelet aggregation	Eye irritation Burning, local and mucous membranes Gastritis Diarrhea (with internal use) Avoid in children <2 years old.	Cream (0.025% or 0.075% capsaicin) topically qid	Warfarin: ↓ platelet aggregation with internal use MAOIs ACE inhibitors Aspirin Cocaine Antacids H₂ blockers Theophylline
Chamomile (*Matricaria recutita, Matricaria chamomilla*)	**GI complaints** **Skin and mucous membrane problems** **Stress and anxiety** Wound healing	Antispasmodic effect Sedative effect Antiinflammatory Carminative	Avoid if allergy to member of daisy family (Asteraceae; e.g., ragweed, asters, chrysanthemums). Contact dermatitis Urticaria	Tea: 3-4 cups per day Capsules: 300-500 mg tid-qid Tincture: 4-6 ml tid Apply topically to affected area	Caution if using with tranquilizers or CNS depressants (?) Warfarin Chemotherapy Cytochrome P450 substrates
Chaste tree (*Vitex agnus-castus*)	**Menstrual problems** **Hyperprolactinemia** Acne Infertility	Hormonal modulator	Rash Headache GI upset Avoid in pregnancy and lactation.	Solution (9 g in 100 ml): 40 gtts qam Dried extract: 4.2 mg qd Must take consistently for several months to see effect	Metoclopramide (Reglan) Contraceptive agents Avoid with dopamine agonists.
Cranberry (*Vaccinium macrocarpon*)	**Urinary tract infections**	↓ Bacterial adherence to bladder endothelium	Diarrhea May increase risk of kidney stones	Prophylaxis: 90 ml qd Treatment: 360-960 ml qd Tincture 0.5-1 tsp tid	Lansoprazole, omeprazole Warfarin Cytochrome P450 substrates

Herb	Indications	Actions	Precautions/Side effects	Dosage	Interactions
Dong quai (*Angelica sinensis*)	**Dysmenorrhea** **Other menstrual disorders** Menopause symptoms Allergies	Phytoestrogen Antimicrobial effects Smooth muscle relaxant IgE inhibition	Photodermatitis Uterine stimulant Carcinogenic constituents Hypersensitivity Excess bleeding and fever Avoid with hormone-sensitive tumors.	Dried root or rhizome: 1-2 g PO or IV tid Tincture (1:5): 3-5 ml tid Fluid extract (1:1): 0.5-2 ml tid	Warfarin Heparin Ticlopidine
Echinacea (*Echinacea* spp)	**Colds and flu** **Immunity** **Upper respiratory infections** **Urinary tract infections** Wound healing (topical) Recurrent candidal vaginitis	Immunostimulant ↑ Macrophage phagocytosis Stimulates lymphocyte activity Antiinflammatory Antimicrobial properties	Avoid in HIV/AIDS, autoimmune disease, collagen vascular disease, MS, and TB. Avoid if allergy to sunflower seeds or member of daisy family (Asteraceae) such as ragweed. (?) Avoid during pregnancy.	Dried root (or as tea): 0.5-1 g Freeze-dried plant: 325-650 mg Juice of aerial portion of *E. purpurea* stabilized in 22% ethanol: 2-3 ml (0.5-0.75 tsp) Tincture (1:5): 2-4 ml (1-2 tsp) Solid (dry powdered) extract (6.5:1 or 3.5% echinacoside): 150-300 mg	Chemotherapy agents Cytochrome P450 substrates Immuno-suppressants
Eleuthero (*Eleutherococcus senticosus*)	**Herpes type II** Fatigue **Athletic performance** Influenza complications	↑ Lymphocyte count Tonifying Immunomodulator Adaptogen	Diarrhea Sleep disturbance Anxiety Alters diabetes control Caution with cardiovascular disorders Avoid during antibiotic treatment of dysentery.	Dried root: 2-4 g Tincture (1:5): 10-20 ml Fluid extract (1:1): 2-4 ml Solid (dry powdered) extract (20:1): 100-200 mg	Caution with antipsychotics, barbiturates, and sedatives Anticoagulants Chemotherapy agents Digoxin Hypoglycemics Kanamycin

(Continued)

TABLE 11-2

Common Herbs in Integrative Medicine—cont'd

Herb	Common Uses*	Activity	Adverse Effects and Contraindications	Doses†	Drug Interactions‡
Ephedra (*Ephedra sinensis, ma huang*)	**Asthma** **Bronchitis** **Cough** **Decongestant** Energy **Weight loss** Diuretic	Sympathomimetic activating α and β_1/β_2 receptors CNS stimulant Stimulates uterine contractions	↑ BP, root ↓ BP, plant above ground Anxiety, restlessness Headaches Irritability Nausea, vomiting Urinary obstruction with BPH Addictive potential Dysrhythmias Alters diabetes control Kidney stones Glaucoma Caution in heart disease, hypertension, diabetes, or thyroid disease	Based on alkaloid content 1%-3% 12.5-25 mg bid-tid 12.5-25 mg bid-tid Crude herb 500-1000 mg tid	Cardiac glycosides Halothane Guanethidine MAOIs Oxytocin Diabetic medication Dexamethasone Ergot derivatives Methylxanthines Reserpine Must be protected from the light
Evening primrose oil (*Oenothera biennis*)	**Fibrocystic breast** **Eczema** Diabetic neuropathy Psoriasis Breast pain Lactation	Source of GLA (gamma-linoleic acid)	Headache GI symptoms Insomnia May exacerbate temporal lobe epilepsy and schizophrenia	Based on 8% GLA content 500-2000 mg tid-qid	Phenothiazines Tamoxifen Anesthetics Anticoagulants

Herb	Uses	Actions	Side effects/Cautions	Dosing	Drug interactions
Feverfew (*Tanacetum parthenium*)	**Migraine prophylaxis and treatment** Dizziness Tinnitis Dysmenorrhea	↓ Platelet aggregation Smooth muscle relaxant ↓ Prostaglandin synthesis and serotonin release from platelets and WBCs Antinociceptive Inhibits serotonin release	Stop 2 weeks before major surgery. Oral ulcers GI upset Rash Rebound migraine Nervousness Avoid in pregnancy and lactation, or if allergy to sunflower seeds or member of daisy family (Asteraceae) such as ragweed.	Depends on adequate level of parthenolide (0.4%-0.66%) Freeze-dried, pulverized leaves: 25-50 mg bid	Warfarin: ↓ platelet aggregation NSAIDs
Flax seed (*Linum usitatissimum*)	**Hyperlipidemia Constipation Cardiovascular risk reduction Systemic lupus erythematosus** Breast cancer risk reduction Irritable bowel; inflammatory bowel disease	↓ Platelet aggregation Antiinflammatory	Diarrhea Allergic reaction Caution with hormone-sensitive cancers Contraindicated with bowel obstruction	Capsule (1 g): 3-6 capsules qd Oil: 1-2 tbsp qd	Mucilage may affect absorption of oral drugs. Anticoagulants Antidiabetic drugs
Garlic (*Allium sativum*)	**Hyperlipidemia Hypertension** Cancer prevention Antimicrobial Atherosclerosis	Inhibits platelet aggregation ↑ Fibrinolysis Antioxidant ↓ Systolic and diastolic blood pressure	Stop 2 weeks before major surgery Heartburn GI upset Flatulence Body/breath odor ↓ Blood glucose	10 mg allicin or 4 g fresh garlic; equivalent to 1-2 cloves/day	May potentiate antithrombotic effect of anti-inflammatories, warfarin, and aspirin Saquinavir Cyclosporin Chlorzoxazone Dipyridamole Ticlopidine Cytochrome P450 substrates

(Continued)

TABLE 11-2

Common Herbs in Integrative Medicine—cont'd

Herb	Common Uses*	Activity	Adverse Effects and Contraindications	Doses†	Drug Interactions‡
Ginger (Zingiber officinale)	**Antiemetic** **Nausea** **Motion sickness** **Morning sickness** **Arthritis** Antiinflammatory Rheumatological	Stimulates intestinal tone and peristalsis Cholagogue Antiinflammatory Antioxidant Positive inotrope Inhibits platelet aggregation	Stop 2 weeks before major surgery. GI upset Caution if patient has gallstones	Dry powder ginger root: 1 g Extract (20% gingerol and shogaol): 100-200 mg tid	Warfarin: ↓ platelet Chemotherapy agents aggregation General anesthetics Heparin Antacids Antidiabetic drugs Antihypertensives Barbiturates H₂ blockers Proton pump inhibitors
Ginkgo biloba (Ginkgo biloba)	**Cerebrovascular insufficiency** **Peripheral vascular disease** **Vascular dementia** **Alzheimer's disease** **Memory** Vertigo Tinnitus Macular degeneration Depression PMS Diabetic neuropathy Raynaud's syndrome Retinopathy Glaucoma Sexual dysfunction associated with SSRIs	Membrane stabilizer Antiplatelet activating factor (PAF) Free radical scavenger Antioxidant ↑ Alpha brain waves ↓ Theta brain waves	Stop 2 weeks before major surgery. GI upset Allergies (whole plant) Spontaneous bleeding problems Headaches Skin rashes Dizziness Palpitations Seizures Avoid in pregnancy	Based on standard extract 25% ginkgo heterosides 40 mg bid-tid up to 80 mg bid-tid Use consistently for at least 12 weeks to determine effectiveness	Warfarin Aspirin (↓ platelet aggregation) MAOIs (↑ effect) Fluoxetin Glyburide Insulin Haloperidol Heparin Metformin Thiazide diuretics Ticlopidine Trazadone Buspirone Cytochrome P450 substrates
Ginseng (Panax ginseng) Ginseng radix (Eleutherococcus senticosus)	**Fatigue** **Weakness** **Energy** Immunity Mentation Diabetes	Immune enhancement Prevention of platelet aggregation Tonic effect	Stop 2 weeks before major surgery. Agitation Insomnia (PM doses) BP Edema	Based on ginsenoside content 4.5-6 g daily Root powder (5% gindenoside): 100 mg qd-tid	Warfarin (↓ platelet aggregation) Corticosteroids (↑ side effects) Digoxin (↑ serum levels)

Herb	Uses	Actions	Cautions	Dosage	Interactions
	Respiratory illnesses Libido Stress induced GI ulcers Postoperative stress		Hypertonia Caution with cardiac problems, diabetes, psychosis, and agitation	May use cyclically for 15-20 days followed by 2-week interval without ginseng	MAOIs, hypoglycemics (↑ effects) Opoids, diuretics (↓ effect) Stimulants Antidiabetic drugs
Goldenseal (*Hidrastis canadensis*)	**Cold** **Immunity** Diarrhea Sore throat Ocular trachoma infections	Antimicrobial (often combined with echinacea) Immune stimulant Activates phagocytes	Avoid in pregnancy, lactation, and diabetes (may lower glucose) Mouth irritation Digestive disorders Avoid in infants.	Dried root or as infusion (tea): 2-4 g Tincture (1:5): 6-12 ml (1.5-3 tsp) Fluid extract (1:1): 2-4 ml (0.5-1 tsp) Solid (powdered dry) extract (4:1 or 8%-12% alkaloid content): 250-500 mg	Antihypertensives Cytochrome P450 substrates Antacids CNS depressants Heparin H_2 blockers Proton pump inhibitors
Grape seed extract (*Vitis vinifera*)	Atherosclerosis **Retinopathy** **Venous insufficiency** Hepatic protective Dental caries	Proanthocyanidins: powerful antioxidants Vascular renewal and stability Collagen support	None known	25-250 mg bid	Tetracycline, doxycycline Warfarin
Hawthorn (*Crataegus laeviagata*)	**Congestive heart failure** **Hypertension** **Angina** Cardiac function	Cardioactive glycosides Positive inotropic ACE inhibition Mild diuretic Collagen stabilizer Dilates coronary vessels ↓ Peripheral resistance ↓ Oxygen consumption	Hypotension GI distress Rash Arrhythmia Avoid in pregnancy.	Berries or flowers (dried): 3-5 g or as infusion Tincture (1:5): 4-5 ml (alcohol may elicit pressor response in some individuals) Fluid extract (1:1): 1-2 ml Freeze-dried berries: 1-1.5 g Flower extract (standardized to contain 1.8% vitexin-4)	May potentiate effects of digitalis drugs Calcium channel blockers CNS depressants Nitrates

(Continued)

TABLE 11-2

Common Herbs in Integrative Medicine—cont'd

Herb	Common Uses*	Activity	Adverse Effects and Contraindications	Doses†	Drug Interactions‡
Horse chestnut (*Aesculus hippocastanum*)	**Venous insufficiency** **Varicose veins** **Nocturnal leg cramps** **Pruritus and swelling of legs** Topically for hemorrhoids, skin ulcers, varicose veins, sport injuries, trauma	Aescin component reduces lysosomal activity, improves venous tone, and inhibits capillary protein premeability. Diuretic	GI irritation ↓ gastric emptying Pruritus Nausea Standardized seed extracts are safe, but whole herb may be fatal. Avoid in pregnancy and lactation, liver disease, renal disease. May cross-react with latex allergy	Based on aescin 90-150 mg initially, followed by 35-70 mg qd	Anticoagulants Antidiabetes drugs
Kava (*Piper methysticum*)	Anxiety **Restlessness** **Insomnia** Anticonvulsant Oral anesthetic Depression Attention deficit hyperactivity disorder	GABA receptor-like actions Limbic system modulation Inhibits voltage-dependent sodium channels in brain Skeletal muscle relaxant	Dermatitis Sedation May impair reflexes and judgment for driving in high doses Avoid in pregnancy and lactation, depression, and Parkinson's disease. Contraindicated in endogenous depression Hepatoxicity *Note:* kava is nonaddictive.	Anxiolytic dose: 45-70 mg kavalactones tid Sedative dose: 180-210 mg 1 hour before bedtime	Alcohol Benzodiazepines Barbiturates Anti-Parkinson's drugs Other psycho-pharmacological agents, general anesthetics Cytochrome P450 substrates
Licorice (*Glyyrrhiza* spp)	Upper respiratory infection Oral and gastric ulcers Infection	Antiinflammatory Expectorant Antioxidant Demulcent Adrenocorticotropin	Avoid in pregnancy. Contraindicated in cholestatic liver disease, cirrhosis, hypertension, hypokalemia, and renal insufficiency	Powdered root: 1-2 g Fluid extract (1:1): 2-4 ml Solid (dry powdered) extract (4:1): 250-500 mg	Furosemide Estrogens Chorothiazide, metalozone Isoniazid Antihypertensives Insulin Risperidone

					Ibuprofen Digitalis glycosides Corticosteroids Cytochrome P450 substrates
Milk thistle (Silybum marianum)	Cirrhosis Alcoholic and viral hepatitis Mushroom poisoning (Amanita) Other hepatotoxins	Cell membrane stabilizer Stimulates ribosomal protein synthesis Free radical scavenger Antioxidant Contraindicated in liver disease Inhibits leukotriene formation Choleretic and lipotropic	GI upset Laxative effect Alcohol-based extracts Contraindicated in liver disease	Based on silymarin content 70-210 mg tid Silybin bound to phosphatidylcholine: 120-240 mg bid	Acetaminophen Butyrophenones Phenothiazines Indinavir Metronidazole Nitrous oxide Chemotherapy Clofibrate General anesthetics Haloperidol Cytochrome P450 substrates
Peppermint (Mentha piperita)	Dyspepsia Irritable bowel syndrome Biliary dyskinesia Digestive aid Myalgia Neuralgia Nasal decongestant Tension headache (topically)	Antispasmodic Cholagogue Menthol is active ingredient. Antibacterial Antiviral Stimulates gastric secretion Coolant ↓ Lower esophageal sphincter tone Carminative	Nonenteric dosage may worsen heartburn in esophageal reflux and hiatal hernia. Caution in pregnancy and in small children (choking from menthol) Allergic reactions Bradycardia Muscle tremor Dermatitis, skin rash Contraindicated in gallstones, achlorhydria, and liver damage	Infusion: 1-2 tsp dried leaves per 8 oz water Enteric-coated capsule (0.2 ml oil/capsule): 1-2 capsules tid Menthol 1.26-16% applied topically up to qid	Antacids Cisapride
Saw palmetto (Serenoa repens)	Benign prostatic hyperplasia (stages I and II) Prostatitis	Antiandrogenic (5α-reductase) Bladder muscle spasmolytic Antiinflammatory	GI side effects Diarrhea Avoid in pregnancy. Potential risk of aggravation of estrogen-sensitive tumors	Crude berries: 10 g bid Liposterolic extract (standardized at 85%-95% fatty acids and sterols): 160 mg bid	Anticoagulants Contraceptives Estrogens

(Continued)

TABLE 11-2

Common Herbs in Integrative Medicine—cont'd

Herb	Common Uses*	Activity	Adverse Effects and Contraindications	Doses†	Drug Interactions‡
			Rule out advanced prostatic hypertrophy and prostate cancer.		
St. John's wort (Hypericum perforatum)	**Depression: mild to moderate** **Anxiety** **Insomnia** Contusions First-degree burns Wound healing Antiinflammatory (topically) Myalgias Eczema	Affects neurotransmitters serotonin, dopamine, catecholamines, and possibly MAOIs; reduction of interleukin-6 Antiviral Antibacterial	Avoid in pregnancy (? uterotonic). GI side effects Photodermatitis Allergy Fatigue Insomnia Headache Restlessness Avoid in bipolar disorder.	Dried flowers: 2-4 g tid Tincture (1:5): 3-6 ml tid Fluid extract (1:1): 1-2 ml tid Standardized fluid extract (0.14% hypericin: 1 mg hypericin/3 ml): 0.5-0.9 ml tid Standardized solid (dry powdered) extract (0.14% hypericin): 600 mg tid Standardized solid (dry powdered) extract (0.3% hypericin): 300 mg tid	Potential interaction with SSRIs, general anesthetics, and benzodiazepines Chemotherapy Cyclosporine Digoxin Indinavir Oral contraceptives Theophylline Trazadone *No longer contraindicated:* use with MAOIs, tyramine-containing compounds, 5-L-dopa, hydroxy-tryptophan
Tea tree oil (Melaleuca alternifolia)	**Skin infections** **Acne** Mucosal and vaginal lesions Fungal infections (skin/nails)	Antibacterial Antiviral Antifungal	Contact dermatitis Allergic reaction Orally may cause significant toxicity; confusion and ataxia	Apply topically to affected area.	None known

| Valerian (*Valeriana officinalis*) | **Insomnia**
Anxiety | GABA domain effects
Improves latency and quality of sleep
Improves slow-wave sleep | Overdose with temporary GI, chest, and CNS symptoms
(?) Use in pregnancy and lactation
Caution in children <12 years old
Odor
Cardiac disturbances
Note: Valerian is not habit-forming. | Dried root (or as tea): 1-2 g
Tincture (1:5): 4-6 ml (1-1.5 tsp)
Fluid extract (1:1): 1-2 ml (0.5-1 tsp)
Solid (dry powdered) extract (4:1): 250-500 mg
Valerian extract (1%-1.5% valtrate or 0.5% valerenic acid): 150-300 mg | Avoid with benzodiazepines, barbiturates, general anesthetics, and alcohol.
Cytochrome P450 substrates |

↑, Increased; ↓, decreased; *g* gram(s); *GI*, gastrointestinal; *PO*, oral; *IV*, intravenous; *SSRI*, selective serotonin reuptake inhibitor; *BP*, blood pressure; *qd*, every day; *bid*, twice daily; *tid*, three times daily; *qid*, four times daily; *qam*, every morning; *HIV*, human immunodeficiency virus; *AIDS*, acquired immunodeficiency syndrome; *TB*, tuberculosis; *MS*, multiple sclerosis; *NSAIDs*, nonsteroidal antiinflammatory drugs; *MAOIs*, monoamine oxidase inhibitors; *ACE*, angiotensin-converting enzyme; *CNS*, central nervous system; *PMS*, premenstrual syndrome; *BPH*, benign prostatic hypertrophy; *IgE*, immunoglobulin E; *WBCs*, white blood cells; *GABA*, gamma-aminobutyric acid.

* The most frequent indications are shown in **boldface** type.

†Dosages vary by preparation. Consult appendix sources listed or expert practitioner.

‡Drug-herb interactions: many interactions as cited are theoretical, based on mechanism of action, pharmacokinetics, or other preclinical data and have not been observed in patients. Although this type of data suggests caution, it may not contraindicate combined use. For in-depth detail on interactions, consult the Natural Medicine Comprehensive Database, other appendix sources listed, or an expert botanical medicine practitioner.

References

Blumenthal M: *The ABC clinical guide to herbs,* Austin, Texas, 2003, American Botanical Council.

Blumenthal M, Goldberg A, Brinckman J: *Herbal medicine: expanded Commission E monographs,* Newton Mass, 2000, Integrative Medical Communications.

Chen J, Chen T: *Chinese medical herbology and pharmacology,* City of Industry, Calif, 2004, Art of Medicine Press.

Davidow J: *Infusions of healing,* New York, 1999, Simon & Schuster, Fireside Press.

Selected Readings

Blumenthal M, Busse WR, Goldberg A, et al: *The complete German Commission E monographs: therapeutic guide to herbal medicines* (American Botanical Council, Austin, Texas), Boston, 1998, Integrative Medicine Communications.

Ernst E, Pittler M, Stevinson C: *The desktop guide to complementary and alternative medicine: an evidence-based approach,* St Louis, 2001, Mosby.

Jellin J, *Pharmacist's Letter,* editor: *Natural medicines comprehensive database,* Stockton, Calif, 2004, Therapeutic Research Faculty.

Lininger S, Wright J, Austin S, et al: *The natural pharmacy,* Rocklin, Calif, 1998, Prima Publishing. (A referenced overview of natural remedies for multiple conditions; refers to herbal, nutritional, homeopathic, and other alternative therapies; a useful CD-ROM may be sampled at www.healthnotes.online.)

Murray M, Pizzorno J: *Encyclopedia of natural medicine,* Rocklin, Calif, 1998, Prima Publishing. (For only $25, an economic and practical guide to naturopathic healing methods, including herbs, nutraceuticals, diet, and lifestyle changes.)

Physicians' desk reference (PDR) for herbal medicines, Montvale, NJ, 1999, Medical Economics. (For their first edition, an effort to give physicians and other health professionals a usable handbook.)

Physicians' desk reference (PDR) for herbal supplements, Montvale, NJ, 2004, Medical Economics.

Pizzorno J, Murray M: *Textbook of natural medicine,* London, 1999, Churchill Livingstone.

Websites

Herb Research Foundation www.herbs.org

American Botanical Council: www.herbalgram.org

Consumer Reports: http://www.consumerreports.org/main/home.jsp/bhfv=7&bhqs=1. (Subscription)

Drug Digest with Drug-Herb Interaction feature: http://www.drugdigest.org/DD/Home

PDA resources, including herbal information: www.epocrates.com (Subscription)

HealthNotes Online: http://www.healthnotes.com/ (Subscription)

Longwood Herbal Task Force: http://www.mcp.edu/herbal/

Natural Medicines Comprehensive Database, including PDA version: www.NaturalDatabase.com (Subscription)

Natural Standard: http://www.naturalstandard.com/ (Subscription)

Office of Dietary Supplements: http://ods.od.nih.gov/Health_Information/IBIDS.aspx

Sloan-Kettering Herb Reference: http://www.mskcc.org/mskcc/html/11570.cfm

University of Texas Medical Branch Alternative and Integrative Medicine Project: http://cam.utmb.edu

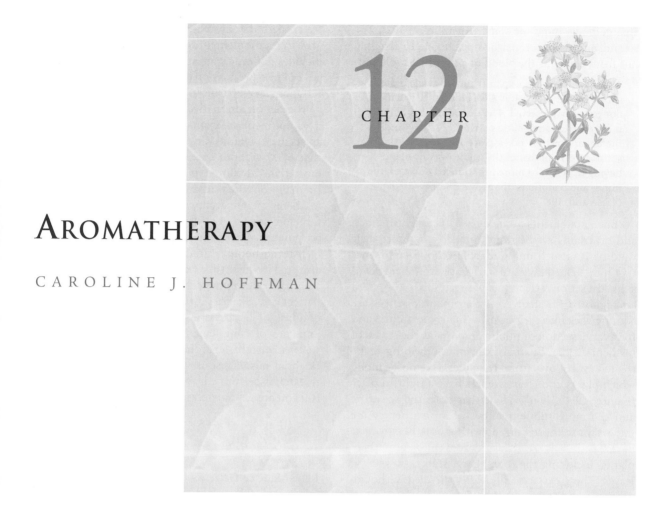

CHAPTER 12

AROMATHERAPY

C A R O L I N E   J .   H O F F M A N

romatherapy is the therapeutic use of essential oils extracted from plants. The term *aromathérapie* was coined by the French chemist René-Maurice Gattefossé in 1928. His book of the same name was published in 1937. Many consider Gattefossé to be the "father of the modern-day scientific use of essential oils."

The food and perfume industries are the largest users of essential oils. Some confusion about the therapeutic potential of aromatherapy may be a result of this link with the cosmetic industry. The dictionary definition of *aromatherapy* is "a method of treating bodily ailments using essential plant oils" (*Chambers Dictionary,* 1988). *Aroma* is defined in chemical terms as belonging to the closed-chain class of organic compounds or benzene derivatives. *Therapy*

is defined as a treatment used to combat a disease or abnormal condition. *Essential oils* are described as oils forming the odiferous part of plants and as ethereal, suggesting not only a chemical constituent but also a "heavenly," spiritlike, or airy quality. On the basis of these definitions, *aromatherapy* is a treatment using a range of organic compounds, of which the odor or fragrance plays an important part.

Jean Valnet, the French physician well known for his invaluable work on aromatherapy, speaks of aromatherapy as the medicinal use of aromatic essences derived from plants (Valnet, 1990). Kusmirek, an aromatherapist based in England, describes aromatherapy as an industry combining perfumery, science, "psychoaromatherapy," and "aromacology," stating that the use of essential oils seeks to influence or change body, mind, or spirit (Kusmirek, 1992). Tisserand, an English aromatherapist, refers to essential oils from plants as the blood of a person, as follows:

> They are not the whole plant, but are whole organic substances in themselves. Like blood they will die if not properly preserved. The essential oil is like the most ethereal and subtle part of the plant, and its therapeutic action takes place on a higher more subtle level than that of the whole organic plant . . . having in general a more pronounced effect on the mind and emotions than does herbal medicine (Tisserand, 1988).

Such statements are not based in scientific fact, and no trials have been performed to support their validity. It is such unfounded, anecdotal comments that have helped keep aromatherapy from being considered a serious science. Valnet states that, forgotten and ignored for many years, aromatic essences are coming back into their own, for many researchers and for a large section of public opinion, as the "stars of medicine." Many patients are now unwilling to be treated except by natural therapies, foremost among which plants and their essences have a rightful place (Valnet, 1990). It is evident that both the scientific and the more subtle qualities of aromatherapy are important to those working with aromatherapy oils.

Essential oils are extracted from different parts of plants, including the roots, bark, stalks, flowers, or leaves. These extracts are mostly distilled, although other methods might be used. Essential oils might be applied to the body through massage with a vegetable oil, inhaled, used as a compress, mixed into an ointment, or inserted internally through the rectum, vagina, or mouth. The latter method is used chiefly by the medical profession in France.

Aromatherapy appears to be one of the fastest-growing complementary therapies in the United Kingdom. Madame Marguerite Maury, born in Austria, brought aromatherapy to the United Kingdom from France. She was the first layperson to study and use the effects of essential oils absorbed through the skin. Her research was based on that of Gattefossé and her own clinical work with her husband, a French homoeopathic doctor. She promoted the modern-day use of massage with essential oils, the *aromatherapy massage,* and began teaching aromatherapy to beauticians. This training has gradually filtered from the cosmetic into the therapeutic domain and is increasingly being used by nurses, physiotherapists, and other health care professionals.

Modern-day aromatherapy is one of the fastest growing complementary therapies. This growth includes not only training and practice of aromatherapy but also production of essential oils. In the United Kingdom it is difficult to pick up a magazine or watch a program on alternative or integrative medicine that does not mention aromatherapy. Trained aromatherapists in the United Kingdom currently number more than 5000, without a central register. In one survey, of more than 21,000 people who responded to a questionnaire on alternative medicine, 7% had used aromatherapy, compared with 25% for osteopathy, 14% for chiropractic, 12% for homeopathy, and 9% for acupuncture (Consumers Association, 1992).

Aromatherapy gradually is becoming more accepted in the orthodox medical field as a treatment to enhance both physical and psychological aspects of patient care. Skeptics might reject the therapy because of a lack of clinical trials—a criticism leveled at other branches of complementary medical treatments—as well as concern regarding the safety and quality of essential oils. These issues will be resolved as more research is performed, and aromatherapy will have its full and appropriate place in modern health care.

HISTORY

René-Maurice Gattefossé was a French chemist and scholar who described aromatherapy as a particular branch of science and therapeutics in 1928. He became interested in the study of essential oils after an accident in his laboratory. Gattefossé burnt his hand badly after a chemical explosion. He applied lavender essential oil that was nearby. The burn healed with remarkable speed and without infection or scarring. Amazed at this result, Gattefossé began to investigate the properties of essential oils. He was the first person to analyze and record the individual chemical components in each oil, classifying the oils according to their properties (e.g., antitoxic, antiseptic, tonifying, stimulating, calming) (Franchomme and Pénoël, 1990).

Gattefossé carried out experiments in military hospitals during World War I. He claimed to achieve remarkable results using essential oils, preventing gangrene, curing burns, and obtaining cicatrization much more quickly than usual. After the war, however, his methods came under professional scrutiny and were largely left behind (Maury, 1964).

Essential oils from aromatic plants were used before 1928. It is uncertain how long *distilled* essential oils have been used. Popular opinion claims that the Arabs discovered the distilling of plants in the Middle Ages, and Avicenna has been given credit for this achievement in the tenth century AD (Arcier, 1990). However, an Italian research party led by Dr. Paolo Povesti, the director of the International Biocosmetic Research center in Milan, found a perfectly preserved terra-cotta distillation apparatus, or "still," in the museum of Taxila at the foot of the Himalayas. It was used for beauty products and dated back 5000 years to the Indus Valley civilization (Williams, 1989).

Aromatic substances, which may or may not include essential oils as prepared today, were used in the ancient civilizations of Egypt, China, Greece, Rome, and Arab countries; in the Middle Ages; during the scientific revolution; and up to the present. The importance of this is captured in the comment of Marguerite Maury (1964): "Perfumes and aromatics have their own history and long past. The latter is so bound up in the story of mankind that it is impossible to separate the two."

In ancient Egypt, Nefertum was the god of perfumes, incense, and fragrant oils. He was the son of Ptah, the creator god, and Sekmet, the goddess of fiery protection, healing, and alchemical distillation. In a hymn to Nefertum, he is described as the "Lord of oils and ungents, the soul of life." Nefertum smells the soul of the lotus and plants and purifies the body. In Egyptian life, fragrance was a means of communication between the gods and humanity, offering health to the living and assisting the dead in the next life (Steele, 1992). The uses of aromatic products for spiritual well-being, health, and beauty somewhat overlapped. King Ramses III reportedly burned 2 million blocks of incense during the 30 years of his reign (Stoddart, 1991). The medicinal properties of aromatic oils were understood by the later Egyptian periods, and a wide range of essential oils was used, including frankincense, myrrh, cedarwood, henna, and juniper. The essence of cedarwood was prepared by heating in clay vessels covered by a layer of woolen fibers. These fibers were then squeezed, allowing the essence to be extracted (Valnet, 1990). When the tomb of Tutenkhamun was discovered in 1922, vases were found in the tomb, which on analysis contained ointments of frankincense in a base of animal fat. The scent was apparently faint but still in evidence (Tisserand, 1988).

The ancient Chinese are well known for their use of herbal medicine, acupuncture, and moxibustion (the burning of mugwort to balance the body's energy), but there seems to be little detail regarding the use of aromatic oils. The Hebrews gained their knowledge of aromatic oils from prisoners held by the Egyptians.

The ancient Greeks used the aromatic essences both for medicine and for perfumes. Hippocrates expounded the virtues of a daily bath and a scented massage to maintain health and well-being. Aristotle argued that pleasant smells contribute to the well-being of humanity. The Roman poet Lucretius described the particles of pleasant smells as being "smooth and round," whereas particles of unpleasant smells were "barbed and prickly."

Biblical evidence of the use of aromatic substances is present in both the old and new testaments. God commanded Moses to make a holy anointing oil of myrrh, cinnamon, calamus, cassia, and olive oil (Exodus 30:22-25); frankincense and myrrh were brought to the birth of Jesus Christ (Matthew 2:11).

The Middle Ages saw a rise in the use of oils both as perfumes and as medicines. Catherine de Medici, married to King Henry II, made the use of aromatic substances for ailments and perfumery fashionable. Her perfumer, Cosimo Ruggieri, not only assisted her with her health and beauty but was also able to prepare much less pleasant substances to help dispose of her enemies. Aromatic oils also were used to block out the smell of poor hygiene and ward off various plagues; pomanders and the fragrant tops on walking sticks were often used for this purpose. In 1589 a German pharmacopeia listed 80 essential oils for treating different conditions, and lavender essence was first prepared in France at this time (Arcier, 1990).

Outside Europe, the Native American shamans also used herbs and aromatics. The *perfumeros,* or healers, bathed their patients in scents and, by the skillful use of perfume, could transform the "auric field," the energetic or emotional envelope that surrounds a person. The blowing of tobacco smoke over a person, combined with a perfume, also was seen as having curative powers. The use of fragrance enabled transformations in religious, magical, and healing rituals. An ancient connection exists between fumigating and perfuming in this culture (Steele, 1992).

The scientific revolution and the manufacturing of synthetic substances that began in the nineteenth century saw the retreat of essential oils until the work by Gattefossé and his followers during the twentieth century. The perfume industry developed separately from the therapeutic field, with the introduction of such names as Coco Chanel, who launched the famous Chanel No. 5 in 1921. It was Chanel who said that the "most mysterious, most human thing," is smell. With the subsequent commercial development of the cosmetic industry, the gap between the cosmetic and the therapeutic use of essential oils became evident. Chanel and her scientific advisers successfully used synthetic products to make modern perfumes. This process separated cosmetics completely from the therapeutic use of essential oils, except perhaps for good feelings experienced by people wearing and experiencing the perfumes.

Marguerite Maury's research into the cutaneous application of essential oils began the teaching of aromatherapy in the 1950s as it is used today. Maury was influenced by the work of Valnet, who was an army physician during World War II. He recognized that essential oils could have been used to alleviate soldiers' infection rather than the massive amounts of penicillin prescribed. He obtained consistent results using essential oils with his wartime patients in Tonkin (Valnet, 1990). Madame Maury identified two uses of aromatherapy in France: (1) as part of allopathy in its use by doctors and (2) as a beauty treatment in the form of massage. She also acknowledged the more subtle aspect of aromatherapy and mentioned its link to vibratory medicine.

DEVELOPMENT

Madame Maury influenced the beginnings of the practice of aromatherapy in the United Kingdom. Micheline Arcier, a well-known aromatherapist in London, met Madame Maury at a beauty conference in 1959. Arcier and three other masseuses asked Maury to run a course for them. Madame Maury had clinics in London, Paris, and Switzerland, and Madame Arcier worked with her in London. Madame Arcier then began working with the oils and teaching small numbers of masseuses in the 1960s and 1970s. She also met Valnet, who worked and consulted from her London clinic. This was the beginning of the development of what is now referred to as the "Anglo-Saxon approach" to aromatherapy.

Aromatherapy was still little known at this time. In fact, this method did not earn widespread popu-

larity until the 1980s. It is interesting to note the recent growth of aromatherapy, and yet, how few people have been responsible for its development over the last few decades.

Since the 1980s, numerous schools of massage and aromatherapy have opened. Again, more than 5000 aromatherapists are registered in the United Kingdom, although not all practice full-time. Training in aromatherapy has continued in schools for lay massage practitioners but has spread to nursing colleges and universities, where the courses may be taken as part of a diploma or degree or master's program. An increasing number of nurses are choosing aromatherapy as a topic for their doctoral research (e.g., Wilkinson, 1995).

The United States has been swift to follow this UK model, and two organizations now represent standards in in aromatherapy training: the National Association of Holistic Aromatherapy, with more than 4000 members, and the Aromatherapy Registration Council, which has set a national examination for registration. As in the United Kingdom, U.S. universities and colleges now offer postgraduate courses in aromatherapy for nurses. Each state develops its own legislation in relation to practice (Buckle, 2003).

The skills of therapeutic massage, usually the Swedish style, were taught to masseuses and physiotherapists as part of their professional training. Massage was part of the curriculum at nursing schools at the turn of the twentieth century but was excluded as their training became more scientific and technically oriented. It is now recognized as a valuable skill in terms of pain management and stress relief and is slowly being reintroduced into nurses' training.

More than 100 books have been published on the topic of aromatherapy in the last 10 years, indicating the rise in its popularity. Unfortunately, these books do not add much new research-based information about essential oils. They often are published for commercial benefit rather than to further the science of aromatherapy. Most books are aimed at both lay and professional audiences, indicating the lack of sophistication in this field. Many books offer recipes of essential oils, losing sight of the fundamental principles involved. The exceptional work by Franchomme and Pénoël (1990) gives detailed chemical analysis of each oil and conditions, indications, and contraindications for each. Other books address this issue by providing more scientific information, including the available research on essential oils, their chemical constituents, and the clinical practice of aromatherapy (Tisserand and Balacs, 1995; Vickers, 1996). There is an increasing amount of research being performed worldwide and in North America, where a study on the inhalation of essential oils for the treatment of respiratory conditions was previously the exception (Boyd and Pearson, 1946).

THEORETICAL BASIS

Essential oils are volatile, fragrant, organic constituents that are obtained from plants either by *distillation,* which is most common, or by *cold pressing,* which is used for the extraction of citrus oils. Oils may be extracted from leaves (eucalyptus, peppermint), flowers (lavender, rose), blossoms (orange blossom or neroli), fruits (lemon, mandarin), grasses (lemongrass), wood (camphor, sandalwood), barks (cinnamon), gum (frankincense), bulbs (garlic, onion), roots (calamus), or dried flower buds (clove). Varying amounts of essential oil can be extracted from a particular plant; 220 pounds of rose petals will yield less than 2 ounces of the essential oil, whereas other plants, such as lavender, lemon, or eucalyptus, give a much greater proportion. This accounts for the variation in price among essential oils. Essential oils come from sources worldwide: lavender from France, eucalyptus from Australia, and sandalwood from India.

Essential oils are typically a mixture of more than 100 organic compounds, which may include esters, alcohols, aldehydes, terpenes, ketones, coumarins, lactones, phenols, oxides, acids, and ethers. There is debate within the aromatherapy community regarding the mechanisms of effects of essential oils. Showing the functional group theory, Table 12-1 lists the major chemical components and the specific therapeutic effects attributed to them (Franchomme and Pénoël, 1990). Within the oils there might be more of some active constituents than others, which gives the oil its particular therapeutic value. For example, oils containing large amounts of esters (50%-70%), such as neroli *Citrus aurantium* ssp. *amara,* are thought to be calming, whereas other oils, such as tea tree *Melaleuca alternifolia* terpineol-4, are regarded as antibacterial, antiviral, and immune system boosters because of the large amounts of alcohol (45%-50%) in their composition. This functional group theory model is now challenged within the international aromatherapy community for failing to take into account the ideas of synergy and antago-

TABLE 12-1

Chemical Components of Essential Oils and Their therapeutic Actions

Chemical Component	Therapeutic Action
Aldehydes	Antiinfectious, litholitic, calming
Kotones	Mucolitic, litholitic, cicatrising, calming
Esters	Antispasmodic, calming
Sesquiterpenes	Antihistamines, antiallergic
Coumarins, lactones	Balancing, calming
C15 and C20	Estrogen-like action alcohols
Acids, aromatic	Antiinfectious, aldehydes, immunostimulants
Phenols, C10 alcohols	Antiinfectious, immunostimulants
Oxides	Expectorant, antiparasitic
Phenyl methyl ethers	Antiinfectious, antispasmodic
C10 terpens	Antiseptic, cortisone-like action

From Franchomme P, Pénoël D. 1990. L'aromatherapie Exactement. Roger Jallois, Limoges.

nism and for essentially being too broad (Tisserand, 1998/99). Critics of aromatherapy may say that the idea of an active ingredient goes against the desire for a whole natural substance. There is a question of the naturalness of any oil removed from a plant because immediately after the flower is cut, chemical changes occur; other chemicals may appear in the oil that were not originally in the plant (Dodd, 1991).

Aromatherapy is used for a wide range of physical, mental, and emotional conditions, including burns, severe bacterial infections, insomnia, depression, hypertension, and arrhythmias. Some of the findings that support these claims are discussed in the research section of this chapter.

The process of liquid gas chromatography is used to identify the quantity of each chemical constituent within the oil. As with grapes grown for wine, the quality of the yield varies according to the climate and other growing conditions of the plant. Lavender oil is popularly thought to be harmless, but according to its chemical type, or chemotype, it might not be suitable for use as an therapeutic oil. True lavender, *Lavandula angustifolia,* grown at approximately

1000 meters in the French Alps, has a high degree of purity and therapeutic constituents, whereas Stoechas lavender, *Lavandula stoechas,* grown at sea level by the Mediterranean, contains high quantities of ketones and therefore may be neurotoxic and abortive and is contraindicated in pregnant women, babies, and children (Franchomme and Pénoël, 1990).

Potential side effects of essential oils include the neurotoxic and abortive qualities already mentioned, as well as dermal toxicity, photosensitivity, allergic reactions, problems with internal use, and liver sensitivity (Franchomme and Pénoël, 1990; Tisserand and Balacs, 1995). Unless oils are labeled with the full botanical data in Latin, it is impossible to tell whether they are dangerous or contraindicated. Lack of legislation over labeling and quality control of essential oils in the United Kingdom has contributed to the unease in some health care settings about their use. The fact that essential oils can be purchased at retail stores also gives the general public a false impression about the relative safety of these oils.

The quality of essential oils also can be affected by their producers, who might add chemicals to extend the oil's capabilities or pesticides to act as contaminants. Gas chromatography will identify the chemical makeup of any oil, but it is not a complete assurance of quality. A certain degree of adulteration is common in the essential oil world, and it is often impossible for the consumer to detect. Reputable oil suppliers who perform their own quality control are currently the only safeguard.

There are few principles for the treatment of aromatherapy. Many aromatherapists discuss the concept of synergy at some length, that the whole natural essence is more active than its principal constituent. Those constituents that form a smaller percentage of the whole are found to be more active than the principal constituent (Valnet, 1990). As early as 1919, Heurre stated that it is not enough to place side-by-side the principal chemical elements that analysis shows to be present in a particular vegetable essence to obtain a product that, therapeutically speaking, is as active as that of the natural essence (Valnet, 1990).

The basis of the action of aromatherapy is thought to be the same as that of modern pharmacology, using smaller doses. The chemical constituents are absorbed into the body, affecting particular physiological processes. Aromatherapy oils are taken into the body through the oral, dermal, rectal, or vaginal routes, or simply by olfaction.

The cutaneous administration of essential oils mixed in a vegetable carrier oil in the form of an aromatherapy massage is a common method of administration in the Anglo-Saxon approach to aromatherapy. Benefits can be gained not only from the oils through the skin but also from inhalation of the vapor and from physical therapy in the form of massage. Once the oil reaches the upper dermis, it enters the capillary circulation, where the oil can be transported throughout the body (Hotchkiss, 1994). In one study a massage oil made with lavender penetrated the skin after 10 minutes (Jäger et al., 1992). Blood samples taken at intervals after massage, when analyzed by gas chromatography, showed that two major constituents of lavender oil, linalool and linalyl acetate, reached maximal concentrations 20 minutes after the massage, although traces had been evident at 5 minutes. Levels returned to baseline after 90 minutes, indicating elimination of lavender from the bloodstream. Other studies support the passage of aromatic compounds through the skin of humans (Bronough, 1990; Collins et al., 1984).

The *oral* administration of essential oils comes from the current French medical approach to aromatherapy and carries more potential risks of poisoning or irritation to the gastric mucosa if administered by unqualified persons. It might be useful for qualified medical practitioners to administer larger doses of essential oils into the body for the treatment of serious infections. A more detailed knowledge of essential oil toxicology is required for administration by the oral route than currently possessed by the average aromatherapist. Interest in this form of administration is growing, and good opportunities are available for training in this style of administration in the English language, particularly in Provence, France, with trainers such as Rhiannon and Bob Harris.

A significantly smaller dose is administered to the body through the skin than when given orally (Tisserand and Balacs, 1995). *Rectal* administration of oils in the form of suppositories may be useful for local problems and to avoid the portal system of the body, thus allowing higher systemic concentrations of the oils to be absorbed. *Vaginal* administration in the form of pessaries or douches also is used for local problems.

Simple *inhalation* of the oils is a method used for respiratory conditions, insomnia, and mood elevation and enhancement, or simply for making an environment more pleasant. It is not surprising that essential oils are absorbed through inhalation, considering that conventional medications such as those for asthma are administered in this way. Steam inhalers can be used for respiratory infections, and a variety of electrical and fan-assisted devices may be used to scent a room. Locomotor activity in mice increased after the inhalation of rosemary oil (Kovar et al., 1987). A rise in serum levels of 1,8-cineole, a major constituent of rosemary, corresponded with the rise in locomotor activity. Aromatic compounds of sandalwood, rose, neroli, and lavender all were present in the blood of mice after inhalation (Buchbauer et al., 1991). Studies also have demonstrated the absorption of aromatic compounds by humans (Falk, 1990; Falk-Filipsson, 1993). Overexposure to oils absorbed by this method can result in headaches, fatigue, or allergic reactions such as streaming eyes and skin problems.

The influence of touch in the form of massage is a major aspect of aromatherapy treatment when the oils are administered *cutaneously*. One study was able to show additional psychological benefit, including reduction in anxiety, to cardiac patients who had aromatherapy massage with the essential oil of neroli (*Citrus aurantium* ssp. *amara*) compared with those who had massage with a plain vegetable oil (Stevensen, 1994). Other studies have shown positive psychological benefits from massage, including positive subjective response (Madison, 1973), the perceived state of relaxation (Longworth, 1982), reported pleasurable feelings (Bauer and Dracup, 1987), and an improvement in the perceived level of anxiety (Dunn, 1992). Physiological results from massage generally have shown no significant difference in heart rate or arterial blood pressure (Bauer and Dracup, 1987; Dunn, 1992; Kaufmann, 1964; Longworth, 1982; Reed and Held, 1988) or in respiratory rate (Bauer and Dracup, 1987; Dunn, 1992; Kaufman, 1964; Longworth, 1982; Reed and Held, 1988). The importance of massage for both relaxation and release of physical and psychological stress should not be underestimated and can be seen only as a positive aid to the administration of essential oils when administered appropriately.

It is suggested that aromatherapy would not have gained its rapid increase in popularity if the oils were not fragrant, thus affecting mood and emotions. Several references have already been made to the inextricable link among the development of human biology,

the sense of smell, and the importance of aromas. Sigmund Freud developed the idea of "organic repression" of the sense of smell. He attributed this to upright gait, which elevates the nose from the ground, where it had enjoyed pleasurable sensations previously (Freud, 1929). This repression may not be complete, but many people have a diminished sense of smell, a sense more vital to the survival of animals than humans. It may be this need to satisfy pleasurable sensations through the sense of smell that is attracting so many people to aromatherapy.

The human response to aromas is associated with olfaction naturally. The neurons of the olfactory system, which are the chemical senses of the body, rest in the section of the midbrain known as the *limbic system*. The structures of the limbic system extend from the midbrain through the hypothalamus into the basal forebrain, which is concerned not only with visceral functions but also with emotional expression. The cortical and medial nuclei of the amygdala, a body situated within this system, receive information from the olfactory system. The basolateral nuclei are involved with the expression of emotion (Shepherd, 1983). Therefore, aromatherapy's effect on emotion and psychological state is not surprising (Hardy, 1992; Stevensen, 1994). The emotional and psychological benefit of aromatherapy is important in many clinical situations, including chronic, life-threatening conditions such as cancer, heart disease, and acquired immunodeficiency syndrome (AIDS).

SETTINGS

Aromatherapy is used in many settings throughout Europe and the United Kingdom. These settings include clinics run by private aromatherapists, clinics attached to general medical practices, and orthodox health care settings used by aromatherapists or other health care professionals who have been trained in aromatherapy. With regard to the practice of aromatherapy, individual member countries of the European Union each have their own regulations.

Under English Common Law a person is innocent until proven guilty. Because there is no law currently stating a minimum level of training and practice in aromatherapy in the United Kingdom, practitioners can perform without attaining a minimum standard of competence. The British Department of Employment has granted funding for a working party to define national occupational standards for aromatherapy, reflexology, homeopathy, and hypnotherapy. A core curriculum for these complementary therapies also is being proposed. Meanwhile, aromatherapists are working toward statutory registration in line with what has existed for osteopaths since 1993.

There is a growing move to regulate complementary and alternative (or integrative) medicine worldwide to safeguard the public and to ensure high standards of clinical practice. For example, in the United Kingdom a report published by a select committee in the House of Lords (2000) outlined the requirements for the field in terms of education, practice, research and regulation. A new committee, the Aromatherapy Consortium, with members representing the various aromatherapy organizations, is promoting the case for statutory regulation of aromatherapy in the United Kingdom.

In other European countries, legislation on the practice of complementary and integrative therapies, including aromatherapy, is different because European law differs from English law. Under the Napoleonic Law developed from the Treaty of Rome, a person is guilty until proven innocent. The practice of complementary therapies in Switzerland, Germany, and France is illegal unless a person is medically qualified, although nonmedical practitioners are tolerated to a certain extent. No therapist in Europe can advertise treatment of any kind or make medical claims except helping stress. *Treatment* is taken to mean a treatment of any physical or mental disorder by medical or physical means. Because of the legal difficulties of calling oneself a therapist in either Switzerland or Germany, practitioners of aromatherapy have coined the term *aromatology* and call themselves *aromatologists* (Ashby, 1993).

Aromatherapists who work in practices with general medical practitioners generally do so on a session-by-session basis. The physician often maintains clinical responsibility for the patient referred to the aromatherapist. Aromatherapy in orthodox health care settings is being provided by lay aromatherapists and increasingly by trained nurses or other health care professionals such as physiotherapists with aromatherapy training. According to the United Kingdom Central Council (UKCC) *Code of Professional Practice* (1992), each nurse is accountable for his or her own actions, including standards of training to ensure competence in practice. The use of aromatherapy

within nursing practice falls into this category. Professional bodies such as the Royal College of Nursing (RCN) will provide insurance for nurses using aromatherapy within their nursing practice. Chartered physiotherapists in the country need to obtain separate insurance for the use of aromatherapy.

Growth in the use of and interest in aromatherapy has developed so rapidly in recent years that professional legislation has struggled to keep up. Aromatherapy and massage are being taught to professional audiences in Southeast Asia, Australia, and North America, while being reintroduced as a modern concept with cutaneous application for the use of health care professionals other than doctors in some European countries.

Box 12-1 lists settings in the United Kingdom where aromatherapy has been adopted, and Box 12-2 provides some of the diverse reasons for the use of aromatherapy in these settings. These listings are not conclusive, and research performed to support

BOX 12-1

Conventional Medical Settings Where Aromatherapy Is Used in the United Kingdom

Intensive care units	Palliative care settings
Coronary care units	Hospices
Renal units	Pediatric units
Neurological units	Midwifery units
HIV/AIDS units	Learning disability settings
Geriatric units	Burn units
Rheumatology units	Wound clinics
Cancer units	

HIV, Human immunodeficiency virus; *AIDS,* acquired immunodeficiency syndrome.

BOX 12-2

Reasons to Administer Aromatherapy in Conventional Medical Settings

Relaxation
Stress and anxiety relief
Pain and discomfort relief
Insomnia and restlessness
Infections and wound healing
Burns
Enhancing self-image
Stimulating immune function
Treatment for constipation

the use of aromatherapy in some of these settings is discussed later.

The United Kingdom is being used as a model for many other countries with regard to legislation regarding the practice of aromatherapy. In the European Union, debate in 1994 focused on the regulation of herbal medicines, including essential oils, in preparation for the single European market. Historically, English practitioners have been able to dispense herbal medicines using special rights afforded them by Henry VIII. In the 1994 debate, no undue pressure was being placed on the United Kingdom to implement the directive, and in line with a discretionary caveat allowing each European member country to amend a directive, Germany chose to exempt herbal medicines from licensing. The British House of Commons tabled a motion on October 27, 1994 (Motion 1672) to discuss this matter. The British government decided that herbal medicines should continue to be exempt from licensing requirements and should not be subject to the new regulations required by the European directive. Notice was made of the valuable contribution of herbal medicines over the centuries, and concern was raised at the large cost of providing the research data necessary to meet the licensing requirements, as well as the cost of licensing each product.

RESEARCH

As with many other complementary and integrative therapies, the research basis for aromatherapy is incomplete. Problems already have been noted regarding the attributes given to some essential oils that have their basis in herbal medicine rather than aromatherapy research. In fact, much of the research performed on the use of essential oils or their individual constituents has been performed in animal models and isolated tissue cultures. There is an increasing number of trials conducted in human subjects under clinical conditions, and this evidence is being reviewed systematically by organizations such as the Cochrane Collaboration in the United Kingdom and the National Institutes of Health (NIH) in the United States (see later discussion).

Kusmirek (1992) identifies the problem with the rapid development of aromatherapy: popular use has outstripped research. Members of the medical profession and those wanting to use aromatherapy in the conventional health care settings have found that this lack of research in essential oils precludes acceptance of aromatherapy in the clinical environment. Little is known about possible interactions with conventional medications or treatments. It is presumed, however, that because the doses of essential oils absorbed in the body generally are small and because there has been no reported incidence of difficulties, essential oils administered in physiological doses are safe given the contraindications mentioned earlier. However, further research is required. This section presents a brief review of aromatherapy research data, with particular emphasis on the action of the essential oils. A more detailed description may be found in Vickers (1996).

Antimicrobial Activity

The effect of essential oils on a wide variety of pathogens is well known. Their chemical constituents of alcohols and aldehydes, terpenes, and phenyl methyl ethers help explain this action. The antimicrobial aspects of essential oils have been the most widely investigated. Janssen and colleagues (1987) performed a useful review of the literature in this field from the 1970s to the early 1980s. They concluded that many essential oils do have antimicrobial effects, but they found this difficult to qualify because of the variation in test methods and the insufficient description of essential oils and microorganisms in some studies. From the different chemotypes or chemical subgroups of *Thymus vulgaris* (common thyme), the strongest antifungal chemotype had eight times the effect of the weakest.

Another investigation reported antibacterial activity of a number of oils, including *Artemisia dracunculus* (tarragon), *Salvia officinalis* L (sage), *Salvia sclarea* (clary sage), and *Thymus vulgaris* L (thyme) (Zani, 1991). Other studies support the antimicrobial actions of essential oils (Baylier, 1979; Panizzi et al., 1993). Evidence also indicates that the constituents of essential oils have antimicrobial properties. The alcohols geraniol, eugenol, menthol, and citral all showed high antibacterial activity in one investigation (Moleyar and Narasimham, 1992).

Animal Models

Buchbauer and colleagues (1991) performed perhaps the most extensive research on essential oils in animal models. After 1 hour of inhaling an essential oil or fragrance compound, mice became sedated by sandalwood, rose, neroli, and lavender. Some of the constituent compounds found to have a sedative effect on inhalation were anethole, bornyl salicylate, coumarin, 2-phenylethyl acetate, benaldehyde, citronella, and geranyl acetate. Compounds that resulted in stimulation after inhalation include geraniol, isoborneol, isoeugenol, nerol, methylsalicylate, α-pinene, and thymol. Lavender oil was found to be a more effective sedative than either of its major constituents (linalool and linalyl acetate) in isolation (Buchbauer, 1991). Again, this supports aromatherapists' claims of synergy within essential oils (Price, 1995; Tisserand, 1988).

Tissue Cultures

Peppermint, commonly known for its benefit in digestive disorders, has been found to inhibit gastrointestinal smooth muscle in tissue models (Taylor et al., 1983) and affects the flow of calcium across the cell wall of the gastrointestinal smooth muscle (Taylor et al., 1984). Large doses of peppermint might have been found to induce spasm. This idea would support findings that large doses in essential oils may produce opposite effects.

Pharmacological Preparations in Animals

The effects of essential oils with pharmacological preparations in animals have been studied. As mentioned earlier, both medical professionals and aromatherapists have expressed concern about the lack of information on interactions between aromatherapy oils and conventional drug preparations in humans. In 1969, Jorich investigated the effects of essential oils on drug metabolism using pentobarbital, a sedative, to induce sleep in rats; 1,8-cineole, an oxide, was found to interfere significantly with pentobarbital. Both the sleeping times and the brain levels of the drug were reduced by about 50% after subcutaneous injection and aerosol inhalation. These effects were persistent even when the 1,8-cineole was administered 36 hours before the pentobarbital. Similar results were reported elsewhere (Wade et al., 1986).

Psychological Effects

In Torri and colleagues' 1988 study, inhalation of various essential oils was found to lead to a change in brain wave activity. The oils were measured for an increase (+) or decrease (−) of brain wave activity (Table 12-2). This study generally supports the claims of stimulation and relaxation made about essential oils, with particular reference to jasmine as stimulating and lavender as relaxing (Tisserand, 1988). Overstimulation from the oils was found to have a lowering effect on brain waves, which is suggested to be the same effect that oil would have in clinical use. If this is true, dosage of essential oils may need closer examination through further trials.

Analgesic Effects

Analgesic properties are attributed to some oils, although the evidence for this is scarce. One study demonstrated that lemongrass leaves produced a dose-dependent analgesia in rats. Both subplantar and oral doses of the constituent myrcene were administered with similar effect. Myrcene, a constituent of oils, including rosemary, lavender, juniper, and lemongrass to a lesser extent, was credited with the effect (Lorenzetti et al., 1991). Undiluted lavender oil is well known as a first-aid remedy for minor burns, both removing pain and promoting healing, as in Gattefossé's laboratory accident.

TABLE 12-2

Effects of Inhalation of Essential Oils on Brain Wave Activity

Oil	Effect	Oil	Effect
Basil	++	Marjoram	−
Bergamot	−	Neroli	+++
Rosewood	+/−	Patchouli	+
Camomile	−	Peppermint	+++
Clove	+++	Rose	++
Geranium	+/−	Sage	+
Jasmine	++	Sandalwood	−
Lavender	−	Valerian	+/−
Lemon	−	Ylang ylang	+++
Lemongrass	+		

+, Increase in brain wave activity; −, decrease in brain wave activity

Clinical Research

Earlier aromatherapy research in conventional health care settings had been undertaken in the United Kingdom by nurses with a particular interest in the field. This is now changing, with increased amounts of clinical research being carried out in different settings in the United States and other countries, including Australia. Areas where early clinical research is being done in the United States (Buckle, 2003) includes the use of peppermint oil instead of ondansetron (Zofran) for children with nausea, frankincense (*Boswellia carterii*) to help with sedation in dying patients, and a reduction in the need for morphine.

In the United Kingdom the evaluation of aromatherapy research has reached a point where there have been three recent scientific Cochrane Reviews, with two in aromatherapy. One examined pain relief in cancer and palliative care (Fellowes et al., 2004), the second examined the effectiveness of aromatherapy for dementia (Thorgrimsen et al., 2004), and the third review examined complementary and alternative therapies for pain management for women in labor, including aromatherapy (Smith et al., 2004). Overall conclusions from all three reviews suggest some therapeutic effects but highlight the need for larger and more rigorously controlled trials in this field.

Osborn and colleagues (2001) performed a survey of aromatherapists to ascertain their treatment of patients with rheumatic disease symptoms and found that aromatherapists frequently prescribed both English and German chamomile (*Anthemis nobilis* and *Matricaria chamomilla*, respectively) to help with pain and inflamed joints.

In addition, considerable work has been performed in Australia examining the wound-healing effects of essential oils in a pilot study performed by Guba (1999) involving the use of six essential oils and aromatic extracts and vegetable oils. The essential oils included were true lavender (*Lavandula angusifolia*), mugwort (*Artemesia vulgaris*), sage (*Salvia officinalis*), and everlasting flower (*Helichrysum italicum* ssp. *serotinum*).

In the United Kingdom, earlier studies have been performed in the intensive care setting, with others performed in the field of midwifery, palliative care, and care of elderly persons. Some of these trials found psychological benefits to the patients from aromatherapy in conjunction with massage. In a ran-

domized controlled trial, 100 cardiac surgery patients in intensive care received the aromatherapy oil of neroli (*Citrus aurantium* ssp. *amara*) in foot massage, and after 4 days, anxiety in particular was reduced more than in patients who were massaged with a plain vegetable oil (Stevensen, 1994). Both groups who had the massage with or without the neroli oil scored significantly better statistically on a modified Spielberger state anxiety questionnaire than did the control groups on the day of massage. The only significant physiological difference between the massage and nonmassage groups was transient and related to respiratory rate immediately after the massage.

Buckle (1993) massaged postcardiotomy patients with two different lavender essential oils, *Lavandula angustifolia* and *Lavandula latifolia*, hoping to show a difference between the effects of the two oils. Although the presentation of the trial lacked detail and the results were insignificant, there was some difference between the two oils, somewhat supporting the conclusion that massage with essential oils proved more beneficial than massage without essential oils. In an unpublished study, Dunn (1992) used intensive care as a setting in a randomized trial to measure the effects of massage with lavender oil compared with plain oil massage and rest in 122 patients. Physiological changes were not significant, but positive psychological changes were better for those massaged with essential oil than for those receiving the plain oil massage and those given the period of rest.

Anecdotal reports from mothers that lavender oil helped relieve perineal discomfort after childbirth were followed with a randomized trial involving 635 women. Each woman was given a bottle of pure lavender oil, a synthetic lavender oil that smelled like the other, or an inert compound, with instructions to add 6 drops to their bath daily. Results were not significant, but pain was slightly reduced in the pure lavender group. That group also had the highest rates of infection (Dale and Cornwall, 1994). This study may demonstrate that anecdotal reports from patients about essential oils are not reliable.

In a study of 51 patients attending a center for palliative care, the effects of three aromatherapy massages given weekly were examined with or without the essential oil of Roman chamomile, *Chamemalum nobile*. Using the Rotterdam Symptom Checklist (RSCL) and State-Trait Anxiety Inventory, posttest scores for all patients improved. These were statistically significant in the aromatherapy group on the RSCL physical symptom subscale, quality-of-life subscale, and state anxiety scale (Wilkinson, 1995). In a small study of four patients on a long-stay elderly care ward, researchers assessed sleep over three consecutive 2-week periods—the first period with night sedation, the second without, and the third with lavender diffused into the air at set intervals. Sleep was poorer in the second week, and in the third week sleep was as good as in the first week (Hardy, 1992). However, this trial was assessed only by observation.

Aromatherapy in clinical research is just beginning in earnest. There are methodological problems with much of the clinical research presented that make results difficult to assess. In the absence of further clinical trials, there also is the problem that aromatherapists are relying on many trials from animal and tissue models for the basis of their practice. There is no guarantee that these results can be replicated in humans. It is likely that, as more and better-quality research is performed in the clinical use of aromatherapy, its appropriate place in the field of complementary and integrative medicine (CIM) will become established. Perhaps because of this history, Europe (including the United Kingdom) is well advanced in aromatherapy. This situation provides another example of the advancement of Europe over the United States in the application and integration of alternative therapies.

CONCLUSION

Compared with other areas of complementary medicine, development of aromatherapy has been relatively recent. Although aromatic substances and oils have been used throughout history, a sound and agreed-on system has yet to be developed for their use, a fact especially evident when comparing aromatherapy to a system such as Chinese medicine. Recent interest in essential oils by both aromatherapists and health care professionals should encourage more rigorous clinical research into the science of aromatherapy so that understanding may be gained as to the importance and worth of this natural therapy. Until a substantive scientific base is ascertained, it is believed that aromatherapy will not take a full place beside the more established complementary and integrative health care systems.

References

Arcier M: *Aromatherapy,* London, 1990, Hamlyn.

Ashby N: Aromatherapy in the balance: aromatherapy in the UK and Europe—an overview by law, *Aromather Q* 37:13-14, 1993.

Bauer WC, Dracup KA: Physiologic effects of back massage in patients with acute myocardial infarction, *Focus Crit Care* 14(6):42-46, 1987.

Baylier MF: Bacteriostatic activity of some Australian essential oils, *Perfumer Flavourist* 4(23):23-25, 1979.

Boyd EM, Pearson GL: The expectorant action of volatile oils, *Am J Med Sci* 211:602-611, 1946.

Bronough RL: In vivo percutaneous absorption of fragrance ingredients in rhesus monkeys and humans, *Food Chem Toxicol* 28(5):369-374, 1990.

Buchbauer G et al: Aromatherapy: evidence for sedative effects of the essential oil of lavender after inhalation, *Z Naturforsch* 46:1067-1072, 1991.

Buckle J: Aromatherapy: does it matter which lavender oil is used? *Nurs Times* 89(20):32-35, 1993.

Buckle J: Aromatherapy in the USA, *Int. J Aromather* 13(1):42-46, 2003.

Chambers dictionary, Cambridge, 1988, R&W Chambers, Cambridge University Press.

Collins AJ, Notarianni LJ, Ring EF, Seed MP: Some observations on the pharmacology of "deep-heat," a topical rubefacient, *Ann Rheum Dis* 43(3):411-415, 1984.

Dale A, Cornwall S: The role of lavender oil in relieving perineal discomfort following childbirth: a blind randomized clinical trial, *J Adv Nurs* 19:89-96, 1994.

Dodd GH: The molecular dimension in perfumery. In van Toller S, Dodd GH, editors: *Perfumery: the psychology and biology of fragrance,* London, 1991, Chapman & Hall.

Dunn C: A report on a randomized controlled trial to evaluate the use of massage and aromatherapy in an intensive care unit, Reading, UK, 1992, Battle Hospital (Unpublished paper).

Falk A: Uptake, distribution and elimination of alpha-pinene in man after exposure by inhalation, *Scand J Work Environ Health* 16:372-378, 1990.

Falk-Filipsson A: d-Limonene exposure to humans by inhalation: uptake distribution, elimination and effects on the pulmonary system, *Toxicol Environ Health* 38:77-88, 1993.

Fellowes D, Barnes K, Wilkinson S: Aromatherapy and massage for symptom relief in patients with cancer, *Cochrane Library* 3, Chichester, UK, 2004, John Wiley & Sons (Cochrane Review).

Franchomme P, Pénoël D: *L'aromatherapie exactement,* Limoges, 1990, Roger Jallois.

Freud S: *The complete psychological works.* Vol 21. Civilization and its discontents (Strachy J, editor), London, 1929, Hogath Press.

Guba R: Wound healing: a pilot study using an essential oil-based cream to heal dermal wounds and ulcers, *Int J Aromather* 9(2):67-74, 1999.

Hardy M: Sweet scented dreams, *Int J Aromather,* 1992.

Hotchkiss S: How thin is your skin? *New Scientist* 141(1910): 24-27, 1994.

House of Commons: Notices of motions 1672, No 150 27, October 1994.

House of Lords Select Committee on Science and Technology: Complementary and alternative medicine, Paper 123, London, 2000, HSMO.

Jäger W, Buchbauerg, Jirovetz L, Fritzer M: Percutaneous absorption of lavender oil from a massage oil, *J Soc Cosmetic Chem* 43:49-54, 1992.

Janssen AM et al: Antimicrobial activity of essential oils: 1976-1986 literature review, *Planta Med* 53(5): 395-398, 1987.

Kaufman MA: Autonomic responses as related to nursing comfort measures, *Nurs Res* 13:45-55, 1964.

Kovar KA, Gropper B, Friess D, Ammon HP: Blood levels of 1,8-cineole and locomotor activity of mice after inhalation and oral administration of rosemary oil, *Planta Med* 53(4):315-318, 1987.

Kusmirek J: Perspectives in aromatherapy. In van Toller S, Dodd GH, editors: *Fragrance: the psychology and biology of perfume,* Barking, UK, 1992, Elsevier.

Longworth JCD Psychophysiological effects of slow stroke back massage in normatensive females, *Adv Nurs Sci,* July 1982, pp 44-61.

Lorenzetti BE, Souza GE, Sarti SJ, et al: Myrcene mimics the peripheral analgesic activity of lemongrass tea, *J Ethnopharmacol* 34(1):43-48, 1991.

Madison AS: Psychophysiological response of female nursing home residents to back massage: an investigation of one type of touch, 1973, University of Maryland (Doctoral thesis).

Maury M: *The secret of life and youth,* London, 1964, Macdonald.

Moleyar V, Narasimham P: Antibacterial activity of essential oil components, *Int J Food Microbiol* 16(4):337-342, 1992.

Osborn CE, Barlas P, Baxter GD, Barlow JH: Aromatherapy: a survey of current practice in the management of rheumatic disease symptoms, *Comp Ther Med* 9(2):62-67, 2001.

Panizzi L, Flamini G, Cioni FL, Morelli I: Composition and antimicrobial properties of essential oils of four Mediterranean Lamiaceae, *J Ethnopharmacol* 39(3): 167-170, 1993.

Price S: *Aromatherapy for health care professionals,* Edinburgh, 1995, Churchill Livingstone.

Reed BV, Held JM: Effects of sequential tissue massage on autonomic nervous system of middle aged and elderly adults, *Phys Ther* 68(8):1231-1234, 1988.

Shepherd GM: Neurobiology, Oxford, 1983, Oxford University Press.

Smith CA, Collins CT, Cyna AM, Crowther CA: Complementary and alternative therapies for pain management in labour, *Cochrane Library* 3, Chichester, UK, 2004, John Wiley & Sons (Cochrane Review).

Steele JJ: The anthropology of smell and scent in ancient Egypt and South American shamanism. In van Toller S, Dodd GH, editors: *Fragrance: the psychology and biology of perfume,* Barking, UK, 1992, Elsevier.

Stevensen CJ: The psychophysiological effects of aromatherapy massage following cardiac surgery, *Complement Ther Med* 2:27-35, 1994.

Stoddart DM: Human odour culture: a zoological perspective. In van Toller S, Dodd GH, editors: *Perfumery: the psychology and biology of fragrance,* London, 1991, Chapman & Hall.

Taylor BA, Luscombe CK, Duthie HL: Inhibitory effect of peppermint oil on gastrointestinal smooth muscle, *Gut* 24:A992, 1983.

Taylor BA, Luscombe CK, Duthie HL: Inhibitory effect of peppermint and menthol on human isolated coli, *Gut* 25:A1168, 1984.

Thorgrimsen L, Spector A, Wiles A, Orrell M: Aroma therapy for dementia, *Cochrane Library* 3, Chichester, UK, 2004, John Wiley & Sons (Cochrane Review).

Tisserand R: *The art of aromatherapy,* Saffron Waldon, UK, 1988, CW Daniel.

Tisserand R: Editorial comment, *Int J Aromather* 9(2):49 1998/99.

Tisserand R, Balacs T: *Essential oil safety,* Edinburgh, 1995, Churchill Livingstone.

Torri S, Fukuda H, Kanemoto H, et al: Contingent negative variation (CNV) and the psychological effects of odour. In van Toller S, Dodd GH, editors: *Perfumery: the psychology and biology of fragrance,* London, 1988, Chapman & Hall, pp 107-121.

United Kingdom Central Council: *Code of professional practice,* London, 1992, UK Central Council of Nursing, Midwifery and Health Visiting.

Valnet J: *The practice of aromatherapy,* Saffron Waldon, UK, 1990, CW Daniel.

Vickers AJ: *Massage and aromatherapy: a guide for health care professionals,* London, 1996, Chapman & Hall.

Wade AE et al: Alteration of drug metabolism in rats and mice by an environment of cedarwood, *Pharmacology* 1:317-328, 1986.

Wilkinson S: Aromatherapy and massage in palliative care. *Int J Palliative Nurs* 1(1):21-30, 1995.

Williams D: Lecture notes on essential oils, 1989, Eve Taylor.

Zani F, Benvenuti S, Bianchi A, Albsini A, Melegari M, Vampa G, Belloti A, Mazza P: Studies on genotoxic properties of essential oils with *Bacillus subtilis* rec-assay and Salmonella/microsome reversion assay. *Planta Med* 57:237-241, 1991.

Suggested Readings

Consumers' Association: Survey: alternative medicine. Which? London, 1992, pp 44-49.

Davis P: *Aromatherapy: A-Z,* Saffron Waldon, UK, 1990, CW Daniel.

Dodd GH, van Toller S: The biology and psychology of perfumery, *Perfumer Flavorist* 8:1-14, 1983.

Van Toller S, Dodd GH, editors: *Fragrance: the psychology and biology of perfume,* Barking, UK, 1992, Elsevier.

13

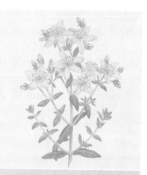

NATUROPATHIC MEDICINE

JOSEPH E. PIZZORNO, JR.
PAMELA SNIDER

The doctor of the future will give no medicine, but will interest his patient in the care of the human frame, in diet and in the cause and prevention of disease.

—THOMAS EDISON

Thomas Edison's insightful prediction is proving true today, as natural medicine finds itself in the midst of an unprecedented explosion into mainstream health care. Consumers are spending more annually out of pocket for alternative medicine than for conventional care. In particular, as a model for integrative primary care natural medicine is undergoing a powerful resurgence. With its unique integration of vitalistic, scientific, academic, and clinical training in medicine, the naturopathic medical model is a potent contributing factor to this health care revolution.

HISTORY*

Although naturopathic medicine traces its philosophical roots to many traditional world medicines, its body of knowledge derives from a rich heritage of writings and practices of Western and non-Western nature doctors since Hippocrates (circa 400 BC). Modern naturopathic medicine grew out of healing systems of the eighteenth and nineteenth centuries. The term *naturopathy* was coined in 1895 by Dr. John

*The authors express their appreciation to George Cody, whose chapter "History of Naturopathic Medicine," in *A Textbook of Natural Medicine* (JE Pizzorno and MT Murray, editors, Seattle, 1995, John Bastyr College Publications), provided the basis for much of this section.

Scheel of New York City to describe his method of health care. However, earlier forerunners of these concepts already existed in the history of natural healing, both in America and in the Austro-Germanic European core. Naturopathy became a formal profession after its creation by Benedict Lust in 1896. The profession has now celebrated its 109th birthday.

Over the centuries, natural medicine and conventional medicine have alternately diverged and converged, shaping each other, often in reaction. During the past hundred years the naturopathic profession progressed through several fairly distinct phases, as follows:

1. Latter part of the nineteenth century: *The Founding by Benedict Lust;* origin in the Germanic hydrotherapy and nature cure traditions.
2. 1900 to 1917: *The Formative Years;* convergence of the American dietetic, hygienic, physical culture, spinal manipulation, mental and emotional healing, Thomsonian/eclectic, and homeopathic systems.
3. 1918 to 1937: *The Halcyon Days;* during a period of great public interest and support, the philosophical basis and scope of therapies diversified to encompass botanical, homeopathic, and environmental medicine.
4. 1938 to 1970: *Suppression and Decline;* growing political and social dominance of the American Medical Association (AMA), lack of internal political unity, and lack of unifying standards, combined with the American love affair with technology and the emergence of "miracle" drugs and effective modern surgical techniques perfected in two world wars, resulted in legal and economic suppression.
5. 1971 to present: *Naturopathic Medicine Reemerges;* reawakened awareness by the American public of the importance of health promotion; prevention of disease; and concern for the environment and the establishment of modern, accredited, physician-level training reestablished public interest in naturopathic medicine, resulting in rapid resurgence. Current projections predict a continuing increase in the number of licensed naturopathic physicians.

> The per capita supply of alternative medicine clinicians (chiropractors, naturopaths and practitioners of Oriental medicine) will grow by 88% between 1994 and 2010, while allopathic physician supply will grow by 16%. . . . The total number of naturopathy graduates will double over the next five years. The total number of naturopathic physicians will triple (Cooper and Stoflet, 1996).

The Founding of Naturopathy

Naturopathy, as a generally used term, began with the teachings and concepts of Benedict Lust. In 1892, at age 23, Lust came from Germany as a disciple of Father Kneipp (the greatest practitioner of hydrotherapy) to bring Kneipp's hydrotherapy practices to America. Exposure in the United States to a wide range of practitioners and practices of natural healing arts broadened Lust's perspective, and after a decade of study, he purchased the term *naturopathy* from Scheel of New York City (who coined the term in 1895) in 1902 to describe the eclectic compilation of doctrines of natural healing that he envisioned was to be the future of natural medicine. Naturopathy, or "nature cure," was defined by Lust as both a way of life and a concept of healing that used various natural means (selected from various systems and disciplines) of treating human infirmities and disease states. The earliest therapies associated with the term involved a combination of American hygienics and Austro-Germanic nature cure and hydrotherapy.

In January 1902, Lust, who had been publishing the *Kneipp Water Cure Monthly* and its German language counterpart in New York since 1896, changed the name of the journal to *The Naturopathic and Herald of Health* and began promoting a new way of thinking of health care with the following editorial:

> We believe in strong, pure, beautiful bodies . . . of radiating health. We want every man, woman and child in this great land to know and embody and feel the truths of right living that mean conscious mastery. We plead for the renouncing of poisons from the coffee, white flour, glucose, lard, and like venom of the American table to patent medicines, tobacco, liquor and the other inevitable recourse of perverted appetite. We long for the time when an eight-hour day may enable every worker to stop existing long enough to live; when the spirit of universal brotherhood shall animate business and society and the church; when every American may have a little cottage of his own, and a bit of ground where he may combine Aerotherapy, Heliotherapy, Geotherapy, Aristophagy and nature's other forces with home and peace and happiness and things

forbidden to flat-dwellers; when people may stop doing and thinking and being for others and be for themselves; when true love and divine marriage and pre-natal culture and controlled parenthood may fill this world with germ-gods instead of humanized animals.

In a word, Naturopathy stands for the reconciling, harmonizing and unifying of nature, humanity and God.

Fundamentally therapeutic because men need healing; elementary educational because men need teaching; ultimately inspirational because men need empowering.

Benedict Lust

According to his published personal history, Lust had a debilitating condition in his late teens while growing up in Michelbach, Baden, Germany, and had been sent by his father to undergo the Kneipp cure at Woerishofen. He stayed there from mid-1890 to early 1892. Not only was he "cured" of his condition, but he became a protégé of Father Kneipp. He immigrated to America to proselytize the principles of the Kneipp Water-Cure (Figure 13-1).

By making contact in New York with other German Americans who were also becoming aware of the Kneipp principles, Lust participated in the founding of the first "Kneipp Society," which was organized in Jersey City, New Jersey, in 1896. Subsequently, through Lust's organization and contacts, Kneipp Societies were also founded in Brooklyn, Boston, Chicago, Cleveland, Denver, Cincinnati, Philadelphia,

Columbus, Buffalo, Rochester, New Haven, San Francisco, the state of New Mexico, and Mineola on Long Island. The members of these organizations were provided with copies of the *Kneipp Blatter* and a companion English publication Lust began to put out called *The Kneipp Water-Cure Monthly*. In 1895 Lust opened the Kneipp Water-Cure Institute on 59th Street in New York City.

Father Kneipp died in Germany, at Woerishofen, on June 17, 1897. With his passing, Lust was no longer bound strictly to the principles of the Kneipp water cure. He had begun to associate earlier with other German American physicians, principally Dr. Hugo R. Wendel (a German-trained "Naturarzt") who began, in 1897, to practice in New York and New Jersey as a licensed osteopathic physician. In 1896, Lust entered the Universal Osteopathic College of New York and became licensed as an osteopathic physician in 1898.

Once he was licensed to practice as a health care physician in his own right, Lust began the transition toward the concept of "naturopathy." Between 1898 and 1902, when he adopted the term *naturopath*, Lust acquired a chiropractic education; changed the name of his Kneipp Store (which he had opened in 1895) to "Health Food Store" (the first facility to use that name and concept in the United States), specializing in providing organically grown foods and the materials necessary for drugless cures; and founded the New York School of Massage (in 1896) and the American School of Chiropractic.

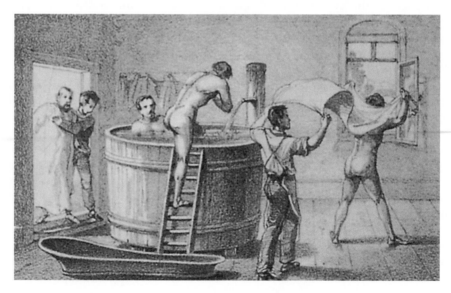

Figure 13-1 Curative baths, one form of hydrotherapy, were a popular form of natural healing in the late nineteenth century. (Courtesy Wellcome Institute Library, London.)

In 1902, when he purchased and began using the term *naturopathy* and calling himself a "naturopath," Lust, in addition to his New York School of Massage and American School of Chiropractic, his various publications, and his operation of the Health Food Store, began to operate the American School of Naturopathy, all at the same 59th Street address. By 1907, Lust's enterprises had grown sufficiently large that he moved them to a 55-room building. It housed the Naturopathic Institute, Clinic, and Hospital; the American Schools of Naturopathy and Chiropractic; the now entitled "Original Health Food Store"; Lust's publishing enterprises; and New York School of Massage. The operation remained in this four-story building, roughly twice the size of the original facility, from 1907 to 1915.

From 1912 through 1914, Lust took a sabbatical from his operations to further his education. By this time he had founded his large estatelike sanitarium at Butler, New Jersey, known as "Yungborn" after the German sanitarium operation of Adoph Just. In 1912 he attended the Homeopathic Medical College in New York, which, in 1913, granted him a degree in homeopathic medicine and, in 1914, a degree in eclectic medicine. In early 1914, Lust traveled to Florida and obtained an MD's license on the basis of his graduation from the Homeopathic Medical College.

From 1902, when he began to use the term *naturopathy,* until 1918, Lust replaced the Kneipp Societies with the Naturopathic Society of America. Then in December 1919, the Naturopathic Society of America was formally dissolved because of insolvency, and Lust founded the "American Naturopathic Association." Thereafter, the association was incorporated in some additional 18 states. Lust claimed to at one time have 40,000 practitioners practicing naturopathy. In 1918, as part of his effort to replace the Naturopathic Society of America (an operation into which he invested a great deal of his funds and resources in an attempt to organize a Naturopathic profession) and replace it with the American Naturopathic Association, Lust published the first *Yearbook of Drugless Therapy.* Annual supplements were published in either *The Naturopath and the Herald of Health* or its companion publication with which *The Naturopath* at one time merged, *Nature's Path* (which began publication in 1925). *The Naturopath and Herald of Health,* sometimes printed with the two phrases reversed, was published from 1902 through 1927, and from 1934 until after Lust's death in 1945.

Benedict Lust's principles of health are found in the introduction to the first volume of the *Universal Naturopathic Directory and Buyer's Guide,* a portion of which is reproduced in Box 13-1. Although the terminology is almost a century old, the concepts Lust proposed have provided a powerful foundation that has endured despite almost a century of active political suppression by the dominant school of medicine.

The Schools of Thought that Formed the Philosophical Basis of Naturopathy

Because of its eclectic nature, the history of naturopathic medicine is among the most complex of any healing art, which explains the unusually large portion of this chapter devoted to this subject. Although the following discussion is divided into distinct schools of thought, this is somewhat artificial because those that founded and practiced these arts (especially the Americans) were often trained in, influenced by, and practiced several therapeutic systems or modalities. However, it was not until Benedict Lust that the many threads were woven together into a unified professional practice, making naturopathic medicine the first Western system of full-scope *integrative* natural medicine based on the *vis medicatrix naturae.* The following presents the formative schools of Western thought in natural healing and some of their leading adherents. Although the therapies differ, the philosophical thread of promoting health and supporting the body's own healing processes runs through them all. These threads are derived from centuries of medical scholarship, both Western and non-Western, concerning the self-healing process.

After a brief overview of Hippocrates' seminal contribution to the natural medicine way of thought, the basic themes are presented in order: healthful living; natural diet; detoxification; exercise, mechanotherapy, and physical therapy; mental, emotional, and spiritual healing; and natural therapeutic agents. Hippocrates and centuries of nature doctors' writings remain empirically rich repositories of observations for future research.

Hippocrates

Ancient peoples believed that disease was caused by magic or supernatural forces, such as devils or angry

BOX 13-1

Principles, Aims, and Program of the Nature Cure System Circa 1918

Since the earliest ages, medical science has been of all sciences the most unscientific. Its professors, with few exceptions, have sought to cure disease by the magic of pills and potions and poisons that attacked the ailment with the idea of suppressing the symptoms instead of attacking the real cause of the ailment.

Medical science has always believed in the superstition that the use of chemical substances that are harmful and destructive to human life will prove an efficient substitute for the violation of laws, and in this way encourages the belief that a man may go the limit in self-indulgences that weaken and destroy his physical system, and then hope to be absolved from his physical ailments by swallowing a few pills, or submitting to an injection of a serum or vaccine, that are supposed to act as vicarious redeemers of the physical organism and counteract life-long practices that are poisonous and wholly destructive to the patient's well-being.

The policy of expediency is at the basis of medical drug healing. It is along the lines of self-indulgence, indifference, ignorance and lack of self-control that drug medicine lives, moves and has its being.

The natural system for curing disease is based on a return to nature in regulating the diet, breathing, exercising, bathing and the employment of various forces to eliminate the poisonous products in the system, and so raise the vitality of the patient to a proper standard of health.

Official medicine has, in all ages, simply attacked the symptoms of disease without paying any attention to the causes thereof, but natural healing is concerned far more with removing the causes of disease, than merely curing its symptoms. This is the glory of this new school of medicine that it cures by removing the causes of the ailment, and is the only rational method of practicing medicine. It begins its cures by avoiding the uses of drugs and hence is styled the system of drugless healing.

The Program of Naturopathic Cure

1. ELIMINATION OF EVIL HABITS, or the weeds of life, such as over-eating, alcoholic drinks, drugs, the use of tea, coffee and cocoa that contain poisons, meat eating, improper hours of living, waste of vital forces, lowered vitality, sexual and social aberrations, worry, etc.
2. CORRECTIVE HABITS. Correct breathing, correct exercise, right mental attitude. Moderation in the pursuit of health and wealth.
3. NEW PRINCIPLES OF LIVING. Proper fasting, selection of food, hydropathy, light and air baths, mud baths, osteopathy, chiropractic and other forms of mechano-therapy, mineral salts obtained in organic form, electropathy, heliopathy, steam or Turkish baths, sitz baths, etc.

Natural healing is the most desirable factor in the regeneration of the race. It is a return to nature in methods of living and treatment. It makes use of the elementary forces of nature, of chemical selection of foods that will constitute a correct medical dietary. The diet of civilized man is devitalized, is poor in essential organic salts. The fact that foods are cooked in so many ways and are salted, spiced, sweetened and otherwise made attractive to the palate, induces people to over-eat, and over eating does more harm than underfeeding. High protein food and lazy habits are the cause of cancer, Bright's disease, rheumatism and the poisons of autointoxication.

There is really but one healing force in existence and that is Nature herself, which means the inherent restorative power of the organism to overcome disease. Now the question is, can this power be appropriated and guided more readily by extrinsic or intrinsic methods? That is to say, is it more amenable to combat disease by irritating drugs, vaccines and serums employed by superstitious moderns, or by the bland intrinsic congenial forces of Natural Therapeutics, that are employed by this new school of medicine, that is Naturopathy, which is the only orthodox school of medicine? Are not these natural forces much more orthodox than the artificial resources of the druggist?

From Lust B: Principles of health. Vol 1, *Universal naturopathic directory and buyer's guide,* Butler, NJ, 1918, Lust Publications.

gods. Hippocrates, breaking with this superstitious belief, became the first naturalistic doctor in western history. Hippocrates regarded the body as a "whole" and instructed his students to prescribe only beneficial treatments and refrain from causing harm or hurt.

Hippocratic practitioners assumed that everything in nature had a rational basis; therefore the physician's role was to understand and follow the laws of the intelligible universe. They viewed disease as an effect and looked for its cause in natural phenomena: air, water, food, and so forth. They first used the term *vis medicatrix naturae,* the "healing power of nature," to denote the body's ability and drive to heal itself. One of the central tenets is that "there is an order to the process of healing which requires certain things to be done before other things to maximize the effectiveness of the therapeutics" (Zeff, 1997). The step order used by Tibetan medicine is also an example of this tenet represented in traditional world medicines.

Hydrotherapy

The earliest philosophical origins of naturopathy were clearly in the Germanic hydrotherapy movement: the use of hot and cold water for the maintenance of health and the treatment of disease. One of the oldest known therapies (water was used therapeutically by the Romans and Greeks), the modern history of hydrotherapy began with the publication of *The History of Cold Bathing* in 1697 by Sir John Floyer. Probably the strongest impetus for its use came from Central Europe, where it was advocated by such well-known hydropaths as Priessnitz, Schroth, and Father Kneipp. They were able to popularize specific water treatments that quickly became the vogue in Europe during the nineteenth century. *Vincent Preissnitz* (1799-1851), of Graefenberg, Silesia, was a pioneer natural healer. Unfortunately, he was prosecuted by the medical authorities of his day and was actually convicted of using witchcraft because he cured his patients by the use of water, air, diet, and exercise. He took his patients back to nature—to the woods, the streams, the open fields—treated them with nature's own forces, and fed them on natural foods. His cured patients were numbered by the thousands, and his fame spread over Europe. *Father Sebastian Kneipp* (1821-1897) became the most famous of the hydropaths, with Pope Leo XIII and Ferdinand of Austria (whom he had walking barefoot in new-fallen snow for purposes of hardening his constitution) among his many famous patients. He standardized the practice of hydrotherapy and organized it into a system of practice that was widely emulated through the establishment of health spas or "sanitariums." The first sanitarium in this country, the Kneipp and Nature Cure Sanitarium, was opened in Newark, New Jersey, in 1891.

The best known American hydropath was J.H. Kellogg, a medical doctor who approached hydrotherapy scientifically and performed many experiments trying to understand the physiological effects of hot and cold water. In 1900 he published *Rational Hydrotherapy,* which is still considered a definitive treatise on the physiological and therapeutic effects of water, along with an extensive discussion of hydrotherapeutic techniques. Drs. O.J. Carroll, Harold Dick, and John Bastyr, among others, brought the use of hydrotherapy techniques forward into modern naturopathic practice.

Nature Cure

Natural living, a vegetarian diet, and the use of light and air formed the basis of the Nature Cure movement founded by *Dr. Arnold Rickli* (1823-1926). In 1848 he established at Veldes Krain, Austria, the first institution of light and air cure or, as it was called in Europe, the *atmospheric cure.* He was an ardent disciple of the vegetarian diet and the founder, and for more than 50 years the president, of the National Austrian Vegetarian Association. In 1891, *Louis Kuhne* (circa 1823-1907) wrote the *New Science of Healing,* which presented the basic principles of "drugless methods." *Dr. Henry Lahman* (ca 1823-1907), who founded the largest Nature Cure institution in the world at Weisser Hirsch, near Dresden, Saxony, constructed the first appliances for the administration of electric light treatment and baths. He was the author of several books on diet, nature cure, and heliotherapy. *Professor F.E. Bilz* (1823-1903) authored the first natural medicine encyclopedia, *The Natural Method of Healing,* which was translated into a dozen languages, and in German alone ran into 150 editions.

Nature Cure became popular in America through the efforts of *Henry Lindlahr,* MD, ND, of Chicago, Illinois. Originally a rising businessman in Chicago with all the bad habits of the "Gay Nineties" era, he became chronically ill while only in his 30s. After receiving no relief from the orthodox practitioners of his day, he learned of Nature Cure, which improved his health. Subsequently, he went to Germany to stay in a sanitarium to be cured and to learn Nature Cure. He went back to Chicago and earned his degrees from the Homeopathic/Eclectic College of Illinois. In 1903 he opened a sanitarium in Elmhurst, Illinois, "Lindlahr's Health Food Store," and shortly thereafter founded the Lindlahr College of Natural Therapeutics. In 1908 he began to publish *Nature Cure Magazine* and began publishing his six-volume series of *Philosophy of Natural Therapeutics.*

One of the chief advantages of training in the early 1900s was the marvelous inpatient facilities that flourished during this time. These facilities provided in-depth training in clinical nature cure and natural hygiene in inpatient settings. Nature cure and natural hygiene are still at the core of naturopathic medicine's fundamental principles and approach to health care and disease prevention.

The Hygienic System

Another forerunner of American naturopathy, the "hygienic" school, amalgamated the hydrotherapy and nature cure movements with vegetarianism. It originated as a lay movement of the nineteenth century and had its genesis in the popular teachings of *Sylvester Graham* and *William Alcott*. Graham began preaching the doctrines of temperance and hygiene in 1830, and published, in 1839, *Lectures on the Science of Human Life;* two hefty volumes that prescribed healthy dietary habits. He emphasized a moderate lifestyle, a flesh-free diet, and bran bread as an alternative to bolted or white bread. The earliest physician to have a significant impact on the hygienic movement and the later philosophical growth of naturopathy was *Russell Trall*, MD. According to Whorton in his *Crusaders for Fitness:*

> The exemplar of the physical educator-hydropath was Russell Thatcher Trall. Still another physician who had lost his faith in regular therapy, Trall opened the second water cure establishment in America, in New York City in 1844. Immediately, he combined the full Priessnitzian armamentarium of baths with regulation of diet, air, exercise and sleep. He would eventually open and or direct any number of other hydropathic institutions around the country, as well as edit the *Water-Cure Journal,* the *Hydropathic Review,* and a temperance journal. He authored several books, including popular sex manuals which perpetuated Graham-like concepts into the 1890's, sold Graham crackers and physiology texts at his New York office, was a charter member (and officer) of the American Vegetarian Society, presided over a short-lived World Health Association, and so on (Whorton, 1982).

Trall founded the first school of natural healing arts in this country to have a 4-year curriculum and the authorization to confer the degree of MD. It was founded in 1852 as a "Hydropathic and Physiological

School" and was chartered by the New York State Legislature in 1857 under the name "New York Hygio-Therapeutic College."

He eventually published more than 25 books on the subjects of physiology, hydropathy, hygiene, vegetarianism, and temperance, among many others. The most valuable and enduring of these was his 1851 *Hydropathic Encyclopedia,* a volume of nearly 1000 pages that covered the theory and practice of hydropathy and the philosophy and treatment of diseases advanced by older schools of medicine. The encyclopedia sold more than 40,000 copies.

Martin Luther Holbrook expanded on the work of Graham, Alcott, and Trall and, working with an awareness of the European concepts developed by Preissnitz and Kneipp, laid further groundwork for the concepts later advanced by Lust, Lindlahr, and others. According to Whorton, Holbrook proposed the following:

> For disease to result, the latter had to provide a suitable culture medium, had to be susceptible. As yet, most physicians were still so excited at having discovered the causative agents of infection that they were paying less than adequate notice to the host. Radical hygienists, however, were bent just as far in the other direction. They were inclined to see bacteria as merely impotent organisms that throve only in individuals whose hygienic carelessness had made their body compost heaps. Tuberculosis is contagious, Holbrook acknowledged, but "the degree of vital resistance is the real element of protection. When there is no preparation of the soil by heredity, predisposition or lowered health standard, the individual is amply guarded against the attack." A theory favored by many others was that germs were the effect of disease rather than its cause; tissues corrupted by poor hygiene offered microbes, all harmless, an environment in which they could thrive.
>
> The orthodox hygienists of the progressive years were equally enthused by the recent progress of nutrition, of course, and exploited it for their own naturopathic doctors, but their utilization of science hardly stopped with dietetics. Medical bacteriology was another area of remarkable discovery, bacteriologists having provided, in the short space of the last quarter of the nineteenth century, an understanding, at long last, of the nature of infection. This new science's implications for hygienic ideology were profound—when Holbrook locked horns with female fashion, for example, he did not attack the bulky, ground-length skirts still in style

with the crude Grahamite objection that the skirt was too heavy. Rather he forced a gasp from his readers with an account of watching a smartly dressed lady unwittingly drag her skirt "over some virulent, revolting looking sputum, which some unfortunate consumptive had expectorated."

Trall and Holbrook both advanced the idea that physicians should teach the maintenance of health rather than simply provide a last resort in times of health crisis. Besides providing a strong editorial voice denouncing the evils of tobacco and drugs, they strongly advanced the value of vegetarianism, bathing and exercise, dietetics and nutrition along with personal hygiene (Whorton, 1982).

John Harvey Kellogg, MD, another medically trained doctor who turned to more nutritionally based natural healing concepts, also greatly influenced Lust. Kellogg was renowned through his connection, beginning in 1876, with the Battle Creek Sanitarium, which was founded in the 1860s as a Seventh Day Adventist institution designed to perpetuate the Grahamite philosophies. Kellogg, born in 1852, was a "sickly child" who, at age 14, after reading the works of Graham, converted to vegetarianism. At the age of 20, he studied for a term at Trall's Hygio-Therapeutic College and then earned a medical degree at New York's Bellevue Medical School. He maintained an affiliation with the regular schools of medicine during his lifetime, owing more to his practice of surgery than his beliefs in that area of health care (Figure 13-2).

Kellogg designated his concepts, which were basically the hygienic system of healthful living, "biologic living." Kellogg expounded vegetarianism, attacked sexual misconduct and the evils of alcohol, and was a prolific writer through the late nineteenth and early twentieth centuries. He produced a popular periodical, *Good Health,* which continued in existence until 1955. When Kellogg died in 1943 at age 91, he had had more than 300,000 patients through the Battle Creek Sanitarium, including many celebrities, and the "San" became nationally known.

Kellogg was also extremely interested in hydrotherapy. In the 1890s he established a laboratory at the San to study the clinical applications of hydrotherapy. This led to his writing of *Rational Hydrotherapy* in 1902. The preface espoused a philosophy of drugless healing that came to be one of the bases of the hydrotherapy school of medical thought in early twentieth-century America.

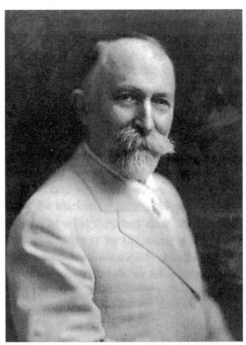

Figure 13-2 Dr. John Harvey Kellogg, brother to the Kellogg of breakfast cereal fame and a physical culture movement proponent. (Courtesy Historical Society of Battle Creek, Battle Creek, Mich.)

Influence on Public Health

It is a little known fact that most of our current and accepted public hygiene practices were brought into societal use by the early Hygienic reformers. Before their efforts, neglect of these basic physiological safety measures was rampant. The Hygienists had a great influence on decreasing morbidity and mortality and increasing life span, as well as the adoption of public sanitation. Orthodox medicine is typically credited with these advances.

Currently, certified professional Natural Hygienists are the proponents of the highest standards of training and supervised clinical fasting and participate in training naturopathic physicians. Naturopathic medicine uses the precepts of Natural Hygiene in reestablishing the basis of health, the first step in the therapeutic order.

Autotoxicity

Lust was also greatly influenced by the writings of *John H. Tilden,* MD (who published between 1915 and 1925). Tilden became disenchanted with orthodox medicine and began to rely heavily on dietetics and nutrition, formulating his theories of "autointoxication" (the effect of fecal matter remaining too long in the digestive process) and "toxemia." He provided the natural health care literature with a 200-plus-page dissertation entitled *Constipation,* with a whole chapter devoted to the evils of not responding "when nature called."

Elie Metchnikoff (director of the prestigious Pasteur Institute and winner of the 1908 Nobel Prize for a contribution to immunology) and Kellogg wrote prolifically on the theory of autointoxication. Kellogg, in particular, believed that humans, in the process of digesting meat, produced a variety of intestinal self-poisons that contributed to autointoxication. As a result, Kellogg widely proselytized that people must return to a more healthy natural state by allowing the naturally designed use of the colon. He believed that the average modern colon was devitalized by the combination of a low-fiber diet, sedentary living, the custom of sitting rather than squatting to defecate, and the modern civilized habit of ignoring "nature's call" out of an undue concern for politeness.

Although the concept of toxemia is not a part of the body of knowledge presented in conventional medical schools, all naturopathic students are presented with this concept. Some of that presentation relies on outdated materials, such as the naturopathic texts of 75 and 100 years ago (e.g., Lindlahr, Tilden). However, modern research and textbooks are beginning to investigate this phenomenon. Drasar and Hill's *Human Intestinal Flora* (1974) demonstrates some of the biochemical pathways of the generation of metabolic toxins in the gut through dysbiotic bacterial action on poorly digested food (Zeff, 1997, 1998). In the last 20 years, our understanding of the concept of toxemia has been significantly updated by practitioners in the newly emerging field of *functional medicine,* a health care approach that focuses attention on biochemical individuality, metabolic balance, ecological context, and unique personal experience in the dynamics of health. Maldigestion, malabsorption, and abnormal gut flora and ecology are often found to be primary contributing factors not only to gastrointestinal disorders but also to a wide variety of chronic, systemic illnesses. Laboratory assessment tools have been developed that are capable of evaluating the status of many organs, including the gastrointestinal tract. These cutting-edge diagnostic tools provide physicians with an analysis of numerous functional parameters of the individual's digestion and absorption and precisely pinpoint what in the colonic environment is imbalanced, thus promoting dysbiosis.

Thomsonianism

In 1822, *Samuel Thomson* published his *New Guide to Health,* a compilation of his personal view of medical theory and American Indian herbal and medical botanical lore. Thomson espoused the belief that disease had one general cause—derangement of the vital fluids from "cold" influences on the human body—and that disease therefore had one general remedy: animal warmth or "heat." The name of the complaint depended on the part of the body that was affected. Unlike the conventional American "heroic" medical tradition that advocated bloodletting, leeching, and the substantial use of mineral-based purgatives such as antimony and mercury, Thomson believed that minerals were sources of "cold" because they come from the ground and that vegetation, which grew toward the sun, represented "heat" (Figure 13-3).

Thomson's view was that individuals could self-treat if they had an adequate understanding of his philosophy *and* a copy of *New Guide to Health.* The right to sell "family franchises" for use of the Thomsonian method of healing was the basis of a profound

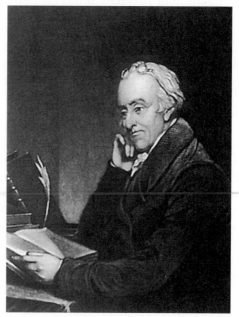

Figure 13-3 Samuel Thomson (1769-1843). (Courtesy National Library of Medicine, Bethesda, Md.)

lay movement between 1822 and Thomson's death in 1843. Thomson adamantly believed that no professional medical class should exist and that democratic medicine was best practiced by laypersons within a Thomsonian "family" unit. By 1839 Thomson claimed to have sold some 100,000 of these family franchises, called "friendly botanic societies."

Despite his criticism of the early medical movement for their "heroic" tendencies, Thomson's medical theories were "heroic" in their own fashion. Although he did not advocate bloodletting or heavy metal poisoning and leeching, botanic purgatives—particularly *Lobelia inflata* (Indian tobacco)—were a substantial part of the therapy.

Eclectic School of Medicine

Some of the doctors practicing Thomsonian, called *botanics,* decided to separate themselves from the lay movement and develop a more physiologically sound basis of therapy. They established a broader range of therapeutic applications of botanical medicines and founded a medical college in Cincinnati. These Thomsonian doctors were later absorbed into the "Eclectic School," which originated with Wooster Beach of New York.

Wooster Beach, from a well-established New England family, started his medical studies at an early age, apprenticing under an old German herbal doctor, Jacob Tidd, until Tidd died. Beach then enrolled in the Barclay Street Medical University in New York. After opening his own practice in New York, Beach set out to win over fellow members of the New York Medical Society (into which he had been warmly introduced by the screening committee) to his point of view that heroic medicine was inherently dangerous and should be reduced to the gentler theories of herbal medicine. He was summarily ostracized from the medical society. He soon founded his own school in New York, calling the clinic and educational facility "The United States Infirmary." However, because of political pressure from the medical society, he was unable to obtain charter authority to issue legitimate diplomas. He then located a financially ailing but legally chartered school, Worthington College, in Worthington, Ohio. There he opened a full-scale medical college, creating the Eclectic school of medical theory based on the European, Native American, and American traditions. The most enduring eclectic herbal textbook is *King's American Dispensary* by *Harvey Wickes Felter* and *John Uri Lloyd*. Published in 1898, this two-volume 2500-page treatise provided the definitive work describing the identification, preparation, pharmacognosy, history of use, and clinical application of more than 1000 botanical medicines. The eclectic herbal lore formed an integral core of the therapeutic armamentarium of the naturopathic doctor (ND).

Homeopathic Medicine

Homeopathy, the creation of an early German physician, *Samuel Hahnemann* (1755-1843), had four central doctrines: (1) the "law of similars" (that like cures like); (2) that the effect of a medication could be heightened by its administration in minute doses (the more diluted the dose, the greater the "dynamic" effect); (3) that nearly all diseases were the result of a suppressed itch, or "psora"; and (4) Hering's law: healing proceeds from within outward, above downward, from more vital to less vital organs, and in the reverse order of the appearance of symptoms (pathobiography).

Originally, most U.S. homeopaths were converted orthodox medical doctors, or *allopaths* (a term coined by Hahnemann). The high rate of conversion made this particular medical sect the archenemy of the rising orthodox medical profession. The first American homeopathic medical school was founded in 1848 in Philadelphia; the last purely homeopathic medical school, based in Philadelphia, survived into the early 1930s (see Chapter 8).

The Manipulative Therapies: Osteopathy and Chiropractic

In Missouri, *Andrew Taylor Still,* originally trained as an orthodox practitioner, founded the school of medical thought known as *osteopathy*. He conceived a system of healing that emphasized the primary importance of the structural integrity of the body, especially as it affects the vascular system, in the maintenance of health. In 1892 he opened the American School of Osteopathy in Kirksville, Missouri.

In 1895, Daniel David Palmer, originally a magnetic healer from Davenport, Iowa, performed the first spinal manipulation, which gave rise to the school he termed *chiropractic*. His philosophy was similar to Still's except for a greater emphasis on the importance of proper neurological function. He formally published his findings in 1910, after having founded a chiropractic school in Davenport (see Chapter 10).

Less well known is "Zone Therapy," originated by *Joe Shelby Riley,* DC, a chiropractor based in Washington, D.C. Zone therapy was an early forerunner of acupressure. It related the pressure and manipulation of the fingers and tongue and percussion on the spinal column according to the fingers' relation to certain zones of the body. (See Chapter 9).

Christian Science and Role of Belief and Spirituality

Christian Science, formulated by *Mary Baker Eddy* in 1879, comprises a profound belief in the role of systematic religious study (which led to the widespread Christian Science Reading Rooms), spirituality, and prayer in the treatment of disease. In 1875 she published *Science and Health with Key to the Scriptures,* the definitive textbook for the study of Christian Science.

Lust was also influenced by the works of *Sidney Weltmer,* the founder of "Suggestive Therapeutics." Weltmer's work dealt specifically with the psychological process of desiring to be healthy. The theory behind Professor Weltmer's work was that whether it was the mind or the body that first lost its grip on health, the two were inseparably related. When the problem originated in the body, the mind nonetheless lost its ability and desire to overcome the disease because the patient "felt sick" and consequently slid further into the diseased state. Alternatively, if the mind first lost its ability and desire to "be healthy" and some physical infirmity followed, the patient was susceptible to being overcome by disease (see Chapter 9).

Physical Culture

Bernarr McFadden, a close friend of Lust's, founded the "Physical Culture" school of health and healing, also known as *physcultopathy.* This school of healing gave birth across the United States to gymnasiums where exercise programs were designed and taught to allow the individual man and woman to establish and maintain optimal physical health.

Although many theories exist to explain the rapid dissolution of these diverse healing arts (which at one time made up more than 25% of U.S. health care practitioners) in the early part of the twentieth century, low ratings in the infamous Flexner Report (which rated all these schools of medical thought among the lowest), the self-application of the blessing "scientific" on allopathic medicine, and growing political

sophistication of the AMA clearly played the most significant role.

All these healing systems and modalities were naturally unified in the field of naturopathic medicine because they shared one common tenet: respect for and inquiry into the self-healing process and what was necessary to establish health.

The Halcyon Days of Naturopathy

In the early 1920s the "health fad" movement was reaching its peak in terms of public awareness and interest. Conventions were held throughout the United States, with one attended by several members of Congress, culminating in full legalization of naturopathy as a healing art in the District of Columbia. Not only were the conventions well attended by professionals, but the public also flocked to them, with more than 10,000 attending the 1924 convention in Los Angeles.

During the 1920s and up until 1937, naturopathy was in its most popular phase. Although the institutions of the orthodox school had gained ascendancy, before 1937 the medical profession had few real solutions to the problems of human disease.

During the 1920s, *Gaylord Hauser,* later to become the health food guru of the Hollywood set, came to Lust as a seriously ill young man. Lust, through application of the nature cure, removed Hauser's afflictions and was rewarded by Hauser's lifelong devotion. His regular columns in *Nature's Path* became widely read among the Hollywood set.

The naturopathic journals of the 1920s and 1930s provide much valuable insight into the prevention of disease and the promotion of health. Much of the dietary advice focused on correcting poor eating habits, including the lack of fiber in the diet and an overreliance on red meat as a protein source. As in the 1990s, we now hear the pronouncements of the orthodox profession, the National Institutes of Health (NIH), and the National Cancer Institute (NCI) that the early assertions of the naturopaths that such dietary habits would lead to degenerative diseases, including cancers associated with the digestive tract and the colon, were true.

The December 1928 volume of *Nature's Path* was the first American publication of the works of *Herman J. DeWolff,* a Dutch epidemiologist. DeWolff was one of the first researchers to assert, on the basis of studies of the incidence of cancer in the Netherlands, that there was a correlation between exposure to petrochemicals and various types of cancerous conditions. He saw a connection between chemical fertilizers and their use in some soils (principally clay) that led to their remaining in vegetables after they had arrived at the market and were purchased for consumption. It was almost 50 years before orthodox medicine began to see the wisdom of such assertions.

Suppression and Decline

In 1937 the popularity of naturopathy began to decline. The change came, as both Thomas and Campion note in their works, with the era of "miracle medicine." Lust recognized this and his editorializing became, if anything, even more strident. From the introduction of sulfa drugs in 1937 to the Salk vaccine's release in 1955, the American public became used to annual developments of miracle vaccines and antibiotics. The naturopathic profession adhered to its vitalistic philosophy and a full range of practice but unfortunately was poorly unified at this time on other issues of standards. This made the profession vulnerable to interguild competition.

Lust died in September of 1945 in residence at the Yungborn facility in Butler, New Jersey, preparing to attend the 49th Annual Congress of his American Naturopathic Association (ANA). Although a healthy vigorous man, he seriously damaged his lungs the previous year saving patients when a wing of his facility caught fire; he never fully recovered. On August 30, 1945, for the official program of that congress, held in October 1945 just after his death, he noted his concerns for the future. He was especially frustrated with the success of the medical profession in blocking the efforts of the naturopaths to establish state licensing laws that would not only establish appropriate practice rights for NDs but also protect the public from the pretenders (i.e., those who chose to call themselves naturopaths without ever bothering to attain formal training). As Lust stated:

> Now let us see the type of men and women who are the Naturopaths of today. Many of them are fine, upstanding individuals, believing fully in the effectiveness of their chosen profession—willing to give their all for the sake of alleviating human suffering and ready to fight for their rights to the last ditch. More power to them! But there are others who

claim to be Naturopaths who are woeful misfits. Yes, and there are outright fakers and cheats masking as Naturopaths. That is the fate of any science—any profession—which the unjust laws have placed beyond the pale. Where there is no official recognition and regulation, you will find the plotters, the thieves, the charlatans operating on the same basis as the conscientious practitioners. And these riff-raff opportunists bring the whole art into disrepute. Frankly, such conditions cannot be remedied until suitable safeguards are erected by law, or by the profession itself, around the practice of Naturopathy. That will come in time (Lust, 1945).

In the mid-1920s, *Morris Fishbein* came on the scene as editor of the *Journal of the American Medical Association* (JAMA). Fishbein took on a personal vendetta against what he characterized as "quackery." Lust, among others, including McFadden, became Fishbein's epitome of quackery. Unfortunately, he proved to be particularly effective politically and in the media.

The public infatuation with technology, the introduction of "miracle medicine," World War II's stimulation of the development of surgery, the Flexner Report, growing political sophistication of the AMA through the leadership of Fishbein, intraprofession squabbles, and the death of Lust in 1945 all combined to cause the decline of naturopathic medicine and natural healing in the United States. In addition, these years, called the *years of the great fear* in Caute's book by that name, were the years during which to be unorthodox was to be un-American.

U.S. courts began to take the view that naturopaths were not truly doctors because they espoused doctrines from "the dark ages of medicine" (something American medicine had supposedly come out of in 1937) and that drugless healers were intended by law to operate without "drugs" (which became defined as anything a physician would prescribe for a patient to ingest or apply externally for any medical purpose). The persistent lack of uniform standards, lack of insurance coverage, lost court battles, a splintered profession, and a hostile legislative perspective progressively restricted practice until the core naturopathic therapies became essentially illegal and practices financially nonviable.

Although it was under considerable public pressure in those years, the ANA undertook some of its most scholarly work, coordinating all the systems of naturopathy under commission. This resulted in the publication of a formal textbook, *Basic Naturopathy* (Spitler, 1948), and a significant work compiling all the known theories of botanical medicine, *Naturae Medicina* (Kuts-Cheraux, 1953). Naturopathic medicine began splintering when Lust's ANA was succeeded by six different organizations in the mid 1950s.

By the early 1970s, the profession's educational institutions had dwindled to one: the National College of Naturopathic Medicine, with branches in Seattle and Portland, Oregon.

Naturopathic Medicine Reemerges

The combination of the counterculture years of the late 1960s, the public's growing awareness of the importance of nutrition and the environment, and America's disenchantment with organized institutional medicine (which began after the miracle era faded, and it became apparent that orthodox medicine has its limitations and is prohibitively expensive) resulted in alternative medicine in general gaining new respect and in the rejuvenation of naturopathic medicine. At this time, a new wave of students were attracted to the philosophical precepts of the profession. They brought with them an appreciation for the appropriate use of science, modern college education, and matching expectations for quality education.

Dr. John Bastyr (1912-1995) and his firm, efficient, professional leadership inspired science and research-based training in natural medicine to begin to reach toward its full potential. Dr. Bastyr, whose vision was of "naturopathy's empirical successes documented and proven by scientific methods," was "himself a prototype for the modern naturopathic doctor, who culls the latest findings from the scientific literature, applies them in ways consistent with naturopathic principles, and verifies the results with appropriate studies." Bastyr also saw "a tremendous expansion in both allopathic and naturopathic medical knowledge, and he played a major role in making sure the best of both were integrated into naturopathic medical education" (Kirchfield and Boyle, 1994).

Responding to the growth in public interest during the late 1970s, naturopathic colleges were established in Arizona (Arizona College of Naturopathic Medicine, 1977), Oregon (American College of Naturopathic Medicine, 1980), and California (Pacific College of Naturopathic Medicine, 1979). None of these three survived. In 1978 the John Bastyr College of Naturopathic Medicine (later renamed Bastyr University) was formed in Seattle by Joseph E. Pizzorno, Jr., ND; Lester E. Griffith, ND; William Mitchell, ND; and Sheila Quinn to teach and develop science-based natural medicine. They believed that for the naturopathic profession to move back into the mainstream, it needed to establish accredited institutions, perform credible research, and establish itself as an integral part of the health care system. Bastyr University not only survived but thrived, and it became the first naturopathic college ever to become regionally accredited. In 1993, Michael Cronin, Kyle Cronin, and Konrad Kail, NDs, founded the Southwest College of Naturopathic Medicine and Health Science in Scottsdale, Arizona. In 1997 the University of Bridgeport with the leadership of Jim Sensenig, ND, founded the University of Bridgeport College of Naturopathic Medicine.

With five credible colleges (including the Canadian College of Naturopathic Medicine in Ontario), active research, an appreciation of the appropriate application of science to natural medicine education, and clinical practice, naturopathic medicine is well on the road to recovery.

A sixth promising naturopathic college, the Boucher Institute of Naturopathic Medicine, was established in January 2000 in Vancouver, British Columbia. Boucher Institute graduated its first class in May 2004.

Recent Influences

A tremendous amount of scientific support for the principles of naturopathic medicine has been conducted at mainstream research centers and increasingly at naturopathic medical schools. In fact, allopathy is turning more to the use of naturopathic methods in the search for effective prescriptions for current intractable and expensive diseases (Werbach, 1996). It is now well established that nutritional factors are of major importance in the pathogenesis of both atherosclerosis and cancer, the two leading causes of death in Western countries, and studies validating their importance in the pathogenesis of many other diseases continue to be published. Much of the research now documenting the scientific foundations of naturopathic medicine practices and principles can be found in *A Textbook of Natural Medicine* (Pizzorno and Murray, 1985-95). This two-volume, 200-chapter work contains 7500 citations to the peer-reviewed scientific literature documenting the efficacy of many natural medicine therapies.

Although the naturopaths were astute clinical observers and a century ago recognized many of the concepts that are now gaining popularity and the support of scientific data, the scientific tools of the time were inadequate to assess the validity of their concepts. In addition, as a group they seemed to have little inclination to the application of laboratory research, especially because "science" was the bludgeon used by the AMA to suppress the profession. This has now changed. In the past few decades a considerable amount of research is now providing the scientific documentation of many of the concepts of naturopathic medicine, and the new breed of scientifically trained naturopaths is using this research to continue development of the profession. The following sections describe a few of the most important trends.

Therapeutic Nutrition

Since 1929, when Eijkman and Hopkins shared the Nobel Prize in medicine and physiology for the discovery of vitamins, the role of these trace substances in clinical nutrition has been a matter of scientific investigation. The discovery that enzyme systems depended on essential nutrients provided the naturopathic profession with great insights into why an organically grown, whole-foods diet is so important for health. Nutritional biochemist Roger Williams' formulation of the concept of "biochemical individuality" in 1955 further developed these ideas and provided great insights into the unique nutritional needs of each individual and how to correct inborn errors of metabolism and even treat specific diseases through the use of nutrient-rich foods or large doses of specific nutrients. Linus Pauling, the two-time Nobel Prize winner, coined the concept of "orthomolecular medicine" and provided further theoretical substantiation for the use of nutrients as therapeutic agents.

Functional Medicine

In 1994, Jeff Bland, PhD, coined the term "functional medicine" to describe the sophisticated, science-based development of therapeutic nutrition in the prevention of illness and promotion of health.

Focusing on biochemical individuality, metabolic balance, and the ecological context, functional medicine practitioners avail themselves of recently developed laboratory tests to pinpoint even slight imbalances in an individual's biochemistry that can set into motion a cascade of biological triggers, paving the way to suboptimal function, chronic illness, and degenerative disease. A broad range of functional laboratory assessment tools in the areas of digestion (gastrointestinal), nutrition, detoxification and oxidative stress, immunology and allergy, production and regulation of hormones (endocrinology), and the heart and blood vessels (cardiovascular system) provide physicians with the information needed to recommend nutritional interventions specific to the individual's needs and to monitor their efficacy precisely.

Environmental Medicine and Clinical Ecology

Although recognition of the clinical impact of environmental toxicity and endogenous toxicity has existed since the earliest days of naturopathy, it was not until the environmental movement and the seminal work of Rachel Carson and others that the scientific basis was established. Clinical research and the development of laboratory methods for assessing toxic load have provided objective tools that have greatly increased the sophistication of clinical practice. Clinical and laboratory methods were developed for the assessment of idiosyncratic reactions to environmental factors and foods.

Spirituality, Health, and Medicine

Naturopathic medicine's philosophy of treating the whole person and enhancing the individual's inherent healing ability is closely aligned with its mission of integrating spirituality into the healing process. Scientific evidence is growing on how spirituality can play a part in healing. Since Descartes separated mind from body in the seventeenth century, medical science has attempted to explain disease independently of mind, in terms of germs, environmental agents, or wayward genes. At present, however, the evidence is not just clinical observation but chemical fact. An explosion of research in the new and rapidly expanding field of psychoneuroimmunology is revealing physical evidence of the mind-body connection that is changing our understanding of disease (see Chapter 15). Scientists no longer question whether but rather *how* our minds have an impact on our health, and the implications of the connections uncovered in only the last 20 years are extraordinary.

In his book *Healing Words,* Larry Dossey, MD, pulls together what he describes as "One of the best kept secrets in medical science": the extensive experimental evidence for the beneficial effects of prayer. Dossey reviews studies that provide evidence for a positive effect of prayer on not only humans but mice, chicks, enzymes, fungi, yeast, bacteria, and cells of various sorts. He emphasizes, "We cannot dismiss these outcomes as being due to suggestion or placebo effects, since these so-called lower forms of life do not think in any conventional sense and are presumably not susceptible to suggestion" (Pizzorno, 1995).

"Cutting-Edge" Laboratory Methods

A final significant influence has been the development of laboratory methods for the objective assessment of nutritional status, metabolic dysfunction, digestive function, bowel flora, endogenous and exogenous toxic load, and liver detoxification function. Each of these has provided ever more effective tools for accurate assessment of patient health status and effective application of naturopathic principles.

Genomics. One of the most exciting recent advances is genomic testing, the ability to evaluate each individual's template for making the enzymes of life. This technology is now allowing a level of objective evaluation of biochemical individuality never before available, greatly strengthening the naturopathic doctor's ability to practice personalized medicine. The ability to assess each individual's unique nutrient needs as well as susceptibilities to environmental toxins promises to change fundamentally the practice of medicine (Pizzorno, 2003).

During the last several years, as America's staggering health care debt accumulates due to increasing chronic disease, these core, traditional naturopathic principles are surfacing widely as central to creating an effective health care system, as follows:

> *Current medical education inculcates many of the dominant values of modern medicine: reductionism, specialization, mechanistic models of disease, and faith in a definitive cure. . . . What is needed is a model of care that addresses the whole person and integrates care for the person's entire constellation of comorbidities. . . . Nothing short of a fundamental redesign of primary care systems is required (Grumbach, 2003).*

PRINCIPLES

> *Although in many ways, modern medicine resembles a science, it continues to be criticized for its lack of unifying theories, and for this reason alone its claim to being a science has remained suspect.*
>
> —BLOIS (1988)

> *What physicians think medicine is profoundly shapes what they do, how they behave in doing it, and the reasons they use to justify that behavior. . . . Whether conscious of it or not, every physician has an answer to what he thinks medicine is, with real consequences for all whom he attends. . . . The outcome is hardly trivial. . . . It dictates, after all, how we approach patients [and] how we make clinical judgments.*
>
> —PELLEGRINO (1979)

> *Medical philosophy comprises the underlying premises on which a healthcare system is based. Once a system is acknowledged, it is subject to debate. In naturopathic medicine, the philosophical debate is a valuable, ongoing process which helps the understanding that disease evolves in an orderly and truth-revealing fashion.*
>
> —BRADLEY (1985)

Naturopathic medicine is a distinct system of health-oriented medicine that, in contrast to the currently dominant disease-treatment system, stresses promotion of health, prevention of disease, patient education, and self-responsibility. However, naturopathic medicine symbolizes more than simply a health care system; it is a way of life. Unlike most other health care systems, naturopathy is not identified with any particular therapy but rather a way of thinking about life, health, and disease. It is defined not by the therapies it uses but by the philosophical principles that guide the practitioner.

Seven powerful concepts provide the foundation that defines naturopathic medicine and create a unique group of professionals practicing a form of medicine that fundamentally changes the way we think of health care. In 1989 the American Association of Naturopathic Physicians unanimously approved the definition of *naturopathic medicine,* updating and reconfirming in modern terms its six core principles as a professional consensus. "The definition and principles of practice provide a steady point of reference for this debate, for our evolving understanding of health and disease, and for all of our decision making processes as a profession" (Snider and Zeff, 1988).

The seven core principles of naturopathic medicine are as follows, with "wellness and health promotion" emerging into the forefront of the scholarly discussion of naturopathic clinical theory:

1. The healing power of nature *(vis medicatrix naturae)*
2. First do no harm *(primum non nocere)*
3. Find the cause *(tolle causam)*
4. Treat the whole person (holism)
5. Preventive medicine
6. Wellness and health promotion (emerging principle)
7. Doctor as teacher *(docere)*

The Healing Power of Nature *(vis medicatrix naturae)*

Belief in the ability of the body to heal itself—the *vis medicatrix naturae* (the healing power of nature)—if given the proper opportunity, and the importance of living within the laws of nature is the foundation of naturopathic medicine. Although the term *naturopathy* was coined in the late nineteenth century, its philosophical roots can be traced back to Hippocrates and derive from a common wellspring with traditional world medicines: belief in the healing power of nature.

Medicine has long grappled with the question of the existence of the *vis medicatrix naturae* (VMN). As Neuberger stated, "The problem of the healing power of nature is a great, perhaps the greatest of all problems which has occupied the physician for thousands of years. Indeed, the aims and limits of therapeutics are determined by its solution." The fundamental reality of the VMN was a basic tenet of the Hippocratic school of medicine, and "every important medical author since has had to take a position for or against it" (Neuberger, 1932, in Kirchfeld and Boyle, 1994).

When standard medicine soundly rejected the principle of the VMN at the turn of the twentieth century, nature doctors, including naturopathic physicians in the United States from 1896 on, diverged from conventional medicine. Naturopathic physicians recognized the clinical importance of the inherent self-healing process; embraced it as their core academic and clinical principle; and developed an entire system of medical practice, training, and research based on it and related principles of clinical medicine.

Naturopathic medicine is therefore "vitalistic" in its approach (i.e., life is viewed as more than just the sum of biochemical processes), and the body is believed to have an innate intelligence or process (the VMN), which is always striving toward health. Vitalism maintains that the symptoms accompanying disease are not typically caused by the morbific agent (e.g., bacteria); rather, they are the result of the organism's intrinsic response or reaction to the agent and the organism's attempt to defend and heal itself (Lindlahr, 1914a; Neuberger, 1932). Symptoms are part of a constructive phenomenon that is the best "choice" the organism can make, given the circumstances. In this construct the physician's role is to understand and aid the body's efforts, not to take over or manipulate the functions of the body, unless the self-healing process has become weak or insufficient.

Although the context and life force of naturopathic medicine is its vitalistic core, both vitalistic and mechanistic approaches are applicable to modern naturopathic medicine. Vitalism has reemerged in current terms in the body-mind-spirit dialogue. Matter, mind, energy, and spirit are each part of nature and therefore are part of medicine that observes, respects, and works with nature. Much of modern biomedicine and related research is based on the application of the theory of mechanism (defined in *Webster's Dictionary* as the "theory that everything in the universe is produced by matter in motion; materialism") in a highly reductionistic, single-agent, pathology-based, disease care model. Applied in a vitalistic context, mechanistic and reductionistic interventions provide useful techniques and tools to naturopathic physicians. The unifying Theory of Naturopathic Medicine, as discussed later, provides clinical guidance for integrating both approaches.

First Do No Harm *(primum non nocere)*

Naturopathic physicians prefer noninvasive treatments that minimize the risks of harmful side effects. They are trained to use the lowest-force and lowest-risk preventive, diagnostic, therapeutic, and co-management strategies. They are trained to know which patients they can safely treat and which ones they need to refer to other health care practitioners. Naturopathic physicians follow three precepts to avoid harming the patient:

1. Naturopathic physicians use methods and medicinal substances that minimize the risk of harmful effects and apply the least possible force or intervention necessary to diagnose illness and restore health.
2. When possible, the suppression of symptoms is avoided because suppression generally interferes with the healing process.
3. Naturopathic physicians respect and work with the VMN in diagnosis, treatment, and counseling because if this self-healing process is not respected, the patient may be harmed.

Find the Cause *(tolle causam)*

Every illness has an underlying cause or causes, often in aspects of the lifestyle, diet, or habits of the individual. A naturopathic physician is trained to find and remove the underlying cause(s) of disease. The therapeutic order helps the physician remove them in the correct "healing order" for the body (see later discussion). As the new science of psychoneuroimmunology is explicitly demonstrating, the body is a seamless web with a multiplicity of brain–immune system–gut–liver connections (see Chapter 15). Not surprisingly, chronic disease typically involves a number of systems, with the most prominent or acute symptoms being those chronologically last in appearance. As the healing process progresses and these symptoms are alleviated, further symptoms then resurface that must then be addressed to restore health. To paraphrase David Jones, MD, and "tack rules": "If you're sitting on a tack, it takes a lot of aspirin to feel better. If you're sitting on two tacks, removing one does not necessarily lead to a 50% improvement/reduction in symptoms."

Treat the Whole Person (Holism)

As noted in the preceding principle, health or disease comes from a complex interaction of mental, emotional, spiritual, physical, dietary, genetic, environmental, lifestyle, and other factors. Naturopathic physicians treat the whole person, taking all these factors into account. Naturopathically, the body is viewed as a whole. Naturopathy is often called *holistic medicine* in reference to the term *holism,* coined by philosopher Jan Christian Smuts in 1926, to describe the *gestalt* of a system as greater than the sum of its parts. A change in one part causes a change in every part; therefore the study of one part must be integrated into the whole, including the community and biosphere.

Naturopathic medicine asserts that one cannot be healthy in an unhealthy environment, and it is committed to the creation of a world in which humanity may thrive. In contrast to the high degree of specialization in the present medical system, which reflects a mechanistic orientation to single organs, the holistic model relegates specialists to an ancillary role. Emphasis is placed on the physical, emotional, social, and spiritual integration of the whole person, including awareness of the impact of the environment on health.

Preventive Medicine

The naturopathic approach to health care helps prevent disease and keeps minor illnesses from developing into more serious or chronic degenerative diseases. Patients are taught the principles with which to live a healthful life, and by following these principles, they can prevent major illness. Health is viewed as more than just the absence of disease; it is considered a dynamic state that enables a person to thrive in, or adapt to, a wide range of environments and stresses. Health and disease are points on a continuum, with death at one end and optimal function at the other. The naturopathic physician believes that a person who goes through life living an unhealthful lifestyle will drift away from optimal function and move relentlessly toward progressively greater dysfunction. Genotype, constitution, maternal influences, and environmental factors all influence individual susceptibility to deterioration, and the organs and physiological systems affected. Box 13-2 lists these and other determinants of health addressed by the naturopathic physician in both treatment and prevention.

The virulence of moribific agents or insults also plays a central role in disturbance, causing decreasing function and ultimately serious disease.

In our society, although our life span at birth has increased, our health span has not, nor has our health expectancy at age 65. We are living longer but as

BOX 13-2

Determinants of Health and Other Factors in Naturopathic Preventive Medicine

Determinants of Health

Inborn
- Genetic makeup (genotype)
- Constitution (determines susceptibility)
- Intrauterine/congenital
- Maternal exposures
  - —Drugs
  - —Toxins
  - —Viruses
  - —Psychoemotional
- Maternal and paternal genetic influences
- Maternal nutrition
- Maternal lifestyle

Disturbances
- Illnesses: pathobiography
- Medical interventional (or lack of)
- Physical and emotional exposures, stresses, and trauma
- Toxic and harmful substances

Hygienic/Lifestyle Factors
- Nutrition
- Rest
- Exercise
- Psychoemotional health
- Spiritual health
- Community
- Culture
- Socioeconomic factors
- Fresh air
- Light
- Exposure to nature
- Clean water
- Unadulterated food
- Loving and being loved
- Meaningful work

disabled individuals (Pizzorno, 1997). Although such deterioration is accepted by our society as the normal expectation of aging, it is not common in animals in the wild or among those fortunate peoples who live in an optimal environment (i.e., no pollution, low stress, regular exercise, and abundant natural, nutritious food).

In the naturopathic model, death is inevitable; progressive disability is not. This belief underscores a fundamental difference in philosophy and expectation between the conventional and naturopathic models of health and disease. In contrast to the disease treatment focus of allopathic medicine, the health promotion focus of naturopathic medicine emphasizes the means of maximizing health span.

Wellness and Health Promotion (Emerging Principle)

Establishing and maintaining optimal health and balance is a central clinical goal. Wellness and health promotion go beyond prevention. This principle represents a proactive state of being healthy, characterized by positive emotion, thought, intention, and action. Wellness is inherent in everyone, no matter what disease is being experienced. The recognition,

experience, and support of wellness through health promotion by the physician and patient will more quickly heal a given disease than treatment of the disease alone.

Doctor as Teacher (*docere*)

The original meaning of the word *docere* is "teacher." A principle objective of naturopathic medicine is to educate the patient and emphasize self-responsibility for health. Naturopathic doctors also recognize the therapeutic potential of the physician-patient relationship. The patient is engaged and respected as an ally and a member of her or his own health care team. Adequate time is spent with patients to diagnose, treat, and educate them thoroughly (see Chapters 1 and 2).

Naturopathic Practice Today

Current naturopathic physicians are licensed primary care providers of integrative natural medicine and are also recognized for their clinical expertise and effectiveness in preventive medicine. Naturopathic doctors (NDs) are trained as family physicians, regardless of elective postdoctoral training or clinical emphasis. This is intentional and consistent with naturopathic principles of practice. NDs are trained to assess causes and develop treatment plans from a systems perspective and with systems skills on the basis of naturopathic principles and, specifically, on the principle "treat the whole person," as follows:

> Naturopathy, in fact, is typically *meta-systematic.* . . . The organism [is] always seen in the context of its physical and social environment. . . . Beyond this, naturopathy, ultimately might even be considered *cross-paradigmatic,* touching inevitably on the economics, politics, history, and sociology of the various healing alternatives, ultimately penetrating to the contrasting philosophies underlying naturopathy and allopathy. Naturopathy results from a guiding philosophy at odds with the dominant mechanistic philosophy undergirding Western industrialized society. Allopathy, in contrast, is clearly derived from these same premises. Or in Eisler's terms, naturopathy embraces a *partnership* model of relationship, while allopathy falls within the *dominator* model. . . . [T]his partnership/dominator model extends not only to the treatment process but to the healer/patient relationship itself (Funk, 1995).

NDs may also practice as specialists, after postdoctoral training in botanical, homeopathic, nutritional medicine, physical medicine, acupuncture, Ayurvedic medicine, Oriental and Chinese herbal medicine, counseling and health psychology, spirituality and healing, applied behavioral sciences, and midwifery. Some NDs choose to focus their practice on population groups such as children, the elderly, or women, or in clinical areas such as cardiology, gastroenterology, immunology, or environmental medicine. These diverse practices are consistent with the eclectic origins of naturopathic medicine and are part of its strength.

In addition to these specialties, at one end of the spectrum are practitioners who adhere to the nature cure tradition and focus clinically only on diet, detoxification, lifestyle modification, hydrotherapy, and other self-healing modalities. At the other end are those whose practices appear to be similar to the average conventional medical practice, with the only apparent difference being the use of pharmaceutical-grade botanical medicines instead of synthetic drugs. However, fundamental to all styles of naturopathic practice is a common philosophy and principles of health and disease: the unifying theory in the hierarchy of therapeutics, or the therapeutic order described in the following section. The therapeutic order is derived from all of the principles and guides the ND's choice of therapeutic interventions.

UNIFYING THEORY: THE HEALING POWER OF NATURE AND THE THERAPEUTIC ORDER

In facilitating the process of healing, the naturopathic physician seeks to use those therapies and strategies that are most efficient and that have the least potential to harm the patient. The concept of "harm" includes suppression or exhaustion of natural healing processes, including inflammation and fever. These precepts, coupled to an understanding of the process of healing, result in a therapeutic hierarchy. This hierarchy (or therapeutic order) is a natural consequence of how the organism heals. Therapeutic modalities are applied in a rational order, determined by the nature of the healing process. The natural order of appropriate therapeutic intervention follows:

1. Reestablish the basis for health.
2. Stimulate the VMN.
3. Tonify and nourish weakened systems.
4. Correct structural integrity.
5. Prescribe specific substances and modalities for specific conditions and biochemical pathways (e.g. botanicals, nutrients, acupuncture, homeopathy, hydrotherapy, counseling).
6. Prescribe pharmaceutical substances.
7. Use radiation, chemotherapy, and surgery.

This appropriate therapeutic order proceeds from least to most force. All modalities can be found at various steps, depending on their application. The spiritual aspect of the patient's health is considered to begin with step 1 (Zeff, 1997; steps 5 through 7 added by Snider).

The concepts expressed in the therapeutic order are derived from Hippocrates' writings and those of medical scholars since Hippocrates concerning the function and activation of the self-healing process. Dr. Jared Zeff (1997) expresses these concepts as the hierarchy of therapeutics in his article "The Process of Healing: a Unifying Theory of Naturopathic Medicine." These concepts are further explored, refined, and developed in *The Textbook of Natural Medicine,* third edition, by Zeff, Snider, and Myers *(A Hierarchy of Healing: the Therapeutic Order—the unifying theory of naturopathic medicine).*

The philosophy represented in the therapeutic order does not determine what modalities are good or bad. Rather, it provides a clinical framework for all approaches and modalities, used in an order consistent with that of the natural self-healing process. It respects the origins of disease and the applications of care and intervention necessary for health and healing with the least intervention.

The therapeutic order exemplifies the concept: use the least force, one of the key tenets of the naturopathic principle "Do No Harm." The therapeutic order schematically directs the ND's therapeutic choices in an efficient order rather than a "shotgun" approach. This common philosophy and theory both distinguishes the field of naturopathic medicine and enables it to consider and incorporate new therapies.

Naturopathic medicine's philosophical approach to health promotion and restoration necessitates a broad range of diagnostic and therapeutic skills and accounts for the eclectic interests of the naturopathic profession. Obviously, at times the body needs more than just supportive help. The goal of the ND in such situations is first to use the lowest-force and lowest-risk clinical strategies (i.e., the least invasive intervention that will have the most effective therapeutic outcome) or, when necessary, to co-manage or refer to specialists and other health care professionals.

Because the goal of the ND is to restore normal body function rather than to apply a particular therapy, virtually every natural medicine therapy may be used. In addition, to fulfill their role as primary care family physicians, NDs may also administer vaccines and use therapies such as office surgery and prescription drugs when less invasive options have been exhausted or found inappropriate. In the restoration of health, prescription drugs and surgery are a last resort but are used when necessary. As Kirschner and Brinkman (1988) said, "The use of petroleum by products and the removal of body parts is a poor first line of defense against disease."

Naturopathic medical school curricula are continually revised in light of these principles. Curriculum integration is built on the science-based educational structure already in place in these colleges. Basic sciences, ND, and non-ND physician faculty are trained in naturopathic philosophy and principles and the therapeutic order as core assumptions that invite scholarly inquiry. Discussion and inquiry concerning the philosophy and theory are stimulated and supported in interdisciplinary faculty teams. The fruits of these endeavors are brought into the classroom to enhance students' critical thinking concerning clinical values and assumptions. Naturopathic research on these principles themselves is a widely embraced priority for the naturopathic profession. In 2004 the Naturopathic Medical Research Agenda (NMRA), a 2-year research project sponsored by the NIH Center for Complementary and Alternative Medicine, identified three key hypotheses as central to the future and the foundations of naturopathic medical research. The third hypothesis states: "The scientific exploration of naturopathic medical practices and principles will yield important insights into the nature of health and healing" (Standish et al., 2004).

DIAGNOSIS

In the naturopathic medicine program at Bastyr University, for example, the principles just discussed and the therapeutic order are translated into a series of questions that drive curriculum development and case analysis and provide guidance to students learning the art and science of naturopathic medicine. These Naturopathic Case Analysis and Management questions (see next section) are integrated with conventional SOAP algorithms (subjective, objective, assessment, plan) as the process of naturopathic case analysis and management, the clinical application of philosophy to patient care. For example, although a conventional pathological diagnosis is made through the use of physical, laboratory, and radiology procedures, it is done in the context of understanding the underlying causes of the pathology and the obstacles to recovery.

NATUROPATHIC CASE ANALYSIS AND MANAGEMENT

I. The Healing Power of Nature (vis medicatrix naturae)
1. **What is the level of the disease process? What is the direction of the disease process? What is the purpose of the disease process?**

2. How is the healing power of nature supported in the case? What therapeutic interventions allow/respect, palliate, facilitate, or augment the self-healing process? How does the therapeutic intervention do this?
3. Is the person in balance with nature?
4. What is being in balance with nature?
5. Is this person in balance with his or her environment?
6. How are you assessing the healing powers of this individual?
7. What is the prognosis for this individual?
8. What is the patient's metaphor for healing? What moves or will move this patient toward healing or recovery?
9. How does the patient see himself or herself healing (the patient process)?
   • Are people helping him or her?
   • Is he or she doing it on his or her own?
   • How long will it take?
   • Is the doctor doing the healing?
   • Is the patient doing the healing?
   • Are the doctor and patient working together?
   • What else is important in this patient's healing process?

II. First Do No Harm (primum non nocere)

1. What is the potential for harm with this particular treatment plan?
2. Are you doing no harm? How?
3. How are you avoiding suppression? Is suppression necessary? Why?
4. What is the appropriate course of action? Is it waiting?
5. What is the appropriate level and force of intervention? Why? How is the least force applied?
6. Identify the appropriate treatment:
   • Level of therapeutic order
   • Modality/substance
   • Dosage
   • Frequency
   • Duration
   Justify the timing of the treatment in terms of short- and long-term management.
7. Are there any obstacles to the patient's recovery? Explain.
8. What referral or co-management strategies are required to ensure patients' optimal outcome?

III. Find the Cause (tolle causam)

1. What level of healing are you aiming toward (i.e., suppression, palliation, cure)?
2. Where and/or what are the limiting factors in this person's life (concept: health is freedom from limitations)?
3. Where is the center of this person's disease (i.e., physical, mental, emotional, spiritual)?
4. What are the causative factors contributing to this patient's condition/state? What is the central cause or etiology? What are other contributing causes? Of these causative factors, which are avoidable or preventable?

IV. Treat the Whole Person (Holism)

1. How are you working holistically?
2. Can you see the person beyond the disease?
3. What aspects of the person are you addressing?
4. What aspects of the person are you not addressing?
5. Would a referral to another health care practitioner assist you in working holistically? When? To whom? If not, why not?
6. What are the patient's goals and expectations in relationship to their health and treatments?
7. What are your goals and expectations for the patient? What are the differences between yours and the patient's? How are they similar?
8. How will the treatment plan help the patient take more responsibility for his or her health and healing?
9. Are you empowering the patient? How?
10. What is the vitality level of this patient?
11. Identify cultural, community, and environmental issues and concerns that need to be included in the assessment.
12. What family/psychological/spiritual/social systems issues need to be included in the assessment?

V. Preventive Medicine

1. What is being done or planned in regard to prevention?
2. Doctor means teacher—what are you teaching this person about his or her health?
3. Have you done a risk factor assessment for this patient? Have all preprimary, primary, secondary, and tertiary interventions and education relevant to life span or gender been identified and addressed?
4. Does this patient do regular health screening self-examinations?

VI. Wellness and Health Promotion (Emerging Principle)

1. What is being done to cultivate wellness?
2. How are you contributing to optimal health in this individual?
3. How can you contribute to optimal health in this individual?
4. What are the patient's goals and expectations in relationship to their own wellness (e.g., creativity, energy, enjoyment, health, balance)?
5. How can these goals be achieved? Are the expectations realistic?

6. How can achievement of these goals be measured?

7. Once achieved, how can the patient maintain an optimal level of wellness?

8. Are you stimulating wellness or treating disease, or both?

9. Is the patient demonstrating positive emotion, thought, and action? If not, why not?

10. Can the patient recall or imagine a state of wellness?

11. Is the patient able to participate in his or her own process toward a state of wellness?

VII. Doctor as Teacher (docere)

1. What type of patient education are you providing? Assess wellness issues and prevention issues for this person. Identify educational needs of this patient regarding (a) therapeutic goals, (b) prevention, and (c) wellness.

2. How can you determine the level of a patient's responsibility?

3. In what ways do you cultivate and enhance your role as teacher?

4. How have you listened to and respected the patient?

5. In what ways are you working to "draw out" the patient's vital force and vitality through the physician-patient relationship?

THERAPEUTIC MODALITIES

Naturopathic medicine is a vitalistic system of health care that uses natural medicines and interventionist therapies as needed. Natural medicines and therapies, when properly used, generally have low invasiveness and rarely cause suppression or side effects. This is because, when used properly, they generally support the body's healing mechanisms rather than taking over the body's processes. The ND knows when, why, and with what patient more invasive therapies are needed based on the therapeutic order and appropriate diagnostic measures. The ND also recognizes that the use of natural, low-force therapies; lifestyle changes; and early functional diagnosis and treatment of nonspecific conditions is a form of preprimary prevention. This approach offers one viable solution for cost containment in primary health care.

Traditional health care disciplines such as traditional Chinese medicine (TCM), Yunani medicine, and homeopathic medicine each have a philosophy, principles of practice, and clinical theory that form a system for diagnosis, treatment, and case management. A philosophy of medicine is, in essence, the rational investigation of the truth and principles of that medicine. The principles of practice form an outline or guidelines to the main precepts or fundamental tenets of a system of medicine. Clinical theory provides a system of rules or principles explaining that medicine and applying that system to the patient by means of diagnosis, treatment, and management. The specific substances and techniques, as well as when, why, and to whom they are applied and for how long, depend on the system. Modalities (e.g., botanical medicine, physical medicine) are not systems but rather therapeutic approaches used within these systems. One modality may be used by many systems but in different ways.

The importance of systems is that efficacy, safety, and efficiency of diagnostic and treatment approaches depend as much on the system as on the effects of the substance on physiology or biochemical pathways. This is exemplified by data in the TCM Work Force Survey conducted by the Department of Human Services in Victoria, New South Wales, and Queensland, Australia. In this study, Bensoussan and Myers (1996) assessed adverse events and length of TCM training for practitioners, as follows:

> The number of adverse events reported were compared to the length of TCM training undertaken by the practitioner. It appears from these findings that shorter periods of training in TCM (less than one year) carry an adverse event rate double that of practitioners who have studied for four years or more.... These practitioners were asked to respond to two questions regarding the theoretical frameworks they used to guide their TCM practice. TCM philosophy is adopted more readily as the basis for practice by primary TCM practitioners than by allied health practitioners using TCM as part of their practice. In answer to the question, "Do you rely more predominantly on a TCM philosophy and theoretical framework for making your diagnosis and guiding your acupuncture or Chinese herbal medicine treatments?" 90% of primary TCM practitioners answered yes in contrast to 24% of non-primary practitioners.

Nonprimary practitioners were typically educated for less than 1 year and were medical doctors.

It is the system used by each of these disciplines that makes it a uniquely effective field of medicine rather than a vague compendium of complementary and integrative (or alternative) medicine (CIM/CAM) modalities. Techniques from many systems are used within naturopathic medicine because of its primary care integrative approach and strong philosophical orientation.

Clinical nutrition, or the use of diet as a therapy, serves as the therapeutic foundation of naturopathic medicine. A rapidly increasing body of knowledge supports the use of whole foods, fasting, natural hygiene, and nutritional supplements in the maintenance of health and treatment of disease. The recognition of unique nutritional requirements caused by biochemical individuality has provided a theoretical and practical basis for the appropriate use of megavitamin therapy. Controlled fasting is also used clinically.

Botanical medicines are also important; plants have been used as medicines since antiquity. The technology now exists to understand the physiological activities of herbs and a tremendous amount of research worldwide, especially in Europe, is demonstrating clinical efficacy. Botanical medicines are used for both vitalistic and pharmacological actions. Pharmacological effects and contraindications, as well as synergetic, energetic, and dilutional uses, are fundamental knowledge in naturopathic medicine (see Chapter 11).

Homeopathic medicine derives etymologically from the Greek word *homeos,* meaning "similar," and *pathos,* meaning "disease." Homeopathy is a system of medicine that treats a patient and his or her condition with a dilute, potentized agent, or drug, that will produce the same symptoms as the disease when given to a healthy individual, the fundamental principle being that *like cures like.* This principle was actually first recognized by Hippocrates, who noticed that herbs and other substances given in small doses tended to cure the same symptoms they produced when given in toxic doses. Prescriptions are based on the totality of all the patient's symptoms and matched to "provings" of homeopathic medicines. Provings are symptoms produced in healthy people who are unaware of the specific remedy they have received. Large numbers of people are tested and these symptoms documented. The symptoms are then added to toxicology, symptomatology, and data from cured cases to form the homeopathic materia medica. Homeopathic medicines are derived from a variety of plant, mineral, and chemical substances and are prepared according to the specifications of the *Homeopathic Pharmacopoeia of the United States.* Approximately 100 clinical studies have demonstrated the clinical efficacy of homeopathic therapies (see Chapter 8).

Traditional Chinese medicine is analogous to naturopathic medicine to the extent that it is a system with principles corollary to working with the self-healing process. According to Bensoussan and Myers (1996):

TCM shares some common ideas with other forms of complementary medicine, including belief in a strong inter-relationship between the environment and bodily function and an understanding of illness as starting with an imbalance of energy. . . . The TCM diagnostic process is . . . particularly holistic in nature [again similar to naturopathic medicine] and is usually contrasted to a reductionistic approach in western medicine. Western medicine often defines disease at an organ level of dysfunction and is increasingly reliant on laboratory findings. In contrast, TCM defines disease as a whole person disturbance.

Quiang Cao, ND, LAC, Bastyr University, explains as follows:

TCM never treats just the symptom, but the individual's whole constitution and environmental conditions; all are considered in a holistic context. The symptom signals constitutional excess or deficiency. The goal is not just to alleviate the symptom but to balance yin and yang, hot and cold, excess and deficiency, internally and externally.

Acupuncture is an ancient Chinese system of medicine involving the stimulation of certain specific points on the body to enhance the flow of vital energy (qi) along pathways called *meridians.* Acupuncture points can be stimulated by the insertion and withdrawing of needles, the application of heat (moxibustion), massage, laser, electrical means, or a combination of these methods. Traditional Chinese acupuncture implies a very specific acupuncture technique and knowledge of the Oriental system of medicine, including yin-yang, the five elements, acupuncture points and meridians, and a method of diagnosis and differentiation of syndromes quite different from that of Western medicine. Although most research in this country has focused on its use for the pain relief and the treatment of addictions, it is a complete system of medicine effective for many diseases (see Chapter 21).

Hydrotherapy is the use of water in any of its forms (e.g., hot, cold, ice, steam) and methods of application (e.g., sitz bath, douche, spa and hot tub, whirlpool, sauna, shower, immersion bath, pack, poultice, foot bath, fomentation, wrap, colonic irrigations) in the maintenance of health or treatment of disease. It is one of the most ancient methods of treatment and has been part of naturopathic medicine since its inception. Nature doctors, before and since Sebastian Kneipp, have used hydrotherapy as a central part of clinical practice. Hydrotherapy has been used to treat disease and injury by many different cultures, including the Egyptians, Assyrians, Persians, Greeks, Hebrews, Hindus, and Chinese. Its most sophisticated applications were developed in eighteenth-century Germany. Naturopathic physicians today use hydrotherapy to stimulate and support healing, for detoxification, and to strengthen immune function for many chronic and acute conditions.

Physical medicine refers to the therapeutic use of touch, heat, cold, electricity, and sound. This includes the use of physiotherapy equipment such as ultrasound, diathermy, and other electromagnetic energy agents; therapeutic exercise; massage; massage energy, joint mobilization (manipulative), and immobilization techniques; and hydrotherapy. In the therapeutic order, correction of structural integrity is a key factor; the hands-on approach of naturopathic physicians through physical medicine is unique in primary care.

Detoxification, the recognition and correction of endogenous and exogenous toxicity, is an important theme in naturopathic medicine. Liver and bowel detoxification, elimination of environmental toxins, correction of the metabolic dysfunction(s) that causes the buildup of non–end-product metabolites—all are important ways of decreasing toxic load. Spiritual and emotional toxicity are also recognized as important factors in restoring health.

Spirituality and health issues are central to naturopathic practice and are based on the individual patient's belief and spiritual orientation; simply, what moves the patient toward life and a higher purpose than himself or herself. Because total health also includes spiritual health, naturopathic physicians encourage individuals to pursue their personal spiritual development. As a plethora of studies in the newly emerging field of psychoneuroimmunology have demonstrated, particularly those examining both the placebo and the nocebo effect, the body is not a mere collection of organs, but rather a body, mind, and spirit in which the mind-spirit part of the equation marshals tremendous forces promoting health or disease.

Counseling, health psychology, and *lifestyle modification techniques* are essential modalities for the naturopathic physician. An ND is a holistic physician formally trained in mental, emotional, and family counseling. Various treatment measures include hypnosis and guided imagery, counseling techniques, correcting underlying organic factors, and family systems therapy.

THERAPEUTIC APPROACH

Respect Nature

We are natural organisms, with our genomes developed and expressed in the natural world. The patterns and processes inherent in nature are inherent in us. We exist as a part of complex patterns of matter, energy, and spirit. Nature doctors have observed the natural processes of these patterns in health and disease and determined that there is an inherent drive toward health that lives within the patterns and processes of nature.

The drive is not perfect. At times, when unguided, unassisted, or unstopped, the drive goes astray, causing preventable harm or even death; the healing intention becomes pathology. The ND is trained to know, respect, and work with this drive and to know when to wait and do nothing, act preventively, assist, amplify, palliate, intervene, manipulate, control, or even suppress, using the principle of the least force. The challenge of twenty-first–century medicine is to support the beneficial effects of this drive and come to a sophisticated application of the least force principle in mainstream health care. This will prevent the last 20 years of life being those of debility from chronic, degenerative disease for the average American and extend the health span throughout the life span.

Because the total organism is involved in the healing attempt, the most effective approach to care must consider the whole person. In addition to physical and laboratory findings, important consideration is given to the patient's mental, emotional, and spiritual attitude; lifestyle; diet; heredity; environment; and family and community life. Careful attention to each person's unique individuality and susceptibility to disease is critical to the proper evaluation and treatment of any health problem.

Naturopathic physicians believe that most disease is the direct result of the ignorance and violation of "natural living laws." These rules are summarized as the consumption of natural, unrefined, organically grown foods; ensuring adequate amounts of exercise and rest; living a moderately paced lifestyle; having constructive and creative thoughts and emotions; avoiding environmental toxins; and maintaining proper elimination. During illness, it is also important to control these areas to remove as many unnecessary stresses as possible and to optimize the chances that the organism's healing attempt will be successful. Therefore, fundamental to naturopathic practice is patient education and responsibility, lifestyle modification, preventive medicine, and wellness promotion.

Naturopathic Approaches to Disease

The ND's therapeutic approach is therefore basically twofold: to help patients heal themselves and to use the opportunity to guide and educate the patient in developing a more healthful lifestyle. Many supposedly incurable conditions respond very well to naturopathic approaches.

A typical first office visit with an ND takes 1 hour. The goal is to learn as much as possible about the patient using thorough history and review of systems, physical examination, laboratory tests, radiology, and other standard diagnostic procedures. Also, the patient's diet, environment, toxic load, exercise, stress, and other aspects of lifestyle are evaluated, and laboratory tests are used to determine physiological function. Once a good understanding of the patient's health and disease status is established (making a diagnosis of a disease is only one part of this process), the ND and patient work together to establish a treatment and health promotion program.

Although every effort is made to treat the whole person and not just his or her disease, the limits of a short description necessitate discussing typical naturopathic therapies of specific conditions in a simplified, disease-oriented manner. The following sections then provide examples of how the person's health can be improved, resulting in alleviation of the disease.

Cervical Dysplasia

The only traditional medical approach to treating cervical dysplasia, a precancerous condition of the cervix, is surgical resection. Nothing is done to treat the underlying causes. The typical naturopathic treatment would include the following:

1. *Education*. The patient should be educated about factors that increase the risk of cervical cancer, such as smoking (risk = 3.0), multiple sex partners (risk = 3.4), and the use of oral contraceptives (risk = 3.6) (Clarke et al., 1985).
2. *Prevention*. Because 67% of patients with cervical cancer are deficient in one or more nutrients (Orr et al., 1985), and serum β-carotene (critical for prevention of cancer of cells such as those in cervix) level is only half that of normal women (Dawson et al., 1984), the woman's nutritional status would be optimized (through diet, especially by increasing intake of fruits and vegetables) and with regard to those nutrients known to be deficient (often a result of oral contraceptive use) in women with cervical dysplasia and the deficiencies of which may promote cellular abnormalities: folic acid (Van Niekerk, 1966), β-carotene (Dawson et al., 1984), vitamin C (Romney et al., 1985), vitamin B_6 (Ramaswarmy and Natarajan, 1984), and selenium (Dawson et al., 1984).
3. *Treatment*. The vaginal depletion pack (a traditional mixture of botanical medicines placed against the cervix) would be used to promote sloughing of the abnormal cells.

The advantages of this approach are (1) the causes of the cervical dysplasia have been identified and resolved, so the problem should not recur; (2) no surgery is used, thus no scar tissue is formed; and (3) the cost, particularly considering that many women with cervical dysplasia have recurrences when treated with standard surgery, is reasonable. More important, however, is that the woman's health has been improved, and other conditions that could have been caused by the identified nutritional deficiencies have now been prevented.

Migraine Headache

The standard medical treatment is primarily to use drugs to relieve symptoms, a costly and recurrent practice. Nothing is done to address the underlying causes. In contrast, the naturopath recognizes that most migraine headaches are caused by food allergies, and abnormal prostaglandin metabolism caused by nutritional abnormalities results in excessive platelet aggregation. The approach is straightforward, as follows:

1. Identify and avoid the allergenic foods because 70% or more of patients have migraines in reaction

to foods to which they are intolerant (Natero et al., 1989).

2. Supplement with magnesium because migraine patients have significantly lowered serum and salivary magnesium levels, which are even lower during an attack (Sarchielli et al., 1992). In one study, 89% of those responding to magnesium showed low pretreatment serum magnesium levels (Mauskop, 1996). In another report, magnesium levels in the brain, as measured by nuclear magnetic resonance (NMR) spectroscopy, were significantly lower in patients during an acute migraine than in healthy individuals (Weaver, 1990, in Gaby, 1998. Several studies have shown the importance of magnesium in reversing the causes of migraine (Johnson, 2001).

3. Reestablish normal prostaglandin balance by decreasing animal fats (high in platelet-aggregating arachidonic acid) and supplementing with essential fatty acids such as fish oils (Woodcock et al., 1984). Omega-3 supplementation has proven effective in adolescents with migraine (Harel et al., 2002).

4. Supplement with riboflavin. "Forty-nine individuals with recurrent migraines were given 400 mg/day of the B-vitamin riboflavin for at least 3 months. The average number of migraine attacks fell by 67% and migraine severity improved by 68%" (Gaby, 1998).

Hypertension

The patients with so-called idiopathic, or essential, hypertension can be very effectively treated if they are willing to make the necessary lifestyle changes, as follows.

1. *Diet.* Numerous studies have shown that excessive dietary salt in conjunction with inadequate dietary potassium is a major contributor to hypertension (Fries, 1976; Khaw and Barrett-Connor, 1984; Meneely and Battarbee, 1976). Further, dietary deficiencies in calcium (Belizan et al., 1983; McCarron et al., 1982), magnesium (Dyckner and Wester, 1983; Resnick et al., 1989), essential fatty acids (Rao et al., 1981; Vergroesen et al., 1978), and vitamin C (Yoshioka et al., 1981) all contribute to increased blood pressure. Also, increased consumption of sugar (Hodges and Rebello, 1983), caffeine (Lang et al., 1983), and alcohol (Gruchow et al., 1985) are all associated with hypertension.

Many studies have shown the antihypertensive effects of increasing fruits and vegetables, key to the dietary recommendations of NDs for over a hundred years (John, et al, 2002).

2. *Lifestyle.* Smoking (Kershbaum et al., 1968), obesity (Havlik et al., 1983), stress (Ford, 1982), and a sedentary lifestyle are all known to contribute to the development of high blood pressure.

3. *Environment.* Exposure to heavy metals such as lead (Pruess, 1992) and cadmium (Glauser et al., 1976) increase blood pressure.

4. *Botanical medicine.* Many herbal medicines are used when necessary for the patient's safety initially to lower his or her blood pressure rapidly until the slower, but more curative, dietary and lifestyle treatments can have their effects. Included are such age-old favorites as garlic *(Allium sativa)* and mistletoe *(Viscum album).*

The causes of high blood pressure are not unknown, but they are generally unheeded.

Lifestyle modification is crucial to the successful implementation of naturopathic techniques—health does not come from a doctor, pills, or surgery but rather from the patients' own efforts to take proper care of themselves. Unfortunately, our society expends considerable resources to induce disease-promoting habits. Although it is relatively easy to tell a patient to stop smoking, get more exercise, and reduce his or her stress, such lifestyle changes are difficult in the context of peer, habit, and commercial pressure. The ND is specifically trained to assist the patient in making the needed changes. This involves many aspects: helping the patient acknowledge the need; setting realistic, progressive goals; identifying and working through barriers; establishing a support group of family and friends or of others with similar problems; identifying the stimuli that reinforce the unhealthy behavior; and giving the patient positive reinforcement for his or her gains.

ACCOUNTABILITY IN NATUROPATHIC MEDICINE

Acceptance of a profession typically is seen to derive from sanctions associated with educational institutions, professional associations and licensing boards.

—ORZACK (1997)

It is extremely important to realize that the establishment of standards and especially credentialling standards is critical for the public to know . . . whatever the discipline is.

—LEVENDUSKI (1991)

Although naturopathic medicine in the early part of the twentieth century was unique, clinically effective, and powerfully vitalistic, it suffered because it had not reached maturity in terms of professional unification, scientific research, and other recognizable standards of public accountability. These goals have finally been achieved during the two decades of 1978 to 2000.

Naturopathic medicine has responded to the need to integrate not only the best that conventional and natural medicine have to offer, but also the issues of public safety, efficacy, and affordability through the following mechanisms:

- Fully accredited naturopathic medical training (regional and professional)
- Standardized science-based naturopathic medical education
- Broad-scope licensing laws
- Nationally standardized licensing examinations
- Professional standards of practice and peer review
- Credentialing and quality improvement plans
- Scientific research and efficacy documentation

These are well-accepted mechanisms for public accountability in all forms of licensed health care. Naturopathic medicine's credibility has resulted in part from these important achievements by a unified profession.

SCOPE OF PRACTICE, LICENSING, AND PROFESSIONAL ORGANIZATIONS

NDs practice as primary care providers. They see patients of all ages, from all walks of life, with every known disease. They make a conventional Western diagnosis using standard diagnostic procedures, such as physical examination, laboratory tests, and radiological examination. However, they also make a pathophysiological diagnosis using physical and lab-

oratory procedures to assess nutritional status, metabolic function, and toxic load. In addition, considerable time is spent assessing the patient's mental, emotional, social, and spiritual status.

Therapeutically, NDs use virtually every known natural therapy: dietetics, therapeutic nutrition, botanical medicine (primarily the European, Native American, Chinese, and Ayurvedic), physical therapy, spinal manipulation, lifestyle counseling, exercise therapy, homeopathic medicine, acupuncture, psychological and family counseling, hydrotherapy, and clinical fasting and detoxification. In addition, according to state law, NDs may perform office surgery, administer vaccinations, and prescribe a limited range of drugs. Because NDs consider themselves an integral part of the health care system, they meet public health requirements and work within a referral network of specialists in much the same way as a family practice medical (allopathic) doctor. This network includes the range of conventional and nonconventional providers.

NDs (or NMDs) are licensed in 14 states (Alaska, Arizona, California, Connecticut, District of Columbia, Hawaii, Kansas, Maine, Montana, New Hampshire, Oregon, Utah Vermont, and Washington), and the two U.S. territories of Puerto Rico and the Virgin Islands. NDs have a legal right to practice in Idaho and Minnesota. Because no licensing standards exist in these two states and NDs also practice in other states without government approval, individuals with little or no formal education are still able to proclaim themselves NDs, to the significant detriment of the public and the profession. The American Association of Naturopathic Physicians (AANP, Washington, DC) assists consumers in identifying qualified NDs (http://www.naturopathic.org/).

The scope of naturopathic practice is stipulated by state law. Legislation typically allows standard diagnostic privileges. Therapeutic scope is more varied, ranging from only natural therapies to vaccinations, limited prescriptive rights, and office surgery. In addition, some states allow the practice of natural childbirth. Many states identify NDs as primary caregivers in their statutes.

In addition to the Council on Naturopathic Medical Education (CNME), two key organizations provide leadership and standardization for the naturopathic profession. The AANP, founded in 1985 by James Sensenig, ND, and others, was established to provide consistent educational and practice standards for the profession and a unified voice for public relations and political activity. Most licensed NDs in the United States are AANP members. The Naturopathic Physicians Licensing Examination (NPLEx) was founded under the auspices of the AANP in 1986 by Ed Hoffman-Smith, PhD, ND, to establish a nationally recognized standardized test for licensing. NPLEx is recognized by all states licensing NDs. All states licensing NDs and all states in the process of attaining licensure have state professional naturopathic associations. The Alliance for State Licensing is an ongoing state licensure effort.

INTEGRATION INTO THE MAINSTREAM

The American public has increasingly turned to alternative practitioners in search of healing for a variety of conditions not ameliorated by conventional medical practices. Such conditions include otitis media, cardiovascular disease, depression, chronic fatigue syndrome, gastrointestinal disorders, chemical sensitivities, recurrent infectious diseases, rheumatoid arthritis, general loss of vitality and wellness, and many other chronic and acute conditions.

> Unquestionably, the health care system is undergoing profound change. . . . Many . . . current aspects of health care have resulted from a period of rapid change in the early part of this century. We are returning to a period of rapid change. . . . What is less certain is exactly where that change will lead. The task . . . is to identify and understand the forces of change and describe these forces so that [we] can make [our] decisions more wisely (Bezold, 1986).

Examples of Integrative Steps

Naturopathic medicine has accomplished important steps in integrating into mainstream delivery systems.

Reimbursement: "Every Category of Provider" Law

In 1993, during health care reform in Washington state, the "every category of provider" law was passed. This law mandated insurance companies to include access to every category of licensed provider in all types of plans in insurance systems for the treatment of all conditions covered in the Basic Health Plan. Washington State Insurance Commissioner Deborah Senn, who vigorously enforced this law, formed the Clinician Working Group on the Integration of Complementary and Alternative Medicine (CWIC), bringing together medical directors, plan representatives, and conventional and CAM providers to identify issues and solutions to integration barriers in insurance systems. This step has been important in increasing consumers' access to the health care providers of their choice, including licensed CIM/CAM professionals, as well as providing a solution focus to valid integration challenges.

Other reimbursement initiatives have also been successful. NDs throughout the United States are being integrated as primary care providers and specialists in traditional and managed care systems. The Pacific Northwest has emerged as a testing ground or model for integration because of the legislative and regulatory environment in the region.

Health Professional Loan Repayment and Scholarship Program

In 1995, Washington State's Department of Health made naturopathic physicians eligible for student loan repayment in the state's Health Professional Loan Repayment and Scholarship Program. Grants are awarded for student scholarships and student loan reimbursement to health care providers qualified and willing to provide health care in underserved areas or to underserved populations. The first and second naturopathic physician grants for loan repayment were awarded in 1998 and 2000.

King County Natural Medicine Clinic

No conventional model or infrastructure now exists in mainstream medicine for the systematic delivery of care that integrates natural and conventional providers. This integrative model is fundamental to naturopathic medicine. The King County Natural Medicine Clinic in Kent, Washington, is the first publicly funded integrative care clinic in the United States and has been a collaboration between Bastyr University and Community Health Centers of King County (CHCKC) with funding provided by the Seattle King County Department of Public Health. This project forms an unprecedented union between three health forms: conventional medicine, natural medicine, and public health. The clinic has successfully applied a co-management model by using an interdisciplinary health care team co-led by naturopathic physicians and medical doctors, including nurse practitioners, acupuncturists, and dietitians. The clinic serves the medically underserved.

The Centers for Disease Control and Prevention (CDC) and independent researchers have conducted research to study the provider-to-provider interactions and their effect on health care, patient satisfaction, and cost-effectiveness. Other studies have compared results from natural and conventional therapies on specific conditions treated using this model.

Co-Management

In *Naturopathic Medical Co-Managemet* in *The Emerging Integrative Care Model,* Milliman and Donovan (1996) describe co-management as follows:

> Naturopathic medical (co-management) is the practice of medicine by a naturopathic physician (N.D.) in concert with other care givers (N.D., M.D., D.O., L.Ac., D.C., etc.) wherein each care giver operates:
>
> • In communication with others, according to established convention
> • Within his licensed scope of practice and acknowledged domain of expertise
> • With respect for the other care giver's autonomy, but with recognition of the ultimate responsibility and, therefore, authority of the patient's primary care giver (PCP)
> • With respect for the other care giver's expertise, but with recognition of the ultimate responsibility and, therefore, final authority of the informed patient's choices and decisions.

Co-management presents an opportunity to educate other providers to naturopathic medicine as well as a chance to learn from them and expand one's information base and diagnostic and therapeutic potential. Most importantly, however, it greatly increases the therapeutic choices and quality of care to patients, often resulting in more supportive and less invasive therapies (minimizing iatrogenic diseases), while promoting healthier lifestyles and overall reduction in health-care dollars spent.

Continuous Quality Improvement

In 1996 the Washington Association of Naturopathic Physicians (WANP) developed a quality assurance program consistent with national accreditation standards. This plan, known as *Continuous Quality Improvement* (CoQI), was completed and adopted by the Washington State Department of Health and was the first naturopathic CoQI plan approved in the United States. This process is used by all health care professions and enables the profession to define and continuously update its own standards of care. Jennifer Booker and Bruce Milliman, NDs, led this effort.

Residencies

Utah is the first state to require a 1-year residency for naturopathic licensure. Residency opportunities for NDs are growing rapidly through sites established by the naturopathic colleges. Cancer Treatment Centers of America offer a growing number of residencies and staff positions to naturopathic physicians. National College of Naturopathic Medicine and Bastyr University offer a growing number of residencies throughout the United States. All naturopathic colleges also offer on-site residencies.

Hospitals and Hospital Networks

A number of hospitals across the United States continue to employ NDs as part of their physician staff in both inpatient and outpatient settings. Examples of the types of treatment centers established over the last 10 years include the following:

- HealthEast Healing Center, a clinic that is part of a larger "hospitals plus provider networks delivery system," employs MDs, an ND, an acupuncturist, and body workers, using a "learning organization" model (Alternative Medicine Integration and Coverage, 1997).
- The Alternative and Complementary Medical Program at St. Elizabeth's Hospital in Massachusetts has a credentialed ND on staff. "The hospital is a teaching center for Tufts University Medical School" (Alternative Medicine Integration and Coverage, 1998).
- Centura Health (CH), the largest health care system in Colorado, is composed of an association of Catholic and Adventist hospitals. CH owns preferred provider organization Sloans Lake Managed Care. NDs are credentialed along with ND homeopaths and many other CAM providers in this hospital-based network (Alternative Medicine Integration and Coverage, 1998).

- American Complementary Care Network (ACCN) has recently placed two NDs in key positions: Medical Director of Naturopathic Medicine and Chair of Quality Improvement (Alternative Medicine Integration and Coverage, 1998). Other networks, such as Wisconsin-based CAM Solutions and Seattle-based Alternare, have integrated ND-credentialed medical directors on staff.

When health systems, insurers, and health maintenance organizations (HMOs) decide to cover alternative medicine, NDs are sought out in licensed states. Even in states without naturopathic licensure, health systems and managed care organizations exploring integration have come to understand and value the depth of training of naturopathic physicians (Weeks, 1998).

EDUCATION

The trend of modern medical research and practice in our great colleges and endowed research institutes is almost entirely along combative lines, while the individual, progressive physician learns to work more and more along preventive lines.

—LINDLAHR (1914)

The education of the ND is extensive and incorporates much of the diversity that typifies the natural health care movement. The training program has important similarities to conventional medical education (science based, identical basic sciences, intensive clinical diagnostic sciences), with the primary differences being in the therapeutic sciences, enhanced clinical sciences, clinical theory, and integrative case management. Naturopathic training places the pathology-based training of conventional physicians into the context of the broader naturopathic assessment and management model inclusive of nature, mind, body, and spirit in health care. To be eligible to enroll, prospective students must first successfully complete a conventional premedicine program that typically requires a college degree in a biological science. The naturopathic curriculum then takes an additional 4 years to complete. Residency opportunities are increasing rapidly throughout the United States, at NCNM Bastyr and SCNM. As noted previously, residency is now required for licensure in the state of Utah.

The first 2 years concentrate on the standard human biological sciences, basic diagnostic sciences, and introduction to the various treatment modalities. The conventional basic medical sciences include anatomy, human dissection, histology, physiology, biochemistry, pathology, microbiology, immunology and infectious disease, public health, pharmacology, and biostatistics. The development of diagnostic skills is initiated with courses in physical diagnosis, laboratory diagnosis, and clinical assessment. The program also covers natural medicine subjects such as environmental health, pharmacognosy (pharmacology of herbal medicines), botanical medicine, naturopathic philosophy and case management, Chinese medicine, Ayurvedic medicine, homeopathic medicine, spinal manipulation, nutrition, physiotherapy, hydrotherapy, physician well-being, counseling and health psychology, and spirituality and health.

The second 2 years are oriented toward the clinical sciences of diagnosis and treatment while natural medicine subjects continue. Not only are the standard diagnostic techniques of physical, laboratory, and radiological examination taught, but what makes the diagnostic training unique is its emphasis on *preventive* diagnosis, such as diet analysis, recognition of the early physical signs of nutritional deficiencies, laboratory methods for assessing physiological dysfunction before it progresses to cellular pathology and end-stage disease, assessment and treatment of lifestyle and spiritual factors, and methods of assessing toxic load and liver detoxification efficacy. The natural therapies, such as nutrition, botanical medicines, homeopathy, acupuncture, natural childbirth, hydrotherapy, fasting, physical therapy, exercise therapy, counseling, and lifestyle modification, are studied extensively. Courses in naturopathic case analysis and management integrate naturopathic philosophy into conventional algorithms using the therapeutic order.

During the last 2 years, students also work in outpatient clinics, where they see patients first as observers and later as primary caregivers under the supervision of licensed NDs.

As previously mentioned, four schools currently exist in the United States and two in Canada: Bastyr University (Bastyr), National College of Naturopathic Medicine (NCNM), the Southwest College of Naturopathic Medicine and Health Sciences (Southwest), the University of Bridgeport College of Naturopathic

Medicine (UBCNM), and in Canada, the Canadian College of Naturopathic Medicine (CCNM) and the Boucher Institute of Naturopathic Medicine. The oldest institution is NCNM, which was established in 1965, in Portland, Oregon. The largest institution and first to receive accreditation is Bastyr University, established in Seattle, Washington, in 1978. Over the years Bastyr has broadened its mission to also include accredited degree and certificate programs in nutrition, acupuncture and Chinese medicine, midwifery, applied behavioral sciences, health psychology, exercise and spirituality and health. Southwest College, established in 1993, has developed an active research department. The University of Bridgeport, established in 1997, is the most recent addition. Like its counterparts in the United States, CCNM in Toronto, Ontario, has a rapidly increasing enrollment. Naturopathic education is accredited by the U.S. Department of Education–recognized Council on Naturopathic Medical Education (CNME). The CNME has granted institutional accreditation to NCNM and accreditation of the Naturopathic Medicine program at Bastyr (Bastyr and NCNM are also accredited by the Northwest Commission on Colleges and Universities), and Southwest is accredited by the North Central Association of Schools and Colleges. All states licensing naturopathic physicians recognize the CNME as the official accrediting agency for naturopathic medicine. The offices of the CNME are located in Portland, Oregon.

RESEARCH

Science clearly is an essential condition of a right decision.

—PELLEGRINO (1979)

However, clinical decisions cannot be solely dependent on science, when, with the best of efforts and with billions of public and private dollars spent, medical research has yielded twenty percent (and in some narrow areas up to fifty percent) of medical procedures and practices as scientifically proven and efficacious.

—OFFICE OF TECHNOLOGY ASSESSMENT (1978)

There is a paucity of theories of medicine. . . . The theory of medicine has lagged seriously behind theories of other sciences . . . any unitary theory of medicine which identifies it exclusively with science is doomed to failure.

—PELLEGRINO (1979)

The primary intellectual problem facing medicine today is that the information base of medicine is so poor. For a profession with a 2,000 year history which is responsible in the United States for 250 million lives and spends over $600 billion a year, we are astonishingly ignorant. We simply do not know the consequences of a large proportion of medical activities. The . . . task is to change our mind set about what constitutes an acceptable source of knowledge in medicine.

—EDDY (1993)

The relationship between scientific research and the study of the healing power of nature, a traditionally vitalistic principle, is important. The scientific method is a well-accepted approach to communicating what we learn about medicine's mysteries to others; however, it has been limited in its development by conventional medicine's approach to research. Orthodox research appears to turn on the premise that the universe functions without *telos*, or purpose. Connections are mechanistic. Clinical relevance is directed toward pharmaceutical disease management by means of a single-agent, placebo-controlled, double-blind crossover trial.

What distinguishes naturopathic medicine's clinical research from that of biomedicine (a term coined to refer to the currently dominant school of medicine) is not the presence or lack of science. It is a collective confidence in the perception of a vital force or life force. The arguments then follow. What is it? What exactly does it do and how? As Dr. John Bastyr noted, "We all have an innate ability to understand that there is a moving force in us, that doesn't necessarily need to be understood mechanistically" (interview, August 1989). Future scientific work and naturopathic medical research on this principle is bound by the shared perception (1) that there is a pattern in health and disease; (2) that there is order in the healing process; and (3) that order is based on the life force, which is self-organized, intelligent, and intelligible. Within this paradigm, we can research the life force.

Confirming and challenging clinical perceptions and even disproving core assumptions is fundamental to naturopathic medicine's core values. Scientific methods must be challenged to find new approaches to test large quantities and types of clinical data, outcomes, and systems from naturopathic practices. So far, the actuality of the "healing power of nature" (*vis medicatrix naturae*) has not been proved or disproved by the single-agent double-blind study. New models (e.g., outcomes research, field and practice-based research, multifactorial models) provide fertile ground for researching the validity of nonconventional medicine and offer new opportunities for research on conventional practices.

Until recently, original research at naturopathic institutions has been quite limited. The profession has relied on its clinical traditions and the worldwide published scientific research, as follows:

Research in whole practices are only recently gaining interest with the development of methodologies in practice-based and outcomes research. There is a lack of research in whole practices like naturopathy, Oriental medicine, or Ayurveda compared to conventional practice whether in a particular disease or in overall health outcomes. Biomedical research methods which are considered gold-standard by the scientific community have been typically developed to provide reliable data on a single therapeutic intervention for a specific Western disease entity. The requirements of these research methods distort naturopathic practice and may render it apparently less effective than it may actually be. The measures may not take account of residual benefits in a patient's other health problems nor on future health and health care utilization.

Compounding the methodological difficulties of research in this medical variant, there are structural obstacles as well. Distinct from the situation in conventional medicine, there is only the beginning of a research infrastructure at the profession's academic centers. Practitioners expert in naturopathic medicine and the individualization of treatment are typically not trained in rigorous comparative trials. Even if the infrastructure and training were in place, sources of funding remain few and small, and most funding agencies make their decisions on the basis of biomedical theories which naturopathy may directly challenge. When research is done on aspects of naturopathic treatment, more studies are done on substances rather than procedures or lifestyle changes. Without the economic incentives which favor the in-depth study of patentable drugs, trials in naturopathic therapeutics, often derived from a long history of human use, are smaller and with fewer replications. Many practices present special methodological or ethical problems for control, randomization, blinding, etc., perhaps making it impossible to perform a study as rigorous as some might wish. Nevertheless, there are numerous studies which yield indications of the effectiveness of individual treatments (Calabrese et al., 1997).

As mentioned earlier, a comprehensive compilation of the scientific documentation of naturopathic philosophy and therapies can be found in *A Textbook of Natural Medicine,* coauthored and edited by Joseph Pizzorno, ND, and Michael Murray, ND. First published in 1985, the *Textbook* was, until 1998, in a looseleaf, two-volume set, published by Bastyr University Publications and updated regularly. The 2006 edition (Churchill Livingstone) consists of more than 220 chapters and references more than 9,000 citations from the peer-reviewed scientific literature. It addresses the philosophy and clinical theories of naturopathic medicine.

In the past 15 years, Bastyr University, NCNM, and Southwest have developed active research departments that have resulted in the publication of original research in several peer-reviewed journals, both alternative and mainstream. In 1994, Bastyr University was awarded a 3-year, $840,000 grant by the NIH Office of Alternative and Complementary Medicine to establish a research center to study alternative therapies for human immunodeficiency virus and acquired immunodeficiency syndrome (HIV/AIDS). Eleven other centers were established in conventional medical schools. The Bastyr group lead by Leanna Standish, ND completed a text on alternative therapies in HIV/AIDS for this series *Medical Guides to Complementary and Alternative Medicine.* The profession published a peer-reviewed journal, the *Journal of Naturopathic Medicine,* founded in 1990 by Peter D'Adamo, ND, of Norwalk, Connecticut, through 1997. It has been succeeded by the *International Journal of Naturopathic Medicine,* founded in 2004.

THE FUTURE

We could have a significant and immediate impact on costly health care problems if the complementary and alternative medicine disciplines and interventions were widely available.

—DOSSEY AND SWYERS (1992)

Naturopathic medicine is enabling patients to regain their health as NDs effectively co-manage and integrate care with pertinent providers, to their patients' and the public's benefit. Today's ND, an extensively trained and state-licensed family physician, is equipped with a broad range of conventional and unconventional diagnostic and therapeutic skills. This modern ND considers himself or herself an integral part of the health care system and takes a full share of responsibility for common public health issues. NDs are healers and scientists, policy makers, and teachers and are active in industry and environmental issues.

The scientific tools now exist to assess and appreciate many aspects of naturopathy's approach to health and healing. Conventional medical organizations that spoke out strongly against naturopathic medicine in the past now often endorse such techniques as lifestyle modification, stress reduction, exercise, consumption of a high-fiber diet rich in whole foods, other dietary measures, supplemental nutrients, and toxin reduction.

These changes in perspective signal the paradigm shift that is occurring in medicine. Emerging knowledge, high health care costs, and unmet health care needs continue to force this shift in perspective into changes in our current health care system. What was once rejected is now becoming generally accepted as effective. In many situations, it is now recognized that naturopathic alternatives offer benefit over certain orthodox practices. In the future, more concepts and practices of naturopathic medicine will undoubtedly be assessed and integrated into mainstream health care.

Historically, emerging bodies of knowledge in health care have formed into schools of thought and professions (with standards) as the public's need for their services increased. Naturopathic medicine's reemergence is no accident or anomaly. Naturopathic medicine has followed the developmental stages that health care professions typically undergo while becoming accountable to the public. Access has increased with increasing research, conceptual unity, and standards.

These models and standards in emerging CIM/CAM fields, including naturopathic medicine, hold answers to issues in health care, its delivery, and the health care system that are as significant as the interventions. With accreditation, licensure, reimbursement, ongoing research, and widespread public acceptance, the naturopathic clinical model is reaching professional maturity today.

References

Belizan J, Villar J, Pineda O, et al: Reduction of blood pressure with calcium supplementation in young adults, *JAMA* 249:1161-1165, 1983.

Bensoussan A, Myers S: *Towards a safer choice: the practice of traditional Chinese medicine in Australia,* Macarthur, Australia, 1996, Faculty of Health, University of Western Sydney, pp 20, 82, 109.

Bezold C: Health trends and scenarios: implications for the health care professions, *Am Ent Inst Stud Health Policy* 449:77-97, 1986.

Blois M: Medicine and the nature of vertical reasoning, *N Engl J Med* 318(13):847-851, 1988.

Bradley R: Philosophy of naturopathic medicine. In *Textbook of natural medicine,* Seattle, 1985, John Bastyr College Publications.

Calabrese C, Breed C, Ruhland J: The effectiveness of naturopathic medicine in disease conditions. Presented at State of the Science in Naturopathic Medicine, Annual AANP Convention, 1997.

Clarke E, Hatcher J, McKeown-Essyen G, Liekrish G: Cervical dysplasia: association with sexual behavior, smoking, and oral contraceptive use, *Am J Obstet Gynecol* 151:612-616, 1985.

Cooper R, Stoflet S: Trends in the education and practice of alternative medicine clinicians, *Health Affairs* 15.3:226, 233, 1996.

Dawson E, Nosovitch J, Hannigan E: Serum vitamin and selenium changes in cervical dysplasia, *Fed Proc* 46:612, 1984.

Dossey L, Swyers J: *Alternative medicine expanding medical horizons,* Washington, DC, 1992, US Government Printing Office.

Dyckner T, Wester O: Effect of magnesium on blood pressure, *BMJ* 286:1847-1849, 1983.

Eddy D: Decisions without information, *HMO Pract* 5(2):58-60, 1993.

Eddy MB: *Science and health with key to the scriptures,* 1875.

Felter HW, Lloyd JU: *King's American dispensary,* 1898.

Ford M: Biofeedback treatment for headaches, Raynaud's disease, essential hypertension, and irritable bowel syndrome: a review of the long-term follow-up literature, *Biof Self-Reg* 7:521-535, 1982.

Fries E: Salt, volume and the prevention of hypertension, *Circulation* 53:589-595, 1976.

Funk J: Naturopathic and allopathic healing: a developmental comparison, *Townsend Lett Doctors Patients,* October 1995, pp 50-58.

Gaby A: Commentary on migraine, 1998 (Unpublished paper).

Glauser S, Bello C, Gauser E: Blood-cadmium levels in normotensive and untreated hypertensive humans, *Lancet* 1:717-718, 1976.

Gruchow HW, Sobocinski MS, Barboriak JJ: Alcohol, nutrient intake, and hypertension in US adults, *JAMA* 253:1567-1570, 1985.

Grumbach K: Chronic illness, comorbidities, and the need for medical generalism, *Ann Fam Med* 1:4-7, 2003.

Harel Z, Gascon G, Riggs S, et al: Supplementation with omega-3 polyunsaturated fatty acids in the management of recurrent migraines in adolescents, *J Adolesc Health* 31:154-161, 2002.

Havlik R, Hubert H, Fabsitz R, Feinleib M: Weight and hypertension, *Ann Intern Med* 98:855-859, 1983.

Hodges R, Rebello T: Carbohydrates and blood pressure, *Ann Intern Med* 98:838-841, 1983.

John JH, Ziebland S, Yudkin P, et al: Effects of fruit and vegetable consumption on plasma antioxidant concentrations and blood pressure: a randomised controlled trial, *Lancet* 359:1969-1974, 2002.

Johnson S: The multifaceted and widespread pathology of magnesium deficiency, *Med Hypotheses* 56:163-170, 2001.

Kershbaum A, Pappajohn D, Bellet S, et al: Effect of smoking and nicotine on adrenocortical secretion, *JAMA* 203:113-116, 1968.

Khaw KT, Barrett-Connor: Dietary potassium and blood pressure in a population, *Am J Clin Nutr* 39:963-968, 1984.

Kirchfield F, Boyle W: *Nature doctors,* Portland, Ore, East Palestine, Ohio, 1994, Medicina Biological/Buckeye Naturopathic Press, p 311.

Kirschner R, Brinkman R: American Association of Naturopathic Medicine Conference, Select Committee on Definition of Naturoapathic Medicine, Billings, Mont, 1988.

Kuts-Cheraux AW: *Naturae medicina,* Des Moines, Iowa, 1953, ANPSA.

Lang T, Degoulet P, Aime F, et al: Relationship between coffee drinking and blood pressure: analysis of 6,321 subjects in the Paris region, *Am J Cardiol* 52:1238-1242, 1983.

Levenduski P: Testimony to US Department of Education, Washington, DC, 1991, National Advisory Committee on Accreditation and Institutional Eligibility (CNME hearing).

Lindlahr H: *Nature cure,* 1914a.

Lindlahr H. Philosophy of natural therapeutics. Vols I, II, and III. *Dietetics,* Maidstone, England, 1914b, Maidstone Osteopathic.

Lust B: *The naturopathic and herald of health,* 1896.

Lust B: *Universal naturopathic directory and buyer's guide,* Butler, NJ, 1918, Lust Publications.

Lust B: Program, 49th Congress of American Naturopathy Association, 1945.

Mauskop A, Altura BT, Cracco RQ, Altura BM. Intravenous magnesium sulfate rapidly alleviates headaches of various types. *Headache* 36:154-60, 1996.

McCarron D, Morris C, Cole C: Dietary calcium in human hypertension, *Science* 217:267-269, 1982.

Meneely G, Battarbee hd: High sodium–low potassium environment and hypertension, *Am J Cardiol* 38:768-781, 1976.

Milliman B, Donovan P: *Naturopathic medical co-management* in *The emerging integrative care model: the best of naturo-*

pathic medicine anthology, Tucson, 1996, Southwest College Press.

Natero G et al: Dietary migraine: fact or fiction? *Headache* 29:315-316, 1989.

Office of Technology Assessment, Washington, DC, 1978, US Department of Commerce National Technical Information Service.

Orr J, Wilson K, Bodiford C, et al: Nutritional status of patients with untreated cervical cancer. II. Vitamin assessment, *Am J Obstet Gynecol* 151:632-635, 1985.

Orzack L: Professions and world trade diplomacy: national systems and international authority. In. *Professions, identity, and order in comparative perspective.* Edited by Vittorio Olgiati, Louis H. Orzack, and Mike Saks. Onati, Spain: Onati Institute for International Study of the Sociology of Law (IISL), 1998.

Pellegrino E: Medicine, science, art: an old controversy revisited, *Man Med* 4:43-52, 1979.

Pizzorno J: Editorial, *Integr Med Clinician J* 2:4, 2003.

Pizzorno JE, Murray MT: *A textbook of natural medicine,* Seattle, 1985-95, John Bastyr College Publications.

Pizzorno LE: Using your mind as healer, *Delicious!,* 1995.

Pizzorno L: The roots of herbalism in America. *Delicious!,* June 1997.

Pruess HG: Overview of lead toxicity in early life: effects on intellect loss and hypertension, *J Am Coll Nutr* 11:608, 1992.

Ramaswamy P, Natarajan R: Vitamin B_6 status in patients with cancer of the uterine cervix, *Nutr Cancer* 6:176-180, 1984.

Rao R, Rao U, Srikantia S: Effect of polyunsaturated vegetable oils on blood pressure in essential hypertension, *Clin Exp Hyperten* 3:27-38, 1981.

Resnick LM, Gupta RK, Laragh JH: Intracellular free magnesium in erythrocytes of essential hypertension: relationship to blood pressure and serum divalent cations, *Proc Natl Acad Sci USA* 81:6511-6515, 1989.

Romney S, Duttagupta C, Basu J, et al: Plama vitamin C and uterine dysplasia, *Am J Obstet Gynecol* 151:978-980, 1985.

Sarchielli P et al: Serum and salivary magnesium levels in migraine and tension-type headaches: results in a group of adult patients, *Cephalgia* 12:21-27, 1992.

Snider P, Zeff J: Select Committee on Definition of Naturopathic Medicine report, House of Delegates, Portland, Ore, 1988, 1989, American Association of Naturopathic Physicians.

Spitler HR: *Basic naturopathy,* Des Moines, Iowa, 1948, American Naturopathic Association.

Standish L, Snider P, Calabrese C, NMRA Core Team: The future and foundations of naturopathic medical science, Report to NIHCCAM on Naturopathic Medical Research Agenda (NMRA), 2004.

Van Niekerk W: Cervical cytological abnormalities caused by folic acid deficiency, *Acta Cytol* 10:67-73, 1966.

Vergroesen A, Fleischman A, Comberg H, et al: The influence of increased dietary linoleate on essential hypertension in man, *Acta Biol Med Germ Band* 37:879-883, 1978.

Weaver K: Magnesium and Migraine. *Headache* 30:168, 1990.

Weeks J: Personal communication, August 1998.

Werbach M: *The American Holistic Health Association complete guide to alternative medicine,* New York, 1996, Werner Books, pp 118, 123.

Whorton J: *Crusaders for fitness,* Princeton, NJ, 1982, Princeton University Press.

Woodcock BE, Smith E, Lambert WH, et al: Beneficial effect of fish oil on blood viscosity in peripheral vascular disease, *BMJ* 288:592-594, 1984.

Yoshioka M, Matsushita T, Chuman Y: Inverse association of serum ascorbic acid level and blood pressure or rate of hypertension in male adults aged 30-39 years, *Int J Vit Nutr Res* 54:343-347, 1981.

Zeff J: The process of healing: a unifying theory of naturopathic medicine, *J Naturopath Med* 7(1):122, 1997.

Zeff J: *J Naturopath Med* 8(1):90, 1998.

Zeff J, Snider P, and Myers A. A hierarchy of healing: the therapeutic order—the unifying theory of naturopathic medicine. In. Pizzorno J and Murray M. *Textbook of natural medicine.* St. Louis, 2006, Churchill Livingstone.

Suggested Readings

Beasley JD, Swift JJ: *The impact of nutrition, environment and lifestyle on the health of Americans,* Annandale-on-Hudson, NY, 1989, The Kellogg Report.

Benjamin H: *Everybody's guide to nature cure,* ed 7, England, 1981, Thorsons.

Bilz FE: *The natural method of healing.* Vols 1 and 2, New York, 1898, International News.

Brown D: *Quarterly Review of Natural Medicine,* Seattle, 1994, NPRC.

Coulter H: *Divided legacy.* Vol II, Washington, DC, 1973, Wehawken Books.

Dejarnette MB: *Technic & practice of bloodless surgery,* Nebraska City, 1939, (Private).

Dossey, L: *Healing Words,* New York, 1997, HarperCollins Publishers.

Filden JH: *Impaired health (its cause & cure),* ed 2, Denver, 1921, (Private).

Garlic has to smell bad to do some good, *Fam Pract News* 22:31, 1992.

Graham RL: *Hydro-hygiene,* New York, 1923, Thompson-Barlow.

Griggs B: *Green pharmacy,* London 1981, Jill, Norman, & Hobhouse.

Hofoss D, Hjort P: The relationship between action and research in health policy, *J Soc Sci Med* 15A:371. 1981

Johnson AC: *Principles & practice of drugless therapeutics,* Los Angeles, 1946, Chir Ed Extension Bureau.

Jones D: Functional medicine application to disorders of gene expression, Fifth International Symposium on Functional Medicine, Hawaii, 1998.

Kellogg JF: *Rational hydrotherapy,* Battle Creek, Mich, 1901, 1902.

Kellogg JH: *New dietetics,* Battle Creek, Mich, 1923, Modern Medical Publishing.

Kuhne L: *Neo-naturopathy (new science of healing),* Butler, NJ, 1918, Lust Publishers (Translated by B Lust).

Lindlahr H: Philosophy, practice, and dietetics of natural therapeutics. Vols I and II, Maidstone, England, 1914-1919, Maidstone Osteopathic.

Lust B: *Universal directory of naturopathy,* Butler, NJ, 1918, Lust Publishers.

MacFadden B: *Building of vital power,* New Jersey, 1904, Physical Culture Publishing.

McKeown T: *The role of medicine: dream, mirage, or nemesis?* London, 1976, Nuffield Provincial Hospitals Trust.

Murray MT: *Natural alternatives to over-the-counter and prescription drugs,* New York, 1994, William Morrow.

Murray MT, Pizzorno JE: *Encyclopedia of natural medicine,* Rocklin, Calif, 1991, Prima Publishing.

Neuberger M: The doctrine of the healing power of nature throughout the course of time, *J Am Inst Homeopath* 25:861-884, 1011-1465, 1932 (Translated by LJ Boyd).

Petkov V: Plants with hypotensive, antiatheromatous and coronary dilating action, *Am J Chin Med* 7:197-236, 1979.

Pizzorno J: *Total wellness,* Rocklin, Calif, 1998, Prima Publishing, p 14.

Pizzorno J, Murray M: *Textbook of naturopathic medicine,* New York, 1999, Churchill Livingstone.

Richter JT: *Nature—the healer,* Los Angeles 1949, (Private).

Riley JS: *Zone reflex,* Washington, DC, 1924, Publications of Health Research.

Shelton H: *Natural hygiene, man's pristine way of life,* San Antonio, 1968, Dr Shelton's Health School, p 8.

St. Anthony's Business Report on Alternative and Complementary Medicine, May 1997, p 5.

St. Anthony's Business Report on Alternative and Complementary Medicine, July 1998, pp 6-7.

St. Anthony's Business Report on Alternative and Complementary Medicine, August 1998, pp 4-5.

Starr P: *Social transformation of American medicine,* New York, 1983, Basic Books.

Trall RT: *Hydropathic encyclopedia* (3 vols), New York, 1880, SR Wells.

Weltmer E: *Practice of suggestive therapeutics,* Nevada, Mo, 1913, Weltmer Institute.

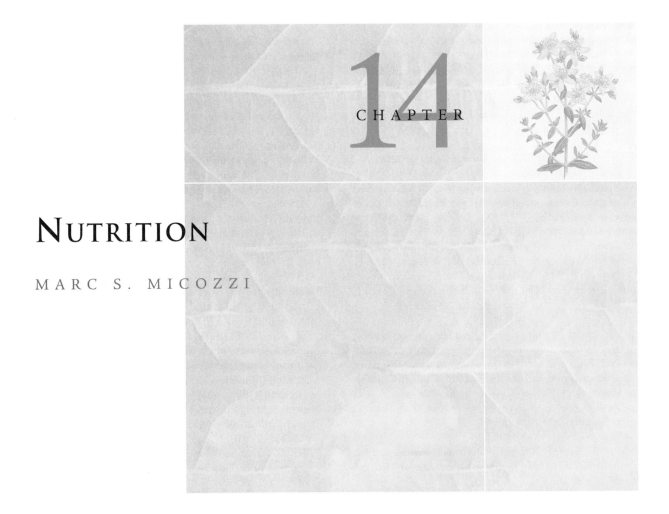

NUTRITION

MARC S. MICOZZI

People eat food, not nutrients. When we rummage through the refrigerator for a snack or cruise the supermarket aisles trying to decide what to fix for dinner, our choices are much more likely to reflect cultural, social, and family patterns than to be based on the federal government's food pyramid and recommended daily allowances.

Food has powerful symbolic meaning and has played a key role in our religious and social rituals for thousands of years. From birthday cake to the bitter herbs of the Passover seder to Thanksgiving turkey to communion wafers, food helps form our social bonds, express our spirituality, and define who we are. Rituals remain powerful even when we no longer recall their origins. For example, Christians worldwide celebrate Easter by eating colored eggs, although few could explain the connection between hard-boiled eggs and Jesus' resurrection.

Substances can have radically different meanings for different groups. For Muslims, Christian Scientists, and members of Alcoholics Anonymous, wine is strictly "taboo," whereas for Catholics, wine is part of a sacrament that is by definition "an outward sign instituted by Christ to give grace." Individuals also bring very different perspectives to the table. For some vegetarians, chicken soup represents cruelty to animals, whereas for many other people, it recalls Mom's tender care during childhood illnesses.

An intellectual understanding of what constitutes good nutrition is no match for the powerful psychological, social, and spiritual forces that have been shaping human eating habits since the Stone Age.

EATING HABITS OF EARLY HUMANS

Humans are omnivores; we can eat almost everything found in nature, and with a few exceptions (e.g., wood, grass), we can extract nutrition from whatever we consume. For hundreds of thousands of years, our early ancestors roamed the forests and plains as hunter-gatherers. The hunters brought home very lean meat; wild game has only 4% to 6% body fat versus the 40% to 60% body fat found in modern domesticated animals. The gatherers collected plants that were high in fiber and complex carbohydrates and provided many necessary vitamins. These early humans obtained calcium from animal bones and other minerals from the dirt that inevitably clung to wild plants and game.

Life was a constant struggle to obtain enough fat and calories, and our ancestors developed a decided preference for foods that tasted rich in these needed nutrients. In the small, hunter-gatherer tribes, food was often allocated on the basis of social status, gender, and age, providing it with significance beyond the satisfaction of hunger. When agriculture was developed 10,500 years ago, diets became more stable. Seasonal crops led to seasonal feasts, adding another layer of cultural meaning to food consumption.

Although even the earliest farmers sought to improve their crops genetically—for example, selecting and sowing the seeds of wheat that had stronger stalks and quicker, more uniform germination—the quality of food did not change much. Humans learned to use yeast (made from microbes, which had been present on the planet for millions of years) to produce bread, beer, and wine; other microbes were used to make cheese and yogurt. These microbes made certain plants and dairy products easier (and more enjoyable) to consume and digest, but humans were still eating the diet that their digestive system and metabolism were designed for: low in fat and high in protein, complex carbohydrates, and fiber, with no refined sugar. Everything in the human diet remained completely natural . . . until modern times.

MODERN ERA: FOOLING MOTHER NATURE

Fast-forwarding to the twentieth century, we find a very different picture of food production and consumption. Early in the century, advances in biochemistry allowed scientists to isolate some of the active ingredients in food. In 1928, for example, it was discovered that limes, the British Navy's traditional method of preventing scurvy, worked by providing sailors with vitamin C. Unfortunately, while vitamin C supplements proved easier to store and dispense, they did not provide the full benefits of the fruit. Later research disclosed that lime pulp contains *bioflavonoids*, which are necessary for absorbing and processing vitamin C. Bioflavonoids also help maintain collagen and capillary walls and protect against infection and cancer. Scientists were discovering that replacing natural products with artificial ones did not always improve on the original.

However, this finding did not stop scientists from trying to improve on nature. Currently, modern technology and agribusiness have "improved" crops by covering them with artificial chemicals, including pesticides, fungicides, ripening agents, and fumigants, all of which make them more efficient to grow, ship, and store. Genetic engineering has changed the biological structure of many plants in ways not yet fully understood. Some plants are irradiated (flooded with "harmless" radiation) to lengthen their shelf life. Animals destined for the table are dosed with antibiotics to prevent disease and with hormones to make them fat and juicy.

Once vegetables, fruit, milk, meat, and eggs leave the farm, they are often "processed" into "food products," such as canned soup and frozen dinners. Processed foods are generally high in fat, salt, and sugar; are lower in nutrients than fresh foods; and contain a host of chemicals to boost flavor, color, texture, and shelf life. Consider the following:

- Pounds of sugar the average American consumed per year in the nineteenth century: less than 10
- Pounds of sugar the average American consumes per year today: 150

Among the many artificial substances used in processed foods are such synthetic sweeteners as aspartame, silicon dioxide, phenylalanine, tribasic calcium phosphate, benzosulfimide, and calcium silicate. The effects of all these chemicals on our bodies are not entirely known, but saccharin, the first widely used artificial sweetener, was shown to cause cancer in laboratory animals. Aspartame (NutraSweet) is now being studied for possible neurological effects. Large quantities of one of its ingredients, methanol, have been shown to cause blindness, brain swelling, and inflammation of the pancreas and heart muscle.

In addition to pseudosugars, we now have "fake fats." Partially hydrogenated oil does not occur in nature but in the laboratory, when liquid vegetable fats are turned into solids by pumping them with hydrogen. This makes them more like animal fats in taste and feel, as well as in their harmful effects on the cardiovascular system; in fact, partially hydrogenated fats have been associated with higher cancer rates than saturated fats. *Trans*-fatty acids (TFAs) are formed when unsaturated fatty acids (the building blocks of fat) are deformed by certain heat or chemical treatments. These deformed fats may be toxic. TFAs in the diet may damage the regulatory machinery of the body, significantly compromising health. Despite these concerns, partially hydrogenated oils and TFAs are found in a wide range of processed foods, including almost all margarines, mass-produced breads, convenience foods, and junk foods, as well as some baby foods.

For a variety of reasons, including productivity, efficiency, convenience, profit, arrogance, and curiosity, we have found abundant ways to change the nature of our diets and the nature of the animals and plants that feed us. As a nation, the U.S. population eats high on the food chain, consuming unprecedented amounts of meat, chicken, fish, dairy products, fat, salt, and sugar. We cover our food with artificial chemicals while it is grown, processed, preserved, and genetically altered in ways that have only recently been introduced on this planet. After hundreds of thousands of years of evolution, during which our bodies became perfectly adapted to drawing nutrition from the natural environment, we have suddenly introduced large quantities of new, artificial substances into our diets, hoping to improve on nature.

How have these "advances" affected our health?

DISEASES OF AFFLUENCE

We have become a nation in which one third of the U.S. population is significantly overweight, and more than one quarter—24% of adult males, 27% of adult females, and 27% of children—are obese. Although this is caused by a variety of factors, ranging from genetics to the introduction of the car (reducing the necessity to move around) and television (reducing the desire to move around), a clear and direct correlation exists between food consumption and excess body weight.

Research has shown an equally clear and direct connection between excess body weight and illness, especially the leading killers in the United States: cardiovascular disease and cancer. Today, 60 million Americans have cardiovascular disease, including high blood pressure, heart disease, and stroke. This year, cardiovascular disease will kill about 1 million Americans, more than 2600 a day, or one death every 33 seconds. Another 1.2 million people will be diagnosed with cancer this year, and almost 600,000 will die of it. Thousands more will suffer from other diseases related to diet: diabetes, gallbladder disease, respiratory disease, sleep apnea, gout, osteoporosis, and a host of other conditions.

For more than a century, the United States Department of Agriculture (USDA) has been trying to improve our eating habits by issuing dietary recommendations. It currently spends $333.3 million per year educating the public about what we should and should not consume and in what quantities (USDA, 1997, 1999). That seems a great expenditure until we consider that America's food manufacturers spend that amount promoting snacks and nuts; their total annual advertising budget is more than $7 billion, most of which is spent promoting highly processed, packaged foods. The fast-paced American lifestyle relies on these convenience foods and on restaurant and take-out fare. We now spend 45% of our food dollars on away-from-home meals and snacks, most of which are higher in fat, salt, and sugar and lower in fiber and calcium than meals prepared at home.

According to the USDA's *Healthy Eating Index*, some small improvements have been made in the American diet. On a scale of 1 to 100, the average U.S. score rose from 61.5 in 1990 to 63.8 in 1995, but it still falls far short of the 80 or above that marks a good diet. Put another way, Americans are earning about a C– in healthy eating practices.

Box 14-1 lists trends in American eating habits in the twentieth century.

WHAT SHOULD WE BE EATING?

Most Americans know (but don't necessarily act on) the basic facts: a healthy diet includes lots of fresh, unprocessed fruits, vegetables, and grains; modest amounts of protein and fat; and very little white sugar and salt. The question of precisely how much of each type of food we need, however, becomes more complicated.

All food provides energy, which is measured in units called *calories*. Nutritionists generally recommend daily intake of 1600 calories for older adults and sedentary women; 2200 calories for children, teenage girls, active women, and sedentary men; and 2800 calories for teenage boys, active men, and very active women. Calories are taken into our bodies as carbohydrates, proteins, and fats (which are known as *macronutrients,* or major constituents of diet). We also require vitamins and minerals (which are effective in small amounts and thus known as *micronutrients*) to process these nutrients and maintain body functions.

Nutritionists, physicians, research scientists, alternative practitioners, food manufacturers, and consumers hold differing views about what percentage of calories we should obtain from each macronutrient. People favoring a largely vegetarian, low-fat diet tend to recommend that we receive about 15% of our calories from protein, 60% from carbohydrates, and 25% from fats. Proponents of high-protein diets often advocate 30% protein, 40% carbohydrates, and 30% fats. The food pyramid, developed by the U.S. Department of Health and Human Services and USDA, sug- gests that we use fat "sparingly" and that our daily fare include 2 to 3 servings of dairy products; 2 to 3 servings of meat, poultry, fish, eggs, beans, and nuts; 3 to 5 servings of vegetables; 2 to 4 servings of fruit; and 6 to 11 servings of bread, cereal, rice, and pasta (Box 14-2).

Although these numbers may provide useful guidelines, they do not address one crucial factor: the *quality* of nutrients in each category. The food

BOX 14-1

American Eating Habits: 1900 to 1980

- Fresh fruit and vegetable consumption drops from 40% to 5% of the diet.
- Sugar consumption rises 50%.
- Beef consumption rises 50%.
- Fat and oil consumption rises 150%.
- Cheese consumption rises 400%.
- Margarine consumption rises 800%.

BOX 14-2

The Changing Shape of U.S. Government Guidelines

Over the years, the U.S. Department of Agriculture has revised its diet recommendations in response to research findings and new concepts of nutrition.

1946 to 1958: the "Basic 7" Daily Food Guide
- Leafy, green, and yellow vegetables: 1 or more servings
- Citrus fruit, tomatoes, raw cabbage: 1 or more servings
- Potatoes and other vegetables and fruits: 2 or more servings
- Milk, cheese, ice cream: children, 1 to 4 cups of milk; adults, 2 or more cups
- Meat, poultry, fish, eggs, dried peas, beans: 1 to 2 servings
- Bread, cereal, flour: 2 or more servings
- Butter and fortified margarine: 2 tablespoons

1958 to 1979: Four Basic Food Groups (per day, for adults)
- Milk group: 2 or more cups
- Meat group: 2 or more servings
- Vegetable and fruit group: 4 or more servings
- Bread and cereal group: 4 or more servings

1979 to 2005 the Food Pyramid (per day)
- Fats, oils, sweets: use sparingly
- Milk, yogurt, cheese: 3 to 5 servings
- Dry beans, nuts, seeds, eggs, meat: 2 to 3 servings
- Vegetables: 3 to 5 servings
- Fruits: 2 to 4 servings
- Bread, cereal, rice, pasta: 6 to 11 servings

2005 MyPyramid
- Customized based on personal characteristics
- Personal plans available at www.mypyraimid.gov

pyramid, which recommends 6 to 11 servings of grain-based foods, fails to distinguish, for example, between the empty calories of frozen waffles, which are composed primarily of white sugar and white flour, and a bowl of whole-grain cereal. It encourages us to use fats "sparingly" but advocates 2 or 3 helpings of cheese and whole milk, which contain at least 8 grams (g) of fat per serving, plus up to 3 servings of meat, which can contain up to 26 g of fat per serving. Is a "Whopper" (40 g of fat) part of a healthy diet? Are PopTarts (20 g of white sugar) giving us the right kind of energy to start the day?

Clearly the numbers alone do not tell the whole story. All carbohydrates are not created equal, nor does everyone need the same amount of them, or of any given nutrient. Our food needs are influenced by many factors, such as age, gender, body size, activity level, and reproductive status, and will change over time. To determine what type of diet is best for our bodies at different stages of our lives, we need some understanding of how the nutrients in food enable our bodies to function.

Carbohydrates

Carbohydrates provide large amounts of quick energy. We obtain carbohydrates from fruits, vegetables, beans, grains, and other plant materials, as well as from dairy products. Our bodies easily transform carbohydrates into *glucose* (blood sugar), which the body needs for fuel, and into *glycogen*, a form of sugar that can be stored in the liver and muscles until needed, then transformed into glucose.

There are two types of carbohydrates: simple and complex. *Simple* carbohydrates, or simple sugars, include white table sugar (sucrose), the sugar in fruit (fructose), and the sugar in milk (lactose). In *complex* carbohydrates, such as whole grains, beans, and vegetables, the sugar molecules are linked together in longer, more complicated chains.

Both types of carbohydrates become blood sugar, but the simple sugars are converted more quickly, elevating insulin levels and providing a "sugar rush" that quickly abates, often leading to feelings of tiredness. Complex carbohydrates are metabolized more slowly, providing a sustained supply of energy. One complex carbohydrate has a different role; fiber is not absorbed into the body at all but helps with digestive and bowel function. One of the disadvan-

tages of an overprocessed, highly refined diet is that foods tend to linger in the body, which can allow carcinogens (cancer-causing substances) to be absorbed or produced by the body. Fiber in the diet has been shown to reduce constipation, which decreases the risk of colon, breast, and other cancers; it also shrinks intestinal polyps (growths), which can lead to cancers. About 25 g of fiber a day is usually sufficient and will occur naturally in a diet that includes a good supply of complex carbohydrates.

Proteins

Protein is essential for the growth, maintenance, and repair of every cell in the body and for the production of hormones, antibodies, and digestive enzymes. When we consume dietary protein, we break it down into amino acids, which are the building blocks we need to make our own proteins.

There are two types of dietary proteins: complete and incomplete. *Complete* proteins, which are found in meat, poultry, fish, eggs, dairy products, and soybeans, provide the full range of essential amino acids we need. *Incomplete* proteins, which include some but not all needed amino acids, are found in grains, beans, nuts, seeds, and leafy green vegetables. However, incomplete proteins can be combined to provide the full range of amino acids our bodies require. For example, brown rice served with beans, nuts, or seeds forms a whole protein.

Protein cannot be stored in the body for future use, so we need to replenish our supply every day. Most Americans consume twice the protein we need. When we take in more than the body can use, the excess is either burned off as energy or stored in the body as fat.

Fats

Fat is the most concentrated form of energy available to us and is necessary for growth and healthy function. As babies and children, we needed fat for brain development. As adults, many of us consume more than we need, leading to weight gain and a national obsession about staying thin, especially for women. Conflicting cultural pressures make it difficult to obtain a realistic picture of the amount and types of fat we need.

Our body's fats are made up of fatty acids, which come in three major types: saturated, polyunsaturated, and monounsaturated.

Saturated fatty acids come from meats (e.g., beef, lamb, veal, pork), egg yolks, dairy products (e.g., cream, whole milk), and a few plant products, including coconut oil and vegetable shortening. The liver turns saturated fat into cholesterol, which is used to make cell membranes, hormones, and vitamin D.

Cholesterol travels through the body in the form of lipoproteins. *Low-density lipoproteins* (LDLs, or "bad cholesterol") contain large amounts of cholesterol, whereas *high-density lipoproteins* (HDLs, or "good cholesterol") carry relatively little cholesterol and help remove excess cholesterol from blood and tissues. If the LDL level is too high for the HDLs to clear away, the excess cholesterol forms plaque on the artery walls, which can lead to heart disease.

Polyunsaturated fatty acids (PUFAs)come from corn, soybean, safflower, and sunflower oils and some fish oils. PUFAs may actually lower "bad" cholesterol levels, but they have a tendency to lower HDLs as well, leaving the body less capable of removing the amounts of cholesterol that are present. Although not as harmful as the saturated type, PUFAs can pose a health risk if too many are used in the diet.

Monounsaturated fatty acids are found in olive, peanut, canola, and other vegetable and nut oils. These fats actually reduce LDLs slightly and do not reduce HDLs, so they may benefit the body when taken in moderation.

Many oils are actually a combination of these different types of fatty acids, but in general, one type predominates, which is how the oil is described on the food label.

Vitamins

In 1913, American biochemist Elmer McCollum became the first scientist to isolate a vitamin. Further research revealed that this substance, which became known as vitamin A, helps maintain skin, teeth, bones, hair, mucous membranes, and reproductive capacity. We can obtain vitamin A from cream, butter, egg yolks, cod liver oil, and some leafy green and yellow vegetables, or we can simply take a pill containing vitamin A. This is the great vitamin debate: for decades scientists have been arguing about whether supplements containing vitamins and minerals are a useful addition to the diet or whether we can and should obtain all the vitamins and minerals we need from the foods we eat.

No one disputes the need for vitamins, which enable us to make use of the energy stored in food to perform a variety of functions, ranging from maintaining the nervous system to forming red blood cells. There are two main categories of vitamins: fat-soluble and water-soluble. The *fat-soluble* vitamins, including A, D, E, and K, can be stored in the body's fat for days or weeks, whereas *water-soluble* vitamins dissolve quickly in the bloodstream and are removed by urine or sweat. Because water-soluble vitamins cannot be stored, these vitamins need to be resupplied on a daily basis. The most essential water-soluble vitamins are B_1, B_2, B_6, B_{12}, folic acid, C, niacin, pantothenic acid, and biotin.

There is some controversy about how much of each vitamin we need to stay healthy. The U.S. Food and Drug Administration (FDA) has issued guidelines based on the National Academy of Science's Recommended Daily Allowances (often listed on supplement labels as RDAs). Some consider these numbers the minimum needed to maintain health, whereas others maintain these are maximum amounts that should not be exceeded.

Vitamin C, one of the most popular and widely debated vitamins, provides a good example of these divergent views. The RDA for vitamin C is 60 mg per day, the amount found in a single orange. Consuming less than this amount compromises the immune system, bones, and skin and even our ability to reproduce. Researchers at the University of California at Berkeley and the USDA's Western Human Nutritional Research Center determined that without 60 mg of vitamin C per day, waste products of metabolism known as *free radicals* can damage deoxyribonucleic acid (DNA). This can lead to cancer, heart disease, and other illnesses in all of us; for would-be fathers, this means sperm may contain genetic mutations that can result in birth defects, genetic disease, and cancer in future children.

Since the amount of vitamin C in a single orange can prevent all that, what can larger amounts do?

Linus Pauling, winner of Nobel prizes for chemistry and peace, would respond that megadoses of vitamin C can fight colds and boost the immune system. He consumes 300 times the recommended amount, about 18,000 mg, every day. Because vitamin C is water soluble, he points out, any excess will wash out harmlessly in the urine. Some scientists argue that our physiology and metabolism may not be equipped to handle micronutrients at levels higher than could be found in nature. Many complementary and integrative (or alternative) medicine (CIM) practitioners take the middle path, advocating 300 to 3000 mg of vitamin C per day.

Then there is the real controversy: are you better off eating oranges or taking vitamin C tablets? To some extent, that depends on where you stand in the dosage debate; eating one orange a day is manageable, 300 are not. As we learned with limes, natural foods are complex arrangements of ingredients that tend to work best together rather than in isolation or synthesized form. We have identified a number of vitamins and their uses but may be far from understanding the full range of benefits we obtain from whole foods. Most physicians recommend receiving vitamins from a healthy diet; this is good advice, but in a nation earning a C– in nutrition, not very realistic. If your intake for the day consists of frozen waffles and coffee for breakfast, a hot dog with fries and cola for lunch, and pizza for dinner, you are probably going to miss a few nutrients. The most practical approach is to eat the best diet possible and take a multivitamin (without iron) as a "backstop," for those days when life is too hectic to squeeze in even a single orange.

Minerals

Minerals are everywhere in nature and range from beneficial (calcium) to poisonous (arsenic). The minerals essential to human function include calcium, phosphorus, potassium, sodium (salt), chloride, and magnesium. In addition, we need a number of trace elements, including iron, zinc, selenium, manganese, copper, iodine, molybdenum, cobalt, chromium, and fluorine. As with vitamins, most physicians recommend obtaining minerals from a healthy diet, whereas many CIM practitioners advocate supplements to ensure a regular supply.

RDAs have only been established for six minerals—calcium, phosphorus, iron, magnesium, iodine, and zinc—and two of those guidelines have recently been questioned. Much recent publicity has surrounded the role of calcium in preventing osteoporosis, the brittle bones that come with age, especially for women. The National Academy of Science recently raised the RDA for calcium from 800 to 1000 mg for

nonpregnant women and from 1200 to 1500 mg for pregnant women. Although this is a step in the right direction, compliance remains doubtful. The old RDAs were not met by 68% of the total population; more significantly, they were not met by 84% of women between ages 35 and 50 and 87% of girls between 15 and 18 years old. With higher standards, these compliance percentages may slip still lower.

The one mineral that medical professionals have been successful in promoting, *iron,* has turned out to be potentially harmful. For many years, while expressing now-discredited concerns about potential dangers from most supplements, the medical profession advocated the use of iron supplements. Vital for the production of hemoglobin, which transports oxygen to the body's cells, iron is also necessary for many immune, growth, and enzyme functions. Lack of iron leads to anemia, especially in pregnant women, and other conditions, including fatigue, fragile bones, and mental disorders. However, because iron is stored in the body, excesses can easily build up, causing the production of free radicals, which have been associated with cancer and heart disease. This author has conducted independent research showing that excess iron can cause cancer. More often, overuse of iron supplements causes digestive discomforts and disorders. Dietary guidelines for iron are now being revised downward.

Exactly how much of any nutrient is needed depends largely on the physical condition of the individual. Pregnant women, athletes, smokers, people with chronic illnesses, and those of various ages and lifestyles all have different dietary requirements. The one dietary requirement that is relatively consistent for all of us is the need for water.

Water

The human body can survive up to 5 weeks without food but rarely lasts beyond a few days without water. Our bodies are almost 70% water, which is vital for every bodily process, including absorption and digestion of food, transporting nutrients throughout the body, and carrying out waste materials. Water is naturally lost through sweat and elimination. Caffeine, alcohol, and other stimulants act as diuretics, which increase urination and further deplete the body's reserves of liquids. To replace all this lost fluid, we need to drink at least eight glasses of water a day. Dry mouth, headache, and fatigue are often signs we are dehydrated. Exercise, massage, and other activities increase our need for water. When we are ill, additional fluids help flush toxins from the body and restore well-being.

DIET AS THERAPY

Although most mainstream Western physicians receive little training in diet and rarely consider it as a therapy, many other health practitioners consider food a vital part of preventing and treating illness (see Chapters 13, 21,25,27).

Traditional Chinese Medicine

Since ancient times, the Chinese have used food for medicinal purposes, and many contemporary medical schools include a classroom kitchen to train students in preparing beneficial foods. Families and some restaurants routinely prepare special dishes to meet the needs of people who are ill, elderly, pregnant, or lactating. Beneficial foods are identified and selected on the basis of such traditional Chinese medical concepts as the five-phase theory and yin and yang, two models for the dynamic processes governing the universe and human bodies. *Yin* is associated with the female principle, and its properties include cold, slowness, darkness, the interior, and deficiency. *Yang* is associated with the male principle; its properties include heat, light, speed, the exterior, and excess. A disease characterized by too much cold would be associated with yin, and a practitioner might prescribe foods and herbs that stimulate yang by enhancing heat or "scattering the cold" (see Chapter 21 and following section on macrobiotics).

Ayurveda

Developed in ancient India, Ayurveda (Sanskrit for "the knowledge of long life") has always incorporated food into its holistic approach to health. In Ayurveda, three *doshas* (vata, pitta, and kapha) define the three basic mind-body or constitutional types. Each dosha finds certain foods and flavors beneficial, whereas others may be harmful if taken in too large a quantity. For instance, people whose dominant dosha is

vata, which is responsible for the body's kinetic energy and associated with the element of air, may suffer from nervous energy and will be soothed by warm, moist, sweet foods and aggravated by pungent, bitter, raw foods. Following an appropriate vata diet can help people avoid or recover from a wide range of vata disorders, such as insomnia, constipation, anxiety, high blood pressure, and arthritis (see Chapters 25 and 27).

Naturopathy

A synthesis and refinement of nineteenth-century "nature cures," naturopathy considers a wholesome diet one of the cornerstones of good health, along with exercise, fresh air, adequate sleep, and a low-stress lifestyle. Naturopaths believe the body has an innate tendency to heal itself and that nourishing food is necessary for the body's self-maintenance and repairs. Practitioners recommend a diet of whole (unprocessed) foods, especially fresh fruits and vegetables, which should be organic (free of chemicals and other additives) if possible. Fasting, including juice fasts, may be prescribed to rid the body of toxins. Naturopaths started the first "health food stores" in America and developed many foods, such as graham crackers, that were revolutionary in their use of whole grains (see Chapter 13).

Macrobiotics

Loosely based on the traditional Chinese concept of yin and yang, the macrobiotic diet was developed in the 1950s by George Osawa, a Japanese educator and philosopher. The name is derived from the Greek *makros* ("big" or "long") and *bios* ("life"), and its practitioners believe a long and healthy life can be achieved through a balanced diet and other beneficial practices. As with traditional Chinese physicians, macrobiotics advocates believe all foods have yin or yang properties. Yin foods, which are thought to be calming, include green vegetables, fruits, nuts, and honey. Yang foods, said to be strengthening, include meat, fish, eggs, and beans. Whole grains, which have balanced yin and yang, form the cornerstone of the diet. Too much yin food can leave a person feeling resentful and worried; an overly yang meal may generate feelings of aggressiveness. Eating the proper foods can help rebalance feelings and restore physical well-being.

Reversing Heart Disease

Heart disease was considered irreversible until the 1980s, when cardiologist Dean Ornish proved that heart patients could restore heart health through diet, exercise, and stress management. Based on the Pritikin diet, Ornish's diet is very low in fat (perhaps too low at 15% of calories) and cholesterol and is high (perhaps too high) in carbohydrates and fiber. It excludes almost all animal products except for skim milk and fat-free yogurt. An occasional glass of wine is permitted; smoking is not. In a rigorous week-long training session, participants are taught how to cook and eat according to Ornish's guidelines and are instructed in exercise, yoga, and meditation. When they go home, they are expected to continue the regimen indefinitely. This approach is not easy to maintain, but when the alternative is heart bypass surgery, possibly followed by another operation in 5 years, participants are motivated; in 99% of cases, those who followed the regimen successfully reversed the course of their heart disease. Many who question the optimal nature of the Ornish diet point to the benefits of social support and stress reduction to help account for their results.

Vegetarian and Vegan

A *vegetarian* does not eat meat, poultry, or fish but does eat eggs and dairy products. Research has demonstrated that a vegetarian diet can reduce the risk of heart disease, high blood pressure, diabetes, osteoporosis, gallbladder disease, colon cancer, and other conditions. A *vegan* diet excludes all animal-based foods, including dairy products, eggs, and honey. Unless supplements are used, vegans risk deficiency of vitamin B_{12}. The vegan diet has been used to treat asthma, arthritis, high blood pressure, and angina.

Raw Foods

In the late nineteenth century, Swiss physician Max Bircher-Benner developed a diet that is 70% uncooked vegetables and fruits; the balance of the diet can include meat, dairy products, grains, nuts, and seeds. He believed that raw foods (1) are more natural and appropriate for the human digestive system, (2) maintain their nutrients better than cooked food, and (3) prolong the life span.

Detoxification

Since ancient times, people have sought to eliminate toxins from the body by fasting and special diets, often in conjunction with other means, such as emetics and enemas. At present, many Americans are concerned about ridding their bodies of waste products that have accumulated because of poor digestion or sluggish elimination or that have resulted from environmental toxins. Practitioners recommend eating only raw fruits and vegetables and drinking large amounts of water; yogurt may also be included in the regimen.

The Atkins Diet

In the 1970s, Robert Atkins developed a diet based on the principle that sugar and refined carbohydrates increase the body's production of insulin, a hormone necessary for the transformation of carbohydrates to blood sugar. Consumption of white bread, pasta, cereal, and other highly processed, low-fat foods causes insulin levels to spike. When the carbohydrates are absorbed and high amounts of insulin are no longer needed, insulin levels drop sharply, reducing energy and encouraging thoughts of a carbohydrate-laden snack. Atkins developed a diet that severely restricts the intake of processed and refined carbohydrates and promotes instead a diet focusing on "nutrient-dense" foods—proteins, fats, and complex carbohydrates—supported by multivitamins and other supplements (Atkins Center, 2004). The Atkins Diet has been demonstrated to be effective for short-term weight loss but the long-term health effects are of concern to some.

The "Zone" Diet

Like Atkins, Barry Sears designed a diet that reduces the intake of processed foods and sugar in order to control insulin. Sears' diet, which he calls "Zone Perfect" and most people know as "The Zone," uses food as a drug to keep insulin levels in the "therapeutic zone" 24 hours a day. According to Sears, every meal and snack should contain a set ratio of macronutrients: 30% protein, 40% carbohydrates, and 30% fats. Sears also suggests adding supplements, such as omega-3 fish oils and antioxidants, to enhance the Zone diet (Zone Perfect, 2004).

FOOD OR DRUG?

Sears and Atkins are not the only people using food's druglike properties to affect the body. Scientists have long been aware that many fruits, vegetables, grains, and beans appear to reduce the risk of heart disease, cancer, and other conditions because they contain *antioxidants* (vitamins, minerals, and enzymes that protect cells from being damaged by oxidation). Now another group of disease-fighting nutrients has been identified as phytochemicals, also known as "nutraceuticals."

Phytochemicals are thought to fight cancer and other ailments by keeping disease-causing substances from latching on to healthy cells and by removing toxins before they can cause harm. There are many thousands of phytochemicals—tomatoes alone contain 10,000 different kinds—each with a slightly different function. Genistein, for example, which is found in soybeans, prevents the formation of the capillaries needed to nourish tumors. Indoles, which increase immune function, are found in members of the Brassica family such as broccoli and cauliflower. The bioflavonoids found in limes prevent certain cancer-causing hormones from attaching to the body's cells. Much as an earlier generation of scientists sought to identify and synthesize vitamins, today's researchers are working to isolate and manufacture phytochemicals. However, it is unlikely that they will be able to reproduce the rich mix of beneficial substances found in a single tomato or a handful of soybeans.

Sometimes we do not need to eat the plant to obtain the benefits of phytochemicals. For example, brewing teas such as green tea can provide a natural mixture of antioxidants to be drunk as a beverage. The antioxidant profile of green tea (from Asia) has been studied extensively in terms of its anticancer effects. A newly popular red tea (from South Africa) has a similar profile of antioxidants, but without the caffeine, while also having anticancer properties.

FOOD ALLERGIES

Soybeans may be bristling with needed nutrients and phytochemicals, but they are among the common foods that trigger allergies. Other major offenders include nuts (especially peanuts), dairy products, fish, shellfish, wheat, eggs, and food additives, especially preservatives and coloring agents.

An *allergy* occurs when the immune system reacts to an ordinary food as if it were a hostile invader, producing an antibody known as IgE (immunoglobin E). This antibody attaches itself to specialized immune cells known as "masts," and when the offending food is encountered again, the antibody causes the mast cell to release chemicals that cause the allergic reaction. The result may be skin disorders (e.g., hives, eczema), respiratory conditions (e.g., allergic rhinitis, asthma), stomach problems (e.g., cramps, diarrhea), or headaches. In severe cases, people may develop anaphylactic shock, causing collapse and possibly even death.

Although no one knows for certain what causes allergies to arise, it is common for them to run in families, although each family member may have a different type. Some theorize a possible psychological component; on some deep level, allergy sufferers may view the world as inherently hostile. "It is fairly common to be sensitive to one or two foods," notes physician Christiane Northrup. "But women with multiple food allergies that are resistant to simple dietary change often have a history of abuse of some type, or they are continuing to live in dysfunctional relationships or to stay in overly stressful jobs" (Northrup, 1994).

Start with the Usual Suspects

The offending substance (known as an *allergen*) can often be identified by a simple skin prick test, in which one after another of the "usual suspects" is injected under the skin to see how the body responds. Another investigative technique is the radioallergosorbent test (RAST), in which blood is drawn, serum containing antibodies is extracted, and possible allergens are added to test for a reaction. Naturopaths favor an *elimination diet,* in which various foods are systematically removed from the menu for 2 weeks. When symptoms disappear, foods are reintroduced one by one until a reaction takes place, indicating which one is causing the allergy.

Herbalists often recommend that the elimination diet be accompanied by immune boosters, such as echinacea and red clover, digestive aids (e.g., slippery elm, marshmallow, hops), and dandelion root to support liver function (see Chapter 11). Yoga practitioners can teach postures designed to aid digestion and overall well-being (see Chapter 26). Nutritionists with expertise in supplements advise taking vitamins and minerals, including zinc, selenium, vitamin C, magnesium, and manganese.

Homeopaths treat allergies with a form immunotherapy in which highly diluted amounts of the allergen are taken with the aim of overcoming the reaction (see Chapter 8). This is similar to the controversial approach known as *desensitization,* in which people are exposed to minute but increasing amounts of the allergen until a higher level of tolerance is achieved. Enzymes have proved effective in treating some milk sugar allergies. For the majority of those with allergies, the most effective treatment is avoiding the allergen in question.

FUNCTIONAL FOODS

The American food industry is currently responding to the public's desire for healthier fare by creating a variety of products that, they claim, provide enhanced health benefits, such as lowering cholesterol and heightening mental abilities. Known as *functional foods,* these products include snacks, cereals, margarines, and salad dressings laced with calcium, vitamins, fiber, and such new constituents as DHA (docosahexaenoic acid), which is currently being used for Japanese schoolchildren and is said to improve concentration.

If you want to achieve the benefits of functional foods, you must eat a large quantity of them. One margarine, for example, must be eaten three times a day for 2 weeks to lower cholesterol by 10%. To obtain their full allotment of vitamins from snack foods, toddlers must eat three and a half cookies a day. Often six times as expensive as standard fare—(e.g., one margarine retails for $17.22 a pound), these functional foods require a level of commitment many families are not prepared to make.

The greatest drawback to many functional foods is the flavor. As *New York Times* food critic William Grimes noted, one cholesterol-controlling apricot and orange cereal bar has the "texture of a rubber eraser, enlivened by a hideously artificial fruit flavor." He noted that a "sugar controller" for diabetic patients, a fudge brownie flavor nutrition bar, "chews like a plug of tobacco, minus the flavor, except for a haylike aftertaste. The chocolate coating seems to be for color only. Nuts depicted on the wrapping fail to show up in the actual bar" (Grimes, 1999). In a taste test of 13 functional foods, five got a "thumb's up," including the bone-building Aviva Instant Hot Chocolate and Viactiv's caramel-flavored soft calcium chews; the majority of products received a "thumb's down." Grimes addresses the "pleasure principle" as follows:

> All food is functional. That's why humans eat three times a day. But unlike animals and insects, they do not eat for function's sake alone. Somewhere in the tortured mental software that governs eating behavior, the pleasure principle lives in more or less uneasy proximity to the efficiency principle. We eat to live, but we also live to eat.

NUTRITION VS. NOURISHMENT

> Food and emotions are very deeply linked in human beings for reasons far older than our current obsession with thinness. For centuries the human race was able to survive because we ate the things our tribes said were okay to eat. We avoided the poisonous berries and ate what Mother said was safe. Food has always been an essential part of the daily ritual of living, and the foods we were fed in childhood have left a very deep impression on us. At an unconscious and conscious level, they help us feel safe and cared for (Northrup, 1994).

One of the reasons diets and food fads are so popular is that we are tribal beings who take our cues about what to eat from those around us. One of the reasons diets so often fail is that they conflict with much deeper cultural programming that comes from our family of origin. If generations of your relatives served beef brisket (or borscht, or macaroni and cheese) for dinner every Sunday, that dish will forever be equated with family gatherings and feelings of belonging. However flawed they may be, our families usually present our strongest links to our past and to others; in a profound way, they represent safety and the sense of being at home.

Unfortunately, the eating patterns of the past do not always work well in the twenty-first century. The rib roast with gravy and buttered potatoes that once nourished our great grandparents on the farm may lead to a heart attack in someone whose most strenuous daily activity is booting up the computer. On the other hand, the food products our contemporary culture urges us to consume—loaded with fat, salt, sugar, artificial ingredients, and chemical additives and stripped of nutrients during processing—are equally unlikely to sustain us into a healthy and advanced old age. Taking a scientific, reductionist approach also is not the answer; obsessing about every calorie and gram of fat on our plate can turn food into an enemy. Eating is one of the most vital ways we connect with our environment and with each other. Treating food as a hostile force is not good for our bodies, our souls, or our relationship with the world.

So, what is the key to healthy eating? Moderation and common sense are a good starting point. Once we understand our basic nutritional needs and which foods we would be wise to avoid when possible, we can move gradually into patterns of eating that provide us with a sense of physical well-being. However, unless we have a medical condition such as diabetes that requires strict dietary controls, healthy eating does not mean abandoning favorite foods forever. Sometimes a piece of grandmother's fried chicken, an ice cream cone on a summer afternoon, or a mug of sugary cocoa after sledding are necessary reminders that being alive is sometimes supposed to be fun, and that sharing food with the people we love can be healthy for our hearts in ways not yet recognized by biomedical science. Food is rich in cultural, social, and personal meaning as well as nutrients, and all these elements are necessary for a balanced diet.

References and Readings

American Cancer Society: *Statistics.* Accessed at www.cancer.org (2004).

American Heart Association: Cardiovascular diseases. In *International classification of diseases,* ed 9, pp 390-459, 745-747. Accessed at www.americanheart.org (2004).

Ames BN: DNA damage from micronutrient deficiencies is likely to be a major cause of cancer, *Mutat Res* 475:7-20, 2001.

Appel LJ: Lifestyle modification as a means to prevent and treat high blood pressure, *J Am Soc Nephrol* 14:S99-S102, 2003.

Appel LJ, Moore TJ, Obarzanek E, et al: A clinical trial of the effects of dietary patterns on blood pressure. DASH Collaborative Research Group, *N Engl J Med* 336: 1117-1124, 1997.

Atkins Center: The Atkins diet: a brief overview. Accessed at www.atkinscenter.com (2004).

Balch JF, Balch PA: *Prescription for nutritional healing,* ed 2, New York, 1997, Avery Publishing Group, pp 8-9.

Calle EE, Rodriguez C, Walker-Thurmond K, et al: Overweight, obesity, and mortality from cancer in a prospectively studied cohort of US adults, *N Engl J Med* 348:1625-1638, 2003.

Carter JP, Saxe GP, Newbold V, et al: Hypothesis: dietary management may improve survival from nutritionally linked cancers based on analysis of representative cases, *J Am Coll Nutr* 12:209-226, 1993.

Convit A, Wolf OT, Tarshish C, et al: Reduced glucose tolerance is associated with poor memory performance and hippocampal atrophy among normal elderly, *Proc Natl Acad Sci USA* 100:2019-2022, 2003.

Enig MG et al: Dietary fat and cancer trends: a critique, *Fed Proc* 37:139-145, 1978.

Feldstein CA, Akopian M, Renauld A, et al: Insulin resistance and hypertension in postmenopausal women, *J Hum Hypertens* 16(suppl 1):S145-S150, 2002.

Ford ES, Giles WH, Dietz WH: Prevalence of the metabolic syndrome among US adults: findings from the third National Health and Nutrition Examination Survey, *JAMA* 287:356-359, 2002.

Foster GD, Wyatt HR, Hill JO, et al: A randomized trial of a low-carbohydrate diet for obesity, *N Engl J Med* 348: 2082-2090, 2003.

Giovannucci E: Tomatoes, tomato-based products, lycopene, and cancer: review of the epidemiologic literature, *J Natl Cancer Inst* 91:317-331, 1999.

Grimes W: But how do they taste? A food critic answers, *New York Times,* Dec 12, 1999, p 16.

Heilbronn LK, Ravussin E: Calorie restriction and aging: review of the literature and implications for studies in humans, *Am J Clin Nutr* 78:361-369, 2003.

Hildenbrand GL, Hildenbrand LC, Bradford K, et al: Five-year survival rates of melanoma patients treated by diet therapy after the manner of Gerson: a retrospective review, *Altern Ther Health Med* 1:29-37, 1995.

Holick MF: Vitamin D: a millenium perspective, *J Cell Biochem* 88:296-307, 2003.

Hu FB, Willett WC: Optimal diets for prevention of coronary heart disease, *JAMA* 288:2569-2578, 2002.

Jenkins DJ, Kendall CW, Marchie A, et al: Effects of a dietary portfolio of cholesterol-lowering foods vs lovastatin on serum lipids and C-reactive protein, *JAMA* 290:502-510, 2003.

Kalmijn S, Launer LJ, Ott A, et al: Dietary fat intake and the risk of incident dementia in the Rotterdam Study, *Ann Neurol* 42:776-782, 1997.

Le Bars PL: Magnitude of effect and special approach to *Ginkgo biloba* extract EGb 761 in cognitive disorders, *Pharmacopsychiatry* 36(suppl 1):S44-S49, 2003.

Li CI, Malone KE, Porter PL, et al: The relationship between alcohol use and risk of breast cancer by histology and hormone receptor status among women 65-79 years of age, *Cancer Epidemiol Biomarkers Prev* 12:1061-1066, 2003.

Liu S, Manson JE, Buring JE, et al: Relation between a diet with a high glycemic load and plasma concentrations of high-sensitivity C-reactive protein in middle-aged women, *Am J Clin Nutr* 75:492-498, 2002.

Luchsinger JA, Tang MX, Shea S, et al: Antioxidant vitamin intake and risk of Alzheimer disease, *Arch Neurol* 60:203-208, 2003.

Luft FC, Weinberger MH: Heterogeneous responses to changes in dietary salt intake: the salt-sensitivity paradigm, *Am J Clin Nutr* 65:612S-617S, 1997.

Messina MJ: Emerging evidence on the role of soy in reducing prostate cancer risk, *Nutr Rev* 61:117-131, 2003.

Micozzi M: Sugar, substitutes, and subsistence, Buies Creek, NC, *Diet Watchers* 2(2):1, 1988.

Micozzi M: Diet and cancer prevention, Buies Creek, NC, *Diet Watchers* 4(2):1, 1992.

Morris MC, Evans DA, Bienias JL, et al: Consumption of fish and n-3 fatty acids and risk of incident Alzheimer disease, *Arch Neurol* 60:940-946, 2003.

Morrow DJ: A medicine chest or a grocery shelf? *New York Times,* Dec 12, 1999, pp 1, 16.

Murray M, Birdsall T, Pizzorno JE, et al: *How to prevent and treat cancer with natural medicine,* New York, 2002, Riverhead Books.

Northrup C: *Women's bodies, women's wisdom,* New York, 1994, Bantam Books, pp 686-724.

Paolisso G, Sgambato S, Pizza G, et al: Improved insulin response and action by chronic magnesium administration in aged NIDDM subjects, *Diabetes Care* 12:265-269, 1989.

Pasternak RC: Report of the Adult Treatment Panel III: the 2001 National Cholesterol Education Program guidelines on the detection, evaluation and treatment of elevated cholesterol in adults, *Cardiol Clin* 21:393-398, 2003.

Pharmaceutical Information Associates: Focus on . . . obesity, *PIA Medical Sciences Bulletin,* Pharmaceutical Information Associates. Accessed at www.pialtd.com (2004).

Reaven GM: Pathophysiology of insulin resistance in human disease, *Physiol Rev* 75:473-486, 1995.

Ridker PM, Buring JE, Cook,NR, et al: C-reactive protein, the metabolic syndrome, and risk of incident cardiovascular events: an 8-year follow-up of 14 719 initially healthy American women, *Circulation* 107:391-397, 2003.

Robbins J, Malkmus G: Food consumption in the USA, based on USDA statistics. Accessed at www.health free.com (2004).

Sacks FM, Svetkey LP, Vollmer WM, et al: Effects on blood pressure of reduced dietary sodium and the Dietary Approaches to Stop Hypertension (DASH) diet. DASH-Sodium Collaborative Research Group, *N Engl J Med* 344:3-10, 2001.

Seshadri S, Beiser A, Selhub J, et al: Plasma homocysteine as a risk factor for dementia and Alzheimer's disease, *N Engl J Med* 346:476-483, 2002.

Stendig-Lindberg G, Tepper R, Leichter I: Trabecular bone density in a two year controlled trial of peroral magnesium in osteoporosis, *Magnes Res* 6:155-163, 1993.

Tabet N, Mantle D, Walker Z, et al: Endogenous antioxidant activities in relation to concurrent vitamins A, C, and E intake in dementia, *Int Psychogeriatr* 14:7-15, 2002.

US Department of Agriculture (USDA), Economic Research Service: Food consumption, prices and expenditures, 1970-1995, Statistical Bulletin 939, August 1997; Food consumption, prices and expenditures, 1970-97, Statistical Bulletin 965; USDA report encourages Americans to remember nutritional needs when eating out, News Release No 0060.99, 1999; America's eating habits: changes and consequences, Agriculture Information Bulletin 750 (AIB-750). Accessed at www.econ.ag.gov (2004).

Valerian D: Fueling for peak performance, Cleveland, *Northern Ohio Live Magazine* 12(6):36, 1992.

Westman EC, Yancy WS, Edman JS, et al: Effect of 6-month adherence to a very low carbohydrate diet program, *Am J Med* 113:30-36, 2002.

Witteman JC, Grobbee DE, Derkx FH, et al: Reduction of blood pressure with oral magnesium supplementation in women with mild to moderate hypertension, *Am J Clin Nutr* 60:129-135, 1994.

Zone Perfect: an overview of the Zone diet. Accessed at www.zoneperfect.com (2004).

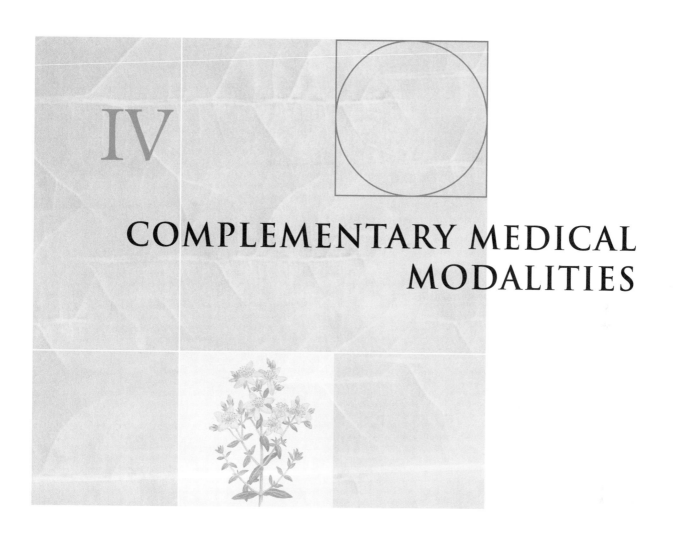

IV

COMPLEMENTARY MEDICAL MODALITIES

Although most forms of complementary and integrative medicine can be seen to draw on a "mind-body" connection, the complementary medical approaches described in this section appear to make use of physiological mechanisms by which mental state may be reflected in direct biological responses. Likewise, although "bioenergy" is invoked in many complementary modalities and integrative medicine therapies, energy medicine itself uses this energetic property as the sole means and primary mode of cure. Ultimately, mind and energy may be reflected in the "consciousness" approach of many complementary and integrative medicine forms of traditional healing. ❧

CHAPTER 15

NEUROHUMORAL PHYSIOLOGY AND PSYCHONEUROIMMUNOLOGY

MARC S. MICOZZI

HAKIMA AMRI

NEUROHUMORAL MECHANISMS

The autonomic nervous system (ANS) maintains homeostasis by a series of humoral and nervous system interactions that continually occur on a subconscious, involuntary level. The ANS sends nervous impulses to all parts of the body as directed by the integration of several complex biofeedback mechanisms.

The information from these biofeedback loops is integrated in the central nervous system (CNS), and appropriate neural directives are passed along to the organs of respiration, circulation, digestion, excretion, and reproduction via the ANS.

Thus the body is maintained in a state of dynamic equilibrium, continually responsive to stimuli from internally monitored systems and environmental influences.

The functional anatomy of the ANS has important implications for therapeutics (Table 15-1). The division of the system into two major parts—sympathetic and parasympathetic—provides a series of checks and balances to regulate body functions. This division enables an ongoing dialogue between the two parts to maintain dynamic equilibrium. The opposition of two vital forces may be likened to the Asian concept of the yin and the yang (see Chapter 21), whereby the interaction of these opposing forces maintains the balance and harmony of humans and the universe. In addition, each of the two forces may take on some characteristics of the other. Thus the sympathetic and parasympathetic divisions are

TABLE 15-1

Sympathetic and Parasympathetic Divisions of the Autonomic Nervous System (ANS)

	Sympathetic	Parasympathetic
Synonym	Adrenergic	Cholinergic
Preganglionic fiber	Short	Long
Neurohumoral agent*	Acetylcholine	Acetylcholine
Ganglion location	Paravertebral	End organ
Postganglionic fiber	Long	Short
Neurohumoral agent*	Norepinephrine	Acetylcholine
Extraautonomic sites	Adrenal medulla	Neuromuscular junction
Evolutionary role	Fight-flight/defense-alarm	Relaxation response
		Vegetative functions
Activators	Multiple	Specific
Blockers	Diffuse	Selective
	Nonspecific	Cholinesterase
Degradative enzymes	Monoamine oxidase	
	Methyltransferase	

*These compounds are referred to as *neurohumoral agents* to the extent that they are present both in the general circulation and within nervous tissue. These compounds are *neurotransmitters* to the extent that they manifest their activity across presynaptic or postsynaptic junctions during transmission of nerve impulses.

antagonistic, with a few notable exceptions. Coronary and pulmonary blood vessels are dilated by both divisions of the ANS, whereas the vessels supplying blood to skeletal muscles may be dilated by the sympathetic system in exercise or by the postganglionic parasympathetic neurotransmitter at rest.

The unique short-term and long-term adaptability of the human organism to environmental stimuli is facilitated by the actions of the ANS. The so-called fight-flight or defense-alarm responses are promulgated by the *sympathetic nervous system,* which raises blood oxygenation and pressure, regulates blood flow to the musculoskeletal system for activity and to the skin for thermal regulation, and causes retention of fluids and electrolytes in a state of arousal. These acute physiological responses are adaptive in the short-term and allow long-term survival of the human organism.

The "relaxation response" is mediated by the dynamic opponent of the sympathetic system—the parasympathetic system. The *parasympathetic nervous system* directs the normative functions of the organism, allowing development of an ongoing state of well-being and physiological equilibrium. The maintenance of vegetative functions has facilitated human development and cultural evolution. The ability to relax has allowed humans to reserve some portion of

physical and mental energy for the pursuit of activities peripheral to primary survival. This ability has given humans their unique cultural attributes, which enable each individual to express the inclination for creativity. The selective responsiveness of the ANS has enabled humans, both as individuals and as a species, to make the successful adaptation to the environment, which has characterized human evolution.

The anatomical divisions corresponding to the functional autonomy of the sympathetic and parasympathetic nervous system can be traced along the length of the brain and spinal column (Figure 15-1). The ANS begins with cranial nerve X, the vagus, a single bundle of parasympathetic nerves that originates from the brain stem and courses throughout the body. Cranial nerves III, VII, and IX also send some parasympathetic fibers to the eyes, nose, and salivary glands. *Vagus* means "wanderer" in Latin, and no other nerve interfaces at so many diverse points along the functional anatomy. Passing down along the spinal cord, the cervical, thoracic, and lumbar divisions send sympathetic nerves throughout the body. Finally, the sacral divisions of the spinal cord send a few parasympathetic nerves to the lower regions of the body.

Each nerve of the ANS has two longitudinal divisions as it passes from the CNS to the end organs.

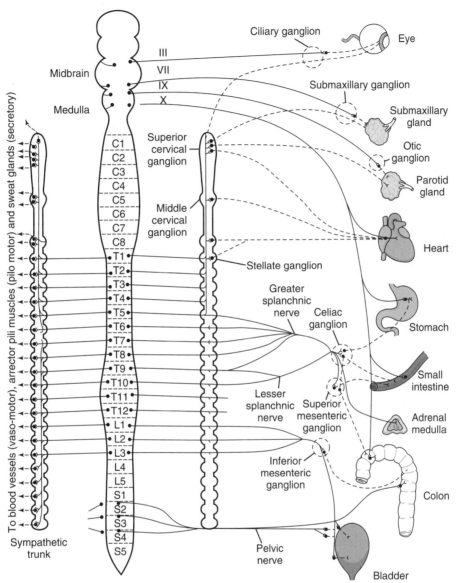

Figure 15-1 Autonomic nervous system and cranial nerves. (From Williams PL: *Gray's anatomy,* Edinburgh, 1995, Churchill Livingstone.)

The initial, or *preganglionic,* nerve fiber originates in the CNS and terminates in a nerve ganglion. Here it synapses with a new continuation—the postganglionic nerve fiber. This *postganglionic* fiber originates in the ganglion and terminates at a site of action. Autonomic nerve impulses travel in a continuum along the preganglionic fiber, through the synapse, and onto the postganglionic fiber to the site of action. In the sympathetic division, the preganglionic fibers are short and end in nearby ganglia, which

occur in chains along the thoracic and lumbar vertebrae. From there, the postganglionic fibers travel to the diverse sites of action. In the parasympathetic system the preganglionic fibers are long and travel into ganglia located near end organs. From there, postganglionic fibers traverse a short distance to the sites of action.

The occurrence of *synapses* in the ganglia, between the preganglionic and postganglionic fibers, is important to therapy. Local anesthetics affect nerve conduction in the nerve fiber. Otherwise, these nerve impulses may be influenced by activities at the synaptic junction site. The interactions that occur in the synapse are a microcosm of neurophysiology and serve to distinguish the sympathetic system functionally from the parasympathetic system. These distinctions are used extensively in therapy. Each of these systems makes use of characteristic neurohumoral agents for the unique transmission of nervous impulses throughout the body. The preganglionic fibers of both divisions use *acetylcholine* as the neurotransmitter across the synapse. The postganglionic parasympathetic transmitter is also acetylcholine, but the sympathetic transmitter is *norepinephrine*. The exclusive postganglionic use of acetylcholine as the parasympathetic and norepinephrine as the sympathetic neurotransmitter holds throughout the ANS, except in the case of sweating of the palms, soles, and axilla, where the autonomic innervation is adrenergic, but the neurotransmitter is acetylcholine. Because these neurohumoral compounds used in the transmission of impulses across the synaptic junction are distinct chemical entities, they tend to accumulate at their sites of release. Such an occurrence would limit effectiveness of the ANS in providing sensitive, instantaneous regulation of body systems. Thus the synaptic sites maintain extensive and sophisticated mechanisms for the reuptake and degradation of released neurohumoral transmitters, and the synaptic junctions are kept clear of accumulated active compounds on an ongoing basis.

Specific enzymes degrade norepinephrine in the sympathetic postganglionic synapses, as well as their metabolic products. The concentration of these metabolites may be increased in certain pathological conditions and detected by analytical chemical techniques.

The enzyme responsible for the breakdown of acetylcholine in the postganglionic parasympathetic synapse is *acetylcholinesterase*. Although acetylcholine itself cannot practically be administered even when its properties are desired, a "functional dose" may be given through inhibition of its breakdown by cholinesterase. Thus, anticholinesterases form the basis for parasympathetic nervous stimulation in clinical therapeutics. A phenomenon known as *denervation hypersensitivity* greatly depends on this system of reuptake and degradation. When the autonomic innervation to an organ is anatomically interrupted (denervation), the postganglionic synaptic site loses its induced degradative enzymes, and the synaptic receptor becomes extremely sensitive (hypersensitivity) to the neurohumoral agent. Thus any amount of the original neurohumoral agent introduced into the site by the circulation, through administration or otherwise, will have a magnified effect because the activity will not be mitigated by action of its appropriate degradative mechanism.

The functional divisions of the ANS have great pathophysiological and therapeutic significance. For example, the entire gastrointestinal (GI) tract is extensively innervated by nerve fibers from both the sympathetic and the parasympathetic division. As previously discussed, the parasympathetic ganglia, where preganglionic fibers synapse with postganglionic fibers, are located near the sites of action in end organs. In the case of the GI tract, the parasympathetic ganglia lie in two areas of the esophageal, gastric, intestinal, and colonic walls: Auerbach's myenteric plexus and Meissner's submucous plexus. These ganglia may be congenitally absent, as in Hirschsprung's disease, or destroyed by a number of pathogenic agents. The resultant disease depends on the location of the deficiency or insult along the GI tract.

With destruction of the parasympathetic ganglia, there is prolonged, unopposed sympathetic stimulation. The characteristic effect is for the diseased segment to become constricted with impaired motility and loss of peristaltic action. The segment of the GI tract proximal to the constriction lesion becomes extensively dilated as a pathological response to the event.

Achalasia of the esophagus is such a condition, where a local area of constriction leads to proximal dilation of the esophagus. It has been thought that achalasia is caused by degenerative disease of the parasympathetic vagus nerve, which innervates this area.

Pyloric stenosis of the gastric outlet is a similar condition. A ganglionic megacolon, or Hirschsprung's disease, is caused by a congenital lack of parasympathetic ganglion cells in the intestinal tract.

Chagas' disease, or South American trypanosomiasis, caused by the parasitic organism *Trypanosoma cruzi,* may be associated with both megaesophagus and megacolon resulting from the toxic degeneration of the intraluminal nerve plexus through *T. cruzi* infection. On the other hand, selective loss of sympathetic activity occurs in Horner's syndrome, with the characteristic triad of ptosis, miosis, and anhydrosis (lid lag, pupillary constriction, and loss of sweating). Horner's syndrome occurs with injury to the cervical sympathetic trunk and unopposed parasympathetic innervation.

Unfortunately, no autonomic therapeutic agents are available for the effective treatment of disorders such as Horner's syndrome or irreversible disorders of the GI tract. However, autonomic drugs to treat diseases of the circulatory and respiratory systems are common therapies in medicine. The same neurohumoral mechanisms involved by medical therapeutics may also be used in a nonspecific manner by many of the "mind-body" techniques of complementary, integrative and alternative medicine.

PSYCHONEURO-IMMUNOLOGY

The Romans' view of *mens sanum in corpore sano*, "a sound mind in a sound body," as well as the Greek philosopher Galen's observation that women suffering from depression had a predisposition toward developing breast cancer, reflected the early recognition of mind-body interactions and their significance in health and disease. However, it was not until studies in the 1950s and 1960s verified the impact of stress on overall health that the mind-body connection became a focus of attention.

In 1964, Solomon and Moos described the interaction between mind and body as a result of stress exposure. George Engel's view that genetics is not the only cause of poor health, and that social and psychological factors have a direct impact on all biological processes, further expanded this new, holistic medical model referred to as "psychoneuroimmunology," or PNI (Engel, 1977; Lutgendorf and Costanzo, 2003). Subsequent research strongly suggested that the higher cognitive and limbic emotional centers are capable of regulating virtually all aspects of the immune system and therefore play a significant role in health and disease (Ader et al., 1991; Blalock, 1994; Reichlin, 1993).

Autonomic and neuroendocrine processes constitute the mind-body pathways of communication.

The ANS innervates the bone marrow, thymus, spleen, and mucosal surfaces, the areas where immune cells develop, mature, and encounter foreign proteins (Felten et al., 1992). This innervation involves sympathetic, parasympathetic, and nonadrenergic noncholinergic (NANC) fibers. As discussed earlier, signal transduction occurs through epinephrine, norepinephrine, acetylcholine, and neuropeptides. These chemical messengers exert tissue-specific inflammatory or antiinflammatory effects on immune target tissues, and nerves and inflammatory cells mutually influence each other in a time-dependent manner (Watkins, 1995). Development and aging of the immune system and ANS appear to be closely related (Ackerman et al., 1989; Bellinger et al., 1988).

The neuroendocrine pathway constitutes the second, indirect communication channel involving the hormonal regulation of immune cell function. Immune cells have surface receptors for endorphins, enkephalins, and the various hormones, such as growth hormone, thyroid-stimulating hormone, sex hormone–releasing hormones, vasopressin, and prolactin (Blalock, 1994; Felten et al., 1992). The release of many of these hormones is intimately related to thoughts and emotions and has a profound effect on immune system function. The "molecules of emotion" therefore govern the immune response through the endocrine system, leading to either suppression or enhancement (Pert et al., 1998).

Because thoughts, feelings, emotions, and perceptions alter immunity (Watkins, 1995), complementary therapies targeted at these areas should affect health and elicit changes in pathological conditions (Watkins, 1994).

Epilepsy illustrates this point (i.e., effect of the mind on the brain). Epileptic seizures can be triggered by stressful events (Fenwick, 1998), and negative emotions exacerbate the condition. A potential mechanism is the activation of the cytokine network (Hullkonnen et al., 2004), which corresponds to seizures activity, but the question of "cause versus effect" remains unclear.

The reverse scenario is reflected in a long-term study involving healthy World War II veterans who were asked to write about their war experiences and themselves. The essays were rated on a scale ranging from extreme optimism to extreme pessimism. When the candidates reached the age of 45, health status positively correlated with optimistic scoring at the beginning of the study (Peterson and Bossio, 1993).

Evidence for PNI Mediating the Effects of Complementary, Integrative, and Alternative Therapies

The use of PNI-related techniques has dramatically increased in the United States. According to a recent survey, 1 in 5 adults reported using one or more therapies during the previous year (Wolsko et al., 2004). Relaxation techniques, guided imagery, hypnosis, and biofeedback are the most frequently used modalities. Patients sought these PNI-related techniques for chronic diseases such as anxiety (34%), depression (26.5%), headaches (18.5%), back or neck pain (18%), heart problems or chest pain (18%), arthritis (14.8%), digestive disorders (12.4%), and fatigue (12.1%). The authors estimated that the absolute numbers of patients using the modalities listed were as follows: for back and neck pain, 11.2 million; for anxiety, 6.3 million; and for fatigue, 6.8 million. Between 29% and 55% of patients found these therapies "very helpful" for their respective health condition.

What is the evidence that complementary, integrative, and alternative therapies work through the previously outlined mind-body pathways? To date, few studies have actually investigated the mechanism of action of these therapies. Some data suggest that the activity of the ANS may be altered by chiropractic intervention (Beal, 1985; Bouhuys, 1963), hypnosis (DeBeneditts et al., 1994; Neild and Cameron, 1985), conditioning (Hatch et al., 1990), and acupuncture (Han et al., 1980; Jian, 1985). Other studies have indicated that the benefit derived from acupuncture (Kasahara et al., 1992) and spinal manipulation (Vernon et al., 1986) might be mediated through endorphin release.

Several studies demonstrate that acupuncture-induced analgesia is blocked by naloxone, an opioid antagonist, indicating that an opioidergic mechanism mediates the acupuncture analgesic response (Mayer et al., 1977, Sjolund and Eriksson, 1979). In electroacupuncture, electrical pulses are applied via acupuncture needles. Opioid and nonopioid pathways govern the antinociceptive effect induced by electroacupuncture; the neural pathways and neurotransmitters involved have not been elucidated. However, the PNI-mediated mechanism in electroacupuncture occurs at the level of neuronal nitric oxide synthase, nitric oxide expression and synthesis in the brain, and the therapeutic response induced by acupoint ST36 (Ma, 2004).

Using state-of-the-art technology (e.g., two-dimensional electrophoresis-based proteomics) and an animal model for neuropathic pain, Sung and colleagues (2004) detected 36 proteins that were differentially expressed in the brain of injured animals when compared to controls. Most interestingly, these proteins were restored after treating the injured animals with electroacupuncture. Of these proteins, 21 have been characterized as playing a role in inflammation, enzyme metabolism, and signal transduction, and this study undoubtedly will elucidate other pathways triggered by acupuncture.

A growing body of evidence suggests that *meditation* alleviates anxiety, fosters a positive attitude, and improves the immune response. A meditation training program known as "mindfulness-based stress reduction" (MBSR) yielded increased left frontal lobe activation in response to both negative and positive emotion induction. When vaccinated after intervention, the meditation group experienced a significantly increased rise in antibody titers. The correlation between the shift toward left-sided brain activation and the elevated immune response demonstrates the relationship between the psychoneuroimmunological system and mediation (Davidson et al., 2003). Similarly, cancer outpatients using the same MBSR technique experienced improved mood, which correlated with a more favorable hormone profile with regard to melatonin, cortisol, dehydroepiandrosterone-sulfate (DHEA-S), and the cortisol/DHEA-S ratio, as well as an enhanced immune response (Carlson et al., 2004).

Yoga has become a popular practice in Western culture. Based on the development and balance of psychophysical energies, yoga has been proven beneficial in pulmonary and cardiovascular conditions, including asthma, chronic bronchitis, and hypertension (Raub, 2002). A recent study investigating the effects of yoga and meditation on psychological profile, cardiopulmonary performance, and melatonin secretion demonstrated increased well-being, improved performance, and elevated plasma melatonin levels (Harinath et al., 2004).

Mind-body anatomic and physiologic pathways are illustrated in Figure 15-2.

Placebo Effect

A *placebo* is an inert substance or a control method used to evaluate the psychological and physiological

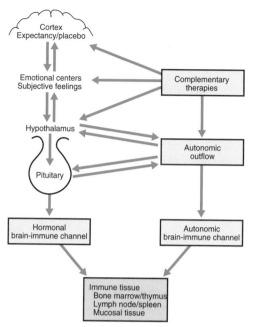

Figure 15-2 Brain-immune pathways of alternative medicine.

implications of a new drug or procedure. Its effect should not exceed that of the experimental drug or method, which would otherwise be considered ineffective. The placebo response is unpredictable, unreliable, and mediated by nonspecific mechanisms that are dismissed as immeasurable and irrelevant.

How does the psychoneuroimmunological complex relate to the placebo effect? It has been argued that every therapeutic intervention, whether complementary, integrative and alternative medicine or allopathic, involves a placebo effect. For example, 50% of the analgesic effect of pain medications is attributed to a placebo response. At the same time, most allopathic physicians consider it unethical or even deceitful to actively encourage a placebo response. PNI research demonstrates that an expectation of recovery can alter subjective feelings of well-being and result in ANS activation and pituitary hormone production. Thus, we have identified specific verifiable pathways by which expectation can alter immunity. However, "expectation" likely has different effects in different individuals, producing large shifts in autonomic balance and hormonal output in some and negligible changes in others, which explains the unpredictability of the placebo response. In addition

to the idea that complementary therapies affect merely "subjective" measures of disease activity, these observations have formed the platform on which allopathic physicians argue that complementary practices are fundamentally flawed and of limited benefit.

Although fallacious, defeatist, and ultimately counterproductive, these arguments persist. The expectation of recovery that promotes a placebo response is separate from any subjective improvement and, incidentally, is also different from hope. It is possible to feel subjectively better without expecting a full recovery. Similarly, it is possible to expect recovery without feeling better at all. Complementary therapies cannot be dismissed as mere placebos, and it is becoming increasingly obvious that they produce substantial subjective and objective clinical benefits unrelated to the placebo effect.

Individuals differ in their responsiveness to the various activation stimuli, whether expectancy, subjective sensations, or complementary therapies. This would explain why complementary therapies that are supposedly mediated by placebo mechanisms, as in allopathic arguments, could outperform placebos in a double-blind trial (Reilly et al., 1994). It would also explain the need to combine a number of complementary approaches to ensure that these pathways are fully activated. The overlap of subjective and objective therapeutic benefits is illustrated in Figure 15-3.

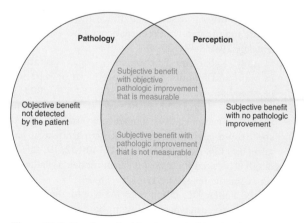

Figure 15-3 Overlap of subjective and objective therapeutic benefit.

CONCLUSION

The medical and scientific communities are showing growing interest in the neurohumoral mechanisms underlying PNI responses to complementary therapies. The studies published to date have been carried out with relatively small groups of subjects and reflect conventional study criteria and design. Although complementary medicine research currently follows the conventional scientific approach to silence critics, the efficacy of various complementary, integrative and alternative modalities may require the development of methodologies based on a new paradigm in order to overcome foreseeable limitations.

References

Ackerman KD, Felten SY, Dijkstra CD, et al: Parallel development of noradrenergic sympathetic innervation and cellular compartmentalisation in the rat spleen, *Exp Neurol* 103:239-255, 1989.

Ader R, Felten DL, Cohen N: *Psychoneuroimmunology,* ed 2, San Diego, 1991, Academic Press.

Beal MC: Viscerosomatic reflexes: a review, *J Am Osteopath Assoc* 85:786-811, 1985.

Bellinger DL, Felten SY, Felten DL: Maintenance of noradrenergic sympathetic innervation in the involuted thymus of the aged Fischer 344 rat, *Brain Behav Immunol* 2:133-150, 1988.

Blalock JE: The immune system: our sixth sense, *Immunology* 2:8-15, 1994.

Bouhuys A: Effects of posture in experimental asthma in man, *Am J Med* 34:470-476, 1963.

Carlson LE, Speca M, Patel KD, Goodey E: Mindfulness-based stress reduction in relation to quality of life, mood, symptoms of stress and levels of cortisol, dehydroepiandrosterone sulfate (DHEAS) and melatonin in breast and prostate cancer outpatients, *Psychoneuroendocrinology* 29:448-474, 2004.

Davidson RJ, Kabat-Zinn J, Schumacher J, et al: Alterations in brain and immune function produced by mindfulness meditation, *Psychosom Med* 65(4):564-570, 2003.

DeBeneditts G, Cigada M, Bianchi A, et al: Autonomic changes during hypnosis: a heart rate variability power spectrum analysis as a marker of sympatho-vagal balance, *Int J Clin Exp Hypnosis* XLII(2):140-152, 1994.

Engel GF: The need for a new medical model: a challenge for biomedicine, *Science* 196:129-136, 1977.

Felten SY, Felten DL, Olschowka JA: Noradrenergic and peptidergic innervation of lymphoid organs, *Chem Immunol* 52:25-48, 1992.

Fenwick PB: Self-generation of seizures by an action of mind, *Adv Neurol* 75:87-92, 1998.

Han JS, Tang J, Ren MF, Zhou ZF: Central neurotransmitters and acupuncture analgesia, *Am J Chin Med* 8:331-348, 1980.

Harinath K, Malhotra AS, Pal K, et al: Effects of Hatha yoga and Omkar meditation on cardiorespiratory performance, psychologic profile, and melatonin secretion, *J Altern Complement Med* 10:261-268, 2004.

Hatch JP, Borcherding S, Norris LK: Cardiopulmonary adjustments during operant heart rate control, *Psychophysiology* 27(6):641-647, 1990.

Hullkkonnen J, Koskikallio E, Rainesalo S, et al: The balance of inhibitory and excitatory cytokines is differently regulated in vivo and in vitro among therapy resistant epilepsy patients, *Epilepsy Res* 59:199-205, 2004.

Jian M: Influence of adrenergic antagonist and naloxone on the anti-allergic shock effect of electro-acupuncture in mice, *Acupunct Electrother Res* 10:163-167, 1985.

Kasahara T, Wu Y, Sakurai Y, Oguchi K: Suppressive effects of acupuncture on delayed type hypersensitivity to trinitrochlorobenzene and involvement of opiate receptors, *Int J Immunopharmacol* 14:661-665, 1992.

Lutgendorf SK, Costanzo ES: Psychoneuroimmunology and health psychology: an integral model, *Brain Behav Immunity* 17:225-232, 2003.

Ma SX: Neurobiology of acupuncture: toward CAM, *Evid Based Complement Altern Med* 1:41-47, 2004.

Mayer DJ, Price DD, Rafii A: Antagonism of acupuncture analgesia in man by the narcotic antagonist naloxone, *Brain Res* 121:368-372, 1977.

Neild JE, Cameron IR: Bronchoconstriction in response to suggestion: its prevention by an inhaled anticholinergic agent, *BMJ* 290:674, 1985.

Peterson C, Bossio L: Healthy attitudes: optimism, hope, and control. In Goldman D, Gurin J, editors: *Mind body medicine,* Yonkers, NY, 1993, Consumer Reports Books, pp 351-366.

Pert CB, Dreher HE, Ruff MR: The psychosomatic network: foundations of mind-body medicine, *Altern Ther Health Med* 4(4):30-41, 1998.

Raub JA: Psychophysiologic effects of Hatha Yoga on musculoskeletal and cardiopulmonary function: a literature review, *J Altern Complement Med* 8: 797-812, 2002.

Reichlin S: Neuroendocrine-immune interactions, *N Engl J Med* 329:1246-1253, 1993.

Reilly DT, Taylor MA, Beattie NGM, et al: Is the evidence for homoeoepathy reproducible? *Lancet* 344:1601-1606, 1994.

Sjolund BH, Eriksson MB: The influence of naloxone on analgesia produced by peripheral conditioning stimulation, *Brain Res* 173:295-301, 1979.

Solomon GF, Moos R: Emotions, immunity, and disease, *Arch Gen Psychiatry* 11(6):657-674, 1964.

Sung HJ, Kim YS, Kim IS, et al: Proteomic analysis of differential protein expression in neuropathic pain and electroacupuncture treatment models, *Proteomics* 4:2805-2813, 2004.

Vernon HT, Dhami MSI, Howley TP, Annett R: Spinal manipulation and beta-endorphin: a controlled study of the effects of a spinal manipulation on plasma beta-endorphin levels in normal males, *J Manipulative Physiol Ther* 9:115-123, 1986.

Watkins AD: The role of alternative therapy in allergic disease, *Clin Exp Allergy* 24:813-825, 1994.

Watkins AD: Perceptions, emotions and immunity: an integrated homoeostatic network, *Q J Med* 88:283-294, April 1995.

Wolsko PM, Eisenberg DM, Davis RB, Phillips RS: Use of mind-body medical therapies, *J Gen Intern Med* 19:43-50, 2004.

MIND-BODY MODALITIES

DENISE RODGERS

HISTORICAL OVERVIEW

Life and healing are inherently mysterious. The essential "stuff" of the universe, including the universe of the mind and body, remains essentially unexplained. The void inside every atom is pulsating with information or unseen intelligence. Molecular biologists and geneticists locate this intelligence within deoxyribonucleic acid (DNA), primarily for the sake of convenience. Life unfolds as DNA imparts its coded intelligence into a sequence where energy and information are interchanged for the purpose of building life from matter.

The reality ushered in by quantum physics made it possible to manipulate the invisible intelligence that underlies the visible world. Einstein taught that the physical body, as with all material objects, is like an illusion, and trying to manipulate it can be like grasping the shadow and missing the substance. The unseen world is a real world, and when we are willing to explore the immense creative power that lies within the mind, we can then access the unseen dimensions of the body.

Although mainstream consciousness seems highly aware of the inherent power of the mind, some of the earliest records of certain mind-and-body techniques were found in Babylonia and ancient Sumer well before the rise of experimental science. In the third century BC, Hippocrates was well versed in the art of mental healing. A serpent coiled around a staff, the Hippocratic symbol is used today to portray the medical/healing profession. History reveals that the coiled serpent symbolizes the healing energy possessed by each of us, lying dormant at the base of the spine, with the staff representing life itself. Eastern philosophy posits that when the serpent is unleashed, healing energy spirals up the spine and out the forehead. This energy, said to be mental in nature, can then be used to heal the physical body.

Most ancient and indigenous medical systems make use of the extraordinary interconnectedness of the mind and body. Native American and the Asian Indian cultures are believed to be in contact with natural healing forces through their dreams, visions, and mystical experiences.

The ancient Greeks were also known for their healing temples. These centers existed for more than 800 years and endured until the rise of the Christian era. Patients would travel long distances to experience one of the Aesculapian healing temples. The first step in seeking a cure was to create inner cleanliness by taking a purifying bath. Patients then were put on a special diet or fast. They would attend one of the great dramas of Euripides or Sophocles, observing the tensions and movements of life. Later they were taken to visit one of the shrines, where healers used imagery to visualize the affected part of the body. During sleep the priests entered the patients' room and touched the diseased parts. Thereafter, patients would dream and were said to awaken healed.

Philippus Aureolus Theophrastus Bombast von Hohenhein, known as Paracelsus, was a Swiss, sixteenth-century Renaissance physician. Although considered the father of modern drug therapy and scientific medicine, he nevertheless opposed the idea of separating the mind from the healing processes of the body. Along with his esteemed medical theories, he held that imagination and faith were the cause of healing power, as follows:

> Man has a visible and an invisible workshop. The visible one is his body, the invisible one is the imagination of the mind. . . . The spirit is the master, imagination the tool, and the body the plastic material. The power of the imagination is the great factor in medicine. It may produce diseases in man and it may cure them. Ills of the body may be cured by physical remedies or by the power of spirit acting through the soul.

Paracelsus believed that physicians could heal by tapping the power of God. He also believed that dreams gave humans clairvoyance and the ability to diagnose illness from long distances.

The philosophies of all these cultures had a common belief in a spiritual center that resides within. They believed in spirit over matter, of mind over body. However, in contrast, modern allopathic medicine has regarded these connections as nonscientific and of secondary importance. Scientific healing, in the form of drug therapy and surgery, has grown to become a dominant Western form of treatment. Since the early 1900s, however, many medical scientists have begun to reinvestigate the role the mind plays in healing. In critical situations, physicians have been known to say, "We've done all we can do—it's in God's hands now," or "It depends on the patient's will to live."

Every physician has witnessed miraculous recoveries unexplainable by scientific understanding. Labeling a recovery as a "spontaneous remission" has become common to describe a healing that cannot be explained by medical standards. Physicians have also long recognized the effectiveness of placebos, substances with no known pharmacological action or benefit. In some cases, placebos can be as much as 70% effective in the treatment of illness, thereby proving the theory that a patient's therapeutic expectation is a contributing factor for healing.

During the past 35 years, the scientific community has made great strides in exploring the mind's capacity to affect the body. This movement has received its impetus from several sources. The rise in incidence of chronic illness over the past few decades and the rapidly increasing costs for treatment have set the stage for deeper exploration of mind-body therapies. These therapies show great promise for mobilizing the body's inherent power to heal itself.

Recent studies have begun to further deepen our understanding of the effects of stress on the body. Convincing evidence supports that the immune system, along with other organs and systems in the body, can be and is often influenced by the mind. These research efforts and clinical experiments suggest that the separation between mind and body, long taken for granted in Western philosophy, is difficult to quantify. These challenges are all part of a new approach to medical science: the challenge of proving that the mind—along with our thoughts and emotions—has a significant impact on the body's health.

For patients, this new synthesis has very practical significance. It suggests that by paying attention to and exerting some control over mental and emotional states, these attempts may actually contribute to prevention of or recovery from disease. The conscious participation of the patient in the process of healing not only offers new insights but also raises new questions about the nature and reality of consciousness.

The predominant fundamental tenet of mind-body medicine is the concept of *treating the whole person*. Another significant tenet is that people can be active participants in their own health care and may be able to prevent disease or shorten its course by taking steps to manage their own mental processes.

Medical researchers are beginning to rediscover what other cultures have historically used in their healing systems, such as meditation, hypnosis, and imagery. Grounded in ancient philosophy, these interventions are capable of stimulating and often facilitating the mind's capacity to affect the body. Experimentation has given practitioners the opportunity to offer nontoxic therapies while examining the specific links between mental processes and autonomic, immune, and nervous system functioning.

Evidence grows that states of mind can affect physiology. No one is promising that people can cure themselves of disease by adjusting their mental attitudes; this is not the message of mind-body interventions. However, mind-body approaches can be used to reduce the severity and frequency of biological symptoms and can potentially help strengthen the body's resistance to disease.

The techniques of mind-body medicine are reasonably well accepted for treating certain chronic and difficult-to-treat medical conditions, from pain syndromes to hypertension. In well-designed studies, relaxation, guided imagery, biofeedback, hypnosis, and related strategies have been proven workable. New evidence is showing that mind-body interventions are consistently effective in improving psychological and medical outcomes after surgery. In a meta-analysis involving 191 studies and more than 8600 patients, psychosocial/behavioral interventions showed reliably moderate effect sizes for improved recovery, pain reduction, and reduced psychological distress (Dreher, 1998). As discussed in this chapter, there is movement on all fronts. Mainstream medical institutions are beginning to take awkward "baby steps" toward implementing them within departments of psychology, psychiatry, oncology, neurology, and rehabilitation. "Mind and body" departments are being established in medical schools and hospitals nationwide. More impressively, both conventional and holistic professionals are beginning to incorporate these approaches into their own personal regimens for greater health and wellness.

This chapter discusses recent evidence that supports mind-body approaches, describes some of the more widely used techniques, and summarizes the results of some of the most effective interventions. The approaches discussed in this section not only demonstrate dramatic results in specific areas but also help form the basis for a new perspective for medicine and healing. From this perspective, it becomes evident that every interaction between physician and patient has the potential to affect the mind and, in turn, the body of the patient.

THE ROLE OF CONSCIOUSNESS

The Dismissal of the Mind

Although ancient mystics believed in the power of the human mind, Western science began to question such matters by the mid-1800s. Until that time, physicians believed the prevailing philosophy that the patient's inner life and social being were vital components of all diagnosis and treatment. They generally believed that medicine should take into account not only biological but also behavioral, moral, psychological, and spiritual factors.

However, these models and methods began to fade by the end of the nineteenth century, and a patient-specific model of treatment gave way to a disease-specific model. During the rise of this era of experimental science, four leading German physiologists (Helmholtz, Ludwig, DuBois-Remond, and Brucke) pledged themselves to account for all bodily processes in purely physiological terms. They determined that any reported connection between mental states and bodily functions was considered biased, subjective, nonmeasurable, and scientifically unreliable (Figure 16-1). More than 15,000 American physicians traveled to Germany to study the fascinating laboratory experimentations being introduced at that time. These innovative breakthroughs were in direct contrast with the style of medicine that had been practiced for centuries. It was believed that proper research could be conducted only in laboratories on isolated constituents—microorganisms, components of blood and urine, tissue, and organs—with the focus on devising universal remedies

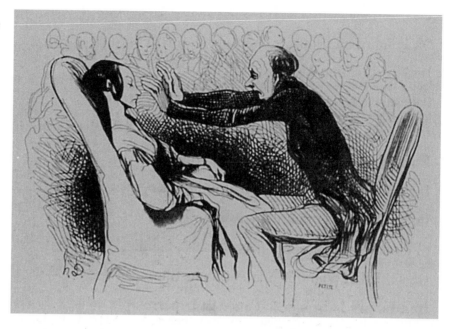

Figure 16-1 Mesmerism and hypnotism were the object of satire and a number of caricatures during the nineteenth century. (Courtesy Bibliothèque Interuniversitaire de Médecine, Paris.)

independent of individual patients. This approach has contemporary medicine in the position of having to learn the scientific basis of something it has known for centuries: that beliefs, thoughts, and feelings affect physiology.

Power of Placebo

The word *placebo* is Latin for "I please." This concept is well illustrated by an anecdote concerning Sir William Osler. One of North America and England's busiest and most famous physicians, Osler brought new light to the power of placebo near the turn of the nineteenth century. Dr. Osler made a house call to a dying boy, who had been unresponsive to any previous treatments. Osler appeared at the boy's bedside dressed in magnificent, scarlet academic robes. After a brief examination, Osler sat down at the boy's bedside, peeled a peach, sugared it, and cut it into pieces. He then fed it, bit by bit, with a fork to the entranced patient, telling him that it was a most special fruit and that if he ate it, he would not be sick.

Osler confided to the boy's father that his chances for survival were slim. He continued to visit the boy daily for more than a month, always dressed in his majestic, scarlet robes and offering the boy nourishment with his own two hands. This dramatic presentation inspired magic and belief well beyond laboratory science and helped catalyze the boy's unexpected and complete recovery.

Eloquently summing up the placebo's power, Osler (1953) wrote the following:

Faith in the gods or saints cures one, faith in little pills another, hypnotic suggestion a third, faith in a plain common doctor a fourth. . . . The faith with which we work . . . has its limitations [but] such as we find it, faith is the most precious commodity, without which we should be very badly off.

Among the early placebo studies documented are those conduced by Dr. Ronald Katz, chairman of the Department of Anesthesiology at the UCLA School of Medicine. Katz reported a series of observations involving patients who were informed that headaches were a complication of spinal anesthesia. At the last minute the patients were told that the choice of anesthesia had been changed from spinal to general. Despite the change, all the patients experienced the symptoms associated with spinal anesthesia (Katz, 1977).

Similar to Katz's study investigating expectations, Dr. J.W.L. Fielding conducted a similar study at the Department of Surgery at Queen Elizabeth Hospital in Birmingham, England. In compliance with informed consent procedure, 411 patients were told they could expect to lose hair as a result of the chemotherapy being administered. Thirty percent of the patients unknowingly received placebos instead of chemotherapy and suffered hair loss even though the pills they had taken contained no medication (Fielding et al., 1983).

Although it has sometimes confounded as much as clarified, the mechanism of pain has provided fascinating clues to investigators of the mind-body healing response. In one landmark study in 1978, dental patients experiencing the aftereffects of an extracted tooth were given a sugar pill and told it was a powerful painkiller. They reported significant pain relief. Then experimenters added another agent: along with the placebo, a separate group of dental patients were given a chemical known to block the action of the brain's own endorphins. The second group experienced significantly less pain reduction than the first group (Levine et al., 1978).

Here was a study that indicated a specific mechanism for placebo—endorphins—without which the magic effect would not have occurred. These studies and many other similar ones led scientists to believe that endorphins mediate much of the mind-body effect, whether that effect is triggered by trauma, placebo, hypnosis, or any other mental agent.

The story does not end there. Two separate studies found that the endorphin-blocker naloxone failed to prevent pain reduction in patients under hypnosis as it had for patients who took a placebo. In another placebo study, however, pain reduction occurred even with naloxone. One plausible explanation is that other forms of endorphins may stealthily bypass the naloxone blockade. There are likely many mind-body routes, with many mechanisms to create similar effects. Therefore, different states of mind may affect the body along different pathways, or the same substances may have multiple effects. In other words, relief of pain may also stimulate immune function because pain-relieving endorphins are key messenger molecules that also "talk" to the immune system.

The natural conclusion emerging from placebo research is that expectation or belief affects biology. The emotional responses of individuals to the world around them, stimulating hopes and joys, fears and anguish, has a potential affect on the physical body. This understanding is fundamental to the treatment of illness. It does not mean that conventional medical treatment should be supplanted by psychological or emotional approaches. The most effective and comprehensive strategy of treatment should be expanded to include the awareness of emotional and psychological factors in concert.

Mind and Emotion Everywhere

Former chief of the Brain Biochemistry Section of the National Institute of Mental Health (NIMH), Candace Pert, PhD, co-discoverer of endorphins, made some startling revelations regarding the existence of neuropeptide receptors throughout the entire body. Pert found that the endocrine system and even the immune system all have these messenger molecules. This means that neuropeptide molecules are involved in a psychosomatic communication network, and that the biochemistry of emotion could be mediating the transference of information flowing throughout the body. Pert maintains that the emotions are the bridge between the mental and the physical, making them prime candidates for a variety of links between thought and healing.

Mind and Immunity

Psychoneuroimmunology (PNI), a term coined by Robert Ader, an experimental psychologist, was first introduced to the scientific community in 1981. Ader had previously conducted experiments with rats that showed the immune system could be conditioned and therefore did not operate autonomously, but was actually under the influence of the brain (see Chapter 15).

In subsequent research at the University of Rochester, Ader and Nicholas Cohen continued to show that the immune system can be trained, or *conditioned*, to respond to a neutral stimulus (placebo). They found that the administration of an immune-suppressing drug and placebo together "conditioned" the immune system to respond to the placebo alone after the drug was discontinued. They also found that by alternating the administration of real medication and placebos, thus conditioning the body's physiological response to the placebo, the conditioning effects of a drug can be increased. They believed that side effects of dependence could be reduced in addition to costs (Ader and Cohen, 1991).

Considering the brief time that PNI has existed as an accepted field of research, a great amount of data has been collected in support of the idea that homeostatic mechanisms are the product of an integrated system of defenses in which the immune system is a critical component. Now that we understand that peptides and receptors are expressed by the nervous system, the digestive system, and the immune system, it is not surprising that immunologic reactivity can be influenced by stressful life experiences (Ader, 2003).

It has become increasingly clear that there must be an intricate network behind spontaneous remissions, which are known to occur in cancer more often than any other disease. Research will likely continue to raise more questions about the mechanics of how the power of the mind actually works. How can the anticipation of a physical effect actually bring about physical change? And if anticipation or attitudes do play a role in creating physical change, how can that knowledge be used to enhance medical treatment or promote good health? If we can answer these questions, can we determine how the human mind converts ideas and expectations into chemical realities? Mind-body practitioners and medical researchers alike must answer these questions.

PSYCHOTHERAPY

The word *psychotherapy* is derived from Greek words meaning "healing of the soul" and refers to treatment involving emotional and mental health, which is interwoven with physical health. Psychotherapy encompasses a wide range of specific treatments, including combining medication with discussion, listening to the patient's concerns, and using more active behavioral and emotional approaches. It should also be understood more generally as the matrix of interaction in which all health professionals operate.

An average of "one in every five people in the United States experiences a major psychological disorder every six months—most commonly anxiety, depression, substance abuse, or acute confusion" (Strain, 1993). It is believed that rate is even greater among patients with a chronic illness and among elderly patients. Approximately three fifths of patients with psychological problems are seen only by primary care physicians, many of whom are not adequately trained in psychotherapy or do not have adequate time to spend with each patient discussing these psychological issues. Despite the enormous need for different forms of psychological care, most people who display the greatest need for such care receive less-than-adequate screening and treatment for their psychiatric conditions.

Research also indicates that primary care physicians recognize cases of depression in only one fourth

to one half of the patients who experience it, and they recognize other types of mental illness in less than one fourth of cases. However, these same physicians write most of the prescriptions for antidepressant and antianxiety drugs and may often prescribe them inappropriately. Clearly, there is a significant need for better recognition and management of the psychiatric conditions that often accompany serious illness.

Methods of Psychotherapy

Mental health professionals are paying more attention to features shared by all effective forms of psychotherapy, especially collaboration between the therapist and patient in developing an account of the patient's emotional life that promotes confidence, heightens well-being, and suggests ways to overcome cognitive or emotional difficulties. The primary aim of psychotherapy is to transform the meaning of the patient's experience by improving emotional state through an intimate relationship with a helpful person. Conventional psychotherapy is conducted primarily through psychological methods such as suggestion, persuasion, psychoanalysis, and reeducation. Although research suggests that the methods do not differ greatly in effectiveness, several hundred types of psychotherapy are available, used individually or in groups. Generally, most forms of psychotherapy fall in the following general categories:

- **Psychodynamic therapy.** Psychodynamic therapy is derived from psychoanalysis and seeks to understand and resolve emotional conflicts that originate in childhood relationships and repeat themselves in adult life. Sessions usually are devoted to exploring current emotional reactions from past situations. This approach works best if the patient's goal is to make fundamental changes in personality patterns rather than to change one specific behavior. Psychodynamic therapy is often called *interpretive therapy* or *expressive therapy*.
- **Behavior therapy.** Behavior therapy emphasizes changing specific behavior, such as a phobia, by stopping what has been reinforcing it or by replacing it with a more desirable response. Sessions are usually devoted to analyzing the behavior and devising ways to change it, carrying out specific instructions between sessions. Behavior therapy is

more effective with focused problems, such as a fear of public speaking.

- **Cognitive therapy.** Cognitive therapy is similar to behavior therapy in changing specific habits; however, it emphasizes the habitual thoughts that underlie those habits. The general strategy is similar to that of behavior therapy, and the two approaches are often used together. Cognitive therapy is effective therapy for treating depression and low self-esteem.
- **Systems therapy.** Systems therapy focuses on relationship patterns, either in couples, between parents and children, or within the whole family. This approach requires that everyone involved attend therapy sessions and often involves experiential practice aimed at changing problem-causing patterns. Systems therapies work well for a troubled marriage or intense conflicts between parent and child, where the problem is in the relationship between them.
- **Supportive therapy.** Supportive therapy concentrates on helping people who are in an intense emotional crisis, such as a deep depression, and may be used in combination with pharmacological support. It focuses on building tools to handle overwhelming day-to-day situations.
- **Body-oriented therapy.** Body-oriented therapy hypothesizes that emotions are encoded in and may be expressed as unexpressed tension and restriction in various parts of the physical body. Various methods of therapy, including breathwork, movement, and manual pressure, are used to help release emotions that are believed to have been held in the muscles and tissues.

Recent research indicates that psychotherapeutic treatment can hasten recovery from a medical crisis and is in some cases the best treatment for it. Brief psychotherapy reduced time spent in hospitals for elderly patients with broken hips by an average of 2 days; these patients returned to the hospital fewer times and spent fewer days in rehabilitation (Strain, 1993). Other studies show that psychotherapy is most effective when begun soon after a patient is admitted to a hospital. At present, however, most psychological problems associated with physical illnesses remain undiagnosed or are not identified until near the end of a hospital stay.

One of the most common psychological problems of medical patients is "reactive" anxiety and depression—the emotional distress stemming from a patient's reaction to diagnosis. Those with serious or terminal illnesses are particularly vulnerable. In other cases, psychiatric symptoms are directly caused by the patient's physical disease. Still other patients experience a shift in their mental or emotional status as a direct result of a specific medication. For example, some patients taking high levels of steroids may react psychotically, whereas others may experience severe depression.

Role of Group Support and Psychological Counseling

Psychologists have known since World War II that social support and group consciousness greatly aids people with their attitudes and emotional resiliency. Over the past 10 years, clinical studies have shown that social support is indeed a significant influence on symptoms of stress for patients with chronic illnesses.

In an earlier yet still impressive study of patients with established coronary artery disease, group support and psychological counseling were combined with diet and exercise. Symptoms such as angina pectoris rapidly diminished or disappeared, and after 1 year the coronary artery obstructions were smaller. This evidence strongly suggested that the most deadly and expensive U.S. health care problem could be potentially reversible through a complementary, non-invasive, diet and behavioral modification approach that emphasizes group psychotherapy (Ornish, 1990).

A landmark case study was conducted in1989 by David Spiegel, MD, a professor of psychiatry and behavioral sciences at Stanford School of Medicine, where he studied the benefits of group support on women with metastatic breast cancer. The women who participated in the group psychotherapy lived an average of 18 months longer than those who did not participate, doubling their survival time. The added survival time was longer than any medication or other known medical treatment could be expected to provide for women with advanced breast cancer. The intense social support the women experienced in these sessions appeared to influence the way their bodies coped with the illness, which suggested that quality of life seemed to affect longevity (Spiegel et al., 1989).

In 1999, Spiegel conducted a multicenter feasibility study to examine the benefits of a supportive-expressive group psychotherapy intervention for recently diagnosed breast cancer patients. One hundred and eleven breast cancer patients within 1 year of diagnosis were recruited from 10 geographically diverse sites of the Community Clinical Oncology Program of the National Cancer Institute (NCI) and two academic medical centers. Each patient who participated in the expressive-psychotherapy group met for 12 weekly sessions for 90 minutes. Results indicated a significant decrease in mood disturbance scores, anxiety and depression (Spiegel et al., 1999).

A similar study was conducted on 102 women with metastatic breast cancer who were randomly selected to receive 1 year of weekly supportive-expressive group therapy and educational materials. Control women received education materials only. Participants who received group therapy showed a significantly greater decline in traumatic stress symptoms and total mood disturbance than controls (Classen et al., 2001).

Recent research suggests that the maintenance of emotional well-being is critical to cardiovascular health. People who feel lonely, depressed, and isolated have been found to be significantly more likely to suffer illnesses and die prematurely of cardiovascular diseases than those who have adequate social support (Williams et al., 1999). Consequently, the development of appropriate interventions to improve emotional health of people with certain psychosocial risk factors has become an important research goal. It is anticipated that such interventions will increase life expectancy of people at risk and may also save millions of dollars in medical care costs.

In a cross-sectional study at Stanford, coping styles of emotional suppression and "fighting spirit" were associated with mood disturbance in 121 cancer patients participating in professionally led, community-based support groups. They concluded that negative affect and an attitude of realistic optimism may enhance adjustment and reduce stress for cancer patients in support groups (Cordova et al., 2003).

Recent studies are beginning to show a convergence of significant psychological, health behavior, and biological effects after a psychological intervention for cancer patients. An Ohio State University study tested the hypothesis that a psychological intervention could reduce emotional distress, improve health behavior, and enhance immune responses;

227 women who had undergone breast cancer surgery were randomized to an intervention that included strategies to reduce stress, improve mood, alter health behaviors, and maintain adherence to cancer treatment. The control group received no intervention. The treatment group met in weekly sessions for 4 months. Patients who attended the weekly support group sessions showed significant lowering of anxiety, improvements in perceived social support, improved dietary habits, and reduction in smoking. Immune responses for the intervention group paralleled their psychological and behavioral improvements. T cell proliferation remained stable or increased in the treatment group, while the responses declined in the control group (Andersen et al., 2004).

Cost-Effectiveness of Psychotherapy

Psychotherapy has been shown to speed patients' recovery time from illness. Faster recovery leads to reduced costs and fewer return visits to medical practitioners. In one study, patients who frequently visited medical clinics were offered short-term psychotherapy, and significant declines were seen in visits to their doctors, days spent in the hospital, emergency department visits, diagnostic procedures, and drug prescriptions. Their overall health care costs were decreased by 10% to 20% in the years after brief psychotherapy (Cummings and Bragman, 1988).

A more specific example of cost-effectiveness was demonstrated in a 1991 study in which 10 group sessions of 90 minutes of psychotherapy and relaxation techniques significantly reduced the severity of pain. In chronic pain patients, those who participated in the outpatient behavioral medicine program had 36% fewer clinic visits than those who did not (Caudill et al., 1991).

In a 1987 study conducted jointly with Mount Sinai and Northwestern, psychiatrist George Fulop of Mount Sinai and his colleagues observed that patients hospitalized for medical or surgical reasons had significantly longer hospital stays if they also had concurrent psychiatric problems, especially if they were elderly. In other words, a patient who had a heart attack and who was also depressed tended to remain in the hospital for more days than a similar heart attack patient whose mood was normal. Fulop's study suggested that treating a medical patient's psychological conditions with psychotherapy in adjunct with medication could not only improve psychological well-being but also affect the patient's physical condition (Fulop et al., 1987).

Another well-known study, published in 1983 by psychologists Herbert J. Schlesinger and Emily Mumford and their colleagues at the University of Colorado School of Medicine, investigated patients with four common chronic diseases: asthma, diabetes, coronary heart disease, and high blood pressure. The researchers examined a group of Blue Cross–Blue Shield patients who underwent some form of psychotherapy after having been identified with one of these physical conditions, then compared them with a control group who did not receive psychological treatment after similar diagnoses were made (Schlesinger et al., 1983). Three years after they received their medical diagnoses, patients who had undergone 7 to 20 mental health treatment visits had incurred lower medical charges than those who did not have psychological treatment. The total charges for the first group, including those incurred for psychotherapy and counseling, were more than $300 less than for the other group. In other words, the savings on medical bills offered by psychotherapy more than compensated for its costs. After 21 sessions the savings began to diminish as the cumulative cost of mental health care increased.

Although this study is often cited as "proof" of psychotherapy's financial advantages for medically ill patients, it was a retrospective study rather than a prospective study. More scientifically controlled studies are needed in which subjects are selected at random from the beginning of treatment and closely followed after treatment. Another limitation of this particular research approach was that the investigators could not clearly define the type of mental health problems the patients experienced or the specific treatment they received. The information gathered encompassed a large variety of psychiatric interventions.

More rigorous research on specific forms of psychotherapy, including precise diagnoses, will be needed to reach firm conclusions about the economic benefits of psychological treatment for medically ill patients. However, there is already sufficient evidence to suggest that this cost/benefit research is important to pursue. For example, one review of 15 studies published between 1965 and 1980 demonstrated that patients who underwent psychotherapy used other medical services 13% less than patients who did not receive psychotherapy.

The concept of what constitutes appropriate areas for psychiatric intervention should be expanded. Many people, including health care professionals and academicians, consider psychotherapeutic intervention in physical illness a peripheral concern. Important research questions regarding unexplained mind-body events have long existed but are generally ignored. However, the studies previously cited suggest that psychological intervention could be most beneficial when used early in the disease process and could affect mortality in certain illnesses.

Although research continues to mount on the effects of psychotherapeutic interventions, further studies are needed to continue researching the interconnectedness of the mind and body and how these methods can offer genuine opportunity to improve health and limit costs simultaneously.

Research on Social Support and Mortality

Thanks to a growing number of large-scale studies, evidence of a link between social support and physical well-being has been prolific. This research shows that having many close social relationships is associated with a lower risk of dying at any age. Research that has looked specifically at sick people shows that once serious illness strikes, social support continues to affect their chances of staying alive.

Internist James Goodwin at the Medical College of Wisconsin studied cancer survival in several thousand patients. The married cancer patients did better medically and had lower mortality rates than the unmarried patients (Goodwin et al., 1987). Similarly, in a study of 1368 patients with coronary artery disease, Redford Williams at Duke University found that having a spouse or other close confidant tripled the chances that a patient would be alive 5 years later (Williams et al., 1999).

In an overview of research concerning mortality and social relationships, James House observed that the relationship between social isolation and early death is as strong statistically as the relationship between dying and smoking or having high serum cholesterol. Therefore the data suggest that it may be as important to one's health to be socially integrated as it is to stop smoking or to reduce one's cholesterol level (House et al., 1988).

In 1990, epidemiologists Peggy Reynolds and George Kaplan at the California Department of Health Services studied the number of social contacts that cancer patients had each day. Women with the least amount of social contact were 2.2 times more likely to die of cancer over a 17-year period than were the most socially connected women (Reynolds and Kaplan 1990).

People who feel lonely, depressed, and isolated have been found to be significantly more likely to suffer illnesses and to die prematurely of cardiovascular diseases than those who have adequate social support (Williams et al., 1999). Naturally, many other potential social factors can account for why one patient survives longer than another. Therefore, most such studies have been careful to eliminate the obvious confounding variables, such as smoking and alcohol use, differences in socioeconomic status, and access to health care. In general, however, the studies still consistently show that more and better social support from family and friends is associated with lower odds of dying at any given age.

Although the relationship between social support and health outcome has been largely underestimated by medical science, two studies recently examined social support and its relationship to mortality. The Department of Community and Preventative Medicine at the University of Rochester School of Medicine found that certain aspects of informal caregiving are important factors in enhancing the survival of frail, nursing home residents. Several social support variables were statistically significant predictors of mortality. Participants whose caregiver was a spouse had a significantly lower risk of mortality compared with those whose caregiver was not a spouse (Temkin-Greener et al., 2004). Researchers at the Mayo Clinic compiled a systematic overview of recent evidence related to the social support network, specifically the role of social support in cardiovascular disease–related outcomes (Mookadam and Arthur, 2004).

A number of studies have demonstrated a relationship between depression and low perceived social support and increased cardiac morbidity and mortality in patients with heart disease. Evidence also suggests that depression increases the risk of acute myocardial infarction and the resulting morbidity and mortality (Malach and Imperato, 2004).

RELAXATION

Stress Management

The popular term *stress* was brought into use by Professor Hans Selye, Director of the Institute of Experimental Medicine and Surgery at the University of Montreal. He determined that stress was "the rate of wear and tear on the body." Confusion and debate continue as to whether stress is the factor that causes the wear and tear or is the resulting damage. Selye termed it "general adaption syndrome" (GAS), which has three phases: an alarm reaction, a stage of resistance, and a stage of exhaustion. A stress cause, or stressor, mobilizes GAS by activating the sympathetic part of the autonomic nervous system. Hormones bring about physiological changes in the body, often referred to as the "fight-or-flight syndrome" (Selye, 1978).

The problem of stress has received wide publicity in the media in recent years. We have also heard the cliché that "stress" was the epidemic of the 1980s and 1990s. Consequently, the term *stress* has become a buzzword that has acquired a highly negative connotation. We have also received much advice over the last few years, from all sorts of sources, about the many different approaches to controlling stress. All the alarmist and negative publicity has stimulated further anxiety and concern in many people's minds— a fear of stress, which in itself can lead to further stress. Having become aware of it, everyone now wants to manage their stress, and many cater to this growing market. This rapidly growing market consists of various experts, consultants, and therapists. Vitamin regimens, herbal supplements, fitness programs, relaxation techniques, and personal development courses are being offered, all in the name of *stress management*. All sorts of experts, both qualified and self-appointed, are convinced that their particular product or service will banish stress for good.

The fact remains that there are no magic cures and no magic bullets. Stress is essentially a result of an interaction between a negative environment, unhealthful lifestyles, and self-defeating attitudes and beliefs. Therefore, unlike what is believed by stress management consultants, no one particular technique, method, program, or regimen of vitamins or herbs can reduce long-term stress.

Stress is most often seen as the outside pressures and problems that encroach on our busy lives: deadlines, excessive workload, noise, traffic, problems with spouse or children, and excessive demands made by others. Stress is the unconscious response to a demand. Stress is not "those things out there," but rather what happens inside our mind and body as we react unconsciously to those things or people. Normally, we experience some degree of stress in everything we do and everything that happens to us.

In *The Magical Child*, Joseph Chiltern Pearce states, "Stress is the way intelligence grows." He explains that, under stress, the brain immediately grows massive numbers of new connecting links between the neurons that enable learning. Although the stressed mind/brain grows in ability and the unstressed mind lags behind, the overstressed brain can collapse into physiological shock. Something is essential to maintain the optimal level of stress, and this is relaxation (Pearce, 1992).

When the stress response is minor, we do not notice any symptoms. The greater the stimulation, the more symptoms we notice. Holmes and Rahe's scale of life changes provides a guide to the amount of stress attached to major events, such as marriage, relocation, emigration, loss of a job, death of a spouse, or birth of a child. These significant life events can quickly overload our ability to cope (Holmes and Rahe, 1967).

In *The Human Zoo*, Desmond Morris posits that modern humans are engaged in the "Stimulus Struggle": "If we abandon it, or tackle it badly, we are in serious trouble." We are trying to maintain the optimal level of stimulation—not the maximum, but that level that is most beneficial, somewhere between understimulation and overstimulation (Morris, 1995).

Stress becomes a problem when it reaches excessive levels, when the demands exceed our ability to respond or to cope effectively. When we are under excessive, prolonged stress and no longer able to cope or adjust, the "stress" becomes "distress." Symptoms then develop that lead to stress-induced illnesses. The physical body "engine" begins to "rev" at high speed, totally absorbing restricted, unproductive energy. Over extended periods, this "wear and tear" begins to take its toll, and disease can creep into the body.

We can learn to control our responses to stress by changing the ways that we think. Stress management is developing the ability to assert control over our behaviors. When we become aware of our ability to control attitudes and behaviors, we naturally begin to assert control over our life's situations that seem to be stressful. It is not the stress itself that is harmful, but our reactions to it that create havoc in the body and mind.

The greatest stressor that most people experience daily is *change*. Challenges, frustrations, conflicting demands and occasional loss, grief, and suffering are among the many unconscious responses to change. These life events are inevitable and require us to adapt to new situations. If we do not adapt to change by altering our attitudes, our minds and bodies suffer. When changes take place in our environment, career, and personal relationships, it becomes essential to learn how to behave, think, and feel differently to cope with the new situation effectively.

We are all continuously adjusting to changing conditions, rather like an air conditioner controlled by a thermostat. As the weather outside changes, the thermostat turns the air conditioner unit on, which begins to bring the interior temperature back to a specified normal level of comfort. The greater the changes outside, the harder the machine has to work to keep up with them. If the external temperature moves into extreme ranges, the machine will be pushed to the limit. If it exceeds its specified limit, it will eventually break down, and the motor will burn out.

So it is with the human machine. Our bodies continuously react to whatever is happening around us or inside of us. We respond physically, mentally, and emotionally to even the most minute changes. This process occurs all the time, whether we are consciously aware of it or not.

Different individuals respond differently to stress. We know people who can remain cool, calm, and collected under the most trying circumstances, and we know others who are unable to cope when faced with even minor situations. The differences are mostly a result of the differences in upbringing, past understandings, present experiences, attitudes, belief structures, family values, perceptions, and coping skills developed over years and generations. Furthermore, when different individuals experience distress, the symptoms they develop are also different; different people seem to channel their excessive stress into different parts of the body. The long-term effects of such different responses include such physical illnesses as ulcers, headaches, chronic backaches, and high blood pressure, which ultimately results in heart disease, cancer, or other chronic disorders.

Decades of research have linked stress, either directly or indirectly, to coronary heart disease, cancer, strokes, lung ailments, accidental injuries, cirrhosis of the liver, immune system deficiencies, and suicide. Stress is often a component of chronic illness, either as a precursor of disease or as an outcome. People who manage stress are more resilient, experience fewer symptoms, and experience an improved quality of life (Kabat-Zinn, 1990).

In looking at 26 randomly control trials testing the effect of cognitive-behavioral techniques (including meditation) on hypertension, Eisenberg and colleagues (1993) found that no single technique appears to be more effective than any other in treating essential hypertension. When prescribed in the absence of other behavioral interventions, cognitive-behavioral techniques were not nearly as effective as standard antihypertensive pharmacotherapy.

Harvard-trained cardiologist Herbert Benson began investigating the benefits of relaxation in the late 1960s and continues to delve into the effects of stress on various disease-specific populations. Benson's group has examined the stress phenomenon and its effect on cardiovascular diseases and neurodegenerative diseases (Esch et al., 2002a, 2000b). They found that stress has a major impact on the circulatory and nervous systems, playing a significant role in susceptibility, progress, and outcome of both cardiovascular and neurodegenerative diseases. However, they also found that some amounts of stress can actually improve performance and thus can be beneficial in certain cases.

According to the American Institute of Stress in New York, workplace stress leads to $300 billion each year in health care costs as a result of missed work (Schwartz, 2004). The Organizational Science and Human Factors Branch of the National Institute for Occupational Safety and Health claims that stressed workers incur health care costs that are 46% higher, an average of $600 more per person, than other employees (Sauter, 2004).

The Relaxation Response

Convinced that the benefits of meditation could potentially lower high blood pressure, Benson continued his research into a variety of psychological and physiological effects that appear common to many mind and body practices. He later identified *the relaxation response,* which elicited a similar response common to meditation, prayer, autogenic training, and some forms of hypnosis (Benson, 1975). He later published his method in a book of the same name.

His research indicated that excessive stress could cause or aggravate hypertension and its related diseases, atherosclerosis, heart attack, and stroke. He then examined the nature of the relaxation response, showing that physiological changes as remarkable as those seen in the fight-or-flight response also occur during true relaxation, including lowering of oxygen consumption, metabolism, heart rate, and blood pressure, as well as increased production of alpha brain waves. A marked decrease in blood lactate was also found. Blood lactate has often been linked with anxiety. According to Benson, the following guidelines can help you achieve the relaxation response:

1. Try to find 10 to 20 minutes in your daily routine; before breakfast is generally a good time.
2. Sit comfortably.
3. For the period you will practice, try to arrange your life so that you will have no distractions. For example, let the answering machine handle the phone, or ask someone to watch the children.
4. Time yourself by glancing periodically at a clock or watch (but do not set an alarm). Commit yourself to a specific length of practice.

Expanding on these guidelines, several approaches can be used to elicit the relaxation response; Benson suggests the following:

Step 1: Pick a focus word or short phrase that is firmly rooted in your personal belief system. For example, a nonreligious individual might choose a neutral word such as "one," "peace," or "love." A Christian person wanting to use a prayer could pick the opening words of Psalm 23, "The Lord is My Shepherd"; a Jewish person could choose "Shalom."

Step 2: Sit quietly in a comfortable position.

Step 3: Close your eyes.

Step 4: Relax your muscles.

Step 5: Breathe slowly and naturally, repeating your focus word or phrase silently as you exhale.

Step 6: Throughout, assume a passive attitude. Do not worry about how well you are doing. When other thoughts come to mind, simply say to yourself, "Oh, well," and gently return to the repetition.

Step 7: Continue for 10 to 20 minutes. You may open your eyes to check the time, but do not use an alarm. When you finish, sit quietly for a minute or so, at first with your eyes closed and later with your eyes open. Then do not stand for 1 or 2 minutes.

Step 8: Practice the technique once or twice a day.

Benson's subsequent research into the relaxation response covered several efficient techniques of relaxation training, including transcendental meditation, Zen and yoga, autogenic training, progression relaxation, hypnosis, and sentic cycles (Table 16-1). He found that these methods had four common elements: a quiet environment, an object to focus the mind on, a passive attitude, and a comfortable position. Some practices are more effective than others, and some are easier to learn and practice than others (Benson, 1993).

Benson's group also found that patients with chronic pain who meditated regularly had a net reduction in general health care costs, suggesting that the effects of relaxation techniques are cost-effective (Caudill et al., 1991).

Deepak and colleagues (1994) found that 11 drug-resistant epileptic patients who practiced Benson's relaxation response for 20 minutes each day experienced a decrease in absolute frequency of seizures, and that the decrease became significant between 6 and 12 months of continued practice. Duration of seizures declined over the 12 months to a more significant degree than did frequency.

The value of Benson's technique for patients with congestive heart failure was evidenced in a study of 57 veterans who received relaxation response training. Approximately half the group reported physical improvements that went beyond disease management and into lifestyle changes and improved relationships (Chang et al., 2004).

Exercise for Stress Reduction

Michael Sacks, MD, professor of psychiatry at Cornell University Medical College, found that various forms of exercise can be powerful methods of relaxation effective for dealing with the stress of daily life. Researchers have found in various studies that exercise can decrease anxiety and depression, improve an individual's self-image, and buffer people from the effects of stress. Not every study has shown the precise benefits researchers were looking for, but taken as a whole, the research strongly supports the common experience that exercise can elevate mood and reduce anxiety and stress (Sacks, 1993).

Although most research has largely focused on the physical benefits of exercise, any exercise can help people feel more focused and relaxed as long as the activity is enjoyable. Regular exercise does seem to affect one aspect in particular: the ability to withstand stress. Exercise and physical fitness can act as a buffer against stress so that stressful events have a less negative impact on psychological and physical health.

TABLE 16-1

Relaxation Response

Technique	Oxygen consumption	Respiratory rate	Heart rate	Alpha waves	Blood pressure	Muscle tension
Transcendental meditation	Decreases	Decreases	Decreases	Increase	Decreases[*]	(Not measured)
Zen and yoga	Decreases	Decreases	Decreases	Increase	Decreases[*]	
Autogenic training	(Not measured)	Decreases	Decreases	Increase	Inconclusive	Decreases
Progressive relaxation	(Not measured)	(Not measured)	(Not measured)	(Not measured)	Inconclusive	Decreases
Hypnosis with suggested deep relaxation	Decreases	Decreases	Decreases	(Not measured)	Inconclusive	(Not measured)

*In patients with elevated blood pressure.

MEDITATION

In 2003 the Centers for Disease Control and Prevention (CDC) announced that chronic diseases affect more than 90 million Americans and account for one-third the years of potential life lost before age 65. The financial burden of treating chronic diseases now accounts for more than 60% of the total medical care costs in the United States. Chronic diseases are those that are "prolonged, do not resolve spontaneously, and are rarely cured completely." Evidence is accumulating that chronically ill patients gain much benefit from using meditation, including a decrease in visits to physicians (Sobel, 1992).

Complementary and alternative (or integrative) medicine (CAM, CIM) defines a broad category of interventions, such as meditation, that are "not taught widely at U.S. medical schools or generally available at U.S. hospitals." In 1997, however, more than 42% of the adult U.S. population used CAM to manage cancer and other chronic diseases, and meditation is one of the most common practices (Eisenberg et al., 2001).

Although the origin of meditation is ancient in its roots, the science of meditation and its physiological effects is in its infancy. Only recently has the concept of meditation been introduced into the realm of modern Western medicine. The Cartesian split between the mind and body in the early seventeenth century resulted in science emphasizing the body and medicine going in the direction of science. The mind-body connection relates to an understanding that the two are not separate (they have always been together) and have an interactive influence on each other. Meditation is said to realign the two, consciousness with the physical body, creating a more harmonious interaction.

Similar to the word *medicine*, the word *meditation* suggests something to do with healing. The physicist and author of *Wholeness and Implicate Order,* David Bohm looks at wholeness as a property of the physical, material world. He points out the root in Latin means "to cure" but that its deepest root means "to measure" (Bohm, 1983). But what does medicine or meditation have to do with measure? The ancient Greeks said, "Man is the measure of all things." According to Jon Kabat-Zinn, PhD, founder and Director of the Stress Reduction Clinic at the University of Massachusetts Medical Center, "It has to do with the platonic notion that every shape, every being, every thing has its right inward measure. In other words, a tree has its own quality of wholeness that gives it particular properties. A human being has an individual right inward measure, when everything is balanced and physiologically homeostatic—that's the totality of the individual at that point in time" (Kabat-Zinn, 1993). He believes that medicine is the science and art of restoring right inward measure when it is thrown off balance. From the meditative perspective and from the perspective of the new mind-body medicine, health does not have a finite or static destination. Health is a dynamic energy flow that changes over a lifetime, with health and illness coexisting together.

Most meditative practices have come to the West from Asian religious practices, particularly those of India, China, and Japan. Others can be traced to the ancient cultures of the world. Although Western meditators practice a contemplative form of meditation, there are also many active forms of meditation, such as the Chinese martial art, t'ai chi, the Japanese martial art aikido, and the walking meditations of Zen Buddhism.

Until recently, the primary purpose of meditation has been religious or spiritual in nature. During the past 20 years, however, meditation has been explored as a means of reducing stress on both mind and body. Many studies have found that various practices of meditation appear to produce physical and psychological changes. Meditation is a self-directed practice for the purpose of relaxing and calming the mind and body. Many methods of meditation include focusing on a single thought or word for a specific time. Some forms of meditation focus on a physical experience, such as the breath or a specific sound or mantra. All forms of meditation have the common objective of stilling the restlessness of the mind so that the focus can be directed inwardly.

Meditation is thus a technique used to calm the mental activity, the endless thoughts, and ways of reacting to our circumstances. As long as these accumulated impressions linger in the inner recesses of the mind, nagging for attention, it remains difficult to experience an inner state of peace, calm, and health. Fast-paced Western society, filled with external stimuli, has conditioned us to push our minds and bodies to the point of exhaustion, often to the detriment of our own well-being. To be still, to experience the peace and contentment that lies within, we must free ourselves from this external materiality.

Meditation is the process of calming and releasing the distractions from the mind for the purpose of opening up and awakening to our true inner natures.

EASTERN TECHNIQUES AND TRANSCENDENTAL MEDITATION

In the mid-1960s, a popular trend in meditation called *transcendental meditation* (TM) began to emerge. The Vedic philosophy and practice was brought from India to the United States by its founder, Maharishi Mahesh Yogi. The Maharishi had eliminated ancient yogic elements that he considered unnecessary in a contemporary environment. Omitting difficult physical postures and mental exercises, his reformed version became more easily understood and practiced by Westerners (see Chapter 27).

TM is relatively simple in application. A student is given a mantra (a word or sound) to repeat silently over and over again while sitting in a comfortable position. The purpose of repeating the sound or word is to prevent distracting thoughts from entering the mind. Students are instructed to be passive and, if thoughts other than the mantra come to mind, to note them and return the attention to the mantra. TM is generally practiced in the morning and in the evening for approximately 20 minutes.

On the Maharishi's first visit to America in 1959, a San Francisco newspaper heralded TM as a "nonmedicinal tranquilizer" and praised it as a promising cure for insomnia. TM soon began to ride a crest of popularity, with almost half a million Americans learning the technique by 1975, and it was embraced by many celebrities of that day, such as the Beatles. It is believed that more than 2 million people currently practice TM.

In 1968, Harvard's Herbert Benson was asked by the Maharishi International University in Fairfield, Iowa, to test TM practitioners on their ability to lower their own blood pressure. Benson initially refused to participate but was later persuaded to do so. Benson's studies and other research showed that TM was associated with reduced health care costs, increased longevity, and better quality of life (Benson et al., 1977); reduced anxiety, lowered blood pressure, and reduced serum cholesterol levels (Cooper and Aygen, 1978); viable treatment of posttraumatic stress syndrome in Vietnam veterans (Brooks and Scarano, 1985); and reduction in chronic pain (Kabat-Zinn et al., 1986).

In a study aimed at linking TM practice to longevity, 73 elders were taught to use TM or mindfulness training. Both groups showed significant reductions in systolic blood pressure compared with those receiving mental relaxation training. As reported by the nursing staff, TM and mindfulness training improved patients' mental health. Longevity was defined as the subjects' survival rate over a 36-month period, which was found to be greater for those using TM than for those in mental relaxation training and control subjects (Alexander et al., 1989).

Additional research showed TM's effectiveness for the reduction of substance abuse (Sharma et al., 1991), blood pressure reduction in African Americans (Schneider et al., 1992), and lowered blood cortisol levels initially brought on by stress (MacLean et al., 1992).

In a follow-up study of 127 African American elders, Schneider again found that both TM and progressive muscle relaxation significantly decreased blood pressure compared with controls, and that TM was significantly more effective than progressive muscle relaxation techniques (Schneider et al., 1995).

In a study to examine the effects of TM on nine women with symptoms of cardiac syndrome X, those who practiced TM for 3 months, results showed an improvement in quality of life, exercise tolerance, and angina episodes (Cunningham et al., 2000). An experiment to determine the effects of TM-based stress reduction on carotid atherosclerosis in 60 hypertensive African Americans used B-mode ultrasound to measure carotid intima-media thickness, a surrogate measure of coronary atherosclerosis, and found that the experimental group showed a significant decrease in thickness versus an increased thickness in control subjects (Castillo-Richmond et al., 2000).

Heron and Hillis broke new economic ground by conducting a quasiexperimental, longitudinal study of the impact of the TM program on government payments to physicians in Quebec. They found a 13.78% mean annual difference in payments between the TM practitioner group and a randomly selected and matched group of other enrollees over a 6-year period. A true experimental design with randomization would be needed to control for social factors that may have confounded study results (Herron and Hillis, 2000).

Western Techniques and Mindfulness Meditations

The term *mindfulness* was coined by Jon Kabat-Zinn, PhD, known for his work using mindfulness meditation to help medical patients with chronic pain and stress-related disorders (1993a, 1993b). As with other mind-body therapies, mindfulness meditation can induce deep states of relaxation, at times directly improve physical symptoms, and can help patients lead fuller and more satisfying lives. Although Asian forms of meditation involve focusing on a sound, phrase, or prayer to minimize distraction, the practice of mindfulness does the opposite. In mindfulness meditation, distractions are not ignored but focused on. This form of meditation practice can be traced originally from the Buddhist tradition and is about 2500 years old. The method was developed as a means of cultivating greater awareness and wisdom, with the aim of helping people live each moment of their lives as fully as possible.

Kabat-Zinn points out that mindfulness is about more than feeling relaxed or stress free. Its true aim is to nurture an inner balance of mind that allows an individual to face life situations with greater clarity, stability, and understanding and to respond more effectively from that sense of clarity.

An integral part of mindfulness practice is to accept and welcome the stress, pain, anger, frustration, disappointment, and insecurity when those feelings are present. Kabat-Zinn believes that acknowledgment is paramount. Whether pleasant or unpleasant, admission is the first step toward transforming that reality.

Kabat-Zinn founded the Stress Reduction Clinic at the University of Massachusetts Medical Center in Worcester, where he is an associate professor of medicine. Established in 1995, the Center for Mindfulness in Medicine is an outgrowth of the clinic. Since the clinic was founded, more than 10,000 medical patients have gone through his mindfulness meditation programs, almost all referred by their physicians.

To date, Kabat-Zinn's Center for Mindfulness has produced 15 peer-reviewed papers on Mindfulness-Based Stress Reduction (MBSR). Current research pursuits of the Center include a prostrate cancer study funded by the U. S. Department of Defense, a cost-effectiveness study, development of an innovative substance abuse recovery program for young, low income, inner city mothers, and a wide variety of other collaborative research endeavors in various states of development.

Unlike standard medical and psychological approaches, the clinic does not categorize and treat patients differently depending on their illnesses. Their 8-week courses offer the same training program in mindfulness and stress reduction to everyone. They emphasize what is "right" with their patients, rather than what is "wrong" with them, focusing on mobilizing their inner strengths and changing their behaviors in new and innovative ways. Facilitators maintain that their programs are not held out as some kind of magical cure when other approaches failed; rather, they provide a sensible and straightforward way for people to experience and understand the mind-body connection firsthand, using that knowledge to better cope with their illnesses.

In the practice of mindfulness, the patient begins by using one-pointed attention to cultivate calmness and stability. When thoughts and feelings arise, it is important not to ignore or suppress them or analyze or judge them by their content; rather, the thoughts are observed intentionally and nonjudgmentally, moment by moment, as events in the field of awareness.

This inclusive noting of thoughts that come and go in the mind can lead to a detachment from them, allowing a deeper perspective about the stresses of life to emerge. By observing the thoughts from this vantage point, one gains a new frame of reference. In this way, valuable insight can be allowed to surface. The key to mindfulness is not the topic focused on but the quality of awareness brought into each moment. Observing the thought processes, without intellectualizing them and without judgment, creates greater clarity. The goal of mindfulness is to become more aware, more in touch with life and its happenings at the time it is happening, in the present.

Acceptance does not mean passivity or resignation. Accepting what each moment offers provides the opportunity to experience life more completely. In this manner, any situation can be responded to with greater confidence and clarity.

One way to envision how mindfulness works is to think of the mind as the surface of a lake or ocean. Many people think the goal of meditation is to stop the waves so that the water will be flat, peaceful, and tranquil. The spirit of mindfulness practice is to experience the waves.

The consistent practice of mindfulness meditation has been shown to decrease the subjective experience of pain and stress in a variety of research settings. One study found a 65% improvement in pain symptoms and an approximate 60% improvement in sleep and fatigue levels from before to after the intervention in a sample of 77 patients with fibromyalgia, an illness known to have psychosomatic components (Kaplan et al., 1993).

Dunn and colleagues (1999) used electroencephalographic (EEG) recordings to differentiate between two types of meditation, concentration and mindfulness, and a normal relaxation control condition. They found significant differences between readings at numerous cortical sites, suggesting that concentration and mindfulness meditations may be unique forms of consciousness and not merely degrees of a state of relaxation.

In a pilot study using mindfulness of movement as a coping strategy for multiple sclerosis, patients attended six individual one-on-one sessions of mindfulness training. Results showed that balance improved significantly compared with controls (Mills and Allen, 2000).

Eighty cancer patients were followed for 6 months after attending a mindfulness meditation group for 1.5 hours each week for 7 weeks. They were also asked to practice meditation at home on a daily basis. Results showed significantly lower mood disturbances and fewer symptoms of stress at the 6-month follow-up for both male and female patients. The greatest improvement, however, occurred on subscales measuring depression, anxiety, and anger. Results of various mindfulness meditation techniques are consistent with other meditation-based interventions (Carlson et al., 2001).

Nurses are often known to make mindfulness practice part of their continuing education. They find that this technique often prevents compassion fatigue and burnout, enhances health, and increases awareness of holism within the self.

HYPNOSIS

Modern hypnosis is said to have begun in the eighteenth century with Franz Anton Mesmer, who used what he called "magnetic healing" to treat a variety of psychological and psychophysiological disorders, such as hysterical blindness, paralysis, headaches, and joint pains. The famous Austrian neuropathologist Sigmund Freud initially found hypnosis to be extremely effective in treating hysteria and then, troubled by the sudden catharsis of powerful emotions by his patients, abandoned its use.

The word *hypnosis* is derived from the Greek word *hypnos,* meaning "sleep." It is believed that hypnotic suggestion has been a part of ancient healing traditions for centuries. The induction of trance states and the use of therapeutic suggestion were a central feature of the early Greek healing temples, and variations of these techniques were practiced throughout the ancient world.

In more recent years, hypnosis has experienced a resurgence. Initially, this form of therapy became popular with physicians and dentists. At present, hypnosis is widely used by mental health professionals for the treatment of addictions, pain control, anxiety disorders, and phobias. During hypnosis a patient enters a state of attentive and focused concentration and becomes relatively unaware of the immediate surroundings. While in this state of deep concentration, people are highly responsive to suggestion. Contrary to popular folklore, however, people cannot be hypnotized against their will or involuntarily. They must be willing to concentrate their thoughts and to follow the suggestions offered. Essentially, all forms of hypnotherapy are actually forms of self-hypnosis.

Hypnosis has three major components: *absorption* (in the words or images presented by the hypnotherapist), *dissociation* (from one's ordinary critical faculties), and *responsiveness*. A hypnotherapist either leads patients through relaxation, mental images, and suggestions or teaches patients to perform the techniques themselves. Many hypnotherapists provide guided audiotapes for their patients so that they can practice the therapy at home. The images presented are specifically tailored to the particular patient's needs and may use one or all of the senses.

Physiologically, hypnosis resembles other forms of deep relaxation. It is known to decrease sympathetic nervous system activity, decrease oxygen consumption and carbon dioxide eliminations, and lower blood pressure and heart rate, and it is linked to increasing or decreasing certain types of brain wave activity.

Hypnotherapy's effectiveness lies in the complex connection between the mind and the body. It is now well understood that illness can affect your emotional state and, conversely, that your emotional state can affect your physical state. For example, stress, an emotional reaction, can make heart disease worse, and heart disease, a physical condition, can cause depression.

Hypnosis carries this connection to the next logical step by using the power of the mind to bring about change in the body. No one is quite sure how hypnosis works, but with more sophisticated imaging techniques, that is changing.

Clinical Applications

One of the most dramatic early uses of hypnosis was for skin disorders. In the mid-1950s an anesthesiologist, Arthur Mason, used hypnosis to effectively treat a 16-year-old patient who had warts. Within 10 days the wart fell off and normal skin replaced it (Mason and Black, 1958). Since that time, hypnosis has been used to improve other skin disorders dramatically, such as ichthyosis.

Depending on the individual's situation, hypnotherapy can be used as a complement to medical care or as a primary treatment. Many people find that hypnotherapy's benefits are enhanced by the use of biofeedback to induce physiological changes. Biofeedback helps patients see that they can control certain bodily functions simply by altering their thoughts, and the added confidence helps them improve more rapidly.

There is little doubt that the regular practice of self-hypnosis is helpful to people with chronic disease. The benefits include reduction of anxiety and fear, decreased requirements for analgesics, increased comfort during medical procedures, and greater stability of functions controlled by the autonomic nervous system, such as blood pressure. Training in self-hypnosis also enhances the patient's sense of control, which is often affected by chronic illness. Hypnotherapy may also have direct clinical effects on certain chronic diseases, such as reducing bleeding in hemophiliac patients, stabilizing blood sugar in diabetic patients, and reducing the severity of asthmatic attacks.

Irritable Bowel Syndrome

For many years, W.M. Gonsalkorale has been researching the benefits of hypnotherapy for irritable bowel syndrome at University Hospital of South Manchester, United Kingdom. In only 3 months, symptoms such as pain and bloating, as well as the level of "disease interference" with life, changed profoundly for most of the 232 participants (Gonsalkorale et al., 2002). Good evidence now supports the long-term benefits for up to 6 years following hypnotherapy. In 204 patients, of the 71% who responded to therapy, 81% maintained their improvements, and the remaining 19% claimed that deterioration of symptoms had been slight (Gonsalkorale et al., 2003). Besides improving physical symptoms, hypnotherapy has also been shown to improve cognitive changes such as anxiety, depression, and quality of life (Gonsalkorale et al., 2004).

Preoperative Therapy

In 1997, Mehmet Oz, a cardiothoracic surgeon at Columbia Presbyterian Medical Center, received a great deal of attention for advocating and using complementary medical approaches in his surgical practice. Before coronary bypass surgery, Oz took 32 patients and randomized them to two groups. One group received instruction on self-hypnosis relaxation techniques before surgery, and the other group received no instruction. Results showed that patients who practiced the self-hypnosis techniques were significantly more relaxed than the control subjects in the days after surgery (Ashton et al., 1997). There was no significant difference between the two groups in length of hospital stay and postoperative mobidity and mortality.

Postoperative Therapy

Carol Ginandes, a Harvard instructor, investigated how hypnotherapy can help people heal more quickly after surgery. Each of 18 women having breast reduction surgery was placed in one of three groups. One group received standard surgery care. The second group received the same care and also received psychological support. The third group underwent hypnosis before and after surgery in addition to standard care. Those who had undergone hypnosis healed more rapidly, felt less discomfort, and had fewer complications (Ginandes et al., 2003).

Ginandes is now researching the use of medical hypnosis to accelerate wound healing. She is currently gathering preliminary evidence from a small trial showing statistically significant improvements 7 weeks after surgery in women who received hypnosis as adjunct therapy.

Pain Control

Hypnosis can also be effective in reducing the fear and anxiety that accompanies pain. Because it is said that anxiety increases pain, hypnotherapy helps a patient gain control over the fear and anxiety, thereby reducing the pain. Many controlled studies have demonstrated that hypnosis is an effective way to reduce migraine attacks in children and teenagers. In one experiment, 30 schoolchildren were randomly assigned a placebo or propranolol (a blood pressure–lowering agent) or taught self-hypnosis. Only the children who used the self-hypnosis techniques had a significant decrease in severity and frequency of headaches (Olness and Gardner, 1988). A study of chronically ill patients reported a 113% increase in pain tolerance among highly hypnotizable subjects compared with a control group who did not receive hypnosis (Debenedittis et al., 1989).

Researchers at Virginia Polytechnic Institute found that during a hypnotic state aimed at bringing about pain control, the prefrontal cortex of the brain directed other areas of the brain to reduce or eliminate their awareness of pain (Gordon, 2004). A technique used for surgery in people with little or no tolerance for chemical anesthesia, called "spinal anesthesia illusion," was developed by Philip Ament, a dentist and psychologist from Buffalo, New York. In this method a deep state of relaxation is induced by having the patient count mentally or focus on a specific image. The patient is given the suggestion that he or she will feel a growing numbness begin to spread from the navel to the toes as he or she counts to a higher and higher number. Once the patient feels numb, the surgery can proceed. After the surgery the therapist gives the patient suggestions that lead to the gradual return of normal sensations.

Dentistry

Some people have learned to tolerate dental work (e.g., drilling, extraction, periodontal surgery) using hypnosis as the sole anesthesia. Even when an anesthetic is used, hypnotherapy can also be used to reduce fear and anxiety, control bleeding and salivation, and lessen postoperative discomfort. Used with children, hypnosis can decrease the chances of developing a dental phobia.

Pregnancy and Delivery

It is believed that Lamaze and other popular breathing techniques used during labor and delivery may actually work by inducing a hypnotic state. Women who have used hypnosis before delivery tend to have a shorter labor and more comfortable delivery than other pregnant women. There are even reports of cesarean sections performed with hypnosis as the sole anesthesia. Women are taught to take advantage of their body's natural anesthetic abilities to make childbirth a less painful, more positive experience.

Anxiety

Hypnosis can be used to establish a new reaction to specific anxiety-causing activities, such as stage fright, airplane flight, and other phobias. Typically the hypnotherapist helps the patient undo a conditioned physiological response, such as hyperventilation or nausea. This method can also be used to help calm athletes who are prepared to compete. Hypnotherapy can be used to quell most any fear, whether associated with examinations, public speaking, or social interactions.

Allergies/Asthma

Ran Anbar, a pediatric pulmonologist at State University of New York's Upstate Medical University in Syracuse, teaches children self-hypnosis to help them control their allergies and asthma (Gordon, 2004).

BIOFEEDBACK

Biofeedback therapies emerged in the 1960s and 1970s, when advances in psychological and medical research converged with developments in biomedical technology. Improved electronic instruments could convey information to patients about their autonomic nervous systems and their muscles in the form of audio and visual signals that patients could understand. The word *biofeedback* became the general term to define the procedures and treatments that make use of these instruments (Green and Green, 1977).

Biofeedback therapy uses special instruments and methods to expand the body's natural internal feedback systems. By watching a monitoring device, patients can learn by trial and error to adjust their thinking and other mental processes to control bodily processes previously thought to be involuntary, such as blood pressure, temperature, gastrointestinal functioning, and brain wave activity. In fact, biofeedback can be used on almost any bodily process that can be measured accurately.

Biofeedback does not belong to any particular field of health care and is used in many disciplines, including internal medicine, dentistry, physical therapy and rehabilitation, psychology and psychiatry, and pain management. As with other forms of therapy, biofeedback is more useful for some clinical problems than for others. For example, biofeedback is a useful treatment in Raynaud's disease, a painful and potentially dangerous spasm of the small arteries, and certain types of fecal and urinary incontinence. It has also become an integral part of the treatment of many other disorders, including headaches, anxiety, high blood pressure, teeth clenching, asthma, and muscle disorders.

More recently, researchers have been experimenting with biofeedback treatments for conditions believed to stem from irregular brain wave patterns, such as epilepsy, attention deficit disorder (ADD), and attention deficit–hyperactivity disorder (ADHD) in children, with promising results.

Biofeedback is successful in helping people learn to regulate many physical conditions partly because it puts them in better contact with specific parts of their bodies. For example, biofeedback can help teach people to tighten muscles at the neck of the bladder to better control impaired bladder function. It can help postoperative patients learn to reuse muscles of the legs and arms. It can help teach stroke patients to use alternative muscles to move a limb if the primary ones can no longer do the job. Biofeedback is also helpful in training patients to use artificial limbs after amputation.

In a normal biofeedback session, electrodes are attached to the area being monitored. These electrodes feed the information to a small monitoring box that registers the results by a sound tone that varies in pitch or on a visual meter that varies in brightness as the function being monitored decreases or increases. A biofeedback therapist leads the patient in mental exercises to help the patient reach the desired result. Through trial and error, patients gradually train themselves to control the inner mechanism involved. Training for some disorders requires 8 to 10 sessions; however, a single session often can provide symptomatic relief. Patients with long-term or severe disorders may require longer therapy. The aim of the treatment is to teach patients to regulate their own inner mental and bodily processes without the help of a machine.

Five Common Forms of Biofeedback Therapy

1. **Electromyographic biofeedback.** Electromyographic (EMG) feedback measures muscular tension. Sensors are attached to the skin to detect electrical activity related to muscle tension in that area. The biofeedback instrument amplifies and converts this activity into useful information, displaying the various degrees of muscle tension. This form of biofeedback therapy is most often used for tension headaches, physical rehabilitation, chronic muscle pain, incontinence, and general relaxation purposes.

2. **Thermal biofeedback therapy.** Thermal biofeedback therapy is used to measure skin temperature, as an index of blood flow changes from the constriction and dilation of blood vessels. Low skin temperature usually means decreased blood flow in that area. A temperature-sensitive probe is taped to the skin, often on a finger. The instrument converts information into feedback that can be seen and heard and can be used to reduce or increase blood flow to the hands and feet. Thermal biofeedback is often used for Raynaud's disease, migraine headaches, hypertension, and anxiety disorders and to promote general relaxation.

3. **Electrodermal activity therapy.** Electrodermal activity therapy is used to measure changes in sweat activity too minimal to feel. Two sensors are attached to the palm side of the fingers or hand to measure sweat activity. They produce a tiny electrical current that measures skin conductance on the basis of the amount of moisture present. Increased sweat can mean arousal of part of the autonomic nervous system. Electrodermal activity therapy can be used to measure the sweat output stemming from stressful thoughts or rapid deep breathing. It is most often used for anxiety and hyperhidrosis.

4. **Finger pulse therapy.** Finger pulse therapy measures pulse rate and force. With this method a sensor is attached to a finger and helps measure heart activity as a sign of arousal of part of the autonomic nervous system. It is most often used for hypertension, anxiety, and some cardiac arrhythmias.

5. **Breathing biofeedback therapy.** Breathing biofeedback therapy measures breath rate, volume, rhythm, and location. Sensors are placed around the chest and abdomen to measure air flow from

the mouth and nose. The feedback is usually visual, and patients learn to take deeper, slower, lower, and more regular breaths using abdominal muscles. This simple form of biofeedback is most often used for asthma and other respiratory conditions, hyperventilation, and anxiety.

Goals and Appeal

The general goal of biofeedback therapy is to lower body tension and change faulty biological patterns to reduce symptoms. Many people can and do reach goals of relaxation without the use of biofeedback. Although biofeedback may not be necessary, it can potentially add something useful to any treatment.

A major reason why many patients find biofeedback training appealing is that, as with behavioral approaches in general, it puts the patient in charge, giving him or her a sense of mastery and self-reliance over the illness. It is believed that such an attitude can play a critical role in shortening recovery time, reducing incidence, and lowering health care costs.

Research Considerations

Biofeedback-assisted relaxation training has been shown to be associated with a decrease in medical care costs, a decrease in the number of claims and costs to insurers in claims payments, reduction in medication and physician use, reduction in hospital stays and rehospitalization, reduction of mortality and morbidity, and enhanced quality of life (Basmajian, 1989).

An unpublished study involving 241 employees of a Siberian metal company showed promising results for the integration of biofeedback training into occupational medicine as a method to increase workers' ability to work with few errors while increasing labor productivity levels. The subjects had initial levels of psychosomatic disorder presenting with symptoms of headaches, sleepiness, and periodic blood pressure fluctuations. Workers attended 10- to 40-minute biofeedback sessions over 2 weeks. The results clearly indicated that the workers were able to control the brain's blood flow. Furthermore, a follow-up biofeedback session was repeated 1 month later and showed that all subjects from the initial group could recall their strategies for producing positive change.

A study involving 30 patients with fibromyalgia syndrome received biofeedback and experienced statistically significant improvements in mental clarity, mood, and sleep (Mueller et al., 2001). However, future research is needed in controlled trials to understand disease mechanisms better.

The use of biofeedback, both sensory and augmented, has been used with some degree of success for patients with fecal incontinence. In 40 women randomly assigned to receive either augmented or sensory biofeedback, after 12 weeks of treatment the augmented form of biofeedback was found to be superior (Fynes et al., 1999).

Biofeedback techniques have also been used with some success to treat epilepsy and attention problems, such as sleeplessness, fatigue, and body pain. Another study compared biofeedback to standard care for fecal incontinence. Results showed biofeedback was not superior to standard care, but those who received biofeedback had significantly improved scores for hospital anxiety and depression (Norton et al., 2003).

More recently, 92 patients with systemic lupus erythematosus were assigned randomly to receive biofeedback-assisted cognitive-behavioral treatment or usual medical care. Those who received biofeedback had significantly greater reductions in pain and psychological functioning over controls. At 9-month follow-up, the biofeedback group continued to exhibit relative benefit compared with controls (Greco et al., 2004).

In a randomized U.K. study, 38 patients were assigned to sphincter repair or sphincter repair plus biofeedback. Although not significant, continence and satisfaction scores improved and were sustained over time. Quality-of-life measures also improved with the biofeedback group (Davis et al., 2004).

The Department of Psychiatry at Robert Wood Johnson Medical School in New Jersey evaluated the effectiveness of heart rate variability (HRV) biofeedback as a complementary treatment for 94 patients with asthma. Compared with the two control groups (placebo and wait list), subjects in both the two biofeedback groups were prescribed less medication, showing that HRV biofeedback may prove to be a useful adjunct to asthma treatment and may help to reduce dependence on steroid medications (Lehrer et al., 2004).

Research on exactly how biofeedback works is somewhat inconclusive. Some studies link its benefits directly to physiological changes that the patient learns to make voluntarily. Other experiments find benefits even for patients who do not make the desired changes in the physiological measures. Biofeedback appears to help some patients increase their sense of control, heighten their optimism, and lessen feelings of hopelessness triggered by chronic health problems (Hatch et al., 1987). It appears that biofeedback used as adjunct therapy could add something useful to an existing therapy.

IMAGERY

Since human societies began analyzing human experiences, philosophers have tried to define and explain the interior processes of the mind—all those experiences that are invisible to another person because they do not have physical referents. Philosophers have speculated at length on the nature of mental imagery, and scientists have found the phenomenon difficult to verify or measure. Behavioral psychologists of the 1920s went so far as to say that mental images simply did not exist.

Since 1960, psychologists have done a great amount of work exploring and categorizing mental imagery and inner processes. Contemporary psychologists distinguish several types of imagery. Probably the most common form of imagery that people experience is *memory*. If a person tries to remember a friend, the bed in his or her room, or what the seats of his or her car feel like, that person immediately perceives an image in his or her mind, the "mind's eye." People refer to this experience as forming a mental picture. Some people believe that they do not "see" the scene but simply have a strong sense of the scene and "know" what it looks like.

Imagery is both a mental process and a wide variety of procedures used in therapy to encourage changes in attitudes, behaviors, or physiological reactions. As a mental process, it is often defined as "any thought representing a sensory quality" (Horowitz, 1983). In addition to the visual, it includes all the senses: aural, tactile, olfactory, proprioceptive, and kinesthetic. *Imagery* is often used synonymously with *visualization*. However, visualization refers only to "seeing" something in the mind's eye, whereas imagery can use one sense or combination of senses to produce an image.

Creating images with the mind is also a way of communicating with the deeper-than-conscious aspects of the mind. This is apparent when considering the dream state, which communicates mainly in images, which are then interpreted to make a story. This communicative quality of imagery is important because feelings and behaviors are primarily motivated by subconscious and unconscious factors.

Imagery can be taught either individually or in groups, and the therapist often uses it to affect a particular result, such as quitting any addictive behavior or bolstering the immune system to attack cancer cells. Because it often involves directed concentration, imagery can also be regarded as a form of guided meditation.

Many practices discussed in this chapter use a component of imagery. Psychotherapy, hypnosis, and biofeedback all use various elements of this process. Any therapy that relies on the imagination to stimulate, communicate, solve problems, or evoke a heightened awareness or sensitivity could be described as a form of imagery.

Numerous early studies indicated that mental imagery could bring about significant physiological and biochemical changes. These findings have encouraged the development of imagery as a health care tool. Imagery was found to have the capacity to affect dramatically the oxygen supply in tissues (Olness and Conroy, 1988), cardiovascular changes (Barber, 1969), vascular or thermal changes (Green and Green, 1977), the pupil and cochlear reflex (Luria, 1968), heart rate and galvanic skin response (Jordan and Lenington, 1979), and salivation (Barber et al., 1984; White, 1978).

Clinical Applications

Communication with the unconscious has previously been the domain of hypnosis, which basically consists of two components: (1) the use of a technique to induce a state of consciousness where there is a freer access to the deeper part of the mind and (2) a method of communicating with that deeper part of the mind. Often this communication will involve making suggestions to the inner depths of the mind, suggesting items or behaviors that the individual desires for his or her betterment. Several different techniques are used to induce the necessary state of consciousness, some quite similar to more common relaxation techniques and to meditation techniques (Jordan and Lenington, 1979).

Self-Directed Imagery

Increased attention is focusing on the ability of individuals to use these principles for their own healing purposes. Through the practice of effective deep relaxation techniques, individuals can bring themselves to a state of consciousness where they have increased access to deeper parts of their minds. Then, using imagery, they can "reprogram" new healthy images (Achterberg, 1985).

Self-directed imagery is another powerful way in which individuals can have more control over their healing processes. Imagery can be used to contribute to the healing of physical problems and has been used extensively in the area of pain control. In one method the individual allows an image for his or her pain to emerge. For example, an individual may create an image that characterizes the area of pain, then create a second image to counteract the pain image. Once the images are formed, the individual uses a relaxation or meditation technique to open access to the levels where his or her self-healing power resides and to imagine the healing image. This process could be repeated as often as necessary, allowing changes in the healing image that might either spontaneously appear or be appropriate if the image associated with the pain were to change.

Self-directed imagery can also be used to stimulate personal growth and change by repeatedly entering a relaxed or meditative state and strongly imaging a new desired behavior. Similarly, by repeatedly imaging oneself as having already achieved a desired goal, the deeper mind gradually accepts this new image and works to bring it into reality.

Carl O. Simonton, MD, often regarded as the grandfather of guided imagery, and his wife, Stephanie, brought the use of meditation and imagery for cancer self-help to popular attention. They emphasized several aspects characteristic of a powerful healing image: (1) that the image be created by the healee himself or herself, (2) that it involve as many sense modalities as possible, and (3) that it have as much dynamism and energy behind it as possible. The image must be vital because that vitality is what stimulates the image to take root (Simonton et al., 1978).

Research Considerations

Early studies suggest a direct impact between imagery and its corresponding effects on the body. These findings include the following:

1. Correlations between various types of leukocytes and components of cancer patients' images of their disease, treatment, and immune system (Achterberg and Lawlis, 1984).
2. Enhanced natural killer cell function after a relaxation and imagery training procedure with geriatric patients (Kiecolt-Glaser et al., 1985) and in adult cancer patients with metastatic disease (Gruber et al., 1988).
3. Specificity of imagery training was suggested by a study on training patients in cell-specific imagery of either T lymphocytes or neutrophils. The effects of training, assessed after 6 weeks, were statistically associated with the type of imagery procedure used (Achterberg et al., 1989).

Of all the many mind and body modalities, the practice of guided imagery appears to be the most widely used and accepted among many nursing departments. The University of Akron College of Nursing conducted a study that demonstrated guided imagery was an effective intervention for enhancing comfort in women undergoing radiation therapy for early-stage breast cancer. In this study, 53 women were randomized to either a control or a treatment group. The experimental group listened to a guided imagery tape once a day for the duration of the study. The guided imagery group demonstrated significantly improved comfort over controls, with the treatment associated with greater comfort over time (Kolcaba and Fox, 1999).

A community-based nursing study was recently conducted in Sydney, Australia, where 56 people with advanced cancer experiencing anxiety and depression were randomly assigned to one of four treatment conditions: (1) progressive muscle relaxation training, (2) guided imagery training, (3) both treatments, and (4) control group. Patients were tested for anxiety, depression, and quality of life. There was no significant improvement for anxiety but significant positive changes for depression and quality of life (Sloman, 2002).

Nurses at Ephrata Community Hospital in Pennsylvania found that offering their patients guided imagery compact discs (CDs) can be effective in a variety of ways. They report that guided imagery (1) helps patients relieve pain and anxiety before and after surgery, (2) helps patients relax and sleep better during evening hours, (3) helps to lower blood pressure, and (4) reduces the need for breathing and respiratory devices. Nurses also report that the CDs are often more effective than sedation for easing confusion in older patients. Each bedside contains a packet of CDs and a CD player with earphones. Each CD focuses on a major component of a successful hospital stay (e.g., health and healing, comfort, peaceful rest, courage, serenity). In addition, all the staff nurses, therapists, social workers, and managers are trained in the use of the CDs and employ them for their personal benefit (Miller, 2003).

Differences in pain and power were examined at Kent State's College of Nursing, where 42 patients were randomly assigned to treatment and control groups. Those who received guided imagery had decreased pain during the last 2 days of the 4-day trial. No differences in power emerged (Lewandowski, 2004).

In 1993 a study was conducted to compare the effectiveness of various types of guided imagery for preoperative patients. Three outcomes were examined: intraoperative blood loss, length of hospital stay, and use of postoperative pain medication. A population of 335 surgical patients was randomly assigned to five groups. Each of the four experimental groups was provided with a guided imagery audiotape created by four different therapists. The control group received an audiotape with a "whooshing" noise with no meaningful physiological effect. Results showed that three of the four audiotapes produced no significant benefits on any of the medical outcomes examined. By contrast, the guided imagery audiotape produced by Belleruth Naparstek, a highly regarded therapist and imagery practitioner, produced highly significant results in two outcomes, blood loss and length of stay. Bennett found that Naparstek's tape was much more sophisticated than the others. Her imagery had been scored with specially composed music designed to highlight and accompany each image, with an emphasis on spiritual connectedness. Naparstek included visualizations of positive outcomes, faster wound healing, less pain, and no nausea (Bennett, 1996).

In two unpublished studies, guided imagery was used to reduce menopausal symptoms. The University Hospital in Linkoping, Sweden, found that menopausal women using guided imagery averaged 73% fewer hot flashes over 6 months and a significant reduction in other symptoms. A study at New England Deaconess Hospital of 33 menopausal women who were not using hormone replacement therapy (HRT) found that these types of strategies offered a significant reduction in hot-flash intensity, tension/anxiety, and depression.

Cleveland Clinic researchers measured 130 colorectal surgery patients for anxiety levels, pain perceptions, and narcotic medication requirements (Tusek et al., 1997). The treatment group listened to guided imagery tapes for 3 days before their surgery, during anesthesia induction, intraoperatively, after anesthesia, and for 6 days after surgery; the controls received routine perioperative care. Patients in the guided imagery group experienced considerably less preoperative and postoperative anxiety and pain, and they required 50% less narcotic medication after surgery than controls.

Not only is guided imagery shown to be effective for reducing pain and anxiety preoperatively and postoperatively, but it is now proving to be cost-effective. In 1999 a cardiac surgery team implemented a guided imagery program to compare cardiac surgical outcomes in those who received guided imagery and those who did not. Patients who completed the guided imagery program had a shorter average length of hospital stay, a decrease in average direct pharmacy costs, and a decrease in average direct pain medication costs, while maintaining high overall patient satisfaction with care and treatment provided (Halpin et al., 2002).

MENTAL HEALING

The idea that consciousness can affect the physical body has a time-honored and respected historical base. The observation that "there is a measure of consciousness throughout the body" is scattered about the 2000-year-old Hippocratic writings. The ancient Persians expounded on this concept, insisting that a person's mind can intervene not just in his or her own body but also in that of another individual located far away. The great Muslim physician Abu Ali ibn Sina (Avicenna in Latinized form, 980-1037 AD) later postulated that it was the faculty of imagination that humans use to make themselves ill or to restore health.

The attitudes of the ancient Greeks and Persians toward the interaction between minds and bodies gave rise to two very different types of healing: local and nonlocal. The Greeks believed that the action of the mind on the body was a "local" event in the here and now. The Persians, however, viewed the mind-body relationship as "nonlocal." They held that the mind was not localized or confined to the body but extended beyond the body. This implied that the mind was capable of affecting any physical body, local or nonlocal.

Implications of Nonlocality

Modern physicists have long recognized the concept of nonlocality. These developments rest largely on an idea in physics called Bell's theorem, introduced in 1964 by the Irish physicist John Stewart Bell, and subsequent experiments. Bell showed that if distant objects have once been in contact, a change thereafter in one causes an immediate change in the other, even if they are separated to the opposite ends of the universe. Thus it is important to realize that nonlocality is not just a theoretical idea in physics, but also that its proof rests on actual experiments.

The idea prevalent in contemporary science is that the mind and consciousness are entirely local phenomenon, localized to the brain/body and confined to the present moment. From this perspective nonlocal healing cannot occur in principle because the mind is bound by the "here and now." Research studies conducted in distant mental influence challenge these modern-day assumptions. Dozens of experiments, specifically conducted over the past 25 years, suggest that the mind can bring about changes in nonlocal physical bodies, even when shielded from all sensory and electromagnetic influences. This suggests that mind and consciousness may not be located at fixed points in space (Braud, 1992; Braud and Schlitz, 1991; Jahn and Dunne, 1987).

Some physicists believe that nonlocality applies not just to the domain of electrons and other subatomic particles but also to our familiar world consisting of dense matter. A growing number of physicists think that nonlocality may apply to the mind. Physicist Nick Herbert, in his book *Quantum Reality,* states, "Bell's theorem requires our quantum knowledge to be non-local, instantly linked to everything it has previously touched" (Herbert, 1987).

For the Western model of medicine, the implications of a nonlocal concept are profound and include the following:

1. Nonlocal models of the mind could be helpful in understanding the actual dynamics of the healing process. They may help to understand why in some patients a cure suddenly appears unexpectedly or when a healing appears to be influenced by events occurring nonlocally.

2. Nonlocal manifestations of consciousness may complicate traditional experimental designs and require innovative research methods because they suggest that the mental state of the healer may influence the experiment's outcome, even under "blind" conditions (Solfvin, 1984).

These assumptions give rise to the idea that consciousness could prevail after the death of the body/brain, suggesting that some aspect of the psyche is not bound to points in space or time. This idea in turn leads toward a nonlocal model of consciousness, which allows for the possibility of distant healing exchange.

This nonlocal model of consciousness implies that at some level of the psyche, no fundamental separations exist between individual minds. Nobel physicist Erwin Schroedinger suggested that at some level and in some sense there may be unity and oneness of all minds (Schroedinger, 1969). In the nonlocal model, distance is not fundamental but is completely overcome. In other words, because of the unification of consciousness, the healer and the patient are not separated by physical distance.

In 1997, Marilyn Schlitz, research director at the Institute for Noetic Sciences, compiled a summary and meta-analysis of 30 formal experiments in which self-reported healers attempted to influence autonomic nervous system activity in a distant person. Results across the experiments showed a significant variation during the distant intentionality periods (Schlitz and Braud 1997).

For 30 years, psychologist Lawrence LeShan investigated the local and nonlocal effects of prayer and healing. He taught these techniques to more than 400 people and ultimately became a healer himself. He maintained that healing changes were observed to have occurred 15% to 20% of the time but never could be predicted in advance of any specific healing (LeShan, 1966).

LeShan found that mental-spiritual healing methods are of the following two main types:

- *Type I (nonlocal).* The healer enters a prayerful, altered state of consciousness in which he or she views himself or herself and the patient as a single entity. There is no physical contact or any attempt to offer anything of a physical nature to the person in need, only the desire to connect and unite. These healers emphasize the importance of empathy, love, and caring in this process. When the healing takes place, it does so in the context of unity, compassion, and love. This type of healing is considered a natural process and merely speeds up the normal healing processes.

• *Type II (local).* The healer does touch the patient and may imagine some "flow of energy" through his or her hands to the patient's area receiving the healing. Feelings of heat are common in both the healer and patient. In this mode, unlike type I, the healer holds the intention for healing.

Research about the origins of consciousness and how it relates to the physical brain are practically nonexistent. Although hypotheses purporting to explain consciousness do exist, there is no agreement among researchers as to its nature, local or nonlocal.

SPIRITUALITY AND HEALING

Throughout the ages, ancient mystical traditions have valued the spiritual qualities of humans over the physical, emphasizing the transcendence of one over the other. In the background of most mystical traditions is the idea that the body is somehow at odds with the spirit. A war wages, and one must battle the war to achieve an enlightened status. Still other theologians postulate that the greatest spiritual achievement of all may lie in the realization that the spiritual and the physical are but one, and that perhaps the ultimate spiritual goal is to transcend nothing but to realize the integration and oneness of our being.

A new quality of spiritual awakening has been emerging worldwide over the past 30 years. This innovative approach encourages people to develop faith in their own capacity to create their own reality in partnership with the "God-force within." In many cultures, both Eastern and Western, prayer-based spiritual healing is an integral part of modern religious practices.

The premise of creating our own reality is, in essence, a spiritual one. This concept is sometimes contrary to many fundamental religious positions that embrace God as an external being because spirituality emphasizes a "God-within" reality. Transcending the boundaries and limitations of specific religions, a spiritual practice honors the relationship between the individual and the God-force as a partnership.

When people consider the possibility that they create their own realities, the question that invariably arises is, "Through what source? What is the source of this power of creation that runs through my being?" The answer to this question is not found externally, but internally. This internal source seeking to understand our own nature is the study of divinity in action, incarnated into each person.

The blending of spirituality with the tenets of alternative, complementary, and integrative therapies provides individuals with a means of understanding how they contribute to the creation of their illness and to their healing. This consideration does not come from a place of self-blame and is not as the result of the will of God but rather results from attempting to understand a spiritual purpose for suffering in a physical body. The relationship that is cultivated ultimately transcends the human value system of punishment versus reward and grows into a relationship based on principles of co-creation and co-responsibility. Therefore the journey of healing for patients, as well as the journey of life, is thereby freed of the burden of feeling victimized by fate, circumstances, or God, free to have faith and hope not only in God but in themselves as well.

Research in the last 10 years has made an indelible mark on the way health care professionals think about the role of spirituality and religion in physical, mental, and social health. Hundreds of studies have explored the relationship between body and spirit. Most studies have been cross-sectional, but some have also been longitudinal. Many studies now document an association between religious involvement and lower anxiety, fewer psychotic symptoms, less substance abuse, and better coping mechanisms. A comprehensive review found that 478 of 742 quantitative studies (66%) reported a statistically significant relationship between religious involvement and better mental health and greater social support. The review also found that almost 80% of those who are religious have significantly greater well-being, hope, and optimism compared with those who are less religious (Koenig et al., 2001).

At Duke University, studies have been conducted examining the effects of religiousness on the course of depression in 850 hospitalized patients over age 60. Results showed that religious coping predicted lower levels of depressive symptoms at baseline and at 6 months after discharge (Koenig et al., 1992).

Koenig's studies and others have shown that spirituality and religiosity are clearly associated with longer survival, healthier behaviors, and less distress and are believed to have an effect on coping (Pargament et al., 1998; Tix and Frazier, 1997), anxiety (Koenig et al., 1993), aging (Crowther et al., 2002), end of life (Daaleman and VandeCreek 2000), and lower cortisol measures in HIV/AIDS patients (Ironson et al., 2002).

Power of Prayer

The use of prayer in healing may have begun in human prehistory and continues to this day as an underlying tenet in almost all religions. The records of many of the great religious traditions, including the mystical traditions of Christianity, Taoism, Hinduism, Buddhism, and Islam, give the strong impression that enlightenment comes when one begins to explore the dynamic qualities of interrelation and interconnection between the self and the source of all beings.

The word *prayer* comes from the Latin *precarious*, "obtained by begging," and *precari*, "to entreat"—to ask earnestly, beseech, implore. This suggests two of the most common forms of prayer: *petition*, asking something for one's self, and *intercession*, asking something for others.

Prayer is a genuinely nonlocal event, not confined to a specific place in space or to a specific moment in time. Prayer reaches outside the here and now; it operates at a distance and outside the present moment. Because prayer is initiated by a mental action, this implies that some aspect of our psyche also is genuinely nonlocal. Nonlocality implies infinitude in space and time because a limited nonlocality is a contradiction in terms. In the West, this infinite aspect of the psyche has been referred to as the *soul*. Empirical evidence for the power of prayer therefore may be seen as indirect evidence for the soul.

Scientific attempts to assess the effects of prayer and spiritual practices on health began in the nineteenth century with Sir Francis Galton's treatise "Statistical Inquiries into the Efficacy of Prayer" (Galton, 1872). Galton assessed the longevity of people frequently prayed for, such as clergy, monarchs, and heads of state. He concluded that there was no demonstrable effect of prayer on longevity. By current scientific standards, Galton's study was flawed. He was successful, however, in promoting the idea that prayer is subject to empirical scrutiny. Galton did acknowledge that praying could make a person feel better. In the end he maintained that although his attempts to prove the efficacy of prayer had failed, he could see no good reason to abandon prayer.

Those who practice healing with prayer claim uniformly that the effects are not diminished with distance; therefore it falls within the nonlocal perspective discussed earlier. Claims about the effectiveness of prayer do not rely on anecdote or single case studies; numerous controlled studies have validated the nonlocal nature of prayer. Moreover, much of this evidence suggests that praying individuals, or people involved in compassionate imagery or mental intent, whether or not it is called "prayer," can purposefully affect the physiology of distant people without the awareness of the "receiver."

The medical community has recently begun to acknowledge the importance of exploring the association between spirituality and medicine. Many medical schools now offer courses in religion, spirituality, and health. According to a 1994 survey, 98% of hospitalized patients ascribe to a belief in God or some higher power, and 96% acknowledge a personal use of prayer to aid in the healing process. In addition, 77% of 203 hospitalized family practice patients believed that their physicians should consider their spiritual needs. In contrast, only 32% of the patients' family physicians actually discussed spirituality with their patients (King et al., 1994).

Anecdotal accounts of the power of prayer are legendary, and countless books on these subjects are available; however, literature containing scientific value is still limited.

The now-famous prayer study involving humans was published in 1988 by Randolph Byrd, a staff cardiologist at San Francisco School of Medicine, University of California, where he randomized 393 patients in the coronary care unit to either a group receiving intercessory prayer or to a control group. Intecessory prayer was offered by interventionists outside the hospital. They were not instructed how often to pray, but to pray as they saw fit. In this double-blind study, the prayed-for patients did better on several counts. Although not statistically significant, there were fewer deaths in the prayer group; they were less likely to require intubation and ventilator support; they required fewer potent drugs; they experienced a lower incidence of pulmonary edema; and they required cardiopulmonary resuscitation less often (Byrd, 1988).

In 1999, W.E. Harris attempted to replicate Byrd's findings at the Mid America Heart Institute in Kansas City. Although he did not achieve significant results, researchers reported that patients received significant benefit, as reflected on a coronary care unit outcome measure (Harris et al., 1999). Critics have charged that controlled studies on prayer are impossible because extraneous prayer cannot be eliminated from the control group.

Other studies have been conducted with intercessory prayer as the intervention for alcohol abuse and dependence (Walker et al., 1997), kidney dialysis (Matthews et al., 2001), and self-esteem (O'Laoire, 1997). A prospective study of 40 patients with class II or III rheumatoid arthritis compared the effects of direct-contact intercessory prayer with prayer. Persons receiving direct-contact prayer showed significant overall improvement at the 1-year follow-up. The distant prayer group showed no additional benefits (Matthews et al., 2000).

The benefits of spiritual healing were examined in 120 patients with chronic pain at the Department of Complementary Medicine at the University of Exeter, United Kingdom. Patients were randomized to face-to-face healing or simulated face-to-face healing for 30 minutes per week for 8 weeks or to distant healing or no healing for the same time. Although subjects in both healing groups reported significantly more "unusual experiences" during the sessions, the clinical relevance of this is unclear. It was concluded that a specific effect of face-to-face or distant healing on chronic pain could not be demonstrated over eight treatment sessions in these patients (Abbot et al., 2002).

Although research problems will be difficult to overcome in evaluating the power of prayer, Byrd's initial prayer study broke significant ground in medical research. Many questions still remain unanswered, and further study is warranted to define the role of intercessory prayer on quantitative and qualitative outcomes and to identify end points that best measure efficacy.

While validated evidence continues to build concerning the efficacy of prayer, Dossey (1993) maintains that some serious questions arise in the wake of these experiments. The evidence clearly shows that mental activity can be used to influence people non-locally, at a distance, without their knowledge. Scores of experiments on prayer also show that it can be used to great effect without the subject's awareness. Therefore the question is whether it is ethical to use these techniques if recipients are unaware that they are being used. This question becomes even more compelling as we consider the possibility that prayer, or any other form of mind-to-mind communication, may be used at a distance to harm people without their knowledge. Institutional review committees, who oversee the design of experiments involving humans and to ensure their safety, have rarely had to consider these types of ethical questions.

COMBINED APPROACHES

While evidence continues to mount regarding the efficacy of mind and body approaches used individually, more and more researchers and clinicians are beginning to combine various approaches to create a synergistic healing process.

Combining hypnosis and guided imagery showed impressive results in dealing with the postoperative course of pediatric surgical patients. Fifty-two children were randomly assigned to an experimental or control group. Children in the experimental group were taught imagery, which included hypnotic suggestions for a favorable postoperative course. Significantly lower postoperative pain ratings and shorter hospital stays occurred for the children in the imagery group. State anxiety was decreased for the guided imagery group but increased for the control group (Lambert, 1996).

A study at the University of Texas (Houston) School of Public Health was conducted to differentiate the effects of imagery and support on coping, life attitudes, immune function, quality of life, and emotional well-being after breast cancer. Forty-seven women were randomly assigned to standard care or six weekly support or imagery sessions. For all women, interferon-gamma increased, neopterin decreased, quality of life improved, and natural killer cell activity remained unchanged. Compared with standard care, both interventions improved coping skills and perceived social support and generally enhanced meaning in life. When comparing imagery with support, imagery participants tended to have less stress, increased vigor, and improved functional and social quality of life (Richardson et al., 1997).

Harvard's Mind/Body Institute randomly assigned 128 college students to an experimental group or a wait-list control. The experimental group received six 90-minute group-training sessions in the relaxation response and cognitive-behavioral skills. Significantly greater reductions in psychological distress, state anxiety, and perceived stress were found in the treatment group (Deckro et al., 2002).

Funded by the U.S. Department of Defense, California Pacific Medical Center conducted a study that examined the outcomes for 181 women with breast cancer. Women were randomized to a 12-week "mind, body, and spirit" support group or to a standard support group. The mind, body, and spirit women were taught meditation, affirmations, imagery, and ritual. The standard group combined cognitive-behavioral approaches with group sharing and support. Both interventions were found to be associated with improved quality of life, decreased depression and anxiety, and spiritual well-being. Only the mind, body, and spirit group showed significant increases in measures of spiritual integration. At the end of the intervention, the mind, body, and spirit group showed higher satisfaction and had fewer dropouts than the standard group (Targ and Levine, 2002).

Kinney and Rodgers (2003) conducted a similar intervention for breast cancer survivors using a mind, body, and spirit self-empowerment program. Fifty-one women attended a 12-week psychospiritual supportive program that included multiple strategies for creating a balance among spiritual, mental, emotional, and physical health. Components included meditation, visualization, guided imagery, affirmations, and dream work. Results showed statistically significant improvements in depression, perceived wellness, quality of life, and spiritual well-being.

Guided imagery and progressive relaxation techniques were the focus of a recent study at New Jersey Goryeb Children's Hospital. Eighteen children between ages 5 and 12 years with chronic abdominal pain were taught guided imagery and progressive relaxation techniques over 9 months. Abdominal pain improved in 89% of the patients, weekly pain episodes decreased, pain intensity decreased, days missed from school decreased, and physician office contacts decreased. In addition, social activities increased and quality of life improved (Youssef et al., 2004).

In a recent Korean study, guided imagery and progressive relaxation techniques were also combined to reduce anticipatory nausea, vomiting, and postchemotherapy nausea and vomiting for 30 patients with breast cancer and to measure their effects on patients' quality of life. Both therapies combined showed improvements on all measures (Yoo et al, 2005).

References

Abbot NC, Harkness EF, Stevinson C, et al: Spiritual healing as a therapy for chronic pain: a randomized clinical trial, *Pain* 91(1/2):79-89, 2002.

Achterberg J: *Imagery in healing: shamanism and modern medicine,* Boston 1985, Shambhala,.

Achterberg J, Lawlis GF: *Imagery and disease: diagnostic tools,* Champaign, Ill, 1984, Institute for Personality and Ability Testing.

Achterberg J, Lawlis GF, Rider MS: The effects of music-mediated imagery on neutrophils and lymphocytes, *Biofeedback Self-Regulation* 114:247-257, 1989.

Ader R: Conditioned immunomodulation: research needs and directions, *Brain Behav Immun* 17(suppl 1):S51-S57, 2003.

Ader R, Cohen N: *Psychoneuroimmunology,* ed 2, San Diego, 1991, Academic Press.

Alexander CN et al: Transcendental meditation, mindfulness, and longevity: an experimental study with the elderly, *J Pers Soc Psychol* 57(6):950-964, 1989.

Andersen BL, Farrar WB, Golden-Kreutz DM, et al: Psychological, behavioral, and immune changes after a psychological intervention: a clinical trial, *J Clin Oncol* 22(17:3570-3580, 2004.

Ashton C, Whitworth GC, et al: Self-hypnosis reduces anxiety following coronary artery bypass surgery: a prospective, randomized trial, *J Cardiovasc Surg* 38:69-75, 1997.

Barber TX: *A scientific approach,* New York, 1969, Van Nostrand.

Barber TX: Changing "unchangeable" bodily processes by hypnotic suggestions: a new look at hypnosis, imaging and the mind/body problem, *Advances* 1(2):7-40, 1984.

Bennett HL: A comparison of audiotaped preparations for surgery: evaluation and outcomes. Paper presented at Annual Meeting of Society of Clinical and Experimental Hypnosis, 1996, Tampa, Fla.

Benson H: *The relaxation response,* New York, 1975, Morrow.

Benson HR: The relaxation response. In Goleman D, Gurin J, editors: *Mind-body medicine,* New York, 1993, Consumer Reports Books.

Benson H, Kotch JB, Crassweller KD: Relaxation response: bridge between psychiatry and medicine, *Med Clin North Am* 61:929-938, 1977.

Bohm D: *Wholeness and implicate order,* London, 1983, Rutledge.

Braud WG: Human interconnectedness: research indications, *ReVision* 14:140-148, 1992.

Braud WG, Schlitz M: Consciousness interactions with remote biological systems: anomalous intentionality effects, *Subtle Energies* 2, 1991.

Brooks JS, Scarano T: Transcendental meditation in the treatment of post-Vietnam adjustment, *J Counsel Dev* 65:212-215, 1985.

Byrd RC: Positive therapeutic effects of intercessory prayer in a coronary care unit population, *South Med J* 81(7): 826-829, 1988.

Carlson LE et al: The effects of a mindfulness meditation-based stress reduction program on mood and symptoms of stress in cancer outpatients: 6-month follow-up, *Support Care Cancer* 9:112-123, 2001.

Castillo-Richmond A, Schneider RH, et al: Effects of stress reduction on carotid atherosclerosis in hypertensive African Americans, *Stroke* 31(3):568-573, 2000.

Caudill M et al: Decreased clinic use by chronic pain patients: response to behavioral medicine intervention, *J Chronic Pain* 7:305-310, 1991.

Centers for Disease Control and Prevention: About chronic disease: definition, overall burden, and cost effectiveness of prevention, 2003 (http://www.cdc.gov/nccdphp/about.htm).

Chang et al, 2004. et al: Relaxation response for veterans affairs with congestive heart failure: results from a qualitative study within a clinical trial, *Prev Cardiol* 7(2):64-70, 2004.

Classen C et al: Supportive-expressive group therapy and distress in patients with metastatic breast cancer, *Arch Gen Psychiatry* 58:494-501, 2001.

Cooper M, Aygen M: Effects of meditation on blood cholesterol and blood pressure, *J Israel Med Assoc* 95:1-2, 1978.

Cordova MJ, Giese-Davis J, Golant M, et al: Mood disturbance in community cancer support groups: the role of emotional suppression and fighting spirit, *J Psychosom Res* 55(5):461-467, 2003.

Crowther MR, Parker MW, Achenbaun WA, et al: Rowe and Kahn's model of successful aging revisited: positive spirituality-the forgotten factor, *Gerontologist* 42(5):613-620, 2002.

Cummings NA, Bragman JI: Triaging the "somatizer" out of the medical system into psychological system. In EM Stern and F Stern, editors: *Psychotherapy and the somatizing patient,* New York, 1988, Hayward Press.

Cunningham C et al: Effects of transcendental meditation on symptoms and electrocardiographic changes in patients with cardiac syndrome X, *Am J Cardiol* 85(5): 653-655, 2000.

Daaleman TP, VandeCreek P: Placing religion and spirituality in end-of-life care, *JAMA* 284:2514-2517, 2000.

Davis KJ, Kumar D, Poloniecki J: Adjuvant biofeedback following anal sphincter repair: a randomized study, *Ailment Pharmacol Ther* 20(5):539-549, 2004.

Debeneditts C, Panerai AA, Villamira MA: Effect of hypnotic analgesia and hypnotizability on experimental ischemic pain, *Int J Clin Exp Hypn* 37:55-69, 1989.

Deckro GR, Ballinger KM, Hoyt M, et al: The evaluation of a mind/body intervention to reduce psychological distress and perceived stress in college students, *J Am Coll Health* 50(6):281-287, 2002.

Deepak KK et al: Effects of meditation on the clinicoencephalographic activity of drug-resistant epileptics, *Biofeedback Self-Reguraltion* 19(1):25-40, 1994.

Dossey L: *Healing words: the power of prayer and the practice of medicine,* San Francisco, 1993, Harper.

Dreher hd: Mind-body interventions for surgery: evidence and exigency, *Adv Mind-Body Med* 14:207-222, 1998.

Dunn BR et al: Concentration and mindfulness meditations: unique forms of consciousness? *Appl Psychophysiol Biofeedback* 24(3):147-165, 1999.

Eisenberg DM et al: Unconventional medicine in the United States, *N Engl J Med* 238(4):246-252, 1993.

Eisenberg DM et al: Perceptions about complementary therapies relative to unconventional therapies among adults who use both: results from a national survey, *Ann Intern Med* 135(5):344-351, 2001.

Esch T, Stefano GB, Fricchione GL, Benson H: Stress in cardiovascular diseases, *Med Sci Monit* 8(5):RA93-RA101, 2000a.

Esch T, Stefano GB, Fricchione GL, Benson H: The role of stress in neurodegenerative diseases and mental disorders, *Neuro Endocrinol Lett* 23(2):199-208, 2000b.

Fielding JWL et al: An interim report of a prospective, randomized, controlled study of adjuvant chemotherapy in operable gastric cancer: British stomach cancer group, *World J Surg* 7:390-399, 1983.

Fulop G, Strain JJ, Vita J, et al: Impact of psychiatric comorbidity on length of stay for medical/surgical patients: a preliminary report, *Am J Psychiatry* 144: 878-882, 1987.

Fynes MM, Marshall K, Cassidy M, et al: A prospective, randomized study comparing the effects of augmented biofeedback with sensory biofeedback alone on fecal incontinence after obstetric trauma, *Dis Colon Rectum* 42(6):753-758, 1999.

Galton F: Statistical inquiries into the efficacy of prayer, *Fortnightly Review* 12:11225, 1872.

Ginandes C, Brooks P, Sando W, et al: Can medical hypnosis accelerate post-surgical wound healing? Results of a clinical trial, *Am J Clin Hypn* 45(4): 333-351 2003.

Gonsalkorale WM, Houghton LA, Whorwell PJ: Hypnotherapy in irritable bowel syndrome: a large-scale audit of a clinical service with examination of factors influencing responsiveness, *Am J Gastroenterol* 97:954-961, 2002.

Gonsalkorale WM, Miller V, Afzal A, et al: Long term benefits of hypnotherapy for irritable bowel syndrome, *Gut* 52(11):1623-1629, 2003.

Gonsalkorale WM, Toner BB, Whorwell PJ: Cognitive change in patients undergoing hypnotherapy for irritable bowel syndrome, *J Psychosom Res* 56(3):271-278, 2004.

Goodwin JS, Hunt WC, et al: The effect of marital status on stage, treatment and survival of cancer patients, *JAMA* 258:3125-3130, 1987.

Gordon D: The fresh face of hypnosis: an old practice finds new uses, *Better Homes & Gardens,* February 2004.

Greco CM, Rudy TE, Manzi S: Effects of a stress-reduction program on psychological function, pain, and physical function of systemic lupus erythematosus patients: a randomized controlled trial, *Arthritis Rheum* 51(4):625-634, 2004.

Green E, Green A: *Beyond biofeedback,* New York, 1977, Delta.

Gruber BL, Hall NR, Hersh SP, Dubois P: Immune system and psychological changes in metastatic cancer patients using relaxation and guided imagery: a pilot study, *Scand J Behav Ther* 17: 25-46, 1988.

Halpin LS, Speir AM, et al: Guided imagery in cardiac surgery, *Outcomes Manag* 6(3):132-137, 2002.

Harris WS, Gowda M, Kolb JW, et al: A randomized, controlled trial of the effects of remote, intercessory prayer on outcomes in patients admitted to the coronary care unit, *Arch Intern Med* 159(19):2272-2278, 1999.

Hatch JP, Fisher JG, Rugh JD: *Biofeedback: studies in clinical efficacy,* New York, 1987, Plenum.

Herbert N: *Quantum reality,* Garden City, NY, 1987, Anchor/Doubleday.

Herron RE, Hillis SL et al: The impact of the transcendental meditation program on government payments to physicians in Quebec: an update, *Am J Health Promot* 14(5):284-291, 2000.

Holmes TH, Rahe RH: *The social readjustment rating scale, J Psychosom Res* 11:213-218, 1967.

Horowitz M: *Image formation,* New York, 1983, Jason Aronson.

House J, Landis KR, Umberson D: Social relationships and health, *Science* 241:540-545, 1988.

Ironson G, Solomon GF, Balbin EG, et al: The Ironson Woods Spirituality/Religious Index is associated with long survival, health behaviors less stress, and low cortisol in people with HIV/AIDS, *Ann Behav Med* 24(1):34-48, 2002.

Jahn RG, Dunn BJ: Precognitive remote perception. In *Margins of reality: the role of consciousness in the physical world,* New York, 1987, Harcourt Brace, pp 149-191.

Jordan CS, Lenington KT: Psychological correlates of eidetic imagery and induced anxiety, *J Ment Imagery* 3:31-42, 1979.

Kabat-Zinn J: *Full catastrophe living,* New York, 1990, Delacorte Press.

Kabat-Zinn J: Meditation. In Flowers BS, Grubin D, Meryman-Bruner E, editors: *Healing and the mind,* New York 1993a, Bantam Doubleday.

Kabat-Zinn J: Mindfulness meditation. In Goleman D, and Gurin J, editors: *Mind-body medicine,* New York, 1993b, Consumer Reports Books.

Kabat-Zinn J: *Wherever you go, there you are: mindfulness meditation in everyday life,* New York, 1993c, Hyperion.

Kabat-Zinn J, Lipworth L, et al: Four-year follow-up of a meditation-based program for the self-regulation of chronic pain, *J Behav Med* 8:163-190, 1986.

Kaplan KH et al: The impact of a meditation-based stress reduction program on fibromyalgia, *Gen Hosp Psychiatry* 15(5):284-289, 1993.

Katz R: Informed consent—is it bad medicine? *West J Med* 126:426-428, 1977.

Kiecolt-Glaser JK, Glaser R, Williger D, et al: Psychosocial enhancement of immunocompetence in a geriatric population, *Health Psychol* 4:25-41, 1985.

King DE, Bushwick B: Beliefs and attitudes of hospital inpatients about faith healing and prayer, *J Fam Pract* 39:349-352, 1994.

Kinney CK, Rodgers DM, Nash KA, et al: Holistic healing for women with breast cancer through a mind, body, and spirit self-empowerment program, *J Holist Nurs* 21(3):260-279, 2003.

Koenig HG, Cohen HJ, Blazer DG, et al: Religious coping and depression in elderly hospitalized medically ill men, *Am J Psychiatry* 149:1693-1700, 1992.

Koenig HG, Ford S, George LK, et al: Religion and anxiety disorder: an examination and comparison of associations in young, middle-aged, and elderly adults, *J Anxiety Disord* 7:321-342, 1993.

Koenig HG, McCullough M, Larson DB: *Handbook of religion and health: a century of research reviewed,* New York, 2001, Oxford University Press.

Kolcaba K, Fox C: The effects of guided imagery on comfort of women with early stage breast cancer undergoing radiation therapy, *Oncol Nurs Forum* 26(1):67-72, 1999.

Lambert SA: The effects of hypnosis/guided imagery on the postoperative course of children, *J Dev Behav Pediatr* 17(5):307-310, 1996.

Lehrer PM, Vaschillo E, Vashchillo B, et al: Biofeedback treatment in asthma, *Chest* 126(2):352-361, 2004.

LeShan L: *The medium, the mystic, and the physicist,* New York, 1966, Viking.

Levine JD, Gordon NC, Fields HL: The mechanism of placebo analgesia, *Lancet* 2:654-657, 1978.

Lewandowski WA: Patterning of pain and power with guided imagery, *Nurs Sci Q* 17(3):233-241, 2004.

MacLean CRK, Walton KG, et al: Altered cortisol response to stress after four months' practice of the transcendental meditation program. Paper presented at 18th Annual Meeting of Society for Neuroscience, Anaheim, Calif, 1992.

Malach M, Imperato PJ: Depression and acute myocardial infarction, *Prev Cardiol* 7(2):83-90, 2004.

Mason AA, Black S: Allergic skin responses abolished under treatment of asthma and hay fever by hypnosis, *Lancet* 1:877-880, 1958.

Matthews DA, Conti JM, Sireci SG: The effects of intercessory prayer, positive visualization, and expectancy on the well-being of kidney dialysis patients, *Altern Ther Health Med* 7(5):42-52, 2001.

Matthews DA, Marlowe SM, MacNutt FS: Effects of intercessory prayer on patients with rheumatoid arthritis, *South Med J* 93(12):1177-1186, 2000.

Miller R: Nurses at community hospital welcome guided imagery, *Dimens Crit Care Nurs* 22(5):225-226, 2003.

Mills H, Allen J: Mindfulness of movement as a coping strategy in multiple sclerosis. A pilot study. Gen Hosp Psychiatry 22(6):425-431, 2000.

Morris D: *The human zoo,* New York, 1995, Oxford University Press.

Mueller HH, Donaldson CC, Nelson DV, et al: Treatment of fibromyalgia incorporating EEG-driven stimulation: a clinical outcomes study, *J Clin Psychol* 57(7):933-952, 2001.

Mookadam F, Arthur HM: Social support and its relationship to morbidity and mortality after acute myocardial infarction: systematic overview, *Arch Intern Med* 164(14):1514-1518, 2004.

Norton C, Chelvanayagam S, et al: Randomized controlled trial of biofeedback for fecal incontinence, *Gastroenterology* 125(5):1320-1329, 2003.

O'Laoire S: An experimental study of the effects of distant, intercessory prayer on self-esteem, anxiety, and depression, *Altern Ther Health Med* 3(6):38-53, 1997.

Olness K, Gardner GG: *Hypnosis and hypnotherapy with children,* ed 2, Philadelphia, 1988, Saunders.

Ornish D: Can lifestyle changes reverse coronary artery disease? *Lancet* 336:129, 1990.

Osler W: *Aequanimitas,* ed 3, New York, 1953, Blakiston.

Pargament KI, Smith BW, Koenig HG, et al: Patterns of positive and negative religious coping with major life stressors, *J Scientific Study Religion* 37:710-724, 1998.

Pearce JC: *The magical child,* New York, 1992, Penguin.

Reynolds P, Kaplan GA: Social connections and risk for cancer: prospective evidence from t he Alameda County Study, *Behav Med* 16(3):101-110, 1990.

Richardson MA, Post-White J, Grimm EA, et al: Coping, life attitudes, immune responses to imagery and group support after breast cancer treatment, *J Altern Ther Health Med* 3(5):62-70, 1997.

Sacks M: Exercise for stress control. In Goleman D, Gurin J, editors: *Mind-body medicine,* New York, 1993, Consumer Reports Books.

Sauter S: Organizational Science and Human Factors Branch of the National Institute of Occupational Safety and Health, *New York Times,* Sept 5, 2004, p A15.

Schlesinger HJ, Mumford E, Glass GV: Mental health treatment and medical care utilization . . . following onset of a chronic disease, *Am J Public Health* 73:422-429, 1983.

Schlitz M, Braud WG: Distant intentionality and healing: assessing the evidence, *Altern Ther Health Med* 3(6):62-73, 1997.

Schneider RH, Alexander CN, et al: In search of an optimal behavioral treatment for hypertension: a review and focus on transcendental meditation. In Johnson EH, editor: *Hypertension,* Washington, DC, 1992, Hemisphere.

Schneider RH, Alexander CN, et al: A randomized controlled trial of stress reduction for hypertension in older African Americans, *Hypertension* 26(5):820-827, 1995.

Schroedinger E: *What is life? And mind and matter,* London, 1969, Cambridge University Press.

Schwartz J: American Institute of Stress, *New York Times,* Sept 5, 2004, p A15.

Selye H: *The stress of life,* New York, 1978, McGraw-Hill.

Sharma HM. Triguna BD, Chopra D: Maharishi Ayur-Veda: modern insights into ancient meditation, *JAMA* 265:2633-2634, 2637, 1991.

Simonton OC, Simonton S, Creighton J: *Getting well again,* Los Angeles, 1978, Tarcher.

Sloman R: Relaxation and imagery for anxiety and depression control in community patients with advanced cancer, *Cancer Nurs* 25(6):432-435, 2002.

Sobel DS: Mind matters and money matters: is clinical behavioral medicine cost effective? Paper presented at Fourth International Conference on the Psychology of Health, Immunity and Disease, Hilton Head, SC, 1992.

Solfvin J: Mental healing. In Krippner S, editor: *Advances in parapsychological research.* Vol 4, Jefferson, NC, 1984, McFarland.

Spiegel D et al: Effect of psychosocial treatment on survival of patients with metastatic breast cancer, *Lancet* 2(8668):888-891, 1989.

Spiegel D et al: Group psychotherapy for recently diagnosed breast cancer patients: a multicenter feasibility study, *Psychooncology* 8:482-493, 1999.

Strain JJ: Psychotherapy and medical conditions. In Goleman D, and Gurin J, editors: *Mind-body medicine,* New York, 1993, Consumer Reports Books.

Targ EF, Levine EG: The efficacy of a mind-body-spirit group for women with breast cancer: a randomized controlled trial, *Gen Hosp Psychiatry* 24:238-248, 2002.

Temkin-Greener H, Bajorska A, Peterson DR, et al: Social support and risk-adjusted mortality in a frail older population, *Med Care* 42(8):779-788, 2004.

Tix AP, Frazier PA: The use of religious coping during stressful life events: main effects, moderation, and meditation, *J Consult Clin Psychol* 66:411-422, 1997.

Tusek D, Church JM, Fazio VW: Guided imagery as a coping strategy for perioperative patients. *AORN J* 66(4):644-649, 1997.

Walker SR, Tonigan JS, Miller WR, et al: Intercessory prayer in the treatment of alcohol abuse and dependence: a pilot investigation, *Altern Ther Health Med* 3(6):79-86, 1997.

White KD: Salivation: the significance of imagery in its voluntary control, *Psychophysiology* 15(3):196-203, 1978.

Williams R, Kiecolt-Glasser J, et al: The impact of emotions on cardiovascular health, 1999, *J Gend Specif Med* 2(5):52-58.

Yoo HJ, Ahn SH, Kim SB, et al: Efficacy of progressive muscle relaxation training and guided imagery in reducing chemotherapy side effects in patients with breast cancer and in improving their quality of life, *Support Care Cancer* (in press), 2005.

Youssef NN, Rosh JR, Loughran M, et al: Treatment of functional abdominal pain in childhood with cognitive behavioral strategies, *J Pediatr Gastroenterol Nutr* 39(2):192-196, 2004.

Suggested Readings

Baskins TW et al: Establishing specificity in psychotherapy: a meta-analysis of structural equivalence of placebo controls, *J Consult Clin Psychol* 71(6):973-979, 2003.

Benson H: *Timeless healing: the power and biology of belief,* New York, 1996, Scribner.

Chopra D: *Quantum healing: exploring the frontiers of mind/body medicine,* New York, 1990, Bantam Books.

Dossey L: *Recovering the soul: a scientific and spiritual approach,* New York, 1989, Bantam.

Green E, Green A: *Beyond biofeedback,* New York, 1977, Dell.

Holbrook A, Goldsmith D. Placebos: our most effective therapy? *Can J Clin Pharmacol* 11(1):e39-40, 2004; Epub Apr 01 2004.

Locke S, Hornig-Rohan M: *Mind and immunity: behavioral immunology,* New York, 1983, Institute for the Advancement of Health.

Moyers B: In Flowers BS, Grubin D, Meryman-Brunner E, editors: *Healing and the mind,* New York, 1993, Bantam Doubleday.

Naperstek B: *Staying well with guided imagery,* New York, 1994, Warner.

Pert CB: *Molecules of emotion,* New York, 1997, Simon & Schuster.

Schlitz M, Amorok T, Micozzi MS, *Consciousness & healing; Integral approaches to mind-body medicine,* St Louis, 2005, Elsevier.

Simonton OC, Henson R: *The healing journey,* New York, 1994, Bantam.

17

ENERGETIC HEALING

MAURIE D. PRESSMAN

Let it start right here, right now, with us—with you and with me—and with our commitment to breathe into infinity until infinity alone is the only statement that the world will recognize. Let radical realization shine from our faces, and roar from our hearts, and thunder from our brains—this simple fact, this obvious fact: that you, in the very immediateness of your present awareness, are in fact the entire world, in all its frost and fever, in all its glories and its grace, in all its triumphs and its tears. You do not see the sun, you are the sun; you do not hear the rain, you are the rain; you do no feel the earth, you are the earth. And in that simple, clear, unmistakable regard, translation has ceased in all domains, and you have transformed into the very Heart of the Kosmos itself—and there, right there, very simply, very quietly, it is all undone.

—KEN WILBER (1999)

BASIC CONCEPTS

Energy Creates

In the beginning was the word—and the word was made flesh.

—JOHN 3:16

More and more we become aware of the fact that the "word" (consciousness) is the source of all energy. We translate "consciousness" energy into material manifestation. All religions, at their core, teach this. It is the expression of Brahma.

The All is Brahma (God, Allah, Chi, Ka). Brahma created; perturbations occurred in the stillness of the Void; and disturbance became existence as we know it.

313

Healthy existence is peaceful presence and requires flow, balance, cooperation, and the realization of being both "One" and "at-One," a part of each other's "One-ness," thus *flow*. Resistance to flow disturbs the harmony of peace, spirit, and love and the return to the Nirvana of true health.

Thus, *energy* is "force," or that which acts to produce, move, and create. *Healing* is the restoration of wholeness, harmony, flow, and easy unity—within each organism and between each creation.

In the tumult of the 1960s, a treasure of ancient philosophy arrived from the East to the West. Alan Watts (1959), who was trained in the East, found a guru teacher in the course of seeking and brought the new/old knowledge as avant-garde instruction to a revolutionary group of youth, ready to receive, experiment, and expand consciousness in various ways. Many at that time, including John Lilly (1972), Stan Grof (1975), and newly arrived teachers such as Yogananda (1971), Muktananda (1994), Râmakrishna (Muller, 1975), and Krishnamurti, (1969), each developed a coterie of followers. They spread this core of ancient teaching, leading to the insight of the basic energy that we are, and from which we descend. Importation from the East was followed by the Western application of these methods to instruction, to physical healing, as in acupuncture for anesthesia, and to the use of biofeedback by Elmer Green (1977) and others. East had met West, and the meld became a practical application to the body, to the world, and to the advance in scientific discovery of this ancient teaching, which had derived from the intense inner inspection of the mind through yoga and meditation.

A Shift in Paradigm

We are engaged in a slow and painful shift in paradigm. Gradually we look away from the primacy of the body to realize the primacy of the mind and its subtle energies.

What are the "subtle energies"? They are the energies that exist in the fields beyond those defined by the five-sense sensory field. They exist in an energetic spectrum that has been defined by Tiller (2001) as in the "magnetic spectrum," beyond the speed of light. Subtle energies exist in the thought realms, otherwise known as the "spiritual" (not religious) realms. This is the whole and vast domain that exists "behind the retina." It obliterates the need for time and space and

allows us to think in less constricted terms. We can begin to understand dimensions more than four "multi-universes" as defined by Kaku (1994), parallel universes of thinking as well as parallel personalities, existing simultaneously.

Accompanying the paradigm shift is an expansion in our understanding of healing. Sigmund Freud taught us about the deeper layers of mind that move us in action, emotion, and even thinking (Strachey, editor, 1953-1974). We are exercised by forces beyond our conscious understanding. This new knowledge leads into the area of mind-body connection, "psychosomatic medicine." This was strongly advocated in the 1940s and 1950s by French and Alexander and later extended, by a greater respect for the power of the mind, to disorder and its counterpart, healing. Further progress gave birth to "psychoneuroimmunology," with an understanding of the effect of mind on the immune system (see Chapter 15). This pointed to a greater understanding of the failure of healing and new approaches to recovery.

With our progress in understanding the boundless realms of mind, we have come to know that mind is greater than cortex; that mind is not enclosed in the body, or calvarium.; mind is a vast consciousness originating as love, light, and energy. Mind both forms us and informs us. It communicates each part of us with the entire other: each cell of our self with other cells, each community of cells with the "body-whole," and each body with the earth and the planetary system with the great forces beyond.

This understanding of mind and energy has been well described by Ken Wilber (1996) as the "Holon." The Holon is a unit that is sufficient unto itself, but at the same time it makes no sense and cannot even exist, except in terms of it being a part of a larger unity. Therefore the cell, the cell within the body, is a complete unit, indeed a universe unto itself, but it cannot exist or have meaning, except in terms of its existence as part of a larger organism: a liver, a human, an entity that lives as part of a community.

We are this wonderful individual, this eternal unit of energy that exists as a conscious, unique, and individual intelligence, and yet we are each a part of the other in a continuum that is ongoing, dynamically interchanging, and internourishing with the others.

And what is healing but the recognition of this unity that we are and that we are a part of? What is healing but a "making whole," a "making balanced," a "making easy flow" of the interchange and dynamic sharing of each part of ourselves with the other, and each self with all other selves.

From the Arcane School, established by Alice Bailey under the tutelage of her teacher Djwahl Kuhl, comes the following prayer:

I am a point of light within a greater light.
I am a strand of loving energy within the stream of Love Divine.
I am a point of sacrificial fire, focused within the fiery will of God.
And thus I stand.
I am a way by which men may achieve.
I am a source of strength, enabling them to stand.
I am a beam of light shining upon their way.
And thus I stand.
And standing thus, revolve and tread this way
The ways of Man and know the ways of God.
And thus I stand. . . . ”

Definitions

Energy

Webster's Unabridged Dictionary (1996) defines "energy" in various ways: first, "the capacity for vigorous activity; available power"; also in physics, "the capacity to do work."

However, energy has a long history. We must realize that energy is that on which we rest. It is that which has created "us" as well as everything else. It is that which maintains us as well as everything else. In ancient religions and their core teachings, energy is equivalent with the force of existence. Energy is Brahma, descending.

Healing

As to healing, *Webster's* has difficulty, defining it as "growing sound; getting well; mending; or the act or process of regaining health."

If we abandon these dictionary words about healing, however, and take a view from above, we will see that restoring health, or healing, is a matter of creating "flow," assisting each unit to integrate well, both within itself and with its context, its "surround," of which it, itself, is but a part.

Subtle Energy

Science has now shown us that we are congealed energy, precipitated energy, a materialized expression of something higher and beyond the five physical senses.

The present model of healing seems to rest on a chemical basis, but we are entering into an era in which we understand that *biophysical energies* are present and are healing. Oschman (2000) has described biophysical energies that are present in and transmitted through connective tissue. In fact, he has pointed us toward the understanding of a *second* nervous system, one transmitted by the central nervous system (CNS) with its peripheral branches, and the other by the connective tissue (Pressman, 2001) Oschman shows that bending of the connective tissue creates piezoelectric energy through which information is transmitted everywhere in the body, including the interior of every cell. I speculate that there may be yet a *third* information system exercised by the subtle energies of the mind, the *visualization energies*. With this system, we witness some of the miraculous cures that have attended visualization, beginning with the work of Carl Simonton (1978).

Subtle energies are therefore the energies that are present and active and transmitted, but not through the material apparatus, not through the CNS, not through the connective tissue, not through anything measurable by the five senses. Instead, subtle energies are beyond the five physical senses and are those that reside in thought ("high thought") and emotions and follow those experiences that lie behind the retina. "Behind the retina" refers to the realm of imagination, thought, abstract thought, dreams, and inspiration.

Referring again to Tiller's energy spectrum, with its fulcrum being the speed of light, the subtle energies lie beyond that fulcrum. Clinically, we gain access to that domain by passing through the gate that the fulcrum defines (Tiller et al., 2001). Passing through this gateway is achieved by emptying the mind, creating silence of mind and body. Then we find ourselves at the place of quietude and peace while expectantly awaiting new phenomena. In this space we receive new wisdom. In this attitude we send forth healing energies.

The gateway to the subtle realm is also denoted by the achievement of "lucid mind." This is the mind in which the waking consciousness of the material realm meets the dream consciousness of the subtle realm. We can experience both these realms in lucid dreaming and in lucid meditation, with its healing effects on the body.

HISTORY

Energy as a force of action, indeed a force of creation, has been known to exist since the beginning of time.

Our concentration on energy as it is applied to "energy healing" has become popular (in the West) only recently and is growing rapidly. We have been focused on the body as a part of our socioscientific orientation toward physical objects. It was a shock when the atom was smashed (until relatively recently thought to be impossible) and when it was found that matter dissolves into waves of energy. This was also seen in quantum physics (by Schroedinger) when light resolved itself into waves or particles according to the conditions set. $E = mc^2$, translated, means not only that we can burn a log but that the energy emitted can be crystallized again into something solid. Our thinking was turned on its head—literally. Heisenberg (1977) further disturbed the world by showing that we cannot stand apart and observe a world. Our mind is constantly active, and that activity itself changes the very thing observed. Mind energy again, and so it goes on and on.

Speculating clinically, however, I wonder if this might not be related to the power of visualization. Visualization can change things in the body, but perhaps things in behavior and performance as well. In 1972 I combined hypnosis with visualization by the athlete of a perfect performance, and the results were immediate and astounding. The more the visualization was practiced, the more stable the result (Pressman, 1978, 1979, 1980). Observing the self (in the subtle body) also has a positive effect if one visualizes health, or a more nearly perfect performance in any respect.

In the West, energy healing began with Freud when he uncovered the power of the "word" in his earliest works, as well as the power of hypnosis. After all, hypnosis is a matter of energy exchange between hypnotist and the "subject." The elevation of an unconscious drive or emotion is accomplished by the energy of the word, or interpretation. Hypnosis, at the time of the Freud's early work, was under intense study by such greats as Pierre Janet (1965), Charcot (1887-1888), and Joseph Breuer. Herbert Silberer (1971) was studying mysticism in an exploration of hidden energetic power.

Freud went on to uncover deeper and deeper layers of the mind, while tracing the foundations of mind to the earliest childhood experience. In early psychoanalysis, there was evidence of memory, *energetic memory,* imprinted on physiology, as described by Phyllis Greenacre (1969) on the trauma of birth, as well as by Otto Rank (1990).

Hypnosis is mind healing, "energy healing," as in the early work of Breuer and Freud. About 1775, Mesmer, whose work is now being validated (Oschman,

2000), indicated that hypnosis was energetic when he labeled it "animal magnetism" (Bloch, translator, 1980). Mesmer considered it a projection of energy from hypnotist to subject. Energy healing was evident in Freud's *Interpretation of Dreams* in 1900 (1933) when he began to realize the mysterious meaning of the dream, thereafter applying interpretation. This is "word energy," a transfer of energy through interpretation. The transfer from interpretation to acceptance and the subsequent integration by the patient is an energetic process. Although we understand a great deal about the neurological function of the brain and the psychopharmacological reactions involved, an important coordination of thought and emotion energies is simultaneously at work. Interpretation and working through the interpretation are healing processes.

APPROACHES TO ENERGETIC HEALING

With energy, "The deeper we go, the higher we go." If we are to enter into the larger territory of the subtle domain, we must find the gate.

Finding and Entering the "Gate"

How do we find the gate? How do we enter the gate?

The "gate" lies at the point of the Tiller fulcrum. It is Alice's mirror (Carroll, 1990). How do we pass through?

We find the gate by allowing inner silence and contemplation. We pass through the gate when we value the products of imagination. We learn to surrender our ego, our preconceptions, and our personal wishes, allowing an open mind and valuing those things that come in as inspiration. We suspend doubt long enough to savor the new products, then permit them to test themselves in the context of living in the material realm. This involves bringing the waking consciousness of the left brain, with its practical-material-scientific functioning, into equal partnership with the world of dreams, imagination, intuition, and inspiration—approving the meld and moving onward in humble appreciation of the guidance we receive. This comes from surrender to the high self and "Spirit," from which we descend.

Is this far-fetched? Look at the work of Hal Puthoff (2002), who discovered the infinite field of Brahma as the source of creation, called the *zero-point field* (ZPF) in physics. The ZPF "bestirs itself," much as does Brahma (God, the All), and allows the disturbance to materialize into creation. Is it so strange that a Frank Lloyd Wright, a Leonardo da Vinci, a Michelangelo, or a Louis Kahn creates new products, although with the help of canvas, blueprints, and subsequent construction engineers? The source of creation is in the imagination of the creator-human. It is imagination that allows itself to arrive and then to be sculpted into action by the practical mind. This is not magic; this is the creative product of the "high mind," the imagination, as we see it today.

Teachers such as Rudolph Steiner (1994), Sri Aurobindo (1972), and Madame Blavatsky of Theosophy (Cranston, 1993) trained themselves to surrender to silence and a belief in the inspired world. Then they brought forth their enlightened teaching.

I was particularly helped by Steiner, who valued the use of mind and thought (high mind, high thought) to deduce the products of the subtle spiritual realm. At an early age, Steiner was appointed to archive the works of the great poet-scientist Goethe. He learned how Goethe had entered into the "being" of things. This meant a surrender on Goethe's part as he entered the plant, became the plant, understood the plant, and saw the plant, not only in its immediate aspect of perhaps full blossom, but the entire process (Steiner, 1988). He realized that there was a higher "something" guiding this process, creating the seed, the stem, the leaf, the blossom, and the seed again. It was a form in the subtle realm, giving process and order to formation, and the possibility of fulfillment of potential as the potential integrated with the material world "surround" of weather, soil, nutrients, location, sun, pollinating insects, and so on.

Thus it is in our world as well. We are created by a higher energy. We descend into manifestation. We allow ourselves to fulfill the "stencil" of potential. We are integrated into this world that we call the "material," and we vary according to our environment as we integrate. We also shape our environment. This is the constant interfusing of energies, the high energies, of thought and art and existence.

This is the way that it works.

As I read Steiner and learned about Goethe's adventure that resulted in his description of the "archplant," I saw it in my mind's eye: Goethe's energy going forth to meet the plant's energy. It was like travel from earth to a space station where two consciousnesses, Goethe's and the plant's, met and communicated with each other on a high plane, after which Goethe brought back new knowledge for description. This is true as well of "high" human transactions. As we relinquish our egos, we meet each other on a more elevated plane, and we bring back a greater understanding to each on this material plane—to be lived and to be lived better. This also means that we not only integrate this new knowledge but train ourselves as well, to live as higher personalities, constantly striving to transcend the primitive, the animal, the selfish, and the childish, and to arrive at a greater appreciation of the other and ultimately all others in nature. We learn to associate in mutual understanding and appreciation, to live with each other, and to enhance others as they enhance us. This is the creation of a "higher order" that leads us, as individuals and as the collective, to the return to the highest orders of creation.

Energy: Its Origin and Destination

"In the beginning was the word, and the word was made flesh." In the beginning God said, "Let there be light, and there was light." Thus the word, "consciousness," was and is precedent to light. The "word" is supervalent even to what Einstein thought was the fastest and nearest to ultimate in creation, "light." Now, researchers in quantum physics discover that there is much beyond the speed of light.

We are gifted with great minds in science, revealing more and more, with deeper understanding, of the way things work in God's world. The further these findings go, the more we see that the *core essentials* of all religion go hand in hand with these advances. This is "spiritual science." Let us consider some of these revelations and their relationship to core spirituality.

Not long ago the hologram was discovered. The hologram is familiar to all of us, seen as three-dimensional ghosts at amusement parks and three-dimensional logos on credit cards. The hologram is such that if we break the photographic plate into a 128 parts, each part will project the whole picture, although in a somewhat more diffuse way than the original. At the same time, all the information is retained. The whole is contained in each part, and each part contains the whole. What can be more descriptive of our relationship with each other in God's world, than the hologram, since it shows that we are truly united? It reveals that we each contain the other within ourselves, and we are similarly contained within our fellow human. Furthermore, the hologram has been used as a model by the great neuroscientist Karl Pribram as a model for the function of the brain. No matter how much of the brain is ablated, function remains; one part of the brain can function for the other. Indeed, there is increasing reason to believe that the mind exists *beyond* the brain. It is suggested that the brain functions as a "tuning station," much like a radio, attuning to the greater mind surrounding us, and that this greater mind is a holographic network of which we are a part. It is a mind in which we participate, a mind into which we can enter in order to know about each other and about things across the world, things in the past and the future, and things beyond our present knowledge and imagination.

Again I refer to the work of Puthoff (2002) and the ZPF, that field of existence and surroundings that occurs when we approach absolute zero. We now have a field of almost infinite potential energy. It is a "soup" in which all *potential* exists. Any disturbance of the field will give rise to energetic perturbations that, when they bump against each other, begin the process of manifestation and creation, then grow by further agglutination and accretion into physical substance. But what does this mean? It means that as the ancient scriptures say, "Brahma" (God, the All Potential, the Void) is everywhere existent around us and is ready to create and does create by disturbance. It is "Consciousness" ready to filter down into manifest existence.

The basic understanding of creation is derived from the ancient teachings of core Judaism, core Christianity, and core scriptures in Hinduism. In the beginning, God decided to create. This was the "Word," or consciousness. This energy, (consciousness) filtered down through seven levels into physical manifestation. It then bounced back to become a rising evolution of development, of a higher and higher consciousness. We see this in the rising evolution from animal to human to high human, as well as in the further development of our nature to become more global and more empathic. If we look into this ancient formula, we can see that that infinite potential discovered by Puthoff is consistent with the "Infinite Potential" whom we regard as the "All."

Oschman's discoveries are consistent with this holographic plan. Again, Oschman (2000) describes how the connective tissue of the body surrounds every organ and cell, then penetrates the wall of the cell through the nucleus, dividing into ever-smaller discriminations. This describes a wonderful communication system within the body: one body, one cell knowing what each part of the body does, a holographic revelation. Furthermore, these emanations transmit through tissue, and while relaying information throughout the body, they extend beyond the body. This is consistent with a silent communication between people, a banding and bonding within the holographic network, an extrasensory (ESP) connection. Thus we see evidence of the "High Mind," the "High Consciousness," which spirituality would want us to have. It is a "consciousness communication" that we feel intuitively when we silence the mind.

In this new and exciting age of discovery, Fritz Popp shows that the cells themselves emanate light, and that this light is a communication between the cells (Chang et al., 1998). This light, too, carries communication from each part of the body to the other, then extends beyond the body to be captured by measurement and to be seen and felt by others. This provides further evidence of a holographic network.

The work of Robert Jahn and Brenda Dunne (1987) shows that the mind can influence material bodies; *psychokinesis* is moving objects with the mind. This work has been extended by Dean Radin (1997) and Roger Nelson (1996), showing that massive mind-energy, such as exists during Superbowl or while awaiting major jury decisions (e.g., O.J. Simpson trial). Such mass attention creates a powerful energy that is measured by the "random event" generator. It is an energy that will change the environment as well.

William Tiller, professor emeritus at Stanford University, has shown that the consciousness of meditators will change the very chemistry of water. This means that we can change the chemistry of the body by consciousness of mind. Further, in Tiller's experiment, it was shown that the environment itself was charged, so that the energy it held would change the pH of water when, subsequently, vials of water were brought in and no meditators were present (Tiller et al., 2001).

Thus we begin to know the power we carry in our minds and consciousness, especially in the "high mind," which is achieved in meditation and prayer. It is the hope for the future because it can change the world around us.

Consciousness creates! "In the beginning was the word, and the word was made flesh."

Now we see a most modern advance in physics, "string theory" (Greene, 2003). This new theory describes how the deeper we go, the nearer we come to the ultimate level, and there, energy is contained in strings, like violin stings. They vibrate at a variety of frequencies that are infinite in their variability. These vibrations give rise to individual, and infinitely varied, manifestations of creation. This is again the work of the mind, of waves of energy of mind, and of the existence of "Consciousness" as it exists in holographic pattern.

These are some of the revelations of modern physics. These are the revelations that I believe God is allowing to unfold. This is the counterpoise to the present darkness in the world. This is the counterpart that exists and grows. It is, I believe, the "Light-Love-Consciousness" energy that may counter the terrorist threats that exist today.

Entry into the Field of Subtle Energy

Tiller (1997) has given us a clear view of the spectrum of energy from the most material to the most sublime. Again, the fulcrum of the energy spectrum exists at the speed of light. That which is on the left side (slower than the speed of light) exists in the *material realm;* it is to be seen and discovered and embraced by our five-sense sensory apparatus. Everything on the other side is in the *subtle realm,* that abstract realm, the thought realm, and even the "beyond-thought" realm. This is the area of imagination, creation, dream formation, and ascent into the superpowers of the mind.

How do we enter into the subtle field? The fact is, we do so each night in the world of the dream. We do so during the day when we float in imagination or speculate in creative problem solving. This is a world full of undreamed-of possibilities, described by Steiner (1994) in many ways as the world in which we (our intelligence, that is) exist after death. According to both Tiller (1997) and Steiner, in this world things are the reverse of what we see in the material realm.

How do we enter into and navigate in this subtle world? There is a mirror of the mind that gives entry. It is the place where the dream consciousness meets the waking consciousness. When we are awake in our dreams, as in lucid dreaming, and when we are awake in our meditations, as in lucid meditation, we have this meeting of the two minds. It is a gate of entry to the realm of creativity and *energy healing.*

The Mind Mirror: Zone of Creativity

The mirror has been used as a zone of transition in many symbolic references: the Harry Potter story, the mirror on the wall in Sleeping Beauty, the Magic Mirror, and Alice in Wonderland falling through to another world;

Raymond Moody (1988) replicated the psychomanteons of ancient Greece, where visitors would come to communicate with the spirits of the departed. Such places existed (as Moody has shown in scholarly research) in many places in the world. They had in common a period of preparation, not unlike meditation, and a dark and highly polished surface into which the person would gaze. The mindset of the Greek society allowed for such experiences. Moody has created a simple replica by erecting a darkened room and having the subject sit looking forward into a mirror. However, the mirror is darkened because it reflects a dimly lit room, and the subject is seated low enough that one's own image is not reflected. Moody, who is the pioneer in near-death experiences, reports that many subjects will actually see and communicate with the spirits that appear in the mirror.

Other equivalents of the mirror include breaking through the "time warp" as a parallel of the mirror, as in *Star Trek.* All these are sensed references to a "state of mind," of creativity, of enlarged insight that lies close at hand. It is the state of mind of lucid dreaming or in lucid meditation. At such times, one is half-awake half-asleep, dreaming, imaging, and receiving inspiration while being consciously aware at the same time, knowing that all this *is* happening. One has passed through the mirror to the other side.

My Model

In my clinical work and in reading the literature on subtle energy, I have been well served by the following model.

In the beginning is the All, the "Ain Sof," the nothingness out of which everything is created. Its infinite energy filters down through seven levels, the fourth level called, in Sanskrit, *Buddhi.* In this domain resides the "Soul," and it is the messenger of the Spirit. The Spirit is the All, the ultimate Creator, and the inhabitant, at the same time, of each thing that is created. In the course of the human journey, the Soul weaves out of itself progressively lower vibrations, which become the thought body (the mental body), the astral body (the emotional body), and then the physical body infused by a life energy called the *etheric net*.

When we meditate and enter into lucid meditation, we arrive at the mirror of the mind. We become creative and receive inspiration. We create the conditions for energy healing both of ourselves and of those we want to help. In this state of mind, visualizing healing becomes a force. It is an energy that calls forth the immune system, and it may well create a new cellular structure for a new and healed body (Pressman, 2001a).

Meditation Finds the Mirror

When we meditate, we prepare the mind so that we can locate the mind mirror.

We find it by making the body comfortable and then forgetting it. We do the same with the emotional body and again with the mental body, letting "mind chatter" drift away until we move into the place of peace, "the zone." This zone is the mirror of the mind. It is here that we transition to an always-present, always-powerful, always-fertile other world—an inner world, the *subtle energy* realm.

Science Validates Brahma (Conscoiusness Energy)

Scientific Basis

With the smashing of the atom and the arrival of quantum physics, the scientific world was turned on its head. As a result, its understanding of waves of energy, instead of particles that contained energy, gave a new approach to science. There was the recognition of "emanations," which were not measurable, observable, or findable as physical objects. "The deeper we go, the higher we go." The deeper we go, as in meditation, the more we enter into the realm of waves of energy. This is Brahma, the exposition of the All, joining with Western scientific experimentation, to make the formerly unthinkable, provable.

Much of the new work of Jahn and Dunne, Puthoff, Radin, Nelson, and Popp is beautifully exposited by the scientific journalist Lynne McTaggart in her book *The Field* (2002). She gives evidence, and a feeling of palpable proof, of the emanations of mind energy, influencing and even creating the physical world. All this, again, is compatible with the basic formula that God creates, and energy descends through various vibrations of lower frequencies, winding up as physical manifestation, which in turn emanates its own energies of a rising form. All this is a condensed and congealed consciousness, or more correctly, a condensed and congealed *intelligence*.

In *Energy Psychology in Psychotherapy,* Fred Gallo states that "thought field is an invisible, non-physical structure in space that binds energetically encoded information in a cohesive structure" (2002, p. 5). He further states the following:

> The structure of thought fields (information fields) is similar to that of molecules and DNA, which are informational structures accepted by the established hard sciences. Psychological disorders have a structure, an implicate order, information. Alleviation of such conditions is achieved by disassembling that structure, collapsing or subsuming such information, disrupting or perturbing the order of the disorder, so that a new healthy order may be installed causing the disorder to reach entropy (Gallo, 2002, p. xxvii).

In my interpretation, this means that dissolving the obstruction of flow allows not only harmony but also availability of new experience; for example, to change a posttraumatic stress disorder–embedded trauma into a review of and a new way of looking at the trauma.

HEALING

The Great Verbal Approaches

How real is real? How real is the world of the "word" and the world of the "subtle energies"?

A reference to Shakespeare by the great and recent philosopher Sri Aurobindo speaks with poetic beauty and great clarity of the power of the world of the subtle energies, within themselves, as well as in our day-to-day lives, as follows:

> Of the latter kind (i.e. imagination persisting in the material world, my interpretation) in a certain country one named Shakespeare created a new world by

the force of his Avidya his faulty of imagining what is not. That world is as real and unreal today as it was when Shakespeare created it. . . . Within the limits of that world, Iago is real to Othello, Othello to Desdemona, and all are real to any and every consciousness which can for a time abstract itself from this world. We are aware of them, observe them, grow in knowledge about them, see them act, hear them speak, feel for their griefs and sorrows; and even when we return to our own world, they do not always leave us, but sometimes come with us and influence our actions (Sri Aurobindo, 1995).

In 1895, in his attempts to establish the basis for his work, and a powerful new paradigm in the world of psychiatry, Freud spoke passionately about the power of the word. I referred to this as follows:

Mind energetics is distinguished from "Energy Psychology" (Gallo, 2002) for we view Energy Psychology as a form of therapy that applies its activity to the physical body. In contrast, Mind energetics deals with the flow of energy that occurs in the course of those transactions that are primarily mind-to-mind, with special emphasis on the verbal and empathic communications. It takes a special interest in dreams and their meaning, and in the manner in which these dream energies are active in life.

We have made great advances measuring the subtle energies emanating from the body, received by the body and transmitted through the body as information, impulse, will and desire. But the ultimate in energy psychology is the study of Consciousness.

Others have pursued the energies of the acupuncture meridia, the healing energies of the Reiki hands, the synchronous electro-encephalograms or electro-magnetograms of the pair of healer-healee as they are in mutual transmission-reception. But all of these will be looked upon as enfolded in a higher discovery when we know more about the healing energies of love, of empathy, of caring intention (Pressman, 2004).

Freud's prescience, as well as his early clinical experience, is well borne out by the emanations that are now studied by the advanced form of electro-encephalography (EEG), *neurofeedback,* as well as the work of such scientists as Puthoff, Oschman, Radin, Jahn and Dunne, Roger Sherman, James Austin (1998), and Arnold Mindell (2000).

I refer again to Tiller's description of the spectrum of energies that exist throughout creation because it is so powerfully enlightening and useful. Energies continue from the lowest frequency to the highest, with the mind point, the fulcrum, being the speed of light. Again, everything on the left side travels at speeds slower than that of light and is part of the three-dimensional world. Everything on the right side, and greater than the speed of light, is in the subtle realm (and the subtle realm is the thinking and "above-thinking" realm). The subtle energies that reside in this domain are those that cannot be seen, touched, or tasted, but that can be discovered by virtue of their effects, much like electricity. The world of the subtle realm is the inverse of the world of the material domain and probably obeys different laws: Time and space do not exist. There are dimensions upon dimensions, parallel universes of astronomy and quantum physics and mind. We see this clinically when we operate on multiple levels at once. Even the familiar experience of giving a well-remembered speech and having your mind drift to the effect on the audience, or perhaps other things as the speech continues, is a simple manifestation of living on multiple planes at once. Let us remember, too, the patient with multiple personalities. Although only one is manifest at a time, the many personalities are present and ready to come forth. They live, multiply and simultaneously (Pressman, personal communication). Other people are able to perform two tasks at once; my wife is able to read a book and listen to a television program at the same time, absorbing both.

Mind-to-mind energies as they are expressed in verbal communication, in ESP, in empathy and intuition, and through mind to body healing are emanations of a higher order, carried by higher frequencies of vibration than the meridian-based energies. Tiller (1997) has pointed out that "deltron" energies exist at the point of transition from material to subtle and are mediated by emotions. This fits clinically because the power of the word is carried by emotion, and life is lived by emotion; interpretation without emotion is meaningless in terms of realization. As one of my respected teachers said, "Emotions flow through the body like blood through the arteries, always during life."

The following exchange with Jim Oschman raised the question of how we could study the power of love, empathy, anger, and even hatred in mind-to-mind transmissions:

Speaking of the healing effect of Reiki, Oschman described a sweeping series of vibratory frequencies that coordinate specifically with those of the various organs of the body. This knowledge lets us know that Reiki supplies the particular vibratory energy that would be healing to the specific organ, according to its unique vibration signature. I told him of my interest in Mind Energetics and the psychotherapeutic transactions that occur during verbal psychotherapy. I wished that there could be a similar study of *thought* energies, love (caring) energies, good-intention energies, spiritual energies as they relate to therapeutic relationships. I reminded him that Bill Tiller had pointed us to the continuum of energies that exist along the electromagnetic spectrum and the ascendancy of those vibrations from emotion to mind to spirit. Accordingly, thought energies and good-intention energies and love energies might be of a higher order, comprising a higher spectrum of vibrations than those of the magnetic range projected from the healing hand. In truth though, I wondered: "Can word energies, love-energies, patient-therapist coherence be studied? Can these things be measured?" This area seems to be neglected in our "subtle energy" investigations. What is the evidence that these energies might be of a higher order? If they are, what is their nature? How can we study them?

Oschman replied as follows:

As you can imagine, I have been giving thought to these questions. I now make a distinction between two kinds of healing. Some therapies focus on one of them, other therapies focus on the other, and some involve both. One kind of healing involves low frequencies, in the ELF range. These are frequencies that are emitted from the hands of the healer who is connected to the earth's rhythms (Schulman resonance), which are constantly changing, sweeping up and down through the biological range, stimulating the activities of various cells (such as skin, capillary, nerve, ligament, bone). By stimulating these cells to be active, the tissue healing process is "jump started." In essence, the body's ordinary tissue repair processes are activated. It takes time for the healing to take place, as cells must migrate to the place that has been injured, and they have to do some work of clearing out debris and building new structures. Once begun, the repair process can take days or weeks to be completed, depending on the extent of the tissue damage. As always, intention is a part of the healing process, and the therapist who has a clear image of what is happening can greatly facilitate the process. There are good ways of studying this energy transfer, by showing the coherence between

two people's heart and brain rhythms. Heart rate variability is a valuable measure for this kind of study. There are also heart tuners that enable two people to maximize their heart to heart coherence.

There is another kind of healing that relies on much higher frequencies and is much faster. This kind of healing involves connecting with the formative process, the process by which the body is created again and again, possibly thousands or millions of times each second. In this kind of healing, living structure is actually replaced in an instant. It is replacement, not repair. The most dramatic evidence that this can happen comes from study of multiple personality disorders in which the organism shifts virtually instantaneously from one form to another. An individual can have several or even many different personalities with different characteristics.

These high frequencies are difficult to study, but it is not impossible. They are the so-called spiritual frequencies; they are well described in the Buddhist literature, for example. This is the real source of our energy, our power, our ability to create the world around us, including other people who populate that world. You said, "An envelope surrounds us, and there is transmission through an environment of peace." This is a good description of a special state that occurs from time to time in a variety of therapies, a state in which anything can happen. I am very interested in exploring this state and the process that can lead to it. It is a key teaching in the Dzong-Chen tradition, for example (Oschman, personal communication).

Deep Relationship

Humans can join in deep relationships, such as deep moments of love between people. I believe this is paralleled in deep moments of psychotherapy, when the patient and therapist are surrounded by an envelope of silence, and there is a "surround," a bubble of energy and a transmission energies from one to the other. Through this tube of communication is passed thought and experience, from one to the other, which can then be raised to the level of cognition and spoken word. This is the achievement not only of a special human relationship, but also of a rising of each individual from the level of body, from the level of primitive emotion, from the level of ordinary thinking to the higher plane wherein dwells the causal body, or "soul" (Pressman, 2001c). When we arrive at that level, we are in the zone of peace, and we partake of larger energies that surround us, not only in the biofield, but also in the cosmic field, which has been alluded to by Carl Gustav Jung in his description of archetypes and the collective mind (Jaffé, editor, 1963). This has also been described by the great poet-scientist Johann Goethe, who entered (mentally) the "being" of the plant (Pressman, 2000). In so doing, he was able to mix his energy-consciousness with the energy-consciousness of the plant and make a great discovery. From this he derived what he called the "archplant" (an archetype), which is a "stencil of potential" that exists in the subtle realm, and which is filled in by the form of the plant: from seed to stem to leaf to blossom to seed again. This form is the *holding energy,* which allows the plant of its species to repeat the cycle. There is a similarity to what I have called an "archform," which gives shape to each of us, as well as our behavior (Pressman, unpublished). It gives shape to our organs and our body configuration. It holds the configuration for our own potential, an ever-widening form of creation. This idea has been further made visible by the premier work of Rupert Sheldrake (1994), who has described "morphogenic fields," fields that give shape to objects: insects, animals, humans, and even behavior as they occur in manifestation.

Thus the powerful energies of the subtle realm allude to and embrace the mental energies, the mind-to-mind energies.

Clinical Manifestations of Mind-to-Mind Energies

Meditation and Hypnosis

I believe that meditation is simple in its basic principles: attention is that which gives life to whatever is observed. It vivifies. As we attend the physical body, we make it more aware in the realm of mind and even in existence. If we remove attention from the body, however, as we do in meditation, it functionally disappears. The same is true of the emotions as we let them quiet down. The same is true again as we let intruding thoughts drift away. The result is that we arrive at a zone of peace, and we are at that point in the "causal body." This is the body of formation, the body that exists between lifetimes, the body that creates from itself emanations that result in the mental

body (the thought body), the astral body (the emotional body) and the physical body.

Meditation, allowing us to arrive at the causal level, also allows us to recreate the flesh and form. It is well known that we recreate body cells every 7 years, but I believe things go beyond this phenomenon. The causal body, by virtue of relationships, desires, lifestyle, and *visualization,* can create and recreate new substance. This is the source of healing, mind to body, through visualization, as described by Simonton (1978). Simonton was pioneer in using visualization to treat cancer, often with surprising results. As mentioned, in 1972 I initiated the use of hypnosis and visualization in training Olympic athletes (ice skaters), helping to create a more nearly perfect performance, with astounding results.

Heart Energy

Joseph Chilton Pearce, a pioneer author and lecturer in the new field of subtle energies, states that the heart is the "fifth brain" in *The Biology of Transcendence* (Pearce, 2002). The heart contains neurons and neurological tissue and communicates with the brain. It is a watershed way station. Its energies can be united with the neocortex to create acts of extraordinary love and benevolence, or it can join with the primitive brain to bring about deeds of primitive evil.

Paul Pearsall's work is also significant in this respect. He has gathered clinical information that indicates more than the physical organ is transplanted during a heart transplant. Additional vibrations that contain the personality of the donor are also given to the recipient, influencing the recipient's disposition in life (Pearsall, 1998). In line with all this is the discovery that the heart is the most powerful source of magnetic energy in the body.

Visualization

Elmer Green, who established the Voluntary Controls department at the Menninger Clinic, told me that visualization can create anything in the body. The work of Simonton and others, as well as my work with Olympic skaters, which has now become popular as visualization training for performance, supports the idea. Visualization must be carried out in a state of quiet mind—and thus the opportunity to reach the causal body. For the most part, this requires time, but there are remarkable instances where visualization under hypnosis has had the immediate effect of having warts drop off, or blisters raised. One of Green's subjects, Jack Schwartz, was famous for being able to pierce himself with a long needle and stop the bleeding with his mental energy. All this is a tribute to the power of visualization. This state of mind is certainly sought and achieved in the advanced martial arts.

CONCLUSION

Energy healing depends on the "alchemy of personality." We evolve from birth to physical death through a rising series of elevations of consciousness, from the material to the abstract and on to the aesthetic and altruistic. It is possible that the Creator is "Love, Light, Consciousness," and that we are condensed energy—congealed consciousness that then rises to higher and higher levels. Thus, love, light, and consciousness may be the secret of our immortality as a personal consciousness, and the energies we acquire through learning may be transmitted to yet another chapter in another lifetime. This may be the hope of society; the more we advance, the more we take pleasure from the helping side of things.

The idea is to relieve the encumbrances of personality that hold back flow and the natural evolution upward. The buoyancy of the soul (the higher part of the personality) is evident in many ways, including meeting tragedy, the natural desire to help in group therapy and the evolution of a greater consideration for others as we mature, with the subsequent transcendence to a higher order of things. We are evolving into the next race of men and women.

Thus we have a "wholistic" and "holographic" picture of the approaches of energetic healing, each performing on many levels, within many universes, acting concurrently, within us and around us, changing obstruction into flow and discordance into harmony.

This is a model for healing, but not only of the individual, but of the collective "whole" called humanity.

References

Arcane School: *http://www.lucistrust.org/arcane/*.

Austin JH: *Zen and the brain: toward an understanding of meditation and consciousness,* Cambridge, Mass, 1998, MIT Press.

Chang JJ, Fisch J, Popp FA, editors: *Biophotons,* Dordrecht, Boston, 1998, Kluwer.

Carroll L: *Alice in wonderland,* Morris Plains, NJ, 1990, Unicorn.

Charcot JM: *Charcot, the clinician: the Tuesday lessons.* Excerpts from nine case presentations on general neurology delivered at the Salpêtrière Hospital in 1887-88 by Jean-Martin Charcot (translated with commentary by CG Goetz).

Cranston SL: *HPB: the extraordinary life and influence of Helena Blavatsky, founder of the modern Theosophical movement,* New York, 1993, Putnam.

Freud S: *The interpretation of dreams,* New York, 1933, Macmillan.

Freud S: *The standard edition of the complete psychological works of Sigmund Freud,* London, 1953-1974, Hogarth Press (Translated from the German under general editorship of J Strachey, in collaboration with A Freud, assisted by A Strachey and A Tyson).

Gallo FP, editor: *Energy psychology in psychotherapy: a comprehensive sourcebook,* New York, 2002, Norton.

Green E, Green A: *Beyond biofeedback,* New York, 1977, Delacorte Press/S Lawrence.

Greenacre P: *Trauma, growth, and personality,* New York, 1969 (1952), International Universities Press.

Greene B: *The elegant universe,* New York, 2003, Vintage Books.

Grof S: *Realms of the human unconscious: observations from LSD research,* New York, 1975, Viking.

Heisenberg W: In Price WC, Chissick SC, editors: *The uncertainty principle and foundations of quantum mechanics: a fifty years' survey,* New York, 1977, Wiley.

Jahn RG, Dunne BJ: *Margins of reality : the role of consciousness in the physical world,* San Diego, 1987, Harcourt Brace Jovanovich.

Janet P: *The major symptoms of hysteria: fifteen lectures given in the medical school of Harvard University,* ed 2, New York, 1965 (1920, 1929), Hafner.

Jung CG: *Memories, dreams, reflections,* New York, 1963, Pantheon Books (Recorded and edited by A Jaffé; translated from the German by R and C Winston).

Kaku M: *Hyperspace,* New York, 1994, Anchor Books.

Krishnamurti J: *Meditations,* Beckenham (Kent), 1969, Krishnamurti Foundation.

Lilly JC: *The center of the cyclone: an autobiography of inner space,* New York; 1972, Julian Press.

McTaggart L: *The field: the quest for the secret force of the universe,* New York, 2002, HarperCollins.

Mesmer FA: *Mesmerism: a translation of the original scientific and medical writings of F.A. Mesmer,* Los Altos, Calif, 1980, Kaufman (Translated and compiled by G Bloch; introduction by ER Hilgard).

Mindell A: *Quantum mind: the edge between physics and psychology,* Portland, Ore, 2000, Lao Tse Press.

Moody RA Jr: *The light beyond,* New York, 1988, Bantam Books (with P Perry; foreword by A Greeley).

Muktananda S: *Play of consciousness: a spiritual autobiography.*

Muktananda S: *Chitshakti vilas,* ed 4, South Fallsburg, NY, 1994, ed 4, SYDA Foundation (introduction by S Chidvilasananda).

Muller FM, editor: *Râmakrishna: his life and sayings,* New York, 1975, AMS Press.

Nelson RD et al: Field REG anomalies in group situations, *J Sci Explor* 10(1):111, 1996.

Oschman JL: Personal communication.

Oschman JL: *Energy medicine: the scientific basis,* New York, 2000, Churchill Livingstone.

Pearce JC: *The biology of transcendence: a blueprint of the human spirit,* Rochester, Vt, 2002, Park Street Press.

Pearsall P: *The heart's code: tapping the wisdom and power of our heart energy,* New York, 1998, Broadway Books.

Pressman MD: Mind over figures, *Skating Magazine,* 1978.

Pressman MD: Psychological techniques for the advancement of sports potential. In Klavora P, Daniel J, editors: *Coach, athlete and the sport psychologist,* Toronto, 1979, University of Toronto.

Pressman MD: Psychological techniques for the advancement of sport potential. In Suinn RW, editor: *Psychology in sports: methods of applications,* Minneapolis, 1980, Burgess Publishing.

Pressman MD: Exploring the invisible realm, *Monthly Aspectarian,* Chicago, September 2000, Lightworks Publications.

Pressman MD: The mind mirror-the zone of creativity, *Monthly Aspectarian,* Morton Grove, Ill, April 2004.

Pressman MD: Our two nervous systems and God's wholistic plan, *Monthly Aspectarian,* Morton Grove, Ill, December, 2001.

Pressman MD: *Visions from the soul: bridging personality to spirit,* Scottsdale, Ariz, 2001, Inkwell Productions.

Pressman MD: Mind energetics: evolution and arrival, *Semin Integr Med* 36-47, 2004.

Pressman MD: Living in the "supermind" (Unpublished manuscript).

Pressman TE: Personal communication.

Radin DI: *The conscious universe: the scientific truth of psychic phenomena,* New York, 1997, HarperEdge.

Rank O: *In quest of the hero,* Princeton, NJ, 1990, Princeton University Press.

Sheldrake R: *The rebirth of nature,* Rochester, Vt, 1994, Park Street Press.

Silberer H: *Hidden symbolism of alchemy and the occult arts,* New York, 1971, Dover (Translated by SE Jelliffe).

Simonton OC, Matthews-Simonton S, Creighton J: *Getting well again: a step-by-step, self-help guide to overcoming cancer for patients and their families,* Los Angeles, 1978, Tarcher (New York, St Martin's Press).

Sri Aurobindo on himself, Pondicherry, 1972, Sri Aurobindo Ashram Trust.

Sri Aurobindo: *The Upanishads,* Pondicherry, 1995, All India Press, pp 36-37.

Steiner R: *Goethean science,* Spring Valley, NY, 1988, Mercury Press.

Steiner R: *How to know higher worlds,* Hudson, NY, 1994, Anthroposophic Press.

Strachey J, editor/translator: *Studies on hysteria: Josef Breuer and Sigmund Freud,* 1953-1974 (In collaboration with A Freud; assisted by James Strachey and Alex Tyson,1957).

Tiller WA: *Science and human transformation: subtle energies, intentionality, and consciousness,* Walnut Creek, Calif, 1997, Pavior.

Tiller WA, Dibble WE Jr, Kohane MJ: *Conscious acts of creation: the emergence of a new physics,* Walnut Creek, Calif, 2001, Pavior.

Watts A: *Beat Zen, square Zen, and Zen,* San Francisco, 1959, City Lights Books.

Wilber K: *A brief history of everything,* Boston, 1996, Shamballa.

Wilber K: As quoted by Joel Metazger on ONN, *Joel@wisdomtalk,* 1999.

Yogananda: *Self-realization,* Los Angeles, Calif, 1971, Fellowship.

BIOPHYSICAL DEVICES AND MODALITIES

MARC S. MICOZZI

There is a biophysical aspect to many healing modalities that have long been observed clinically. Contemporary fundamental physics is now in the process of providing explanatory models, mechanisms, and paradigm for the biophysical basis for many healing phenomena. These biophysical characteristics extend beyond the currently established basis of biomedical science in reductionist biochemical, molecular biological, and anatomical terms. Further, biophysics is consistent with many biomedical observations in whole-organism biology, physiology, and homeostasis.

Contemporary biophysics is important for understanding the basis of many contemporary diagnostic and therapeutic approaches. Biophysics, rather than biochemistry or molecular biology, may better pro-vide explanatory mechanisms for the observed effectiveness of such clinical practices as acupuncture, homeopathy, touch, and meditation (Duer, 1998).

For example, nonthermal, nonionizing electromagnetic fields in low frequencies have been observed to have the following effects on the physical body: stimulation of bone repair, nerve stimulation, soft tissue wound healing, treatment of osteoarthritis, tissue regeneration, immune system stimulation, and neuroendocrine modulation (National Institutes of Health, 1993).

Contemporary biophysically based modalities include electrodermal screening, applied kinesiology, bioresonance, and radionics. Utilization of these approaches involves the availability of devices and practitioners.

HISTORY AND BACKGROUND

Many well-established historical healing traditions have drawn on diagnostic and therapeutic approaches that may now be interpreted in light of contemporary biophysics. The ancient and complex healing traditions of China and India make reference to and utilize practices based primarily on biophysical modalities. Acupuncture, acupressure, Jin Shin Do, t'ai chi, reiki, qi gong, tui na, and yoga may be seen today to operate on a biophysical basis, but these have developed over three millennia in widespread clinical practice and observation. Contemporary outcomes-based clinical trials are demonstrating the efficacy of these modalities in many medical conditions (Wootton and Sparber, 2003). In addition, Asian medical systems have used sound, light, and color for their healing properties, which may be seen in biophysical perspective (Chapter 2).

U.S. Schools of Thought and Practice

Biophysical medical modalities have also been prominent in the history of American medicine. Several schools of thought were created in the United States, or brought from Europe, that center around healing approaches which we may now associate in whole or in part with emerging biophysical explanations. Such schools and their founders have often influenced each other through time (Box 18-1)

In addition, interpretations of herbal, nutritional, and even pharmacological therapies have been extended to include "vibrational energy" as a mechanism of action.

There have been many adherents, practitioners, and clinical observations over time of these schools of thought and practice. They have been outside the realm of regular medical practice partially because the mechanisms of action of these approaches have not been explained within the biomedical paradigm. Hypnosis is an example of an effective therapeutic modality with widespread effectiveness and acceptance within medicine (Temes, 1998). However, there remains no explanation for its mechanism of action. An alternative approach to explaining hypnosis has been developed on a statistical basis, describing the profile of clients

---

BOX 18-1

Chronological Order of Schools and Founders with Influence on Development of Biophysical Devices

- Homeopathy (Samuel Hahnemann, Germany, 1830-1860)
- Faith Healing (Phineas Quimby, 1830-1860)
- Christian Science (Mary Baker Eddy, 1861-1880)
- Theosophy (Blavatksy/Olcott, 1861-1880)
- Movement Therapy (Matthias Alexander, 1861-1880)
- Iridology (Liljequist, von Peczely, 1861-1900)
- Zone Therapy–Reflexology (William Fitzgerald, 1901-1920)
- Anthroposophical Medicine (Rudolph Steiner, 1901-1920)
- Polarity Therapy (Randolph Stone, 1921-1940)
- Bach Flower Remedies (Edward Bach, 1921-1940)
- Electro-Magnetism (Semyon and Valentine Kirlian, 1921-1940)
- Movement Therapy (Moshe Feldenkreis, 1941-1960)
- Shiatsu (Tokujiro Namikoshi, 1941-1960)
- Jin Shin Jitsu (Jiro Murai, 1941-1960)
- Orgone Therapy (Wilhelm Reich, 1941-1960)
- Structural Integration (Ida Rolf, 1960-1980)

---

and conditions likely to benefit and developing "hypnotic susceptibility scales." This same approach is available for the clinical study of any therapeutic modality with observable outcomes in the absence of a "mechanism of action." Mechanism is always bounded by the prevailing scientific paradigm and may not be the most clinically useful question (Chapter 5). With the development of new scientific observations, a new paradigm emerges that is more inclusive in its explanation of observed phenomena.

Individual Practitioners

In addition to the fairly widespread, organized schools of thought and practice, there are many intuitive healers whose practices are highly individuated and highly eclectic. These practitioners represent important approaches used by many clients. The knowledge and practices represented by such gifted healers must be passed on or will be lost. This represents a situation in the contemporary United States that is analogous to concerns about herbal remedies in the rain forest. Environmentalists are rightly concerned about the loss to biodiversity of unique plants; ethnobotanists are concerned about the loss of the peoples whose cultural knowledge only can convert the rain forest plants to cures.

Empirical Assumptions of Biophysically Based Modalities

1. The human body has a biophysical component.
2. What has been scientifically defined as the "mind" is biophysically linked to the human body.
3. Every part of the human body is biophysically linked to every other part of the body.
4. Mental states (thoughts, emotions) generate physiological responses in the human body through neurological, hormonal, and immunological mechanisms (pyschoneuroimmunology).
5. Biophysically based modalities are noninvasive by currently measurable and clinically observable criteria.

NONINVASIVE BIOPHYSICAL DEVICES FOR DIAGNOSIS AND TREATMENT

Practitioners using biophysical modalities employ a number of noninvasive devices (i.e., devices that do not penetrate the skin) to measure electrical charges and magnetic fields of particular low frequencies. Such devices are also believed to promote healing by interacting with the body.

Biophysical properties of the body have long been observed and utilized in healing. For example, these properties have been known as *chi* in traditional Chinese medicine, *prana* in Ayurvedic medicine, and *vital force* in homeopathy. Acupuncturists, homeopathic doctors, chiropractors, and practitioners of biophysical medicine and magnetic field therapy (including medical doctors) are among the practitioners who use noninvasive devices to detect and influence biophysical properties of the body.

While conventional medicine recognizes the presence of electrical charges and magnetic forces in the body, certain biophysical properties, also referenced as "subtle energy," have not generally been studied or utilized by Western science and medicine.

Unlike other medical devices regulated by the U.S. Food and Drug Administration (FDA), many of the noninvasive devices used to detect and influence these biophysical properties fall into a gray area from a regulatory standpoint. In 1976 the FDA set standards for the regulation of acupuncture needles as an experimental device, and the needle was reclassified as a therapeutic device in 1996 partially based on clinical evidence published in a series of articles in the new *Journal of Alternative and Complementary Medicine: Research on Paradigm, Practice and Policy*, during 1995. The FDA team working on reclassification specifically requested the editor of the journal at that time (the editor of this textbook) to provide lists of references in order to accelerate the review process. That FDA action occurred prior to the NIH Consensus Conference on Acupuncture in 1997. However, FDA did not adopt standards for electroacupuncture devices, a major category of biophysical devices. One of the challenges continues to be the inability of Western science to measure these biophysical properties. As a result, such devices, when cleared by the FDA, are generally approved for use for "investigational" purposes, as in research studies, but not in the diagnosis or treatment of illness.

The following sections list proposed categories of devices: (1) electrical and magnetic devices used in conventional medicine for conventional purposes, (2) conventional devices used in innovative applications, (3) conventional devices used for both innovative and conventional applications, and (4) unconventional devices.

Electrical and Magnetic Devices Used in Conventional Medicine

Devices that measure the electrical and magnetic properties of the physical body have been used in conventional medicine for many years. These electrical devices include the ECG, EEG, and EMG, used to measure heart, brain, and muscle activity, respectively, for diagnostic purposes. The electrocardiogram (ECG, EKG) reads the electrical rhythms of the heart, the electroencephalogram (EEG) records electrical brain waves, and the electromyogram (EMG) measures electrical properties of the muscles, which may be correlated to muscle performance. The EMG is often used in physical (rehabilitative) medicine to diagnose conditions that cause pain, weakness, and numbness.

In addition to the use of devices that measure electrical charges, conventional medicine has made increasing use of magnetic resonance imaging (MRI) for diagnostic purposes. MRI measures the magnetic fields of the body to create images for the diagnosis of physical abnormalities. Another device, the superconducting quantum interference device (SQUID), combines magnetic flux quantization and Josephson tunneling to measure magnetic heart signals complementary to ECG signals.

Conventional Medical Devices for Innovative Applications

Some of the devices just described have also been used in innovative ways (not as originally intended) for treatment purposes, such as the use of the ECG and EEG in biofeedback to monitor subconscious processes and "feed back" this information to support behavioral change. The ECG is also the basis of Flexyx neurotherapy, an innovative approach to modulate central perception and processing of afferent signals from the physical receptors in the body (pressure, pain, heat, cold).

MRI, used to diagnose a variety of medical abnormalities, is also being used in a number of innovative ways, as in neuroscience to show brain activity during different tasks, such as reading or language, and procedures during acupuncture. At the National Institutes of Health (NIH), basic science researchers are currently investigating innovative uses of MRI to measure physiological changes, such as eye movement or brain activity.

Conventional Devices Used for Treatment in Both Conventional and Biophysical Medicine

Some devices that utilize electrical charges and magnetic fields are being used by both conventional and biophysical medical practitioners.

Superconducting quantum interference device. In addition to its use in conventional medicine, SQUID has also been used to measure weak magnetic fields of the brain. In other studies, it has been used to measure large, frequency-pulsing biomagnetic fields that emanate from certain practitioners, such as polarity therapists. This biomagnetic field is thought to trigger biological processes at the cellular and molecular levels, helping the body repair itself.

Transcutaneous electrical nerve stimulation unit. Developed by Dr. C. Norman Shealy, the transcutaneous electrical nerve stimulation (TENS) unit is used by both conventional medicine and biophysical practitioners for pain relief. The FDA approved the TENS unit as a device for pain management in the 1970s. The electronic unit sends pulsed currents to electrodes attached to the skin, displacing pain signals from the affected nerves and preventing the pain message from reaching the brain.

TENS has been suggested to stimulate the production of endorphins as one proposed mechanism of action. In 1990, TENS was the subject of a study in the *New England Journal of Medicine*. Although it was found ineffective in this study, other studies have found TENS helpful for mild to moderate pain. TENS may have better results with skin and connective tissue pain than with muscle or bone pain.

Electro-Acuscope. Using a lower electrical current than the TENS unit, the Electro-Acuscope device reduces pain by stimulating tissue rather than by stimulating the nerves or causing muscle contractions. It is thought to relieve pain by running currents through damaged tissues. Medical doctors, chiropractors, and physical therapists use the Electro-Acuscope for treatment of muscle spasms, migraines, jaw pain, bursitis, arthritis, surgical incisions, sprains and strains, neuralgia, shingles, and bruises. As with the TENS unit, the Electro-Acuscope has been approved by the FDA as a device for pain management.

Diapulse. The Diapulse device emits radio waves that produce short, intense electromagnetic pulses that penetrate the tissue. It is said to improve blood flow, reduce pain, and promote healing. The Diapulse is used in a variety of health care settings, especially in the treatment of postoperative swelling and pain.

Unconventional Devices Used in Biophysical Medicine

The following devices are some of the more popular devices used in biophysical medicine. The FDA has not set standards for these devices, but some may be registered with the FDA as "biofeedback" devices.

Electroacupuncture Devices

Dermatron. Voll, a German physician, introduced the Dermatron in the 1940s. Voll believed that acupuncture points have electrical conductivity, and he used this device to measure electrical changes in the body. This technique became known as "electroacupuncture according to Voll" (EAV) and is currently known as *electroacupuncture biofeedback*. Used for diagnosis, the Dermatron became the basis for a number of devices manufactured in Germany, France, Russia, Japan, Korea, the United Kingdom, and the United States.

Vega. Another modified electroacupuncture device similar to the Voll device, the Vega works much faster and is also used for diagnosis. Based on the belief that the first sign of abnormality in the body is a change in electrical charge, this device records the change in skin conductivity after the application of a small voltage. Computers have been added to recent models under different names, such as the Computron.

Mora. Franz Morel, MD, a colleague of Voll, developed the Mora, another variation of the Voll device. Morel believed that electromagnetic signals could be described by a complex waveform. The Mora reads "wave" information from the body. Proponents believe that the Mora can relieve headaches, migraines, muscular aches and pains, circulation disorders, and skin disease.

Other devices. Modern variations of Voll's electroacupuncture devices include the Accupath 1000, Biotron, Computron, DiagnoMetre, Eclosion, Elast, Interro, LISTEN System, Omega AcuBase, Omega Vision, Prophyle, and Punctos III.

Devices Using Light and Sound Energy

Cymatic instruments. In addition to the electroacupuncture biofeedback treatment and other devices that measure electrical charges described above, there are also therapeutic *cymatic* devices, in which a sound transducer replaces the electrodes of the EAV devices. Each organ and tissue in the body emits sound at a particular harmonic frequency. The cymatic device recognizes and records the emitted sound patterns associated with each body part and bathes the affected area with sound to balance the disturbance. These devices are used for diagnosis and treatment.

Sound probe. This device emits a pulsed tone of three alternating frequencies. The sound probe is thought to destroy bacteria, viruses, and fungi that are not in resonance with the body.

Light beam generator. This device is thought to work by emitting photons of light that help restore a normal energy state at the cellular level, allowing the body to heal. The light beam generator is believed to promote healing throughout the body and help correct such problems as depression, insomnia, headaches, and menstrual disorders.

Infratronic QGM. This device uses electroacoustical technology to direct massage-like waves into the body. The Infratonic QGM is used as an effective pain management tool in China, Japan, Taiwan, Singapore, France, Spain, Mexico, and Argentina. The FDA has approved this device for therapeutic massage in the United States.

Teslar watch. Named after the researcher Nikola Tesla, the Teslar watch was developed to modulate the harmful effects of "electronic" pollution from modern sources, such as computers, cell phones, televisions, hair dryers, and electrical blankets. It is believed that these products create magnetic energy that may destabilize the body's electromagnetic field. Although this energy is created from extremely low frequencies (ELFs), which range from 1 to 100 hertz, it is believed to affect humans adversely over time.

Kirlian camera. This device records and measures high-frequency, high-voltage electrons using the *gas visualization discharge* (GVD) technique, also called the "corona discharge." The most experienced researchers in this technique are Russian; Seymon and Valentina Kirlian pioneered this research in the 1970s. Other contributors include Nikola Tesla in the United States, J.J. Narkiewich-Jodko in Russia, and Pratt and Schlemmer in Prague. In 1995, Korotkov and his team in St. Petersburg developed a new Kirlian camera using a Crown TV.

References

Duer H: (Interview with Hans Duer in *Meridians* (Summer 1998), publication of the Traditional Acupuncture Institute, Columbia, MD. Dr Duer is professor emeritus and former director of the Max Planck Institute and former chair of the Werner Heisenberg Institute of Physics in Munich.)

National Institutes of Health: *Alternative therapies: expanding medical horizons*, Bethesda MD, 1993.

Temes R (ed.): *Medical hypnosis: an introduction and clinical guide*, New York and London: Churchill Livingstone, 1998.

Wootton JC, Sparber, A: Surveys of complementary and alternative medicine usage: A review of general population trends and specific patient populations. *Semin Intgr Med* 1:10-24, 2003.

Resources

Professional Organizations

BioElectroMagnetics Institute
John Zimmerman, PhD, President
2490 W Moana Lane
Reno, NV 89509-7801
Phone: 702-827-9099

John E. Fetzer Institute
9292 West KL Ave
Kalamazoo, MI 49009
Phone: 616-375-2000
Fax: 616-372-2163
Website: *www.fetzer.org*

Institute of Noetic Sciences
Attention: Marilyn Schlitz, PhD
PO Box 909
Sausalito, CA 94966
Phone: 415-331-5650
Fax: 415-331-5673

International Society for the Study of Subtle Energies and Energy Medicine (ISSSEEM)
11005 Ralston Road, #100 D
Arvada, CO 80004
Phone: 303-425-4625
e-mail: *issseem@compuserve.com*

Books

Becker RO: *Cross currents: the perils of electropollution, the promise of electromedicine,* Los Angeles, 1990, Tarcher, Perigee.
Becker RO, Selden G: *The body electric: electromagnetism and the foundation of life,* New York, 1985, Quill, Morrow.
Blank M, editor: *Electromagnetic fields: biological interactions and mechanisms,* Washington, DC, 1995, American Chemical Society (includes two chapters of particular interest on health effects of bioelectromagnetic fields).
Gerber R: *Vibrational medicine: new choices for healing ourselves,* Santa Fe, NM, 1988, Bear.
Oschman JL: *Energy medicine: the scientific basis of bioenergy therapies,* New York, 2000, Churchill Livingstone.
Schlitz M, Amorok T, Micozzi M: *Consciousness and healing: integral approaches to mind-body medicine,* St Louis, 2005, Elsevier, Churchill Livingstone.

Journal Articles

Galantino ML, Eke-Okoro ST, Findley TW, Condoluci D: Use of noninvasive electroacupuncture for the treatment of HIV-related peripheral neuropathy, *J Altern Complementary Med* 5, April 1999.
Lytle CD, Thomas BM, Gordon EA, Krauthamer V: Electrostimulators for acupuncture: safety issues, *J Altern Complementary Med* 6, February 2000.
Naeser MA: Carpal tunnel syndrome: clinical outcome after low-level laser acupuncture, microamps transcutaneous electrical nerve stimulation, and other alternative therapies, *J Altern Complementary Med* 5, February 1999.
Patterson MA, Patterson L, Patterson SI: Electrostimulation: addiction treatment for the coming millennium, *J Altern Complementary Med* 2, Winter 1996.
Richards TL, Lappin MS, Acosta-Urquid J, et al: Double-blind study of pulsing magnetic field effects on multiple sclerosis, *J Altern Complementary Med* 3, Spring 1997.
Walleczek J: Bioelectromagnetics: the question of subtle energies, *Noetic Sci Rev* 28, Winter 1993.

Website

International Society for the Study of Subtle Energies and Energy Medicine (ISSSEEM) *www.ISSSEEM.org*

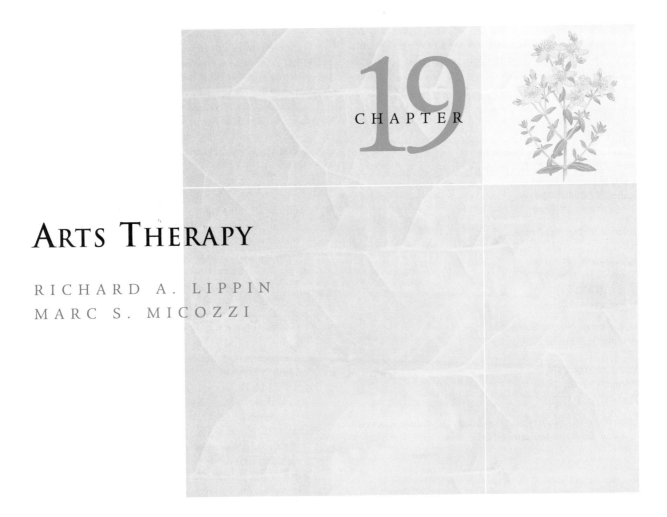

CHAPTER 19

ARTS THERAPY

RICHARD A. LIPPIN
MARC S. MICOZZI

The capacity for the arts to enhance health has been known since antiquity. We are currently experiencing a resurgence of interest in this topic based on several megatrends in medicine. Among these megatrends are a shift from reductionism to holism and a shift from paternalism to consumerism. Other fundamental factors contributing to the serious study of the relation of the creative and the healing arts are major scientific advances in neuroscience and the concurrent growth of so-called mind-body medicine and the resurgence of interest in the application of physics, including energy concepts, to human health. Passive exposure to the arts alone, including music, dance, painting, sculpture, poetry, and drama, has proven health-giving properties, and interestingly, passive exposure to live or original arts can be differentiated from exposure to electronic or printed reproductions.

The central theme of this chapter, however, is the relationship of "expressive" or "active" creative arts therapies to human health and well-being, where patients actively engage in one or more of the creative arts. This creative process enhances or augments the life force through classic biophysiological responses such as movement, relaxation, and emotional catharsis, as well as through self-discovery and awareness; increased self-esteem, pleasure, hope, and optimism; and the achievement of transcendence, which enhances our spiritual selves. Perhaps most important, the creation of beauty itself is a profound and powerful source of health and well-being.

HISTORY

Contemporary physician Michael Samuels has stated that art, prayer, and healing all come from the same source. Other scholars have said that every child, every adult, and every culture gives form to its feelings and ideas through art. Even before objective language was used in science with conceptual thought, it is believed that early, preliterate humans naturally embodied feelings, attitudes, and thoughts in symbols. Thus, some believe that the metaphorical use of language preceded the literal and scientific. Many anthropologists who study prehistory have hypothesized that singing and dancing preceded the development of verbal interchange among humans. Eighteenth-century Italian philosopher Giambattista Vico has suggested that humans danced before they walked and that poetry came before prose. This is echoed by social theorist Jean-Jacques Rousseau, who believed that musical sounds accompanied or preceded speech as we know it.

The most basic roots of the impact of the arts on health may be traced to the dawn of *Homo sapiens* and humans' unique awareness of themselves. This existential jolt of separateness or aloneness and awareness of mortality has been a driver of artistic expression ever since. The early cave drawings in Southern France may have served many purposes for early humans. Through them, for example, humans communicated and thus connected with fellow humans, mastered and taught others about a vast and potentially hostile environment by rendering it in artistic form, recorded their accomplishments and existence, and simply enjoyed the pleasures of beautiful images, rhythmic sound, and elegant movement. All these behabiors represented individual and collective cultural survival mechanisms and were "health giving" in the broadest sense.

The ancient Greeks recognized the connection between healing and the arts by their building of aesculapia, or temples of medicine, constructed in places of natural beauty, where, among other interventions, arts played a prominent role in the healing process. According to Aristotle, Pythagoras began the daily practice of singing and playing as the means by which the soul achieved catharsis. Homer told of his hero Ulysses being treated for hemorrhage with both bandages and incantation. Anathaneum reported a cure for sciatica in which flutists were hired to play music in the Pythagorean mode for the affected area.

In other non-Western traditions, as early as the Han dynasty, Chinese scholars began to realize that music could affect the human body, not only psychologically but physiologically, and during the Tsin dynasty (265-420 BC), music was known and used as a means of cultivating pleasant personality and positive mood.

During the Renaissance, music as one art form pervaded medieval medical practice and theory. Music prescribed was not only for good digestion and for bodily preparation before surgery but also as a stimulus to wound healing, a mood changer, and a critical accompaniment to bloodletting. Specifically composed medical music (the shivaree) graced the wedding chamber to ensure erotic coupling at the astrologically auspicious moment.

In the modern era, although highly creative individuals in the arts and health continue to make individual contributions, the roots of the modern application of the arts to medical science belong to the professional *creative arts therapy* movement. Stimulated by the growth of modern mental health science after World War II, art therapists, music therapists, dance or movement therapists, poetry therapists, and drama therapists have provided meaningful therapeutic opportunities for people of all ages in a wide variety of settings, but with a particular emphasis on mental health settings.

The creative arts therapists have established a solid professional base through education, training, professional publications (including journals), credentialing mechanisms, and scientific research. There are currently more than 5000 music therapists, 10,000 dance therapists, 3000 art therapists, and several hundred drama and poetry therapists in the United States. The arts therapy movement now includes more than 140 undergraduate and postgraduate degree programs. At least 10 professional associations are in existence in various creative arts therapies, and several professional journals are being published.

The growth of the application of the arts in medicine owes a debt to this creative professional community. It is noteworthy that two hearings were held in 1991 and 1992 under the jurisdiction of the U.S. Senate's Select Committee on Aging dealing with the healing power of music, the visual arts, and dance in the aging population. These hearings led to changes in the Older Americans' Act that enhanced insurance coverage for the creative arts therapies and provided increased professional credibility and acceptance of these interventions.

Also, a hospital arts movement continues to grow. This successful movement emphasizes improving the environmental quality of health care institutions through the architectural design, interior design, and placement of fine art in strategic health care setting locations and performances in a variety of hospital arts settings, such as lobbies, waiting rooms, patient rooms, and high-tech intervention venues. These individuals and organizations generally do not state that they are engaging in "therapy," but they have a general belief in the salutary effect of aesthetic environments on patients, visitors, family members, staff, and the overall health care institution community. Among the leading organizations in this important new field are the Society for the Arts in Healthcare, the Foundation for Hospital Arts, Art that Heals, Arts as a Healing Force, the British Healthcare Arts Centre, and the Center for Health Design and Aesthetics. Collaboration with the professional architectural and interior design community provides exciting opportunities. Some professionals have begun incorporating not only performance but also specific sounds into the holistic health care environment. For example, Annette Ridenour, President of Aesthetics, Inc., worked with a composer whose music integrates with the architecture, the color, and the intention of the selected space. Patients and staff often participate in the production of such art and performances (Ridenour 1999). Again, these activities are not categorized as therapeutic per se, but leaders in the field are encouraging at least some outcome measurement studies, which economics may demand.

In recent years there has been a growing interest in the application of the arts to all specialties of medicine, in addition to the previous emphasis on the application of the arts in psychiatry. In part, this trend relates to the recognition of the problems associated with excessive pharmacological and surgical intervention. Calls for the formation of a new medical specialty known as "Arts Medicine" seek to explore the many synergistic relations amongst the healing and the creative arts (Lippin, 1985). The arts could be explored for their etiological, diagnostic, educational, therapeutic, and environmental impact on health. Also in recent years, creative arts and expressive arts therapists are expanding their emphasis on applying their work in mental health settings to other medical specialties, most notably pediatrics, gerontology,

oncology, cardiology, physical medicine and rehabilitation (physiatry), and thanatology (death and dying). For several reasons, there appears to be differential capacity to apply these interventions to pediatric populations, geriatric populations, and to other "special" populations, as explored later in this chapter.

Definitions

Arts: For this chapter the definition is limited to music, dance, visual arts, poetry, and drama. (A case can be made that all human activities, such as avocational cooking and gardening or work for pay, can be engaged in artistically when aesthetics becomes an "ontology," or way of being.)

Creativity: Mihali Csikszentmihaly (1996) defines creativity as "the ability to produce something that changes the existing patterns and thoughts in a domain."

Creative arts therapy: The National Coalition of Arts Therapies Associations (NCATA) states that creative arts therapies include art therapy, dance/movement therapy, drama therapy, music therapy, psychodrama, and poetry therapy. These therapies use arts modalities and creative processes during intentional intervention in therapeutic, rehabilitative, community, or educational settings to foster health, communication, and expression and promote the integration of physical, emotional, cognitive, and social functioning, enhancing self-awareness and facilitating change.

Arts medicine: The International Arts Medicine Association states that arts medicine studies the relationship of human health to the arts. Arts and artistic activities are explored for their etiological, diagnostic, educational, therapeutic, and environmental potential.

Expressive therapies: Natalie Rogers, a leader in this field, states that expressive therapies are the use of the expressive arts in a supportive setting to facilitate awareness, growth, and healing. Various art modes interrelate simultaneously in what Rogers (1993) calls the *creative connection*.

Imagery and visualization: Imagery is both a mental process and a wide variety of procedures used in therapy to encourage changes in attitudes, behavior, or physiological reactions. As a mental process, it can be defined as "any thought representing a

(Continued)

sensory quality which might include the visual, oral, tactile, olfactory, proprioceptive and kinesthetic." Whereas *visualization* refers to "seeing something in the mind's eye" only, procedures for *imagery* fall into at least three major categories: evaluation or diagnostic imagery, mental rehearsal, and therapeutic intervention.

Leaders in the creative arts therapies field and others have introduced more recent terms, such as *musicmedicine, medical art therapy,* and *medical dance therapy,* reflecting the increasing use of the creative arts therapies in medical settings other than mental health settings. Of particular note is the pioneering work of Drs. Ralph Spintge and Roland Droh, who founded the International Society for Music in Medicine after studying music's anxiolytic and analgesic properties in thousands of surgical patients in a hospital wired throughout for music in Ludenscheid, Germany (Spingte and Droh, 1989).

THEORETICAL CONSIDERATIONS AND MECHANISMS OF ACTION

Before discussing the various types, current practices, and research in expressive or creative arts therapies, consideration of general theory and possible mechanisms of action seems appropriate. Expressive arts therapies are often categorized as "mind-body therapies" or embracing the "holistic model" of medicine. Fueled by advances in neuroscience, mind-body or holistic medicine recognizes that the entire universe and everything in it, including one's perceptions of it through the human brain, affect human physiology and medical outcomes, ranging from accidents to dysfunction and disease to wellness and peak performance.

One fundamental shift that is gaining credibility is support for a transformation from our current pathology-based health care system to a health care system that embraces a fundamental view of humans as good and empowered to seek and achieve increasingly higher levels of health or wellness. The arts play an essential role in realizing the preceding health care model, because the arts promote the salutary effects of freedom, self-esteem, growth, pleasure, communication, love, a sense of community, and the connectedness to a universal life force.

Another fundamental concept associated with the expressive arts therapies is that humans can deterministically choose to perceive the innate and abundant beauty of themselves and the universe and can incorporate this beauty into their lives on a conscious decision basis. Therefore, one role of the health professional or healer is to recognize, validate, nurture, support, and facilitate the expression of the innate goodness and beauty of the patient and the universe. In this model, physicians and other health professionals do not direct behavior or provide interventions; instead, they allow or provide permission to enjoy the beauty and bounty of human existence. Thus they do not extinguish negative behaviors as much as they encourage innate positive ones.

Also, humans have an innate ability to counter both individual and collective destructiveness and decay (entropy)—in short, to choose life over death. Engaging in the arts is thus life affirming and life enhancing. Neurosurgeon Michael Salcman (1992 has stated "at the heart of both the arts and the sciences is a desire to leave the world marginally better than one finds it. Thus the will to create and heal is the moral force and guiding principal of the medical profession."

Another fundamental theoretical consideration is the growing call for the "democratization of the arts." Thus, everyone may engage in the arts without fearing shame, ridicule, derision, or embarrassment and in a safe environment that allows patients to cast off their "inner critic." Such concepts have been described as the emergence of a new paradigm of "medical optimism" (Lippin, 1985, 1991). This paradigm is essentially based on a love of life, self-determination, and responsibility, in contradistinction to our current predominant medical paradigm of pathology and paternalism, which is based on a fear of death, dependency, and victimhood. A proven and potential biological mechanism of action for arts interventions includes muscular movement, which is a central feature of expression in all the arts. Furthermore, engaging in the arts can induce relaxation and pleasure. The arts can also lead to self-knowledge, self-discovery, mood change, and emotional catharsis (e.g., weeping, laughing, sexual activity). Finally, the arts can elicit and augment spiritual and transcendental states and their associated psychological and physiological benefits.

Musculoskeletal Movement

Artistic creation involves musculoskeletal movement, which is a reaffirmation and augmentation of life force itself, because movement is central to the living state. To some degree, all expressive arts involve muscular movement. Although the most obvious expression is dance, movement is also involved in the making of music, singing, painting, sculpting, drama, and even the act of writing. Musculoskeletal movement involved in the creation of art may have special relevance to pediatric and geriatric populations and those categorized as having disorders of movement, regardless of the specific cause.

In addition to the basic musculoskeletal and cardiopulmonary benefits of movement, from a psychiatric perspective, movement "frees up" and allows the discharge of suppressed emotions and trapped energy from psychic and somatic blocks. Such an energy release facilitates new levels of perception that may lead to integration of body, mind, and spirit. Dance therapists have stated that movement is our primary realm of expression on which all other means depend. For example, the movement impulse can be transformed into words, tones, lines, and color. Our inner experience is externalized through movement to some material separate from ourselves.

From a musculoskeletal or exercise perspective, the demands of ballet are said to exceed those of professional football. For example, in dance, the deceleration of the "rigid" body is of the order of 40 g. At the professional level, virtually all forms of art require an extraordinary level of sensorimotor control, precision, speed, endurance, and strength. For example, forearm blood flow changes in pianists increase over basal blood flow rates, and cardiac index increases at the highest stages of piano playing. Increases in heart rate and blood pressure can be achieved, demonstrating not only that forearm activity is significant in piano playing, but that it is truly a "total body" experience. One of the theories also associated with the noted longevity of orchestral conductors is the amount of musculoskeletal movement or aerobic exercise in which conductors routinely engage as they practice their art.

In singing, so-called classical (opera quality) and "belting" (e.g., Ethel Merman) singing techniques have been analyzed by electromyography, measuring both intrinsic and extrinsic muscles associated with the act of singing.

Many studies have demonstrated the antidepressant effect of musculoskeletal movement in exercise. Exercise has been proven to be time and cost-effective compared with psychotherapy and drug treatment for depression and is potentially useful as a preventive measure for future depressive episodes. Hence exercise, including movement in the arts, may become a primary treatment of choice. Also, exercise is probably safer than a lifelong commitment to pharmacotherapy.

Relaxation Response

Herbert Benson's classic description of the relaxation response did not specifically reference the arts. His emphasis was on mental focusing devices and a passive attitude toward distracting thoughts (Benson et al., 1974). However, other authors believe that the arts, either passively experienced or actively pursued, can elicit the relaxation response. Steven Halpern has documented music's impact on the relaxation response through what he calls his "antifrenetic alternative" music, which he contrasts with other forms of New Age music. In Western culture a passive relaxation response can be supplemented with what some have called *active meditation,* in which engaging in the arts produces a timeless experience associated with deep relaxation and neurophysiological changes. Psychiatrist and music therapist John Diamond, for example, refers to the arts as the "royal yoga" or the supreme meditation.

There are three explanations for how music promotes a relaxation response. *Biochemical theory* states music is the sensory stimulus processed through the sense of hearing. Sound vibrations are transformed into neurological impulses that activate biochemical changes either through the sympathetic or parasympathetic nervous system. *Entrainment theory* suggests that oscillations produced by music are received by the human energy field, and various physiological systems entrain with or match the hertz or oscillation frequency of the music. *Metaphysical theory* suggests that music is divine in nature and puts us in touch with or augments our spiritual selves, thus inducing a highly relaxed state.

Emotional Catharsis

Among the healing capacities of the arts is its ability to stimulate or augment emotion and the biological and behavioral concomitants of emotions. These range from simple mood alteration to full-blown emotional catharsis. In addition to a body of serious psychiatric literature on the complex topic of emotional catharsis, listed among stress-releasing techniques are the "weep response" (crying), the "mirth response" (laughing), and the "sexual response" (orgasm) (Lippin, 1985).

It is becoming increasingly clear that the arts can both stimulate and augment weeping, laughing, and sexual behaviors. The physiology of all three of these important human behaviors and their benefit is being increasingly studied and validated by the scientific community.

Music, poetry, and photographs can be used to stimulate conscious memories or may subconsciously precipitate sad and wistful mood changes leading to weeping. Laughing can be stimulated through all of the arts, but especially through the joy of dancing, music, theater, clowning, and popular singing (e.g., barbershop quartets).

The capacity for stimulating healthy sexuality through various forms of artistic expression is well known, especially as it relates to the stimulatory effect of visual depictions of sexuality and physical beauty of the human form, as well as the enhanced libido associated with dancing.

Self-Discovery

Knowledge of oneself has been defined as a cornerstone of health in most cultures. Some authors believe it is the most important goal of any psychotherapeutic intervention. This can be characterized as a lifelong intrapsychic discovery or "self-diagnostic process" for everyone. It is theorized that only through self-knowledge can rational, hence healthy, choices be made.

Carl Rogers, developer of person-centered psychotherapy, incorporated the belief that each individual has worth, dignity, and the capacity for expression and self-direction (Rogers, 1951). Rogers' philosophy is based on a trust in the inherent impulse all human beings have toward growth and his faith in the innate capacity of each person to reach toward his or her full potential. This tenet is a major theoretical foundation for the value of expressive arts therapy as developed by Rogers' daughter, Natalie Rogers. She enhances her father's theory of creativity by using the fundamental person-centered principles as the foundation for expressive arts as a healing process. A critical component to this theory is that individuals or groups must have a safe, accepting, empathetic, and supportive environment in order to develop this full potential (Rogers, 1993).

Carl Rogers' research revealed that when a person feels accommodated and understood, emotional healing occurs. This basic truth is so simple yet so profound that it is often overlooked or misunderstood. The creative process is easily squashed in a judgmental atmosphere. Creating a nonjudgmental, permissive, stimulating environment for expression of self is essential to emotional healing. Furthermore, Sigmund Freud believed that love and work are central to health ("the purpose of life is to love and to work") .

Noted sociologist Jean Houston describes "entelechy," or the discovery and dynamic unfolding of our essence of who we are and who we are meant to be, our "essence" (Houston, 1982). It has long been known that the arts can play a key role in the self-discovery process. Engaging in the creative arts can provide a safe, direct path to both the "personal unconscious" and the "universal collective unconscious" as described by Carl Jung. It also provides a path to spiritual discovery. For example, the more one regularly creates, the more one will notice an image often repeated in various ways. This is described as "the true self made visible." Not only specific organs but also physiological processes may have the capacity to stimulate the production of psychic images meaningfully related to the type of physical disturbance and its location. This phenomenon may arise from electrical and chemical messages from the diseased part of the body to the brain, which are interpreted as mental images. We may comprehend that, through wordless communications and in his or her own idiom (the arts), a person can and does convey both somatic and psychological conditions. Somatically, pictures may point to events in the past relevant to anamnesis (recall), early diagnosis, and prognosis. During a period of creative acitivity from 1986-1995, The National Museum of Health and Medicine in Washington, DC, mounted an exhibition on "Headache Art" in which headache sufferers depicted their affiflictions through visual representations. Psychologically, we may observe what happens deep in the mind (e.g., how drawings can help express hopes, fears, and forebodings through past or ongoing traumas).

Furthermore, drawings can serve as bridges between the health provider and the patient, the family, and the surrounding world. Indeed, their meaning and what it implies could guide the healing professions to assist especially critically ill patients in living as near to his or her essential being as possible, whether in recovery, in the midst of illness, or close to death.

Finally, we may ask how it could be that spontaneous drawings may reflect the total situation of a person (e.g., as dreams may). D'Arcy Hayman (1969) has stated that the expressive arts "give voice to the self," the highest form of individuality. Natalie Rogers, one of the founders of expressive arts therapies, says we express our inner feelings by creating outer forms; "expressive art" refers to using the emotional, intuitive aspects of ourselves in various media. To use the arts expressively means going into our inner realms to discover feelings and to express them through visual art, movement, sound, writing, or drama. In the therapeutic model based on humanistic principles, the term *expressive therapy* has been reserved for nonverbal and metaphorical expressions. *Humanistic* expressive arts therapy differs from analytical or the medical model of arts therapies, in which the arts are used to diagnose, analyze, and "treat" people. Many have already discovered some aspect of expressive art as being helpful in our daily lives. One may doodle as one speaks on the telephone and find it soothing. One might write or keep a personal journal and find that as one writes, feelings and ideas change, perhaps as one writes down one's dreams and looks for patterns and symbols. One might paint or sculpt as a hobby and realize that the intensity of the experience transports oneself out of everyday problems, or perhaps one sings in the shower, while driving, or going for long walks. These activities exemplify self-expression through movement, sound, writing, and art to alter one's state of being. These are ways to release one's feelings, clear one's mind, raise one's spirits, and bring oneself into higher states of consciousness. This process is indeed therapeutic (Rogers, 1993).

When using the arts for self-healing, or therapeutic purposes, the expressive arts therapist is not concerned about the beauty of the visual art, the grammar or the style of writing, or the harmonic flow of the song. The expressive arts therapist uses the arts to "let go," to express, and to release. We can also gain insight by studying the symbolic and metaphorical messages. Art speaks back to us if we take the time to let in those messages. In regard to music, it may bypass the intellectual defenses and go to the nexus that connects the body, mind, emotion, and spirit. People are often afraid to experience themselves fully because of the possible pain they may discover. Music is a nonverbal form through which we can explore aspects of ourselves on a multisensory level.

The expressive arts thus may lead into the unconscious as they allow us expression of previously unknown facets of ourselves. This brings to light new information and awareness.

Creativity

Because it is believed to be increasingly strategic in the business world and is supported by scientific discovery, much has been written recently on the topic of creativity. Little, however, is known about the fundamental biology and health impact of creativity. Noted psychologist Abraham Maslow believed that creativity is a fundamental characteristic inherent in humans at birth. Carl Rogers, aforementioned founder of person-centered psychotherapy, stated that from the nature of the inner condition of creativity, it is clear that it cannot be forced but must be permitted to emerge. A limited amount of early childhood research has shown that exposure to and involvement in the arts has a potential trophic or growth influence on the brain and on the body.

In expressive arts therapies, although the expressive product itself may have value and can provide important feedback cybernetically to the individual, it is the process of creation that can be profoundly transformative. Norman Cousins observed cellist Pablo Casals literally transformed from a frail and slow 90-year-old to a vibrant, thoroughly engaged musician while playing the cello, demonstrating extraordinary intellectual and physiological performance. Cousins attributed this to Casals being thoroughly engaged in his own creativity and his desire to accomplish a specific purpose, not merely a physical exercise of playing the cello (Cousins, 1979).

Creativity expert Mihaly Csikszentmihalyi references the term *flow* and describes creative individuals as having the personality traits of independence, self-confidence, unconventionality, alertness, ambition, commitment to work, willingness to confront hostility, inquisitiveness, a high degree of self-organization, and the ability to work effectively for long periods without sleep. Their cognitive style, the way they think, rather than their native intelligence, seems to set creative individuals apart from their peers. Intrinsic factors (a passion for pursuing a particular activity for the sake of the activity itself) rather than extrinsic factors (e.g., fame, fortune, status, prizes) seem to motivate creative individuals (Csikszentmihalyi, 1990, 1996).

Some believe a correlation exists between creativity and mental illness or emotional pain. However, most experts would argue that it is unlikely that mental illness could be routinely advantageous to the creative process because the concentration required for creative endeavors is likely to be hampered by symptoms of the illness that would make creative "flow" difficult to achieve. A high rate of psychosis and neurosis among artists and performing artists does not mean that emotional turmoil is the source of creativity. Instead, most people who have serious mental illness, including major mood disorders, show little evidence of creativity.

Neurobiology of the Creative Process

The therapeutic benefits of activities that involve the experience of creativity provide powerful evidence for a biologically adaptive function that may be independent of any specific kinesthetic, visual, or musical art form. University of Tennessee ethologist Neil Greenberg believes that important insights into the nature of creativity can be obtained by looking into its biological causes and consequences. He has drawn on his work into the neuroendocrine aspects of behavior to develop a model of creativity as a highly evolved mechanism for coping with stress. In his view, creativity is part of the ensemble of neurobehavioral mechanisms that enable organisms to respond to real or perceived needs of varying urgency (Greenberg, 1997). In other words, creativity is a key mechanism for coping with possible challenges to the dynamic balance within itself and between itself and its environment. The fullest expression of creativity involves contributions from systems that mediate affect, motivation, and cognition and that are orchestrated largely by the neural and endocrine mechanisms of the stress response. The needs that these mechanisms address range from coping with life-threatening emergencies to resolving cognitive dissonance.

The well-studied selective effects of the stress response on different forms of learning and on pathologies associated with creativity (e.g., depression, temporal lobe epilepsy) provide a framework for examining the roles of ancient and recently evolved brain mechanisms in creativity.

Creativity is energized and focused by neural mechanisms linked to hormonal responses that evolved to cope with stress and that are woven throughout the nervous system. Specific patterns of neuroendocrine responses evoked are determined by the duration and intensity of a stressor and apparent prospects for its control. Furthermore, the way the stress response is activated can determine whether creative work will be impaired or enhanced. Specific neural mechanisms involved in creativity thought to be affected by elements of the stress response include heightened reactivity, long-term potentiation, perceptual restructuring, and selective memory.

The study of creativity has been handicapped by its traditional focus on one or another element of the dynamic ensemble of underlying processes. Furthermore, the concept is torn between two points of view: (1) that creativity is only rarely expressed, and then only in gifted individuals, and (2) that it is so ubiquitous as barely to deserve special comment. Drawing on the work of Margaret Boden and working with Bruce MacLennan, a University of Tennessee computer scientist specializing in neural connectionism, Greenberg is working to bridge the gap and build a framework for understanding when and why creativity is manifest.

Tinin has written about neurophysiology and the aesthetic response. He puts forth a theory of the aesthetic response to explain why it is so resistant to verbal analysis. There is a mimetic response to art that is not available for verbal reflection not only because it is automatic and unintended, but also because its nonverbal, cerebral initiative is actively denied by consciousness, which reflexively owns all mental initiative (Tinin, 1990, 1991, 1992). Human perception of nonverbal communication, including art, is an active, unconscious process in which the receiver creates the perception by active mimicry. The viewer's response to a picture, for example, begins with an active, nonverbal experience that is largely outside of consciousness and involves kinesthetic and visceral mimicry preceding verbal interpretation. The viewer circumscribes the lines and volumes with movement of the scanning eyes while mimetic movement of other body parts follows the contours of the figure. The listener's response to music is played out with movement by the head, shoulders, and other body parts. Observers of sculpture unknowingly imitate the implied movement of the sculpture. This kinesthetic imitation is automatic and unintended, and it predicts the person's pleasure in the art. Thus, is it the sensation produced by mimetic motor activity combined with an emotional pattern of visceral arousal that constitutes the aesthetic experience? Any inhibition of either kinesthetic or autonomic mimicry determines the pleasure of the response to the artistic stimuli. This resistance is universal and is a necessary consequence of the ego's requisite maintenance of mental unity.

Arieti (1976) defined creativity as the "magic synthesis" of primary process and secondary process thinking into what he called "tertiary process," thus building on Freud's topographical model of the mind as consisting of conscious and unconscious portions, each with different systems of logic. In addition to Arieti's "magic synthesis," other theorists have put forth proposals to account for creativity in terms of the conscious/unconscious dichotomy, including sexual sublimation, regression in the service of the ego, freedom from neurosis, schizophrenic thinking, and a race against the human awareness of mortality.

Pleasure and Play

There has been increasing societal awareness in modern Western culture that pleasure is not a sin, although societal values increasingly reward work and not play for most Americans.. The role of physicians as "finger waggers," admonishing patients not to succumb to their "basic instincts," is changing. Rather, physicians can trust their patients or even encourage them to engage in responsible pleasures that do not harm others or society. A new role of the physician is to give permission, even encouragement, to enjoy the beauties and bounties of life (including the arts) without guilt. The inclusion of pleasure and creativity into life is part of a prescription for total health.

On an intuitive and anecdotal basis, the capacity for the arts to induce pleasure is well known. Although explanation of the neurophysiology of human pleasure is still in its infancy, this topic is being studied more carefully. Using research findings in the fields of medicine, biology, and psychology,

Robert Ornstein and David Sobel, MDs, in their book *Healthy Pleasures* have been pioneers in articulating the crucial role of pleasure in health. Dr. Sobel has defined pleasure as having a central role in human evolution in that pleasure can serve as a guide to survival behaviors (Ornstein and Sobel, 1989).

Creativity expert Mihaly Csikszentmihalyi (1990, 1996) states that eight main elements were reported repeatedly to describe how it feels when an experience is pleasurable: (1) clear goals every step of the way (e.g., musician knows what note to play next); (2) immediate feedback to one's actions (e.g., artist sees what color he has placed on the canvas); (3) a fine balance and congruence between challenge and skills; (4) action and awareness are merged; (5) abstractions are excluded from consciousness, that is, there is total engagement (e.g., musician becomes the music, dancer becomes the dance); (6) no worry of failure, and self-consciousness disappears; (7) sense of time becomes distorted (in a positive sense) (e.g., dancers and figure skaters may report that a quick turn seems 10 times as long); and (8) the activity becomes "autotelic," that is, something that becomes an end in itself. Although the arts can provide gains in money and status, most people engaging in the arts do so because of the sheer pleasure.

Related to pleasure is the concept of *play*. Because stress is proven to be linked with ill health, engaging playfully in music, art, dance, poetry, and drama can move a person from puritanical emphasis on "doing something productive" into becoming a receptive being. In this state there is increased activation of the parasympathetic nervous system, which is one of the reasons why play could be so essential to health.

We may seek creative experience because it is pleasurable, but pleasure, like creativity itself, exists not for its own sake but because it serves the needs of organisms to thrive and reproduce. Pleasure is nevertheless an ardently sought emotion. Michel Cabanac derived the equation *pleasant = useful* from his extensive review of responses of people to external thermal stimuli when they possess differing internal thermal states (Cabanac, 1971). Pleasure, Robert Wright reminds us, is *not* the end purpose of life; contrary to some traditional views, such as that of J.S. Mill, *pleasure is a device for steering the organism in the right direction*. Our seeking of pleasure, Wright believes, is "sponsored by [our] genes, whose primary goal . . . is to make us prolific, not lastingly happy." Pleasure is addictive; "we are designed to feel that the next great goal will bring bliss, and the bliss is designed to evaporate shortly after we get there."

Nesse and Berridge (1997) also emphasize the adaptive function of pleasure in their interpretation of our vulnerability to addiction. Pleasure is an emotional experience, and emotions "are coordinated states, shaped by natural selection, that adjust physiological and behavioral responses to take advantage of opportunities and to cope with threats that have recurred over the course of evolution. . . . Thus, the characteristics and regulation of basic emotions match the requirements of specific situations that have often influenced fitness. Emotions influence motivation, learning and decisions and, therefore, influence behavior and, ultimately, fitness."

Optimism and Hope

Hope is currently viewed as a significant determinant of health and health outcomes. Again, however, we are in the early stages of understanding the physiology of these feelings.

In *Learned Optimism* (1990), psychologist Martin Seligman explores the limited research on optimism's impact on the immune system. The relationship of hope and optimism to health is linked also to the concept of meaning in life (Frankl, 1963). Palomore (1995) studied social factors such as work satisfaction and predictors of longevity, and Wong (1989) described the need for personal meaning in successful aging. Engaging in the arts can provide a person with a sense of hope and meaning by actively expressing the self, producing a beautiful product, and sharing it with loved ones or the public.

The most important function of the arts from a medical standpoint, however, may be its *revitalization* function, in which the creative process itself reaffirms and augments the desire of humans to choose life over death consciously and deterministically in this critical and tenuous period in the history of human culture and civilization.

Spirituality and Transcendental States

The arts are playing an increasing role in the Western world's spiritual renewal. Addressing the National Coalition of Arts Therapies Associations (NCATA) in Washington, DC, in November 1990, renowned psychoanalyst Rollo May described art therapists as "harbingers or sparks of a new world—a new religion based on man's endless search for beauty and the joy of human beings helping other human beings."

The excesses of materialism and alienation, rebellion, and shock seen in modern art (the so-called culture of transgression) may be seen by some as yielding to a postmodern emphasis and rebirth of arts that connect us to our spiritual selves, with an emphasis on enduring values, including beauty and harmony within ourselves and within the universe. For many, engaging in the arts is fundamentally a spiritual path or transformational process, a way of being, a shift from scientism and materialism to the treatment of the soul. Michael Samuels and colleagues believe that the arts free the body's own internal healing mechanisms, uniting body, mind, and spirit as art is produced; no interpretation or therapy is necessary. The creative process itself is the healer (Samuels, 1991). In music, Reverend Cynthia Snodgrass quotes Biblical passages on the need to reclaim our sound traditions. From the Genesis passages of creation to the collapsing walls of Jericho to the healing of King David with the melodies of the harp, we may see revival in those testimonies from the Hebrew scriptures that stand as witness to music's power.

Deep within us, Samuels believes we have a memory of the beautiful place where our spirit was given breath by traveling inward, and only through art we can experience this spiritual essence, this loving and healing force. Thus, art is the voice of the spirit and is the energy of healing. The artist and the healer are feeling the rebirth of these ancient traditions. At the source, "they" and "we" are all connected. In the place of birth is a universal land of awesome power and beauty. From it comes painting of stars, of swirls of light, of radiance; from that universal realm comes early movement and the softest sounds: "ohm," "amen," or "mama" (Chapter 26). Closer to the surface we find radiant colors, still abstract, and in the next world we see the birth of archetypal symbols and dream figures; finally, upward we are in "body land" and the so-called material world.

Because art acts at the level of the spirit, energy is involved (Chapter 17). Art therapist Shaun McNiff says whenever illness is associated with the loss of soul, the arts emerge spontaneously as remedies, or "soul medicine." Creation is interactive, and all the players are instruments of the soul's instinctual process of ministering to the self (McNiff, 1981, 2004). Art historian and psychiatrist Hans Prinzhorn has believed that patients' art was a natural antidote to schizophrenic disintegration and alienation. Louise Montello, a music therapist, writes about the loss of self or the loss of one's connection to the "divine child," which she believes is the root of much chronic illness (Montello, 1992, 1994, 2002). "Once the self, however, is awakened through the arts which is some sort of playful and/or prayerful activity, the healing process is awakened from within. Once self is established, then the soul can be consciously cared for," states Montello. Thomas Moore, in his famous book *Care of the Soul,* says, "Art is not about the expression of talent or the making of pretty things—it is about the preservation and containment of soul." Art captures the eternal in the everyday, and it is the eternal that seeds the soul. In Montello's description of working with emotionally disturbed ("soul-starved") children, she states that these children hunger for beauty, love, and goodness that art can provide.

McNiff (1992) states that art as a medicine is in a postheroic phase in art's history. Individual heroics are replaced by the individuation of expression within a group that supports each member's natural and spontaneous emanations. Connection exists between our life force, our inner core or soul, the essence of all things. Therefore, as we journey inward to discover our essence or wholeness, we discover our relatedness to the outer world. The shamanic community of the creator is in our genes, is waiting to be released. This collective involvement is yet another shamanic element that survives to manifest itself in every aspect of the current application of art as medicine. Painters influence and stimulate one another with their images, as do musicians improvising with related sounds. Participants become what the romantic poets call "agencies of the flying sparks." Soul moves about through charges and countercharges.

In this world, pathology and health are not limited to patients; they are in all of us. Tribal societies knew how to make use of those who were possessed by emotional upheavals. In contemporary Western society, we do not. By trying to fix them, improve them, eliminate them, drug them, and/or cure them, we are demonstrating that we have not grasped how they can help us. McNiff says that the best medicine one can offer to a troubled person is a sense of purpose, the feeling that what he or she is going through

may contribute to the vitality of the community and that the process is reciprocal. During the Biblical age of prophets, harp players would perform special pieces of music to produce a mental state in which extrasensory powers were thought to be activated, and it is said of Elisha—"and it came to pass when the minstrel played that the hand of the Lord came upon him." David played for King Saul to help him recover from depression and paranoia. In this spiritual renaissance, especially among so-called Evangelicals, the arts are playing an increasing role in religioius services throughout the world. Thus, making a joyful noise unto the Lord becomes increasingly manifest in such phrases as "God respects you when you work. He loves you when you sing." Many believe the basic purpose of the creative or expressive arts therapies is to access the deepest centers of the spirit and bring back the abducted soul from the excesses of a modern, excessively materialistic and increasingly uncivil society.

CURRENT PRACTICE AND GOALS

The goals of *dance and movement therapy* are numerous and vary according to the population served. For emotionally disturbed persons, the goals are to uncover and express feelings, gain insight, and develop therapeutic bonds and attachments. For physically disabled patients, the goals are to increase movement and self-mastery and esteem, have fun, and heighten creativity. For the elderly population, the goals are to maintain a healthy body, enhance vitality, develop relationships, and express fear and grief. For mentally retarded persons, the goals are to motivate learning, increase bodily awareness, and develop social skills. An underlying goal in dance and movement therapy is that visible movement can affect total biopsychosocial potential and function, promoting healing by altering mood, reawakening stored feelings and memories, organizing thoughts and actions, reducing isolation, and establishing rapport. Total body movement stimulates functions of body systems such as circulation, respiration, and skeletal and neuromuscular activity, including the use of muscles and joints to reduce body tension and body armoring. Other known clinical effects are the reduction of chronic pain, depression, and suicidal ideation.

Music therapy goals include physical and emotional stimulation for those in chronic pain and those with impaired movement. The neurological mechanisms by which music decreases pain awareness were discussed earlier. Music can evoke a wide range of emotional responses and has both sedative and stimulant qualities. Music is also a unique form of communication. Music can be used with patients who are nonverbal or who have difficulty communicating, such as in autism, where music can facilitate social interaction. Music has been used effectively in the treatment of eating disorders. Music can be used to express a wide range of emotions, from anger and frustration to affection and tenderness. Selecting music from an individual's past may evoke memories of times, places, events, and persons. Such memories can contribute additional information to the individual's treatment.

Art therapy can be effectively used as a therapy and especially as a diagnostic tool. Patients may focus on parts of their bodies that unconsciously concern them and that they have been unable to verbalize. Patients may draw images about their disease processes and explore all the medical and psychological manifestations of their disorder.

Poetry therapy uses poetry for the purposes of healing and personal growth. The participant's own creative writings are viewed as avenues toward self-discovery. Poems used as a method of a life review and reminiscence have been particularly effective in assisting elderly persons. A "life review" involves the person writing his or her own autobiography using photo albums, letters, memoirs, and interviewing techniques to gather and integrate a person's life experiences into a meaningful whole. Telling one's own "story" through poems, songs, and journals produces vital narrative material for the therapeutic process. The special goals of poetry therapy are to increase the patient's spontaneity and capacity for playing with words and ideas; to strengthen communication, particularly listening and speaking and writing skills; and to help the patient experience the life-giving and nourishing qualities of beautiful writing. Poems serve as catalysts to evoke feelings within and can help focus on the other person's reaction to the words. Poetry enables individuals to express experiences they may be unable to say in any other way, which may be the first step in speaking about shameful and taboo subjects. The most powerful poetic device is symbolic representation through *metaphor*. When patients externalize feelings into poetry, the product is a tangible, literally black-and-white, testament to feelings and thoughts previously without literal form. The externalization gives participants a feeling of mastery and allows them to view their own feelings from a different perspective. Patients often are comforted by a poem, which they can literally carry on their persons as they do with biblical and other quotes. Poetry may have layers of meaning with an ability to conceal and reveal, thus providing both psychological closeness and distance when necessary. Reading poetry aloud together, as with prayer, can build cohesion, boost ego, and enable individuals and groups to respond to the rhythm and beauty of the poem together.

Practices that use the techniques of *imagery* include biofeedback, systematic desensitization, counterconditioning, echosynthesis, neurolinguistic programming, Gestalt therapy, rational-emotive therapy, meditation, relaxation techniques, and hypnosis. Procedures for imagery fall into at least three major categories: (1) evaluation or diagnostic imagery, (2) mental rehearsal, and (3) therapeutic interventions. Techniques used in evaluation or *diagnostic imagery* involve asking the patient to describe his or her condition in sensory terms. *Mental rehearsal* is an imagery technique used before medical techniques, usually in an attempt to relieve anxiety, pain, and side effects that are exacerbated by a heightened emotional reaction. Surgery or a difficult treatment is rehearsed before the event so that the patient is prepared and is rid of any unrealistic fantasies.

Imagery as a *therapeutic intervention* is based on the concept that images have either a direct or indirect effect on human physiology and health outcomes. Patients are taught how to use their own flow of images about the healing process, or they are guided through a series of images that are intended to soothe or distract them to reduce sympathetic nervous system arousal or generally enhance relaxation.

Whether imagery is merely an antidote to feelings of helplessness or whether the image itself has the capacity to induce the desired physiological effect is still unclear. Existing research suggests that both conclusions are justified, depending on the particular situation being studied. Among the research accomplishments in imagery, there is a great emphasis on immunology. Findings include correlations between various types of leukocytes and components of cancer patients' images of their disease, treatment, and immune system, as follows:

- Enhanced natural killer cell function after relaxation and imagery training procedure with geriatric patients and in adult cancer patients with metastatic disease.
- Altered neutrophil adherence or margination and white blood cell count after an imagery procedure.
- Increased secretory immunoglobulin A (IgA) after training in location activity and morphology of IgA after 6 weeks of daily imaging.

The specificity of imagery training was suggested in patients with cell-specific imagery of either T lymphocytes or neutrophils.

MEDICAL ART THERAPY

A special issue of *Art Therapy* on the topic of art and medicine (1993) noted the term *medical art therapy* and stated that distinct differences exist between art therapy conducted in the psychiatric milieu and art therapy conducted in a medical setting because of the environmental realities and goals of each. Also, the physical conditions of patients determine how often therapy can be presented and used. Healing is not only defined by improved laboratory values, x-ray films, or the eradication of a tumor. Healing is the process of "being made whole," physically, psychologically, and spiritually. Healing can take place even as the body weakens and dies. Thus it is said that although the body may not be cured, it may be healed.

The greatest impact of engaging in the art of expressive therapies could be their potential to synthesize and integrate patient issues such as pain, loss, and death; the art therapies assist patients through art making and the creative process. *Medical art therapy* is defined as the use of art, expression, and imagery with individuals who are physically ill, experiencing trauma to the body, or undergoing aggressive medical treatment such as surgery or chemotherapy. In some cases, as when the patient is fragile and susceptible to infection, the therapist must be cognizant of maintaining a sterile environment through the appropriate use of art therapy media and tools. At other times the patient may be unable to participate actively without physical adjustments, such as arranging for the therapist to be at the bedside or creation of special devices to assist the patient in the creative act. Other art therapists have discussed necessary adaptations in art experiences for patients with dementia and for pediatric patients who have experienced serious burns. Art therapy with pediatric cancer patients may be offered in the hospital waiting room, where children await chemotherapy and radiation treatments or checkups. Family, including siblings, may be present and may become part of the art therapy. However, confidentiality is not easily maintained in this type of open environment, where patients come and go at will and where art therapy essentially takes place in a quasipublic arena, such as a waiting area or at a bedside.

RESEARCH

Advances in neuroscience, psychoneuroimmunology, and psychoneurocardiology have provided necessary tools to engage in solid scientific research on creative and expressive arts therapies. The impact of music in particular on human physiology has been well studied and demonstrates great promise (Chapter 27). For example, music's capacity as an analgesic or anxiolytic agent is well documented, as is its impact on mood. Music has been studied with burn patients, terminally ill patients, and those with cerebral palsy, stroke, and Parkinson's disease. The impact of music on the immune system has also been studied, including the impact on patients with acquired immunodeficiency syndrome (AIDS) and other immune disorders.

Bittmen (2001), for example, demonstrated significant modulation of neuroendocrine-immune parameters in normal subjects through group drumming a form of music therapy. Furthermore, music has been studied extensively among elderly patients as a means to improve quality-of-life measures. Mickey Hart, one of two drummers with the former San Francisco Bay Area band, the Grateful Dead, has advocated this type of work. Other studies have demonstrated the effect of music on physiological measures such as galvanic skin response, vasoconstriction, muscle tension, respiratory rate, heart rate variability, pulse rate, and blood pressure. Music has been used to relieve anxiety and depression in coronary care units and to promote recovery from heart attacks. It has also been shown that listening to different types of music can lower levels of the stress hormones cortisol, adrenaline, and noradrenaline and increase levels of atriol and natriuretic peptide, a potent antihypertensive hormone produced by the atria of the heart.

Neurophysiology researchers have postulated that music affects brain function in at least two ways: (1) it acts as a nonverbal medium that can move through the auditory cortex directly to the limbic system (an important part of the emotional response system), and (2) it may stimulate the release of endorphins, thereby allowing these polypeptides to act on specific brain receptors. This theory is supported by direct recording of neuronal discharge rates while listening to music. However, because music can alter mood and emotional states, it is also likely that the immune and hormonal changes seen after subjects listen to music are mediated by the autonomic nervous system. The Institute of Heart and Math previously investigated the effects of music on autonomic activity with powered spectral density analysis of heart rate variability and of immunity, measuring levels of secretory IgA from saliva samples. This work demonstrated a relationship between increased autonomic activity and increased salivary IgA.

The term "designer music" was introduced by the music industry to describe a new genre of music designed to affect the listener in specific ways. This term has also been used in the scientific literature to specify this type of music. Research and clinical studies have shown that so-called designer music produces a significant effect on listeners' physiological and psychological status. As mentioned earlier, after U.S. Senate hearings in 1991 on the impact of music on elderly persons, the Older Americans Act Amendments of 1992 listed music therapy as both a supportive and preventive medical service. Furthermore, among the initial grants of the National Institutes of Health (NIH) Office of Alternative Medicine (now the National Center for Complementary and Alternative Medicine) was one to investigate the effects of specific music therapy interactions on empirical measurements in persons with brain injuries.

In the visual or "plastic" art therapy field, research has been done on psychiatry and burn patients; on patients with eating disorders, chemical addictions, deafness, aphasia, and autism; and as a prognosticator in childhood cancer, in childhood bereavement cases, and in sexually abused adolescents. The visual arts, because they produce a permanent visual "record," lend themselves to high-quality research in art as a diagnostic tool.

Dance therapy research has demonstrated clinical efficacy in ameliorating depression, decreasing bodily tension, expressing anger, reducing chronic pain, and enhancing circulatory, respiratory, and musculoskeletal function.

Although music and the other arts have been used successfully as treatment modalities for mood and other psychiatric disorders and medical conditions, uncertainty remains as to how such effects are mediated within the brain. There is speculation that benefits are achieved through music's ability to modify directly the neuronal substrates (neurological loci) of affective states, which then have widespread effects on the autonomic, hormonal, and immunological mechanisms of the body. Studies could be done to quantify specific components of dance, including exercise, social contact, bonding, spontaneous versus instructional dance, male-female relationships versus male-male or female-female dancing versus group dancing, touch versus no touch dancing, and with and without music. Manfred Clynes postulated "essentic forms," which he describes as "biologically given expressive dynamic forms for a specific emotion" and theorizes that the neurobiological process of recognition of pure emotion essentic forms may release specific substances in the brain, which then act to transmit and activate those specific emotional experiences (Clynes, 1982). The "iso principle," first described in 1948, seeks to match the patient's musical mood, which helps the patient gain insight into internal thoughts and memories. These concepts require further research.

Entrainment, as noted earlier, is an aspect of sound that is closely related to rhythm and the way these rhythms affect humans. Powerful rhythmic vibrations of one object will cause the less powerful vibrations of another object to "lock in step" and oscillate at the same frequency. The music potential ("rider") is based on the hypothalamus having strong connections to the limbic system. Thus the connection between music and health is likely to have a mechanism involving a "neural" hypothalamic–frontal limbic loop and a neuroendocrine hypothalamic-immunological loop.

New research is beginning to explain the physiology of hope and positive expectations. In one series of studies, patients entering the hospital for open-heart surgery or surgical repair of a detached retina were evaluated before and after surgery. Those who expressed greater optimism regarding surgical results, confidence in the ability to cope with the surgical outcome, and trust in their surgeon recovered more quickly. Among patients undergoing heart surgery, death rates were lower. Hopeful expectations may also predict who will develop cancer of the cervix. The more optimistic the woman, the less likely she is to have cervical cancer.

A study of patients with advanced breast and skin cancer revealed that a joyful attitude and optimistic style were the strongest psychological predictors of how long patients would remain cancer free before the disease returned. *Webster's Dictionary* defines optimism as "an inclination to anticipate the best possible outcome; a tendency to seek out, remember and expect a pleasurable experience." Optimists have a high level of "locus of control" and feel challenged, not threatened, by the current environment and the future. Also related to optimism is the capacity for love. Siegel (1987) stated that if he teaches AIDS patients to love themselves and others fully, there is an automatic increase in the immune globulins and killer T cells.

In the aesthetic paradigm, where the arts are used, the fundamental goal of the artist is to communicate, share, or even love, unlike the athletic or militaristic paradigm, where the fundamental purpose of the athlete or soldieris to compete or kill.

Pennebaker and Francis (1992) of Southern Methodist University in Dallas indicated that individuals who wrote about upsetting personal events displayed significant changes in psychometric surveys.

Research issues in creative or expressive arts therapies for the future generally could include the following:

1. What is the impact of aesthetic stimuli, including color, form, sound, rhythm, movement, words, and beauty itself, on human physiology?
2. Specifically, how does the human brain perceive, process, integrate, and react to aesthetic stimuli?
3. What is the neurophysiological nature of creativity and its relationship to human health?
4. What are the biopsychosocial characteristics of living and performing and of visual artists as related to a more complete understanding of the limits of human capacities?
5. How can the study of highly successful elderly artists and performers contribute to understanding the role of the arts in the aging process?
6. How can the arts be effectively used to enhance early brain development and early childhood education?
7. How can the arts contribute to the development of individual and cultural self-esteem, in that self-esteem is increasingly viewed as central to the development of mental health and cultural well-being?
8. How can the arts be used to improve diagnostic and prognostic capabilities in medicine?
9. Which already-developed models are most promising for the successful integration of the arts to improve the environmental quality of health care settings?
10. What specific steps must be taken to ensure inclusion of arts medicine topics in formal art or medical curricula?

SPECIAL POPULATIONS

Although the expressive arts therapies can be applied to most patients in most medical settings, these therapies are of special value to the following special subgroups:

- *Pediatric patients.* Children are more freely expressive and in the early years are less verbal than other medical populations. Children also can engage in creative play more easily.
- *Geriatric patients.* The geriatric population is especially vulnerable to the excesses of pharmacological and surgical interventions. The arts can serve as an alternative or supplement. Also, musculoskeletal movement associated with expressive arts in older persons can be a fundamental therapeutic goal. Disorders of the central nervous system, especially those associated with memory loss (e.g., Alzheimer's disease) seem to be differentially benefited by creative or expressive arts therapies. Verghese and colleagues (2003), for example, specifically identified dance as the only primary physical activity to confer some protection against cognitive decline.
- *AIDS patients.* Since the AIDS epidemic became manifest in the early 1980s, the expressive arts have

played a key role in assisting patients, their loved ones, and their families in dealing with this devastating disease. Much art has been produced by and for patients with AIDS, partly because of the effect of this syndrome on the artistic workforce sector. The famous AIDS quilt project is an example of this phenomenon.

- *Health professionals.* Health professionals have always been subject to physical and psychological stresses inherent in their profession. Increased incidences of serious forms of psychopathology, sociopathy, and burnout are seen in these populations. Also, disabled or ill health professionals can cause significant harm to patients in their charge. In recent years a massive transition in the enterprise of health care has added additional transition and career stresses to health professionals. On the positive side, some studies have demonstrated that physicians in particular possess differential creative skills. Therefore, health professionals are encouraged to engage in the arts, especially as a stress reduction technique or for stress prevention. Also, when physicians engage in the arts, they share and demonstrate their common humanity with their patients. Contemporary physician/poet John Graham-Pole (1997) stated, "Such self-revealing [writing poetry] opens my vulnerability to others, helps me lick my wounds without leaving a scar, washes me clean, releases my tensions, redresses my balance, captures painful and delicious sense, validates me as a sentient human being."

- *Patients with chronic diseases and chronic pain.* Engaging in the arts provides hope, pleasure, and beauty and enhances the quality of life for individuals coping with chronic disease and chronic pain syndromes.

- *Dying patients.* Faced with the realization of imminent mortality, dying patients often seek to resolve lifelong psychosocial issues and, importantly, spiritual issues. This can be greatly facilitated and enhanced through artistic expression. Dying patients often express lifelong conflicts and desires through artistic expression. Also, the creation of artistic products allows the dying patient to leave something of value to loved ones, friends, and society. The product of self-generated art adds beauty, joy, and meaning to the last days of the dying patient's life. Also, dying patients often are depressed and may be in pain, and the arts can assist with these conditions as well.

CONCLUSION

As the excesses of the predominant scientific and theoretical paradigms in medicine yield to the new and emerging paradigms, the application of the arts will play an increasing role in *health* in the broadest sense of the term. We are entering into an era where art is viewed as a major positive force able to unlock each person's potential for goodness and individual growth, as reflected in a healthier society composed of revitalized, healthier people.

The arts will continue to unfold as a major cost-effective contribution to individual, institutional, and societal health. Researchers, educators, and practitioners and the payers and regulators of these endeavors will increasingly appreciate the role that the arts can play in producing healthy individuals, healthy families, healthy communities, healthy schools, healthy workplaces, and a healthy planet.

Acknowledgments

We wish to acknowledge the following individuals and organizations for their help in the preparation of this chapter: Natalie Rogers, author of *The Creative Connection*; Neil Greenberg, University of Tennessee; Susan Kleinman, Chair of NCATA; Alicia Seeger, Administrator of NAPT; Eric Miller of Expressive Therapies Concepts; and the creative arts therapy community, on whose shoulders the modern arts-medicine movement stands; our physician colleagues within the arts-medicine movement, including John Graham-Pole, John Diamond, Michael Samuels, Patch Adams, Michael Salcman, Eric Avery, Joel Elkes, Ralph Spintge, Yoshihito Tokuda, and Itzhak Siev-Ner; also, David Hinkamp from the ACOEM Section on Arts-Medicine and Naj Wikoff from the C. Everett Koop Institute at Dartmouth University; from the hospital arts movement, Janice Palmer and John Feight; Drexel University's Hahnemann Creative Arts in Therapy Program Directors Ronald Hayes, Paul Nolan, and Sherry Goodill; And to Karen Barton, Robert Hand, and Roberta Dougert for assistance in the preparation of this manuscript.

References

Arieti D: *Creativity: the magic synthesis,* New York, 1976, Basic Books, pp 16-20.

Benson H, Beary JF, Carol MP: The relaxation response, *Psychiatry* 37:37-46, 1974.

Bittman B et al: Composite effects of group drumming music therapy on modulation of neuroendocrine-immune parameters in normal subjects, *Altern Ther Health Med* 7(1):38-47, 2001.

Cabanac M: Physiological role of pleasure. *Science* 173:1103-1107, 1971.

Clynes M, editor: *Music, mind, and brain: the neurophysiology of music,* New York, 1982, Plenum.

Cousins N: *Anatomy of an illness as perceived by the patient,* New York, 1979, Norton, pp 72-87.

Csikszentmihalyi M: *Flow: the physiology of optimal experience,* New York, 1990, Harper & Row.

Csikszentmihalyi M: *Creativity: flow and the psychology of discovery and invention,* New York, 1996, HarperCollins, pp 58-76, 110-113.

Frankl VE: *Man's search for meaning: an introduction to logotherapy,* New York, 1963, Simon & Schuster.

Graham-Pole J: Why I write poetry, *Int J Arts Med* 5(1):34-39, 1997.

Greenberg N: Creativity: the adaptationist view, University of Tennessee University Studies Colloquy on Creativity (working paper), 1997. http://utk-biogw.bio.utk.edu/Neils.nsf/.

Hayman D: *The arts and man: a world view of the role and function of the arts in society,* Englewood Cliffs, NJ, 1969, Prentice Hall.

Houston J: *The possible human: a course in enhancing your physical, mental, and creative abilities,* Los Angeles, 1982, Tarcher.

Lippin R: Arts medicine: a call for a new medical specialty, *Philadelphia Med* 81:14-15 1985.

Lippin R: A message from the president of IAMA, *Int J Arts Med* 1(1):4-7, 1991.

McNiff S: *The arts and psychotherapy,* Springfield, Ill, 1981, Charles C Thomas.

McNiff S: *Art as medicine: creating a therapy of the imagination,* Boston, 1992, Shambhala, pp 1, 14-17, 22, 25.

McNiff S: *Art heals: how creativity cures the soul,* Boston, 2004, Shambhala.

Montello L: Arts medicine, *Int J Arts Med* 1(2):33-34, 1992.

Montello L: Arts medicine editorial, *Int J Arts Med* 3(2):34-35, 1994.

Montello L: *Essential musical intelligence: using music as your path to healing, creativity and radiant wholeness,* Wheaton, Ill, 2002, Quest Books.

Ornstein R, Sobel D: *Healthy pleasures,* Menlo Park, Calif, 1989, Addison-Wesley, pp 168-169, 277-282.

Palmer J, Nash F: The hospital arts movement, *Int J Arts Med* 1(1):34-38, 1991.

Palomore EB: Physical, mental and social factors in predicting longevity, *Am Psychol Assoc* 9(2, pt 1):103-108, 1995.

Pennebaker JR, Francis ME: Putting stress into words: the impact of writing on physiological, absentee, and self-reported emotional well-being measures, *Am J Health Promot* 6(4):280-287, 1992.

Ridenour, A., Designing a healing clinical office environment: Creating healing spaces, In Micozzi, MS, Current Review of Complementary Medicine, Philadelphia: Current Science Press, pp. 125-130, 1999.

Rogers CR: *Client-centered therapy: its current practices, implications, and theory,* New York, 1951, Houghton Mifflin.

Rogers N: *The creative connection: expressive arts as healing,* Palo Alto, Calif, 1993, Science & Behavior Books, pp 1-9, 50-64, 86-90.

Salcman M: Presidential address: the education of a neurosurgeon—the two cultures revisited, *Neurosurgery* 31(4):686-696, 1992.

Samuels M: Art as a healing force, Bolinas Museum, March-April 1991 (Published for exhibition "Art as Healing Force").

Seligman M: *Learned optimism,* New York, 1990, Knopf, pp 168-177.

Siegel B: Images in disease and healing. In *Love, medicine, and miracles,* New York, 1987, Harper & Row, pp 50-51, 157-160.

Spingte R, Droh R, editors: *Music medicine,* Proceedings of International Society for Music in Medicine. IV. International MUSICMEDICINE Symposium, Rancho Mirage, Calif, October 1989.

Tinnin L: Biologic processes in nonverbal communication and their role in the making and interpretation of art, *Am J Art Ther* 29:9-13, 1990.

Tinnin L: Creativity and mental unity, *Perspect Biol Med* 34:347-354, 1991.

Tinnin LW: The neurophysiological process of mimicry as a model for the aesthetic response. Presented at MedArt International World Congress on Arts and Medicine, New York, February 1992.

Verghese J et al: Leisure activities and the risk of dementia in the elderly, *N Engl J Med* 348(25):2508-2516, 2003.

Wong PTP: Personal meaning and successful aging, *Can Psychol* 30:3, 1989.

Suggested Readings

Achterberg J: *Imagery and healing: shamanism and modern medicine,* Boston, 1985, New Science Library.

Ackerman D: *A natural history of the senses,* New York, 1990, Random House, pp 175-285.

Anonymous: Alternative medicine: expanding medical horizons. Report to National Institutes of Health on Alternative Medical Systems and Practices in the United States, Workshop on Alternative Medicine, Chantilly, Va, September 1992, pp 25-30.

Anonymous: AIDS and the arts, *Newsweek,* Jan 18, 1993, pp 16-23.

Benson H, Stuart EM: *The wellness book,* New York, 1992, Birch Lane Press, pp 33-65, 121.

Bertman SL: *Facing death: images, insights, and interventions—a handbook for educators, healthcare professionals, and counselors,* New York, 1991, Hemisphere, pp 1-9, 169-200.

Bonny H: Music listening for intensive coronary care units: a pilot project. In *Music Rx,* Port Townsend, Wash, 1978, Institute for Consciousness and Music (tape set with accompanying booklet).

Campbell D: Music: *Physician for times to come,* Wheaton, Ill, 1991, Quest Books.

Campbell DG: *The roar of silence: the healing powers of breath, tone, and music,* Wheaton, Ill, 1989, Theosophical Publishing House.

Davis W, Thaut M: The influence of preferred relaxing music on measures of state anxiety, relaxation, and physiological responses, *J Music Ther* 26:168-187, 1989.

Estill J: Belting and classic voice quality: some physiological differences, *Med Probl Perform Artists* 3(1):37-43, 1988.

Fox J: The healing pulse of poetry: the life-giving power of your own words, *The Quest,* Autumn 1992, pp 65-70.

Goodill SW, Morningstar DM: The role of dance/movement therapy with medically involved children, *Int J Arts Med* 2(2):24-27, 1993.

Gorelick K: Poetry on the final common pathways of the psychotherapies: private self, social self, self-in-the-world, *J Poetry Ther* 3(1), 1989.

Hanna JL: The power of dance: health and healing, *J Altern Complementary Med* 1(4):323-331, 1995.

Hanser S: Music therapy with depressed older adults. In Spingte R, Droh R, editors: *Music medicine.* Proceedings of International Society for Music in Medicine. IV. International MUSICMEDICINE Symposium, Rancho Mirage, Calif, October 1989.

Harvey A, Rapp L: Music soothes the troubled soul . . . , *Ad Nurse,* March-April 1988, pp 19-22.

Higgins JM: *Escape from the maze: 9 steps to personal creativity,* New York, 1997, New Management.

Johnson DR: Introduction to the special issue—creative arts therapists as contemporary shamans: reality or romance? *Arts Psychother* 15:269-270, 1988.

Laws K: Physics and the potential for dance injury, *Med Probl Perform Artists* 1(3):73-79, 1986.

Laws K: The physics and forces of partnered lifts in dance, *Med Probl Perform Artists* 3(3):88-93, 1988.

Leedy JJ: *Poetry as healer: mending the troubled mind,* New York, 1985, Vanguard, pp 200-212.

Lerner A, Mahlendorf UR, editors: *Life guidance through literature,* Chicago, 1991, American Library Association.

Malchiodi, Calif: Introduction to special issue: art and medicine, *Art Ther* 10(2):66-69, 1993.

Malchiodi, Calif: Medical art therapy: contributions to the field of arts medicine, *Int J Arts Med* II(2):28-31, 1993.

Malchiodi, Calif: Commentary on "Art for Recovery": using art to humanize the medical milieu, *Int J Arts Med* 3(1):24-25, 1994.

McCraty R, Barrios-Choplin B, Atkinson M, Tomasino D: The effects of different types of music on mood, tension, and mental clarity, *Altern Ther* 4(1):75-84. 1998.

Moore N: Alternatives, *Altern Ther* 4(1):37-40, 1998.

Nachmanovich S: *Free play: improvisation in life and arts,* New York, 1990, Penguin Putnam.

Nemetz LD: Dance/movement therapy: speaking the language of self, *Int J Arts Med* 4(2):26-31, 1995.

Panksepp J, Bekkedal MYV: The affective cerebral consequence of music: happy vs sad effects on the EEG and clinical implications, *Int J Arts Med* 5(1):18-27, 1996.

Parr SM: The effects of graduated exercise at the piano on the pianist's cardiac output, forearm blood flow, heart rate, and blood pressure, *Med Probl Perform Artists* 3(3):100-104, 1988.

Pratt RR: The history of music and medicine. In Pratt RR, editor: *The Third International Symposium on Music in Medicine, Education, and Therapy for the Handicapped,* Lanham, Md, 1985, University Press of America, pp 237-268.

Pratt RR: Healing and art, *Int J Arts Med* 1(2):3, 1992.

Pratt RR: The new interface between music and medicine. In Spingte R, Droh R, editors: *Music medicine,* St Louis, 1992, MMB Music.

Pratt RR, Tokuda Y, editors: *Arts medicine,* Proceedings of First US/Japan Arts Medicine Leadership Conference (Tokyo, 1993), St Louis, 1997, MMB Music,

Reiter S: Enhancing the quality of life for the frail elderly: Rx: the poetic prescription, *J Long-Term Home Health Care* 13(2), 1984.

Rogers CR: *On becoming a person,* Boston, 1961, Houghton Mifflin.

Rogers CR: *A way of being,* Boston, 1980, Houghton Mifflin.

Sataloff RT, Brandfonbrener AG, Lederman RJ, editors: *Textbook of performing arts medicine,* New York, 1991, Raven Press, pp 30-31.

Schindler AG: Contemplating creativity. In *Encyclopedia Britannica,* 1997 Medical and Health Annual, Chicago, 1996, pp 44-61.

Spencer MJ: *Live arts experiences: their impact on health and wellness—a work in progress,* New York, 1996, Hospital Audience, pp 49-72.

Spingte R: Psychophysiological surgery preparation with and without anxiolytic music. In Droh R, Spingte R, editors: *Angst, Schmerz, Musik in der Anasthesie,* Basel, 1982, Editiones Roche, pp 77-88.

Standley J: Meta-analysis of research in music and medical treatment effect size as a basis for comparison across multiple dependent and independent variables. In Spingte R, Droh R, editors: *Music medicine,* Proceedings of International Society for Music in Medicine. IV.

International MUSICMEDICINE Symposium, Rancho Mirage, Calif, October 1989, pp 364-378.

Stoll B: Art therapy: from isolation to international visibility, *Int J Arts Med* 1(1):27-32, 1991.

Storr A: *Music and the mind,* New York, 1992, Ballantine, pp 12-13.

Taylor D: *Biomedical foundations of music as therapy,* St Louis, 1997, MMB Music, pp 51-118.

Turner SS: Expression through dance for the well-elderly. In Spingte R, Droh R, editors: *Music medicine,* Proceedings of International Society for Music in Medicine. IV. International MUSICMEDICINE Symposium, Rancho Mirage, Calif, October 1989.

Wikström BM, Theorell T, Sandström S: Psychophysiological effects of stimulation with pictures of works of art in old age, *Int J Psychosom* 39(1-4):68-75, 1992.

Zhuo D: The tradition of music therapy in the People's Republic of China, *0* 1(2):4-6, 1992.

20

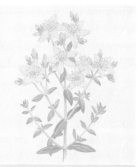

Humor

PATCH ADAMS, WILLIAM F. FRY,
LEE GLICKSTEIN, ANNETTE GOODHEART,
CHRISTIAN HAGESETH III, RUTH HAMILTON,
ALLEN KLEIN, VERA M. ROBINSON,
PATTY WOOTEN

The arrival of a good clown exercises a more beneficial influence upon the health of a town than of twenty asses laden with drugs.

—THOMAS SYDENHAM, MD
(SEVENTEENTH-CENTURY PHYSICIAN I [ADAMS])

Before tackling what humor therapy might be, I [Adams] would like to introduce where I think it fits into complementary and integrative medicine in a discussion on wellness or preventive medicine. Allopathic medicine has generally ignored this field. What could be more complementary to any system of disease care than a sound emphasis on being well? As the economic crisis in medicine worsens, it seems both prudent and inevitable that we focus much greater attention on living healthful lives. The complementary therapies have all had a greater emphasis on wellness partly because they fit into their more holistic approaches (see

Chapter 1). Often, in spending more time with patients, the intimacy that happens leads toward a compassionate desire to help the patient feel better. The primary care health provider clearly sees the difference in the way healthy people on a wellness program respond to illness from the way people respond to illness who do not do wellness care for their health. We also see less frequent illness in people on wellness programs.

WELLNESS—RECOGNIZING WHOLE POTENTIAL

Exercise and recreation are as necessary as reading. I will say rather more necessary because health is worth more than learning.

—THOMAS JEFFERSON

The practice of family medicine can be an exercise in frustration. Current medical education focuses on disease care: a patient comes to the doctor sick, does the prescribed treatment, and returns to the world. Why he or she got sick in the first place is glossed over with a few quick questions, partly because in the short dialogue between physician and patient, there is no time to address the patient's lifestyle. I have chosen to spend long hours with patients for these past 25 years to try to understand the processes that lead to illness. In medical school, "health" was defined as the absence of disease, so those not complaining of symptoms were healthy. Yet, so few adults I have spoken with speak of life as a wondrous zestful journey, and most illnesses seen by a family doctor have a huge lifestyle component, frustrating the physician because they could have been prevented with self-care.

Health

Health is obviously so much more than a disease-free interlude. To be healthy is to have a body toned to its maximum performance potential, a clear mind exploding with wonder and curiosity, and a spirit happy and at peace with the world. Most adults, however, exist in a gray area between health and sickness, a zone where people say, "I'm fine," when asked how they feel. This "fine" can be chock full of disease as diverse and inhibiting as (1) the chronic fatigue or "blah" experienced by those labile fluctuations in blood sugar as a result of a high-sugar diet, (2) the foot problems that come from wearing shoes geared for fashion, not fitness, and (3) the distraction and anger that linger on after poor communication with a spouse or friend. In fact, our lifestyle is assaulting us now and anticipating future expression in disease in hundreds of silent ways.

Because wellness is the summation of all factors leading us to being healthier, this chapter can only touch, ever so briefly, on some of those of paramount importance, ideally stimulating a thirst in each person to discover individual parameters. In the wellness model, patients become responsible for their own health because health results from an active participation that only the self can give. The health professional's role then shifts from that of mechanic fixing the breakdowns to a gardener nurturing growth.

Much of illness, from minor to profound, has a powerful stress component. The intention of the well-

ness movement is to offer many insights and paths to eliminate unhealthy stress and make good use of positive stress. It is time to "lighten up" and live life in deepest appreciation of all its gifts.

Wellness is a great investment with many repercussions. A long-term investment in good health opens the door to a lifetime of quality living for the investor. The physical body becomes the vehicle for indulging in every activity one desires, never limited because of being out of shape. However, the benefits of wellness extend far beyond the self. Family life can become a rich, creative, and happy experience on the train of communication and cooperation. The workplace can become a fun place, as a well-dressed attitude and personality help make all employees a team and every task a delight. Separating self, family, and work is arbitrary and possibly even dangerous, because the health of one so obviously has an impact on all the others. People who are at maximum health will be happier and more loving in all their relationships and thus prepared to give their best work performance. An individual striving to be healthy, full of caring and curiosity, brings loving management and creativity to the workplace. A body in tone and at proper weight is ready for the tasks at hand. If any of these areas is ignored in one's pursuit of health, the others will suffer. Studies have shown that emphasizing a human-centered, healthy workplace and providing space and time to exercise and be more personal cuts absenteeism and turnover and increases honesty and productivity.

Unfortunately, one of life's ironies is that wisdom mostly comes with age. By the time we realize that a habit has profoundly hurt us, we feel helpless to change the habit, even justifying it as intrinsic to our nature. Luckily the design of a great organism is such that it can recover remarkably well; in fact, it begins to repair itself as soon as we alter the unhealthy habit. Wellness is not some kind of "end product"; it is a process, a journey, where each day presents its unique face, and we must choose from many choices which paths to follow. We cannot rest on the health of our past, because it must be renewed each day.

Life is a cascade of choices, and we are an expression of both the short-term and the long-term choices we make. To manage the number of choices we have to make daily, we fall into habits, and a routine substitutes for a choice. These habits can be a double-edged sword: Although it is true we do not have to concern ourselves any longer with an immediate choice, once entrenched, a habit is incredibly hard to break. When the habit is an unhealthy one and we want to break it, the task is arduous. Wellness seems like an emerging system to help people restructure or balance habits, so how we live becomes healthy, not as a task of effort but simply as a collection of positive, intentional habits. As medical practitioners focus on the causes and prevention of illness, they are finding that many major diseases could have been prevented or dramatically postponed through lifestyle changes. Most of this information has been reiterated throughout medical literature from Hippocrates to the present.

Nutrition

Take nutrition, for example. Simplified, we are a sack of water with chemicals in solution. How these chemicals interact determines what we are to be, but in many of the interactions, chemicals are used up or altered and must be replenished. Nutrition consists of the proper consumption and assimilation of foods containing those necessary chemicals. Because few foods contain all or most of the needed nutrients, we have to obtain them in a variety of foods. As people have moved further from food sources, and as food companies have changed the foods grown to have longer shelf life, our diets have changed dramatically. For about the last 100 years, synthetic chemicals, refined foods, sugar, and salt have replaced many of the natural foods our ancestors ate.

Refined simple sugars so dominate our lives that they are ubiquitous, present even in table salt. In the United States 100 years ago, we consumed 3 pounds of sugar per person per year; we now consume 140 to 180 pounds. Many believe this has had a profound effect on our health. Certainly it plays a major role in one of the most devastating diseases—obesity. The federal government has stepped in to encourage some nutrition changes: (1) dramatic cutbacks in sugar and salt consumption, (2) increase in foods containing fiber, and (3) vast decrease in milk products and other animal fat products. I would expand on this to say eat mostly whole grains, fresh fruit, and vegetables and, if eating meats, eat mostly fish and poultry.

Exercise

If nutrition is the fuel, exercise is the "toner" for the body. Modern civilization has changed few things in

our lives as severely as the amount of exercise we get. We have never been as sedentary as we are today, and this, combined with dietary changes, has made much of our adult population overweight and flabby. There is a popular quip that says, "If you do not use it, you lose it." The interplay of muscles, bones, tendons, ligaments, and joints demands consistent stimulation to stay in tone. Being in shape does not mean simply being slender but having all the muscles trained.

There are four types of exercise to consider. The body's internal toner in *heart-lung (aerobic)* exercise strengthens the heart, exercises the bellows to supply oxygen to the body and rid it of carbon dioxide, and tones the muscles used in exercise, all giving the body endurance. Joint *flexibility exercises*, such as stretching or yoga-style exercises, keep the body limber and relaxed. *Strength exercises* are important to tone those muscles not covered in the heart-lung exercises. *Balancing exercises*, such as dance, gymnastics, or circus skills, add another dimension to maximum performance.

Being in shape has obvious rewards in being physically able to do whatever you want to do, and regular exercise has other benefits. It has been shown to lower blood pressure, to have a positive effect on mental health, to diminish stress, and to aid digestion. I believe that regular exercise does such good for the body that it appears to slow the aging process.

Emotional Life

Just as we must exercise our bodies to be fit, so must we exercise our minds to keep awake and alert. The greatest instruments for the mind's stimulation are wonder and curiosity. Boredom is a major disease, eroding the health of many adults who over time narrow their spheres of interest. Wonder and curiosity are the tools that all children carry with them in their interactions with the world. In fact, that wonder and curiosity are what make kids seem so alive. For adults, somewhere along the line, sunsets become routine and life's pace too hectic. But wonder and curiosity can be recaptured. There are no stimulants that begin to awaken a person like a new interest captivating one's life or consuming ongoing exploration. The next time a person is excited about something, instead of turning it off, jump right into it and share in their interest. Carry your wonder and curiosity into your older years and you take your youth with you. Often, having such a vibrant interest is a major impetus and motivation for staying healthy, so the exploration goes unimpeded.

It goes without saying that love is the most important wellness factor in sustaining a healthy, happy life. Love, that passionate abstract, has captured the arts from the beginning as they attempt to define and elucidate it. As a healing force, *love* can be defined as that unconditional surrender to the overwhelming wonderful feeling experienced in giving to or receiving from an object. We most often express love toward family, friends, God, self, lovers, pets, nature, or hobbies. By "surrender" I mean to lose oneself in awe, trust, respect, fun, and tenderness for the object of surrender. In striving for maximum wellness, one could pursue love in all the parameters just mentioned. It appears that the more one submits to unconditional love toward one object, the easier it is to do so for others. The unconditional aspect is so important because without it, love is often lost to expectations, doubts, and fears.

If love is the foundation for happiness, then fun, play, and laughter are the vehicles for its expression. The great physician Sir William Osler said that laughter is the "music of life." Humor and laughter are the subject of this chapter.

Faith

Faith is the cornerstone of our inner strength. Faith is a personal, passionate, immutable belief in something of inexhaustible power and mystery. Whenever we have to face any kind of devastating change without some kind of solid belief, we become prey to confusion, fear, and panic. Often these present crises present questions that have no answers; the discomfort arising from this uncertainty is healed in the domain of our beliefs. Faith has no physical characteristics, no external requirements; it is not a commodity. To acquire a belief, one simply needs to have an interest and a willingness to submit to its mystery. Although there are many great religious traditions that promote a common interpretation of belief, I think the truth is that each person has to find an individual, meaningful faith. Faith is not summarized by a label but expressed by an inner experience of strength that lives in each of us, day by day.

Nature

Whereas faith is intangible, requiring sweet surrender, nature is a physical, sensual thing. Our relationship with nature has had great historical significance as part of our healthy life. It is little surprise that most symbols in early religions were from nature. Our moods are often described in terms of nature: a synonym for "happy" is "sunny." The first warm bright day after winter heightens spirits as few days of the year do. Love has a metaphorical connection to the moon. Most early celebrations grew out of ties with and reliance on the seasons. We have such strong needs to connect with nature that billions of dollars are spent to bring nature into our homes in the form of pets and house plants. Medical literature is currently peppered with the therapeutic significance of putting pets in the lives of elderly and mentally ill patients.

Flowers are a major communication of love at sick beds, deaths, marriages, and special occasions. The few weeks we take during a year to relax on vacation are mostly spent with a natural setting in mind: the beach or the mountains, for instance. Let's face it—nature is the mother of wonder. If we are to be fully well, we need a daily communion with nature, both in the spectacular sunset and in the tenacious blade of grass as it pushes up through the sidewalk.

Creativity

Our imagination, hands, and senses are the tools for the next major wellness factor—creativity. Life is experienced as a rich journey if we believe we have a creative hand in its passage. Creativity is not just expressed through hobbies and arts but can touch every aspect of our life: our work, family, and even how we wait in line. The importance seems to be in the enjoyment of the process rather than in the quality of the final product. Creativity works like our muscles: the more it is exercised, the greater its tone. Explore the next idea, activity, or interest in your life that catches your eye. Whenever exploring, do not settle for one point of view; set it aside and insist on other perspectives. Explore the spontaneous. The key here is to be open and susceptible. Do not catalogue your hobbies and interests as indulgences; respect them as major medicines. Our interests often decline with age, and this can be deadly. Try to see each day as a building block to the next. Be sure to take advantage of all the human creativity in existence, because the arts give such a sense of well-being.

Service

As soon as people recognize how fortunate they are to be well, there arises the urge to give thanks. The healthy expression of that thanks is in service. Unless individuals believe they live a life of service, in whatever form suits them, I believe that they will have a difficult time feeling life is ultimately fulfilling. John Donne wrote, "No man is an island," acknowledging that we are all connected in some way. It is through helping others that we find this deepest interdependence. It is important that this service be done out of thanks in the joy of giving, because service can easily slide into a debit-and-credit mentality. Service can take many forms, from simply being a loving friend or parent to stopping to help someone in need. These are very personal forms of service. I suggest that there is also an important wellness connection to our community and our planet.

Synergy

To these components of wellness could be added passion, hope, relaxation, wisdom, and peace. In the wellness lifestyle, each of these components suggests a context in which men and women can live their lives so that they can feel healthy, as well as a context that dramatically softens the experience when they do become sick. I think it safe to say that these components of wellness, regularly practiced, are healthy to individuals and families. When these two are healthier, it helps make the community and society healthier.

All these wellness components act uniquely in each person within a specific culture, and they all act together in a person at the same time without a measurement of relative value.

Most of these wellness components are dramatically affected by the others; for example, humor is different in a jolly, friendly person than in an angry, lonely one. If one were to use these in a therapeutic way, it would make sense to have the medical environment exude these qualities to create a context of love, wonder, curiosity, and humor. This atmosphere would have a positive health effect on patients, staff, and visitors, whether in an office or in a hospital.

The examination of these wellness qualities, until modern times, has not been by science, but rather by art, philosophy, and religions. However, some of the most exciting research in medicine today is finding the connections in biochemistry and physiology between the mind and its thoughts on the health of the body. This new field is evolving and is now popularly called *mind-body medicine* or *psychoneuroimmunology* (see Chapter 15).

HUMOR

This chapter looks at one component of wellness—humor. Many of the wellness components are difficult to measure (e.g., love, passion, faith) with some scientific precision or standard. Humor is believed to be different because it has a handle to measure it—laughter. Laughter has wide variation within genders, ages, and cultures, making actual studies point to a direction rather than establish a fact. This is one area of study in which anecdotal experience may have to count as science. I do not think one who uses humor in therapy does so because he or she found that laboratory studies showed value. Humor therapy is not a static regimen of memorized jokes and numbers of chuckles per hour. Humor therapy comes out when therapists decide to let their humorous parts join the interaction with a patient. This can be in many forms, such as laughter, theater, verbal, and physical play. With humor, the one who practices (whether laugher, funny person, clown, or comic) the craft—the laboratory—is the patient, audience, or friend. All of one's past experience in that laboratory is brought to the spontaneous act with the patient, and if it is effective, smiling and laughter occur. This positive feedback is the determining feature in reproducing the gesture, statement, or behavior that elicited the laughter. When a patient says, "My doctor has a good bedside manner," he or she is not speaking about expertise but of qualities of interaction. A friendly, playful sense of humor is at the core of a good bedside manner. The patient's appreciation perpetuates the behavior. Friendship is the safest context for humor to work in, so when humor has missed its mark, instead of offense, forgiveness is felt.

A merry heart doeth good like a medicine.

—PROVERBS 17:22

History

There is little history of the use of laughter therapy; much of it is being made now. However, there is a large body of comments on humor and laughter from philosophy, religion, and the arts.

Arthur Koestler summarizes a fraction of these comments in his book *The Act of Creation:*

> Among the theories of laughter that have been proposed since the days of Aristotle, the "theory of degradation" appears as the most persistent. For Aristotle himself laughter was closely related to ugliness and debasement; for Cicero "the province of the ridiculous . . . lies in certain baseness and deformity"; for Descartes laughter is a manifestation of joy "mixed with surprise or hate or sometimes with both"; in Francis Bacon's list of laughable objects, the first place is taken by "deformity" (Koestler, 1964).

The essence of the "theory of degradation" is defined in Hobbes's *Leviathan:*

> The passion of laughter is nothing else but sudden glory arising from a sudden conception of some eminency in ourselves by comparison with the infirmity of others, or with our own formerly.

Bain, one of the founders of modern psychology, largely followed the same theory:

> Not in physical effects alone, but in everything where a man can achieve a stroke of superiority, in surpassing or discomforting a rival, is the disposition of laughter apparent.
>
> For Bergson laughter is the corrective punishment inflicted by society upon the unsocial individual: "In laughter we always find an unavowed intention to humiliate and consequently to correct our neighbor." Max Beerbohm found "two elements in the public's humour: delight in suffering, contempt for the unfamiliar." McDougall believed that "laughter has been evolved in the human race as an antidote to sympathy, a protective reaction shielding us from the depressive influence of the shortcomings of our fellow men."
>
> The first to make the suggestion that laughter is a discharge mechanism for "nervous energy" seems to have been Herbert Spencer. His essay on the "Physiology of Laughter" (1860) starts with the proposition: "Nervous energy always *tends* to beget muscular motion; and when it rises to a certain intensity always does beget it. . . . Emotions and sensations tend to generate bodily movements, and . . . the movements are violent in proportion as the emotions or sensations are intense." Hence, he concludes, "when consciousness is unawares transferred from great things to small" the "liberated nerve force" will expand itself along the channels of least resistance, which are the muscular movements of laughter.

One wonders where in their descriptions appears something useful in helping patients or caregivers in the delivery of care. For this we turn to research done in the twentieth century.

Research

According to Ruxton (1988), humor can help establish rapport and verbalize emotionally charged interpersonal events. Using humor, patients may find it easier to bring embarrassing or frightening parts of their history, and with nurses using funny anecdotes and being more vulnerable with a patient, it appears to strengthen the staff-patient bond.

Coser (1959) looked closely at a hospital's social structure and found that humor helped relieve tension, reassure, transfer information, and draw people together. Norman Cousins (1979) put humor back on the therapeutic map when he laughed himself well from a profound painful, chronic illness, dramatically reducing the pain of his ankylosing spondylitis. He spent the rest of his life working at the University of California School of Medicine investigating the positive emotions and their relationship to health. Dr. William Fry studied humor for 30 years and believes it is an exercise for the body. Mirthful laughter exercises the diaphragm and cardiovascular systems, initially causing an increased heart rate and blood pressure but after a short while a much longer lasting decrease in heart rate and blood pressure, a relaxation response. Paskind (1932) showed that skeletal muscle tone was diminished during mirthful laughter in muscles not actually participating in the laughter. Lloyd (1938) showed an expiratory predominance with mirthful laughter manifesting in a decrease in residual air in the lungs and increased oxygenation of the blood. From work done by Schachter and Wheeler (1962) and Levi (1965), catecholamine levels appear to be elevated with mirthful laughter. Lee Berk describes later the body's immune response to laughter.

Freud suggests that the psychotherapeutic use of humor causes a release of stress, tension, and anxiety. Psychotherapists use humor to facilitate insight (through metaphor, joke, or story) and offer a sense of detachment or perspective. Humor can build a tighter relationship between therapist and patient. Humor can be offered as a tool for coping with life's troubles. Mahrer and Gervaize (1974) looked at their review of the research literature on laughter in psychotherapy and found that strong laughter is a valuable indication of the presence of strong feelings and is seen by most therapeutic approaches as a desirable event. Strong laughter seems to correlate with increased self-esteem and heightened experiencing.

Although no research has conclusively shown a release of endorphins with mirthful laughter, the anecdotal literature about laughter's pain-killing properties is massive. Cousins (1979) opened this door. The Clemson nurses program did a study with elderly residents in a long-term care facility. The residents were divided into two groups. One group watched a comedy video nightly for 6 weeks; the other watched a serious drama. The nurses checked the need for analgesics. There were fewer requests for painkillers from the comedy group. Texas Tech Medical School did another test. Research participants were shown comedy or serious material for just 20 minutes. Relaxation therapy was given to another group. The researchers then determined the participants' pain thresholds using inflated blood pressure cuffs. The comedy group had the greatest pain tolerance of these groups.

I would like to relate a powerful story of a time when humor quite clearly was a painkiller.

Context

I have been doing street clowning almost daily for 30 years, increasingly all over the world. In my 25 years of being a physician, I have always practiced in a humorous context. With a group called Gesundheit Institute, we are building the first hospital to fully incorporate humor. Although disconcerting at first, in the many lectures to lay and medical audiences I have given for the last 8 years about our work, when asked which ward they would choose—a serious, solemn one or a fun, silly one—more than 85% have chosen the fun one. Few people need more than their personal experience to be completely convinced that humor is necessary for their personal health and the health of their relationships.

The primary practice of medicine is a delicate balance between science and art. Ideally, this relationship is one of friendship in which, although radically different in approach, there is a mutual appreciation for the value of all parties involved and a thankfulness and a necessity that they can work together in harmony. Science and art play different roles in the healing interaction. Medical science works at tackling the disease (the organ or systems afflicted) using a well-mapped out series of thought processes, tests, and treatments. The "art of medicine" is concerned with how the disease affects the patient, the family, and their society—the larger repercussions of the disease. These concepts are beautifully discussed in *The Illness Narratives* (Kleinman, 1988) and *The Nature of Suffering* (Cassell, 1991). The art of medicine comes from the intuition and inherent magic found in compassion, love, humor, wonder, and curiosity. For these reasons, one is hard put to break down the components or mechanics of what is working in the art of medicine. Simply put, science serves reductionism, and art serves holism. For this reason, when I do clowning, I am free to explore all these healing abstractions. I use all of these in a multitude of combinations, not because they are well mapped out but because they can more freely arise within the clown persona.

I am both a professional clown and a physician. Each discipline took about the same number of years to master. The difficulties in becoming each were also similar. In one I had to master information and the ability to synthesize information to make responsible decisions, and in the other I had to master the art of spontaneity and freedom of behavior. I could never say which parts of my clown persona did the trick in a healing interaction, and I bet the patient could not either. I can only say that my character brings a blatant expression of love, innocence, fun, joy, and friendliness to which people readily respond.

I believe humor and love are at the core of good bedside manner, burnout prevention, and malpractice prevention, and for these alone, humor deserves a central place in a medical practice, but let us not deny its value in just raw fun. Despite my long, deep experiences with humor, I still can be brought to tears of joy over its power.

This was all brought home to me in November 1991 in a children's burn unit in a hospital in Tallinn, the capital of Estonia.

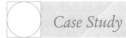

Case Study

For 4 years I have taken a group of clowns to the former Soviet Union to promote good relations between our countries, to spread good cheer, and to provide a 2-week seminar in clowning for both beginners and professionals. We clown in hospitals, orphanages, prisons, and schools, and we perform a tremendous amount in the street. Everywhere we go, patients, staff, and clowns are tremendously uplifted; at times it even seemed to help their medical problems.

Estonia was the footnote to a trip that normally just visits Moscow and St. Petersburg. I added it in 1991 so that we could explore a new country. We arrived 25 clowns strong at the burn hospital, where right off I noticed a woman crying outside a closed door. My medical training told me that this was a mother crying agonizingly over a severely ill child. I knew that to touch her pain I should not clown with her—but with her child. Against strong protestations from the smiling staff, I went inside the room.

I walked in on three women (one physician and two assistants) who had just begun to change dressings and perform debridement on a 5-year-old boy, Raido, with at least 60% third-degree burns solid from ears to knees on both sides of his body. He was in his third week of recovery. I was first struck by the medical supply and pharmaceutical shortages so devastating in the Soviet Union in the winter of 1991. There were no masks or gloves and no strong painkillers, but the work had to be done. With the utmost in loving tenderness on the staff's part and commanding bravery on the boy's part, I watched the bandages come off his wound, revealing a bloody exudative, meaty field, slowly healing from the edges with no evidence of grafts. The silence was punctuated by Raido's screams with each tug of the bandages. At first I felt the horror of a parent for his suffering. From this came a gushing empathy moving the clown to act instinctively; to love, comfort, care for, and bring forth laughter. Without fear.

I watched only for the first third of removal because I was not sure how to proceed. Raido's neck involvement prevented him from looking up at me. When they took a short break, I went over, dressed in full clown regalia, bent over him, and smiled. Spontaneously he looked surprised and delighted and said in Estonian, "You look beautiful." My heart was captured. I immediately went around to the head of his stretcher and spent the next hour stroking his face and hair, smiling and laughing and talking with him. We played. He stopped screaming entirely. I was only 1 foot from his small, unburned face, and I fell in love with him (having a 4-year-old son myself). I had never seen humor's power so raw. I kept telling him he was beautiful and strong and that he was going to live.

It is clear that the child is the one who changed himself from being sad to being cheerful. I was my clown self. His response "you're beautiful" came as a surprise. My character is not "beautiful." It was his willingness to let me inside that made me be of value to him. Another child could have been spooked and cried. Unlike an operation, the impact of humor on the patient wholly has to do with the patient.

I cannot say what I did that was, in this case, the catalyst for a pain-free experience. Was it the sparkle in my eye, the duck hat on my head, the soothing stroking of his head, the words of love and encouragement—or was it simply skilled diversion?

Raido asked me to come back to his room, so I wheeled his mummified body (bandages already bloody) back to his bed. There for 1 hour I entertained him with clown silliness, still peering into his sky-blue eyes and stroking his face. I don't know who benefited more, because my whole body shook, thrilled for being there. I left most of my toys with Raido, even dressing up his dad like a clown while Raido laughed heartily. It was hard to leave him; I felt like he had given me so much. ✍

Humor as Therapy

So what is humor therapy? In its broadest sense it is whatever one does to put mirth into a patient encounter or hospital setting. This is a brand new field, and many are exploring how to add humor to the medical setting.

Ruth Hamilton has been using humor carts at Duke University Medical Center since 1989. Peggy Bushey is a nurse who has used the same carts in the intensive care unit at Medical Hospital of Vermont for several years. These carts have comic videos and cassettes, funny and cartoon books, props, makeup, costumes, and a host of volunteers called in on consultation for patients or staff who request it. Patients have given wonderful feedback on the painkilling and relaxing results of cart use. There is a suggestion that they improve communication, help visitors to hospitals to relax, and even increase motivation in rehabilitation programs. Greater staff relaxation may also be a factor.

Other hospitals, such as Dekalb near Atlanta, have created lively rooms, similar to an expanded cart, with all the same items and a place to use them. Carts and rooms do not make humor, however, so the volunteer becomes the key.

In 1990, Michael Christensen of the Big Apple Circus started taking clowns into children's hospitals to make regular, three-times-a-week rounds to the children. What started out as a whim for him has become a full-time passion. He now has 45 clowns in six hospitals in New York City. Clowns who have worked for him have since set up similar programs in France, Germany, and Holland. The wonderful, positive feedback by staff, patients, and family keeps this program alive.

Others, like Annette Goodheart, insist they do "laughing therapy," not humor therapy. There are laughter meditations and workshops on laughter and play. For many the decision has simply been how to bring more laughter, play, and levity to the medical setting. I suggest a broader view for humor therapy. In our society that harbors alienation, depression, anxiety, and boredom one could decide to be indiscriminately humorous and joyous to try to add these elements to every human encounter. I believe it would help our general societal health.

Humor therapy could include a loud bow tie, singing on the ward, word play, cartoons put up around the hospital, and even inviting comedians to come into the hospital. One note of caution: some believe humor can be harmful in some situations, especially in psychotherapy. I would certainly suggest humor that is not racist or sexist. I suggest first becoming quite close to your patients and have them be sure of your tenderness and sincerity so that if a funny situation or joke hurts, someone can simply apologize. It behooves the medical history taker to make an exploration into the patient's sense of humor and act on it. Because humor in therapy is so new to medicine, I asked a dozen of the leading voices in humor today to make a few statements about their place in the use of humor. I encourage people considering putting more humor in their practice to contact the resources at the end of this chapter for greater depth.

HUMOR THERAPY IN PRACTICE

Big Apple Circus Clown Care Unit

The Big Apple Circus Clown Care Unit (CCU) is a community outreach program of the Big Apple Circus, a not-for-profit performing arts organization presenting the finest classic circus in America. The CCU transforms the performance of classic circus arts to aid in the care and healing of hospitalized children and teens, their parents, and caregivers.

Since classic circus defines a specific body of knowledge, so too does classic clowning. The classic clown types, White, Auguste, and Eccentric, appeared as horsemen, acrobats, jugglers, dancers, musicians, and of course, actors and actresses. Using all these skills, they had a singular focus: to make people laugh. To this end, they used parody. They parodied all circus acts, rules, structures, and authority as symbolized in one circus figure: the black-booted, top-hatted, red-coated, riding-cropped ringmaster.

For the Big Apple Circus CCU the hospital room replaces the circus ring; the physician replaces the ringmaster; and all the rules, charts, formulas, procedures, machines, and straight-laced, white-washed corridors of the hospital become the source of endless parody. The focus is still to bring laughter to patients' hearts.

Using juggling, mime, music, and magic, 35 specially trained "doctors of delight" bring the joy and excitement of classic circus to the bedsides of hospitalized children 2 and 3 days each week, 50 weeks per year. The Big Apple CCU makes "clown rounds," a parody of medical rounds in which the healing power of laughter is the chief medical treatment. Using sophisticated medical-clown techniques (including red-nose transplants, rubber chicken soup, and kitty cat scans), professional CCU performers work one-on-one with hospitalized children, their parents, and caregivers to ease the stress of serious illness by reintroducing laughter and fun as natural parts of life.

In the Beginning

The CCU was created in 1986 by Michael Christensen, Director of Clowning at the Big Apple Circus, in cooperation with the medical staff at Babies & Children's Hospital of New York at Columbia–Presbyterian Medical Center. The first CCU clowns, "Dr. Stubs" and "Disorderly Gordoon," learned that they could reduce children's fears about their hospital experiences by using medical instruments as props (e.g., blowing bubbles through a stethoscope) or performing silly medical procedures that echo real medical procedures (e.g., chocolate milk transfusions). The "red-nose transplant," for example, was created specifically to ease the fears of heart transplant patients at Babies & Children's Hospital.

At every CCU host hospital the medical staff has recognized the healing effect of the CCU—how joy and delight relieve the stress of pediatric patients and their worried parents; how music, magic, and mayhem in the halls make patients easier to treat and enhance the effectiveness of the medical staff; and how a happy child appears to get better faster. Dr. Driscoll, Chairman of Pediatrics at Babies and Children's Hospital of New York, stated in a news article, "When a child begins to laugh, it means he's probably beginning to feel better. I see the clowns as healers. When someone gets around to studying it, I wouldn't be at all surprised to see a connection between programs like the CCU and shorter hospital stays."

In addition to numerous news articles and television features, Michael Christensen and the CCU have received wide public recognition for their innovative work in the field of health and humor, including the prestigious *Raoul Wallenberg Humanitarian Award*, the *Red Skelton Award*, and the Northeast Clown Convention's annual *Gold Nose Award*.

Resident Hospital Programs

The Big Apple Circus currently operates CCU programs in seven prominent metropolitan hospitals: Babies & Children's Hospital of New York at Columbia-Presbyterian Medical Center, Harlem Hospital Center, The Hospital for Special Surgery, Memorial Sloan-Kettering Cancer Center, Mount Sinai Medical Center, New York University Medical Center, and Schneider Children's Hospital of Long Island Jewish Medical Center. Each CCU clown team works under the direct supervision of the hospital's chief of pediatrics.

In addition, the CCU is resident each summer at Queens Hospital Center and Paul Newman's Hole in the Wall Gang Camp for children with cancer and chronic blood diseases.

Working in close partnership with the medical staff at each hospital, the CCU tailors its activities to meet the special needs of each facility. The supervising clown consults daily with nurses, child life staff, and chief residents on the status of individual children. The clown team visits children in all areas of the hospital, including at their bedsides in wards, in intensive care units, and in clinic and acute care waiting rooms. The CCU clowns also visit specialty clinics such as the bone marrow transplant unit at Memorial Sloan-Kettering Cancer Center and the HIV/AIDS clinic at Harlem Hospital.

All CCU clowns are professional performers who have been auditioned and selected for their professionalism, artistry, and sensitivity. They undergo a rigorous CCU training program to prepare them for working safely and appropriately in the hospital environment. The CCU continually improves its level of quality through rehearsals, continuing education, and procedural and artistic reviews.

The CCU has plans to expand to preeminent children's hospitals in major cities throughout the country. Affiliate programs begun by Big Apple Circus CCU-trained performers currently operate in Paris, France; Sao Paulo, Brazil; and Wiesbaden, Germany.

If you would like further information about the CCU, please contact us:

Big Apple Circus Clown Care Unit
35 West 35th Street, 9th Floor
New York, NY 10001
(212) 268-2500

THE GROWING WORLD OF HUMOR

When I first started my humor studies in 1953, there was a vast dearth of scientific investigation of the subject. Literary analyses of humor and comedy abounded, and there was ample hypothesizing and theorizing, particularly about the identity of the crucial element of humor that precipitates the mirthful reaction. Also, a few psychological and anthropological studies had carried out examinations of humor preferences, humor values, interactive uses of humor, communication, and humor; this was as close as we got to science. Mind you, it was not a complete wasteland, but it looked like an Edward Hopper canvas; it certainly was not Times Square at midnight on New Year's Eve.

I had entered the field through the gate of humor and communications, as a member of ethnologist Gregory Bateson's research team. The research team had been originally assembled by Gregory to explore the roles of the "paradoxes of logical type" in communication (Fry, 1971). As a psychiatrist, I was the team member with training most closely related to the so-called hard sciences, with university classes in a large variety of chemistries, physics, embryology, bacteriology, laboratory technology, physiology, and biochemistry. The scientific method had been portrayed to me as the criterion for research purity and rigor.

I did and still do hold the scientific method in high respect. During my psychiatric residency, I had exercised my understanding of scientific discipline by designing, conducting, and reporting in the literature a postdoctoral psychophysiological study of schizophrenia.

In the 1950s a certain excitement had been stirred in the humor studies field by psychologist D.E. Berlyne, a very talented and innovative scholar. Up to the time of his contributions, humor theory was strongly dominated by the views Freud had adopted from philosopher Herbert Spencer's "discharge of energy" postulate (Bainy, 1993). This dominance directed most views of humor to observing it primarily as a cathartic phenomenon, a sudden diminution of repressed psychic energy involving a release from inhibition. Berlyne's contribution shifted emphasis to the state of arousal, which he proposed to be the dominant element of the humor response: "laughter . . . is restricted to situations in which a spell or moment of aversely high arousal is followed by sudden and pronounced arousal reduction" (Berlyne, 1972). Needless to say, this attempt to supplant Freud's doctrine aroused much controversy and energy. Some of the energy was channeled into research procedures aimed at proving or disproving one or another of the main themes and their various corollaries. As these experiments proceeded and were reported in the scientific literature, I became increasingly distressed by what I perceived as defective protocols, in that much of the test ratings were based on subjective and vaguely defined and arbitrary criteria; in many instances, test results were measured by degrees of humor identified as "much," "moderate," or "slight," or by some similar system. I believed that conclusions based on these studies were flawed by deficiencies of objectivity. I agonized over this scientific design issue for many months, even several years into the 1960s.

I finally came to the conclusion that the best readily available source of objectivity in humor experimentation would be the physiological phenomena that both the Freudians and the Berlynians agreed accompany the perception of humor and the experiencing of reactive mirth. A National Institutes of Mental Health Small Grant in 1963-1964 made it possible for me to develop an answer to the question of whether it is possible to observe experimentally the somewhat ephemeral physiology of mirth in such artificial and rigid environments as those that often develop in scientific pursuits (when the fun of science is lost sight of or is ignored). The outcome of my feasibility exploration was "certainly yes," and after wasting months during the Vietnam War buildup futilely trying to obtain financial support from government scientific agencies (when armaments had so much greater priority than laughter), I got to work on designing and carrying out a series of basic science studies of the physiology of mirth and laughter. That research program continued during the following approximately 15 years.

I am (I hope not immodestly) proud that I and my colleagues in those studies were able to perform contributive research in most of the human body's major physiology system areas (Fry, 1994). We have been able to demonstrate significant impacts of mirth and mirthful laughter in the cardiovascular, respiratory, muscular, immune, endocrine, and central nervous systems. With that basic science information being established and disseminated, many other professional persons subsequently have found it possible and desirable to extend their speculations and practice outside spheres of scholarly study into many directions, much of it relating to health issues, both in prevention of disease and in uses of humor as adjunctive therapy to traditional treatment procedures.

During the years in which I was absorbed in that research adventure (the 1960s, 1970s, and early 1980s), several other themes and ventures were forming, developing, building, expanding, and arousing the interest and participation of more and more persons throughout North America, in the United Kingdom, and to a certain extent in Europe, especially in France, The Netherlands, and Belgium. This process was a vital component of a truly revolutionary movement throughout the world. The worldwide movement has been designated by several different titles, depending on the specific location or years being designated. Broader titles identify this movement as a modern renaissance, a new style of life, and the Deconstruction era; more specific titles designate the Hippy Revolution, the Free Speech Movement, and an overturning of old values. The period for awhile was named The Age of Aquarius. Other, less enthusiastic designations characterize the new era as being a time of Satan's dominance over humankind or an ascendancy of evil and libertine practices. Whatever the values ascribed, there is little argument over the presence of new beliefs and values and social practices, over the revolutions of social customs, garb, artistic expression, communication, lifestyles, music, interpersonal interactions of many varieties, and religious practices. This revolution undoubtedly was built on the shoulders of earlier times, as is the way of the world. However, this was a watershed era, a parametric cultural shift.

Tons of paper and miles of words have been exchanged during the past 35 years regarding this parametric revolution. Discussion of the underlying implications, dealing with issues of the past and future of humanity, is beyond the scope of this contribution. Suffice it to say that a vast proportion of the revolutionary changes has been associated with what can be called the "pragmatics" of human life and human behavior. Changes brought during these turbulent years have been more in the everyday ways of humans, less so in consideration of the many and deep implications of the turbulence and its innovative consequences. To be sure, these implications have received some attention, but to large extent in the more traditional manner of analysis and consideration. The changes of lifestyle and performance have been huge and have been little inhibited by the paucity of reflective attention turned toward them. There has been much change in daily ways of life, but not only in so-called developed cultures; the revolution has been universal over the globe, with varied intensities and varied specifics of behavior.

Returning to the issues of humor in health care, it is apparent that a part of the revolution has been a process of reshaping the pragmatics of health care, making it possible to consider many new features of health care, including interrelationships between health care and humor, wherein humor takes adjunctive roles such as cited previously. Underlying the pragmatics that predominate with this mutation is new emphasis on the principle of one's personal responsibility for one's own health care (Cousins, 1979). More so than many other products of the revolutionary era, this issue of health care responsibility received more and more attention during the 1970s and 1980s. With this expanding orientation and under the title of holistic medicine, implementation of adjunctive roles in healing and health care for humor, as well as many other alternative, complementary, and integrative nontraditional medical practices, became not only possible but realized. Many uses of the opportunity for using humor and mirthful laughter have been instituted and operated

successfully. Physician Patch Adams is one of the luminous pioneers in this humor movement. The movement is spread throughout areas of the world where humans attempt to improve the quality of their lives, both in health and at times of disease.

The nature of many humor–health care innovations is such that adjunctive use of humor, mirth, and laughter is having increasingly interesting application. Facilities have been established in hospitals, convalescent homes, day care centers, long-term care units, and rehabilitation centers in which sources of humor are made available. This availability is usually intended primarily for the patient or resident, but this practice has also brought forth recognition that benefits of humor can be experienced by others in the broader health care environment. As studies have demonstrated, staff members, patients' family members, volunteers, and community contacts all have benefited by having humor "tonics" available at times when they are beset by the various "negative emotions" so common in such circumstances. Patient benefits are demonstrated to come doubly, both from direct impact and from the energizing and positive effects on those who are participating with the patient in his or her struggle for return to or maintenance of health. It has been indicative of this "double value" that much of the encouragement for humor facility establishment in health care institutions has come from nursing staffs, who experience the greater degree of patient-provider interaction, both in terms of quantity and intensity.

This use of humor in health care facilities as adjunctive therapy to other, more traditional medical procedures and practices does not stand alone in the new orientation about humor in health care. A rising enthusiasm for humor in wider use, beyond institutional use and beyond the age-old popularity of humor as an important source of entertainment and amusement, is fueling spread of humor forms among populations throughout the world (Berger, 1993). This enthusiasm has broken down many of the customary prejudices against humor, which have previously characterized humor as frivolous, unimportant, or vulgar and reprehensible. People have shaken the sense of guilt or shame or flippancy that earlier restricted their access to their natural, genetically inculcated sense of humor (Morreall, 1983). Individuals in their inner lives, in their relationships with family members, in the workplace, and in their public activities increasingly avail themselves of this element of their biological inheritance for enriching their existence and for making unexpected discoveries about the complexities of life (Blumenfeld and Alpern, 1994; Klein, 1989). Workshops, seminars, lectures, and discussion groups throughout the world explore new and beneficial values of humor and laughter for leading healthful lives, for helping patients recover from illness, and for helping patients maintain higher quality of life during illness. Humor has even been admitted into the quiet privacy of psychotherapy and counseling (Fry and Salameh, 1993).

Humor continues to be a major source of entertainment, a major component of the array of pleasures to be enjoyed in this world. All evidence indicates sturdy continuation of that status. Humor and laughter, with new knowledge and new attitudes about their values and benefits, now increasingly spread their magic into areas of human experience not previously visualized as appropriate places for their presence.

LAUGHING SPIRIT LISTENING CIRCLES

The potential for healing laughter bubbles deep within us like natural hot springs. It just is. For me, humor therapy is about providing the safe space that allows us to erupt in our uniquely unpredictable, often socially unacceptable way, fluidly carrying warm chuckles, hot guffaws, and tender tears to the places within and without that serve our body, our soul, and our community.

The laughter that is the best medicine is that which lies beneath seriousness and respects gravity, sadness, fear, frustration, and anger. It is not the surface, over-the-counter, diluted gigglery we call "lightening up."

Robust tears are no less potent than lusty laughter, and when "lightening up" is even slightly more valued over "getting heavy," therapy is dead and community is crippled.

I practice humor therapy in a form I call *laughing spirit listening circles*. Each participant in a group of 6 to 10 gets equal time to receive absolute positive, silent attention, first for 3 minutes, then for 5 minutes. The guidelines are "dare to be boring." You do not even have to speak. When you do, just tell the truth without trying to be funny. Stay in connection with individuals when you speak. *Receive* your support, rather

than trying to give. The first time around is often serious, even grave, as people feel the safety and respect and build the integrity of the community. By the second time around, laughter and tears often flow, sometimes interchangeably.

THREE MYTHS ABOUT LAUGHTER THAT KEEP US FROM LAUGHING

The first major myth about laughter that prevents us from laughing as much as we need to is that "we must have a reason to laugh." The people who respond to my opening laughter with great seriousness at my workshops may feel that there is no reason for me to be laughing, or if there is, they missed it. Not only must we have a reason to laugh, according to this myth, but the reason must be so good that when someone challenges us with "Why are you laughing? What's so funny?" when we explain it, they too will laugh. If they do not laugh, very often we are presented with a puzzled face and a remark, such as, "That was it? Boy, do you have a weird sense of humor!"

Many of us unconsciously censor our laughter because at some level we think our reason for laughing is not good enough. It is important to note here that the reality is that laughter is unreasonable, illogical, and irrational. I propose that we do not need a reason to laugh. When we see a 6-month-old baby laughing, we do not demand, "What's so funny?" but rather delight in the response and often join in. We can do so with adults. Insisting on a reason to laugh is an excellent way of stopping someone, or ourselves, from laughing. This is important to remember when we are in situations in which laughter is inappropriate. We may want to ask ourselves, "Why am I laughing right now?" so that we can stop, for example, if you get the giggles when pulled over by a policeman for speeding or some other infraction of the law.

The *second major myth* about laughter is that "we laugh because we are happy," when the reality is we are happy because we laugh. I ask my groups how many feel better after they have laughed, and there is always a unanimous show of hands. At this point I remark that if laughter came out of happiness, we would not feel better after laughing—we would have already felt better before laughing.

I think that laughter has been assigned the job of indicating happiness because we have been so desperate for some outward sign of this vague, undefined, but treasured state. Actually, most people (I am certainly one of them) do not know what happiness is. We know that the Declaration of Independence mandates us to pursue it, but judging by our national behavior, we are somewhat confused about where happiness lies. If we feel better after we laugh, laughter must come from a source other than happiness.

Those of us who have laughed until we have cried know that in the middle of the process, we cannot tell which is which. We do not laugh because we are happy and cry because we are sad; we laugh or cry because we have tension, stress, or pain. Laughter and tears rebalance the chemicals our bodies create when these distressed states are present, so we feel better after we have laughed or cried.

The *third major myth* is that "a sense of humor is the same thing as laughter." I suggest that even though the two terms are used interchangeably, they are very different processes. The reality is that you do not need a sense of humor to laugh. Again, when we see a 6-month-old baby laughing, we do not remark, "Doesn't that baby have a wonderful sense of humor!" A sense of humor is learned; laughter is innate. A sense of humor is an intellectual process, whereas laughter spontaneously engages every major system in the body.

There is absolutely no agreement on what a sense of humor is or what makes something funny. Senses of humor vary according to culture, age, ethnic or economic background, race, gender, and so on. I remarked to one of my groups that women in the ladies' room laugh at different things than men in the men's room. A man raised his hand and said, "Men don't laugh in the men's room." I didn't realize this, having spent very little time in the men's room. (Later on, a man came up to me and said he knew why men didn't laugh in the men's room. . . . It is hard to laugh and aim at the same time.)

A sense of humor does not guarantee laughter in the person to whom we give that designation. Many people with great senses of humor do not laugh. Groucho Marx was known to have laughed only once, publicly or privately. Often, people who make other people laugh do so because they can control when the laughter will occur. The emphasis on humor diverts us from the broad scope of laughter that is available, making laughter a specialty that is then possible only occasionally.

A DEFINITION OF HUMOR

A clear understanding of what constitutes humor and what does not, as listed next, is a necessary starting point to prevent the inevitable misunderstandings that arise when the subject is considered.

1. Humor is *not* the equivalent of laughter. Humor may or may not stimulate laughter; sometimes it is merely a quiet smile or even an inner glow of delight. Laughter may accompany humor, but it also accompanies aggression, surprise, and even grief.
2. Joking makes up a minor percentage of humor experience. Only about 4% of the adult population admit to remembering and telling jokes well, whereas more than 90% consider that they "have a pretty dog-gone good sense of humor." Humor is conveyed between persons much more nonverbally, such as in the eye twinkle and the smile.
3. Humor is not a form of therapy. It is a perspective and an appropriate behavior integrated in the overall conduct of our lives.
4. Humor does *not* cure cancer, baldness, or major depression. Humor is a marvelous adjunct to the overall conduct of one's psychological life, especially when confronting illness, tragedy, or death.
5. Although the observational evidence is intriguing, humor as yet has *not* been demonstrated conclusively to release endorphins. ("Endorphins": Small children without parents who live in the house all the time.)

Humor is a mature psychological response to stress in which the stressful issue is maintained in conscious, without distortion, and is responded to with amusement when double meanings, ironies, or some other inconsistency is noted. Humor does not increase the discomfort of the individual nor those in his company.

Until the 1970s, humor was looked down on in the conduct of medicine as being unprofessional or uncaring or even as beneath the standard of care. Such an attitude was in response to immature psychological defenses masquerading as humor (e.g., passive aggression, schizoid fantasy, projection).

Applying humor with kindness, compassion, and empathy is the key. For the most part, humor in medical practice should take the form of gentle amusement, twinkling eye contact, and only in the rarest situations, jokes.

The following is a short listing of specific guides to the conduct of humor (Hageseth, 1988).

- Five mature ego mechanisms of defense (after Vaillant):
  1. Altruism
  2. Humor
  3. Anticipation
  4. Suppression
  5. Sublimation
- Three pathways to a humor experience (Hageseth):
  1. Nonverbal interactive (e.g., smiling, eye twinkle)
  2. Stimulation of forbidden subjects
  3. Jokes and other forms of verbal humor
- Four elements to successful communication of humor:
  1. Relationship
  2. Rapport
  3. Setting
  4. Timing

THE LAUGH MOBILE PROGRAM

Carolina Health and Humor Association is an educational service organization dedicated to promoting humor in health care and for personal growth. As founder and executive director, I started the Duke Humor Project with the department of Duke Oncology Recreation Therapy in 1986. At Duke University Medical Center in Durham, North Carolina, oncology patients may come for as long as 6 weeks for various cancer treatments. One difficulty with recreational programming is that patients must feel well enough to attend a group craft or entertainment program. Often the patient is too ill to leave the room during the intensive treatments. The Laugh Mobile was created to bring humorous media bedside to these patients. Volunteers from Carolina Health and Humor Association use the Laugh Mobile to deliver bedside laughs and to initiate a *humor intervention*. A humor intervention may be described as a plan to promote joy and laughter in the treatment program for patient care.

The Duke Humor Project continues to bring joy bedside to cancer patients at Duke Medical Center. The Laugh Mobile delivers humorous media bedside to patients and family twice weekly. Humor volunteers engage in yo-yo demonstrations, guitar playing, and practical jokes. For example, the patient may want to set up a "whoopee cushion" under the covers of his or her bed and then invite the doctor "to have a seat and take a load off." Water guns are also dispensed to allow the patient a way to fight back. It is all in the interest of building fun-loving relationships, and the staff is highly receptive to any humor statements from the patient, especially practical jokes.

One of the evolving aspects of the Duke Humor Project and the Laugh Mobile Program is the referral procedure used for targeting the patients. The professional oncology recreation staff attends grand rounds and gathers information about the patients that may be most receptive to humor. Background information is reported in a notebook that goes with the Laugh Mobile. This reports pertinent information on the patient and suggestions for the best approach. For example, the staff may relate that the patient is hard of hearing or that the patient may enjoy learning to juggle scarves. The humor volunteer comes in and sees each patient on referral. A comment by the volunteer reports back to the staff about how the humor intervention worked. This gives the hospital staff an opportunity to follow up between Laugh Mobile visits.

As a designer of humor programs such as the Laugh Mobile Program, I see humor and intentional laughter programs expanding to reach patients in all stages of recovery. I believe that to be effective, I must continue to volunteer with the cancer patients and the Laugh Mobile Program weekly. I am now opening new avenues for spreading the humor programming by the design of programs for bone marrow transplant and cardiac care patients. Each illness seems to have its own set of humorous episodes and strategies. It is my challenge to explore with the patient the areas that need more humor and to suggest funny coping strategies. Perhaps my greatest challenge is continually to seek new ways for the "humor impaired" to laugh and to invite the medical staff to enjoy more playfulness. I am confident that community-based groups such as Carolina Ha Ha, which offers both trained volunteers and professional program implementation, will continue to plant the seeds of comic caring and loving laughter.

IT MAY BE SERIOUS BUT IT NEEDN'T BE SOLEMN

*These healing hot springs of holistic "laughtears" are what
I'm after in humor therapy.
I try to be playful but others won't respond.
If I ever needed humor it is now.
I want to smile and laugh, but that upsets my family.*

—HOSPICE PATIENTS' COMMENTS (AMERICAN JOURNAL
OF HOSPICE CARE, 1990)

A couple of years ago my father-in-law was very ill. Once, when he came home from the hospital, it was his and my mother-in-law's wedding anniversary. I suggested that they invite a few friends over for dinner and I would cook a turkey.

Jimmy managed to get out of bed to join us. He enjoyed the meal, but the strain of feeding himself and the presence of guests were obviously tiring him. Noticing this and knowing that he could not hear very well, my mother-in-law wrote a note and passed it to me to give to him. I read it and got hysterical. She remembered what she just wrote and laughed out loud, too.

The note said, "Happy Anniversary dear. Do you want to go to bed?"

Jimmy read what his wife had written, looked up across the table, and with a twinkle in his eye and a smile on his face slowly said to her, "I would love to dear, but we have company."

It was only a brief moment of levity in his difficult last days, but it was a moment that was long remembered after he was gone.

Looking for humor in the not-so-funny world of serious illness may seem like a disrespectful thing to those who are suffering. However, situational humor, which inevitably arises during stressful times, is very appropriate. Because of humor's ability to give a new perspective to any situation, it is an important coping tool for everyone involved in the dying process, including the physician.

Laughter is a powerful tool in powerless situations. It can give hope and an upper hand to patients, who are experiencing both physical and mental loss, as well as to physicians who cannot change that loss or stop the demise of the patient.

The safest way for a physician to find that laughter is first to establish a rapport with the patient, then look for humor by listening to what the patient jokes about. Above all, do not go into a patient's room with a battery of jokes. First, jokes can be offensive, and second, when you enter a patient's room, you have no knowledge whether they will be receptive to your kidding around. Keep in mind that humor is a wonderful bonding tool, but it can also backfire and create alienation.

My friend, Patty Wooten ("Nancy Nurse"), once told me a story about the time she was bathing a patient who had a rather large surgical scar down her front. The patient said, "Nurse, look at my scar. It looks just like Market Street in San Francisco." Puzzled by this remark, Patty questioned, "What do you mean, 'Market Street in San Francisco?'" "Well," replied the patient, "it goes from Twin Peaks to the waterfront." (Indeed, Market Street in San Francisco does run from Twin Peaks to the waterfront.)

Patty and the patient laughed uproariously together. Then, months later, Patty was bathing another woman who had a similar scar and told her this joke. The patient got highly insulted.

In the first case, humor came from a woman who was comfortable enough to laugh at what she had experienced; the second patient was not.

The best way to find humor when working with seriously ill patients is to listen to what they are saying. The patient is the one who will often give you the laugh lines.

One example comes from a friend of mine who had AIDS for 8 years. One day I walked into Rick's house and found a star of David, a crucifix, and a picture of Buddha on the wall.

"Rick," I said, "you are a Quaker, why do you have these opposing religious items around?" Rick, who never missed a moment for some levity, replied, "Well, you never know who's right. I'm covering all bases!"

Rick was someone with whom I could joke about his illness because he would be the first one to poke fun at his difficulties. Your patients are the ones who will let you know if it is OK to kid around with them, supply you with laughs, and help you see death as less of a grave matter.

HUMOR IN HEALTH CARE

We think of humor as just fun and play—not serious. Yet, it is one of the most healthy, healing phenomena humans have. It is a cognitive, emotional, and physical response to stress. Humor gives us balance and a perspective and provides a comic relief and survival from all the seriousness of living.

Within the health care arena, which is probably one of the most stressful and craziest areas in which we live, humor is a major coping mechanism for patients and staff and a powerful tool for healing. It is the perfect mind-body connection! The humor, verbal or nonverbal, stimulates the feeling of mirth and the laughter, which researchers have found produces a healthy biochemical response in the body.

As an indirect form of communication, humor facilitates all the relationships and manages all the delicate situations that occur. It conveys messages and helps us get in touch with our feelings. And, when we laugh, we release those associated feelings.

Humor reduces all the social conflicts inherent in health care, and it facilitates change and survival in the system. As a major relief mechanism, humor reduces anxiety, provides a healthy outlet for anger and frustration, and is a healthy denial of all the heaviness of crises, tragedy, and death.

Humor is also a major source of coping for the caregiver and for the prevention of burnout. The health professional who can accept and value his or her need for laughter and comedy can then be comfortable using and encouraging humor with clients.

As a communication tool, humor should be an integral part of the total healing/caring process. Humor conveys our concern, understanding, warmth, and caring. As one patient said, when staff laughed and joked with him, he knew they cared.

For the health professional, the key to the therapeutic use of humor is being sensitive to whose needs are being met and being sensitive to the right time, the right place, and the right amount, like a judicious dose of good medicine. And always, it must be used in the context of caring, a laughing *with* and not a laughing "at."

HUMOR—ANTIDOTE FOR STRESS

Humor is a perceptual quality that enables us to experience joy even when faced with adversity. Health professionals work in stress-filled environments that place demands on their physical, emotional, and spiritual well-being (Maslach, 1982). Most caregivers are compassionate and sensitive individuals working with people who are suffering. This too can be a source of stress. Caregivers can experience what is known as *compassion fatigue*—feeling that they have very little left to give (Ritz, 1995). Finding humor in our work and our life can be one way to replenish ourselves from compassion fatigue (Ritz, 1995; Robinson, 1991; Wooten, 1995). This can be an effective self-care tool.

In his book *Stress without Distress*, Selye (1974) clarified that a person's interpretation of stress does not depend solely on an external event, but also on their perception of the event and the meaning they give it; how you look at a situation determines whether you will respond to it as threatening or challenging (Kobassa, 1983). In this context, humor can be an empowerment tool because it gives us a different perspective on our problems, and with an attitude of detachment, we feel a sense of self-protection and control in our environment (Klein, 1989; McGhee, 1994). As comedian Bill Cosby is fond of saying, "If you can laugh at it, you can survive it."

There is a type of humor called "gallows humor" (McGhee, 1994; Robinson, 1991) that is unique to people who deal with tragedy and suffering. Those outside the caregiving professions often do not understand our sometimes desperate need to laugh and may not appreciate this type of humor. The term *gallows humor* supposedly came into being when two brothers were being executed by hanging. Both were standing on the gallows, and one brother was already hanged when the other brother said, "Look at my brother there, making a spectacle of himself. Pretty soon we'll be a pair of spectacles."

This laughing bravado, in the face of death, is what caregivers also use to maintain their sanity amidst the horror. It is well documented that there is more laughter in the intensive care unit (ICU), emergency room, and operating room than in other places in the hospital setting. Much of the humor is sexual, obscene, or jokes directly about the tragedy and suffering (Ritz, 1995; Rosenburg, 1991; Wooten, 1995). This appears to be a psychological game one plays with oneself and others, hoping to communicate: "See, I'm doing okay amidst all this horror. Really. See? I'm laughing!"

An ICU nurse shared with me a sign that the staff had placed in the visitor waiting area to explain what might be overheard and misunderstood (Box 20-1).

We attempt to maintain balance by offsetting tragedy in our lives with comedy. Another true story

BOX 20-1

Laughter in the Intensive Care Unit

If you are waiting . . .
You may possibly see us laughing; or even take
note of some jest;
Know that we are giving your loved one our care at
its very best!
There are times when tension is highest;
There are times when our systems are stressed;
We've discovered humor, a factor in keeping our
sanity blessed.
So, if you're a patient in waiting, or a relative or
friend of one seeing,
Don't hold our smiling against us, it's a way that
we keep from screaming.

Sincerely,
The ICU Staff (anon)

of this cathartic activity was shared by Wayne Johnston, an emergency room nurse:

> You saw me laugh after your father died. . . . To you I must have appeared calloused and uncaring. . . . Please understand, much of the stress health care workers suffer comes about because we do care. Sooner or later we will all laugh at the wrong time. I hope your father would understand, my laugh meant no disrespect, it was a grab at balance. I knew there was another patient who needed my full care and attention . . . my laugh was no less cleansing for me than your tears were for you (Johnston, 1985).

> Laughter can provide a cathartic release, a purifying of emotions, and a release of emotional tension. Laughter, crying, raging, and trembling are all cathartic activities that can unblock energy flow (Goodheart, 1996).

An ability to laugh at our situation or problem gives us a feeling of superiority and power. We are less likely to succumb to feelings of depression had helplessness if we are able to laugh at what is troubling us. Humor gives us a sense of perspective on our problems. Laughter provides an opportunity for the release of uncomfortable emotions, which, if held inside, may create biochemical changes that are harmful to the body.

As the famous American humorist Mark Twain once said:

> Humor is the great thing, the saving thing. Afterall, the moment it arises, all our hardnesses yield, our

irritations and resentments slip away, and a sunny spirit takes their place (Klein, 1989).

References

Bainey M: *Why do we laugh and cry?* West Ryde, Australia, 1993, Sunlight Publications.

Berger AA: *An anatomy of humor,* New Brunswick, NJ, 1993, Transaction Publishers.

Berlyne DE: Humor and its kin. In Goldstein JH, McGhee PE, editors: *The psychology of humor,* New York, 1972, Academic Press.

Blumenfeld E, Alpern L: *Humor at work,* Atlanta, 1994, Peachtree Publishers.

Cassell E: *The nature of suffering,* New York, 1991, Oxford University Press.

Coser RL: Some social functions of laughter: a study of humor in a hospital setting, *Hum Relations* 12:171-182, 1959.

Cousins N: *Anatomy of an illness as perceived by the patient,* New York, 1979, Norton.

Fry WF: Laughter: is it the best medicine? *Stanford MD* 10(1):16-20, 1971 (Stanford Medical Alumni Association).

Fry WF: The biology of humor. *Humor Int J Humor Res* 7(2):111-126, 1994.

Fry WF, Salameh W: *Advances in humor and psychotherapy,* Sarasota, Fla, 1993, Professional Resources Press.

Goodheart A: *Laughter therapy,* Santa Barbara, Calif, 1996, Stress Less Press.

Hageseth CM: *A laughing place,* Ft. Collins, Colo, 1988, Berwick Publishing.

Johnston W: To the ones left behind, *Am J Nurs* 85(8):936, 1985.

Klein A: *Healing power of humor,* Los Angeles, 1989, Tarcher.

Kleinman A: *The illness narratives,* New York, 1988, Basic Books.

Kobassa SC: Personality and social resources in stress resistance, *J Pers Soc Psychol* 45:839, 1983.

Koestler A: *The act of creation,* New York, 1964, Macmillan.

Levi L: The urinary output of adrenaline and noradrenaline during pleasant and unpleasant states, *Psychosom Med* 27:80-85, 1965.

Lloyd EL: The respiratory rate in laughter, *J Gen Psychol* 10:179-189, 1938.

Mahrer A, Gervaize P: An integrative review of strong laughter in psychotherapy: what it is and how it works, *Psychotherapy* 21:510-516, 1974.

Maslach C: *Burnout—the cost of caring,* Upper Saddle River, NJ, 1982, Prentice Hall.

McGhee P: *How to develop your sense of humor,* Dubuque, Iowa, 1994, Kendall-Hunt.

Morreall J: *Taking laughter seriously,* Albany, NY, 1983, State University of New York Press.

Paskind HA: Effect of laughter on muscle tone, *Arch Neurol Psychiatry* 23:623-628, 1932.

Ritz S: Survivor humor and disaster nursing. In Buxman K: *Humor and nursing,* New York, 1995, Von Publishers.

Robinson V: *Humor and the health professions,* ed 2, Thorofare, NJ, 1991, Slack.

Rosenburg L: Clinical articles: a qualitative investigation of the use of humor by emergency personnel as a strategy for coping with stress, *J Emerg Nurs* 17(4), 1991.

Ruxton SP: Humor deserves our attention, *Holistic Nurs Pract* 2(3):54-62, 1988.

Schachter S, Wheeler L: Epinephrine, chlorpromazine, and amusement, *J Abnorm Soc Psychol,* 1962.

Selye H: *Stress without distress,* New York, 1974, Lippincott & Crowell.

Wooten P: Interview with Sandy Ritz, *J Nurs Jocularity* 5(1):46-47, 1995.

Suggested Readings

Ader R, Felten DL, Cohen N, editors: *Psychoneuro-immunology,* ed 2, San Diego, 1991, Academic Press.

Arieti S: New views on the psychology of wit and the comic, *Psychiatry* 13:43-82, 1950.

Averill JR: Autonomic response patterns during sadness and mirth, *Psychophysiology* 5(4):399-414, 1969.

Baron RA, Ball RL: The aggression-inhibition influence of nonhostile humor, *J Exp Soc Psychol* 10:23-33, 1974.

Barra JM: High kicks in the ICU, *RN* 49:45-46, 1986.

Baudelaire C: The essence of laughter. In *Essays,* New York, 1956, Meridian Books.

Bergson H: *Laughter: an essay on the meaning of the comic,* New York, 1911, Macmillan.

Berk LS et al: Modulation of human natural killer cells by catecholamines, *Clin Res* 32(1):1984.

Berk LS et al: Eustress of mirthful laughter modifies natural killer cell activity, *Clin Res* 37(1), 1989.

Berk LS et al: Neuroendocrine and stress hormone changes during mirthful laughter, *Am J Med Sci* 296(7):390-396, 1989.

Berkowitz L: Aggressive humor as a stimulus to aggressive responses, *J Pers Soc Psychol* 16:710-717, 1970.

Beyondananda S: *When you see a sacred cow . . . milk it for all it's worth,* Lower Lake, Calif, 1993, Aslan Publishing.

Bhargava KP: An overview of endorphins' probable role in health and disease. In Dhawan BN, editor: *Current status of centrally acting peptides,* Oxford, 1982, Pergamon.

Blair W: What's funny about doctors, *Perspect Biol Med* 21(1):89-98, 1977.

Bloch S, McGrath G: Humor in group psychotherapy, *Br J Med Psychol* 56:88-97, 1983.

Blumenfeld E, Alpern L: *The smile connection,* Englewood Cliffs, NJ, 1986, Prentice Hall.

Bokun B: *Humour therapy,* London, 1986, Vita Books.

Boston R: *An anatomy of laughter,* London, 1974, Collins.

Brill AA: The mechanism of wit and humor in normal and psychopathic states, *Psychiatr Q* 14:731-749, 1940.

Brody MW: The meaning of laughter, *Psychoanal Q* 19:192-201, 1950.

Burton R: *The anatomy of melancholy,* New York, 1927, Tudor Publishing.

Buxman K: Humor in therapy for the mentally ill, *J Psychol Nurs* 29(12):15-18, 1991.

Byrne DE: The relationship between humor and the expression of hostility, *J Abnorm Soc Psychol* 53:84-89, 1956.

Byrne DE, Terril S, McReynolds P: Incongruence as a predictor of response to humor, *J Abnorm Soc Psychol* 62:435-438, 1961.

Cassell E: *The healer's art,* Boston, 1986, MIT Press.

Cassell J: The function of humor in the counseling process, *Rehabil Counsel* 17:240-245, 1974.

Chapman AJ: An experimental study of socially facilitated humorous laughter, *Psychol Rep* 35:727-734, 1974.

Chapman AJ, Foot HC, editors: *It's a funny thing, humor,* International Conference on Humor and Laughter, Oxford, 1976, Pergamon.

Dana B, Laurence P: *The laughter prescription,* New York, 1982, Ballantine.

Dearbom GVN: The nature of the smile and the laugh, *Science,* 1900.

Dillon KM et al: Positive emotional states and enhancement of the immune system, *Int J Psychiatry Med* 15(1):13-18, 1985-1986.

Domis J, Fierman E: Humor and anxiety, *J Abnorm Soc Psychol* 53:59-62, 1956.

Elliot-Binns CP: Laughter and medicine, *J R Coll Gen Practitioners* 37(277):364-365, 1985.

Erdman L: Laughter therapy for patients with cancer, *Oncol Nurs Forum* 18(8):1359-1363, 1991.

Euck JJ, Forter E, Whitley A, editors: *The comic in theory and practice,* New York, 1960, Appleton-Century-Crofts.

Fairbanks D: *Laugh and live,* New York, 1917, Britton Publishing.

Feibleman J: *In praise of comedy,* New York, 1970, Horizon Press.

Flugel JC: Humor and laughter. In Lindsay G, editor: *Handbook of social psychology,* Cambridge, Mass, 1954, Addison-Wesley.

Freud S: *Jokes and their relationship to the unconscious,* New York, 1964, Norton.

Fry WF Jr: *Sweet madness: a study of humor,* Palo Alto, Calif, 1963, Pacific Books.

Fry WF Jr: *Make 'em laugh,* Palo Alto, Calif, 1975, Science and Behavior Books.

Fry WF Jr: Humor and the cardiovascular system. Paper presented at 2nd International Conference on Humor and Laughter, Los Angeles, August 1979.

Fry WF Jr, Rader C: The respiratory components of mirthful laughter, *J Biol Psychol* 19:39-50, 1977.

Fry WF Jr, Stoft PE: Mirth and oxygen saturation levels of peripheral blood, *Psychother Psychosom* 19:76-84, 1971.

Gaberson KB: The effect of humorous distraction on preoperative anxiety, *AORN J* 54(6):1258-1264, 1991.

Greenwald H: Humor in psychotherapy, *J Contemp Psychother* 7:113-116, 1975.

Grotjahn M: *Beyond laughter,* New York, 1956, McGraw-Hill.

Haller B, Zarai R: *Rire c'est la sante,* Geneva, 1986, Editions Soleil.

Harlow HF: The anatomy of humor, *Impact of Science on Society,* 1969.

Hassett J, Schwartz GE: Why can't people take humor seriously? *New York Times Magazine,* February 1977.

The healing power of laughter and play: uses of humor in the healing arts, PO Box 94305, Portola Valley, Calif, 1983, IAHB (12 tapes).

Herth KA: Laughter: a nursing Rx, *Am J Nurs* 84(8):991-992, 1984.

Heuscher J: The role of humor and folklore themes of psychotherapy, *Am J Psychiatry* 137:1546-1549, 1980.

Holden R: *Laughter is the best medicine,* London, 1993, Thorsons.

Holland N: *Laughing: the psychology of humor,* New York, 1982, Cornell University Press.

Joubert L: *Treatise on laughter,* Birmingham, 1970, University of Alabama Press.

Kaplan H, Boyd I: The social functions of humor on an open psychiatric ward, *Psychiatr Q* 39:502-515, 1965.

Keller D: *Humor as therapy,* Wauwatosa, Wis, 1984, Med-Psych Publications.

Klein A: *The healing power of humor,* Los Angeles, 1989, Tarcher.

Kubie LS: The destructive potential of humor in psychotherapy, *Am J Psychiatry* 127:861-886, 1971.

Lefcourt H, Martin R: *Humor and life stress,* New York, 1986, Springer-Verlag.

Leiber DB: Laughter and humor in critical care, *Dimens Crit Care* 5(3):162-170, 1986.

Levine J: Humor as a form of therapy. In Chapman AJ, Foot HC, editors: *It's a funny thing, humor,* Oxford, 1976, Pergamon Press.

McConnell J: Confessions of a scientific humorist. In *Impact of Science on Society,* 1969.

McGhee P, Goldstein JH, editors: *Handbook of humor research.* Vol 1, *Basic issues;* Vol 2, *Applied studies,* New York, 1983, Springer-Verlag.

McHale M: Getting the joke: interpreting humor in group therapy, *J Psychol Nurs* 27(9):24-28, 1989.

Metcalf CW, Felible R: *Lighten up,* Reading, Mass, 1992, Addison-Wesley.

Mind H: The use and abuse of humor in psychotherapy. In Chapman AJ, Foot HC, editors: *Humor and laughter: theory, research and application,* New York, 1976, Wiley & Sons.

Mindess H: *Laughter and liberation,* Los Angeles, 1971, Nash.

Mindess H: Laughter and humor in medical practice, *Behavioral Medicine,* 1979.

Mindess H et al, editors: *The Antioch humor test,* New York, 1985, Avon.

Moody RA Jr: *Laugh after laugh: the healing power of humor,* Jacksonville, Fla, 1978, Headwaters Press.

Nussbaum K, Michaux WW: Response to humor in depression: a predictor and evaluator of patient change, *Psychiatr Q* 37:527-539, 1963.

O'Connell WE: The adaptive functions of wit and humor, *J Abnorm Soc Psychol* 61:263-270, 1960.

O'Connell WE: Humor and death, *Psychol Rep* 22:391-402, 1968.

Pasquali EA: Learning to laugh: humor as therapy, *J Psychol Nurs* 28(3), 1990.

Pirandello L: *On humor,* Chapel Hill, NC, 1974, University of North Carolina Press.

Poland WS: The place of humor in psychotherapy, *Am J Psychiatry* 28:635-637, 1971.

Potter S: *The sense of humor,* Middlesex, England, 1954, Penguin Books.

Powell BS: Laughter and healing: the use of humor in hospitals treating children, *Assoc Care Child Hosp J* IV:10-16, 1974.

Professional Resource Press, Sarasota, Fla, 1993.

Robinson V: *Humor and health.* In Goldstein JH, McGhee P, editors: *Handbook of humor research,* New York, 1983, Springer-Verlag.

Robinson VM: Humor is a serious business, *Dimens Crit Care* 5(3):132-133, 1986.

Rosenheim E: Humor in psychotherapy: an interactive experience, *Am J Psychother* 28:584-591, 1974.

Samra C: *The joyful chant: the healing power of humor,* San Francisco, 1986, Harper & Row.

Schaller CT: *Rire pour gai-rire,* Geneva, 1994, Editions Vivez Soleil.

Spenser H: The physiology of laughter, *Macmillan's Magazine,* 1860.

Vaillant G: *Empirical studies in ego mechanisms of defense,* Washington, DC, 1986, American Psychiatric Press.

Vaillant G: *The wisdom of the ego,* Cambridge, Mass, 1993, Harvard University Press.

Vergeer G, MacRae A: Therapeutic use of humor in occupational therapy, *Am J Occup Ther* 47(8), 1993.

Williams H: Humor and healing: therapeutic effects in geriatrics, *Gerontion* 1(3):14-17, 1986.

Wooten P, editor: *Heart, humor, and healing,* Mt Shasta, Calif, 1994, Commune-A-Key Publishing.

Zillman D et al: Does humor facilitate coping with physical discomfort? *Motivation Emotion* 17(1), 1993.

Health and Humor Resources: Individuals, Organizations, and Publications

Alan Agins, PhD, Asst Professor of Nursing, University of Virginia, School of Nursing, McLeod Hall, Charlottesville, VA 22903-3395, (804) 924-1647.

Steve Allen, Jr, MD, 8 LeGrand Ct, Ithica, NY 19850, (607) 277-1795, physician lecturer on humor.

Al's Magic Shop, 1012 Vermont Ave, Washington, DC 20005, (202) 789-2800.

Dale Anderson, MD, 2982 West Owasso Blvd, Roseville, MN 55113, (612) 484-5162, physician doing humor programs.

Lee Berk, 11645 Wiley St, Loma Linda, CA 92354, (909) 796-4112, research into biochemistry and physiology of laughter, especailly neuroimmunology.

Steve Bhaerman, "Swami Beyondananda," PO Box 110, Burnet, TX 78611, (512) 756-2791, lectures, workshops, books, tapes.

Michael Christensen, Clown Care Unit, Big Apple Circus, 35 W 35th St, New York, NY 10001, (212) 268-2500, clowns who visit pediatric wards.

Clown Hall of Fame, Museum & Gifts, 212 E Walworth, Delavan, WI 53115, (414) 728-9075.

Eric de Bont, Bont's Adventures in Clown Arts, Pardoestheater, postbus 419, 6800 AK Arnheim, The Netherlands, center for learning clown arts.

Mouton DeGruyter, W DeGruyter Inc, 200 Saw Mill River Road, Hawthorne, NY 10532, publishes humor.

Glenn C Ellenbogen, Wry-Bred Press, Inc, 10 Waterside Plaza, New York, NY 10010, (212) 689-5476, 1985, published directory of humor magazines and organizations in America and Canada.

Fellowship of Merry Christians, Cal Samra, PO Box 895, Portage, MI 49081, network of Christian humorists, publishes *The Joyful Noiseletter*.

Laura Fernandez, Die Clown Doktoren, Klaren Thaler Str 3, 65197 Wiesbaden, Germany, 0611-9490981, clown who created hospital clown units in Germany.

William Fry, 156 Grove St, Nevada City, CA 95959, (916) 265-5125, physician researcher on humor.

Cathy Gibbons, Fun Technicians, PO Box 160, Syracuse, NY 13215, (315) 492-4523, fax 469-1392, *Laughmaker's Magazine*.

Leslie Gibson, RN, The Comedy Connection, 323 Jeffords St, Clearwater, FL 34617, (813) 462-7842, lectures and creates hospital humor carts.

Lee Glickstein, Center for the Laughing Spirit, 288 Juanita Way, San Francisco, CA 94127, (415) 731-6640.

Art Gliner, Humor Communications, 8902 Maine Ave, Silver Spring, MD 20910, (301) 588-3561, lectures and workshops.

Annette Goodheart, PO Box 40297, Santa Barbara, CA 93103, (605) 966-4725, laughter therapist, lectures and workshops.

Joel Goodman, The Humor Project, 179 Spring St, Box L, Saratoga Springs, NY 12866, quarterly newsletter *Laughing Matters*, lectures, workshops, and annual humor conference.

Christian Hageseth, MD, 1113 Stoneyhill Dr, Ft Collins, CO 80525, psychotherapist doing humor programs.

Ruth Hamilton, Carolina Health and Humor Association, 5223 Revere Road, Durham, NC 27713, (919) 544-2370, newsletter and workshops.

International Humor Institute, 32362 Saddle Mt Road, Westlake Village, CA 91361, (818) 879-9085.

International Laughter Society, 16000 Glen Una Dr, Los Gatos, CA 95030, (408) 354-3456.

Steve Kissel, 1227 Manchester Ave, Norfolk, VA 23508-1122, (804) 423-3867.

Alan Klein, *The Whole Mirth Catalog*, 1034 Page St, San Francisco, CA 94117, catalog of books and toys.

Karen Lee, The Laughter Prescription, 7720 El Camino Real B-225, Carlsbad, CA 92009, (800) RxHUMOR.

Paul McGhee, The Laughter Remedy, 380 Claremont Ave, Montclair, NJ 07042, (201) 783-8383, researcher and lecturer.

CW Metcalf, The Humor Option, 2801 S Remington, Suite 2, Ft Collins, CO 80525, (303) 226-0610, workshops and presentations on humor.

Jeff Moore, Orthopedic Coordinator, Physical Medicine, Saint Paul Medical Center, 5909 Harry Hines Blvd, Dallas, TX 75235, (214) 879-3848, entertains patients.

Jim Pelley, Laughter Works, PO Box 1076, Fair Oaks, CA 95628, (916) 863-1593, workshops and newsletter.

Dr Karen Peterson, 1320 S Dixie Hwy, Coral Gables, FL 33146, (305) 662-2654.

Caroline Simonds, Le Rire Medecin, 75 Ave Parmenitier, 7509 Paris, France, 42-58-39-91, French version of clown care units.

Dhyan Sutorius, MD, Secretariat of the Center In Favor of Laughter, Jupiter, 1008, NL-1115 TX, Duivendrecht, Holland, 31-0-20-690028.

Christian tal Schaller, 15 Francois Jacquier CH1235 Chene-Bourg, Geneva.

Tumor Humor, Uniquest, PO Box 97391, Raleigh, NC 27624.

Lex Van Someren, Batstangveien 81, 3200 Sandefjord Norway, 034-59644, "The Mystic Clown," teacher of workshops.

Joan White, Joygerms, PO Box 219, Syracuse, NY 13206, (315) 472-2779, spreader of good cheer, resources.

Patty Wooten, RN, "Nancy Nurse," PO Box 4040, Davis, CA 95617, (916) 758-3826, author of *Humor, Heart & Healing*.

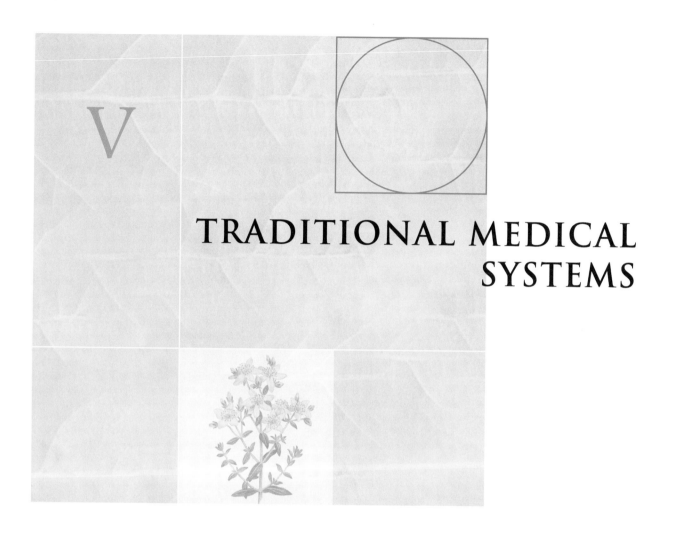

V

TRADITIONAL MEDICAL SYSTEMS

T his section provides a survey of the fundamentals of global health traditions that form integrated systems of thought and practice, following from an explanation of their relevant world views. Although this book aims to present a unified body of the theories and practices of alternatives, many healing traditions throughout the world are marked by significant heterogeneity, consistent with their historical evolution and their underlying philosophies. ∾

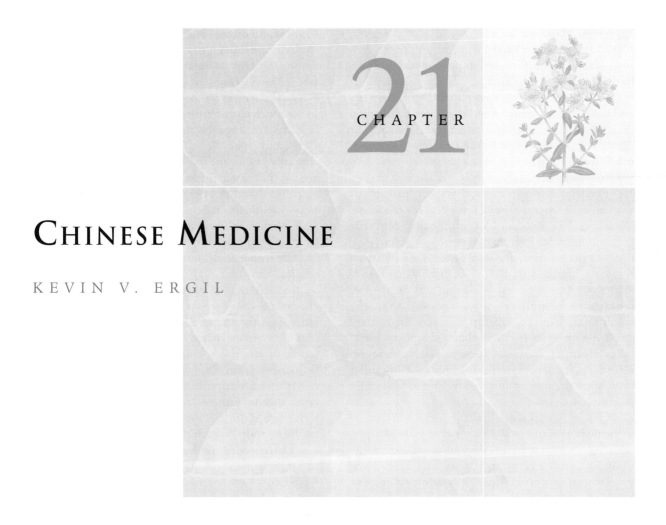

CHAPTER 21

CHINESE MEDICINE

KEVIN V. ERGIL

CHINA'S TRADITIONAL MEDICINE IN CULTURAL PERSPECTIVE

Certain considerations are important to understanding ethnomedical systems in general and Chinese medicine in particular. Medicine is a human endeavor and as such is shaped by the considerations of the humans using and practicing it. These considerations sometimes have very little to do with curing disease in the most simple and efficient way and a great deal to do with economics, politics, and culture. Ideology, belief, and even simple ignorance have influenced the practice of medicine more than rationality. A medical historian or a physician might perceive medicine to be a steady march from ignorance to the light, but these are typically revisionist histories. Medicine is a

human enterprise embedded in and intersected by myriad other human projects. Even the choice of how to conduct a medical procedure or what type of health care to choose may have more to do with habit or economics than with rationality or efficacy.

For example, American gynecologists position their patients for maximum visual exposure during routine examinations, whereas physicians in the United Kingdom allow the patient to lie on her side, assuming a more relaxed posture during the examination (Payer, 1988). An example more relevant to this chapter is the case of a Chinese patient choosing traditional herbal medicine to manage painful and debilitating kidney stones. Although the treatment was ultimately efficacious, the patient's choice was not motivated by a desire for efficacy. Undergoing surgery would have meant that the patient would have been classified as an "invalid" on the work papers and therefore barred from advancement. As a final example, a hospital in California closes its doors to the practice of acupuncture, even though acupuncturists in the state are licensed medical practitioners and their services are routinely requested by hospital patients. In each instance, considerations that are not directly linked to the rational and effective delivery of medical care influence medical choices.

Our own perspectives on medicine and our experience of our own medical systems provide us with ideas of what is normal or typical for medicine. We respond to aspects of a traditional system that correspond with our expectations. We imagine Chinese herbal medicine as a gentle therapy using nontoxic ingredients. Its use of highly toxic substances or drastic purgative therapies is easily overlooked. It is unlikely, for example, that the traditional form of Tibetan therapeutic cautery applied with a hot iron will elicit substantial interest as a form of alternative therapy. Naturalistic and rational elements of systems intrigue us. Unfamiliar or magical diagnostic and therapeutic modes cause us concern.

It is easy to make intellectual errors when dealing with medical systems. We forget that our own perspectives may prevent us from understanding the meaning and use of practices that have been developed within another culture. That failure to account for our own needs and biases also can lead to the overenthusiastic acceptance of ideas whose genesis and application we really do not understand.

If we want to avoid these errors, we must think about medical systems as being embedded in their respective cultures. Each system's structure and elements are vital to their practice in a particular cultural context. "Culture," in this sense, does not imply an all-embracing system of meaning subscribed to by all members of a community, country, or ethnicity. Culture is a complex network of signification, elements of which might resonate only in a local sense, whereas other aspects have almost global relevance. This does not mean that the medical ideas and practices of one society cannot or will not be successfully appropriated by another, but rather that aspects of a system that are meaningful to one group of people might not be meaningful at all to another.

For example, the concept of neurasthenia *(sheng jin shuai ruo)* is an important syndrome in traditional Chinese medicine and Chinese psychiatry, even though this diagnosis has fallen into disrepute among Western psychiatrists and is no longer classified as a disease entity in diagnostic manuals. Neurasthenia was an exceptionally popular diagnosis in the nineteenth century during periods of extensive medical exchange between the United States and China and Japan. The diagnosis has continued to be clinically important in China because it fits well into certain traditional medical models and responds well to cultural and political concerns about mental illness (Kleinman, 1986). Americans and Europeans who encounter neurasthenia within the corpus of Chinese medicine sometimes find it an unusual or obscure concept despite its relevance for Chinese medical practice.

Sometimes, on encountering a new idea, we choose to think about it in familiar terms. One example is the use of the word *energy* to express the idea of qi. An extension of this is the frequent translation of the therapeutic method of draining evil influences from channels as "sedation." Neither energy nor sedation has much to do with the concepts that underlie qi and draining; however, these terms are more familiar to us and make Chinese medicine more accessible. Unfortunately, this practice can obscure the breadth of meaning in these terms (Wiseman and Boss, 1990).

We try to make sense of the world from our position in it, historically as well as culturally. We tend to view history as progressing, as if by design, to a specific end. Events of the past, viewed from the perspective of the present, offer tempting opportunities for reinterpretation in relation to current experience. For example, in the context of current perspectives on disease causation, Wu You Ke's statements that "miscellaneous qi" could cause epidemic disease and his concept of "one disease, one qi" (Wiseman, 1993) have led contemporary sources in China to suggest that coming before the invention of the microscope, such an insight is quite remarkable (Wiseman et al., 1995). The implication that Wu You Ke's observation represented a precursor of germ theory is attractive to Chinese practitioners who are trying to find a place for traditional practices in an increasingly biomedicalized world. In fact, the concept of miscellaneous or pestilential qi has been used extensively in adapting traditional theory to the management of human immunodeficiency virus (HIV) infection. However, as Wiseman points out, it never was explored in relation to the causation of disease by microscopic organisms, nor was it ever conceived as a basis for such an exploration. Its relation to the concept is a retrospective interpretation.

The preceding points are generally relevant to almost any system or collection of medical practices. Some additional points are crucial to understanding the progression of medical thought in China. Although we tend to think that Chinese medicine has been practiced without significant change for millennia, this is simply not true. Chinese medicine has undergone significant change and development over the centuries. Ideas that once were important are now almost invisible, and ideas that were left by the wayside for centuries found favor in later times. Recent ideas have been relatively significant in the organization of the system. Changes in technology, for example, have broadened the clinical use of acupuncture and increased its safety. Ideas, substances, and medical practices have come to China from all over the world, some of which have become significant parts of traditional Chinese medicine, and some of which remain only as observations in ancient texts.

Within China itself, many competing ideas have existed side-by-side. Old theories have been rejected or discovered anew and accorded even more importance than they had at their conception. Some ideas found more fertile ground in other Asian countries, as with the transmission of acupuncture and Chinese herbal medicine to Japan, where particular aspects of the Chinese tradition were emphasized and adapted.

Historian and anthropologist Paul Unschuld critiques the perspective of Chinese medicine as a homogenous monolithic structure, as follows:

> Proponents of this view depict "Chinese Medicine" as an identifiable, coherent system, the contents of which they attempt to characterize. Such an approach is both ahistorical and selective. It focuses on but one of the many distinctly conceptualized systems of therapy in Chinese history, that is the medicine of systematic correspondence, and it neglects both the changing interpretations of basic paradigms offered by Chinese authors through the ages and the synchronic plurality of differing opinions and ideas that existed for twenty centuries concerning even fundamental aspects of this therapy system such as pulse-diagnosis (Unschuld, 1985).

This is a particularly important point, because it is extremely tempting to encounter medical systems with the expectation that they be possessed of an internal logic that reconciles all their aspects. Although many aspects of Chinese medicine can be applied with complete consistency, other aspects or concepts seem to be quite contradictory. This trait leads us to what has been probably the most important aspect of Chinese medicine throughout its history: it is a medical tradition that never threw anything away. Certain medical practices might have been relegated to the attic, but they were available if necessary. A striking example of this is the work of Zhang Zhong Jing, whose system of diagnosis and therapy did not attract much attention during his lifetime but became highly influential centuries after his death. Later, authors believed his theory to be incomplete and broadened its perspective, but his theories and these new theories that emerged in response to them are still important to the contemporary clinician. In the West an incomplete theory is rejected and disappears. In the history of Chinese medicine, theories, practices, and concepts may fade, but they do not entirely disappear. A new theory can exist beside the one that it sought to correct. Clinicians can choose to apply the perspective that they believe is most applicable. In this way, conflicting concepts of cause, systems of diagnosis, and treatment have continued to exist side-by-side.

Unschuld considers this one of the basic characteristics distinguishing traditional Chinese thought from modern Western science (Unschuld, 1985). It also is the aspect of Chinese medicine that is most challenging to Western students. The extent to which deductive reasoning and its necessary condition of "either this or that but not both" are pervasive in our society have made it difficult to approach a medical tradition that dispenses with what we view as a necessary precondition of valid human knowledge. Even European or American advocates of Chinese medical traditions sometimes err and insist that only certain theoretical perspectives or therapeutic methods are correct or authentic.

Years earlier, Lin Yutang wrote that systematic metaphysics or epistemology were alien to traditional Chinese thought, as follows:

> The temperament for systematic philosophy simply wasn't there, and will not be there so long as the Chinese remain Chinese. They have too much sense for that. The sea of human life forever laps upon

the shores of Chinese thought, and the arrogance and absurdities of the logician, the assumption that "I am exclusively right and you are exclusively wrong," are not Chinese faults, whatever other faults they may have (Lin, 1942).

The history of Chinese medical thought also includes many individuals who thought that they were exclusively right. However, the breadth of traditional Chinese medical thought was sustained by an intellectual climate that retained all possible ideas for use and exploration. A given philosopher or clinician might reject an idea, but the idea itself would remain available for future use.

For example, during the Ming dynasty, Wu You Ke (circa 1644) was the leading exponent of the "offensive precipitation sect" *(gong xia pai)* of physicians whose tenets included a distinctive set of ideas concerning the management of epidemic disease and a wholehearted rejection of many established ideas in Chinese medicine (Wong and Wu, 1985). He was subsequently viewed alternatively as a contributor to Chinese medical thought, a proponent of a divergent and uninformed theory, and finally (as noted previously) as the intellectual antecedent of Koch, the discoverer of the tuberculosis bacillus. At no point were his ideas discarded.

Interestingly, in modern China, where the sheer volume of information and the nation's health care needs makes it necessary to teach a standard curriculum to thousands of students each year, this tolerance for varying clinical perspectives continues. For example, certain herbal physicians are known as Minor Bupleurum Decoction *(Xiao Chai Hu Tang)* doctors because their prescriptions are organized around one formula from the *Treatise on Cold Damage (Shang Han Lun)*, an early text on diagnosis and herbal therapy written during the Han dynasty (206 BCE-220 CE). Also, some herbal physicians reject traditional formulas entirely and use contemporary perspectives on the Chinese pharmacopeia to organize their prescriptions.

Some acupuncturists may have a clinical focus dedicated almost entirely to six acupuncture points and may use computed tomography scans to plan clinical interventions. At the same time, two floors down in the same hospital, physicians base their selection of acupuncture points on obscure and complex aspects of traditional calendrics and systems such as the "Magic Turtle."

Once it is understood that Chinese medicine is a large and varied tradition with many manifestations and philosophies, it is possible to begin its exploration.

HISTORY

Chinese medicine has an extensive history. As with most medical traditions, this history can be approached from several perspectives. There is the ancient mythology of Chinese medicine, which attributes the birth of medicine to the legendary emperors Fu Xi, Shen Nong, and Huang Di. There is the history that can be deduced from the careful study of available ancient texts and records, which indicate, for example, that there is no reference to acupuncture as a therapeutic method in any Chinese text before 90 BCE, and that the oldest existing text to discuss medical practices resembling current Chinese medicine dates from the end of the third century BCE (Unschuld, 1985). Finally, there are the more extravagant interpretations of archaeological evidence and textual materials that seek to establish the ancient character of certain Chinese medical practices. An example is the frequent assertion that the stone "needles" excavated at different times in various parts of China were remnants of ancient acupuncture (Chuang, 1982; Wang, 1986). This assertion is based on references to the ancient surgical application of sharp stones in texts from later periods and morphological similarities between the excavated stones and later metal needles.

Legendary Origins

The origins of Chinese medicine are mythically linked to three legendary emperors: Fu Xi, Sheng Nong, and Huang Di. Fu Xi, or the Ox Tamer (ca 2953 BCE), taught people how to domesticate animals and divined the *Ba Gua*, eight symbols that became the basis for the *Yi Jing*, or *Book of Changes*.

Shen Nong, or the Divine Husbandman, also known as the Fire Emperor, is said to have lived from 2838 to 2698 BCE and is considered the founder of agriculture in China. He taught the Chinese people how to cultivate plants and raise livestock. He also is considered the originator of herbal medicine in China, having learned the therapeutic properties of herbs and substances by tasting them. Later authors would attribute their work to Shen Nong to indicate the antiquity and importance of their text. The *Divine Husbandman's Classic of the Materia Medica (Shen Nong Ben Cao Jing)* is a case in point. The text probably was written in 220 CE and reconstructed in 500 CE by Tao

Hong Jing. Given that all historical evidence points to the ancient character of herbal medicine in China, it is appropriate that Shen Nong is considered its originator (Figure 21-1).

Huang Di, the Yellow Emperor (2698-2598), is known as the originator of the traditional medicine of China. He also is seen as the "Father of the Chinese Nation." He is credited with teaching the Chinese how to make wooden houses, silk cloth, boats, carts, the bow and arrow, ceramics, and the art of writing. Legend has it that he gained his knowledge from visiting the immortals. Most important to this discussion is his work *Yellow Emperor's Inner Classic (Huang Di Nei Jing)*, in which the traditional medicine of China is first expressed in a form that is familiar to us today. The text is divided into two books. *Simple Questions (Su Wen)* is concerned with medical theory, such as the principles of yin and yang, the five phases, and the effects of seasons. The *Spiritual Axis (Ling Shu)* deals predominantly with acupuncture and moxibustion. The texts are written as a series of dialogues between the Emperor and his ministers. Qi Bo, the most famous among the ministers, is said to have tested the actions of drugs, cured people's sickness, and written books on medicine and therapeutics.

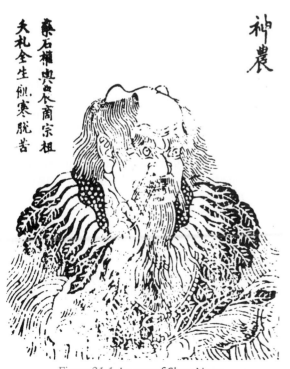

Figure 21-1 Image of Shen Nong.

QI BO EXPLAINS THE ORDERLY LIFE OF TIMES PAST

The first book of *Simple Questions* begins with the Yellow Emperor asking Qi Bo why peoples' life spans are now so short when in the past they lived close to a hundred years. Qi Bo explains that in the past people maintained an orderly life. "In ancient times those people who understood Dao patterned themselves upon the yin and the yang and they lived in harmony with the arts of divination" (Veith, 1972).

It is generally agreed now that the *Yellow Emperor's Inner Classic* was first compiled around 200 BCE. Both in terms of legend and practice, it remains a text that is critical to Chinese medicine.

Ancient Medicine: 2205 to 206 BCE

Little is actually known about the practice of medicine in China before 200 BCE. The Shang dynasty (1766-1121 BCE) is the first dynasty of which there exists clear archaeological evidence. It appears likely that before the Shang, nomadic cultures were scattered across Northern China. Interaction among these groups eventually led to the development of the Shang. This dynasty left the first traces of some form of therapeutic activity. In addition to developing the first Chinese scripts, the Shang had clearly defined social relations. There was a king and nobility, and perhaps most importantly, the people were no longer nomadic.

The Shang response to illness is documented by archaeological finds and writings from the succeeding Zhou dynasty (1122-221 BCE). During this period, ideas developed that would be central to Chinese culture; specifically, a relationship between the living and the dead developed into a ritualized veneration of ancestors. Ancestors could be consulted concerning a variety of issues, including the cause of illness, through the use of oracle bones. Tortoise shells and the scapula of oxen were heated and rapidly cooled, causing them to crack. The resulting patterns would be used for guidance in resolving questions. Often the question posed to the ancestors would be inscribed on the bone itself. Bones could be used for more than one divination. One tomb has yielded more than 100,000 oracle bones, displaying questions such as "Swelling of the abdomen. Is there a curse? Does the deceased Chin-wu desire something of the king?" (Unschuld, 1985). The ancestors were appropriately placated according to the response. Natural causes of illness also were encountered, but these appear to have been addressed through the intervention of ancestors as well.

The Zhou dynasty resulted from a political conflict with a group of Chinese-speaking descendants of the same neolithic peoples who had settled to form the Shang. The defeat of the Shang established one of China's longest dynasties, as well as a pattern of governance that would characterize Chinese society—a central government working in relation to smaller principalities.

The Zhou continued the practices of the Shang rulers, consulting tortoise shell oracles with the aid of *wu,* or shamans. The *wu* acted as intermediaries between the living and the dead, played important ritual roles in court activities and the weather, and were called on to combat the demons who caused illness. During this period the shamanic activity of chasing evil spirits away from towns and homes with spears might have been transferred to the human body, and the practice of acupuncture emerged. Later accounts (eighth century CE) describe the needling techniques used by the physician Bian Qu (fifth century BCE) to drive out demons. However, we have no clear evidence of this.

The Warring States period, toward the close of the Zhou, was marked by political strife and social upheaval. This era saw the emergence of two philosophers, Kong Fu Zi (Confucius) and Lao Zi, whose ideas about social and natural order were to have a lasting impact on Chinese culture. A similar trend occurred within medicine: the human body no longer was seen as subject only to the whims of spirits and demons, but as a part of nature, and subject to discernible natural relationships. Those ideas were elaborated on during the Han dynasty.

The Flowering of Chinese Medicine: 206 BCE to 907 CE

In 206 BCE the empire was reunited under the Han. The Han (206 BCE-219 CE) created a stable aristocratic social order, expanded geographically and economically, and spread Chinese political influence throughout Vietnam and Korea. The Chinese people currently refer to themselves as the Han. This dynasty was a period of great development for the Chinese, including the integration of the Confucian doctrine, elements of yin and yang, and the five-phase theory into the political picture. Textual evidence reveals the emergence of a medicine that is similar to current Chinese medicine.

The earliest texts available were recovered from three tombs dating to 168 BCE that were excavated at Ma Wang Dui in Hunan province (Unschuld, 1985). These texts discuss magical and demonological concepts, as well as some ideas about yin and yang in relation to the body. The texts present an early concept of channels in the body, but in a less developed fashion than the later *Yellow Emperor's Inner Classic.* Ma Wang Dui texts mention moxibustion and the use of heated stones, but they do not speak about acupuncture or specific points on the body, implying that the idea of acupuncture had not yet emerged.

A biography written by a contemporary in 90 BCE describes Chun Yu Yi, the first known physician to record personal observations of clinical cases. Interestingly, he also was tried for malpractice because of his use of the apparently unfamiliar method of acupuncture to change the flow of qi (Unschuld, 1985).

The *Divine Husbandman's Classic of the Materia Medica (Shen Nong Ben Cao Jing),* mentioned earlier, appears during this era as well. This text is the first known formal presentation of individual medicinal substances, the first in a long line of such texts.

The *Classic of Difficult Issues (Nan Jing)* was compiled sometime during the first or second century CE, although its authorship is attributed to the legendary physician Bian Qu. This text has had and continues to have a marked influence on the practice of Chinese medicine and, to an even greater extent, on the practice of Chinese medicine in Japan. It marks a drastic shift in medical thinking, systematically organizing the theory and practice of therapeutic acupuncture in terms of body structure, illness, diagnosis, and treatment. It is almost entirely devoid of magical elements. The author(s) of the *Classic of Difficult Issues* reconciled the contradictions of the *Inner Classic,* in addition to providing many new observations. Although thought to have been written as an independent text, *Classic of Difficult Issues* met with so much resistance because of its radical organization that it became known as a commentary on the *Inner Classic.*

The *Treatise on Cold Damage (Shang Han Lun)* and the *Survey of Important Elements from the Golden Cabinet* and *Jade Container (Jin Gui Yao Lue)* were written in the second century CE by Zhang Zhong Jing, also known as Zhang Ji (142-220 CE). Chinese medical texts of this period were primarily philosophical, but as with the authors of the *Classic of Difficult Issues,* Zhang studied disease from a clinical standpoint, emphasizing the physical signs, symptoms, and course of disease; the method of treatment; and the action of the substances used. He was interested especially in fevers because most of the people in his village died from fever epidemics (possibly typhoid). Although published during the Han dynasty, these texts remained relatively obscure until the Sung dynasty (after 960 CE), when medical thinkers realized that the concepts of diagnosis and therapy presented reflected their own concerns. These texts enormously influenced the practice of herbal medicine in Japan. We examine an herbal formula derived from the *Treatise on Cold Damage* later in this chapter.

Hua Tou (110-207 CE), acupuncturist, herbalist, and surgeon, is a near-legendary figure in Chinese medicine. Besides reportedly using acupuncture and herbs, his adaptation of animal postures is one of the early forms of Qigong. He is said to have used the anesthetic properties of plants to render a patient insensible to pain, enabling him to practice surgery successfully.

Despite Hua Tou's reputation, his surgical innovations seem to have departed with him. Chinese medical history reveals the practice of a variety of minor surgical interventions for growths, hemorrhoids, and wound healing, but none of the significant abdominal surgeries attributed to Hua Tou. The surgical castration used to produce eunuchs for the imperial court was medically significant, and there is textual evidence of Chinese exposure to the surgical practices developed in India for the treatment of cataracts, but these did not form surgical traditions per se.

Huang Pu Mi (215-286 CE) wrote the *Systematic Classic of Acupuncture (Zhen Jiu Jia Yi Jing),* which exercised substantial influence over the acupuncture traditions of China, Korea, and Japan. This text presented and reorganized material from the *Inner Classic* and earlier texts.

It is important to realize that the histories of individual physicians and the texts that have come down to us reflect the medicine of the literate elite of China more than the medical traditions of that nation as a whole. About 80% of the total population consisted of farmers, peasants, and farming villages. These people lived at a level of bare subsistence and worked extremely hard to stay there, entirely dependent on the soil and the weather. They were not exposed to formal education and typically were illiterate. Very little is known of what these people knew or thought at any particular time. Their traditions were regionally oriented and full of folk superstition, historical legend, and aspirations dominated by the hope of survival.

Some authors, especially compilers of materia medica texts, did explore the nonliterate traditions of the Chinese people, but the first systematic publication of this material did not occur until late in the Qing dynasty (Unschuld, 1985). Folk herbal and medical traditions were most systematically explored under the guidance of the postrevolutionary government of China. Texts such as *The Barefoot Doctor's Manual* reflect the inclusion of this type of material.

In 220 CE, after approximately 30 years of strife and religious rebellion by Daoist sects, the Han dynasty fell. After the Han there was another long period of division in China, although not as violent or as divisive as the Warring States period after the Zhou dynasty. In 589 CE the Sui dynasty reunified China and soon was succeeded by the Tang dynasty, considered by many to be the height of China's cultural development. The Tang dynasty spread China's influence as far as Mongolia, Vietnam, Central Asia, Korea, and Japan. During this period, both Buddhism and Daoism strongly influenced medical thought.

Sun Si Miao (581-682), a famous physician of the period, was a prolific author and a productive scholar who was well versed in both Daoist and Buddhist practice. His works include *Thousand Ducat Prescriptions (Qian Jin Yao Fang),* a text on eye disorders, and *The Classic of Spells,* a guide to magic in medicine. The *Thousand Ducat Prescriptions* contains a section titled "On the absolute sincerity of great physicians" that established him as China's first medical ethicist. He addresses the need for diligent scholarship, compassion toward the patient, and high moral standards in the physician, which remain pertinent and seem to speak directly to current medical issues.

SUN SI MIAO EXPLAINS THE INCURABLE NATURE OF PHYSICIANS

Finally, it is inappropriate to emphasize one's reputation, to belittle the rest of the physicians and to praise only one's own virtue. Indeed, in actual life someone who has accidentally healed a disease, then stalks around with his head raised, shows conceit and announces that no one in the entire world could measure up to him. In this respect all physicians are evidently incurable (Unschuld, 1979).

Academic Medicine and Systematic Therapeutics: 960 CE to 1368 CE

By the time of the Sung dynasty the practice of medicine had become more specialized, and efforts were made to integrate past insights systematically. The number of texts published in this dynasty may have exceeded the number written during all the previous dynasties. In 1027, Wang Wei Yi oversaw the casting of two bronze figures that he designed to illustrate the location of acupuncture points. One of these was used in the Imperial Medical College. The bronzes were pierced at the location of the acupuncture points, covered with wax, and filled with water. When a student found the hole under the wax with a needle, water would drip out, indicating it to be the correct spot.

During the Sung dynasty, great advances occurred in herbal therapeutics, and several complete herbal texts with illustrations were published under imperial decree. Tastes and properties were assigned to herbs according to their yin or yang nature, and functions were assigned based on the herb's nature and its ability to treat specific symptoms. Efforts were made to systematize herbal therapeutics. The writings of Zhang Zhong Jing received great interest because of his systematic application of traditional theoretical principles to the use of herbal medicine. The revival of the *Treatise on Cold Damage* influenced medicine for the next several hundred years because it precipitated warm-induced disease theory *(wen bing xue)* during the Ming dynasty.

During the Sung dynasty the education of physicians became more formal. The Imperial College, which had provided for the training of the emperor's physicians, was expanded. In 1076 the Imperial Medical College was founded, with an enrollment of 300 students. There were regional schools as well.

The Jin and the Yuan dynasties saw the continuation of specialized medical thought and independent inquiry. Much of what we recognize as Chinese medicine today—and what we discuss in the section on fundamental concepts—stems from the Sung, Jin, and Yuan dynasties. Physicians of this period developed ideas involving the elaboration of therapeutic approaches on the basis of early theory. They espoused the application of five-phase theory in relation to seasonal influences, supplementing the body, purging the body to eliminate evil influences, and supplementing the yin.

Medicine in the Ming and Qing Dynasties: 1368 to 1911

Physicians continued to pursue lines of inquiry pursued in preceding dynasties, such as the far-reaching naturalistic explorations of Li Shi Zhen (1518-1593). His *Grand Materia Medica (Ben Cao Gang Mu)* included discussions of 1892 substances and, among its topics, described the use of kelp and deer thyroid to treat goiter.

The exploration of more precise linkages between factors in disease causation and therapeutics continued, and a number of medical sects emerged. During a virulent epidemic that struck from 1641 to 1644, Wu You Ke (Xing) (1592-1672) used an unorthodox method that was highly successful. His text, *Discussion of Warm Epidemics (Wen Yi Lun),* explored the theoretical basis for his treatment.

Some authors consider the Ming dynasty to be the peak of the cultural expression of acupuncture and moxibustion in China (Qiu, 1993). This period saw the production of numerous texts on the subject. One of the most influential acupuncture texts, *The Great Compendium of Acupuncture and Moxibustion (Zhen Jiu Da Cheng),* was written by Yang Ji Zhou toward the end of the Ming dynasty.

Intellectual trends of the Ming continued into the Qing dynasty. *The Discussion of Warm Disease (Wen Re Lun)* by Ye Tian Shi complemented Zhang Zhong Jing's method of diagnosing and treating diseases caused by cold with an equally systematic method of diagnosing and treating those caused by heat.

Political, economic, and social trends during the Qing dynasty exacerbated the isolation of the Manchu rulers of the time and exposed the Chinese to the power of Western knowledge, technology, and science. The broadening of cultural horizons and the broadening of medical inquiry combined to shake the classical underpinnings of Chinese medical thought. In 1822, acupuncture was formally eliminated from the Imperial Medical College (Qiu, 1993).

By the close of the Qing dynasty in 1911, political and cultural institutions were in a state of decline. The scattered practitioners of traditional Chinese medicine found themselves increasingly under fire from the advocates of a new and modern China and a new and modern medicine.

The collapse of the Qing and the formation of the Republic laid traditional medicine open to the conquering influence of Western medicine. The Imperial College of Physicians was eliminated (Wong and Wu, 1985), and the Western-educated proponents of reform began to work toward the elimination of the traditional medicine of China and the establishment of Western medicine as the dominant medical system.

From 1914 through 1936 a series of encounters and clashes occurred over the regulation, establishment, or elimination of practitioners of Chinese medicine (Wong and Wu, 1985). The traditional medicine of China, or "medicine" *(yi)* as it had been known, came to be termed "Chinese medicine" *(Zhong Yi)*. Both nationalist and Marxist reformers intensely disliked Chinese medicine.

SO-CALLED CHINESE MEDICINE

Initially the external threat reduced the internal spectrum of competing Chinese interpretations of the classics. The great diversity of individual efforts to reconcile insights from personal experience with the ancient theories of yin yang and the five phases, as well as with other older views about the structure of the body, disappeared behind the illusion of a so-called Chinese medicine *(chung-I [zhong yi])*, supposedly well defined and with theory easily converted into practice. This situation, in turn, has given rise to the historically misleading impression that these diverse elements, like the concepts and practices of Western medicine, constituted a unified, coherent system (Unschuld, 1985).

A critical feature of this new Chinese medicine was its rejection of practices that were manifestly "unscientific," represented in the creation of *Zhong Yi*. This disciplined form of medicine has emerged today as traditional Chinese medicine.

The aspects of the traditional medicine of China that were secured in *Zhong Yi* were later appropriated by the Chinese Marxists in an effort to build a strong medical infrastructure for substantial populations in the face of economic and technical limitations. Chairman Mao's declaration in 1958 that "Chinese medicine is a great treasure house! We must uncover it and raise its standards!" (Unschuld, 1985) inspired efforts to rehabilitate the traditional medicine of China and to "discover" a primitive dialectic within the theoretical underpinnings of the system. The *Revised Outline of Chinese Medicine* stated that "Yin-yang and the five phases *(wu-hsing [wu xing])* are ancient Chinese philosophical ideas. They are spontaneous, naive materialist theories that also contain elementary dialectic ideas" (Sivin, 1987).

The development of Chinese medicine as a system parallel to Western medicine was under way by the time of Mao's declaration. In 1956, four colleges of Chinese medicine were created, with many more to follow. At present, *Zhong Yi* exists as a parallel medical system, integrating necessary biomedical elements while retaining fidelity to the traditional concepts of Chinese medicine. Educational programs emphasize acupuncture and herbal medicine and range from an undergraduate technical certificate to doctoral programs. Most independent practitioners enter the field with a 5-year medical baccalaureate degree (MB/BS) that is earned after high school (Ergil, 1994). In this system, both inpatient and outpatient medical care is delivered from large, well-equipped hospitals, as well as private clinics and pharmacies.

FUNDAMENTAL CONCEPTS

Yin and Yang

The philosophy of Chinese medicine begins with yin and yang. These two terms can be used to express the broadest philosophical concepts, as well as the most focused perceptions of the natural world. Yin and yang express the idea of opposing but complementary phenomena that exist in a state of dynamic equilibrium. The most ancient expression of this idea seems to have been that of the shady and sunny sides of a hill (Unschuld, 1985, p. 55; Wilhelm, 1967, p. 297). The sunlit southern side was the yang, and the shaded northern side was the yin. The contrast between the bright and dark sides of a single hill portrayed the yang and the yin, respectively. If you imagine, for a moment, the different environments that exist on either side of this one hill, you can begin to get an idea of yin and yang. On the bright, sunny side, plants and animals that enjoy light are more prevalent, the air is drier, and the rocks are warm; on the dim, shaded side, the air seems moist and cool.

Yin and yang are always present simultaneously. The paired opposites observed in the world gave tangible expression to the otherwise uncontemplatable Dao of ancient Chinese thought (Box 21-1).

The *Book of Changes (Yi Jing)*, which sought to explore the myriad manifestations of yin and yang, expressed the idea as follows: "That which lets now the dark, now the light appear is tao" (Wilhelm, 1967).

The *Yellow Emperor's Inner Classic*, the oldest text to discuss the medical application of yin and yang in a comprehensive way (Unschuld, 1985, p. 56), states that "yin and yang are the way of heaven and earth" (Wiseman et al., 1985). This text showed how yin and yang were to be used to correlate the body and other phenomena to the human experience of health and disease.

THE INNER CLASSIC ON YIN AND YANG

As to the yin and yang of the human body, the outer part is yang and the inner part is yin. As to the trunk, the back is yang and the abdomen is yin. As to the organs, the viscera are yin whereas the bowels are yang. The liver, heart, spleen, lung, and kidney are yin; the gallbladder, stomach, intestines, bladder, and triple burner are yang (Wiseman et al., 1993).

It is important to note that the preceding quote is taken from the translation of an important contemporary textbook of Chinese medicine. Many ideas expressed in the *Yellow Emperor's Inner Classic* are taught and applied routinely in the contemporary clinical practice of Chinese medicine.

Yin and yang were used to express ideas about both normal physiology and pathological processes. They were applied to the organization of phenomena in many ways, for example, to organize phenomena in terms of the emergence of its dominant yin or yang character. Summer was yang within yang, fall was yin within yang, winter was yin within yin, and spring was yang within yin. Thus the coldest, darkest, and most yin period was yin within yin, whereas spring, when the yang began to emerge from the yin, was yang within yin.

There is a distinctly ecological orientation to the world view that is supported by yin and yang; each phenomenon is seen in relation to its surroundings, and it is expected that each phenomenon will exert an influence on its surroundings that is balanced by an equal but opposing influence (Table 21-1). Just as the language of ecology is the language of interrelation and interdependence, the language of Chinese medicine is a language of interrelation and interdependence. The external landscape, or human environment, is understood to be in profound and dynamic relationship with the internal landscape, or human organism. This idea becomes clearer when we explore disease causation later.

The ancient Chinese understood humans to have a nature and structure inseparable from yin and yang and as such inseparable from the world around

---

BOX 21-1

Origins of Yin and Yang

Out of Tao, One is born;
Out of One, Two;
Out of Two, Three;
Out of Three, the created universe.
The created universe carries the yin at its back and the yang in front;
Through the union of the pervading principles it reaches harmony (Laozi in Lin, 1942).

TABLE 21-1

Yang and Yin Correspondences

Yang	Yin
Light	Dark
Heaven	Earth
Sun	Moon
Day	Night
Spring	Autumn
Summer	Winter
Hot	Cold
Male	Female
Fast	Slow
Up	Down
Outside	Inside
Fire	Water
Wood	Metal

them—a structure that is to be understood by the same rules that guide us in understanding the world in which we live. Life on the shaded side of a mountain has characteristics that differ from those on the sunny side. Finally, the comprehension and adjustment of life in relation to yin and yang would support life itself. Thus it was said, "To follow (the laws of) yin and yang means life; to act contrary to (the laws of yin and yang) means death" (Unschuld, 1985).

Within the traditional medical community of contemporary China, there is debate over the actual nature of yin and yang. Some exponents of a more scientific, less traditional perspective on Chinese medicine want yin and yang to be used as concepts to organize phenomena. Others who express a less modern perspective emphatically state that yin and yang are actually tangible phenomena (Farquhar, 1987). Although it is probably easiest to think about *yin* and *yang* as descriptive terms that help the Chinese physician organize information, it should be remembered (especially in traditional pharmaceutics) that the yin and yang constituents of the body are actual things that can be reinforced by specific substances or actions.

A useful analogy for thinking about yin and yang in this way is that of a candle. If one considers the yin aspect of the candle to be the wax and the yang aspect to be the flame, one can see how the yin nourishes and supports the yang and how the yang consumes the yin and thus burns brightly. When the wax is gone, so is the flame. Yin and yang exist in dependence on each other.

The Five Phases

Another idea that has played a significant part in the development of some aspects of Chinese medicine is that of the five phases (*wu xing*). The five phases are earth, metal, water, wood, and fire. In Chinese *wu* means "five" and *xing* expresses the idea of movement, "to go." For a time the *wu xing* were translated as "the five elements." This translation conveys little of the dynamism of the Chinese concept, instead focusing on the apparent similarities between the *wu xing* and the elements of medieval alchemy. This is an example of the translation problem in which we use the familiar to understand the new. However useful this method may be at first, it can lead to some confusion in the long run. *Wu xing* may include the implication of material elements, but in general, the five phases refer to a set of dynamic relations occurring among phenomena that are organized in terms of the five phases. This philosophy can cover almost every aspect of phenomena, from seasons to odors (Table 21-2).

TABLE 21-2

Correspondences of the Five Phases

Category	Wood	Fire	Earth	Metal	Water
Viscus	Liver	Heart	Spleen	Lungs	Kidney
Bowel	Gallbladder	Small intestine	Stomach	Large intestine	Urinary bladder
Season	Spring	Summer	Late summer	Autumn	Winter
Time of day	Before sunrise	Forenoon	Afternoon	Late afternoon	Midnight
Climate	Wind	Heat	Damp	Dryness	Cold
Direction	East	South	Center	West	North
Development	Birth	Growth	Maturity	Withdrawal	Dormancy
Color	Cyan	Red	Yellow	White	Black
Taste	Sour	Bitter	Sweet	Pungent	Salty
Sense organ	Eyes	Tongue	Mouth	Nose	Ears
Odor	Goatish	Scorched	Fragrant	Raw fish	Putrid
Vocalization	Shouting	Laughing	Singing	Weeping	Sighing
Tissue	Sinews	Vessels	Flesh	Body hair	Bones
Mind	Anger	Joy	Thought	Sorrow	Fear

Qi and the Essential Substances of the Body

Apart from the ideas of yin and yang and the five phases, no concept is more crucial to Chinese medicine than *qi*—the idea that the body is pervaded by subtle material and mobile influences that cause most physiological functions and maintain the health and vitality of the individual. This idea is not typical of biomedical thinking about the body. It is not unusual to see the idea of qi translated with the term *energy*, but this translation conceals its distinctly material attributes. Furthermore, although energy is defined as the capacity of a system to do work, the character of qi extends considerably further.

The Chinese character for qi is traditionally composed of two radicals; the radical that symbolizes breath or rising vapor is placed above the radical for rice (Figure 21-2). Qi is linked with the concept of "vapors arising from food" (Unschuld, 1985). Over time this concept broadened but never lost its distinctively material aspect. Unschuld favors the use of the phrase "finest matter influences" or "influences" to translate this concept. Some phenomena labeled as qi do not fit conventional definitions of substance or matter, further confusing the issue (Wiseman et al., 1995). For this reason, many authors prefer to leave the term *qi* untranslated.

The idea of qi is extremely broad, encompassing almost every variety of natural phenomena. Many different types of qi are in the body. In general, the features that distinguish each type derive from its source, location, and function. There is considerable room for debate in this area, and exploration of a wide range of materials can suggest different ideas about categories of qi. In general, qi has the functions of activation, warming, defense, transformation, and containment (Table 21-3).

The qi concept is important to many aspects of Chinese medicine. Organ qi and channel qi are influenced by acupuncture. In fact, one characteristic feature of acupuncture treatment is the sensation of obtaining the qi, or *de qi*. *Qigong* is a general term for the many systems of meditation, exercise, and therapeutics that are rooted in the concept of mobilizing and regulating the movement of qi in the body. Qi is sometimes compared with wind captured in a sail; we cannot observe the wind directly, but we can infer its presence as it fills the sail. In a similar fashion, the movements of the body and the movement of substances within the body are all signs of the action of qi.

In relation to qi, blood and fluids constitute the yin aspects of the body. *Blood* is produced by the construction qi, which in turn is derived from food and water. Blood nourishes the body. Blood is understood to have a slightly broader and less definite range of actions in Chinese medicine than it does in biomedicine. Within the body, qi and blood are closely linked because blood is considered to flow with qi and to be conveyed by it. This relationship often is expressed by

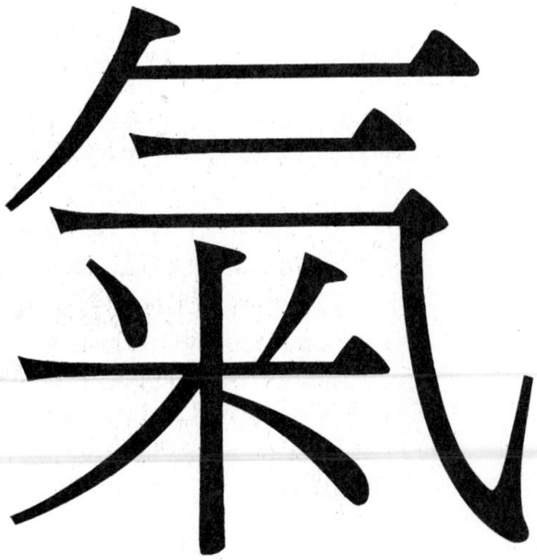

Figure 21-2 The character *qi*.

TABLE 21-3

Types of Qi

Type	Category	Function
Ying qi	Construction qi	Supports and nourishes the body
Wei qi	Defense qi	Protects and warms the body
Jing qi	Channel qi	Flows in the channels (felt during acupuncture)
Zang qi	Organ qi	Flows in the organs (physiological function of organs)
Zong qi	Ancestral qi	Responsible for respiration and circulation

the Chinese saying "qi is the commander of blood and blood is the mother of qi," and some suggest that qi and blood are linked as persons and their shadow are linked.

Fluids are a general category of thin and viscous substances that serve to moisten and lubricate the body. Fluids can be conceptually separated into humor and liquid. *Humor* is thick and related to the body's organs; its functions include lubrication of the joints. *Liquid* is thin and is responsible for moistening the surface areas of the body, including the skin, eyes, and mouth.

Essence and Spirit

Together with qi, essence and spirit make up the *three treasures* in Chinese medicine. In brief, essence is the gift of one's parents, and spirit is the gift of heaven. *Essence* is the most fundamental source of human physiological processes, the bodily reserves that support human life and that must be replenished by food and rest, and the actual reproductive substances of the body. *Spirit* is the alert and radiant aspect of human life. We encounter spirit in the luster of the eyes and face in healthy persons, as well as in their ability to think and respond appropriately to the world around them. The idea expressed by spirit, or *shen* in Chinese, encompasses consciousness and healthy mental and physical function.

The relation of the mind to the body in Chinese medicine does not include the notion of a distinct separation. It is understood that the psyche and soma interact with each other and that aspects of mental and emotional experience can have an impact on the body, and vice versa. In this sense, spirit is linked both to the health of the body and to the health of the mind. Similarly, aspects of human experience that are understood as predominantly mental in a biomedical frame of reference are linked to specific organs in Chinese medicine. For example, anger is related to the liver, obsessive thought to the spleen, and joy to the heart.

Viscera and Bowels (*Zang* and *Fu*)

The ancient Chinese understood human anatomy in ways not dissimilar from their European contemporaries, up to the seventeenth century. Chinese history includes cases of systematic dissection, but none of these reached the extensive explorations into the structure of the body that characterized European medicine by the fifteenth century. Instead, the Chinese medical perspective of the body, although rooted in familiar anatomical structures, represented a system in which organs serve as markers of associated physiological functions rather than actual physical structures.

The physician of Chinese medicine encounters a body in which 12 organs function. These organs are divided into the "viscera," which include six *zang* or solid organs, and the "bowels," which include six *fu* or hollow organs. These organs often are related to the physical structures that we associate with conventional biomedical anatomy. The six viscera are heart, lungs, liver, spleen, kidneys, and pericardium. The six bowels are the small intestine, large intestine, gallbladder, stomach, urinary bladder, and the "triple burner" *(san jiao)*. These organs have physiological functions that often are similar to those associated with them in biomedicine, but that also might be very different. The liver is said to store blood and to distribute it to the extremities as needed. The spleen is understood as an organ of digestion. The Chinese understood the physical structure and location of most of the organs, but because systematic dissection was not extensively pursued, the close observation of physiological function was more often the basis of medical thought.

For example, circulation and elimination of fluids were observed and attributed to an organ that was said to have a name, but no form was established. This organ, the "triple burner," is considered either the combined expression of the activity of other organs in the body or a group of spaces in the body. This example clearly expresses the idea that physiological function, rather than substance, establishes an organ in Chinese medicine. At the same time, the triple burner has always been surrounded by debate because it does not have a clear anatomical structure.

The organs of viscera and bowel are paired in the yin and yang, or *interior-exterior relationship*. The heart is linked with the small intestine, the spleen with the stomach, and so on. Each viscus and each bowel has an associated channel that runs through the organ, through the paired organ, within the body, and across the body's surface, then connects with the channel of the related organ.

Historical evidence suggests that the idea of channels is more ancient than the idea of specific acupuncture points. Although disagreement surrounds the location of specific points, research in the People's Republic of China recently led to the publication of a number of texts dedicated to resolving historical, philological, and anatomical questions about acupuncture points. At this time, 12 primary channels and eight extraordinary vessels are understood to exist. The 12 channels are classically organized in terms of a sixfold yin-and-yang organizational scheme, although they can also be organized in terms of five-phase theory. Qi is understood to flow in these channels, making a rhythmical circuit.

Along the pathways of 14 of these channels (the 12 regular channels and two of the extra channels) lie 361 specific points. In addition, a large number of "extra" points have been derived from clinical experience but are not traditionally considered part of the major channel systems. Beyond this, various individual elaborations of acupuncture theory suggest new points. There are also local microsystems of acupuncture points that have postulated numerous points on the ear, scalp, hand, foot, and other areas of the body.

Acupuncture points appear at many locations on the body. Most often they are located where a gentle and sensitive hand can detect a declivity (slope) with slight pressure on the skin surface. Points are located at the margins or bellies of muscles, between bones, and over distinctive bony features that can be detected through the skin. Methods used to locate points vary. In general, points are found by seeking anatomical landmarks, by proportionally measuring the body, and by using finger measurements; the first method is considered the most reliable. With time and clinical experience, some practitioners can be less formal in their approach to locating acupuncture points, but this topic interests even advanced practitioners. In Japan, clinicians gather regularly to hone their point location skills. In China, point location in relation to classical sources, anatomical study, and empirical evidence is an area of advanced study.

As with qi, the actual term and use of the Chinese expression that we translate as "point" is important. The character *xue*, which has been translated as "point," actually means "hole" in Chinese. A hole often is part of the clinician's subjective experience of the acupuncture point. *Xue* are holes in which the qi of the channels can be influenced by inserting a needle or by other means. Imagining the channel system as a vast subcutaneous waterway, with caves and springs punctuating its course as it flows to the surface, provides a concept of the holes similar to the way the Chinese thought of them for many centuries (Box 21-2).

Holes, or points along the channels, have been categorized and organized in myriad ways. One of the oldest and most well known is a system of categories based on the idea of *shu*, or transport points. This system of point categories applies exclusively to points on the forearm and lower leg, which embody the image of qi welling gently from a mountainous source at the fingertips and gradually gaining strength and depth as it reaches the seas located at the elbow and knee joints.

In reading the preceding brief discussion of the essential anatomy and physiology of Chinese medicine, it is important to remember that this anatomy forms a general reference for physiological function rather than an anatomy of direct links between discrete categories of tissue and specific physiological processes. A strength of Chinese medicine is that its theory allows for generalizations about complex physical processes, in addition to responding to signs and symptoms whose origins are obscure. Also, the distinction between mind and body is not present in Chinese medicine. Although Chinese physicians may display a disconcerting lack of interest in contemporary psychotherapy or its patients, they are quick to posit a link between affect and physiological process, in a manner that might intrigue a contemporary psychobiologist. On this basis, we can proceed to examine how illness manifests in the body.

BOX 21-2

Set of Acupuncture Points: Leg Three Li

- *Location:* 3 cun (body inch) below the depression below the patella, one fingerbreadth from the anterior crest of the tibia.
- *Indications:* Stomach pain, vomiting, abdominal distention, indigestion, diarrhea, constipation, dizziness, mastitis, mental disorders, hemiplegia, pain in knee joint and leg.
- *Depth of needle insertion:* 0.5 to 1.3 inches.

The Causes of Disease

Ultimately, all illness is a disturbance of qi within the body. Its expression as a pathological process displaying specific signs and symptoms depends on the location of the disturbance. Contemporary formal discussions on disease causation use the ideas of Chen Yen (1161-1174), who wrote *Prescriptions Elucidated on the Premise that All Pathological Symptoms Have Only Three Primary Causes (San Yin Qi Yi Bing Cheng Fang Lun)*, and an additional idea of Wu You Ke, that each disease has its own qi.

The three categories of disease are organized in terms of external causes of disease, internal causes, and causes that are neither external nor internal (Wiseman et al., 1995) (Box 21-3). The first category includes six influences that are distinctly environmental: wind, cold, fire, dampness, summer heat, and dryness. When they cause disease, these six influences are known as *evils*. If the defense qi is not robust or the correct qi is not strong, or if the evil is powerful, the evil may enter the surface of the body and, under certain conditions, penetrate to the interior.

The nature of the evil and its impact on the body were understood through the observation of nature and the observation of the body in illness. The clinical meaning of the causes of disease does not lie, for the most part, in the expression of a distinct etiology, but in the manifestation of a specific set of clinical signs. In this sense, the biomedical distinction between etiology and diagnosis is somewhat blurred in Chinese medical theory.

For example, the evils of wind and cold often are implicated in the sudden onset of symptoms associated with the common cold: headache, pronounced aversion to cold, aching muscles and bones, fever, and a scratchy throat. Wind is expressed in the sudden onset of the symptoms and in their manifestation in the upper part of the body, and cold is displayed in the pronounced aversion to cold and the aching muscles and bones. Whether the patient had a specific encounter with a cold wind shortly before the onset of the symptoms is not particularly relevant. Although a patient may mention being outside on a chilly and windy day before the onset of a cold, such exposure could easily result in signs of "wind heat" as well, that is, a less marked aversion to cold, a distinctly sore throat, and a dry mouth. The six evils are not agents of specific etiology but agents of specific symptomatology. These ideas developed in a setting where the possibility of investigating a bacterial or viral cause was nonexistent. Rather, careful observation of the body's response to disease provided the information necessary for treatment.

Each of the evils affects the body in a manner similar to its behavior in the environment. Images of these processes observed in nature and society were inscribed on the body to permit its processes to be readily understood. The human body stood between heaven and earth and was subject to all their influences in a relationship of continuity with its environment. Although these six evils are identified as environmental influences that attack the body's surface, it also is clearly understood they may occur within the body, causing internal disruption.

In the second category of disease causation, "internal damage by the seven affects" refers to the way in which mental states can influence body processes. However, such a statement expresses a separation not implied in Chinese medicine. Each of the seven affects, or internal causes, can disturb the body if it is strongly or frequently expressed. As discussed earlier, each of the mental states—joy, anger, anxiety, thought, sorrow, fear, and fright—is related to a specific organ.

In the third category, nonexternal, noninternal causes encompass the causes of disease that do not result specifically from environmental influences or mental states. These include dietary irregularities, excessive sexual activity, taxation fatigue, trauma, and parasites. "Excessive sexual activity" suggests the possibility that too frequent emission of semen by the male can cause illness. This can occur because semen is directly related to the concept of essence, which is considered vital to the body's function and difficult to replace. This category also includes possible damage to the essence through excessive childbearing or

---

BOX 21-3

The Three Causes of Disease (San Yin)

- *External causes,* or "the six evils": Wind, cold, fire, dampness, summer heat, and dryness.
- *Internal causes,* or internal damage by the "seven affects": Joy, anger, anxiety, thought, sorrow, fear, and fright.
- *Nonexternal, noninternal causes:* Dietary irregularities, excessive sexual activity, taxation fatigue, trauma, and parasites.

bearing a child when the mother is too young or too old.

"Taxation fatigue" expresses the dangers of engaging in a variety of activities for a prolonged period. This category includes both the idea of over-exertion and the idea of inactivity as possible causes of disease. All the concepts included within taxation fatigue reflect the essential thought of Chinese medicine that moderation is the key to health. Lying down for prolonged periods damages the qi, and prolonged standing damages the bones. From the moment that the Yellow Emperor asked Qi Bo why people now die before their time and received his answer, the images of balance, harmony, and moderation have informed Chinese medicine.

Each of the causes of disease, from prosaic causes such as dietary irregularities to exotic notions such as wind evil, disrupts the balance of yang and yin within the body and disrupts the free movement of qi. The next step is to determine the precise pattern of imbalance.

Diagnosis

Diagnostics in Chinese medicine is traditionally expressed within four categories: inspection, listening and smelling, inquiry, and palpation. The fundamental goal is to collect information that reflects the status of physiological processes, then analyze this information to determine which impact a disorder has on that process.

The first of the four diagnostic methods, *inspection (wang)*, refers to the visual assessment of the patient, particularly the spirit, form and bearing, the head and face, and substances excreted by the body. Inspection uses a large body of empirically derived information and theoretical considerations. The color, shape, markings, and coating of the tongue are inspected. For the patient attacked by wind and cold, the examiner would expect to see a moist tongue with a thin white coating, signaling the presence of cold. If heat were present, the examiner might expect a dry mouth and a red tongue. The observation of the spirit, which is considered very important in assessing the patient's prognosis, relies on assessing the overall appearance of the patient, especially the eyes, the complexion, and the quality of the patient's voice. Good spirit, even in the presence of serious illness, is thought to bode well for the patient.

The second aspect of diagnosis, *listening and smelling (wen)*, refers to listening to the quality of speech,

breath, and other sounds, as well as being aware of the odors of breath, body, and excreta. As with each aspect of diagnosis, the five-phase theory can be incorporated into the assessment of the patient's condition. Each phase and each pair of viscus and bowel have a corresponding vocalization and smell.

The third aspect of diagnosis, *inquiry (wen)*, is the process of taking a comprehensive medical history. This process has been presented in many ways, but perhaps best known is the system of 10 questions described by Zhang Jie Bin in the Ming dynasty. The questions were presented as an outline of diagnostic inquiry and included querying the patient about sensations of hot and cold, perspiration, head and body, excreta, diet, chest, hearing, thirst, previous illnesses, and previous medications and their effects. For example, the examiner might expect the patient who has wind and cold symptoms to report an aversion to exposure to cold, headache, body aches, and an absence of thirst.

This step is considered critical to a good diagnosis. Although pulse diagnosis is sometimes regarded as a central feature of Chinese medicine and is rightly regarded as an art, it should not form the sole basis of a complete diagnosis, as follows:

> The *simple questions* expresses the following idea: If, in conducting the examination, the practitioner neither inquires as to how and when the condition arose nor asks about the nature of the patient's complaint, about dietary irregularities, excesses of sleeping and waking, and poisoning, but instead proceeds immediately to take the pulse, he will not succeed in identifying the disease (Wiseman et al., 1995).

Contemporaries of Li Shi Zhen, the author of *The Pulse Studies of Bin Hu (Bin Hu Mai Xue)*, placed great emphasis on the pulse. Although considered an expert, he rejected the idea that one would place an unequal emphasis on any aspect of the diagnostic process.

Palpation (qie), the fourth diagnostic method, includes pulse examination, general palpation of the body, and palpation of the acupuncture points. *Pulse diagnosis* offers a range of approaches and can provide a remarkable amount of information about the patient's condition. The process of pulse diagnosis is carried out on the radial arteries of the left and right wrists. The patient may be seated or lying down and should be calm. The pulse is divided into three parts. The middle part is adjacent to the styloid process of the radius and is called the "bar" position; the "inch"

TABLE 21-4

Pulse Positions

Position	Left		Right	
	Deep	Superficial	Deep	Superficial
Nan Jing				
Inch	Heart	Small intestine	Lung	Large intestine
Bar	Liver	Gallbladder	Spleen	Stomach
Cubit	Kidney	Urinary bladder	Pericardium	Triple warmer
Contemporary Chinese Sources				
Inch	Heart		Lung	
Bar	Liver	Gallbladder	Spleen	Stomach
Cubit	Kidney	Urinary bladder	Kidney	Urinary bladder

is distal to it, and the "cubit" is proximal. The *inch position,* which is nearest the wrist, can indicate the status of the body above the diaphragm; the *bar position* indicates the status of the body between the diaphragm and the navel; and the *cubit position* indicates the area below the navel. Beyond this simple conceptual structure, each pulse position can be interpreted to determine the status of the organs and the channels.

Table 21-4 summarizes two models of what can be felt at each pulse position. The first chart is derived from the *Classic of Difficult Issues,* which first presented this type of pulse diagnosis in a systematic way, and the second chart shows a less elaborate, contemporary pattern. Some authors suggest that the pattern associated with the *Classic of Difficult Issues* is related more to the use of pulse diagnosis in the practice of acupuncture, whereas the later pattern is more relevant to the herbalist (Maciocia, 1989). Not all herbalists or acupuncturists make use of the pulse, but certain styles of acupuncture rely quite heavily on it. There are many possible approaches to the pulse, making it a rich area for the clinician and a vexing area for the biomedically oriented researcher (Birch, 1994).

The pulse allows the clinician to feel the quality of the qi and blood at different locations in the body. Table 21-5 provides a list of 29 pulse qualities and possible associations (Wiseman, 1993). Pulse qualities are organized on the basis of the size, rate, depth, force, and volume of the pulse. The overall quality of the pulse and the variations in quality at certain positions can become quite meaningful to the clinician after several years of close attention. The patient

afflicted with a "wind cold" evil might display a floating and tight pulse, signaling the presence of a cold evil on the surface of the body.

After carrying out the diagnostic process, the practitioner of Chinese medicine must make sense of the information derived. The practitioner constructs an appropriate image of the configuration of the disease so that it can be addressed by effective therapy. Central to this process is the concept of *pattern identification (bian zheng),* which involves gathering signs and symptoms through the diagnostic process and using traditional theory to understand their impact on the fundamental substances of the body, the organs, and the channels. Many intellectual aspects of the diagnostic processes of Chinese medicine, especially when applied to the practice of herbal medicine, are as analytical as a biomedical clinical encounter. The physician must elicit signs and symptoms from the patient and then use them to understand the disruption of underlying physiological processes.

The first step of pattern identification is the localization of the disorder and the assessment of its essential nature, using the *eight principles* that are an expansion of yin and yang correspondences: yin, yang, cold, hot, interior, exterior, vacuity, and repletion.[*]

---

[*]Although many authors continue to use the terms *excess* and *deficiency* to express the Chinese expressions *shi* and *xu,* I prefer Wiseman's "repletion" and "vacuity" as a translation. The use of "excess" simply is incorrect because of the existence of other Chinese terms that convey this idea exactly. "Deficiency" is problematic because it implies measurable quantity, which is not a consideration in the Chinese concept (Wiseman and Boss, 1990). Unschuld uses *depletion* and *repletion* instead.

TABLE 21-5

Pulse Types

	English	Chinese	General Association
1	Normal	zheng chang mai	Normal pulse
2	Floating	fu mai	Exterior condition
3	Deep	chen mai	Interior condition
4	Slow	chi mai	Cold and yang vacuity
5	Rapid	shuo mai	Heat
6	Surging	hong mai	Exuberant heat, hemorrhage
7	Faint	wei mai	Qi and blood vacuity desertion
8	Fine	xi mai	Blood and yin vacuity
9	Scattered	san mai	Dissipation of qui and blood, critical
10	Vacuous	xu mai	Vacuity
11	Replete	shi mai	Exuberant evil with right qi strong
12	Slippery	hua mai	Pregnancy, phlegm, abundant qi and blood
13	Rough	se mai	Blood stasis, vacuity of qi and blood
14	Long	chang mai	Often normal
15	Short	duan mai	Vacuity of qi and blood
16	Stringlike	xian mai	Liver disorders, severe pain
17	Hollow	kou mai	Blood loss
18	Tight	jin mai	Cold, pain
19	Moderate	huan mai	Slower than normal not pathological
20	Drumskin	ge mai	Blood loss
21	Confined	lao mai	Cold, pain
22	Weak	ruo mai	Vacuity of qi and blood
23	Soggy	ru mai	Vacuity of qi and blood with dampness
24	Hidden	fu mai	Deep lying internal cold
25	Stirred	dong mai	High fever, pregnancy
26	Rapid, irregular	cu mai	Debility of visceral qi or emotional distress
27	Slow, irregular	jie mai	Debility of visceral qi or emotional distress
28	Regularly intermittent	dai mai	Debility of visceral qi or emotional distress
29	Racing	ji mai	Heat, possible vacuity

Data from Wiseman N, Ellis A, Zmiewski P, Li C: *Fundamentals of Chinese medicine,* Brookline, Mass, 1995, Paradigm.

As with many other aspects of contemporary Chinese medicine, the eight principles originated in the Sung dynasty. Kou Zong Shi proposed a structure that organized disease into eight essentials: cold, hot, interior, exterior, vacuity, repletion, evil qi, and right qi (Bensky and Barolet, 1990). These were improved on in 1732, in the text *Awakening the Mind in Medical Studies (Yi Xue Xin Wu)* (Sivin, 1987). The original source was written, in the spirit of the times, to create a formal diagnostic structure for herbs that could be conceptually integrated with the ideas already in use for acupuncture. Today this formal structure is applied to both acupuncture and herbal medicine.

The "wind cold" patient had these symptoms: marked aversion to exposure to cold, headache, body aches, absence of thirst, a moist tongue with a thin white coating, and a floating and tight pulse. In terms of the eight principles, this would be an exterior, cold, repletion pattern. The principles of yin and yang would not directly apply.

What does this mean? The eight principles serve fundamentally to localize a condition. When Chinese physicians say that a condition is "external," they mean that it has not yet penetrated beyond the skin and channels to the deeper parts of the body. In this case, a cold condition betrays itself through the body's expression of cold signs. To say a condition is "replete" is to say that the evil attacking the body is strong, or that the body itself is strong.

The eight principles are typically the first step in developing a clear pattern identification, especially if the patient has organ involvement. The eight principles are the application of a yin and yang–based theoretical structure.

A single biomedical disease entity can be associated with several Chinese diagnostic patterns (Box 21-4). For example, viral hepatitis is associated with at least six distinct diagnostic patterns, and lower urinary tract infection might be related to one of four patterns (Ergil, 1995a, 1995b). Each of these patterns would be treated in different ways, according to the saying "one disease, different treatments." The patient whose clinical pattern is "wind cold" has the common cold and a headache, but the same disease could manifest in other patterns.

Also, many different diseases may be captured within one pattern, thus the saying "different diseases, one treatment." One contemporary text lists such diverse entities as nephritis, dysfunctional uterine bleeding, pyelonephritis, and rheumatic heart disease under the diagnostic pattern of "disharmony between the heart and kidney" (Huang et al., 1993, p. 79).

This comparatively precise diagnostic linkage begins to be broadly appreciated in the historical trends of the Sung, Jin, and Yuan dynasties. The six-channel pattern identification proposed by Zhang Zhong Jing is one of many patterns currently used. The patient who has encountered a wind cold evil would, under Zhang Jong Jing's system, be categorized as having tai yang disease. There is considerable room for overlap within the available methods of pattern identification.

Therapeutic Concepts

Once a diagnosis has been determined and, when relevant, a pattern has been differentiated, therapy begins. Therapeutics in Chinese medicine is fundamentally allopathic; that is, it addresses the pathological condition with opposing measures, as follows:

> Cold is treated with heat, heat is treated with cold, vacuity is treated by supplementation, and repletion is treated by drainage (*Inner Classic* [Wiseman et al., 1985]).

Within the realm of acupuncture, moxibustion, and herbal medicine, three fundamental principles of therapy are understood: (1) treating disease from its root, (2) eliminating evil influences and supporting the right, and (3) restoring the balance of yin and yang. These refer to approaches that are appropriate to the patient's condition. It would be appropriate to eliminate the cold evil and support the right qi of the wind cold patient. In a patient with symptoms that reflect a complex underlying pattern, the physician might attempt to treat the root of the patient's condition. For example, functional uterine bleeding caused by a disharmony of the heart and kidney would be addressed primarily by harmonizing the heart and kidney; treating the root of the condition would adjust its symptoms. Treatment methods vary widely; Box 21-5 provides the simplest expression of their organization.

BOX 21-4

Types of Diagnostic Patterns

- Eight principles
- Six evils
- Qi and blood and fluids
- Five phases
- Channel patterns
- Viscera and bowels
- Triple burner
- Six channels
- Four levels

BOX 21-5

Methods of Treatment

- Diaphoresis
- Clearing
- Ejection
- Precipitation
- Harmonization
- Warming
- Supplementation
- Dispersion
- Orifice opening
- Securing astriction
- Settling and absorption

THERAPEUTIC METHODS

This section discusses the therapeutic methods of acupuncture and moxibustion, cupping and bleeding, Chinese massage, qi cultivation, Chinese herbal medicine, and dietetics.

Although acupuncture and moxibustion can be used independently, they are so deeply interrelated in Chinese medicine that the term for this therapy is *zhen jiu,* meaning "needle moxibustion." To capture the distinctively composite character of this phrase, some authors translate the expression as "acumoxa therapy." This close linkage is based on the ancient origins of these methods, and moxibustion apparently was the form of therapy first applied to the channels and holes to treat problems on or within the body. Both acupuncture and moxibustion are used to provide a discrete stimulus to points that lie along channel pathways or to other appropriate sites.

Acupuncture

The therapeutic goal of acupuncture is to regulate the qi. Qi and blood flow through the body, its organs, and the channel pathways. When it flows unimpeded, the body is in a state of health. When some cause, such as an evil, mental state, or trauma, interrupts the flow of qi, illness results and pain can occur. Pain is directly linked to an injury or an interruption of the flow of qi. Acupuncture is used to remove the obstruction. The technique may be used to remove the evil, to direct qi to where it is insufficient, or to cause qi to flow where it previously had been obstructed.

The *Spiritual Axis* of the *Inner Classic* describes nine needles for use in acupuncture (Figure 21-3). With the exception of the needle with a specifically surgical application, the remaining needle types are still in use, either in original or adapted form. Acupuncture is performed today with a wider variety of tools and methods. The *filiform* needle, or fine needle, is the typical acupuncture tool, and it can vary significantly in terms of structure, diameter, and length.

A typical acupuncture needle has a body or shaft that is 1 inch long and a handle of approximately the same length (Figure 21-4). The distinctive part of an acupuncture needle is its tip, which is rounded and moderately sharp, much like the tip of a pine needle. The acupuncture needle is solid and gently tapered; it

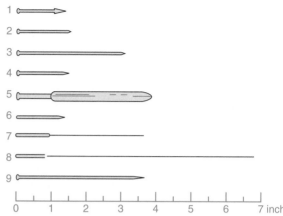

Figure 21-3 The nine needles according to the *Spiritual Pivot.* (From Qiu ML: *Chinese acupuncture and moxibustion,* Edinburgh, 1993, Churchill Livingstone, p 184.)

does not have the lumen or cutting edge of the hypodermic needle used for injection. Its diameter typically is 0.25 mm.

Once the site for insertion has been determined, the needle is inserted rapidly through the skin and then adjusted to an appropriate depth. Although other considerations affect the angle and depth of insertion, methods of manipulation, and the length of retention, this is the basic procedure. A twelfth-century text, *Ode of the Subtleties of Flow,* states, "Insert the needle with noble speed then proceed (to the point) slowly, withdraw the needle with noble slowness as haste will cause injury" (Shanghai College of Traditional Chinese Medicine, 1981).

The essential aim of the acupuncturist is to obtain qi at the needling site. The physician seeks either an objective or a subjective indication that the qi has arrived. Qi can become manifest to the practitioner through sensations experienced by the hands as the needle is manipulated, through observation, or through reports from the patient. The sensation of the arrival of qi often is felt by the practitioner as a gentle grasping of the needle at the site, as if a fishing line has suddenly been seized by the fish. The patient senses the arrival of qi as a sensation of itching, numbness, soreness, or a swollen feeling. The patient

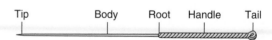

Figure 21-4 The structure of the filiform needle. (From Qiu ML: *Chinese acupuncture and moxibustion,* Edinburgh, 1993, Churchill Livingstone, p 186.)

might experience local temperature changes or a distinct "electrical" sensation. Acupuncture points in different areas of the body respond differently; these variations in response can be an important diagnostic indicator. It is not unusual for a clinician to retain a needle in an acupuncture point where the qi has not arrived until the characteristic sensation occurs.

Once a point has been correctly located, needled, and qi obtained, the clinician may choose to manipulate the needle to achieve a desired therapeutic effect. Styles of needle manipulation have inspired extensive discussions in both ancient and modern texts. Methods may range from simply putting the needle in place, then leaving it there, to engaging in complex manipulations that involve slow or rapid insertion of the needle to greater or more shallow depths. These techniques might create a distinctive sensation along the channel pathway. This needle may be withdrawn promptly after qi arrives, or a short fine needle (known as an *intradermal*) may be retained in the site for several days. In all cases the goal of the clinician is to influence the movement of qi.

One simple style of needle manipulation involves adjusting the direction of the needle to supplement or drain the qi at the particular channel point. If one thinks of the acupuncture point as a hole where the channel qi can be touched and moved, this operation can either cause the qi to become secure and increased in the channel (supplementing) or cause the qi to spill out (draining).

For our patient experiencing the symptoms of wind cold, an acupuncturist might choose to needle several acupuncture points, including Wind Pool (*Feng Chi* GB 20), located on the back of the neck below the occipital bone; Union Valley (*He Gu* LI 4), located in the fleshy area between the base of the thumb and forefinger; and Broken Sequence (*Lie Que* LU 7), on the forearm just above the styloid process of the radius. These particular points could all be treated with a draining method because, in this patient, the channels are replete with the influences of the external evils of wind and cold. Wind Pool is often used to drain wind from the surface of the body and to relieve headache and neck pain. Union Valley is an important acupuncture point used to influence the upper part of the body and to control pain. In the wind cold patient the point is used because of its ability to course wind, resolve the exterior, and treat headache and sore throat. Broken Sequence is said to dispel cold and to diffuse the lung. It courses the

channels and can be used to treat sore throat and headache.

Practitioners use various methods to select acupuncture points for treating a particular patient. One of the most traditional methods is an empirically derived understanding of what points work best for a given condition. Each acupuncture point has numerous indications associated with it based on the accumulated experience of generations of acupuncture practitioners.

Ancient and contemporary texts abound with descriptions of specific sets of acupuncture points that may be used to treat a condition successfully. Broken Sequence and Leg Three Li (*Zu San Li* St 36) are described by the *Song of Point Applications for Miscellaneous Disease* as useful for rapid breathing and dyspnea (Ellis et al., 1991, p. 84) (see Box 21-2).

Besides choosing points on the basis of their indications and the experience and descriptions accumulated in texts, acupuncturists also can apply specific theoretical considerations to traditional acupuncture point categories. For example, they can choose acupuncture points on the basis of their theoretical associations with the five phases. An inference concerning the relative status of the five phases and the organs is made based on the pulses and presenting symptoms. If the patient displays signs of vacuity of the water phase, points could be chosen from the transport points along the kidney channel associated with water to supplement the water phase.

Points also may be chosen on the basis of the actual trajectory of the channel on which the points lie. Union Valley is considered an important point for the head and face because it lies on the pathway of the large intestine channel, which traverses that area of the body. Similarly, points on the lower extremity that lie on the urinary bladder channel, which traverses the entire back, often are used for back pain (Figure 21-5).

Finally, points often are selected entirely on the basis of their sensitivity to palpation or based on a variation in texture perceived by the practitioner. Often a number of suitable acupuncture points in a specific area may be assessed to determine which would be most suitable for needling. In some cases, points that do not lie on specific channels or form part of the collection of recognized extra points can be identified by their tenderness. These points are known as *ah shi*, or "ouch, that's it," points and are an important part of clinical acupuncture's traditional history and contemporary practice.

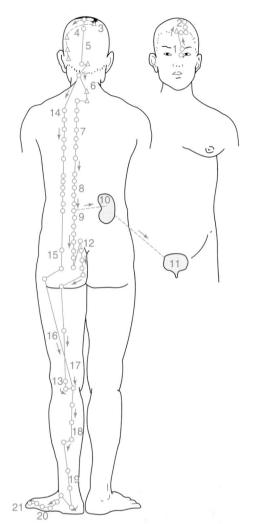

Figure 21-5 The course of the urinary bladder channel of the foot taiyang. (From Qiu ML: *Chinese acupuncture and moxibustion,* Edinburgh, 1993, Churchill Livingstone, p 103.)

With many acupuncture points to choose from and multiple methods on which to base that choice, it is not surprising that many clinicians focus on a few specific methods or a particular collection of points. Some clinicians restrict their approach so that they can focus on adjusting the application of treatment.

Moxibustion *(Jiu Fa)*

Moxibustion *(jiu)* refers to the burning of the dried and powdered leaves of *Artemesia vulgaris (ai ye),* either

on or in proximity to the skin, to affect the movement of qi in the channel, locally or at a distance. *A. vulgaris* is said to be acrid and bitter and, when used as *moxa,* to have the ability to warm and enter the channels. References to moxa appear in early materials, such as the texts recovered from the excavated tombs at Ma Wang Dui (Unschuld, 1985). These texts discuss a number of therapeutic methods, including moxibustion, but do not mention acupuncture. The *Treatise on Moxibustion of the Eleven Vessels of Yin and Yang (Yin Yang Shi Yi Mai Jiu Jing)* describes the application of moxa to treat illness by doing moxibustion on the channels (Auteroche et al., 1992).

Moxibustion can be applied to the body in many ways: directly, indirectly, pole, and warm needle method. *Direct moxibustion* involves burning a small amount of moxa, about the size of a grain of rice, directly on the skin. Depending on the desired effect, larger or smaller pieces of moxa can be used, and the moxa fluff can be allowed to burn directly to the skin, causing a blister or a scar, or it can be removed before it has burnt down to the skin. Such techniques are used to stimulate acupuncture points where the action of moxibustion is traditionally indicated or where warming the point seems to be the most appropriate response. Older texts described the use of direct moxibustion on Leg Three Li and other acupuncture points as a method of health maintenance and prevention.

Indirect moxibustion involves the insertion of a mediating substance between the moxa fluff and the patient's skin. This gives the practitioner greater control over the amount of heat applied to the patient's body and offers the patient increased protection from burning, allowing for the treatment of delicate areas such as the face and back. Popular substances include ginger slices, garlic slices, and salt. The mediating substance is often chosen on the basis of its own medicinal properties and how it combines with the properties of moxa. Ginger might be selected in patients with vacuity cold, whereas garlic is considered useful for treating hot and toxic conditions. Figure 21-6 shows a patient being treated for facial paralysis with indirect moxibustion using ginger slices.

During *pole moxibustion* cigar-shaped roll of moxa wrapped in paper is used to warm the acupuncture points gently without touching the skin. This is a safe method of moxibustion that can be taught to patients for self-application.

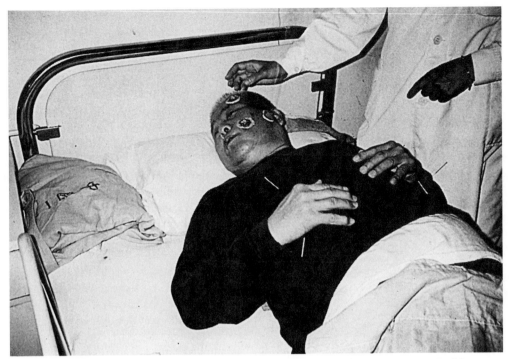

Figure 21-6 Patient receiving indirect moxa. (Courtesy Wind Horse, Marnae Ergil.)

The *warm needle method* is accomplished by first inserting an acupuncture needle into the point and then placing moxa fluff on its handle. After the moxa is ignited, it burns gradually, imparting a sensation of gentle warmth to the acupuncture point and channel. This method is especially useful for patients with arthritic joint pain.

Combined Therapy with Acupuncture

Together, moxibustion and acupuncture are used to treat, or at least ameliorate, a wide range of conditions and symptoms. On the basis of the simple premise that all disease involves the disruption of the flow of qi and that acupuncture and moxibustion regulate the movement of qi, all disease theoretically can benefit from these methods. A brief review of acupuncture texts provides ample evidence of the range of conditions for which acupuncture is considered appropriate. Over the years, efforts have been made outside of China to parse the range of conditions treatable by acupuncture, including a World Health Organization (WHO) Interregional Seminar in the late 1970s (Bannerman, 1979). More recently the WHO established selection criteria for evaluating reports of controlled clinical trials of acupuncture as a basis for reporting on the use of acupuncture in the treatment of various diseases and disorders; Boxes 21-6 and 21-7 list partial results (WHO, 2002). Although comparatively short compared with a clinical manual or acupuncture textbook, these lists are informative in terms of the routine application of acupuncture in China and elsewhere. It is also instructive to compare these two lists with the report of the NIH Consensus Conference discussed later.

Cupping and Bleeding

Two methods important to the practice of Chinese medicine are cupping and bleeding. These may be used separately or together and are often used with other methods, such as moxibustion and acupuncture. *Cupping* involves inducing a vacuum in a small glass or bamboo cup and promptly applying it to the skin surface. This therapy brings blood and lymph to the skin surface under the cup, increasing local circulation. Cupping is often used to drain or remove cold and damp evils from the body or to assist blood

BOX 21-6

*Diseases and Disorders Effectively Treated with Acupuncture**

Adverse reactions to radiotherapy and/or chemo-
  therapy
Allergic rhinitis (including hay fever)
Biliary colic
Depression (including depressive neurosis and
  depression following stroke)
Dysentery, acute bacillary
Dysmenorrhea, primary
Epigastralgia, acute (in peptic ulcer, acute and
  chronic gastritis, and gastrospasm)
Facial pain (including craniomandibular
  disorders)
Headache
Hypertension, essential
Hypotension, primary
Induction of labor
Knee pain
Leukopenia
Low back pain
Malposition of fetus, correction of
Morning sickness
Nausea and vomiting
Neck pain
Pain in dentistry (including dental pain and
  temporomandibular dysfunction)
Periarthritis of shoulder
Postoperative pain
Renal colic
Rheumatoid arthritis
Sciatica
Sprain
Stroke
Tennis elbow

From World Health Organization: *Acupuncture: review and analysis of
reports on controlled clinical trials,* Geneva, 2002, WHO. www.who.
int/medicines/library/trm/acupuncture/acupuncture_ trials.doc.
*Diseases, symptoms, or conditions for which acupuncture has been
proved—through controlled trials—to be an effective treatment.

circulation. *Bleeding* is done to drain a channel or to remove heat from the body at a specific location. Unlike the bloodletting practiced by Western physicians throughout the nineteenth century, this method expresses comparatively small amounts of blood, from a drop to a few centiliters. Figure 21-7 shows a patient receiving cupping and bleeding at an acupuncture point on the urinary bladder channel associated with the lungs.

Chinese Massage (Tui Na)

Literally "pushing and pulling," *Tui Na* refers to a system of massage, manual acupuncture point stimulation, and manipulation that is vast enough to warrant its own chapter. These methods have been practiced at least as long as moxibustion, but the first massage training class was created in Shanghai in 1956 (Wang et al., 1990, p. 16). At present, this field of study can serve as a minor component of a traditional medical education or an area of extensive clinical specialization.

A distinct aspect of Tui Na is the extensive training of the hands necessary for clinical practice. The practitioner's hands are trained to accomplish focused and forceful movements that can be applied to various areas of the body. Techniques such as pushing, rolling, kneading, rubbing, and grasping are practiced repetitively until they become second nature (Figure 21-8). Students practice on a small bag of rice until their hands develop the necessary strength and dexterity.

Tui Na often is applied to limited areas of the body, and the techniques can be quite forceful and intense. Tui Na is applied routinely to orthopedic and neurological conditions. It also is applied to conditions not usually viewed as susceptible to treatment through manipulation, such as asthma, dysmenorrhea, and chronic gastritis. Tui Na is used as an adjunct to acupuncture to increase the range of motion of a joint or instead of acupuncture when needles are uncomfortable or inappropriate, such as pediatric applications.

As with all aspects of Chinese medicine, regional styles and family lineages of massage practice abound. The formal Tui Na curriculum available in Chinese programs is extensive but probably not a complete expression of the range of possibilities.

Qi Cultivation (Qigong)

Qigong is a term that literally embraces almost every aspect of the manipulation of qi by means of exercise, breathing, and the influence of the mind, as discussed later and in Chapter 22. Qigong includes

BOX 21-7

Diseases and Disorders Showing Therapeutic Effects of Acupuncture[*]

Abdominal pain (in acute gastroenteritis or due to gastrointestinal spasm)	Neuralgia, postherpetic
Acne vulgaris	Neurodermatitis
Alcohol dependence and detoxification	Obesity
Bell's palsy	Opium, cocaine, and heroin dependence
Bronchial asthma	Osteoarthritis
Cancer pain	Pain due to endoscopic examination
Cardiac neurosis	Pain in thromboangiitis obliterans
Cholecystitis, chronic, with acute exacerbation	Polycystic ovary syndrome (Stein-Leventhal syndrome)
Cholelithiasis	Postextubation in children
Competition stress syndrome	Postoperative convalescence
Craniocerebral injury, closed	Premenstrual syndrome
Diabetes mellitus, non–insulin-dependent	Prostatitis, chronic
Earache	Pruritus
Epidemic hemorrhagic fever	Radicular and pseudoradicular pain syndrome
Epistaxis, simple (without generalized or local disease)	Raynaud syndrome, primary
Eye pain due to subconjunctival injection	Recurrent lower urinary tract infection
Female infertility	Reflex sympathetic dystrophy
Facial spasm	Retention of urine, traumatic
Female urethral syndrome	Schizophrenia
Fibromyalgia and fasciitis	Sialism, drug-induced
Gastrokinetic disturbance	Sjögren syndrome
Gouty arthritis	Sore throat (including tonsillitis)
Hepatitis B virus carrier status	Spine pain, acute
Herpes zoster (human [alpha] herpesvirus 3)	Stiff neck
Hyperlipemia	Temporomandibular joint dysfunction
Hypo-ovarianism	Tietze syndrome
Insomnia	Tobacco dependence
Labor pain	Tourette syndrome
Lactation deficiency	Ulcerative colitis, chronic
Male sexual dysfunction, nonorganic	Urolithiasis
Ménière disease	Vascular dementia
	Whooping cough (pertussis)

From World Health Organization: *Acupuncture: review and analysis of reports on controlled clinical trials,* Geneva, 2002, WHO.
www.who.int/ medicines/library/trm/acupuncture/acupuncture_trials.doc.
*Diseases, symptoms, or conditions for which the therapeutic effect of acupuncture has been shown but for which further proof is needed:

practices ranging from the meditative systems of Daoist and Buddhist practitioners to the martial arts traditions of China. Qigong is relevant to medicine in three specific areas. First, it allows the practitioner to cultivate demeanor and stamina to perform the strenuous activities of Tui Na, to sustain the constant demands of clinical practice, and to quiet the mind to facilitate diagnostic perception. Second, Qigong cultivates the practitioner's ability to transmit qi safely to the patient. Practitioners may direct qi to the patient either through the needles or directly through their hands. This activity may be the main focus of treatment or an adjunctive aspect, in which case the qi paradigm is expanded to include direct interaction between the patient's qi and the clinician's qi. Third, patients may be taught to do specific Qigong practices that are useful for their illness.

Qi cultivation makes extensive use of the principles of TCM, and its history is intertwined with that of famous physicians. The history of qi cultivation practices is considered to extend back into antiquity and to indicate the early recognition of the

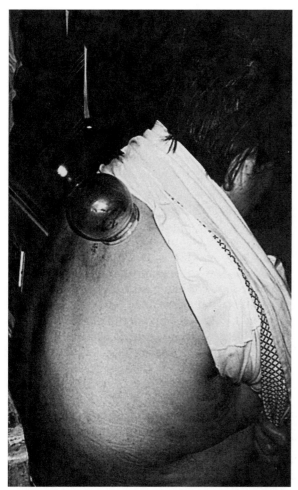

Figure 21-7 Cupping and bleeding. (Courtesy Wind Horse, Marnae Ergil.)

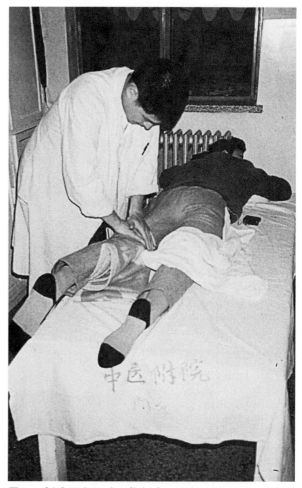

Figure 21-8 Tui Na in clinical practice. (Courtesy Wind Horse, Marnae Ergil.)

importance of exercise to the health of the body. In Lu's *Spring* and *Autumn* annals, the following famous aphorism relates the importance of movement to the maintenance of health and function (Engelhardt, 1989):

> Flowing water will never turn stale, the hinge of the door will never be eaten by worms. They never rest in their activity: that's why.

Within this text, Lu described the role of dance and movement in correcting the movement of qi and yin within the body and benefiting the muscles (Zhang, 1990).

Descriptions of qi cultivation practices and exercises are attributed to the early Daoist masters. Zhuang Zi, writing in the fourth century BCE, reveals the role of breathing and physical exercise in promot-

ing longevity and describes a sage intent on extending his life (Despeux, 1989), as follows:

> To pant, to puff, to hail, to sip, to spit out the old breath and draw in the new, practicing bear hangings and bird-stretches, longevity his only concern (Watson, 1968).

Among the texts recovered at Ma Huang Dui are a series of illustrated guides to the practice of conduction *(dao yin)* that provide guidance to the physical postures and therapeutic properties of this form of qi cultivation (Despeux, 1989, p. 226).

The famous physician of second-century China, Hua Tou, is credited with the creation of a series of exercises. These were based on the movements of the tiger, the deer, the bear, the monkey, and a bird and were to be practiced to ward off disease.

Zhang Zhong Jing, in his Golden Cabinet Prescriptions, recommended the practices of *dao yin* or conduction and Tui Na or exhalation and inhalation to treat disease.

A wide variety of forms of qi cultivation were developed over the centuries, and many have achieved great popularity. Since the 1950s, Qigong training programs have been implemented and sanatoria built, specializing in the therapeutic application of Qigong to the treatment of disease (see Chapter 22).

Fundamental Concepts

Qi cultivation rests on several fundamental principles intended to support activity to enhance the movement of qi and to increase health. Most discussions of qi cultivation address the relaxation of the body, the regulation or control of breathing, and the calming of the mind. Qi cultivation generally is performed in a relaxed standing, sitting, or lying posture. Once the correct position is achieved, the practitioner begins to regulate breathing in concert with specific mental and physical exercises.

For example, one form of Qigong involves the action of visualizing the internal and external pathways of the channels and imagining the movement of the qi along these channels in concert with the breath. As the practice develops, the practitioner begins to experience the sensation of qi traveling along the channel pathways. Traditionally, it is considered that the mind guides the qi to a specific area of the body and that the qi then guides the blood there as well, improving circulation in the area. From this point of view, this particular exercise trains the qi and blood to move freely along the channel pathways, leading to good health.

Another exercise involves the use of breath, visualization, and simple physical exercises to benefit the qi of the lungs. This therapeutic exercise is recommended for bronchitis, emphysema, and bronchial asthma. It is begun by assuming a relaxed posture, whether sitting, lying, or standing. The exercise is begun by breathing naturally and allowing the mind to become calm. The upper and lower teeth are then clicked together by closing the mouth gently 36 times. As saliva is produced, it is retained in the mouth, swirled with the tongue, and then swallowed in three parts while one imagines that it is flowing into the middle of the chest and then to an area about three fingerbreadths below the navel (the *dan tian*, or cinnabar field). At this point, one imagines that one is sitting in front of a reservoir of white qi that enters the mouth on inhalation and is transmitted through the body as one exhales, first to the lungs, then to the *dan tian*, and finally out to the skin and body hair. This process of visualization is repeated 18 times.

This process makes use of the relationship between the mind and qi to strengthen the function of the lungs and to pattern areas of the body associated with the area where the qi that governs the lungs and respiration is stored. This area is associated with the acupuncture point *dan zhong*, or chest center (ren 17), which is located in the middle of the chest. Next the qi is directed to the cinnabar field, which is associated with another location on the ren channel *qi hai*, or sea of qi (ren 6), just below the umbilicus. This area is considered to be important in the production and storage of the body's qi and to the lungs on exhalation.

This exercise typifies the three aspects of a Qigong exercise described previously: relaxation, mental tranquility, and breath control. It induces relaxation through mental concentration, because the exercise of focusing on breathing and the visualized process help remove distracting thoughts from the mind, and the patterning of the breath with visualization controls and regulates the breathing.

It should be stressed that although many forms of Qigong exist, they share general principles of application and a relationship to Chinese medicine concepts.

Chinese Herbal Medicine (*Zhong Yao*)

Since the legendary emperor Shen Nong tasted herbs and guided the Chinese people in herbal use, diet, and therapeutics, herbal medicine has been an integral part of Chinese culture and medical practice. The traditional Chinese materia medica includes much more than herbs; minerals and animal parts are listed as well. The number of substances currently identified is 5767, as recorded in the *Encyclopedia of Traditional Chinese Medicinal Substances (Zhong Yao Da Ci Dian)* published in 1977 by the Jiangsu College of New Medicine (Bensky and Gamble, 1986). This publication is the latest in a long line of definitive discussions of materia medica that have been produced in China over the millennia. The earliest known is the

Divine Husbandman's Classic of the Materia Medica, reconstructed by Tao Hong Jing (452-536 CE). This text classified herbs into upper, middle, and lower grades and discussed the tastes, temperatures, toxicities, and medicinal properties of 364 substances.

Currently, substances are categorized systematically as expansions of the eight methods of therapy discussed earlier (Box 21-8). Subcategories exist within the basic categories into which substances are organized. Prescribing rules take into account the compatibilities and incompatibilities of substances, the traditional pairings of substances, and their combination for specific symptoms.

Both the Ma Wan Dui texts and the *Inner Classic* provide recommendations for the therapeutic combination of substances. Zhang Zhong Jing's work in systematizing herbal prescriptions as therapeutic approaches to specific diagnostic patterns based on yin and yang correspondences was unusual for its time. It was not until physicians of the Sung dynasty became interested in relating herbal practice to a systematic theory and organizing diagnostics accordingly that interest was renewed in the *Treatise on Cold Damage.* This book remains a significant resource for the current practitioner of Chinese herbal medicine.

One of the most comprehensive English-language compilations of Chinese herbal prescriptions derives approximately 20% of its formulas from this source (Bensky and Barolet, 1990).

Not all herbal prescriptions or texts discussing application followed the lead of Zhang Zhong Jing. Many texts offered herbs or prescriptions for specific symptoms without reference to distinct theoretical structures or diagnostic principles. The general population probably applied herbs in exactly this manner. Even today, despite the prescription of herbal formulas being primarily driven by traditional diagnostic theory and pattern diagnosis, extensive compilations of empirically derived herbal formulas with symptomatic indications are published.

Contemporary compilations of formulas are organized similar to substances. The result is that both substances and formulas are organized in a manner that makes them accessible in terms of traditional theories (Box 21-9).

Let us examine the formula and its constituent substances that might be provided to our patient who has encountered a "wind cold evil" or who, in the pattern identification system described in the *Treatise on Cold Damage,* would be said to have a "tai yang stage

---

BOX 21-8

Fundamental Categories of Chinese Materia Medica

- Exterior-resolving
- Heat-clearing
- Ejection
- Precipitant
- Wind-dispelling
- Water-disinhibiting dampness-percolating
- Interior-warming
- Qi-rectifying
- Food-dispersing
- Worm-expelling
- Blood-rectifying
- Phlegm-transforming cough-suppressing panting-calming
- Spirit-quieting
- Liver-calming wind-extinguishing
- Orifice-opening
- Supplementing
- Securing and astringing
- External use

BOX 21-9

Formulas for Chinese Herbal Medicine

- Exterior-resolving
- Heat-clearing
- Ejection
- Precipitant
- Harmonizing
- Dampness-dispelling
- Interior-warming
- Qi-rectifying
- Dispersing
- Blood-rectifying
- Phlegm-transforming cough-suppressing panting-calming
- Spirit-quieting
- Tetany-settling
- Orifice-opening
- Supplementing
- Securing and astringing
- Oral formulas for sores
- External use

pattern." In either case, ephedra decoction (*Ma Huang Tang*) would be an appropriate choice, particularly if the patient had a slight cough as well. The constituents and dosage of the formula are 9 grams (g) of ephedra (*ma huang*), 6 g of cinnamon twig (*gui zhi*), 9 g of apricot kernel (*xing ren*), and 3 g of licorice (*gan cao*). These ingredients are cooked together in water to make a slightly concentrated tea, which is drunk in successive doses. The tea is taken warm to induce sweating, a sign that the qi of the surface of the body that had been impeded by the cold evil is free to move and throw off the evil. The patient stops drinking the tea once sweat arrives.

A traditional system of organizing a formula is to identify ingredients as the ruler, minister, adjutant, and emissary. In this case the *ruler* of the formula is ephedra. The ruler sets the therapeutic direction of the formula. Acrid and warm, ephedra promotes sweating, dispels cold, and resolves the surface. (We examine ephedra again in the discussion of herbal research.) Cinnamon twig is the *minister,* working to assist the ruler in carrying out its objectives. In addition to the effects described for ephedra, it also is said to warm the body. Apricot kernel is the *adjutant,* so it addresses the possible involvement of the lung and moderates the acrid flavor of the other two substances. Because the lung is the organ most immediately affected by wind cold or wind heat, the formula addresses the organ. Finally, licorice is the *emissary,* serving both to render the action of the other herbs harmonious and to distribute it through the body.

The previous example is brief and simple but illustrates fundamental concepts. Chinese herbal therapeutics can be complex. Its practice is broad, and the range of conditions addressed is more extensive than with acupuncture. In terms of complexity and the diagnostic acumen required of the practitioner, it resembles the practice of internal medicine. Herbal therapy also encompasses the external applications of herbs and a variety of methods of preparation. Besides the traditional water decoction, or tea, substances may be powdered or rendered into pills, pastes, or tinctures.

Dietetics

Traditional dietetics encompasses the practice of herbal therapy but also addresses traditional Chinese foods in terms of the theoretical constructs of Chinese medicine. Five-phase theory has been applied to foods since the time of the *Inner Classic*. It is not unusual to see a classroom in a college of Chinese medicine equipped as a kitchen. In larger cities, special restaurants prepare meals with specific medicinal purposes. The practices of this field are deeply rooted in the cultural practices of China and cultural beliefs about diet. Many of the foods organized for use in therapy also are routinely prepared by families when seasons change and when illness strikes, as well as to strengthen a woman after birth, to cause milk to fill the breasts of a new mother, or to nourish elderly persons in their declining years.

CHINESE MEDICINE IN OTHER COUNTRIES

China's traditional medicine is practiced in various forms all over the world. Sometimes its practice follows the contemporary patterns of *traditional Chinese medicine* (TCM, or *zhong yi*). Sometimes its practice is deeply informed by local custom, preference, or regional elaborations.

Chinese Medicine in Korea

A close relationship exists between China and Korea. Chinese medicine arrived in Korea during the Qin dynasty (221-207 BCE). However, the textual basis of Korean medicine in the literary tradition of Chinese medicine seems to have been established during the Han and Tang dynasties (Hsu and Peacher, 1977), during a period of political domination by the Chinese. The closeness between China and Korea during the Kingdom of Silla (400-700 CE) facilitated this exchange of ideas. Formal medical instruction by government-appointed physicians began in 693 CE. Texts such as the *Systematic Classic of Acupuncture* were important to the development of the tradition. With the formation of the Liao dynasty (907-1168), Korea established its independence from Chinese rule, but cultural and medical exchange continued. During the Li dynasty (1392-1910), many texts, including the *Illustrated Classic of Acupuncture Points as Found on the Bronze Model,* reached Korea (Chuang, 1982). Widely used techniques of acupuncture point selection based on five-phase theory have emerged from Korea, including those of the Buddhist priest Sa-am (1544-1610).

At least two comparatively recent innovations based on Chinese medicine have been developed in Korea and have become well known in other parts of the world. Korean *constitutional diagnosis* was developed initially by Jhema Lee (1836-1900) and based a system of herbal therapeutics on a system of diagnostic patterning that used the four divisions of yin and yang. In 1965, Dowon Kuan expanded the system to an eightfold classification and applied it to acupuncture (Hirsch, 1985). *Koryo Sooji Chim,* the system of Korean *hand and finger acupuncture,* was developed by Yoo Tae Woo and published in 1971. The system maps the channel pathways and acupuncture points of the entire body onto the hands, where they are stimulated using very short, fine needles and magnets. This system has gained a significant level of international exposure.

Chinese Medicine in Japan

The history of cultural exchange between China and Japan dates to at least 57 CE. Kon Mu was the first physician to go to Japan and use Chinese methods; he was sent in 414 CE by the king of Silla, in southeast Korea, to treat the emperor Inkyo Tenno. This interaction continued; in 552 a Korean delegation brought a selection of Chinese medical texts to Japan (Bowers, 1970). In 562, Zhi Cong came from southern China with more than 100 books on the practice of Chinese medicine (Huard and Wong, 1968), including the *Systematic Classic of Acupuncture* (Chuang, 1982). By the early eighth century the influence of Chinese medicine was well established. With the adoption of the Taiho code in 702, provision was made for a ministry of health composed of specialists, physicians, students, and researchers (Lock, 1980). In 754 a Buddhist priest, Chien Chen, brought many medical texts from China to Japan. His influence was memorialized in a shrine in Nishinokyo (Chuang, 1982).

Chinese influences on Japanese medicine were derived primarily from the *Classic of Difficult Issues* and *Systematic Classic of Acupuncture.* A revisionist movement in the late seventeenth century established *The Treatise on Cold Damage (Shokanron)* as the core text of herbal medicine, or *kanpo* (Chinese method), in Japan (Lock, 1980).

Several factors have influenced the development of Chinese medicine in Japan, giving it a somewhat unique appearance. The scarcity of ingredients for the preparation of Chinese herbal formulas has led to an emphasis on lower doses in herbal prescriptions than are typical in China. An emphasis on palpatory diagnosis involving channel pathways and the abdomen also became well established. The use of finer-gauge needles and shallow insertion became typical of Japanese acupuncture.

In the mid-seventeenth century, Waichi Sugiyama, a blind man, began to train the blind in acupuncture using very fine needles and guide tubes. Because it had become customary in the earlier part of the Edo period for blind persons to do massage, both massage and acupuncture now became associated with blind practitioners. This contributed to a lower social position for acupuncture practitioners and to specialization in medical practice. Kanpo physicians became primarily practitioners of herbal medicine (Lock, 1980).

This trend toward specialization has continued to the present, with the division of acupuncture, moxibustion, and massage into separately licensed practices (although many individuals hold all three licenses) and the actual practice of herbal medicine being retained in the hands of medical physicians. Interestingly, many Chinese herbal prescriptions are recognized as appropriate therapy for certain medical conditions according to regulations governing health care in Japan.

Japan has seen both focused specialization in and the innovative exploration and expansion of traditional acupuncture. The *Classic of Difficult Issues* often has been the focus for movements to revive the practices of traditional acupuncture. Its influence has contributed heavily to the comparatively recent development of groups of acupuncturists advocating *meridian therapy (keiraku chiryo)* based on the application of concepts in the *Classic of Difficult Issues* and their subsequent interpretation by later Chinese authors. A distinctive feature of meridian therapy is the application of five-phase theory to the transport points, a practice that has influenced the perception and adoption of five-phase theory by European practitioners (Kaptchuk, 1983).

The pioneering work of Yoshio Manaka also has contributed dramatically to the practice of acupuncture. Manaka, a physician who experimented with acupuncture principles when medical supplies were absent during World War II, became convinced of the efficacy and physiological relevance of traditional theories and continued to experiment and develop them throughout his life.

Japanese acupuncture practitioners have a broad range of practices and interests. Although some are particular partisans of specific schools of thought, including some based on contemporary Chinese medicine perspectives, many practitioners have adopted a comparatively eclectic approach.

Chinese Medicine in Europe

The history of Chinese medicine in Europe, particularly acupuncture, is both long-standing and broadly developed. The medical use of acupuncture in Europe dates from the middle of the sixteenth century (Peacher, 1975). The work of Willem Ten Rhyne (1647-1690) in this area culminated in the publication in 1683 of *Dissertatio de Arthritide: Mantissa Schematica: de Acupunctura: et Orationes Tres,* based on information gathered during his service in Japan as a physician for the Dutch East India Company. The German physician Kampfer, who also traveled with the Dutch East India Company and spent time in Japan, contributed his observations.

In France the Jesuit Du Halde published a text that included a detailed discussion of Chinese medicine in 1735 (Hsu, 1989). Soulie de Morant's publication of *L'acupuncture Chinoise* was an extensive discussion of the practice of acupuncture based on direct translation, observation, and actual practice by the author. Published in 1939, the text was rooted in de Morant's exposure to the medicine of China in that country from 1901 to 1917.

England saw the publication of J.M. Churchill's *A Description of Surgical Operations Peculiar to Japanese and Chinese* in 1825. Among early notable English acupuncturists are Drs. Felix Mann and Sidney Rose-Neil, both of whom began their explorations of acupuncture in the late 1950s and who have influenced its development substantially in English-speaking countries. J.R. Worsley, a physical therapist, began his studies of acupuncture in 1962 and had a substantial impact on the perceptions of many English and U.S. practitioners. He visited Hong Kong and Taiwan for a brief period and then became a part of the study group established by Rose-Neil (Hsu and Peacher, 1977). Worsley went on to create the British College of Traditional Chinese Acupuncture and two U.S. schools.

Chinese Medicine in the United States

In 1826, Bache became one of the first American physicians to use acupuncture in his practice (Haller, 1973). Ten Rhyne's text was a part of Sir William Osler's library (Peacher, 1975), and in his *Principles and Practice of Medicine,* Osler prescribes acupuncture for lumbago (Osler, 1913).

Although only occasionally explored by the conventional U.S. medical community, the traditional medicine of China has been practiced in the United States since the middle of the nineteenth century. Herbal merchants, entrepreneurs, and physicians accompanied the Chinese who sold their labor in the United States. The practice of the China Doctor of John Day, Oregon, Doc Ing Hay, is one of the most famous (Barlow and Richardson, 1979). Ah Fong Chuck, who came to the United States in 1866, became the first licensed practitioner of TCM in the United States in 1901, when he successfully won a medical license through legal action in Idaho (Muench, 1984). With the strengthening of medical practice acts throughout the United States, the interruption of the herb supply from China, and the advent of World War II, these practices disappeared or retreated into Chinatowns nationwide.

Substantial attention was focused on acupuncture, the traditional medicine of China, and its regional variants, as a result of James Reston's highly publicized appendectomy and postoperative care in 1971 and the subsequent opening of China by Nixon. As a result, medical practices largely confined to Asia and the Chinatowns of America gained visibility throughout the United States. Increased visibility led to substantial public interest in acupuncture and gradually to the licensure and development of training programs in many states. Currently, 41 states (including the District of Columbia) license, certify, or register the practice of acupuncture and a range of other activities, including herbal medicine by nonphysicians. More than 57 U.S. programs offer training in acupuncture and Oriental medicine.

Americans have a clear interest in the available range of expressions of Chinese medical tradition. In the United States, European interpretations of the application of five-phase theory, Korean constitutional acupuncture, TCM (acupuncture, herbs, Qigong, Tui Na), Japanese meridian therapy, and special family lineages within the Chinese tradition all are taught and practiced. This willingness to accept and explore the traditional and contemporary interpretations of traditional Chinese medicine has led to the emergence of the concept of "Oriental medicine" as an umbrella term for the global domain of practice in this area.

The extent to which the practice of Chinese medicine has come to be viewed as an established therapeutic practice in the United States was recently illustrated by a regulatory action taken by the U.S. Food and Drug Administration (FDA). After a series of reports of adverse events surrounding the use of ephedra-containing supplements in support of weight loss regimens and athletic training, neither of which can be considered to constitute the practice of Chinese medicine, the FDA was compelled to act. In February 2004 the FDA issued a final rule prohibiting the sale of dietary supplements containing ephedrine alkaloids (ephedra), "because such supplements present an unreasonable risk of illness or injury" (FDA, 2004). Intriguingly, it was specifically stated that the "scope of the rule does not pertain to traditional Chinese herbal remedies." Although the logistics of honoring this exemption have yet to be worked out, it is a definite acknowledgment of the professional practice of Chinese herbal medicine in the United States.

Practice Settings

In general, TCM is practiced in a range of clinical settings. Large hospitals entirely devoted to its practice are common in China. In this setting, acupuncture, herbal medicine, and Tui Na are provided on both an inpatient and an outpatient basis. It is not unusual to see a large outpatient facility treating 20 patients simultaneously in the same space. Other settings include smaller practices and even roadside stands. Herbal prescriptions can be obtained from a Chinese herb store in most countries with a significant Chinese population. In Japan, small hospitals, large clinics, and private offices are typical settings.

Wherever TCM is practiced, the delivery settings are not significantly different from the environment in which biomedical services are provided, unless the practitioner wants to emphasize the distinctive character of the practice, or if the practice is marginalized through lack of regulation. In the United States,

record-keeping processes, insurance billing, biomedical screening, and concerns about office hygiene often produce a setting that—except for such peculiarities as acupuncture needles, moxa fluff, and herbs—looks very much like a typical physician's office.

RESEARCH AND EVALUATION

Aspects of Chinese medicine have been the focus of concerted research efforts in China and Japan since the mid-twentieth century, or earlier if one considers research into Chinese herbal medicine in Japan. Recently, substantial research initiatives in this area have been undertaken in the United States and Europe as well, developing rapidly in terms of quality and quantity in the last 20 years. The actual and perceived quality of such research, in both the East and the West, can vary widely. As is the case for medical systems, research standards, and even scientific research, are subject to cultural influences. The randomized, placebo-controlled, and double-blind clinical trial is the definitive standard for an unambiguous biomedical recognition of efficacy, but not all societies require or encourage their medical communities to secure knowledge in this manner. In addition, the simple accessibility of research data is influenced by the language and location of publication. These problems can pose obstacles to the availability and use of research information. Therefore, research that is meaningful to the scientific communities of China, Japan, Europe, or the United States can vary in its relevance to and impact on other communities.

Study design is another problem that emerges with clinical research in Chinese medicine. Problems with research methods have arisen as the Chinese medicine community in the United States and Europe has participated more in research and as the biomedical community has become better educated about various modalities of Chinese medicine.

Efforts by the Office of Alternative Medicine (OAM), created in 1991 under the National Institutes of Health (NIH), have substantially contributed to this process within the United States. The OAM has hosted several conferences dealing with methodological considerations in the field of alternative medicine, and each event has addressed aspects of TCM.

Other OAM-supported projects have included funding of numerous small research grants, many in the area of Chinese or Oriental medicine.

The OAM also sponsored a workshop on acupuncture in cooperation with the FDA. In April1994, members of the acupuncture medical and scientific community gave presentations detailing the safety and the apparent clinical efficacy of acupuncture needles. These presentations became the core of a petition that led, in March 1996, to the reclassification of acupuncture needles by the FDA from a class III, or experimental, device to a class II, or medical, device for use by qualified practitioners with special controls (sterility and single use).

In November 1997 the NIH convened a Consensus Development Conference on the safety and efficacy of acupuncture for the treatment of specific conditions. Acupuncture experts presented evidence to a scientific panel who reached the following formal conclusion:

> Acupuncture as a therapeutic intervention is widely practiced in the United States. While there have been many studies of its potential usefulness, many of these studies provide equivocal results because of design, sample size, and other factors. The issue is further complicated by inherent difficulties in the use of appropriate controls, such as placebos and sham acupuncture groups. However, promising results have emerged, for example, showing efficacy of acupuncture in adult postoperative and chemotherapy nausea and vomiting and in postoperative dental pain. There are other situations such as addiction, stroke rehabilitation, headache, menstrual cramps, tennis elbow, fibromyalgia, myofascial pain, osteoarthritis, low back pain, carpal tunnel syndrome, and asthma, in which acupuncture may be useful as an adjunct treatment or an acceptable alternative or be included in a comprehensive management program. Further research is likely to uncover additional areas where acupuncture interventions will be useful (NIH, 1997).

Considering that less than 2 years earlier, acupuncture needles were still considered an experimental device in the United States, this finding marked significant progress.

In late 1998 the OAM was established as the National Center for Complementary and Alternative Medicine (NCCAM) and was provided with a significant increase in funding (Box 21-10). Since its inception, OAM/NCCAM has continued to refine and develop its approach to fostering research into complementary and alternative medicine (CAM). One strategy is the funding of CAM research centers with developed institutional resources. At present, these specialty centers number 22; many have developed or proposed research that includes aspects of TCM (Boxes 21-11 and 21-12). Some centers, such as the Center for Alternative Medicine Pain Research on Arthritis at the University of Maryland School of Medicine, have built their centers around long-term and sustained research efforts in specific areas. This has allowed them to make substantial strides as increased funding became available because of interest in CAM therapies. Recently, traditional acupuncture and Oriental medicine programs have begun to emerge as visible partners in research initiatives. The New England School of Acupuncture (NESA) has partnered with Harvard in a research collaboration.

Other organizations, such as the Society for Acupuncture Research (SAR), have emerged from the broad-based community of acupuncturists, physicians, and researchers interested in the range of research issues posed by this field. The SAR holds annual meetings and publishes its proceedings. Among its objectives are scholarly exchange between researchers in acupuncture and other modalities related to Oriental medicine, encouragement of research activities by acupuncturists, and clarification of methodological issues related to research in these areas. In 1996, two SAR officers, Stephen Birch and Richard Hammerschlag, compiled a definitive summary of the most successful, well-designed, controlled clinical trials produced to date.

Research into Specific Areas of Chinese Medicine

Research on fundamental concepts, or what might be called *fundamental theory,* includes the exploration of whether concepts such as qi, the channels, acupuncture points, the diagnostic aspects of the pulse, and aspects of pattern diagnosis actually can refer to a reproducibly identifiable and quantifiable phenomenon. All these areas have been or are being actively pursued in a number of countries. This research resembles basic research in physiology and relies on the development of sophisticated models and the design of instrumentation to test these models.

BOX 21-10

Acupuncture Studies Funded by National Center for Complementary and Alternative Medicine (NCCAM)

Acupuncture and Hypertension
Acupuncture and Moxa: A RCT for Chronic Diarrhea in HIV Patients
Acupuncture for Shortness of Breath in Cancer Patients
Acupuncture for the Treatment of Chronic Daily Headaches
Acupuncture for the Treatment of Hot Flashes in Breast Cancer Patients
Acupuncture for the Treatment of Post-Traumatic Stress Disorder (PTSD)
Acupuncture in Cardiovascular Disease
Acupuncture in Fibromyalgia
Acupuncture in the Treatment of Depression
Acupuncture Needling on Connective Tissue by Ultrasound
Acupuncture Safety/Efficacy in Knee Osteoarthritis
Acupuncture to Prevent Postoperative Bowel Paralysis (Paralytic Ileus)
Acupuncture to Reduce Symptoms of Advanced Colorectal Cancer
Acupuncture vs. Placebo in Irritable Bowel Syndrome
Efficacy of Acupuncture for Chronic Low Back Pain
Efficacy of Acupuncture in the Treatment of Fibromyalgia
Efficacy of Acupuncture with Physical Therapy for Knee Osteo-Arthritis
Interaction between Patient and Healthcare Provider: Response to Acupuncture in Knee Osteoarthritis
A Randomized Study of Electroacupuncture Treatment for Delayed Chemotherapy-Induced Nausea and Vomiting in Patients with Pediatric Sarcomas
Use of Acupuncture for Dental Pain: Testing a Model

Research questions derived from the search for the physiological basis of Chinese medical concepts have been pursued for some time in China. One such study investigated the nature of kidney yang and concluded that patients displaying a diagnostic pattern associated with kidney yang vacuity showed low levels of 17-hydroxy corticosteroids in their urine, ultimately suggesting a relationship between the concept of kidney yang and the adrenocortical system (Hao, 1983).

Research on the correlation between the force and waveforms of the radial artery and the diagnostic perceptions of clinicians and physical status of patients has long been pursued in China, the United States, Japan, and Korea (Broffman and McCulloch, 1986; Takashima, 1995; Zhu, 1991). Typically, this research depends on the use of pressure sensors that are pressed against the skin overlying the radial artery in a manner and location that replicates that of the finger position of the traditional clinician. Pulse patterns are recorded and correlated to observations made by the clinician in an effort to determine the physical basis that must be present for a diagnostic perception. Preliminary results are intriguing, but methodological questions concerning population size and standardization of measurement remain.

Research concerning channels and acupuncture points has relied on a variety of techniques, including the measurement of electrical resistance, thermography, tracing the pathways of injected radioisotopes, and dissection. Dissection has not produced particularly interesting results; the so-called Bonghan corpuscles, identified on dissection by Kim Bong Han in Korea, once were proposed as the anatomical basis of acupuncture points. This research has not been replicated, and although occasionally referred to in contemporary materials (Burton Goldberg Group, 1993), it generally is not perceived as credible.

More interesting are the discussions that propose or demonstrate an archaic or cellularly mediated signaling system that uses the bioelectrical properties of the body to propagate information. Early contributors in this area include Robert O. Becker, an orthopedist whose interest in the body's bioelectric properties and bone healing led him to explore the electrical properties of acupuncture points and channel pathways (Becker, 1985; Reichmanis et al., 1975). A component of this hypothesis is the measurable, lowered electrical resistance of the skin at acupuncture points. This unusual electrical property is characteristic of many acupuncture points (Pomeranz, 1988).

BOX 21-11

NCCAM Research Centers Examining Aspects of Chinese Medicine

Center of Excellence for the Neuroimaging of Acupuncture Effects on Human Brain Activity
Specialty: Acupuncture
Massachusetts General Hospital
Charlestown, MA
Investigating the neural basis for the effects of acupuncture through the use of functional magnetic resonance imaging.

NESA-Harvard Acupuncture Research Collaborative
Specialty: Acupuncture
New England School of Acupuncture
Watertown, MA
This Developmental Center for Research will bring together leaders from the Oriental medicine (OM) and conventional medicine communities to critically evaluate the efficacy and safety of acupuncture and to develop sound methodologies for acupuncture research.

Center for CAM Research in Aging and Women's Health
Specialty: Aging and Women's Health
Columbia University
College of Physicians and Surgeons
New York, NY
Studies include a basic science evaluation of various biological activities of a Chinese herbal preparation to help assess its safety for women with or at risk for breast cancer.

Center for Alternative Medicine Research on Arthritis
Specialty: Arthritis
University of Maryland School of Medicine
Baltimore, MD
The Center will investigate the cost-effectiveness of and long-term outcomes following acupuncture treatment for osteoarthritis of the knee; the mechanism of action and effects of electroacupuncture on persistent pain and inflammation; and the mechanism of action of an herbal combination with immunomodulatory properties.

CAM Research Center for Cardiovascular Diseases
Specialty: Cardiovascular diseases
The University of Michigan Taubman Health Care Center
Ann Arbor, MI
The Center will assess the impact of traditional Chinese medicine techniques of Qi Gong on post–coronary artery bypass grafting (CABG) pain, healing, and outcome.

Center for CAM in Neurodegenerative Diseases
Specialty: Neurodegenerative diseases
Emory University School of Medicine
Atlanta, GA
Current projects include the investigation of the effect of the Chinese mind-body modalities of Tai Chi Chuan and Qi Gong on motor disabilities associated with Parkinson's disease.

Yoshio Manaka, a Japanese surgeon and acupuncturist, hypothesized the presence of an archaic signaling system he called the "X-signal system," based on information theory concepts of biological systems, texts such as the *Inner Classic* and *Classic of Difficult Issues,* and experimental observations in his acupuncture clinic (Manaka and Itaya, 1994). Manaka's perspective grew out of exploration of both Chinese and Japanese needling methods and the use of the gentler needling techniques associated with the school of meridian therapy that arose in Japan.

BOX 21-12

NCCAM-Supported Studies in Chinese Medicine Modalities

Chinese Herbal Medicine

Alternative Medicine Approaches for Women with Temporomandibular Disorders

Consistency of Traditional Chinese Medicine Diagnoses and Herbal Prescriptions for Rheumatoid Arthritis

Herbal Treatment of Hepatitis C in Methadone Maintained Patients

Tai Ji Quan

Alternative Stress Management Approaches in HIV Disease

Complementary/Alternative Medicine for Abnormality in the Vestibular (Balance) System

Tai Chi Chih and Varicella Zoster Immunity

Qi Gong

Qigong Therapy for Heart Device Patients

Chinese Exercise Modalities in Parkinson's Disease

In his extensive discussion of the biophysical basis of acupuncture phenomena, James Oschman observes that the solid-state phenomena and the piezoelectric properties of the body's connective tissues provide a potential structure and mechanism that would allow for the existence of a signaling system similar to the role of the channels and points described in traditional literature (Oschman, 1993). Oschman goes on to explore a rich range of topics, including the measurable emission of electromagnetic fields from the hands of Qigong practitioners (Seto et al., 1992). Recently, Helene Langevin's work on the relationship between connective tissue and acupuncture phenomena such as *de qi* has demonstrated a mechanism that may support some of the hypotheses advanced by Oschman (Langevin et al., 2002).

All these explorations are preliminary. Even when research has been carried out and replicated, as in the case of lowered electrical resistance over acupuncture points, continued exploration is needed. It is unlikely that we will see a precise validation of the concepts of Chinese medicine in these areas, but rather a validation of the physiological basis for the existence of such concepts. The genius of Chinese medicine in these areas may lie in its ability to generalize about the manifesta-

tions of incredibly complex biological phenomena in an articulate and useful fashion. Given the preliminary findings on the possible nature of acupuncture points and channels, or on the variety of mechanisms that seem to be involved in acupuncture as a therapeutic phenomena, it seems increasingly likely that a concept such as "qi," or the therapeutic effects of an acupuncture point, must represent the action of many discrete and identifiable physiological processes. The likelihood is that aspects of these processes, observed as a whole, are the basis of the traditional concept.

Materia Medica and Traditional Pharmacology

Investigations of materia medica and traditional pharmacology have been ongoing since the early part of the twentieth century, in both China and Japan. The quality of research work is generally high, and the availability of translated literature is comparatively extensive. because this research can be divided into two areas of examination: the pharmacological properties of traditional materia medica and the clinical efficacy of traditional pharmacology. The first area does not differ from the typical concerns of pharmacological research. In vitro studies and exploration of traditional use can suggest the potential usefulness of certain substances. If one becomes aware of a substance that is alleged to have pharmacological properties, it is comparatively easy to conduct studies to assess the presence of these properties and to isolate apparently active compounds.

A famous case in point is the first herb listed in the Chinese materia medica: *Herba Ephedra*, known botanically as *Ephedra Sinica* Stapf *(ma huang)*. Herba Ephedra is recorded in the *Divine Husbandman's Classic of Materia Medica*. Its chief active component was isolated in 1887 in Japan but remained largely unexplored for 35 years, until C.F. Schmidt and K.K. Chen began to explore its pharmacological effects at the Peking Union Medical College, where the department of pharmacology was beginning a systematic exploration of the Chinese materia medica (Chen, 1977).

These explorations revealed that ephedrine was a sympathomimetic with properties of epinephrine, causing an increase in blood pressure, vasoconstriction, and bronchodilation. Clinically, ephedrine had several distinct advantages over epinephrine; ephedrine could be used orally, had a long duration of action, and was less toxic. It also was found to be useful in the management of bronchial asthma and hay fever and to support the patient's vital signs during the administration of spinal anesthesia. In subsequent years it became possible to synthesize ephedrine. This product of the Chinese materia medica currently is found in a number of pharmaceuticals, including over-the-counter products such as Sudafed and Actifed.

Historically and clinically, *Herba Ephedra* has been applied in a similar fashion in Chinese medicine, except for spinal anesthesia. As mentioned earlier, it is a principal ingredient in the herbal formula Ephedra Decoction. This herb also figures prominently in formulas that are applied to presentations that relate to asthma and allergy. *Herba Ephedra* represents an early and impressive example of pharmacological research in the Chinese materia medica. Other examples in which the traditional clinical applications of single herbs is supported in recent clinical experimentation include *Herba Artemisiae (yin chen hao)* for hepatitis and *Caulis Mu Tong (mu tong)* for urinary tract infections. Extensive compilations discussing identified active constituents, clinical studies, and toxicity of large numbers of substances have been prepared (Chang, 1986).

Explorations of traditional pharmacology are somewhat more complex, although they too are amenable to the methods of double blinding and placebo control that are critical to recognition in the biomedical world. However, given the breadth of possible substances that may be applied clinically (more than 5000) and the number of possible permutations for their combination in formula, the scope of the inquiry becomes quite large. In addition, there is the question of whether to include the traditional considerations that surround diagnosis and pattern identification in the process of prescription and selection of herbal formulas for investigation. Some contemporary studies are designed to take this into account, with the traditional clinician being able to assign individuals to specific treatment groups on the basis of symptoms while still being blinded in relation to the actual constituents of the substances administered to the patient. A recent example of this approach can be seen in a randomized clinical trial of Chinese herbal medicine for the treatment of irritable bowel syndrome conducted by Alan Bensoussan under the auspices of the Research Unit for Complementary Medicine, University of Western

Sydney. This study, in which patients were randomized to three treatment groups: placebo, standard formula, and individualized formula, showed that Chinese herbal medicine provided significant reduction in the symptoms of irritable bowel syndrome (Bensoussan et al., 1998). Research in this area has been extensive both in China and Japan and is emerging in the United States.

Acupuncture

> Disappointingly little has been achieved by literally hundreds of attempts to evaluate acupuncture. Major methodological flaws are apparent in the vast majority of studies (Vincent, 1993).

Although the pessimism of Vincent's statement is captured in the NIH Consensus Panel's conclusions concerning the methodological problems that continue to plague acupuncture studies, the Panel's remarks concerning the range of promising results in specific areas speaks to the development of research standards over the intervening years.

Vincent was speaking to a concern that continues to be shared by many individuals working in the area of acupuncture research. Despite the relatively early interest in acupuncture as a form of alternative and complementary medicine, comparatively few studies have been designed in a way that renders their results useful to other researchers, clinicians, or policy makers.

Over time an increasing number of well-designed studies have emerged. Many of the studies presented at the Workshop on Acupuncture sponsored by the OAM were also presented to the Consensus Panel of Acupuncture convened by the NIH. For the most part, the best clinical research can be clustered into five specific areas that seem to represent the best and most positive research related to acupuncture: (1) antiemesis treatment, (2) management of acute and chronic pain, (3) substance abuse treatment, (4) treatment of paralysis caused by stroke, and (5) treatment of respiratory disease. In addition, acupuncture can show good clinical results in such areas as female infertility, breach version, menopause, depression, and urinary dysfunction (Birch and Hammerschlag, 1996).

The use of acupuncture for the treatment of pain is an area of long-standing medical interest. *Pain control* is the one application of acupuncture that has been used repeatedly by the traditional medical community in Europe and the United States for many years. This area became visible in the 1970s as a result of Chinese reports on acupuncture anesthesia. As a result, this is one of the most widely researched applications of acupuncture. However, it also is one of the most problematic.

Some of the problems that are typical of researching acupuncture treatments for pain, as well as acupuncture therapy in general, are exemplified by the results of two meta-analyses[*] examining acupuncture in the management of chronic pain. The first was conducted by pooling data from 14 studies that used randomized and controlled trials of acupuncture to treat chronic pain and that measured their outcomes in terms of the number of patients whose condition was improved (Patel et al., 1989). This study reached a number of conclusions concerning the relationship of study design to research outcomes and concluded that acupuncture compared favorably with placebo and conventional treatment.

A second meta-analysis reviewed 51 studies and compared the quality of published controlled clinical trials on the basis of research designs and specific factors, including randomization, single and double blinding, and numbers of subjects. This meta-analysis concluded that of the studies reviewed, those favorable to acupuncture were more poorly designed than those that associated negative results with acupuncture. The evidence suggested that the efficacy of acupuncture as a treatment for chronic pain is doubtful (ter Riet et al., 1990).

A careful review of the ter Reit meta-analysis by Delis and Morris suggested that its authors had "included studies which did not meet their criteria," such as a study that was not controlled or in which laser light was used instead of acupuncture needles (Delis and Morris, 1993). This finding prompted them to conduct their own analysis and to reanalyze the studies examined by ter Riet in relation to a number of factors, including investigator training and the appropriateness of treatment. Their meta-analysis showed a trend toward improvement in study design over time, suggesting that many poorly designed acupuncture studies might be viewed best as preliminary efforts by investigators who were sufficiently familiar with the modality to design effective studies.

All three of these meta-analyses pointed out significant issues in relation to acupuncture study design. Besides questions concerning randomization, blinding, placebo control, and sample size, a variety of questions emerged pertinent to the practice of acupuncture as a distinct modality. Is the investigator trained in acupuncture? Is the acupuncture treatment appropriate for the condition? Does the study allow for adjusting the treatment to the individual patient's needs according to traditional diagnostics? Are outcome measures clear? Is placebo or sham acupuncture used, and how will it be administered?

Of all the debated areas in acupuncture research, this last question may receive the most attention. The problem of how to provide a sham treatment in acupuncture is a vexing one. In herbal studies a capsule of inert material that appears similar to the capsule of the medication being investigated can be provided to the patient. Because the patient cannot tell the difference between the two capsules, he or she is effectively blind to the use of a placebo. In acupuncture the problem is more complex because patients receiving treatment definitely know whether they have been stuck with needles or not. Proposed solutions vary from comparing real acupuncture to other modalities to carefully selecting a treatment with few effects (Vincent, 1993) or selecting acupuncture points that are entirely irrelevant (BRITS method) to the conditions being treated (Birch, 1995). In addition, methods of providing simulated acupuncture have been successfully used (Lao et al., 1999).

The potential importance of traditional diagnostic and therapeutic considerations in trial design has been raised by a number of authors (Coan et al., 1980; Ergil, 1995a, 1995b; Jobst, 1995; Hammerschlag, 2003). Some researchers and physicians reject the potential importance of these ideas. Vincent tells us that traditional ideas need to be understood in outline but that questions about efficacy can be asked without considering them in detail. The treatment may be effective whether the theory is valid or not (Vincent, 1993). Hans Agren attempted to make this distinction 30 years ago to identify suitable research agendas, arguing that only the simple empirical observations of Chinese medicine should be an object of medical inquiry (Agren, 1975). The question emerging from the work of various researchers is whether some aspects of traditional theory are, in fact, relevant to the delivery of effective treatment and consequently the inquiry. This question is most

---

[*]A meta-analysis is a research method that pools the results of many studies in an effort to try to reach a more powerful conclusion than an individual study might provide.

recently and eloquently presented by Hammerschlag when he asserts the need to "reassess the importance of a central tenet of evidence based medicine: that acupuncture should outperform placebo" (2003, p. 34) and suggests that it is time to consider research "that considers whole systems of care rather than modalities."

The control of pain is considered to be a major area for the clinical application of acupuncture, and although some of the research in this area has been problematic, a number of studies strongly indicate the importance of acupuncture in pain management. As we have seen, one of the conclusions of the NIH Consensus Panel was that acupuncture could be demonstrated as efficacious for postoperative dental pain. One study showed that acupuncture patients required less postoperative analgesia after oral surgery than a group receiving a sham acupuncture treatment (Lao et al., 1995).

Among the more notable studies in the area of pain management are a clinical trial involving 43 women with menstrual pain, in which women receiving acupuncture treatment had considerably less pain than the placebo and control groups (Helms, 1987). A controlled trial of acupuncture in the management of migraines involved 30 patients who had chronic migraines. Acupuncture was significantly effective in controlling the pain of migraine headaches (Vincent, 1989). Several studies of the management of various types of back pain also have shown acupuncture to be helpful. However, a recent systematic review of randomized controlled trials (RCTs) has determined, "Acupuncture for acute back pain has not been well studied," and that the value of acupuncture in treating chronic back pain "remains in question" (Cherkin et al., 2003, p. 905).

Over the years a number of studies have suggested that the pain of osteoarthritis seems to respond well to acupuncture (Dickens and Lewith, 1989; Junnila, 1982; Thomas et al., 1991). One study suggested a significant cost benefit when the use of acupuncture removes the need for surgical intervention (Christensen et al., 1992). The implications of these studies have lead to the increased commitment of resources to the investigation of the potential role of acupuncture in the management of osteoarthritis and the production of promising clinical data (Berman et al., 1999).

The NIH Consensus Panel concluded that acupuncture had been demonstrated to be effica-cious for the treatment of adult postoperative and chemotherapy nausea and vomiting. Research in the area of antiemesis revolves around the use of the acupuncture point Inner Gate (*neiguan*, P6) to control nausea and vomiting. The use of this point in acupressure to control nausea and vomiting is well known, and its use to control the nausea of pregnancy with pressure bands has been determined to be effective (Aloysio and Penacchioni, 1992). Even consumer products are available that exploit this effect. The point also has been investigated in relation to its use in controlling perioperative emesis that resulted from premedication and anesthetic agents (Ghaly et al., 1987) and in relation to cancer chemotherapy (Dundee et al., 1989).

On the basis of clinical experiences in China, acupuncture is used extensively in the United States for the management of symptoms associated with withdrawal from a variety of substances, including alcohol and cocaine. The summary conclusion of presenters at the Workshop on Acupuncture, Panel on Substance Abuse, indicated that early trial and empirical findings suggest positive treatment effects (Kiresuk and Culliton, 1994).

Acupuncture has been studied clinically in the West in relation to the management of a variety of specific medical conditions, including pulmonary disease and paralysis subsequent to stroke. An extensive review of acupuncture in pulmonary disease led the author to conclude that acupuncture produced favorable effects in the management of patients with bronchial asthma, chronic bronchitis, and chronic disabling breathlessness (Jobst, 1995). A study of 16 patients with right-sided paralysis who had experienced an ischemic infarction of the left hemisphere showed acupuncture produced a good response in patients whose lesion affected no more than half the motor pathway areas (Naeser et al., 1992).

Although the volume of published research on acupuncture in the West has been relatively low—only 200 randomized controlled trials, 42 review articles, and four meta-analyses available in 1995 by one count (Foreman, 1995)—and although there has been substantial growth in the decade since then, the amount of research conducted in China and Japan in the areas discussed previously and in other areas is vast. Although study and publication quality can be a problem and design issues are still present, acupuncture research in China must be regarded as a significant resource. Emerging trends in study design and analysis observed at conferences in China and in recent publications suggest that the trend toward improved research design observed by Delis in the West is at work in the East as well.

Qi Cultivation

Considerable numbers of intriguing studies of qi cultivation have been conducted in China and are beginning to be explored in the United States. Qi cultivation has been examined in relationship to an increase in immunocompetence, as measured through lymphocyte profiles (Ryu et al., 1995) and by changes in electroencephalographic patterns. Qi cultivation has been explored as a tool for managing gastritis, and numerous Chinese studies have suggested that it might be a promising method for treating hypertension.

Unfortunately, many of the problems that have confronted acupuncture research also surround research into qi cultivation. In addition, although there is great interest in qi cultivation in the West, there has not been the equivalent enthusiasm for resolving methodological problems and beginning to establish strong research initiatives.

Research in qi cultivation that investigates the role of the practice of qi cultivation exercises in the beneficial alteration of physiological processes is similar, in many respects, to the investigation of the effects of meditation, yoga, guided imagery, and what Benson termed the *relaxation response*. The challenge here is developing an effective control and ruling out other variables that may influence the results.

Attempts to examine the effects of externally transmitted qi have led to special problems. In some cases, as discussed earlier, it is believed that this phenomenon involves measurable portions of the electromagnetic spectrum. In cases where investigators hypothesize qi as an existent, but presently unmeasurable, phenomenon, they seek to establish the presence and effect of externally transmitted qi by examining its apparent effects on other systems that can be directly observed.

Given the extensive range of phenomena under investigation and the range of claims for the healing potential of qi cultivation, there is a certain amount of skepticism about the field as a whole. Even in China there is some question as to whether qi cultivation should be established as a standard method of treatment within the corpus of Chinese medicine. There is also the belief that some of the practices associated with qi cultivation have the potential for abuse and charlatanism (Tang, 1994).

Qi cultivation remains a challenging part of the broad fabric of China's traditional medicine. Researchers within the field hope that over time it will be possible to increase the availability of well-designed and accessible studies in the field (Sancier, 1996).

Acknowledgments

As is apparent from the text, this presentation owes a heavy debt to the work of Paul Unschuld and Nigel Wiseman. The scholarship and enterprise of these two individuals is reflected in their work and the help that they have provided to students of Chinese medicine such as myself. Marnae Ergil, my wife and colleague, contributed enormously by reviewing text, answering questions, and being willing to check technical points in Chinese language materials at any hour of the day or night. This project would not have been possible without the institutional commitment to scholarship and the support provided by the Pacific College of Oriental Medicine, and later by Touro College.

References

Agren H: A new approach to Chinese traditional medicine, *Am J Chin Med* 3(3):207-212, 1975.

Aloysio DD, Penacchioni P: Morning sickness control in early pregnancy by Neiguan point acupressure, *Obstet Gyenecol* 80(5):852-854, 1992.

Auteroche B, Gervais G, Auteroche M, et al: *Acupuncture and moxibustion: a guide to clinical practice,* Edinburgh, 1992, Churchill Livingstone.

Bannerman RH: The World Health Organization viewpoint on acupuncture, *World Health,* December 1979, pp 24-29.

Barlow J, Richardson C: *China doctor of John Day,* Portland, Ore, 1979, Binford & Mort.

Becker RO: *The body electric: electromagnetism and the foundation of life,* New York, 1985, Quill, William Morrow.

Bensky D, Barolet R: *Chinese herbal medicine: formulas and strategies,* Seattle, 1990, Eastland Press.

Bensky D, Gamble A: *Chinese herbal medicine: materia medica,* rev ed, Seattle, 1986, Eastland Press.

Bensoussan A, Talley NJ, Hing M, et al: Treatment of irritable bowel syndrome with Chinese herbal medicine: a randomized clinical trial, *JAMA* 280(18):1585-1589, 1998.

Berman BM, Singh BB, Lao L, et al: randomized trial of acupuncture as an adjunctive therapy in osteoarthritis of the knee, *Rheumatology (Oxford)* 38(4):346-354, 1999.

Birch S: A historical study of radial pulse six position Diagnosis: naming the unnameable, *J Acupunct Soc NY* 1(3/4):19-32, 1994.

Birch S: A biophysical basis for acupuncture. In Birsh S, editor: *Proceedings of the Second Symposium of the Society for Acupuncture Research*, Boston, 1995, Society for Acupuncture Research, pp 274-294.

Birch S, Hammerschlag R: *Acupuncture efficacy: a summary of controlled clinical trials*, Tarrytown, NY, 1996, National Academy of Acupuncture and Oriental Medicine.

Bowers JZ: *Western medical pioneers in feudal Japan*, Baltimore, 1970, The Johns Hopkins University Press.

Broffman M, McCulloch M: Instrument-assisted pulse evaluation in the acupuncture practice, *Am J Acupunct* 14(3):255-259, 1986.

Burton Goldberg Group: Acupuncture. In Strohecker J, editor: *Alternative medicine: the definitive guide*, Puyallup, WA, 1993, Future Medicine, pp 37-46.

Chang HM: Pharmacology and applications of Chinese materia medica. Singapore, 1986, World Scientific (Translated by SC Yao, LL Wang, and CS Yeung).

Chen KK: Half a century of ephedrine. In Kao FF, Kao JJ, editors: *Chinese medicine—new medicine*, New York, 1977, Neale Watson Academic, pp 21-27.

Cherkin DC, Sherman KJ, Deyo RA, Shekelle PG: A review of the evidence for the effectiveness, safety, and cost of acupuncture, massage therapy, and spinal manipulation for back pain, *Ann Intern Med* 138(11):898-906, 2003.

Christensen BV, Iuhl IU, Vilbe KH, et al: Acupuncture treatment of severe knee osteoarthritis, *Acta Anaesthesiol Scand* 36:519-525, 1992.

Chuang Y: *The historical development of acupuncture*, Los Angeles, 1982, Oriental Healing Arts Institute.

Coan R, Wong GT, Ku S-L, et al: The acupuncture treatment of low back pain: a randomized controlled study, *Am J Chin Med* 8(2):181-189, 1980.

Delis K, Morris M: Clinical trials in acupuncture. In Birch S, editor: *Proceedings of the First Symposium of the Society of Acupuncture Research*, Boston, 1993, Society for Acupuncture Research, pp 68-71.

Despeux C: Gymnastics: the ancient tradition. In Kohn L, editor: *Taoist meditation and longevity techniques*, Ann Arbor, 1989, Center for Chinese Studies, University of Michigan, pp 225-262.

Dickens W, Lewith G: A single-blind, controlled and randomised clinical trial to evaluate the effect of acupuncture in the treatment of trapeziometacarpal osteoarthritis, *Comp Med Res* 3:5-8, 1989.

Dundee JW, Ghaly RG, Fitzpatrick KTJ, et al: Acupuncture prophylaxis of cancer chemotherapy induced sickness, *J R Soc Med* 82:268-271, 1989.

Ellis A, Wiseman N, Boss K: *Fundamentals of Chinese acupuncture*, Brookline, Mass, 1991, Paradigm.

Engelhardt U: Qi for life: longevity in the tang. In Kohn L, editor: *Taoist meditation and longevity techniques*, Ann Arbor, 1989, Center for Chinese Studies, University of Michigan, pp 263-296.

Ergil KV: Chinese specific condition review: urinary tract infections, *Protocol J Botan Med* 1(1):130-133, 1995a.

Ergil KV: Where tradition matters: identifying epistemological and terminological issues in research design. In *Proceedings of the Second Symposium of the Society of Acupuncture Research*, 1995b, pp 59-69.

Ergil MC: Medical education in China, *CCAOM News* 1(1): 3-5, 1994.

Farquhar J: Problems of knowledge in contemporary Chinese medical discourse, *Soc Sci Med* 24(12):1013-1021, 1987.

Food and Drug Administration: FDA issues regulation prohibiting sale of dietary supplements containing ephedrine alkaloids and reiterates its advice that consumers stop using these products, *FDA News*, February 2004, pp 4-17.

Foreman J: What the research shows, *Boston Globe*, 22/5, 25, 27, 1995.

Ghaly RG, Fitzpatrick KTJ, Dundee JW: *Anesthesia* 42:1108-1110, 1987.

Haller JS: Acupuncture in nineteenth century Western medicine, *NY State J Med*, 1973.

Hammerschlag R: Acupuncture: on what should its evidence be based? *Altern Ther* 9 (5):34-5, 2003.

Hao LZ: An attempt to understand the substance of kidney and its disorders, *J Am Coll Tradit Chin Med* (3):82-97, 1983 (Translated by CS Cheung).

Helms JM: Acupuncture for the management of primary dysmenorrhea, *Obstet Gynecol* 69(1):51-56, 1987.

Hirsch RC: Korean constitutional nutrition, *J Am Coll Tradit Chin Med* (1):24-37, 1985.

Hsu E: Outline of the history of acupuncture in Europe, *J Chin Med* 29(1):28-32, 1989.

Hsu H, Peacher W: *Chen's history of Chinese medical science*, Taipei, 1977, Modern Drug Publishers.

Huang B, Di F, Li X, et al: Syndromes of traditional Chinese medicine. Heilongjiang, 1993, Heilongjiang Education Press (Translated by D Ma, W Guo'en, S Sun, and H Cao).

Huard P, Wong M: *Chinese medicine*, New York, 1968, McGraw Hill, World University Library.

Jobst K: A critical analysis of acupuncture in pulmonary disease: efficacy and safety of the acupuncture needle, *J Altern Complement Med* 1:57-86, 1995.

Junnila SYT: Acupuncture superior to Prioxicam in the treatment of osteoarthritis, *Am J Acupunct* 10: 341-346, 1982.

Kaptchuk TJ: *The web that has no weaver: understanding Chinese medicine*, New York, 1983, Congdon and Weed.

Kiresuk TJ, Culliton PD: Overview of substance abuse acupuncture treatment research, 1994, Workshop on Acupuncture.

Kleinman A: *Social origins of distress and disease: depression, neurasthenia, and pain in modern China,* 1986, New Haven, Conn, Yale University Press.

Langevin HM, Churchill DL, Wu J, et al: Evidence of connective tissue involvement in acupuncture, *FASEB J* 16(8):872-874, 2002. http://www.fasebj.org/cgi/reprint/16/8/872.

Lao L, Bergman S, Hamilton GR, et al: Evaluation of acupuncture for pain control after oral surgery: a placebo-controlled trial, *Arch Otolaryngol Head Neck Surg* 125(5):567-572, 1999.

Lao L, Bergman S, Langenberg P, et al: Efficacy of Chinese acupuncture on postoperative oral surgery pain, *Oral Surg Oral Med Oral Pathol Oral Radiol Endod* 79:423-428, 1995.

Lee JK, Bae SKB: Korean acupuncture, Seoul, 1981, Ko Mun Sa.

Lin Y: Laotse, the book of Tao. In Lin Y, editor: *The wisdom of China and India,* New York, 1942, Modern Library, pp 578-624.

Lock M: *East Asian medicine in urban Japan: comparative studies of health systems,* vol 4, Berkeley, 1980, University of California Press.

Maciocia G: *The foundations of Chinese medicine,* Edinburgh, 1989, Churchill Livingstone.

Manaka Y, Itaya K: Acupuncture as intervention in the biological information system, *J Acupunct Soc NY* 1(3/4):19-32, 1994.

Muench C: One Hundred Years of Medicine: The Ah-Fong physicians of Idaho. In Schwarz HG, editor: *Chinese medicine on the Golden Mountain: an interpretive guide,* Seattle, 1984, Washington Commission for the Humanities, pp 51-80.

Naeser MA, Michael PA, Stiassny-Eder D, et al: Real versus sham acupuncture in the treatment of paralysis in acute stroke patients: a CT scan lesion study, *J Neurol Rehabil* (6):163-173, 1992.

National Institutes of Health: Acupuncture, NIH Consensus Statement, 15(5):1-34, 1997.

Oschman J: A biophysical basis for acupuncture. In Birch S, editor: *Proceedings of the First Symposium of the Society for Acupuncture Research,* Boston, 1993, Society for Acupuncture Research, pp 141-220.

Osler W: *The principles and practice of medicine,* New York, 1913, Appleton.

Patel M, Gutzwiller F, Paccand F, Marazzi A: A meta-analysis of acupuncture for chronic pain, *Int J Epidemiol* 18(4):900-906, 1989.

Payer L: *Medicine and culture: varieties of treatment in the United States, England, West Germany, and France,* New York, 1988, Henry Holt.

Peacher W: Adverse reactions, contraindications and complications of acupuncture and moxibustion, *Am J Chin Med* 3(1):35-46, 1975.

Pomeranz B: Scientific basis of acupuncture. In Stox G, editor: *The basics of acupuncture,* New York, 1988, Springer-Verlag, pp 4-37.

Qiu XI: *Chinese acupuncture and moxibustion,* New York, 1993, Churchill Livingstone.

Reichmanis M, Marino AA, Becker RO: Electrical correlates of acupuncture points, *Intern J Acupunct Electrother* 17:75-94, 1975.

Ryu H, Jun CD, Lee BS, et al: Effect of Qigong training on proportions of T lymphocyte subsets in human peripheral blood, *Am J Chin Med* 23:27-36, 1995.

Sancier K: Medical applications of Qigong alternative therapies. 2(1):40-46, 1996.

Seto A, Kusaka S, Nakazatio W, et al: Detection of extraordinary large bio-magnetic field strength from human hand, *Acupuncture and Electro-Therapeutics Research International Journal* 17:75-94 1992.

Shanghai College of Traditional Chinese Medicine: *Acupuncture: a comprehensive text,* Seattle, 1981, Eastland Press (Translated by J O'Connor and D Bensky).

Sivin N: Traditional medicine in contemporary China. In *Science, medicine and technology in East Asia,* vol. 2, Ann Arbor, 1987, Center for Chinese Studies, University of Michigan.

Takashima M: Personal communication: pulse research, 1995.

Tang KC: Qigong therapy—its effectiveness and regulation, *Am J Chin Med* 22:235-242, 1994.

ter Riet G, Kleijnen J, Knipschild P: Acupuncture and chronic pain: a criteria-based meta-analysis, *J Clin Epidemiol* 43:1191-1199, 1990.

Thomas M, Eriksson SV, Lundeberg T: A comparative study of diazepam and acupuncture in patients with osteoarthritis pain: a placebo controlled study, *Am J Chin Med* 19:95-100, 1991.

Unschuld P: *Medical ethics in Imperial China: a study in historical anthropology,* Berkeley, 1979, University of California Press.

Unschuld P: *Medicine in China: a history of ideas,* Berkeley, 1985, University of California Press.

Veith I, translator: *The Yellow Emperor's classic of internal medicine,* Berkeley, 1972, University of California Press.

Vincent CA: A controlled trial of the treatment of migraine by acupuncture, *Clin J Pain* 5:305-312, 1989.

Vincent CA: Acupuncture as a treatment for chronic pain. In Lewith GT, Aldridge D, editors: *Clinical research methodology for complementary therapies,* London, 1993, Hodder and Stoughton, pp 289-308.

Wang G, Fan Y, Guan Z: Chinese massage. In Zhang E, editor: *A practical English-Chinese library of traditional Chinese medicine,* Shanghai, 1990, College of Traditional Chinese Medicine, Publishing House of Shanghai.

Wang X: Research on the origin and development of Chinese acupuncture and moxibustion. In Xiangtong Z, editor: *Research on acupuncture, moxibustion and acupunc-*

ture anesthesia, New York, 1986, Springer-Verlag, pp 783-799.

Watson B: *The complete works of Chuang-tzu,* New York, 1968, Columbia University Press.

Wilhelm R: *The I Ching,* Princeton, NJ, 1967, Princeton University Press (Translated by CF Baynes).

Wiseman N: A list of Chinese formulas, Taiwan, 1993 (Unpublished paper).

Wiseman N, Boss K: *Glossary of Chinese medical terms and acupuncture points,* Brookline, Mass, 1990, Paradigm.

Wiseman N, Ellis A, Zmiewski P, Li C: *Fundamentals of Chinese medicine,* Brookline, Mass, 1985, Paradigm.

Wiseman N, Ellis A, Zmiewski P, Li C: *Fundamentals of Chinese medicine,* Taipei, 1993, SMC.

Wiseman N, Ellis A, Zmiewski P, Li C: *Fundamentals of Chinese medicine,* 1995, Brookline, Mass, Paradigm.

Wong CK, Wu TL: *History of Chinese medicine: being a chronicle of medical happenings in China from ancient times to the present period,* Taipei, 1985, Southern Materials Center.

World Health Organization. Acupuncture: review and analysis of reports on controlled clinical trials, Geneva, 2002, WHO. www.who.int/medicines/library/trm/acupuncture/acupuncture_trials.doc.

Zhang E: Clinic of traditional Chinese medicine. I. In Zhang E, editor: *A practical English-Chinese library of traditional Chinese medicine,* Shanghai, 1990, College of Traditional Chinese Medicine, Publishing House of Shanghai.

Zhu B: Personal communication: pulse research in China, 1991.

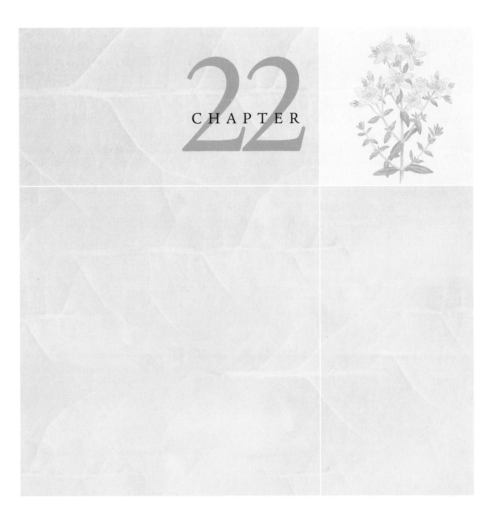

CHAPTER 22

QIGONG

AMY L. AI

This chapter provides an introduction to qi gong, or *Qigong* (also qigong, Qi Gong, QiGong), a type of energy-based health practice based on an energy-centered worldview (Ai et al., 2001). Along with herbs, acupuncture, and other therapeutic approaches, Qigong is one aspect of traditional Chinese medicine (TCM), with a rich history spanning thousands of years. This chapter's primary goal is to summarize its important components and to help the reader better understand this ancient healing art.

It is impossible to understand Qigong's rationale without knowledge of its primary guiding philosophy, *Daoism* (Taoism). In its Chinese character, *dao* refers to the way, or the universal order, to be followed in life and in nature (Ai, 2003). In a cosmic sense, dao refers to the ultimate, indefinable principle underly-

ing all movements—the process involving every aspect in the universe. This chapter therefore begins with the concepts and basics of Qigong, then introduces the philosophical foundation, Daoism, and next presents its influence on TCM and Qigong. Finally, the contemporary scientific investigation of Qigong is summarized.

DEFINITION

Qigong is the phonetic juxtaposition of two Chinese characters: *qi*, meaning "flow of air" in a more literal sense or "vital energy" in a more symbolic sense, and *gong*, meaning "perseverant practice" (Ai, 2003). The translation of the concept of Qigong has been influenced by different perspectives. Trained by Chinese teachers, American Qigong master Cohen (1997) referred to it as "working with the life energy, learning how to control the flow and distribution of qi to improve the health and harmony of mind and body." Shen (1986) considered Qigong as an ancient therapeutic martial art. An advocate of the scientific study of Qigong in China and the American-trained leading physicist there, Qian (1982) defined Qigong as an ancient system for self-development that involves movement, breathing exercises, and conscious control of body energy. Integrating these perspectives, I consider Qigong as an energy-based health practice and healing process involving deep breath and meditation with movement (internal or external) that may provide potential medical benefits.

Notably, the idea of the flowing vital energy is shared among many non-Western legacies, as well as in the shamanic tradition in Western culture, which is traced back to ancient Egypt (Graham, 1990). Some indigenous people in Africa call it "num," whereas Native American tribes speak of the "Holy Wind" (Cohen, 1997). Indians term it "prana," and Russians name it "bioplasma" (Willis, 1991). The uniqueness of the Chinese concept *qi* lies in (1) its focus on holistic health in terms of multilevel energy patterns rather than solely on the physical body or on an external divinity or ghostlike spirit, (2) its pathway of qi circulation *(i.e.,* the acupuncture channel system consisting of several hundred points) (Shen, 1986), and (3) its rationale, resembling an accepted tenet of quantum theory in modern physics (Capra, 1991). In this view, relations and activities of energy patterns are seen as fundamental in both human nature and the universe. The term *qi* refers not only to the essence of all material objects, but also to their interactions in terms of the rhythmic alternation of two fundamental forces, *yin* and *yang,* similar to positive and negative charges in modern chemistry. This ying-yang relation is elaborated further in the next section.

HISTORY

The inclusion of the qi system in health and healing was documented 4000 to 5000 years ago in the classic book of TCM, *Hung De Nei Jing Su Wen* (*Nei Jing,* or *The Yellow Emperor's Classic of Internal Medicine*) (Liao, 1992). The Nei Jing system viewed the human in both cosmic and geographical terms. It explicitly rejected earlier supernatural and magical healing and instead described illness and therapies as a consequence of pernicious and emotional disturbance. This system is based on principles describing the movement of qi in the human body and its relationships to physical and mental health. *Nei Jing* recommended the earliest documented Qigong, Dao-Yi, as a healing exercise to cure chills and fevers and to achieve the state of a tranquilly content, sagelike person who is full of vital spirit (Cohen, 1997).

In many early forms of Qigong performance, slow-moving dance following animal postures were used to promote animal-like vitality, balance, grace, and strength. The founder of Daoist philosophy, Lao Zi, first described basic Qigong principles that had been followed by practitioners for centuries, such as concentration, emptiness of desire, quiescence, flexibility, and infant-like breath. In the fourth century BC, Zhuang Zi, Lao Zi's follower, wrote about the role of infant-like breathing and physical exercise in promoting longevity and described a sage intent on extending his life (Despeux, 1989). In the second century AD the TCM doctor Hua Tuo was known by both his famous anesthetic herb formula, Ma Fu San, and his Qigong practice, Five Animal Plays, based on the movements of the tiger, deer, bear, monkey, and bird. Throughout the Chinese history, many forms of Qigong have been developed among Daoists, Buddhists, TCM practitioners, and martial artists (Shen, 1986).

According to Cohen (1997), Qigong first reached Europe in the late eighteenth and early nineteenth centuries. In 1779 the Jesuit P.M. Cibot translated Daoist Qigong exercise and respiratory techniques in terms of Cong-Fou (Kong-Fu) into French with illustrations. His translated text later became influential for Per Henrik Ling (1776-1839), who founded medical gymnastics on the basis of a vital energy theory to promote health. Described by Dally as "a sort of photographic image of Taoist kung-fu" (Cohen, 1997), Ling's theory and practice laid the foundation of contemporary physical education. The idea of vital energy, however, was dropped in the clash with modern materialistic science.

In the East, by contrast, the culturally rooted legacy of qi has never been abandoned, despite the rapid changes of political regimes in China during the twentieth century. The initial use of Qigong in formal medical profession began in the 1950s, when some Qigong-rehabilitation institutes established by the Chinese government demonstrated the therapeutic effects of internal Qigong in treating hypertension and neurasthenia. The late 1970s witnessed a true renaissance in the practice of medical Qigong or Qigong therapy for the purpose of medical care and rehabilitation. An influential advocate was an elderly master, Guo Lin, who had persistently practiced Daoist Qigong since she developed advanced uterine cancer in her 30s (Shen, 1986). She and her students used Qigong to heal diseases with diagnoses in Western medicine, especially cancer. Since then, numerous styles of Qigong therapy have been invented. However, they all share the essential principles in ancient Daoism and its manifestation in TCM theories.

Current Classification and Development

In practice, Qigong consists of two foundational forms: (1) *dynamic* or *active Qigong*, which involves visible movement of the body, typically through a set of slowly enacted exercises, and (2) *meditative* or *passive Qigong*, which entails still positions with inner movement of the diaphragm. Essential to both are precise control of abdominal breathing, alert concentration, and a tranquil state of mind. The most well-known dynamic Qigong in the Western world is *Tai Ji* (t'ai chi). Dynamic Qigong should also include varied forms of martial Qigong (Kong-Fu, kung-fu), which focus on the development of physical capacity. In contrast to Western exercise, however, dynamic Qigong focuses on flexibility and inner strength rather than masculinity and body size. Based on different philosophical foundations, affiliated intentionality, and spiritual goals, intellectually and spiritually Qigong can also be classified into Daoist, Buddhist, and Confucianist aspects (*Dao Jia* Gong, *Fa Jia* Gong, and *Ru Jia* Going).

From a clinical perspective, Qigong therapy can be classified into two systems (Sancier, 1996). *Internal Qigong* aims to control internal qi flow, to promote one's own health, or to self-heal illness by an individual's own practice. *External Qigong* attempts to achieve healing by manipulating or transmitting another's qi, based on the idea that energy can be led outside or travel through a therapist's body and be conducted to other living and nonliving systems. This form of therapy is performed by a Qigong master whose practice has reached an advanced level or who has an inherent talent in this respect (Qian, 1982). A healer can provide qi through projection without direct contact or through other methods with contact, such as touching acupoints, massage, and osteopathic adjustments. Diseases treated by internal Qigong in China include cardiovascular diseases, such as essential hypertension, coronary heart disease, heart arrhythmia, rheumatic heart disease, and stroke, as well as other functional and organic diseases (Cohen, 1997; Eisenberg, 1985; Sancier, 1996; Shen, 1986).

Public interest in Qigong spurred basic and clinical research in China during the 1980s and some international interests in its role and mechanisms in the 1990s (Cohen, 1997; Hisamitsu et al., 1996; Sancier, 1996; Shen, 1986; Tiller et al., 1995). However, relatively few clinical studies on Qigong's efficacy have been conducted outside China. Moreover, less documentation has been found, even in China, about the clinical research of external Qigong, except for a single case report on its experimental use as anesthesia. Heise (1993) discussed the effectiveness of Tai Ji and Qigong in the treatment of psychosomatic disorders in Germany. McGarry (1996) advocated the integration of Eastern perceptions of the bioenergy field into Western belief systems and approaches to therapeutic interventions in Australia.

The practice of Qigong became known in the United States during the 1990s. *New York Magazine* reported Dr. Oz's experiments using American therapists during heart transplantation surgery at the Columbia-Presbyterian Medical Center (Brown, 1995). An acupoint known as Yongquan (Boddling Spring or KI-1), at the beginning part of the kidney meridian located on the soles of the feet, was used in the application of "energy medicine." At the dawn of the new millennium, the National Institutes of Health began to fund scientific investigations on Qigong efficacy (Ai et al., 2001; Wu et al., 1999). To date, the randomized controlled trials (RCTs) conducted on external Qigong remain pioneer work in nature with potential influence outside the United States (see later discussion).

Philosophical Differences Underlying Western vs. Eastern Medicine

Because of the different worldviews underlying the TCM modality and modern medical sciences, RCTs are not easy tasks. The fundamental difference stems from a philosophical perspective that distinguishes aspects of Eastern and Western cultures. For the most part, the operative philosophy of science is embodied in Aristotelian empirical materialism, in which the knowledge of antiquity was systematically organized into the scheme that underlies much of the Western view of the universe. The formulation of a Cartesian mind/matter (*res cogitans/res extensa*) dualism in the seventeenth century also helped bring about the birth of modern science (Ai, 1996). In this paradigm, matter as the observed object is completely separated from the scientist as an observer. Biomedicine, as the offspring of this outlook, focuses primarily on the material structure of the body, which is further broken down into systems, organs, tissues, cells, chromosomes, genes, and molecules. In this biomedical model the heart, for example, is treated as a pump, a mechanical organ with regular outputs. The diagnosis and treatment of heart disease are centered on aspects of the material organ or other levels of structure: physical, physiological, biochemical, and genetic.

In TCM, however, the heart means more than an anatomical organ. Strangely, the energetic concept of heart, often referred to as "heart qi" in TCM, also contains some function of the mind (Ai, 1996). In a modern view, this involves the brain-heart relationship, which is more explainable in relation to the heart-related functions involving neuroendocrinology, immunology, and the pituitary-hypothalamic-adrenal axis. Without these scientific concepts, the ancient Chinese perspective organized all these phenomena in a system of vital energy movement. The circulation of qi within the human body and its interactions thus became essential to the TCM theory. Accordingly, the Qigong modality was built on an energy-centered worldview, a Daoist view that differs remarkably from that supporting contemporary Western medicine, both ontologically and epistemologically.

DAOIST DIALECTIC VIEW OF THE WORLD AND HUMANS

Energy-Centered Outlook

More than 2000 years ago, Daoism crystallized one of many ancient intellectual legacies of the Chinese culture. The emergence of Daoism echoes the historical environment of its founder, Lao Zi, believed to have lived between 571 and 471 BC during the Spring and Autumn Period of the late Zhou Dynasty, which lasted for 242 years. This historical period was marked by chaotic and ceaseless battles among hundreds of warring dukes and by schools of varied philosophies. Reality was perceived by Daoists in complex relations; the truth in human nature and in universal phenomena was nothing short of ambiguity, paradox, and contradiction. Ancient Daoists sought to achieve a conscious awareness and philosophical understanding of universal principles, or the manner and process of change that underlies all cosmological processes. By the invisible but perceivable image of "flow of air," the word *qi* was used as a vivid metaphor to illustrate the changing energy patterns in universal processes.

In ancient Greece, Aristotle described the world as a systematic structure, and Democritus pioneered the concept of atoms as the basic unit of natural substances. These philosophical perspectives set the fundamental materialistic worldview underlying all modern sciences, in particular classic physical theory. Ancient Daoists, however, were more interested in mastering the order of ever-changing patterns that explained the interactive phenomena at multiple levels in nature, including humans (Ai, 2003). Concurrently, they observed that the transformation of energy is the unifying principle or force among all beings. The ontological difference between the outlooks of the Greek and Chinese traditions was noted by a modern physicist, Fritjof Capra. In *The Tao of Physics*, he suggests that the Daoist ontology resembles that of quantum physics (Capra, 1991). Both traditions propose that all forms of substance are nothing but the materialization of energy. Both view the dynamic patterns of energy as the primary and continual forces in nature, whereas substantive aspects are secondary.

Nonbeing as the Fundamental

Without scientific terminology, Lao Zi used *nonbeing*, or *wu* in Chinese, and *being*, or *you*, to summarize the energetic and substantive aspects of all things. An original energy in the pure form of nonbeing was considered as the primary force that generated the materialistic universe, the sum of all being. In his world-famous *Dao Te Jing*, Lao Zi wrote: "All things are born of being; *being is born of nonbeing*. All living things are formed by being, and shaped by their environment, growing if nourished well by virtue, the being from nonbeing" (emphasis added by the author). In other words, an invisible energetic force as the origin of the world existed before all material substances emerged. Accordingly, the Daoist worldview considers invisible energy movements as constant, ultimate reality, whereas visible materialistic aspects of the world as transit phenomena in a cosmos sense. For example, each human body has its circle between life and death, but the energetic movement of its particles would continue at different levels beyond this circle.

The Chinese character *you* can be translated as *something exists*. In contrast, *wu* can be translated or interpreted as *nothing exists* or *nothingness*. The latter interpretation is somewhat similar to the Buddhist *nothingness* or *emptiness*. Both concepts refer to images of reality, mean that "nothing exists," and are perceived through intuition rather than empirical observation. However, the Daoist nonbeing tends to differ from the Buddhist emptiness in both perspective and content. The Daoist concept concerns the nature of ultimate reality itself. It conceptualizes the origin of the universe or all objective being in the form of energetic nonbeing, or *wu*, or in modern terms, a void field filled with energetic movement. The Buddhism concept *emptiness* involves subjective reflection to that ultimate reality. It offers a cognitive solution as detachment to human suffering through the emptiness of the mind. Taking Lao Zi's dialectic view, therefore, *nothingness* could imply something within, such as moving energy, or Daoist *qi*, or the awareness of spiritual truth through Buddhist liberation, or *Nirvana*, and enlightenment. This ontological difference shapes the different focus of meditative Qigong, as described later.

Daoist Dialectical Epistemology

Furthermore, the being versus nonbeing relation in the Lao Zi excerpt implies not only the Daoist ontology concerning the nature of the universe, including humans, but its dialectical epistemology as well. Capra (1991) noted that the Eastern tradition appreciates intuitive thinking above rational thinking more than its Western counterpart. Despite their basic outlook shared with modern physicists, Daoists do not employ *form* logical thinking, empirical obser-

vation, and deductive reasoning. Rather, their way of knowing is based on dialectical thinking, intuitive imagery, and cyclical patterning. Because of their puzzling dialectics and multiplicity of meaning, some Daoist passages seem to be logically incomprehensible. As Lao Zi said in *Dao Te Jing*: "When living by the Tao, awareness of self is not required, for in this way of life, the self exists, and is also non-existent, being conceived of, not as existentiality, nor as non-existent." Stated abstractly, in this passage, fact *A* holds with both *B* and *non-B*. Seemingly contradictory arguments such as this are expressed throughout his book, because paradox and mutuality are a part of truth in the Daoist philosophy.

The Daoist dialectic way of circular reasoning presents a stark contrast to the laws of *form logic* tracing back to ancient Greek, particularly Aristotelian reasoning (Peng and Nisbettm, 1999). Central to the latter are three laws: *identity, noncontradiction,* and *the excluded middle.* The first law claims that everything must be identical with itself. The second law insists that no statement can be both true and false. The third law declares that *A* is either *B* or *non-B*. For example, in *The Republic*, Plato recorded a conversation about beauty and ugliness with Socrates, clearly differing from the previous Lao Zi passage: "Since fair is the opposite of ugly, they are two." "Of course." "Since they are two, isn't each also one?" "That is so as well." "The same argument also applies then to justice and injustice, good and bad, and all the forms" (Bloom, 1968). Accordingly, at least until recently, the order of the world in the Western perspective has tended to follow a path of *certainty, specification,* and *a linear logic that links cause to effect.* (For example, if *A* leads to *B* and *B* leads to *C*, then *A* also leads to *C*.) Form logic defines the relative truth concerning the contingent reality in structures, enabling natural law to be comprehensible within specified domains. It eventually paved a way to the emergence of modern science that nourished current medical science.

Central to Daoist dialectics, by contrast, are three different but interrelated principles: *change, contradiction,* and *holism* (Peng and Nisbettm, 1999). The first principle claims that reality is *in constant flux.* The second principle states that reality is full of paradoxes. The last principle declares that all things are interdependent and interactive. The order of the world, including human health, therefore tends to follow a path of *uncertainty, mutuality,* and *the circling logic that links an individual part to the whole.* This last principle is the essence of dialectical thinking as the consequence of the first two. The truth thus is often presented in a liquid sense in reference to its context, or as opposite but related aspects, rather than in an isolated and absolute stage. As Lao Zi said, "We cannot know the Tao itself, nor see its qualities directly, but only see by differentiation, which it manifests. Thus, that which is seen as beautiful is beautiful compared with that which is seen as lacking beauty."

Three Basic Principles

Corresponding to this last principle, *holism,* Daoists believe that all things in the world are interrelated and affect every other thing in mutually interactive and cyclical ways. The parts become meaningful only in relation to the whole context. Accordingly, ancient Daoists summarized the absolute truth concerning the ultimate reality in a mysterious web of complex energy systems, which appears to be incomprehensible as the whole. However, its manifestation in the form of changing patterns, such as health, is perceivable in comparison and in connection with opposing and multiple aspects within all phenomena. Daoist dialectics did not lead to classic science or its structurally detailed modern medical diagnosis and intervention, but it can be a helpful lens in comprehending the dynamic energetic totality, such as with TCM and modern physics. Daoists, however, present natural law through different paths than those of scientists. Their energy system was shown in interactive images, symbols, and metaphors. To demonstrate the universal part-whole dynamics of energetic patterns, the Daoist Tai Ji symbol is shown in a half-black and half-white round pattern, a sign of two interactive cosmic forces, *yin* and *yang,* or a dynamic union of two forces generating the vital energy, *qi.*

Corresponding to the second principle, *contradiction,* the polarized yin and yang aspects define each other in all paradoxical relations, such as being and nonbeing, energy and substance, spirit and matter, or mind and body. The S curve dividing line between the yin-yang halves in the Tai Ji symbol implies the constant cyclical movement in contradictive pairs, mutually creating, controlling, and penetrating. Both sides can influence and transform into each other in certain ways, such as in the relationship between health and illness. From this relativist perspective, the metaphor of the qi and the yin-yang relation can be used to describe the energetic and functional relationship of both physical nature and human phenomena. Metaphorically, at an atomic level, this relation can be understood as one between positive and negative particles. At a physical and physiological level, each person has both yin and yang sides at multiple levels, such as the relation of invisible functions to solid organs. At the basic neuropsychological level, all humans have both a rational left hemisphere and an intuitive right hemisphere (Ai, 2003).

Daoism respects nature and emphasizes a harmonic relationship with nature, as do many ancient traditions such as Buddhism, Hinduism, and Native American thought. (Ai, 2003) Yet, corresponding to the first principle, *change,* Daoists were uniquely interested more in the constant movements in the *nonbeing* aspect of nature rather than in the visible (e.g., physical landscape) or invisible (e.g., the spirit) properties in its *being* aspects. The universal principle of all change is presented by a single word, *dao,* the law inherent in nature rather than that created by a creator. The law of nature is not perceived in a fixed order but in a continuous flow in the constant movement of both *nonbeing* and *being* aspects within a hierarchical system, for example, from a higher level of the universe to a lower level of humans. This basic idea is stated by Lao Zi in *Tao Te Jing*: "When the consistency of the Tao is known, the mind is receptive to its states of change. Man's laws should follow natural laws, just as nature gives rise to physical laws, whilst following from universal law, which follows the Tao." The law of universe, not of human logic, is what Daoism intends to comprehend philosophically, to appreciate aesthetically, or to worship spiritually (Crosby, 2002).

I Ching: a Coding System for Universal Changes

Daoism uniquely employs mathematics to predict changing patterns in nature and humans. Unlike scientists, however, even the mathematical patterns of such principles are displayed in symbolic manners. This manner can be traced back 5000 years to an ancient book, *I Ching,* or *The Book of Changes,* which has had profound influence on the Eastern tradition, including TCM and Qigong. The book is entirely devoted to the basic ordering principles and was used to calculate predictable changing patterns in ancient times. The 64 hexagrams of the *I Ching* are considered an oracle (Capra, 1991). Each of these 64 figures is composed of six lines, as shown in Figure 22-1. A line disconnected in the middle, "– –," represents yin and a complete line, "—," represents yang. The 64 hexagrams register the maximum possible combinations of yin and yang, in six lines. Yin and yang, therefore, are the two basic codes in this complex patterning system, including human health. This dichotomized coding system resembles, but emerged thousands of years before, the zero-one language used in computer science. Capra (1991) praises the book in *The Tao of Physics*: "Because of its notion of dynamic patterns, the *I Ching* is perhaps the closest analogy to S-matrix theory in Eastern thought. In both systems, the emphasis is on the process rather than object."

DAOIST INFLUENCES ON TCM AND QIGONG PRACTICE

Energetic Function–Centered Organ System

Throughout Chinese history, Daoism has been the most influential intellectual tradition underlying the development of TCM and Qigong. Concurrent with Daoist ontology, TCM in theory becomes function and health centered, rather than a structure- and disease-oriented system. Each person is considered as an energetic cosmos in miniature. Health phenomena are viewed in light of a complex hierarchical web of qi rather than in merely isolated physical matters. One's energy movement manifests the same pattern as does the universe. As shown in Figure 22-2, the physical

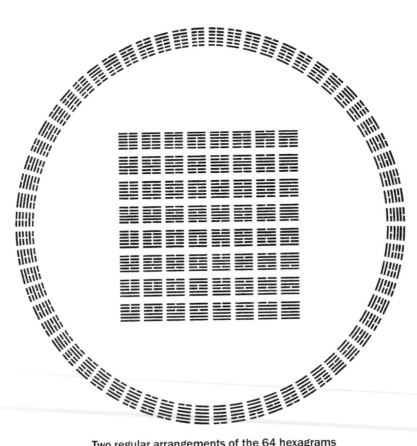

Two regular arrangements of the 64 hexagrams

Figure 22-1 The 64 hexagrams of the *I Ching*.

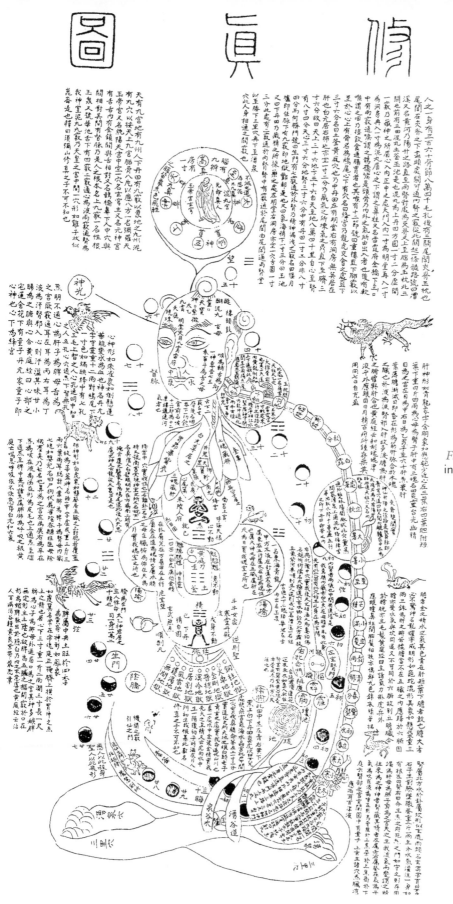

Figure 22-2 An ancient figure in practice.

parts and major acupoints of an ancient figure in practice was illustrated and described in accordance with moon images and other symbols, indicating that qi patterns in human are corresponding to those in seasonal changes and cosmic movements.

Because the energetic *nonbeing* is more fundamental than the substantive *being*, TCM and Qigong focus primarily on the holistic processes of multilevel energy patterns and their interrelations rather than on the material structure of body parts, as does Western medicine. Even organs *(zhang fu)* are primarily described in terms of qi, referring to interactive functions within each one and among all, rather than their exact anatomical structures, because organs are the reservoir of qi in TCM. Likewise, Qigong exercise places more emphasis on the internal movement via breath technology to cultivate essential qi, rather than on external movement via muscular training to build up body size, as do Western physical exercises. However, Daoist healing systems do not deny physical aspects of human health. Instead, these phenomena are integrated into the primary energetic process.

Identified in their physical structures, the 12 TCM organs are not too distant from their placement by European contemporaries in biomedical anatomy. These organs are divided into the viscera, including six *zang* or solid organs, and the bowels, including six *fu* or hollow organs. The organs of viscera (heart, lungs, liver, spleen, kidneys, pericardium) and bowel (small intestine, large intestine, gallbladder, stomach, urinary bladder, "triple burner" [*san jiao*]) are paired in terms of *interior-exterior* (yin-yang) relationship. Besides the "triple burner," in TCM the major physiological functions of these organs are close to those associated with organs similarly named in biomedicine.

Unique to the TCM system, however, are two energy-oriented concepts essential to Qigong practice. One is san jiao, which has no corresponding anatomical structure. This concept refers to the three energetic locations at the middle of chest, diaphragm, and abdomen, which express the functional connection and interaction among paired organs. Another concept relates to acupuncture *meridians*, a circulation system of qi, which also has no identifiable anatomical structure. It consists of 12 primary channels corresponding to the six pairs of yin-yang organs and an additional set of eight extraordinary vessels. Along the pathways of 14 of these channels (the 12 regular channels and two of the extra channels) lie

361 specific acupuncture points. Qi flows along these channels, making a rhythmic circuit over 24 hours daily. Each channel has its own peak energetic time in a daily circle, which can be explained in the fluctuation of the immune and neuroendocrinology system through the 24 hours daily. To cultivate vital energy, some Daoist Qigong styles emphasize meditation on certain acupoints and qi pathways at certain times every day according to the temporal order of daily qi flow *(zi wu liu zu)*.

In principle, health and illness conditions in TCM and Qigong theories follow the coding system in *I Ching*, by matching multilevel energetic components of each individual. Ancient Greeks used four elements—*water, fire, earth*, and *air*—to represent the basic qualities of natural phenomena. Similarly, since the Han Dynasty about 2000 years ago, a five-element system—*wood, fire, earth, metal,* and *water*—was introduced into TCM (Maciocia, 1989). The energetic interaction among the five elements follows the mutual generating and controlling processes. The five-element theory was combined with the yin-yang system in *I Ching* to register the complex energetic interplay among multilevel phenomena that are associated with health (Ai, 2003). Paired organs, tissues, meridians, some acupuncture points, pulse, tongue status, sounds, tastes, colors, time, seasons, directions, planets, temperament, herbs, food, and external pathogens are all coded by these integrated categories along with interconnected relations (Maciocia, 1989; Unschuld, 1985). Organized by the five-element theory, seven emotions or psychic elements (joy, anger, anxiety, concentration, grief, fear, fright) are also linked with the energetic patterns of all functional organs.

Based on this system, the "qi flow of human" becomes a relatively predictable phenomenon, corresponding to the similarly ordered energetic phenomena in the universe.

Health: Holistic Balance in Ever-Changing Qi Processes

Concurrent with Daoist epistemology, the TCM and Qigong theory is literally a systematic elaboration on the changing patterns of qi with respect to the intrarelationship and interrelationship of body, mind, and spirit, as well as their interaction with the energetic environment, in terms of nature, society, and cosmos. Health is maintained only in the internal and external energetic qi contexts of each individual and is perceived with constant changes, contradictions, and holism. Because of the principle of *holism*, illness conditions are often individualistically assessed and addressed with multiple principles concerning the whole energy system rather than with the standardized diagnosis and for structural abnormality. Because of the principle of *contradiction*, health is not viewed in the state of opposition to or absence of disease but rather in an uncertain process of constantly balancing normal and abnormal qi patterns. Because of the principle of *change*, health and illness can be transformed into each other, depending on the interaction between the ailment stage and health practice by an individual. Accordingly, Qigong practice should be integrated into one's lifestyle, which then can boost overall energy, balance the effect of illness, and allow the natural healing capacities to prevail constantly and to transform an ill state into a healthy process.

Such Daoist essence is reflected in the Chinese character of TCM, *zhong yi*. *Yi* means "medicine," and *zhong* usually means "middle," but it also refers to the internally balanced "golden medium." According to an expert on *I-Ching, zhong yi*, or TCM, does not mean the "medicine of middle kingdom," or of China, but refers to the "medicine for inner balance" (Yuan, 1997). Inner balance lies in the harmonic pattern of ever-changing qi in relation to the interplay between ying and yang at all levels of human function, as well as one's habits and environment. This perspective enables TCM and Qigong practice to focus on the prevention of illness conditions through sensitive recognition and management of qi and to emphasize the treatment of preillness stages before ailments are manifest. A TCM classic, *Nan Jing*, or the *Classic of 81 Difficult Medical Issues*, established over 2000 years ago, presented many TCM therapeutic principles for achieving an excellent doctor who can prevent substantive illnesses from the state of pathology and mortality (Wang and Yan, 1988).

Each individual therefore must take the responsibility for his or her own healthy lifestyle, harmonic attitude, and energy exercise, Qigong. Following TCM's preventive essence, Qigong as an energy-oriented practice becomes an art of health, healing, and holistic life, integrating body, mind, and spirit, not a "magic bullet" for specific diseases.

Breathing Meditative Practice: Balanced Energy and Mind-Body Connection

The spirit of Daoism also guides Qigong practice with a heavy emphasis on breathing technique as one approach to holistic health. Lao Zi stated in *Tao Te Jing*:

> Maintaining unity is virtuous, for the inner world of thought is one with the external world of action and of things. The sage avoids their separation, by breathing as the sleeping babe, and thus maintaining harmony. . . . From constancy, there develops harmony, and from harmony, enlightenment. It is unwise to rush from here to there. To hold one's breathe causes the body strain; exhaustion follows when too much energy is used, for this is not the natural way.

Held in the posture of standing, sitting, or lying, the meditative Daoist Qigong practice appears to be similar to the Zen Buddhist approach. Both aspects emphasize deep breathing, concentration, and relaxation. However, these two approaches differ from each other in terms of goals and techniques. Buddhism stresses the experience of awakening from the illusion of life (enlightenment), whereas Daoism emphasizes cultivating energy and spirit *(shen)* as well as promoting health and longevity. Buddhist practice tends to center on the emptiness of mind (detachment), whereas some Daoist practices guide consciousness to follow the qi flow passively along a certain meridian system, such as "heavenly circulation" *(zhou tian)* around the middle line in front and back of the body. Daoist Qigong practice also tends to concentrate on the most important energy center, the cinnabar field *(dan tian)* at about three finger-widths below the navel. This area is considered as the "ocean of qi," where the root of vital energy and longevity reside.

In modern terms, Qigong is essentially a mind-body practice and also a spiritual cultivation. As with early Hippocratic medicine, the approach of TCM and Qigong is psychosomatic and does not follow a soma and psyche dualism (Hammer, 1990; Temkin, 1991). Physical health and ailments are seen not only inseparable from but also as internal responses to emotional stimuli and the environmental stress. From a perspective joining the TCM theories and psychiatric diagnoses, Hammer (1990), an American psychiatrist, devoted an entire book to an explanation of the nature of the qi movement in relation to emotion and illness. When any type of affect becomes overwhelming, emotions become internal agents of illness. Conversely, the dysfunction of organs will be manifested not only in somatic symptoms but also in certain types of emotional distress. For example, in TCM the heart is classified as the "fire" element: an "emperor" organ that houses the individual's spirit (shen) and mental energy, with a tendency to be excessive. It is related to the color red and the emotion of joy. Indeed, in light of modern neuroendocrinology, the heart beats faster because of the increased secretion of adrenal hormones in an ecstatic emotional status, and many patients with cardiovascular disease also have depression and anxiety (Ai, 1996). Interestingly, some American physicians also speak of this mind-body aspect of the heart in terms of "dual rheats" in a human: first a pulsating of muscle in the chest and a precious second cable of communicating neurons that create feeling, longing, and love (Lewis et al., 2001). This view recognizes the important role of neuroendocrinology and immune systems in the organ-brain or body-mind communication, an ancient idea essentially expressed in the concept of qi and Qigong practice.

Qigong practice thus emphasizes the guidance of mind for the qi flow through constant meditative breathing exercise, which in turn spontaneously affects the bodily function. Following Daoist dialectics, no type of emotion is seen as absolutely positive or completely negative. For example, even excessive joy is believed to cause harm to one's energetic balance, as do negative emotions such as anger. This situation can be understood in current terms. For example, a person with coronary heart disease could get sudden cardiac arrest at the time of attending his or her birthday or another holiday party, or of watching a sport game. This attack may result from excessive joy or excitement that also leads to extra stress that the diseased heart could not stand. The key to health in this Qigong perspective lies in the integration and balancing of overall energetic functions rather than in the pursuit of extremity.

Likewise, Daoist Qigong practice does not deny sexuality as a sinful desire, nor does it encourage extreme sexual play in the spirit of hedonism. Rather, sexual energy and behaviors are inseparable parts of health, emotion, and longevity, but they also may be related to illness in malpractice. Some Qigong support techniques promote healthy sexuality in relation to physical and emotional heath. Returning to the "fire" organ example, the qi of pericardium, a parallel "fire" organ to the heart, is to facilitate sexual functioning. A defective pericardium function is believed to impact human activity in varied ways, ranging from hyposexuality to hypersexuality, as well as impacted joy. Currently, this view may also be explainable by neuroendocrinology and psychology. Qigong practice helps maintain the tranquil qi balance in these "fire" organs, readjust dysfunction of both organs and emotions, and restore the healthy energetic patterns in related sexuality.

CLINICAL STUDIES OF QIGONG EFFICACY AND EFFECTIVENESS OUTSIDE THE UNITED STATES

Despite the public interest and theories behind the practice, whether Qigong practice can "cure" medically diagnosed diseases remains an underinvestigated question by Western standards (Ai et al., 2001). As mentioned earlier, studies conducted in China during the 1980s were mostly on the role of internal Qigong, and very few were reported in peer-reviewed journals in English. Sancier (1996) and Cohen (1997) reported some studies from Chinese sources with limited information about the research designs. These facts have made it difficult to gather sufficient data in this area. From these and other Chinese sources, the studies synthesized in this section serve only as a sample of existing Qigong research with some methodological information, not as a comprehensive review. The studies on cardiovascular diseases presented better designs than those on other chronic conditions. Given the focus of this chapter, investigations of the nature or mechanism of qi are not reported here.

Effects on Hypertension and Cardiac Function

Sancier (1996) gathered more than 10 Chinese reports about the effectiveness of Qigong on hypertension. The preventive role of practicing Qigong in relation to stroke and mortality was highlighted. Cohen (1997) mentioned one large sample studying combined Qigong practice with biofeedback devices in the treatment of 639 patients with essential hypertension. At the eighth week, 85.1% of the sample attained significantly lower levels of blood pressure. Patients also reported improved mental health, appetite, sleep, and overall health. During the next 3 years, 97.7% remained stable, and lower levels of blood pressure were maintained despite biofeedback no longer being used. However, no control group was mentioned in this study.

Another randomized controlled study followed 204 hypertensive patients (Kuang et al., 1991; Sancier and Hu, 1991). At the 6-month follow-up, the combination of Qigong and antihypertension medication showed 19% more effectiveness than medication alone. The Qigong group showed reduced plasma dopamine-β-hydroxylase (DBH) activity, increased plasma high-density lipoprotein (HDL), and improvement of blood viscosity and platelet aggregation abnormalities. Hyperresponse of blood pressure to stress was also decreased. At the 6-year follow-up, the clinical effectiveness was 87% ± 3% and 68% ± 1% for the Qigong and control groups, respectively. The total and stroke mortality rates were 17.3% and 11.5% in the Qigong group, compared with 32.0% and 23.0% in the control group.

The most interesting controlled trial tracked 242 patients for 30 years (Cohen, 1997). Both the Qigong and the control groups used standardized antihypertension medication. Significant differences were found in mortality rates (25.41% in Qigong group, 47.76% in controls), stroke rate (20.49% in Qigong group, 40.83% in controls), and stroke-related mortality rate (15.57% in Qigong group, 32.50% in controls).

According to Sancier (1996), Chinese researchers also examined the effect of Qigong practice on the cardiac function of 120 male subjects (ages 55 to 75) by dividing them into three groups: (1) hypertensive subjects with heart-energy deficiency in TCM terms, (2) hypertensive subjects without heart-energy deficiency, and (3) subjects with normal blood pressure. Echocardiography indicated increases of left ventricular ejection fraction, mitral valve diastolic closing velocity, and mean velocity of circumferential shortening, while the total peripheral resistance decreased for the group of 46 hypertensive patients with "heart-energy deficiency." The groups without such a deficiency did not show significant improvement. The deficiency group also showed a decrease in nail fold microcirculation, evaluated by multiple quantitative evaluation, after practicing Qigong for 1 year. However, how "heart-energy deficiency" was measured remains unclear. Furthermore, a related report showed multiple quantitative evaluation of nail fold disturbance in microcirculation of these groups by observing 10 indices of abnormal conditions: configuration of micrangium, micrangium tension, condition of blood flow, slowing of blood flow, thinner afferent limb, effect and afferent limb ratio, color of blood, hemorrhage, and petechiae. Before Qigong practice, the incidence of microcirculation obstruction for the three groups was (1) 73.9%, (2) 26.5%, and (3) 17.5%. After practice for 1 year, group 1 showed a decrease in nail fold microcirculation obstruction from 73.9% to 39.3%. No significant change was found in group 2.

This research team also investigated the effects of Qigong practice on the blood chemistry of hypertensive patients (Kuang et al., 1991; Sancier and Hu, 1991). Improvement was found in plasma coagulation fibrinolysis indices, blood viscosity, erythrocyte deformation index, plasma level of tissue-type plasminogen activator, plasminogen activator inhibitor, factor VIII–related antigen, and antithrombin III. Changes in the activities of two messenger nucleotides (cyclic adenosine monophosphate [cAMP] and cyclic guanosine monophosphate) were also reported.

Some studies of healthy subjects showed the beneficial Qigong effects on cardiac function, microcirculation, and cardiovascular diseases (Chu et al., 1988; Ma, 1983; Mo et al., 1993; Qin, 1988; Wang et al., 1990, 1993). A group of 66 young men were divided into a Qigong exercise group and a regular exercise group. Both groups practiced their exercises for 4 weeks before suddenly entering a highland area. Symptoms of altitude sickness and physiological changes were measured for both groups before and after the experiment. The Qigong group showed less altitude stress than did the controls, as indicated by blood pressure, heart rate, oxygen consumption, microcirculation on the apex of the tongue and nail fold, and temperature at the Laogong acupoint (P8) in the palm of the left hand (Mo et al., 1993a). Another group examined microcirculation disorders of 40 air force pilots before and after entering the highland area (Mo et al., 1993b). Of them, 22 practiced Qigong and 18 did physical exercise for 8 weeks. The abnormalities were significantly less in the Qigong group than in the controls after the altitude change.

Effects on Other Chronic Conditions

Several other studies reported by Cohen (1997) examined Qigong effects on chronic conditions of the respiratory and digestive systems. One study assessed the lung function in 14 elderly patients with cardiac or pulmonary diseases. After 18 months of Qigong practice, their vital capacity, the exhaustive volume of exhaling air after a full inhalation, increased by an average of 3.31%, and their total lung capacity, the volume of air in the lungs after the deepest inhalation, increased by an average of 7.34%. The most significant gain was observed in forced vital capacity, the volume of air exhaled with maximum effort and speed, which increased by an average of 16.11% (p <.001).

Another study reported a standardized training of practice for 2 to 3 months, including a sitting position, deep relaxation, meditation, tranquil breathing for 20 to 30 minutes twice per day, concentration on certain acupoints, and self-massage (Cohen, 1997). After 4 years, 93 patients with bronchial asthma, of the initial sample of 99, reported significant improvement in terms of less frequency, severity, and duration of attacks; less medication use; and better capacity for physical labor. Neither this study nor the previous lung function study described controls.

Cohen (1997) also mentioned several large sample projects concerning Qigong effects on gastric and duodenal ulcer at several hospitals. These reports provided only a description of high percentages of cure rates without any information on research design. A study of 127 patients with various advanced malignant cancers had a relatively better design: 97 patients who underwent chemotherapy and practiced Qigong for 2 hours per day for 3 months were compared with 30 patients who underwent chemotherapy only (Cohen, 1997). Favorable outcomes were observed in terms of symptoms, body weight, and standard immunological indices for those who practiced Qigong in addition to chemotherapy. Despite the similar reports in replicated samples, no detailed information was available about the control design and assessment of outcome measures.

Overall, the conclusions of these studies remain problematic because of the weak research design and such issues as small sample size, heterogeneous subjects, no adequate controls, and lack of objective outcome measures.

Effects on Some Experimental Parameters

During the 1980s, Chinese researchers conducted laboratory tests on the role of external Qigong, or qi emission, in altering the parameters of physical structure or physiological process. Feng and colleagues (1982) suggested that there are two types of external qi: one depresses the growth of coliform bacillus and has a destructive effect, and another promotes growth and has an enhancing effect. Chen showed that qi emission reduced the growth rate of cultured BEL 7402 human liver cancer cells (Sancier, 1996). Liu, Shen, and Wang (1990) demonstrated qi's effects on inhibition of cancer growth in mice. Others reported that qi directed at peripheral blood in vivo induced an increase of plasma cAMP and enhanced the phagocytic function of macrophages (Li et al., 1983; Liu et al., 1982). Jia and Jia (1988) demonstrated the effect of qi on experimental mice with broken bones. Still other studies showed that qi emission protects neurons from damage caused by hydroxyl free radicals. However, there has been no report of such effects on human subjects.

Some Chinese experiments have showed the antiaging effects of internal Qigong practice. One study used a control group to examine the role of Qigong exercise in bone density (Kuang et al., 1991). The design of the control group was not reported. After 1 year of practicing Qigong, 18 male subjects (ages 50 to 59) increased their bone density from 0.627 ± 0.040 to 0.696 ± 0.069 g/cm^3. Among 12 older subjects (ages 60 to 69), bone density increased to a lesser degree. However, the increases of both groups exceeded that of the normal control group at the same age ranges.

A better-designed study examined the levels of active enzyme superoxide dismutase (SOD) that protects cells against damage from superoxide (Cohen, 1997). Two hundred subjects were evenly divided into Qigong and control groups with 50 males and 50 females in each group. The Qigong group practiced Qigong exercise, relaxation, and self-massage for a minimum of half an hour per day over about 1 year. The level of active SOD increased significantly in Qigong exercisers compared with controls (p <.001). Ye and colleagues also showed a significant increase in SOD activity in 116 subjects after Qigong practice for 2 months (Cohen, 1997). However, the use of a control group was not mentioned in this study.

Kuang, Wang, Xu, and Qian (1991) examined the role of Qigong exercise in plasma levels of sex hormones among 70 men (ages 40 to 69) and women (ages 51 to 67). After 1 year's practice, the estradiol level decreased for men and increased for women. An auxiliary study used 24-hour urine estradiol levels as indicators in 30 men (ages 50 to 69) (Xu and Wang, 1994). Qigong practice for 1 year decreased both the estradiol level and the estradiol:testosterone ratio. The change was accompanied by symptom changes of kidney deficiency in the TCM theory (e.g., soreness, dizziness, insomnia, hair loss, impotence, incontinence). Ye and colleagues (1990) reported similar changes in plasma levels of estradiol but not of testosterone in 77 Qigong exercisers compared with 27 controls after 2 months of practice.

Effects on Electroencephalogram (EEG)

Chinese researchers identified a unique brain wave pattern present in the majority of tested healthy Qigong practitioners, especially long-term practitioners (Cohen, 1997). The Qigong GEEK pattern involves four types of brain waves. First, the slowest type, *delta* (0.5-4 Hz), tends to be prevalent during infancy or in deep sleep of adults. However, it was recorded at times in Qigong healers when they were awake. This phenomenon seems to be concurrent with Lao Zi's statement of "breathing like a sleeping babe." Second, the next slowest type, *theta* (4-8 Hz), is normally present during drowsy, barely conscious states, and is likely accompanied with dreamlike images. However, it was present in trained practitioners in a fully awaking but relaxing state. The third, quicker type, *alpha* (8-13 Hz), can be produced by most people by closing the eyes and in relaxation. It is most frequently produced during meditative Qigong. Finally, the quickest type, *beta* (13-26 Hz or higher), is mostly associated with waking consciousness in adults. During practice of Qigong, brain waves slow down from beta to alpha, theta, or a combination of alpha and theta. Particularly, alpha changes from the appearance of ripples on a pond on the EEG to a preponderance of high-amplitude, high-crested ocean waves. This indicates that more brain tissues are acting in the same way simultaneously. More powerful alpha waves in the left hemisphere of the brain characterize the practitioner's attentive meditation on an object. Those in the right hemisphere occur during silent awareness with no object in meditation. In addition, increased alpha and theta waves tend to be recorded in the frontal portions of the brain during the practice. The coherence among these types of waves produced by various parts of the brain also increases. This pattern may lend support for the yin-yang balance theory in TCM and Qigong.

Effects on Mental Health

Studies on mental health outside the United States tend to have design flaws. In China, Wang (1993) assessed type A behaviors among 89 persons who practiced Qigong and 144 persons who did not. Type A traits were shown in 22.43% of the Qigong group and 51.39% of the controls. However, there was no mention of the randomization of these groups or of baseline sociodemographics and health conditions that might have contributed to the difference. In the comparison of 155 Qigong practitioners, 119 individuals with more than 2 years of experience demonstrated considerably better mental health than did those with less than 2 years (Wang, 1993). Outcomes were shown in measures for obsessive-compulsive traits, anxiety or phobic anxiety, depression or psychosis, general mental health, and interpersonal sensitivity on standardized instruments. The cross-sectional nature and the lack of information regarding the sample made causal conclusions somewhat questionable. In Japan, Hayashi (1995) conducted a descriptive survey concerning the effect of *Ru-Jing* (entering into a meditative status of mental void and calmness during practice) on emotional well-being among 226 Japanese Qigong practitioners. Positive mental health benefits included improved emotional stability, increased joy of life, decreased selfishness, and more open-mindedness, enthusiasm, willpower, and care for others. This study did not mention prepractice conditions and did not use standardized instruments in assessment.

Some researchers also investigated a rare side effect of inadequate Qigong practice, called *Qigon deviation* (QD) in modern China (Ai, 2003). QD manifested at a functional level in some aspect of mental health, but its clinical characteristics could not be clearly classified into existing psychiatric disease diagnoses. In 1994 the term *Qigon psychotic reaction*, the U.S. term for QD, was included in the *Glossary of Culture-Bound Syndromes* in the *Diagnostic and Statistical Manual of Mental Disorders (DSM-IV)* of the American Psychiatric Association. Using standardized psychiatric rating scales (Brief Psychiatric Scale, Hamilton Depression and Anxiety Scales, Improved Minnesota Multiphasic Personality Inventory), one study assessed 109 patients (ages 18-69, 89% males) with mental disorders occasioned by Qigong (Shan et al., 1989). Of them, 74 were self-taught learners of Qigong, mostly for self-healing. Patients who experienced QD presented abnormalities in perception, thinking, and behavior in varying degrees. Most of them also experienced specific QD physical symptoms. Patients with QD were categorized into two groups: the schizophrenic type (47 cases) and the neurotic type (62 cases). Most of the QD patients, however, recovered in a short time with no recurrence of attention disorder, delusion, hallucination, depression, anxiety, or behavior disturbances. Therefore, Qigong-triggered mental health disorders are considered temporary.

CLINICAL INVESTIGATIONS OF EXTERNAL QIGONG IN THE UNITED STATES

The enthusiasm over Qigong studies vanished in China about a decade ago, leaving some interesting data, especially on hypertension, for future research, as well as other, inconclusive results due to weak research design. This pioneer work provided valuable hypotheses for further testing of Qigong effects and perhaps the potential for international collaboration on a new wave of Qigong research in the West. At the dawn of the new millennium, the surging public interest in complementary, alternative, and integrative medicine in the United States has stirred two randomized controlled trials (RCTs) funded by the National Institutes of Health (NIH). Both investigated the role of external Qigong in medically diagnosed conditions with a higher standard of clinical research design. Both involved multidisciplinary collaborations and standardized clinical assessments of physical and mental health outcomes, as discussed later (Ai et al., 2001; Wu et al., 1999). A recent article in the *Archives of Internal Medicine* reported a systematic review of 47 studies, including nine RCTs

selected from 11 computerized English and Chinese databases, about Tai Ji effects on health outcomes (Wang et al., 2004). This information is not reported here because modern Tai Ji training, as with the popular Yoga, tends to be a slow form of physical exercise without emphasis on meditative breathing techniques of Qigong.

First NIH-Funded RCT on External Qigong

The first small-scale RCT, funded by the National Center of Complementary and Alternative Medicine (NCCAM), was an interdisciplinary effort using multiple-session assessments (Wang et al., 2004). With one Qigong experimental group and one placebo control group, this trial employed comprehensive evaluation of late-stage complex regional pain syndrome at baseline and at several follow-up stages during the experiment. All patients who completed trials underwent several mental health and domestic functioning tests using the Symptom Check List 90, Sickness Impact Profile, Beck Depression Inventory, and Cognitive-Somatic Anxiety questionnaire. The results of this study did not show any significant difference in domestic functioning or pain relief during the targeted sessions, partially because of the underpowered sample size. Nonetheless, mental health measures did reveal that anxiety in the experimental group was reduced more than in the control group, even within such a small sample. This report suggests that by using a sound research design, it may be possible to provide valid scientific evidence of Qigong effects on mental health and quality of life. The results of this trial have been published by *Alternative Therapy*.

Questions about "Placebo" Control in Qigong Trials

In designing the second NCCAM-funded large sample Qigong trial, Ai and colleagues (2001) argued about the limitation of using the classic RCT, on the basis of materialistic scientific philosophy, to assess the role of invisible bioenergy in terms of qi or other forms. A unique question arises about both the role of the adequate placebo and the appropriate comparison. Unlike pharmaceutical trials, where a placebo tablet looks identical to the medicine but does not contain the active ingredient, a placebo treatment for energy healing trials cannot be so well defined. A basic difference between drug and energy-healing trials is that the former does not involve a living person as the tool of intervention, so researchers do not need to worry about the type of interpersonal influence that occurs in the latter case. Although both clinicians and patients could not distinguish a placebo from a real drug, Qigong masters cannot be blind as to whether or not they are conducting real therapy. From a conventional perspective, the very notion of energy healing appears to fall into the category of what allopathic medicine terms the "placebo effect," which seems to be created from nothing other than the expectations of physicians or patients.

To address this interpersonal influence in assessing external Qigong, the *first* solution is simply to make the placebo aspect of healing invisible (Ai et al., 2001). The investigated therapy can take place with unconscious individuals (those asleep or anesthetized) or with the therapist behind a wall, a screen, or even at a considerable distance. The *second* solution, when this invisible form is implausible, is to conduct the assessment with two control groups, such as with a "treatment" versus both "no treatment" and "sham" (mimic) therapy design. Comparison groups must be designed so that expectations on the part of the research participants can be held constant. If benefits still occur for participants in the actual treatment group, the researcher can conclude that effects were not simply caused by expectations. The *third* solution is to reconsider the effective role of the placebo or expectations in the design rather than ignore or eliminate them. As in psychotherapy, confidence in or hope for the efficacy a therapist-involved treatment may be more important than any particular technique. Qigong researchers should take the historical lesson of Franz Anton Mesmer's claims of the miraculous cure brought about by his redistribution of animal magnetism in people's bodies in eighteenth-century Europe (Wyckoff, 1975). Despite the court's intent to trivialize the cures as resulting from patients' expectations, techniques of mesmerism have survived as hypnotism and are considered legitimate for medical use today. Thus the so-called placebo effect in Qigong healing and similar therapies, such as other types of energy healing, can still be seen as part of a real cure and should be examined in its own right.

Second NIH-Funded RCT on External Qigong

Holding the position of both the second and the third solution just described, the second NCCAM-funded, large-sample Qigong trial is examining its role in the in-hospital rehabilitation of midlife and older patients after cardiac surgery (Ai et al., 2001). The study design combined the methodology of RCT design in clinical medicine and that of a multiwave survey in social sciences to achieve multiple interrelated objectives. The RCT part had three, layered goals. The first goal was to design a conventional efficacy trial on Qigong. The second goal was to test the mechanisms of action in Qigong, such as the energy alternation that occurs in physiological factors. This potential energy alternation may mediate the effect of Qigong on postoperative wound healing and pain control in this study. The third goal was to test the placebo effect. Researchers randomized 360 cardiac surgery patients into three groups, who received (1) no treatment, (2) mimic Qigong by trained actors, or (3) real Qigong by a master. Qigong efficacy was assessed by measures of wound healing, pain relief, use of pain medication, and length of hospitalization. To address the placebo effect further, patients were asked after their participation in the trial if they believed they had received the effective (real) treatment. It was hypothesized that there would be no improvement in the no treatment group, some minimal improvement in the mimicked group, and more improvement in the real-Qigong group.

In addition, this study also examined the influence of spirituality in cardiac recovery, corresponding to TCM theories concerning the connection between the heart organ and the spirit of an individual. Using multiple standardized instruments, a multiwave survey was combined with this clinical trial. Multiple end points and assessments were employed at multiple periods (2 weeks before hospitalization, day before surgery, during postoperative 4 days in the hospital, and 2 months, 6 months, and 2 years after surgery). This survey was specifically designed to explore Qigong effects on mental health, such as depression, anxiety, fatigue, and general distress, as common predictors in the prognosis of coronary heart disease.

Currently, the data are undergoing analysis at the University of Michigan Integrative Medicine

Program. The author anticipates that some aspects of therapeutic and placebo effects will be revealed because of the sufficient statistical power with a relatively large sample. However, as with the first study, this second trial is collecting complicated measures on some difficult conditions, such as wound healing and pain, within only a few days of hospitalization, immediately after severe surgical trauma. This means that Qigong healers have no more than 4 days to deliver their treatment. These conditions tend not to be within the norm of regular treatment using complementary, alternative, and integrative medicine (CAM, CIM), including Qigong, which primarily focuses on the prevention of diseases and maintenance of maintaining health rather than on the treatment of medical diseases. These conditions should be taken into account with the outcome measures. This means that the short-term Qigong efficacy in this study may be affected by the "dosage" (length or intensity) needed by these difficult conditions.

If only a placebo effect is supported in these outcome measures, interesting questions could be raised about the nature of such an effect. Unlike psychotherapy theories that only address the mind, Daoism and TCM theories assume the energetic interaction with respect to the exchange of qi between humans. Even without verbal communication, this energetic contact exists in both Qigong and mimicked therapies, because only dead persons possess no qi. Under the circumstance of a placebo qi efficacy, the further examination of energy healing must move beyond the test of optimal expectations to the assessment of the hypothesized bioenergetic activities in the TCM and Qigong theory. Exploration of this new dimension, however, is beyond the scope of this chapter, which is limited to the introduction of Qigong basics.

Finally, for the interested reader, the author must leave more historical documentation, practical instructions, and a scientific exploration of the nature of qi and other biofield phenomena to specialized books, with the pathology of the qi system discussed in Chapter 21.

CONCLUSION

Ai and colleagues (2001) have stated the implications of these new investigations on Qigong for clinical sciences at the end of their research article, as follows:

Inquiry into controversial issues surrounding Qigong does not arise only from the need to improve the quality of research design on energy healing trials. It is also a call for continuing innovation of research methodology to address the unique challenge of evaluating the complicated framework of CAM modality. Through close cooperation between researchers and CAM practitioners, standardized approaches to valid research protocols can be developed. By scientific testing of plural pathway models, the blossoming of research on energy healing may eventually enrich methodologies used in clinical research on other types of health care (p. 99).

Acknowledgments

The author has been supported by the National Institute on Aging Training Grant, T32-AG0017, National Institute on Aging Grant, R03-AGO-15686-01, National Center for Complementary and Alternative Medicine Grant P50-AT00011, a grant from the John Templeton Foundation, and the John Hartford Faculty Scholars Program. Amy L. Ai, PhD, is Associate Professor at the University of Washington, Seattle, and an affiliated researcher at the University of Michigan Health System Integrative Medicine Program. Address correspondence to Amy L. Ai, Ph.D., University of Washington, 4101 15th Ave NE, Seattle, WA 98105-6299, 206-221-7781 (phone), 206-543-1228 (fax), amyai@u.washington.edu, or amyai@umich.edu.

References

Ai AL: Psychosocial adjustment and health care practices following coronary artery bypass surgery (CABG), *Diss Abstr Int Sci Eng* 57(6B):4078, 1996.

Ai AL: Assessing mental health in clinical study on Qigong: between scientific investigation and holistic perspectives, *Semin Integr Med* 1(2):112-121, 2003.

Ai AL, Peterson C, Gillespie B, et al: Designing clinical trials on energy healing: ancient art encounters medical science, *Altern Ther Health Med* 7:83-90, 2001.

American Psychiatric Association: Glossary of culture-bound syndromes. In *Diagnostic and statistical manual of mental disorders (DSM-IV)*, 1994, Washington, DC, p 847.

Bloom A: *The republic of Plato: translated with notes and an interpretive essay*, New York, 1968, Basic Books.

Brown C: The experiments of Dr. Oz, *New York Magazine*, July 30, 1995, pp 20-23.

Capra F: *The Tao of physics*, ed 3, Boston, 1991, Shamabhala.

Chu W et al: Changes of blood viscosity and RCG in 44 cases with cardiovascular diseases after Qigong exercises. In *Proceedings of the First World Conference for Academic Exchange of Medical Qigonq,* Beijing, 1988, pp 57-58.

Cohen KS: *The way of Qigong: The art and science of Chinese energy healing,* New York, 1997, Ballantine Books.

Crosby DA: *A religion of nature,* Albany, 2002, State University of New York Press.

Despeux C: Gymnastics: the ancient tradition. In Kohn L, editor: *Taoist meditation and longevity techniques,* Ann Arbor, 1989, Center for Chinese Studies, University of Michigan, pp 225-262.

Eisenberg DM: *Encountering qi,* Havmonds Worth, England, 1985, Penguin Books, p 210.

Feng LD, Qian JC, Li SY, et al: Effect of emitted qi (external qi) on gram negative bacilli, *Nature* 5:163, 1982.

Graham H: Ancient perspectives on healing; Eastern perspective on healing. In *Time, energy and psychology of healing,* London, 1990, Jessica Kingsley Publishers.

Hammer L: The fundamental energy constructs of Chinese medicine; The traditional five elements system: emotion and the disease process. In *Dragon rises, red bird flies: psychology, energy and Chinese medicine,* Barrytown, NY, 1990, Station Hill Press.

Hayashi S: *Qigong and mental health: the positive effects of the state of Rujing (tranquillity).* Paper presented at Fourth International Conference on Qigong, Vancouver, BC, Canada, 1995, pp 26-27.

Heise TE: Taiji quan and qigong: extended body oriented therapeutic approaches based on the model of traditional Chinese medicine, *Praxis Psychother Psychosom* 38:255-262, 1993 (in German).

Hisamitsu T, Seto A, Nadazato S, et al: Emission of extremely strong magnetic fields from the head and whole body during oriental breathing exercises, *Acupunct Electrother Res* 21:219-227, 1996.

Jia L, Jia J: Effect of emitted qi on healing of experimental fracture. Paper presented at First World Conference for Academic Exchange of Medical Qigong, Beijing, 1988, pp 13-14 (Chinese Institute of Sports Medicine).

Kuang AK, Wang, RY, Xu DH, Qian XR: Research on "anti-aging" effect of qigong, *J Tradit Chin Med* 11(2):153-158, 1991.

Kuang AK, Wang RY, Xu DH, Qian XR: Research on "anti-aging" effect of qigong, *J Tradit Chin Med.* 11(3):224-227, 1991.

Lewis T, Amini F, Lannon R: *A general theory of love,* New York, 2001, Vintage Books, p 122.

Li CX, Jing L, Zhao K: Study of Qigong Waigi on phagocytic function of mouse peritoneal macrophages, *Nature* 6:910, 1983.

Liao SJ: Acupuncture for low back pain in *Huang Di Nei Jing Su Wen* (Yellow emperor's classic of internal medicine book of common questions), *Acupunct Electrother Res* 17:249-258, 1992.

Liu D, Shen X, Wang C: Study of the effect of external qi in natural killer cell activity on mice with tumors. Paper presented at Third International Symposium on Qigong, Shanghai, 1990, p 73.

Liu S, Huang RS, Wang, XT, et al: Preliminary experimental observations of the effect of Qigong Wai Qi (external qi) on the plasma cAMP, *Nature* 5:165, 1982.

Ma YZ: Hypertension treatment with Qigong, *Qigong Sci* 4:11, 1983.

Maciocia G: The five elements. In *The foundations of Chinese medicine: a comprehensive text for acupuncturists and herbalists,* New York, 1989, Churchill Livingstone.

McGarry J: Applications of Eastern and Naturalistic philosophy in the modification of Western belief systems, *Aust J Clin Hypnother Hypn* 7(2):779-790, 1996.

Mo F, Xu Y, Lu Y, Xu G: Study of prevention of cardiac function disorder due to immediate entry into highlands by Qigong exercise. In *Proceedings of the Second World Conference on Academic Exchange of Medical Qigong,* Beijing, 1993a, p 78.

Mo F, Wan L, Jia Z, Xu G: Study of prevention of microcirculation disorders of pilots on highlands by Qigong. In *Proceedings of the Second World Conference on Academic Exchange of Medical Qigong,* Beijing, 1993b, p 78.

Peng K, Nisbettm EN: Culture, dialectics, and reasoning about contradiction, *Am Psychol* 54:741-754, 1999.

Qian XS: Some theoretical ideas on the development of basic research in human body science, *PSI Res* 1:4-15, 1982.

Qin C et al: Bidirectional adjustment of blood pressure and heart rate by Daoying Tuina on the arterial blood and heart rate. In *Proceedings of the First World Conference on Academic Exchange of Medical Qigong,* Beijing, 1988, p 107.

Ruggie M: Investigating CAM: what works? In *Marginal to Mainstream: Alternative Medicine in America,* New York, 2004, Cambridge University Press, pp 168-169.

Sancier KM: Medical applications of Qigong, *Altern Ther Health Med* 2:40-46, 1996.

Sancier KM, Hu BK: Medical applications of Qigong and emitted qi on humans, animals, cell cultures, and plants: review of selected scientific research, *Am J Acupunct* 19:367-377, 1991.

Shan HH, Yan HQ, Xu SH, et al: Clinical phenomenology of mental disorders caused by Qigong exercise, *Chin Med J* 102(6):445-448, 1989.

Shen GJ: Study of mind-body effects and Qigong in China, *Advances* 3:134-142, 1986.

Temkin O: The medicine of the body and the medicine of the soul: epilogue. In *Hippocrates in a world of pagans and Christians,* Baltimore, 1991, Johns Hopkins University Press.

Tiller W, Greene G, Parks P, Anderson S: Towards explaining the anomalous large body voltage surges on exceptional subjects, *J Sci Explor* 9:355-383, 1995.

Unschuld PU: Taoism and pragmatic drug therapy: from antifeudal social theory to individualistic practices of longevity. In *Medicine in China: a history of ideas,* Berkeley, Calif, 1985, University of California Press.

Wang C, Xu D, Qian Y, Kuang A: Beneficial effect of Qigong on improving the heart function and relieving multiple cardiovascular risk factors. In *Proceedings of the Third World Conference for Academic Exchange of Medical Qigong,* Beijing, 1990, p 40.

Wang C, Xu D, Qian Y, Shi W: Effects of Qigong on preventing stroke and alleviating the multiple cerebrocardiovascular risk factors: a follow-up report on 242 hypertensive cases over 30 years. In *Proceedings of the Second World Conference for Academic Exchange of Medical Qigong,* Beijing, 1993, p 126.

Wang C, Collet J, Lau J: The effect of tai chi on health outcomes in patients with chronic conditions, *Arch Intern Med* 164(8):493-501, 2004.

Wang HT, Yan GH, eds. *Nan Jing,* 1988, pp 103-106 (in Chinese).

Wang JS: Role of Qigong on mental health. In *Proceedings of the Second World Conference for Academic Exchange of Medical Qigong,* Beijing, 1993, p 93.

Willis C: Why new age medicine is catching on, *Time* 138:68-76, 1991.

Wu WH, Bandilla E, Ciccone DS, et al: Effects of Qigong on late-stage complex regional pain syndrome, *Altern Ther Health Med* 5(1):45-54, 1999.

Wyckoff J: *Franz Anton Mesmer: between God and devil,* Englewood Cliffs, NJ, 1975, Prentice.

Xu D, Wang C: Clinical study of delaying effect on senility of hypertensive patients by practicing "Yang Jing Yi Shen Gong." In *Proceedings of the Fifth International Symposium on Qigong,* Shanghai, 1994, p 109.

Yuan CH: "Chinese medicine" is not the abbreviation of the medicine of China: *I-Ching* expert Lui Dajun's definition of "Chinese medicine," *Chinese News* 28:23, 1997 (in Chinese).

Zi L: *Tao Te Jing* (Translated by S Rosenthal) (http://web.clas.ufl.edu/users/gthursby/taoism).

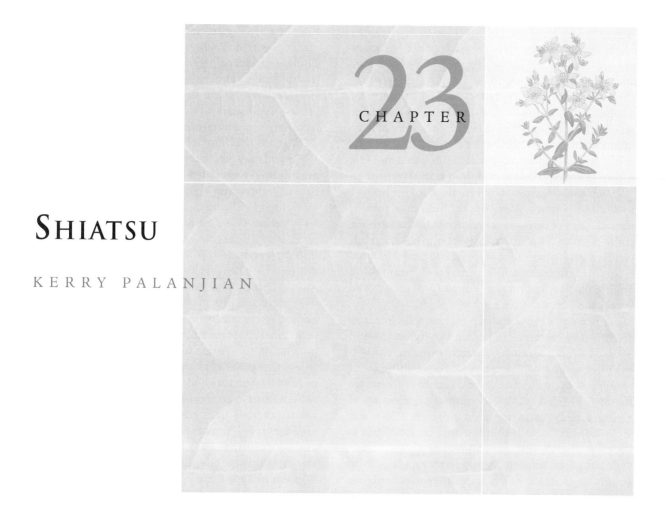

CHAPTER

23

SHIATSU

KERRY PALANJIAN

Simple yet profound, the experience with shiatsu, whether a single session or an ongoing therapeutic relationship between therapist and client, brings the wisdom of ancient civilizations to our Western model of life, thought, and medicine. Shiatsu, which is reinforced by Western and Eastern clinical research and receives official Japanese government sanction, is regarded by many as a life-changing experience. Shiatsu's practice, as a modality for fully clothed recipients, is allowing its growth not only in the private sector, but more importantly as an easy-to-implement research tool in numerous clinical settings and hospitals.

HISTORY

The literal meaning of the Japanese word *shiatsu* (she-AAHT-sue) is "finger pressure" or "thumb pressure."

Over the centuries, Asian medicine, massage therapy, and twentieth-century advancements have combined to yield "modern" shiatsu.

The word *massage* comes from the Arabic word for *stroke*. The practice of massage dates back 3000 years to China. A tomb found in modern Egypt, determined to be from 2200 BC, depicts a man receiving a foot massage. In the fourth century BC, Hippocrates, known as the father of modern medicine, wrote that "the physician must be experienced in many things, but most assuredly in rubbing" (Ballegaards et al., 1996). Further support for the use of touch and massage as healing tools is noted in ancient Egyptian, Greek, Persian, Roman, and Asian manuscripts (Yamamoto and McCarty, 1993).

During the Middle Ages, there was decreased visibility of massage as a healing tool in the West, principally because of the position of the church, which viewed the manipulation of the body to be the work of the devil. Massage was often depicted as a tool of prostitution, a prejudice that still lingers today among uninformed people. In the thirteenth century the German emperor Frederick II seized a number of newborns and did not allow caretakers to cuddle or talk to the infants. All died before they were able to talk. The historian Salimbene described this "experiment" in 1248 when he wrote, "They could not live without petting" (Colt and Hollister, 1997).

People instinctively recognize the need for human touch and contact. From the rubbing of a painful shoulder to the physical act of intimacy, the need for connection and human touch not only feels good but yields many physical and psychological benefits. These benefits are gaining increased recognition among laypeople and are enjoying a substantial increase in support from scientific studies that document numerous broad-based positive effects (see later section on research). The University of Miami Medical School's Touch Research Institute (TRI) is gaining widespread acceptance as a pioneer of research supporting the medical benefits of massage therapy. TRI has published numerous studies and review articles, with more in progress (Colt and Hollister, 1997). Evidence presented in these studies supports the clinical use of massage therapy for a wide range of ailments. Massage therapy has been shown to facilitate weight-gain in preterm infants, reduce stress hormone levels, alleviate symptoms of depression, reduce pain, positively increase measurable immune system functions, and alter electroencephalogram readings in the direction of heightened awareness. The studies also suggest benefits for patients with conditions such as Alzheimer's disease, arthritis, cancer, depression, fibromyalgia, job stress, and premenstrual syndrome (PMS), while additionally documenting benefits related to maternity and labor (http://www. miami.edu/touch-research) (Colt & Hollister, 1997).

Shiatsu's history lies within the antecedents of Asian medicine, as was clearly stated 2000 years ago in *The Yellow Emperor's Classic of Internal Medicine*, a text discussed in *The Art of Shiatsu* (Cowmeadow, 1992). Others suggest that Chinese medical practice was derived from techniques originally developed in India and adapted to China.

Shiatsu has evolved within the genre of touch and massage therapies, as well as within Asian medicine's juxtaposition to ancient and modern Japanese cul-

ture. As a healing art or treatment, shiatsu grew from earlier forms of *Anma* in Japan (*Anmo* or *Tuina* in China) (Lundberg, 1992). *An* denotes "pressure" and "nonpressure," and *ma* means "rubbing" (Yamamoto and McCarty, 1993). This method, which was well known 1000 years ago in China, found its way to Japan and was recognized as the safest and easiest way to treat the human body (Masunaga and Ohashi, 1977). In Japan, shiatsu was used and taught by blind practitioners who relied on their hands to diagnose a patient's condition (Cowmeadow, 1992). Anma was recognized by the medical authorities in Japan in the Nara period (710-784 AD), but subsequently lost its popularity before gaining more widespread use in the Edo era (1603-1868) (Yamamoto and McCarty, 1993), during which doctors were actually required to study Anma. During the Edo period, most practitioners were blind and provided treatments in their patients' homes. An extensive handbook on Anma was published in 1793, and Anma was considered one component of the Asian healing arts, a reputation it enjoys today. Anma's "understanding and assessment of human structure and meridian lines" were and are believed to be important distinctions that separate shiatsu therapy from other healing models and massage therapies (Yamamoto and McCarty, 1993). One author states that European physicians and missionaries from the sixteenth century onward introduced Western anatomy and physiology to Japan (Young, 2004), whereas others suggest Western massage was introduced to Japan in the late 1880s, when the many vocational schools that taught Anma were dominated by blind instructors. However, this very limitation stopped the further development of Anma and led to the evolution of what we recognize today as shiatsu therapy (Yamamoto and McCarty, 1993). The practitioner, Tamai Tempaku, is credited with developing shiatsu as a separate therapy in the early 1900s (Young, 2004).

Modern shiatsu, as noted previously, is therefore a product of twentieth-century refinements and evolution that produced the form of therapy used today. Shiatsu began its modern evolution in the 1920s (the Taisho period) when Anma practitioners adopted some of the West's hands-on techniques, including those of chiropractic and occupational therapy (Yamamoto and McCarty, 1993), as well as the additional merging of *ampuku* (abdominal massage), *do-in* (breathing and self-massage practices), and Buddhism. Tamai Tempaku is credited with establishing shiatsu in Japan and worldwide. The Shiatsu Therapists Association was formed in 1925 (Annussek, 2004).

The practice of shiatsu received much attention and growth from studies conducted after World War II, as described in the following quotation from Saito:

> After World War II, U.S. General Douglas MacArthur directed the Japanese Health Ministry. There were more than 300 unregulated therapies in Japan at that time. MacArthur ordered all 300 to be researched by scientists at the Universities, to document which ones had scientific proof of merit; and which did not. At the end of eight years, the Universities reported back; and "Shiatsu" was the only one therapeutic practice which received scientific approval (Saito, 2001).

In 1955 the Japanese parliament adopted a bill on "revised Anma," which gave shiatsu official government endorsement. This endorsement allowed shiatsu to be legally taught in schools throughout Japan (Yamamoto and McCarty, 1993). Shiatsu received further official Japanese government recognition as a therapy in 1964 (Harmon et al., 1999) through the efforts of Tokujiro Namikoshi and his son, Toru, who emphasized the application of pressure on neuromuscular points to release pain and tension (Young, 2004). In the early 1970s, shiatsu began spreading to the West and rapidly gained widespread acceptance (Cowmeadow, 1992). Although shiatsu and its distant cousin acupuncture are considered medically sound and are "accepted methods of treatment for over one-quarter of the world's population," the United States and many other Western nations consider both techniques experimental (Yamamoto and McCarty, 1993). This is interesting, considering that these "experiments" have been conducted successfully for more than 2500 years (Cowmeadow, 1992). However, several U.S. hospitals now allow the use of acupuncture, and medical and nursing students are beginning to be taught the theories and practice of acupuncture, shiatsu, and macrobiotics. These gains suggest that an environment has been established for rapid, ongoing change in the West. There is a growing acceptance and use of these practices among Western-trained physicians and health care providers.

Shiatsu can be described as a synthesis of Eastern and Western medicine, quickly gaining recognition for its success as an adjunctive healing therapy. "The foundations for modern ideas and techniques in the healing realm come from ancient civilizations. In the West it was Greece and Rome. And in the East it was China, India, and Persia. These foundations are the basis of present scientific methods [of healing]" (Yamamoto and McCarty, 1993). Shiatsu's foundations, and therefore shiatsu itself, are a part of the growing trend and movement toward complementary and integrative medicine (CIM).

PRINCIPLES AND PHILOSOPHY

Many followers of Eastern traditions believe that the natural state of humanity is to be healthy. Yamamoto and McCarty (1993) describe it this way:

> With observation we can see that there is a definite and distinct order in nature. Nature's power guides all things. When we do not follow nature's order we can become sick. We are often reminded of nature's order by the presence of sickness. Sickness can be our teacher. From a traditional point of view the specific name of an illness is not so important. Physical ailments such as headache, gallbladder pain, emotional states such as anger, depression, irritability; and mental conditions such as paranoia, lack of concentration, and forgetfulness; are all various states of disequilibrium or disease. Theoretically there is no disease that is incurable, if we are able to change the way we think, eat, and live. Of course this is easier said than done.

They also write, "The simple understanding that humans are equipped to heal themselves and that [they] can also help others, [forms] the underlying foundation of Shiatsu. Shiatsu [simply] acts like a spark or catalyst to the human body [and] the combination of treatment and way of life suggestions form the basis of total care" (Yamamoto and McCarty, 1993).

The major underlying principle of shiatsu, derived from the tenets of Asian medicine, is actually a reflection of scientific thought. Simply stated, "Everything is energy." When considered in the context of molecular structure, all matter is a manifestation of energy. Shiatsu interacts directly with this energy, and therefore with life itself.

From the perspective of classic Asian medicine, energy moves along 14 distinct pathways in the body; these pathways are called *meridians* or *channels* (*kieraku* in Japanese, *jing* in Chinese) (Yamamoto and McCarty, 1993). The meridians were discovered by accident when certain acupoints (specific locations along the meridians) were stimulated and beneficial results were observed. For example, asthmalike symptoms caused by certain types of battle wounds were relieved when the corresponding acupoint was touched, and menstrual pain was reduced when a heated rock from a fireplace accidentally brushed against a point on the inner thigh (Schlager et al., 2000). Although many in the West may attempt to deny or discount the existence of the meridian network, modern research conducted by biophysicists in Japan, China, and France has documented its existence. Yamamoto and McCarty describe some of this research in the following excerpt from *Whole Health Shiatsu:*

> Many studies have been conducted by biophysicists in Japan, China, and France. They postulated that a measurement of acu-point electricity would be a biophysical index that would illustrate the objective existence of the meridian system. They discovered that acu-points have a lower skin resistance. When an electrical current is passed through a classical acu-point, it has a higher electrical conductance, which is a lower resistance, than the surrounding area. They also discovered that when disease or illness is present, pathological changes take place in the body while changes are found in the resistance of relevant meridians and acu-points. Similar internal changes are also reflected by the acu-points. In other words, imbalance in the organs affect the acu-points, imbalance in the acu-points affect the organs. Researchers also found that the external environment, such as temperature, season, and time of day, changed the resistance of acu-points.
>
> In the Lanzhou Medical College in China a test of the acu-points of the Stomach meridian showed significant variations in conductance when the stomach lining was stimulated by cold or hot water, either before or after eating. In Beijing, ear acu-point research learned that low resistance points on the outer rim of the ear were elevated either in the presence of disease or following long-term stimulation of a corresponding internal organ (Yamamoto and McCarty, 1993).

In addition to the scientific support developed thus far, the benefits of shiatsu are supported by the experiences of clients and practitioners alike. Asthmatic clients experience volatility (pain and sensitivity) along their lung meridian. Clients with lower digestive track symptoms such as constipation experience this same sensitivity along their large intestine meridians. Women with PMS symptoms are sensitive on the lower leg along both the bladder and the kidney meridian, which, according to Shiatsu theory and

literature, are associated with reproductive energy. When clients experience these connections, which are common in shiatsu, they are quick to convert or more readily accept the principles of Asian medicine and to accept the validity of the meridian network. Not only has research documented scientific evidence to support the theory behind shiatsu, but the body's own level of pain along related organ meridian lines makes a client's enlightenment regarding the existence of meridians, based on their own personal experience with shiatsu therapy, difficult to deny.

It is believed that meridians evolved from energy centers in the body called *chakras* (SHOCK-ras) and that our organ systems subsequently evolved from the meridian network. There are 10 meridians directly related to internal organs, two indirectly related, and two related to systems not recognized by Western medicine.

Along the meridian lines are points called *tsubos* (SUE-bows), or *acupuncture points,* of which there are believed to be about 600 (Annussek, 2004). Yamamoto and McCarty describe tsubos in the following excerpt from *Whole Health Shiatsu:*

> The word *Tsubo* or *acu-point* derives from the Oriental characters meaning hole or orifice, and position—the position of the hole. Traditionally, the word hole was combined with other terms such as hollow, passageway, transport, and Ki [Key, or energy, also described in other cultures as Chi, Qi, and Prana]. This suggests that the holes on the surface of the body were regarded as routes of access to the body's internal cavities. The acu-points are spots where Ki comes out.
>
> There are three phases in the historical development of the concept of these holes or acu-points. In the earliest phase people would use any body location that was painful or uncomfortable. Because there were no specific locations for the points, they had no names.
>
> In the second phase, after a long period of practice and experience, certain points became identified with specific diseases. The ability of distinct points to affect and be affected by local or distant pain and disease became predictable. . . .
>
> In the final phase, many previously localized points, each with a singular function, became integrated into a larger system that related and grouped diverse points systematically according to similar functions. This integration is called the *meridian* or *channel system* (Yamamoto and McCarty, 1993).

Although the analogy is not completely accurate, shiatsu is often called "acupuncture without needles." To alter a client's internal energy system or pattern, an acupuncturist inserts needles in tsubos used by a shiatsu practitioner. The most significant difference between the two disciplines is that whereas acupuncture is invasive and is performed by extensively trained doctors, shiatsu is noninvasive and can be practiced by either a professional therapist or a layperson. Shiatsu is also a whole-body technique versus one that is limited to the insertion of needles at specific tsubos. Acupuncture is generally considered more symptom oriented in that people are much less likely to go to an acupuncturist without a specific complaint, whereas clients often equate shiatsu with health maintenance and go for treatments without particular "problems." Although some consider shiatsu a cousin to acupuncture, others suggest a "distant cousin" relationship. The distinctions between the two disciplines are worth noting (Table 23-1). It is also important to note that simple shiatsu can be practiced with little or no understanding of the underlying principles. The practitioner does not have to agree with the principles or understand them to provide shiatsu; however, the techniques are part of a more complicated healing system that, when adhered to and studied, provides more effective results.

Although not all acupuncturists agree with all these distinctions, they form a basis for comparison. All shiatsu practitioners and acupuncturists practice according to their own interpretations and belief systems, so Table 23-1 should not be interpreted as a rigid, fixed framework.

A simple and accurate analogy for understanding the meridian pathways and tsubos in relation to the body's internal organ systems is that tsubos are similar to a system of volcanoes on the earth's surface. We know that a volcano's real energy is not at the surface, but rather is found deep inside the earth. A volcano is a superficial manifestation of the underlying energy. Similarly, a tsubo can be thought of as a manifestation of the underlying energy of the organ system. This does not imply that the therapist should ignore the area of pain a shiatsu client may describe. However, a classically trained shiatsu practitioner looks past sore shoulders, ligaments, and tendons (unless the cause of the pain is trauma to these structures) and focuses on the related organ system through the meridian network. Philosophically, shiatsu practitioners would have a tendency to relate health to the condition of the related "vital" organs (i.e., those associated with the meridian system). Although shiatsu is noninvasive and appears to deal with external or surface pain, according to shiatsu theory and the experience of those who practice and receive the art, it stimulates, sedates, and balances energy *inside* the body as a way to address the root causes of surface and bodily discomfort.

The principles of Asian medicine evident in shiatsu theory and practice state that two types of energies exist in the universe. These two types of energy, called *yin* and *yang*, exist side by side and are considered both complementary and opposing. Unlike Western medicine, which uses more dualistic terms such as "good and bad," Eastern or Asian medicine looks at health more as a manifestation of balance between yin and yang and how an imbalance may *allow* infection or disease to manifest. An effective way to comprehend this

TABLE 23-1

Distinctions between Shiatsu and Acupuncture

Category	Shiatsu	Acupuncture
Movement	Free flowing	Systematic
Focus	Intuitive	Adheres to laws
Theoretical inclination	Taoist	Confucian
Quality	Feminine	Masculine
Tools	Practitioner's body	Needles
Treatment goal	Balance by becoming whole	Balance by alleviating symptoms
Patient interacts with treater	Yes	No
Encourages independence	Yes, immediately	Yes, after treatment series
Physically strengthens:		
Receiver	Yes	Sometimes
Treater	Yes	No

internally is to apply the principles of yin and yang to diet through macrobiotics. When a person's health and metabolism adjust to what Eastern medicine and macrobiotic practitioners consider universal guidelines, natural harmony occurs from "the inside out." Varying states of yin and yang are experienced by the body but are not necessarily comprehended by the mind. This experience can be made manifest by dedication (not necessarily lifelong) to the practice of using food according to the various energetic principles long understood by the Chinese, Japanese, and followers of macrobiotic theory.

In defining yin and yang, bear in mind that a continuum exists between the extremes of each. In shiatsu, major organs are paired together under one of the five major elements. Each pair has both a yang and yin organ. One organ is more compact and tighter (yang), whereas the other is more open and vessel-like (yin). The five elements—wood (tree), fire, earth (soil), metal, and water—proceed in a clockwise manner within the five-element wheel used in Asian medicine (Table 23-2).

According to shiatsu principles, an organ is fed by its opposite energy. For the shiatsu practitioner, pressing and rubbing movements proceed in the direction energy travels along each respective meridian. Shiatsu texts often use the term *structure* to describe an organ, whereas acupuncture texts may describe the same organ in terms of the energy that *feeds* it through the meridian. A yang organ is fed by yin energy. A shiatsu practitioner generally describes the compact kidney as yang because of its *structure* (compared with its paired, more hollow and open yin organ, the bladder). A classically trained acupuncturist generally describes the kidney as yin because it is *fed by* yin energy that flows *up* the body on the kidney meridian. Such differences between the two disciplines in terms of descriptive language can be confusing, although little difference in application of goals, practice, or theory really exists.

Another major principle applied to the practice of shiatsu involves the concepts of *kyo* (KEY-o) and *jitsu* (JIT-sue). Kyo is considered *empty* or *vacant*, whereas jitsu is considered *full, excessive,* or *overflowing*. A jitsu condition along the gallbladder meridian may be a manifestation of a gallbladder imbalance, resulting perhaps from recent consumption of a large pizza and two dishes of ice cream. A kyo or empty condition along the lung meridian (and within the lung itself) may exist in an individual who does not exercise and rarely expands his or her chest cavity or heart. Understanding and finding these energy manifestations is critical to diagnosis in shiatsu practice and is an ongoing, lifelong learning experience for the serious shiatsu practitioner. Although it is generally easy to find jitsu, or excess, it is much more difficult to find emptiness or vacancy (kyo) within the meridian network. One of the keys to doing highly successful or refined shiatsu is the ability to find specific kyo within the body or the organ's meridian network and then to manipulate it effectively.

Shiatsu practitioners may follow the practice of macrobiotics, a set of universal dietary and spiritual guidelines originally brought to the attention of the modern world by George Ohsawa. As David Sergel writes:

> The ultimate goal of macrobiotic practice is the attainment of absolute freedom. The compass to reach this goal is an intimate understanding of the forces of Yin and Yang; a comprehension of an order common to all aspects of the infinite universe. The foundation of this freedom lies in our daily diet.... Since the same cultural soil gave form to both shiatsu and macrobiotics, we might expect to see strong possibilities of a harmonious integration between the two. In fact as we delve deeper, we see evidence that shiatsu arose from a macrobiotic mind and is thus according to this view, from its foundation, a macrobiotic practice (Sergel, 1989).

It would be more accurate to state that shiatsu developed out of a society whose dietary pattern reflected the modern perspective and application of macrobiotics. Shiatsu evolved as a result of day-to-day living and thinking in terms of yin and yang, as did almost everything else in these earlier Asian societies, such as feng shui, art, and even politics.

Macrobiotics is a philosophical practice that incorporates the universal guidelines of yin and yang into

TABLE 23-2

Five Elements of Asian Medicine

Element	Yin	Yang
Wood (tree)	Gallbladder	Liver
Fire	Small intestine	Heart
Earth (soil)	Stomach	Spleen
Metal	Larger intestine	Lungs
Water	Bladder	Kidney

daily life. With diet as its cornerstone, macrobiotic theory posits that these guidelines can be applied to all people, subject to their condition, constitution, lifestyle, environment, and most notably, the latitude at which they live. Food choices are governed by season. Macrobiotics is *not* a diet; it is a philosophy that advocates cooked whole grains as the predominant staple food, to be supplemented by other yang foods such as root vegetables and occasional fish, and yin foods such as leafy greens and occasional seasonal fruit. Extreme yin foods include white sugar, honey, caffeine, most drugs, and alcohol. Examples of extreme yang foods are animal proteins such as red meat, chicken, tuna, and shellfish. Dietary choices are adjusted according to an individual's constitution, environment, work, lifestyle, the season, and where the person lives (especially global latitude). When used indiscriminately, extreme yin and yang foods are more difficult to balance and affect energy, as manifested along the meridian network. For example, eating tropical fruit in Pennsylvania in January when the temperature is 10° F on a daily basis is seen as "eating out of balance."

Macrobiotic philosophy therefore relies on nature, from which it finds ample support. Although we are able to ship foods thousands of miles from where they are grown, nature may not have intended us to consume such foods regularly in an environment that does not support their growth or cultivation. When applied in this way, the philosophies of shiatsu and macrobiotics touch on and address what is viewed as human arrogance by suggesting that when clear-cut guidelines presented by nature are ignored, health consequences can result. Nature demonstrates that the foods that grow and *can* grow in the latitudes where we live are the foods that support our health most fully. This philosophy also states that consumption of root vegetables (i.e., those that produce more heat in the body) is important in the winter, whereas leafy greens and occasional fruit (foods that cool the body) are needed in summer. Interestingly, we intuitively follow this practice to some extent. People who live in locations where the climate varies from season to season tend to eat more salads and fruit in the summer and more cooked and salty foods in the winter. However, macrobiotic philosophy examines this practice more closely and looks at these specific distinctions of yin and yang as being crucial to creating balance in the body, as well as the cornerstone of addressing such imbalance issues such as cancer.

Shiatsu incorporates macrobiotic philosophy into its theory and philosophy regarding the movement of energy along the meridian pathways. A simple explanation of shiatsu philosophy states that the meridians can be seen as circulatory or "plumbing" channels. As long as energy moves freely (i.e., is not too weak or too strong and is not stagnated), health is maintained. If there is a blockage along the channel, the resulting disturbance can lead to minor aches and pains or a major health imbalance. It is possible to observe imbalances of energy flow in specific meridian lines and acupuncture points or tsubos. By applying pressure to a blocked meridian line or tsubo, an overactive or underactive organ system can be directly sedated or stimulated.

Shiatsu massage is not viewed by its practitioners as a panacea. Shiatsu philosophy is very clear in reinforcing the need for dietary and lifestyle guidance and changes to complement and support a shiatsu session (or series of sessions). The choices made by the recipients of treatment are their choices. Many recipients are content to stay at the level at which shiatsu is simply used for pain reduction and for producing a "calmed sense of revitalization." However, others who are open to the underpinnings of shiatsu philosophy may be willing to take additional steps suggested by a classically trained shiatsu practitioner regarding diet and behavior modification.

With sufficient training, the shiatsu practitioner learns to view the energy manifesting at major tsubos on the surface of the skin as indicative of the underlying condition of the organ to which the tsubo is related and connected. For example, a client may think shoulder pain is caused by how he or she sleeps or sits at a desk. A classically trained shiatsu practitioner does not ignore these factors but looks *past* them to the underlying organ system and the foods that affect that organ system. The practitioner attempts to change the energy pattern not just by working at the proximate points of client complaint and distress, but also by working along the entire meridian (or set of meridians). Dietary suggestions may be offered. If the concept that "everything is energy" can be accepted, it may be possible to accept not only that the specific energies of foods can have an effect on organ systems and ultimately on health, but that this effect can produce effects formerly believed to be unrelated to the internal metabolic state as well as the related surface pain or discomfort.

Shiatsu training touches on the principles of Asian medicine because the nature of the organ systems and their related energy should be understood for effective treatment to occur, although, as mentioned previously, this knowledge is not an absolute requirement to practice shiatsu. How far this education goes, particularly in relation to the underlying effects of specific foods and their yin and yang effects on various organs and the body as a whole, depends on the quality of the school, the knowledge of the instructor, and the interest of the students.

The Japanese Ministry of Health and Welfare demonstrated its support of shiatsu's efficacy when it stated, "Shiatsu therapy is a form of manipulation administered by the thumbs, fingers, and palms, without the use of any instrument, mechanical or otherwise, to apply pressure to the human skin, correct internal malfunctioning, promote and maintain health, and treat specific diseases" (Masunaga and Ohashi, 1977).

DIAGNOSIS

The art of Asian diagnosis is a lifelong learning process in the practice of shiatsu. Subtle yet specific, Asian diagnosis is an ongoing and evolving pursuit that a practitioner is continually mastering and learning again from scratch. Modern diagnostic techniques are a relatively recent development in the history of medicine. Powerful, precise, and accurate to a large extent, these techniques' contribution to the improvement of the human condition cannot be denied. However, diagnostic procedures in Western medicine use a disease-oriented model and tend to focus on parts (e.g., cells, tissues, organs) rather than on the whole organism. For example, Louis Pasteur (1822-1895) believed that microbes were the primary cause of disease. Although this theory has proved correct and is applicable to a large number of cases, germs are not the sole cause of disease. Although Asian diagnosis has been practiced for thousands of years, Western medicine has largely ignored its value. However, this is changing with the increased integration of Eastern and Western diagnostic methods.

In Asian medicine and shiatsu, there are two underlying levels of diagnosing humans: constitutional and conditional. Simply stated, an individual's *constitution* is what he or she was born with. Along with inherited traits, the quality of life, energy, and

food intake experienced by the mother while a person is in utero are all considered factors that make up a person's constitution. A person's *condition* is the sum of his or her experience, which includes diet. In classic shiatsu diagnosis, both constitution and condition are assessed according to the methods listed next.

The following four methods of observing "phenomena" are used in Asian medicine (Masunaga and Ohashi, 1977):

1. *Bo-shin:* diagnosis through observation
2. *Bun-shin:* diagnosis through sound
3. *Mon-shin:* diagnosis through questioning
4. *Set su-shin:* diagnosis through touch

Each day, whether we realize it or not, we use the first three methods of observation extensively in our interactions with others and the environment. We all have experienced a funny feeling in our stomachs when we enter a room that has recently been the site of some tension related to human interaction. We choose partners based on many factors, including some innate sense of *energy* recognition we find compatible with our own. Although we are unaware that we use aspects of Asian diagnosis in our everyday lives, we nonetheless make assessments and judgments based on these principles. Without these "diagnostic skills," we would not survive. Shiatsu uses the first three methods liberally, while also relying heavily on the fourth.

In a traditional shiatsu session, diagnosis begins with the first contact between client and practitioner, whether in person or on the telephone. The client's tone of voice, speed of delivery, and choice of words give clues to the trained ear regarding the condition and constitution of the shiatsu client.

On meeting a client for the first time, constitutional and conditional assessments are made. How did the client enter the room? Did she walk upright? Did he smile or frown? Was her handshake strong or weak? Was his hand wet, damp, dry, hot, or cold? The client is often unaware that a classically trained shiatsu therapist begins work with the first contact and continues the assessment as a face-to-face meeting begins. Visual diagnosis and verbal questioning continue as the first meeting between client and therapist proceeds.

To arrive at a constitutional diagnosis, the therapist looks at various physical attributes. No single factor observed gives a total picture, but a *macro* assessment takes the various *micro* elements into account. Size of ears, shape and size of head, distance between the eyes, size of mouth, and size of hands are fundamental observations made in constitutional diagnosis before any physical treatment begins.

Factors considered in conditional assessment are slightly different but work in tandem with the overall assessment. The stated reason for the visit is a factor. In addition, tone and volume of the client's voice, pupil size, eye color, color and condition of the tongue, condition of the nails, and response to palpation along specific points on the hands and arms may be used. Pulse diagnosis, the act of reading distinctly differently levels of heartbeats near the wrists on both hands, may be used, depending on the practitioner's level of training. Generally, pulse diagnosis is more the tool of an acupuncturist, but it has been and can be used by a properly trained shiatsu provider.

The four diagnostic methods (observation, sound, questioning, and touch) are used to develop a singular yin-yang analysis (Ballegaards et al., 1996). At its basic level, Asian diagnosis sets out to determine whether a person is *vibrationally,* or *energetically,* more yin or more yang because these two opposing but complementary states of energy affect each of us.

The diagnostic assessment process continues along specific lines, as follows:

Yang diagnosis: Excess body heat and desire for coolness; great thirst and desire for fluids; constipation and hard stools; scanty, hot, dark urine.

Yin diagnosis: Cold feeling and desire for warmth; lack of thirst and preference for hot drinks; loose stools; profuse, clear urine; flat taste in mouth; poor appetite (Yamamoto and McCarty, 1993).

The key is not in being able to see the yin and yang extremes described in the excerpt. The key is in determining not only what tendency within an individual may be contributing to his or her state, but also the particular organ or organs that have a jitsu or kyo condition, and then working those organs' meridians to change that state. This is the point at which the movement from external or initial diagnosis of constitution and condition ends and treatment begins.

At this point, the practitioner's hands become the primary diagnostic tools. Although diagnosis is an ongoing process during treatment, traditional shiatsu first assesses by palpation of the major organs located in the client's *hara,* or abdomen. Alternatively, some styles of shiatsu begin a treatment session with touch diagnosis on the upper back, an area that also yields a vast amount of information regarding a person's condition. Assessment and diagnosis include observations through palpation that describe the following physical properties: tightness or looseness, fullness or emptiness, hot or cold, dry or wet, resistant or open, and stiff or flexible.

Diagnosis in a shiatsu session does not cease after an initial assessment. Diagnosis is an ongoing process of observation, listening, feeling, and changing focus based on continuously revealed information. The ability to make an accurate diagnosis quickly can be extremely helpful to a practitioner and client in their mutual attempt to create energetic change for the receiving partner. However, shiatsu can be effective in the hands of a relatively unskilled diagnostician. By following the simple concept of paying attention to what is going on underneath one's hands, a layperson, with relatively little training, can provide an effective, relaxing, and enjoyable shiatsu treatment for family and friends in a nonprofessional setting.

PRACTICES, TECHNIQUES, AND TREATMENT

Unlike some disciplines, shiatsu is easy to learn. It is not possible for a layperson to practice chiropractic, acupuncture, or osteopathy, because medical professionals need not only training but also time and continuing education to master techniques and improve skills. Shiatsu also requires a disciplined approach, constant practice, and continuing study to develop in-depth understanding. However, the *basic* practice remains simple, effective, and safe. Shiatsu techniques can be learned and safely applied by anyone, typically resulting in positive effects for both the recipient and the provider. It can be performed anywhere, takes place fully clothed, and requires no special tools, machines, or oils.

Sergel (1989) states, "While ki may indeed emanate from the giver's fingertips it may not be in this way or only in this way that shiatsu works. Masunaga's approach is to emphasize another side, that the healing ki of *shiatsu lies within the quality or spirit of the touch in itself,* as compared with the idea of some invisible current that emanates from the touch." More than 150 years ago Shinsai Ota, in a book on Ampuku (hara, or abdominal) shiatsu, emphasized that "honest, sincere, and simple Shiatsu is much better than merely technique-oriented professional Shiatsu" (Masunaga and Ohashi, 1977). Indeed, shiatsu training often emphasizes that the most important element is to be in touch with what is going on *under one's hands*. Experts agree, indicating that when a practitioner applies pressure and stimulation, he or she should then react and follow up based on an intuitive sense of and reaction to internal changes within the recipient (Yamamoto and McCarty, 1993). A traditionally trained shiatsu practitioner, knowledgeable in the food-energy fundamentals of yin and yang and applying those principles in his or her life, is arguably better suited to respond intuitively to the client. It is believed that *intuition* is enhanced by being in harmony with nature, a condition achieved by following the guidelines of living within nature's principles—earth's rhythms of yin and yang. Harmony in the body is achieved by being in harmony with the universe. Eating large amounts of animal protein and simple carbohydrates, which in their cultivation and processing exploit and pollute the earth, does not yield a calm and focused mind that can easily tap into human intuition. If a person is not in harmony with the natural order, the theory states, he or she is less likely to be able to tap into his or her intuition and tune in to another person's needs and internal energies (Sergel, 1989). Experienced shiatsu practitioners would typically agree.

Although a successful shiatsu session may be based more on intuition than technical understanding, it still is necessary to outline the techniques and preparation needed for a successful shiatsu treatment. Shiatsu recipients are fully clothed. Although shiatsu techniques can be adapted to other massage styles and may be performed on bare skin, traditional shiatsu is applied to a fully clothed person. Clients should be dressed in loose-fitting cotton fiber clothing. Blends containing polyester or other synthetics are thought to block or interrupt the natural transmission of energy between the caregiver and the recipient. Static electricity builds up around synthetic fibers. Because, from an Asian perspective, *everything is energy,* unnatural fibers, which may produce unnatural energies, should not be worn during a shiatsu session.

Because shiatsu requires no special tools or environment, it can be performed anywhere at any time. However, traditional shiatsu is generally performed on a cotton floor futon or shiatsu mat. Shiatsu techniques may be adapted to a table, but this is considered a deviation from the classic perspective. Although shiatsu can take place at any time of day, because the energetic effects of shiatsu differ dramatically in many ways from other methods, practitioners may encourage new clients to schedule a session early in the day, preferably before noon. Because shiatsu can yield a "calmed sense of revitalization," the combination of being relaxed *and* energized is an experience that should be savored throughout the day. Americans often equate "calm and relaxed" with an *inactive* state. Although shiatsu yields different results for different people, one of the most unique effects experienced by most clients is indeed this "calmed sense of revitalization." When treated by a competent practitioner, a new shiatsu client may report that "I never felt this way before."

One reason for the difference in the energetic effects of shiatsu as opposed to other techniques (often called *regular massage* by the general public) is easy to explain. In many forms of therapeutic massage a technique described as *effleurage* or *stroking* (sweeping the skin with the hands) is used. The many benefits of this type of movement on the skin include stimulation of blood flow and the movement of lymph. Although this technique is beneficial, one of its effects is often a feeling of lethargy as cellular waste is moved through the lymphatic system. Because the effects of shiatsu are realized more on the underlying blockage of energy related to the body's organ systems than on the lymphatic system, a shiatsu session can yield a feeling of increased short-term and long-term energy. This is why chair massage using shiatsu techniques is so appropriate and considered by many superior to other techniques in the corporate setting. Employees do not experience the short-term negative energetic effects (lethargy) of effleurage, but rather the energetic boost, the *calmed sense of revitalization,* often associated with effective shiatsu technique. Masunaga and Ohashi (1977) described this difference in the following way:

> Anma and European massage directly stimulate blood circulation, emphasizing the release of stagnated blood in the skin and muscles and tension and stiffness resulting from circulatory congestion. On the other hand, Shiatsu emphasizes correction and maintenance of bone structure, joints, tendons, muscles, and meridian lines whose malfunctioning distort the body's energy and autonomic nervous system causing disease.

Shiatsu, as with other methods, is best received with an empty stomach. This may not always be possible, and recent food consumption is no reason not to receive shiatsu. However, practitioners and recipients should bear in mind that when the body's energies are focused *inward* toward digestion, a shiatsu session, with its attempt to change the body's energies, is somewhat compromised and therefore will be less effective.

In some ways the beginning of a shiatsu session is similar to other massage styles. The room used should be simple, clean, and quiet. A thorough history of the client and his or her concerns should be taken. Questions may relate to sleep patterns, lifestyle, eating habits, and work history. A high level of trust should be established quickly. Often a client is seated in a chair or on a floor mat as the shiatsu practitioner observes and asks questions regarding the client's expectations and level of understanding. Diagnostic techniques to determine the client's constitution and condition are undertaken. The hands, eyes, tongue, and coloration along the upper and lower limbs may be examined. Several deep breaths to begin the process may be suggested. A well-trained shiatsu practitioner obtains a complete history to uncover any risk factors affecting the appropriateness of shiatsu treatment. Clinical experience and training, coupled with good references regarding a therapist's skills and practice, should be the determining factors in selecting a shiatsu practitioner.

A shiatsu session usually begins in one of two ways. In classic shiatsu, the practitioner may use hara, or abdominal massage, to determine which organ or organ system meridians may require treatment. Because this type of probing may not be appropriate or well received by many new shiatsu clients, some practitioners start with the client seated in a chair or on a floor mat and make an initial assessment of the client's energies from the upper back and shoulder region. This gives the practitioner immediate feedback on the client's condition and also helps the client relax. Most people are aware of tension in their upper back, shoulder, and neck and respond rather quickly to the process of relaxation so necessary for successful shiatsu.

These early assessments of client condition, coupled with a practitioner's best understanding and synthesis of the client's overall constitution, dictate the direction in which the therapist moves. Classic shiatsu texts state that "kyo and jitsu must first be found in the meridian lines by touching or kneading" to allow the direction of the shiatsu to be most effective (Masunaga and Ohashi, 1977). However, even when kyo or jitsu is not accurately determined at the outset, effective treatment may still be provided; these conditions can be addressed during the session without any specific perception or awareness of these qualities.

Whether treatment begins in a chair or on a floor mat, most of the session takes place with the client lying down. Applying various techniques along the meridian network, the practitioner attempts to create a better energy balance for the shiatsu recipient. Techniques used include rocking, tapotement (pounding), rubbing, and stretching. A shiatsu practitioner employs his or her entire body to apply pressure. Feet, elbows, knees, fingers, and palms are used as appropriate. A client may be face-down or face-up or may lie on the side, as directed or moved by the practitioner.

Although certain techniques such as rubbing and kneading may be used at this point and throughout a shiatsu session, the application of more stationary pressure by the palms, thumbs, forearms, and elbows usually begins early in a session. The muscles at the base of the occiput may be kneaded with the fingers and thumbs. Often the head is rotated with one hand while maintaining a stationary base of support at the neck with the other hand. Although shiatsu providers generally use similar methods, every practitioner is different.

When the techniques applied to the upper back, shoulders, and neck are completed, the client generally reclines to the floor mat in a position the therapist deems most beneficial. This may be the prone, supine, or side position. Certain individuals may use the side position exclusively because of size, pregnancy, or specific issues.

If the client is placed in a prone position, the therapist may use his or her feet to rock the client's hips or to apply graduated pressure to the legs and feet. This "barefoot shiatsu" technique is used extensively by Shizuko Yamamoto and is a very powerful adjunct to the use of the hands, knees, elbows, and forearms. The stretching of the arms and legs and their rotation at the shoulders and hips, respectively, is not uncommon.

Depending on their relative sizes, the practitioner may also walk on the client. Caution is clearly in order when using this rarely practiced technique, but it is sometimes appropriate and beneficial.

Shiatsu sessions typically take place with the provider on his or her knees next to the client. Pressure is applied along distinct meridian lines with the palms and thumbs. Knees, elbows, and forearms may also be used along these specific channels. To access the energy of the various organs through their respective meridians, the client's position changes to side or supine as the session proceeds.

Generally, conversation is minimized or absent during a shiatsu treatment. Music may be played based on the joint needs and desires of giver and receiver. Blood pressure and breathing rates generally decrease during a session. A shiatsu recipient may feel some cold sensations as he or she begins to relax, a natural reaction of the body's autonomic nervous system. Shiatsu can be performed through a cotton blanket, which most practitioners have available. A shiatsu session can be of any length, although a 60-minute duration is common. Sessions often end where they began, at the base of the client's neck or head with gentle kneading or massaging of neck or facial muscles. Shiatsu recipients are generally asked to remain quiet and still for several minutes after a session.

Most people can receive shiatsu. People with sprains and sports injuries who are seeking *direct* treatment of specific areas of trauma are best referred to massage therapists specifically trained to address these issues. However, gentle and focused shiatsu for these types of injuries can be applied to areas not directly related to the affected area to produce positive results by removing pressure and tension that the body may have created by compensating for the injury. Shiatsu can be used during pregnancy if provided by a practitioner trained in the specific meridians and tsubo points that should be *avoided* during a session. Shiatsu is effective during pregnancy as long as common sense and the specific training and experience of the therapist are taken into account. Both supine and side positions are typically used, as appropriate and comfortable during pregnancy.

Because stationary and perhaps deeper application of pressure is a major part of shiatsu technique, caution should be exercised when treating people who bruise easily, have low platelet counts, or have leukemia, lymphoma, or extensive skin or other cancers. Clients who have an acute or chronic cystic condition must clearly communicate their complete history to reduce any potential risk. Although burn victims have benefited from massage therapy, the application of shiatsu at or near a burn site is not appropriate. In theory or in practice, however, shiatsu should not be considered a painful massage therapy; quite the opposite is the norm.

The previous description of a shiatsu session should be considered generic in nature. There are many variations to the basic techniques, and numerous schools that teach specific shiatsu practices offer a more distinct focus to the underlying themes presented. For a more thorough description and expansion on the practice of Shiatsu, readers are directed to *Shiatsu: Theory and Practice* (Beresford-Cooke, 2001).

The American Organization of Body Therapies of Asia (AOBTA) notes 12 specific areas of Asian technique. Six major schools of Asian practice often described by shiatsu practitioners are described in the following sections, as noted on the AOBTA website.

Acupressure

Acupressure is a system of balancing the body's energy by applying pressure to specific acupoints to release tension and increase circulation. The many hands-on methods of stimulating the acupressure points can strengthen weaknesses, relieve common ailments, prevent health disorders, and restore the body's vital life force.

Five-Element Shiatsu

The primary emphasis of five-element shiatsu is to identify a pattern of disharmony through use of the four examinations and to harmonize that pattern with an appropriate treatment plan. Hands-on techniques and preferences for assessment varies with the practitioner, depending on their individual background and training. The radial pulse usually provides the most critical and detailed information. Palpation of the back and/or abdomen and a detailed verbal history serve to confirm the assessment. Considerations of the client's lifestyle and emotional and psychological factors are all considered important. Although this approach uses the paradigm of the five elements to tonify, sedate, or control patterns of disharmony, practitioners of this style also consider hot or cold and internal or external symptoms and signs.

Japanese Shiatsu

Shiatsu literally means finger *(shi)* pressure *(atsu)*, and although shiatsu is primarily pressure, usually applied with the thumbs along the meridian lines, extensive soft tissue manipulation and both active and passive exercise and stretching may be part of the treatments. Extensive use of cutaneovisceral reflexes in the abdomen and on the back is also characteristic of shiatsu. The emphasis of shiatsu is the treatment of the whole meridian; however, effective points are also used. The therapist assesses the condition of the patient's body as treatment progresses. Therapy and diagnosis are one.

Macrobiotic Shiatsu

Founded by Shizuko Yamamoto and based on George Ohsawa's philosophy that each individual is an integral part of nature, macrobiotic shiatsu supports a natural lifestyle and heightened instincts for improving health. Assessments are through visual, verbal, and touch techniques (including pulses) and the five transformations.

Treatment involves noninvasive touch and pressure using hand and barefoot techniques and stretches to facilitate the flow of *qi* and to strengthen the body-mind. Dietary guidance, medicinal plant foods, breathing techniques, and home remedies are emphasized. Corrective exercises, postural rebalancing, palm healing, self-shiatsu, and Qigong are included in macrobiotic shiatsu.

Shiatsu Anma Therapy

Shiatsu Anma therapy uses a unique blending of two of the most popular Asian bodywork forms practiced in Japan. Dr. Kaneko introduces traditional Anma massage therapy based on the energetic system of traditional Chinese medicine in long form and contemporary pressure therapy, which is based on neuromusculoskeletal system, in short form. *Ampuku,* abdominal massage therapy, is another foundation of Anma massage therapy in Kaneko's school.

Zen Shiatsu

Zen shiatsu is characterized by the theory of kyo-jitsu, its physical and psychological manifestations, and its application to abdominal diagnosis. Zen shiatsu theory is based on an extended meridian system that includes as well as expands the location of the traditional acupuncture meridians. The focus of a Zen shiatsu session is on the use of meridian lines rather than on specific points. In addition, Zen shiatsu does not adhere to a fixed sequence or set of methods that are applied to all. It uses appropriate methods for the unique pattern of each individual. Zen shiatsu was developed by Shizuto Masunaga.

The extended meridian network described and taught by Masunaga is a highly regarded part of shiatsu education. It is taught in quality schools as an integral part of shiatsu theory, diagnosis, and style. A practitioner often learns the extended meridian network toward the end of shiatsu education as an *extension* to the classic meridian network, in the same manner that Master Masunaga explored this expansion in shiatsu thinking, theory, and practice (AOBTA).

TRAINING AND CERTIFICATION

There are currently no federal regulatory standards in the United States for shiatsu practitioners or any massage therapists. As of May 2005, *Massage Magazine* stated that 34 states, plus the District of Columbia and four Canadian provinces, have regulations governing massage therapy, with almost 100,000 credentialed practitioners.

Numerous schools of massage offer certificate programs in shiatsu or more broad-based programs that include shiatsu massage. These programs may be weekend seminars of 1 or 2 days or may provide 600 or more hours of training particular to shiatsu. Schools may offer 350 to 500 hours of training in classic shiatsu with an additional 150 hours in anatomy and physiology. There appears to be a growing trend for internships in all schools of massage.

The American Organization for Bodywork Therapies of Asia (formerly the American Asian Body Therapy Association) is the largest and most prevalent organization particular to the practice of shiatsu. Certified Practitioner applicants must complete a 500-hour program, preferably at a school or institution recognized by AOBTA.

The American Massage Therapy Association (AMTA) is a general association of massage practitioners; it does not actively focus on shiatsu therapy. This highly respected association meets regularly with the AOBTA as a federated massage-supporting organization. The AMTA's mission is to develop and advance the art, science, and practice of massage therapy in a caring, professional, and ethical manner to promote the health and welfare of humanity.

The American Bodywork and Massage Professionals (ABMP) is another highly respected association of massage professionals. Unlike the AOBTA and the AMTA, the ABMP is a for-profit organization.

The National Certification Board for Therapeutic Massage and Bodywork (NCBTMB) is a nationally recognized credentialing body formed to set high standards for those who practice therapeutic massage and bodywork. It accomplishes this through a nationally recognized certification program that evaluates the competency of its practitioners. Since 1992, more than 40,000 massage therapists and bodyworkers have received their certification. The NCBTMB examination is now legally recognized in more than 20 states and in many municipalities. The NCBTMB represents a diverse group of massage therapists, not just shiatsu practitioners. A minimum of 500 hours of formal massage education and successful completion of a written examination are the basic requirements for certification. Practitioners must be recertified every 4 years.

A person considering the use of any massage therapy as an adjunct to health maintenance should carefully select the provider of that therapy. In addition to personal references, it is important to evaluate the practitioner's training, experience, professional affiliations, and certification.

RESEARCH

The results of a number of randomized controlled trials (RCTs) on shiatsu therapy have recently been published. The following sections provide a brief listing of these shiatsu studies, grouped by category.

Cancer and Sleep Disturbances

A study was recently completed at the Joan Karnell Cancer Center at Pennsylvania Hospital to evaluate the effectiveness of shiatsu therapy for treating sleep disturbances in cancer patients. Results are forthcoming. Preliminary data suggest that Shiatsu therapy effectively increased both the quality and the hours of sleep in patients with cancer.

Cardiovascular System

A blind RCT in a university-affiliated hospital documented a decrease in systolic, diastolic, and mean arterial pressure, as well as heart rate and skin blood flow, when acupoints were stimulated by pressure. Researchers concluded that acupressure can significantly and positively influence the cardiovascular system (AOBTA).

A single-blind, pretest-posttest, crossover study in which patients were taught how to self-administer acupressure concluded that real acupressure was more effective than sham acupressure for reducing dyspnea and was minimally effective for relieving decathxis (Felhendler and Lisander, 1999).

Sixty-nine patients with severe angina pectoris were treated with acupuncture, shiatsu, and lifestyle adjustments. Invasive treatment was postponed in 61% of patients because of clinical improvement, and the annual number of in-hospital days was reduced 90%, which was calculated to be an annual savings of $12,000 for each patient in the study. The researchers concluded that this combined treatment may be highly effective for patients with advanced angina (Ballegaards et al., 1996).

Maternity

In a Boston Study, postterm women who used shiatsu were more likely to undergo labor spontaneously than those who did not. The shiatsu group had a significantly lower rate of inductions and slightly fewer cesarean births and instrumental deliveries (Yates, 2004).

Nausea with Breast Cancer Chemotherapy

Finger pressure applied bilaterally to two "major" acupressure points during the first 10 days of a chemotherapy cycle reduced the intensity and experience of nausea among women undergoing therapy (Maa et al., 1997).

Nausea and Vomiting

The use of acupressure at the P6 acupoint was shown to reduce the incidence of nausea and vomiting within 24 hours of anesthesia from 42% to 19% compared with placebo (Dibble et al., 2000).

The use of acupressure at the P6 point was shown to reduce the incidence of nausea and vomiting after cesarean birth compared with placebo (Harmon et al., 1999).

Acupressure bands placed at the P6 points on subjects receiving general anesthesia for ambulatory surgery experienced less nausea (23%) versus the control group (41%), suggesting this method as an alternative to conventional antiemetic treatment (Harmon et al., 2000).

The incidence of postoperative vomiting in children was significantly lower (20%) than in the placebo group (68%) when stationary acupressure was applied to the Korean K-K9 point for 30 minutes before and 24 hours after undergoing strabismus surgery (Fan et al., 1997).

The stimulation of the P6 (Neiguan) acupoint was determined to prevent nausea and vomiting in adults, although no antiemetic effects were noted in children undergoing strabismus surgery. However, it was determined that prophylactic use of bilateral acuplaster in children reduced the incidence of vomiting from 35.5% to 14.7% in the early emesis phase, 58.1% to 23.5% in the late emesis phase, and 64.5% to 29.4% overall. Researchers concluded that the use of acuplaster reduced vomiting in children undergoing strabismus correction (Schlager et al., 2000).

References

American Organization for Body Therapies of Asia: *General definition and scope of practice*, www.aobta.org/definitions.htm.

Annussek G: *Shiatsu*, Thomson Organization, 2004, www.ehendrick.org/healthy/0016420htm.

Ballegaards S, Norrlelund A, Smith DF: Cost benefit of combined use of acupuncture, shiatsu and lifestyle adjustments for treatment of patients with severe angina pectoris, *Acupunct Electrother Res* (United States) 21(3-4):187-197, 1996.

Beresford-Cooke C: *Shiatsu: theory and practice*, ed 2, New York, 2001, Churchill Livingstone.

Chen ML, Lin LC, Wu SC, et al: The effectiveness of acupressure in improving the quality of sleep of institutionalized residents, *J Gerontol A Biol Sci Med Sci* 54A(8):M389-M394, 1999.

Colt GW, Hollister A: The magic of touch, *Life Magazine*, August 1997, pp 55-62.

Cowmeadow O: *The art of shiatsu*, Rockport, Mass, 1992, Element Books.

Dibble SL, Chapman J, Mack KA, et al: Acupressure for nausea: results of a pilot study, *Oncol Nurs Forum* 27(1):41-47, 2000.

Fan CF, Tanhui E, Joshi S, et al: Acupressure treatment for prevention of postoperative nausea and vomiting, *Anesth Analg* 84(4):712-714, 821-825, 1997.

Felhendler D, Lisander B: Effects of non invasive stimulation of acupoints on the cardiovascular system, *Complement Ther Med* 7(4):231-234, 1999.

Harmon D, Gardiner J, Harrison R, et al: Acupressure and the prevention of nausea and vomiting after laparoscopy [see comments], *Br J Anaesth* 82(3):387-390, 1999.

Harmon D, Ryan M, Kelly A, et al: Acupressure and prevention of nausea and vomiting during and after spinal anaesthesia for caesarean section, *Br J Anaesth* 84(4): 463-467, 2000.

Lundberg P: *The book of shiatsu*, New York, 1992, Simon & Schuster.

Maa SH, Gautheir D, Turner M: Acupressure as an adjunct to a pulmonary rehabilitation program, *J Cardiopulm Rehabil* 17:268-276, 1997.

Masunaga S, Ohashi W: *Zen shiatsu: how to harmonize yin and yang for better health*, New York, 1977, Japan Publications.

Saito K: *This is the shiatsu from Japan*, 2001, Japan Shiatsu Association of Canada, www.oyayubi.com/ shiatsu/ story.html.

Schlager A, Boehler M, Puhringer F: Korean hand acupressure reduces postoperative vomiting in children after strabismus surgery, *Br J Anaesth* 85(2):267-270, 2000.

Sergel D: *The Macrobiotic way of zen shiatsu*, New York, 1989, Japan Publications.

Yamamoto S, McCarty P: *Whole health shiatsu*, New York, 1993, Japan Publications.

Yates S: Wellmother.org, 2004, www.midwifery.today.com/articles/shiatsu,asp.

Young J: *Healthy living: complementary medicine—other therapies, shiatsu*, 2004, www.bbc.co.uk/health/complementarytherapies_shiatsu.shtml.

Suggested Readings

Kushi M: *Basic shiatsu*, Becket, Mass, 1995, One Peaceful World Press.

Liechti E: *The complete illustrated guide to shiatsu: the Japanese healing art of touch for health and fitness*, Bement, Ill, 1998, Bement Books.

Namikoshi T: *The complete book of shiatsu therapy*, Tokyo, 1994, Japan Publications.

Namikoshi T: *Shiatsu: Japanese finger-pressure therapy,* Tokyo, 1995, Japan Publications.

Ohashi W, Deangelis P: *The Ohashi bodywork book: beyond shiatsu with the Ohashiatsu method,* Tokyo, 1997, Kodansha International.

Sergel D: *The natural way of Zen shiatsu,* Tokyo, 1999, Japan Publications.

Touchpoints (quarterly newsletter). University of Miami Medical School, Touch Research Institute, 2004 (see Resources).

Yamamoto S: *Barefoot shiatsu: whole-body approach to health,* New York, 1998, Putnam.

Yamamoto S, McCarty P: *The shiatsu handbook: a guide to the traditional art of shiatsu acupressure,* New York, 1996, Putnam.

Resources

Associations

American Organization for Bodywork Therapies of Asia (AOBTA)

1010 Haddonfield-Berlin Road, Suite 408
Voorhees, NJ 08043-3514
Phone: 856-782-1616
Fax: 856-782-1653
Website: www.aobta.org
E-mail: office@aobta.org

AOBTA is a national not-for-profit professional association of practitioners of Bodywork Therapies of Asia. All forms that are recognized by AOBTA originally had their roots in China. Over the centuries, China, Japan, Thailand, and Korea, and more recently, North America and Europe, have changed and evolved these forms into separate and distinct modalities. The AOBTA recognizes *12 forms of Asian Bodywork Therapy.* The AOBTA was formed in 1989 with the coming together of a number of associations, which represented individual disciplines of Asian Bodywork Therapy. AOBTA currently has 1400 active members in the United States and abroad.

Associated Bodywork & Massage Professionals (ABMP)

1271 Sugarbush Dr
Evergreen, CO 80439-9766
Phone: 800-458-2267, 303-674-8478
Fax: 800-667-8260
E-mail: expectmore@abmp.com
Website: www.abmp.com

ABMP is a membership organization serving the massage, bodywork, somatic, and esthetic professions. ABMP competes effectively for members by providing the best value and most responsive, knowledgeable service. Their business philosophy is summed up by their credo: expect more.

American Massage Therapy Association (AMTA)

820 Davis St, Suite 100
Evanston, IL 60201-4444
Phone: 847-864-0123
Fax: 847-864-1178
Website: http://www.amtamassage.org

British Columbia Acupressure Therapists' Association

www.acupressurebc.org
E-mail: bcata@acupressurebc.org

Commission on Massage Therapy Accreditation

1007 Church St, Suite 302
Evanston, IL 60201
Phone: 847-869-5039
Fax: 847-869-6739
http://www.comta.org
E-mail: infor@comta.org

Copenhagen

www.shiatsu.dk/

European-Shiatsu-Association (ESI)

German Shiatsu Association
http://www.shiatsu-gsd.de/

International Macrobiotic Shiatsu Society (IMSS)

2807 Wright Ave
Winter Park, FL 32789
Website: www.imss.macrobiotic.net

A forum for friends interested in the Healing Arts of Macrobiotics and Shiatsu. This dynamic combination is based on the teaching of *Shizuko Yamamoto.* Macrobiotics is a natural approach to living that includes a whole-foods diet. The Yamamoto macrobiotic style is also known as Barefoot Shiatsu. IMSS is a membership organization. All are welcome to join us.

Founded in 1986, after almost five decades of experience by shiatsu master Shizuko Yamamoto, the IMSS promotes a natural approach to living. Macrobiotic Shiatsu uniquely combines the power of natural foods in the *macrobiotic diet* with the traditional Asian healing techniques of *shiatsu.* As all things belong to nature, it is natural to be healthy and happy. When imbalances arise, simple techniques can help to correct them. In a practical manner, Macrobiotic Shiatsu unifies body, mind, and spirit.

AOBTA-Approved Schools

Arizona

Arizona School of Acupuncture and Oriental Medicine
David Epley, LAc President
4646 E Ft Lowell Road, Suite 104
Tucson, AZ 85712
Phone: 520-795-0787
Fax: 520-795-1481
E-mail: admissions@asaom.edu

Desert Institute of the Healing Arts
Margaret Avery-Moon, Director
639 N Sixth Ave
Tucson, AZ 85718
Phone: 520-882-0899
Fax: 520-624-2996
E-mail: margaret@diha.org
Website: www.desertinstitute.org

California

Acupressure Institute of America
Michael Reed Gach, or Joseph Carter
1533 Shattuck Ave
Berkeley, CA 94709
Phone: 800-442-2232; 510-845-1059
Fax: 510-845-1496
Website: www.acupressure.com
E-mail: info@acupressure.com & Jcarter@acupressure.com

Heartwood Institute
Chela Burger, Director
220 Harmony Lane
Garberville, CA 95542
Phone: 877-936-9663
Fax: 707-923-5010
Website: www.heartwoodinstitute.com

International Professional School of Bodywork (IPSB)
Eugenie Newton, Dean of Faculty
1366 Hornblend St
San Diego, CA 92109
Phone: 858-272-4142
Fax: 858-272-4772
E-mail: info@ipsb.edu

Mueller College of Holistic Studies
Penny Youngberg, Dir. of Administration
4607 Park Blvd
San Diego, CA 92116
Phone: 619-291-9811; 800-245-1976
Fax: 619-543-1113
Websites: www.MuellerCollege.com
info@MuellerCollege.com

Pacific College of Asian Medicine
Jack Miller, President
7445 Mission Valley Road, Suite 105
San Diego, CA 92108
Phone: 800-729-0941
Fax: 619-574-6641
E-mail: admissions-sd@PacificCollege.edu

The Jin Shin Do® Foundation
Iona Marsaa Teeguarden, Director
PO Box 416

Idyllwild, CA 92549
Phone: 951-659-5707
E-mail: teegers@earthlink.net
Website: www.jinshindo.org

Maryland

Baltimore School of Massage
6401 Dogwood Road
Baltimore, MD 21207
Phone: 410-944-8855
Fax: 410-944-8859
E-mail: dee@bsom.com

Massachusetts

Acupressure Therapy Institute
Barbara Blanchard, Director
1 Billings Road
Quincy, MA 02170
Phone: 617-497-1477
Fax: 617-253-2156
E-mail: bblanch@mit.edu

Chjarles River School of Shiatsu
Patricia Carusone, Director
585 Massachusetts Ave, 4th Floor
Cambridge, MA 01239
Phone: 617-868-4585
E-mail: info@charlesrivershiatsu.com

Minnesota

Center Point Massage & Shiatsu Therapy School & Clinic
Cari Johnson Pelava and Jackson Petersburg, Directors
1313 5th St SE #336
Minneapolis, MN 55414
Phone: 612-617-9090
Fax: 612-617-9292

New Jersey

Rizzieri School of Healing Arts
Laureen Pladdys, Assistant Director
3001 C West Lincoln Dr
Marlton, NJ 08053
Phone: 856-810-7548
Fax: 856-983-1680
E-mail: RizzMassageEdu@aol.com

New York

Swedish Institute, Inc
School of Massage Therapy & Allied Health Science
Paula J. Eckardt, Director

226 W.26th St
New York, NY 10001
Phone: 212-924-5900
Fax: 212-924-7600

New York College of Health Professions
Lisa Pamintuan, J.D., President
6801 Jericho Turnpike
Syosset, NY 11791
Phone: 800-9-CAREER
Fax: 516-364-6645
E-mail: info@nycollege.edu

Pennsylvania

International School of Shiatsu
Saul Goodman, Director
10 South Clinton St, Suite 300
Doylestown, PA 18901
Phone: 215-340-9918
Fax: 215-340-9181
E-mail: info@shiatsubo.com

Texas

Academy of Oriental Medicine
Jim Coombs, President
Pamela Ferguson, Dean of Asian Bodywork
2700 W Anderson Lane, Suite 204
Austin, TX 78757
Phone: 512-454-1188
Fax: 512-454-7001
E-mail: info@aoma.edu

COSP Candidate Schools

American Institute of Alternative Medicine
Dehui Wang, Dean
6685 Doubletree Ave
Columbus, OH 43229
Phone: 614-825-6278
Fax: 614-825-6279
E-mail: info@aiam.edu

Additional Educational Institutions and Links

Acupuncture/Acupressure Internet Resources
http://www.holisticmed.com/www/acupuncture.html

Living Earth School of Natural Therapies
401 Richmond St West, Studio 1
Toronto, Ontario M5V 3A8 Canada

www.livingearthschool.com
Phone: 416-591-0400
Fax: 905-303-8724
E-mail: shiatsuinfo@livingearthschool.com

The Ohashi Institute (Ohashiatsu®)
147 West 25th St, 8th Floor
New York, NY 10001
Phone: 800-810-4190; 646-486-1187
Fax: 646-486-1409
Website: http://www.ohashi.com/
E-mail: ohashiinst@aol.com
The Institute is a nationally respected and internationally recognized nonprofit educational organization dedicated to the promotion and understanding of the Asian healing arts. Their stated mission is to serve the planet by bringing excellence to the art of healing and serenity to the art of living. Their motto, "Touch for peace."

Natural Healers.com
Detailed information on finding a school; excellent link.
http://www.naturalhealers.com/find.shtml

The Watsu Institute School of Shiatsu and Massage
PO Box 889
Middletown, CA 95461
Phone: 707-987-3801
Fax: 707-987-9638
Website: www.schoolofshiatsuandmassage.com

The British School of Shiatsu Do
3 Farnham Park Dr
Upper Hale, Farnham, Surrey
GU9 0HS, England, UK
Phone: +44 (0) 1252 724059
E-mail: registrar@farnham.shiatsu-do.co.uk
Website: www.shiatsu-do.co.uk
David M Winter, Principal (Farnham)
Tel/fax: 01252-724059

Worldwide Aquatic Bodywork Association (Watsu)
Website: www.waba.edu

Jin Shin Do Foundation for Bodymind Acupressure
PO Box 416
Idyllwild, CA 92549
Fax: (909) 659-5707
Website: www.jinshindo.org

Touch Research Institutes (TRI), University of Miami School of Medicine
PO Box 016820
Miami, FL 33101
Phone: 305-243-6781
Fax: 305-243-6488
E-mail: tfield@med.miami.edu

http://www.miami.edu/touch-research/

Considered the pioneer of, and premium research institute for massage therapy, the first Touch Research Institute was formally established in 1992 by Director Tiffany Field, PhD, at the University of Miami School of Medicine via a startup grant from Johnson & Johnson. The TRI was the first center in the world devoted solely to the study of touch and its application in science and medicine. The TRI's distinguished team of researchers, representing Duke, Harvard, Maryland, and other universities, have successfully improved the definition of define touch as it promotes health and contributes to the treatment of disease. Research efforts that began in 1982 and continue today have shown that touch therapy has numerous beneficial effects on health and well-being. A second TRI is located in the Philippines. A group of neonatologists there have replicated earlier studies showing that preterm infants' weight gain can be facilitated by massage therapy. A third TRI is located at the University of Paris and studies the role of touch in perception, learning, and psychopathology. A fourth TRI is located at the UCLA Medical School Pediatric Pain Center and is focused on the use of touch therapies with children's pain syndromes.

National Certification Board for Therapeutic Massage and Bodywork (NCBTMB)

8201 Greensboro Dr, Suite 300
McLean, VA 22102
Phone: 800-296-0664; 703-610-9015
Fax: 703-610-9005
E-mail: info@ncbtmb.com
Website: www.ncbtmb.com

Massage Magazine

1636 W First Ave #100
Spokane, WA 99204
Phone: 800-533-4263, 509-324-8117 (Outside US)
Website: www.massagemag.com

Covers the massage trade, with articles on technique, research and laws, profiles, and industry news. In publication since 1985, circulated internationally, bimonthly.

The Shiatsu Society (UK)—United Kingdom

Eastlands Court, St Peters Road

Rugby CV21 3QP
Phone: 0845 130 4560
Fax: 01788 555052
E-mail: admin@shiatsu.org
Website: www.shiatsu.org

The Shiatsu Society is a nonprofit umbrella organization for all types and styles of shiatsu. The Society sets standards in training which are implemented by Registered Teachers through its Assessment sub-Committee. The Society maintains a Register of Qualified Practitioners who have passed the Society's Assessment. The Society was set up in 1981 to facilitate communication within the field of shiatsu and to inform the public of the benefits of this form of natural healing. Since then the Society has grown to form a network linking interested individuals, students, and teachers and to fulfill the role of Professional Association for Shiatsu Practitioners.

Shiatsu Therapy Association of Ontario (STAO)

STAO is a nonprofit organization that represents professionally trained Certified Shiatsu Therapists (CST) in Ontario, across Canada, and internationally. The association is a self-regulatory body mandated to protect the interests of the public by setting the highest standards of training and practice in North America.

Phone: 416-923-7826 (STAO, Toronto); toll-free (Canada & US): 877-923-7826
E-mail: info@shiatsuassociation.com

Other Links

http://www.psychotherapiepraxis.at/shiatsuI.htm. Great site for numerous links to shiatsu and related information.

http://articleindex.com/cgi-bin/odp/main.cgi?search=Shiatsu. Article link index for Shiatsu On-Site.

http://www.shiatsu.8m.com/workshops.htm. Shiatsu information pages, numerous links.

http://www.rianvisser.nl/shiatsu/e_index.htm. Shiatsu links: Netherlands.

http://www.kushiinstitute.com. Kushi Institute: macrobiotic educational link.

http://www.google.com. Always a great search engine; enter "Shiatsu," or "Shiatsu Research," etc.

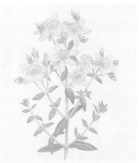

24

TIBETAN MEDICINE

KEVIN V. ERGIL

HISTORICAL AND CULTURAL PERSPECTIVE

Practitioners of the Tibetan system of medicine, the *Science of Healing* (gso.ba.rig.pa), can trace a lineage of practice and precept back through the centuries. As with many aspects of Tibetan cultural practices, the Tibetan medical system displays the thoughtful mixture of aspects of Indic traditions and those of other cultures with indigenous practices. Tibetan medicine is deeply rooted in the worldview of Buddhism and is organized primarily around concepts of the body, which it shares with Ayurveda (India's *Science of Life*). Tibetan medicine is a rich and literate tradition (since the eighth century AD), with diverse practice lineages, specialized knowledge, and regional variation.

Tibetan medicine manifests a remarkable syncretism and adaptability, and its spiritual history, with its links to the origins of Buddhism, reminds its practitioners of the fundamental meaning of the practice of medicine: *compassion*.

From a historical perspective, the circumstances that shaped Tibetan medicine are to a great extent a circumstance of geopolitical factors. Our understanding of the development of Tibetan medicine should begin with a sense of the unique geography of the Tibetan plateau.

Tibet is isolated both by mountain ranges that surround it on three sides and by its own elevation (Figure 24-1). The capital of Tibet, Lhasa, lies at 11,975 feet. The southern border of Tibet is formed by the Himalayan Mountains. Bhutan, Nepal, and

456

Copyright © 2006 Kevin Ergil.

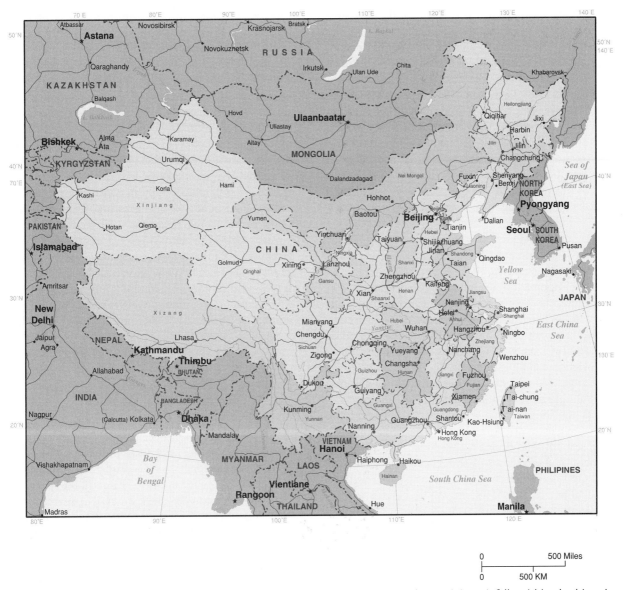

Figure 24-1 The Tibet Autonomous Region, China, literally The Western Storehouse (Xizang) falls within the historic boundaries of Tibet. www.mapresources.com

India are to the south of Tibet. The Tibetan plateau rises as one moves north from the Himalayas. The Kun Lun and the Dang La mountains form a northern border, and beyond them lie Mongolia and China. To the west, as one moves toward Pakistan and Afghanistan, are the Karakoram and Ladakh mountains. The eastern border is formed by the Mekong and Salween as these rivers flow from the north and ultimately form deep gorges to the southeast. Tibet

proper is surrounded on all sides by challenging landscapes that have provided natural barriers.

Geographically, the region known as Tibet lies to the south of what became known as the "silk road." By the second century BC, this route allowed materials of value to be traded along its length. Precious medicinals, such as rhubarb, found their way West to Greece and Rome. This trading route, which provided markets for silk, spice, medicines, produce, gold, and gemstones, also furnished a conduit for the exchange of knowledge and ideas between East and West. The volume of trade along its length fluctuated depending on the security afforded its travelers by local rulers. By the thirteenth century the silk road was not as important to East-West trade as safer and more profitable sea routes had become established. During China's Tang Dynasty (618-907 AD), however, the route was an important link between the West and the cosmopolitan East. Ch'ang-an (just northwest of modern Xian) was a walled city and the western terminus of the silk road for the Chinese. By the eighth century it was a huge city of almost 2 million. A census completed in 754 AD described the presence of some 5000 foreigners in the city, including Turks, Iranians, and Indians who had traveled East to come to this trading center.

It is important to recognize that in the absence of any more rapid form of communication, these trading centers and the individuals who moved between them were the sole conduits for the transmission of information as well as goods. Travelers seeking knowledge, religious pilgrims, and physicians would exchange information and further enhance the cosmopolitan character of this region.

To the south of this cultural nexus, in geographic Tibet, lived dispersed bands of nomadic pastoralists and settled communities under the rule of minor princes or feudal lords. Although little is known of Tibetan history before the sixth century AD, tradition holds that a lineage of 31 kings preceded this period.

In the early seventh century, Namri Songtsen (gnam.ri.srong.btsan) (circa 570-619) the thirty-second king of Tibet, secured the loyalty of warriors in his region and began the process of forming disparate clans of skilled riders into a mobile force who could swiftly project devastating military force into surrounding territories. Under the reign of his son, the thirty-third king, Songtsen Gampo (srong.btsan.gam.po) (ca 609-649), the Tibetan empire began its expansion (Figure 24-2). Building on the military successes of his father, Gampo's forces threatened Xian and compelled the Tang emperor Tai Zong to grant him a Chinese princess in marriage. The gesture, a way used to secure détente by creating family relationships, gained Songtsen Gampo one of his two most famous treaty wives. Gampo's incursions to the south resulted in his marriage to a Nepalese princess as well. These two wives are credited with bringing some of the first Buddhist texts to enter Tibet and guiding the

king toward establishing Buddhism as a state religion (a process that would take more than a century).

The reign of Songtsen Gampo is an extremely significant period in Tibetan history that displays an imperial thirst for knowledge, as well as territory and wealth. At this time the written language of Tibet was developed from Gupta script by the scholar Thonmi Sambhota. The creation of a written alphabet designed for the Tibetan language (and to facilitate the transliteration of Sanskrit) was important. It supported the development of Tibetan record keeping and scholarship, facilitated the transliteration and translation of Sanskrit texts, and made manifest a distinct cultural separation between Tibet and China. Although the ongoing interest of the Tibetans in Chinese texts, and the work of various scholars suggest that it was very likely that Tibetan nobles were literate in Chinese (Gunther 1974), the establishment of a distinctive written language, one which displayed a linguistic commitment to India,

A Note on Transliteration and Translation

This chapter presents the names of Tibetan personages, places, and texts primarily in their conventional English orthography and supplies in parentheses the transliteration of the actual Tibetan according to the Wylie system, for example, "Drukchen" and ('brug.chen). The author is responsible for the translations provided in this text unless otherwise attributed (Ergil, 1983, 1987). In the case of the translated excerpts from Padma Karpo (pad.ma.dkar.po), the fourth Drukchen Rinpoche (1527-1592), the author has enhanced the readability of his translation by providing clarifying expressions and amendations to the typically brief Tibetan material. In addition, some elements (where the original deviated substantially) have been brought into concordance better known (in English) versions of the three roots. Choices concerning the translation, presented here, of specific therapies and medicinals have been made, in some cases, with dependence on the work of Jeffrey Hopkins and Allan Wallace.

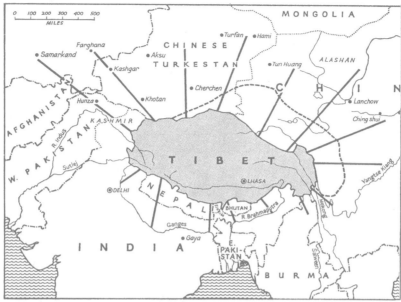

TIBET AND ITS NEIGHBOURS: POLITICAL AND ETHNOGRAPHIC

Shaded area: Political Tibet
Broken line: Limits of Ethnographic Tibet
Radiating lines: Extent of Tibetan influence in 6th to l0th centuries

Figure 24-2 Limits of Tibetan territorial expansion: sixth through tenth centuries.
(From Richardson HE: *A short history of Tibet,* New York, 1962, Dutton.)

was an important sign of the cultural orientation intended for Tibet by its ruler. From this time on, medical scholars in Tibet had a language in which to record their own knowledge, and that obtained from other lands.

King Songtsen Gampo's Chinese wife brought with her a medical text, *Great Analytical Treatise on Medicine* (Kunzang, 1973, p. 15). In addition, Songtsen Gampo sent messengers out across the region (and along the silk route) to summon expert physicians to what is now known as the first conference of learned physicians. Three doctors came to Tibet from India, China, and Persia. Each of the invited physicians brought texts that were then translated into Tibetan. Galenos, a Persian, is said to have remained as a court physician and stayed on to father three sons, who carried his medical lineage to different parts of Tibet.

By this time, following the fall of Rome in the fifth century and the isolation of learned Greek culture in Byzantium, the Persian and Arabian physicians were continuing to practice and expand on the Greco-Roman medical traditions established by figures such as Galen and Dioscorides. During this period, while medieval Europe was increasingly isolated from ancient

centers of learning and restricted in its inquiries by the political turmoil following the fall of Rome and the pre-occupations of the Church, Persians and Arabs were free to explore the wealth of Greco-Roman medical knowledge preserved within Byzantium and to incorporate it into their own cultures. In all likelihood, Galenos, the Persian physician who had adopted the name of Galen for himself, would have been an exponent of what is known throughout the Near East as "Unnani Tibb," or Greek medicine.

As its ruler reached out to the known world for medical knowledge, the cosmopolitan character of the Tibetan medical tradition began to be established. With Xian to the north, India to the south, and the knowledge of the Galenic traditions moving toward Asia from the west, rich information resources were available to the developing empire.

In the eighth century, as Tibet continued to exercise its influence throughout the region, its thirty-seventh king came to the throne. Trisong Detsen (tri.srong.lde.btsan) (ca 741-798 AD) reigned from 754 through 797 and was successful in establishing Buddhism as a state religion.

Two highly significant events occurred during his reign in relation to the development of the medical tradition. The second conference of learned physicians was convened, and the "Four Tantras" were translated and brought to Tibet.

Trisong Detsen sent messengers out with gifts of gold to bring physicians from different parts of the known world. Doctors came from India, Kashmir, China, Persian, Guge (a nearby kingdom), and Nepal. They were invited to translate texts from their own traditions and languages and rewarded with gifts to help them establish themselves in Tibet. The Chinese physician remained in Trisong Detsen's court.

The conferences of learned physicians were opportunities to share knowledge and demonstrate medical acumen. According to one famous version of the events, a patient was placed behind a drawn curtain, and a thin string was wrapped around her wrist and then pulled out through an opening in the curtain. When the string was pulled tight, the vibration of her pulse could be felt through it. Each of the visiting physicians was asked to pull the string taut and to make a diagnosis based on the vibration of the pulse alone, without examining the patient. The winner of this contest was rewarded with land and gold.

Even as the practical skills of diverse physicians were being shared in Tibet, the text that would become the basis for the organized study and practice of Tibetan medicine arrived in Tibet. This text, known today as the "Four Tantras," or *Gyu She* (rgyud. bzhi.), may have been composed in India in about 400 AD. It was both a medical text and a developed expression of the scripture of Northern Buddhism (*Mahayana,* or the Great Vehicle) in relation to medicine.

The understanding within Tibetan medicine concerning the origins of medical knowledge in general and of the knowledge contained within the Four Tantras in particular is intriguing. It is an understanding that simultaneously asserts the primacy of Buddhist medical knowledge and implicitly asserts that all healing traditions share the ultimate goal of providing compassionate care to suffering beings. Because of the importance of Buddhism to the development of Tibetan medicine and the Four Tantras, it is helpful to have a general understanding of the relationship of the teaching contained in the Four Tantras to the life of the Buddha in the sixth century BC.

Buddhism and the Four Tantras

The historical Buddha, Gautama Buddha, or Sakyamuni Buddha, was a privileged prince of the Sakya clan growing up near what is now Lumbini, Nepal. It is said that as a young man he was struck by the understanding that disease, old age, and death are the common fate of all beings and that he committed himself to find a method of releasing himself from the suffering that is the consequence of living. Winning through to enlightenment, a state that is free from the experience of birth and death and the suffering attendant on them, the Buddha then taught to help others free themselves.

His teachings persist to this day in the texts and practices of various traditions, originally delivered orally and only recorded in writing in about 100 BC. Buddhist traditions that emerged from Buddha's teachings included the teachings of the Great Vehicle, or the *Mahayana,* which are often referred to as "Northern Buddhism," because they were so influential in the development of Buddhism in China, Japan, Mongolia, and Tibet. Northern Buddhism scriptures from the first century BC portray a Buddha whose activities and manifestations transcend those initially attributed to the purely historical figure, Gautama Buddha.

These scriptures state that during his lifetime, Gautama Buddha manifested the form of the *Medicine Buddha* (Sskt. Baishajya Guru; Tibetan, sangs.rgya. sman.blha.) in a celestial palace of medicine, Tanadug (Figure 24-3). The Medicine Buddha appeared in the form traditionally associated with a peaceful Buddha. His skin is the deep blue of lapis lazuli and emanates a radiant blue light. In his right hand he holds a branch of myrobalan *(Terminalia chebula)* in the gesture of granting blessings, and in his left hand, which is held in the posture of meditation, he holds a bowl of life-giving nectar. This vivid diety appears in a palace that is surrounded on all sides by medicinal substances.

To the south of the Medicine Buddha lies the mountain known as the "Thunderbolt." It has the power of the sun and is covered in medicines such as pomegranate, long pepper, and capsicum. These medicines are hot tasting, sour, and salty and have the qualities of heat and acridity and thus are said to treat diseases caused by cold. To the north is the "Snow-clad Mountain," which has the power of the moon, and medicines such as sandalwood and camphor grow on it. These medicines are bitter, sweet, and astringent in taste and have the quality of coolness, thus relieving ailments caused by heat. On the east rises the "Fragrant Mountain," which is covered in a forest of myrobalans, and on the west is "Cool Mountain," on which grow medicines such as bamboo, saffron, clove, nutmeg, and cardamoms. It is said that the meadows surrounding the palace are filled with the fragrance of incense and many animals that provide medicinal substances.

Seated in the center of the palace, the Medicine Buddha was surrounded by Rishis, Buddhists, non-Buddhists, and gods. If you imagine a divine and radiant being seated on a throne in a great palace, surrounded by all the great medicines of Asia and their aromas and attended by gods, Hindu scholars, sages, and Buddhists, you can capture something of the image conveyed by the Medicine Buddha's mandala (Figure 24-4).

According to the tradition, each group of disciples in attendance on the Medicine Buddha received different teaching according to their dispositions and needs. Rabgay's translation of the text "Ba. Jung.Don.Gong.'Thad" states the following:

> For the sake of beings, the Sugata through his manifestation, taught the methods of compounding medication in India, moxa and vein clearing in China; and blood letting in Dolpo (North to Tibet). To the assembly of Gods, he taught the "Verses of Healing" and to the Rishis he taught the "Eight works of Charaka," while to the Non Buddhists he

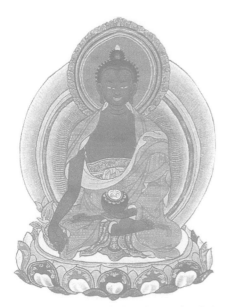

Figure 24-3 Medicine Buddha holding the fruit of the chebulic myrobalan in his right hand and a bowl of life giving nectar in his left. (From Parfionovitch Y, Dorje G, Meyer F, editors: *Tibetan medical paintings: illustrations to the Blue Beryl treatise of Sangye Gamtso,* New York, 1992, Abrams.)

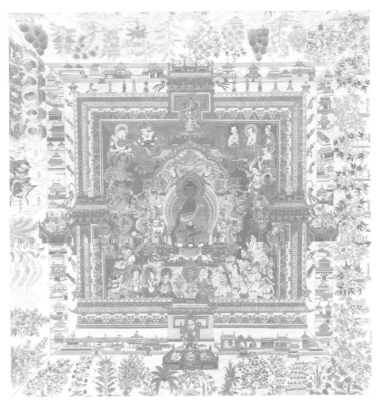

Figure 24-4 Medicine Buddha mandala surrounded by gods and sages as he teaches the four tantras. (From Parfionovitch Y, Dorje G, Meyer F, editors: *Tibetan medical paintings: illustrations to the Blue Beryl treatise of Sangye Gamtso,* New York, 1992, Abrams.)

taught "Krishna Ishvara Tantra." To the Buddhists he taught "The Teachings of the Three Protectors" (Rabgay, 1981 p. 7).

Within the Buddhist tradition it is well understood that an enlightened being teaches according to the requirements and capabilities of the audience. So accordingly, medicine was taught within the traditions that reflected the interests of each group.

While teaching according to the propensities of those assembled, the Medicine Buddha simultaneously emanated two divine beings (further manifestations of the Buddha). From his heart appeared the *Sage Rigpay Yeshe* (rig.pai.ye.shi) and from his tongue the *Sage Yilay Kye* (yid.las.skyed.). The dialogue that ensued as Yilay Kye posed questions and Rigpay Yeshe answered them ultimately became the source of the text, the *Four Tantras,* that would, from at least the twelfth century, exist simultaneously as sacred texts and as a guide to the practice of medicine, delineating the fundamentals of the Tibetan approach to healing.

Among all those in attendance, only the Sage Yilay Kye heard the teaching of the Four Tantras. According to the tradition, these were written down on gold in lapis lazuli ink and preserved in a sacred realm, the Dakini Palace in Uddiyana. Preserved there by dakinis (feminine agents of wisdom and transformation), the texts would be transmitted to the fourth-century author of the Four Tantras as a revealed scripture and, about three centuries later, would be translated into Tibetan.

What should this vivid imagery suggest as we read these words centuries later, embedded in a culture that trains us to be, at best, skeptical of dakini palaces and divine manifestations? There are two important interpretations of the words and images of the text, if we take them metaphorically, rather than taking them literally or dismissing them as esoteric scripture. Consider that within the commentaries on this scripture, the Medicine Buddha is shown to be providing instruction in every form of medicine in Asia. "Moxa and vein clearing" is nothing other than the practice of acupuncture. For centuries, India was the land of medicinal chemistry. The *Caraka Samitha* is one of the most revered texts of Ayurveda. In all these instances the Medicine Buddha is shown as teaching the fundamentals of all the great medical traditions of Asia.

On one level, we might understand this as Mahayana Buddhist one-upmanship ("our tradition trumps your tradition"), and there are elements of this within the history of Northern Buddhsim. For example, one Buddhist tradition asserts the mythological primacy of Buddhism even in relation to the sacred origins of Ayurveda.

Dash states, "According to Indian mythology, Ayurveda was first perceived (not composed) by Brahma and he taught this science to Daksa prajapati, who taught it to the Asvini kumaras, and they taught it to Indra" (1976, p. 28). The tradition extant in Tibet explains that Brahma, in fact, simply remembered the teachings on medicine given to him by Kasyapa Buddha (Kunzang, 1973, p. 9). In this manner the primacy of the Buddhist lineage of medical teachings can be asserted, even though the history of Ayruveda precedes that of Gautama Buddha. Similarly, the Mahayana scripture can be read as establishing the Buddhist roots of every great medical tradition. Given the rivalry and tradition of debate between Buddhist and non-Buddhist schools of thought in India, it is not difficult to see this as a scriptural assertion of primacy.

The other available interpretation (in both these cases) is quite profound. It suggests that from the point of view of a Buddhist or a Buddhist physician, there is no form of medicine that is not ultimately contained within the Buddhist healing tradition, and there is no medicine that is not an expression of the Buddha's compassion.

With this last interpretation in mind, we also have to consider that a distinguishing feature of the tradition of Northern Buddhism was an emphasis on the possibility of participating in the activities of the world while seeking enlightenment. The early Buddhist scriptures that guided monastic conduct forbade monks from the practice of medicine (prescribing of medicines and minor surgery) as an occupation or means of livelihood. These later scriptures suggest that the application of many of the healing methods of Asia represents the application of the teachings of the Buddha.

The description of the origins of the Four Tantras shows medical systems belonging to other traditions and cultures originating from the Buddha's teachings. This establishes the authority and significance of the Buddha as a teacher of medicine. It also expands the range of techniques and traditions that can be included under the heading of "Buddhist medicine." In a similar manner, ascribing the origin of Ayurveda to Kasapya effectively permits all Ayurvedic traditions to be understood as Buddhist medicine.

The Four Tantras in Tibet

A clear conception of an unbroken lineage is critical to Tibetan Buddhists and within the medical tradition as well. The linkage between the historical Buddha and these fourth-century scriptures is provided by the divine manifestation of the Medicine Buddha and establishes these texts as living within the lineage of Northern Buddhism.

The Four Tantras came to Tibet during the reign of Trisong Detsen, the thirty-seventh king (754-797 AD). It is said that they were translated by Vairochana, a disciple of Padmasambhava, one of the important teachers of Buddhism in Tibet. Vairochana visited India and received teachings on the Four Tantras from the pandit Candrabhinanda. On his return from India, Vairochana was instructed by his teacher Padmasambhava to secrete the text and its translation in a pillar at Samye Monastery. The Elder Yuthog Yontan Gonpo (708-833), who was among the court physicians at this time, "not only clarified this work, but also wrote eighteen supplements to it" (Tsarong, 1981, p. 6). The Elder Yuthog is also credited with the founding of Tanadug Medical College in Kongpo Menlung (Tsarong, 1981, p. 95), said to be the first medical school established in Tibet.

The comprehensive revision of the Four Tantras was carried out by the extremely famous descendant of the Elder Yuthog Yontan Gonpo, the Younger Yuthog Yontan Gonpo (1112-1203 AD). He rewrote the work and is thus responsible for the Four Tantras as they currently appear (Finckh, 1979, pp. 2-3; Tsarong, 1981, p. 6). The actual title of the text generally referred to as the "Four Tantras" is *The Ambrosia Heart Tantra: The Secret Oral Teaching on the Eight Branches of the Science of Healing* (bdud.rtsi.snying.po.yan.lag.brgyad.pa.gsang. ba.man.ngag.gi.rgyud.). While there are many texts within the Tibetan medical tradition, the Four Tantras are fundamental in terms of the role they play in medical education and in shaping the practice of medicine. It is also important to recognize that for centuries these texts also guided and informed the medical practices of neighboring Buddhist cultures, such as Mongolia, Ladakh, Sikkim, and Bhutan.

Organization and Content of the Four Tantras

The Four Tantras are the essential texts of the Tibetan medical tradition. They are still the intellectual platform on which a physician's medical training is conducted. Customarily, a student undertakes the study of medicine by memorizing the first tantra, or *Root Tantra* (rtsa.rgyud); the second tantra, or *Explanatory Tantra* (bshad. rgyud); and the fourth tantra, or *Final Tantra* (phyi. rgyud). The third tantra, or *Oral Instruction Tantra* (man.ngag.rgyud), is generally studied later in the curriculum because it presents in great detail the different illnesses, their symptoms, and treatments and often requires commentary. After memorization, a teacher instructs the student on the meaning of the text and elaborates on the material.

This traditional approach to Tibetan medical education was the rule through 1959 and has continued to this day as the practice for formal instruction within the exile community at such schools as the Tibetan Medical Center, in Dharamsala.

The first tantra, or *Root Tantra,* comprises six chapters and is considered to be the essence of the entire Four Tantras. The first two of the six chapters address the way in which the teachings were delivered by the Medicine Buddha and provide a discussion of the divisions of medical knowledge in relation to the entire content of the Four Tantras. The next three chapters address principles of etiology, diagnosis, and treatment in summary. The sixth chapter presents a metaphorical structure: "the three roots," which establishes the three areas of etiology, diagnosis, and treatment as the three roots of a tree. The roots, trunks, branches, and leaves of the tree allow the student to organize all the fundamental aspects of medical knowledge using the image of the tree as a mnemonic device (Figure 24-5). As the text is structured, the third, fourth, and fifth chapters provide the content that forms the leaves of the tree. For a medical tradition that requires students to commit its major texts to memory, this is a valuable tool. It is also an image that can help us understand a great deal about this system. The image and the content of the tree are discussed in detail later and are used to illustrate the essential structure and concepts of Tibetan medicine.

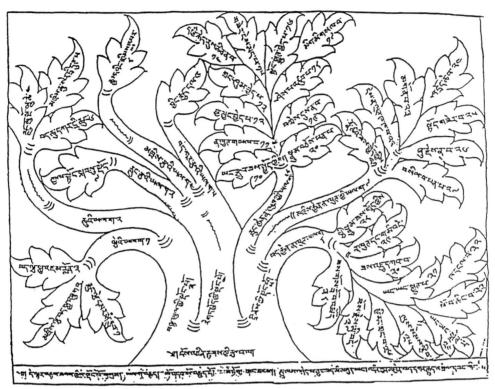

Figure 24-5 The root of diagnosis (dos.la.dzin.rtags.kyi.rtsa.ba.la). Copy of a block print in the possession of Ngo.drup Tsering.

The second tantra, or *Explanatory Tantra,* contains 31 chapters that are said to address the 11 principles of medicine. This tantra expounds the theories and principles of Tibetan medicine in great detail. The third tantra, or *Oral Instruction Tantra,* provides 92 chapters giving detailed guidance to the practice of the 15 divisions of medicine. The fourth and *Final Tantra* provides information on the practice of pulse diagnosis, urine diagnosis, the preparation of medicines, and the use of mild and drastic therapies.

Historically, the Four Tantras have been the object of substantial scholarship in Tibet. Many scholar physicians have written commentaries over the years, including the Fourth Drukchen, Padma Karpo (1527-1592); his version of the three roots is provided in translation throughout this chapter. Collections of vivid scroll paintings *(Thangkas)* were commissioned to illustrate the three roots and many of the chapters of the tantras.

Later Developments

With the gradual growth of Buddhism, Tibetan interest in military affairs waned. After a series of regicides around the ninth century, the line of Songtsen Gampo ended. Tibet became a collection of principalities. Lamas (religious teachers) were often given support by the princes, thus achieving a measure of secular authority. This state of affairs was altered by a series of relationships between the Mongolian khans and various lamas, which began with an attempt to avoid a potential invasion of Tibet by Chingis Khan in 1107 AD. These relationships added a new element to the competition for secular power between lamas and their Tibetan patron princes. Finally, in 1642, the Fifth Dalai Lama, Ngawang Lobzang Gyatso, was established as the religious head of Tibet by Gusri Khan. By virtue of having a saintly and reincarnating ruler with a firm grasp on the country, Tibet emerged as a theocratic state with an operational division between secular and religious authorities. The reign of the Fifth Dalai Lama also saw the creation of a patronage relationship between the emergent Qing (Manchu) Dynasty and religious rulers of Tibet.

The reign of the Fifth Dalai Lama was a period of notable achievements in the history of Tibet. Many of these occurred under the guidance of his regent, Sangye Gyatso (sangs rgyas. rgya.mtsho). It was during this period that the Potala Palace was built outside Lhasa (Figure 24-6).

The Fifth Dalai Lama also established three medical schools during his reign. Sangye Gyatso selected the site for the third school: a mountain named "Iron Mountain," or *Chagpori* (chags.po.ri), a prominent peak outside Lhasa. The regent's decree established that from that time on, each of the large monasteries near Lhasa, as well as those in surrounding districts, would receive a physician of its own from the *Mentsikhang* (sman.rtsi.khang), literally "house of medicine and astrology." These events are viewed the beginning of an organized, state-supported approach to public health in Tibet.

Sangye Gyatso was a devoted scholar and proponent of medicine. In 1688 he wrote the famous commentary to the Four Tantras, the *Blue Beyrl* (bai.du.rya.sngon.po), which remains influential to this day.

During the reign of the Thirteenth Dalai Lama (1895-1933), Kyenrab Norbu (khyen.rab.nor.bu) (1882-1962), a gifted physician and scholar, founded the Lhasa Mentsi Khang in 1928. This new college provided a place for one student from each provincial monastery to study, as well as offering opportunities for private students.

A Culture in Exile

Tibet's geographic and political isolation through the late nineteenth and early twentieth centuries made its traditions an object of curiosity and speculation in the West. Tibetan culture became the purview of military adventures, arcane scholarship, and intrepid explorers. Ultimately, Tibet's isolation would work to its disadvantage.

The events surrounding the establishment of the People's Republic of China in 1949 and the subsequent efforts of the Chinese government to assert an unprecedented political sovereignty over the land and people of Tibet shattered the cultural and political life of Tibet. The occupation of Tibet by the forces of the People's Liberation Army in 1951 culminated in violent military action that led to the flight of His Holiness the Fourteenth Dalai Lama from Tibet to Nepal in 1959 and the establishment of the Tibetan government in exile in northern India. Tibet's historic medical college Chagpori was destroyed by Chinese artillery fire. The medical school established by Sangye Gyatso in the mid-seventeenth century had provided medical training to Tibetans for 300 years, and its presence, high on a promontory overlooking

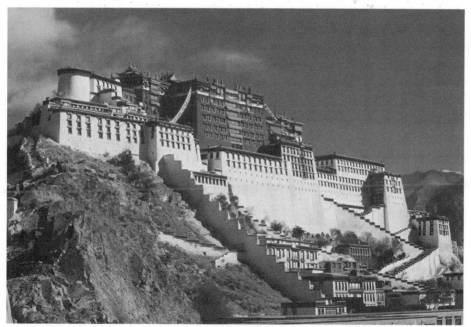

Figure 24-6 Potala Palace, Lhasa, Tibetan Autonomous Regions. (Corbis.)

Lhasa, the capital of Tibet, was testimony to his ongoing impact on the Tibetan medical tradition.

The mass exodus of Tibetans in 1959 created a perilous situation for traditional Tibetan cultural practices. This was further worsened by the excesses of the cultural revolution. During this period (1966-1976), much of the material culture of Tibet was destroyed, and traditional Tibetan culture was actively suppressed by the Chinese government. Since 1959, Tibetans in exile have made substantial efforts to protect and nurture the cultural and spiritual traditions developed in their society for more than a millennium. These efforts are ongoing.

However, Tibetan medicine is a tradition in exile and in flux. Although every effort is made by Tibetans, both outside and inside Tibet, to retain the knowledge and practices of the tradition, the profoundly devastating consequences of the "liberation" of Tibet on this tradition cannot be undone.

Outside of what is now known as the Tibetan Autonomous Region (TAR) of the People's Republic of China (PRC), most efforts to preserve the tradition are coordinated by the Tibetan Government in Exile and particularly by the *Mentsi Khang* (the Tibetan Medical and Astrological Institute), which was established on March 23, 1961, in Dharamsala, Himachal Pradesh. Drs. Yeshi Dhonden and Ven Lodoe Gyatso served as the first heads of the medical and astrological sections, respectively. The preservation of medical teachings and the sponsorship of medical training by Tibetans living outside of the PRC are undertaken by a number of teachers, physicians, and centers throughout India and other parts of the world.

Within the PRC, Tibetan medicine falls under the purview of the State Ethnic Affairs Commission and the State Administration for Traditional Chinese Medicine (SATCM), which in recent years have made an effort to establish several colleges of Tibetan medicine and hospitals that provide training and practice resources for Tibetan medicine. Although the development of Tibetan medicine outside Tibet faces the challenge of a lack of economic and political resources, the tradition within the TAR faces the challenge posed by the profound relationship between the religious components of the medical system, which are fundamental to understanding aspects of Tibetan medicine. Because the practice of Buddhism in Tibet is viewed as a potential focal point for political resistance by the Chinese government, and because many of the major religious figures of Tibet are in exile, the integration of religious perspectives into what is intended to be a state-sponsored approach to indigenous medicine poses a vexing problem to the Chinese administrators charged with preserving indigenous cultural traditions and to the practitioners of Tibetan medicine (Adams, 2001). Chinese efforts to preserve a tradition by integrating it into its national model for the management of traditional medical systems presents the tradition with the same challenge posed to Tibetan culture by China's efforts to populate the Tibetan plateau with Han Chinese settlers and expand transportation corridors into the region. On the one hand, there are unprecedented levels of new available resources and the potential for development that accompanies it, and on the other hand, the initiative and the terms on which the development is conducted lie outside the control of the culture affected by it.

All training, clinical practice, and drug production initiatives, both outside and inside China, represent an effort to remain faithful to tradition while struggling with the demands of modernity and political and social realities. In some cases, as discussed at the conclusion of this chapter, the changes that have occurred reflect tendencies that had already emerged, to some extent, in Tibet before 1959; in other cases, these changes represent entirely new directions for the medical system.

THEORY AND PRACTICE

This section discusses the theory and practice of Tibetan medicine according to the Four Tantras and the perspectives of physicians who have been trained in the tantras and who have put their precepts into action. An exhaustive discussion of all aspects of this topic is beyond the scope of this chapter. My goal is to provide a structured overview of the core theoretical and clinical elements of the system, with particular attention to the way in which core concepts link conceptions of the body, diagnosis, and therapeutics.

The discussion begins with an examination of the fundamental view of the world as composed of the five elements, the basis for understanding the body from the perspective of Tibetan medicine. Then, the metaphorical structure of the three roots of Tibetan medicine is used to organize a discussion of the core concepts and practices of the medical system.

The Five Elements: Sources of Phenomena

The universe and the body both are a result of the interplay of the five elements. The Tibetan term *byung ba* (jung wa) can be translated as "element." It also has the sense of a source or a place of origin. This latter sense is important because the five elements are, in effect, the source of all phenomena. Wind, fire, water, earth, and space are the constituents of the universe and all that is contained within it (Table 24-1).

Because of this, the five elements are fundamental to understanding much of what is done in Tibetan medicine. Each is represented by a set of qualities and is used to describe given organs, functions, tastes, seasons, and so on. Thus, *earth* gives rise to the olfactory organs, *fire* permits the process of digestion, rough and light tastes have a preponderance of the *wind* (or air) element, and *water* dominates the winter season. *Space* provides the area in which the other four elements interact, and it provides openings and cavities within structures formed out of the other four elements. The elements permit interactions between phenomena to be understood in terms of their elemental composition. Consequently, a variety of interesting relationships can be perceived.

It is important to remember that while the Tibetan tradition presents elements as material entities (especially in philosophical discussions), the concepts are employed *qualitatively* and can be easily understood from this perspective. Tsarong represents the elements as energies, or "dynamic forces which deal more with their inherent energetical function rather than their actual state" (1981, p. 10). Elements are neither discrete nor isolatable substances in the sense that the elements of the periodic table are. One finds all five elements in any substance. They are, however, present in different proportions; therefore, when it is said that

something is composed of the fire element, this means that the fire element predominates and that the phenomenon manifests its qualities most distinctly.

At the same time that we understand the elements from a qualitative point of view, it is important to remember that they are not immaterial or abstract. The elements are the constituents of all tangible matter and of very subtle substances as well.

The distinction that can be made between the relative tangibility and perceptibility of phenomena within the Tibetan schema is important. Thus, substance and structures may be gross, subtle, or very subtle, and these distinctions pertain to the ease with which structures and substances may be experienced on the basis of gross sensory perception or using meditative insight.

In the mythical tradition that informs the Tibetan worldview, the earth is said to be supported by a subterranean ocean. Underneath this is a great fire, which is fanned and kindled by a region of wind below it. This image depicts the five elements (space is the matrix) permitting the "emergence of the material world out of an immaterial ground" (Paul, 1982, p. 71). In this universe the change of climate with the seasons is caused by the activity of the winds, which stirs up the fire. This heats the ocean waters, producing spring and summer.

Just as the universe has its basis in the activity of these elements, so do we. The human body is formed from them. In the Buddhist view of conception, the body of a human is formed when the red seed of the mother, the white seed of the father, and the very subtle mind and wind cojoin (Hopkins, 1979, p. 60). This occurs during sexual intercourse. The "very subtle mind and wind" is the transmigrating consciousness of a being who, in this case, is to take birth as a human (Hopkins and Rinbochay, 1979, p. 49). From a Buddhist view, the very subtle mind is the aspect of

TABLE 24-1

Qualities and Functions of the Five Elements

Element	Quality	Function
Earth	Solidity	Formation and stability
Water	Fluidity	Conglomeration and integration
Fire	Warmth	Maturation and transformation
Wind	Motility	Growth and transportation
Space	Spaciousness	Room for growth and movement

consciousness that bears, from life to life, the effects of previous actions. At death, it absorbs the less subtle aspects of mind that are most familiar to an ordinary consciousness.

The various stages of fetal development are dealt with extensively in Tibetan medical texts. For our purposes here, it is only necessary to deal with a few aspects of the process. Latent in the subtle mind and wind are the five elements: earth, water, fire, air, and space, in their subtle state (Hopkins and Rinbochay, 1979, p. 60). It is these five elements, under the influence of *karma*, the actions committed in past lives, that bring about the human body.

> The father's sperm forms the bones, brain and spinal cord, and the mother's blood forms the flesh, blood, solid organs and hollow organs. The (five) sense consciousnesses arise from one's own mind (i.e., the mind of the being who enters the mother's womb). The flesh, bones, organ of smelling and odours are formed from the earth element. The blood, organ of taste, tastes, and the moisture (in the body) arise from the water element. The warmth, clear coloration, the organ of sight and form are formed from the fire element. The breath, organ of touch and physical sensations are formed from the wind element. The cavities in the body, the organ of hearing and sounds are formed from the space element (Donden, 1977, p. 49).

The five elements constitute the body that is the object of the physician's concern and the medicines that the physician will use to cure it.

> Everyone living on this planet has taken birth in dependence upon the five elements. We rely upon them for the necessities of life, and likewise, all medicines are composed of the five elements (Donden, 1977, p. 111).

Even death takes on a pattern derived from the interaction of the five elements, or in this case, four elements, since space is an optional member of the set. Space provides an environment for the activity of the other elements.

> Death begins with the sequential dissolution of the winds associated with the four elements—earth, water, fire, and wind. "Earth" refers to the hard factors of the body such as bone, and the dissolution of the wind associated with it means that wind is no longer capable of serving as a mount or basis for consciousness. As a consequence of its dissolution, the capacity of the wind associated with "water"—

the fluid factors in the body—to act as a mount for consciousness become more manifest. The ceasing of this capacity in one element and its greater manifestation in another is called "dissolution"; it is not, therefore, a case of gross earth dissolving into water (Hopkins and Rinbochay, 1979, p. 15).

This pattern of dissolution continues through all the elements. As death occurs, the five elements are experienced sequentially as their subtle aspects are absorbed before the departure of consciousness from the body.

The interaction of the four elements in the matrix provided by the fifth, space, is a powerful metaphor for the experience of "emptiness" *(sunyata)*, which can be equated with the absorption of all phenomena into an egoless, spacelike awareness of unconditioned selflessness. The experience of emptiness is a prerequisite for the gradual attainment of enlightenment in the Buddhist tradition. "If you take a handful of earth and put it in water it dissolves; if you heat up water with fire, it vaporizes; if you blow excessive wind on the fire, the fire goes out; and when the wind is still, then there is nothing" (Paul, 1982, p. 71).

From their relation to the universe, conception, fetal development, the essential components of the body, death, and medicine, we can see that the five elements are fundamental to all phenomena and their processes. On this basis we can begin to understand the way in which Tibetan tradition views the body and the practice of medicine.

The Situation of the Body

> The first root, the actual situation of the body has two trunks: the trunk of the state of the body uncharacterized by disease and the trunk of the state of the body characterized by disease.

The first trunk, the state of the body uncharacterized by disease, has three branches: the humors, which cause disease, the bodily constituents, and the impurities. Three branches arise from the first trunk and twenty five leaves are produced.

The first branch is the humors and has fifteen leaves. Five of the leaves represent the divisions of wind: life supporting, upward moving, pervasive, fire accompanying, and downward moving. Five more leaves represent the divisions of bile: digesting, radiance controlling, accomplishing, seeing, and color shining. The last five leaves represent the divisions of phlegm: supporting, decomposing, experiencing, satisfying, and connecting.

The second branch of bodily constituents has seven leaves: chyle (nutriment), blood, flesh, fat, bone, marrow, and regenerative fluid.

> The third branch is the impurities (excretions) and has three leaves: feces, urine, and sweat.
> —The "Three Roots," from Padma Karpo's commentary on the Four Tantras

The "Root of the Actual Situation of the Body" has two trunks. The first trunk describes the components of a body in a balanced state, uncharacterized by disease. However, the very nature of the vital substances of the body is a tendency toward imbalance and disturbance. Thus the first branch of the first trunk presents the *three faults* (nyes.pa.gsum), and it is literally the "disease" or "disorder" (nad) branch. The three faults are *wind* (Tibetan, rlung; Sanskrit, vayu), *bile* (mkhris.pa, pitta), and *phlegm* (bad.kan, kapha). They are regarded by Tibetan medicine as discrete physical substances performing functions and having specific locations in the body (Table 24-2).

One may encounter the term *nyes.pa* or its Sanskrit counterpart *dosa* in translation as "humor." This occurs because of the recognizable similarities between the four humors of Greco-Roman medicine (black bile, yellow bile, blood, and phlegm) and the three faults of the Ayurvedic and Tibetan traditions. Given that the roots of "humor" lie in the concept of fluid, there are many advantages to using this common and recognizable expression. However, neither the Tibetan nor the Sanskrit on which the Tibetan is based conveys this sense. Instead, the terms *dosa* and *nyes.pa* suggest the notion of something that is "faulty" or whose character is inherently "defective." In this sense, "fault" more clearly reveals the meaning within the tradition because these vital substances—wind, bile, and phlegm—are faulty by their very nature. They are exceptionally prone to increase, decrease, and disturb, which results in disease. For this reason, the branch that describes them is called the "disorder branch," despite that it represents the 15 divisions of the "faults" in a state of *healthy* function. This becomes clearer as the modes of disease causation are examined.

The five elements form the basis of the three humors in the following manner: earth and water are

TABLE 24-2

Names and Locations of Five Divisions of Three Faults or Humors

Tibetan	Sanskrit	English	Location
Rlung	*Vata*	*Wind*	
srog-'zhin	Prana	Life supporting	Crown
gyen-rgya	Udana	Upward moving	Horacic
khyab-byed	Vyana	Pervasive	Heart
me-mnyam	Samana	Fire equalizing	Stomach
thur-sel	Apana	Downward moving	Perineum
Mkhris-ba	*Pitta*	*Bile*	
'ju-byed	Pachaka	Digesting	Stomach
mdangs-sgyur	Ranjaka	Color regulating	Liver
sgrub-byed	Sadhaka	Accomplishing	Heart
mthong-byed	Alochaka	Seeing	Eyes
mdog-gsal	Brajaka	Color shining	Skin
Bad-kan	*Kapha*	*Phlegm*	
rten-byed	Avalambaka	Supporting	Thorax
myad-byed	Kledana	Decomposing	Epigastric
myong-byed	Bodhaka	Experiencing	Tongue
tshim-byed	Tarpaka	Satisfying	Head
'byor-byed	Shleshaka	Connecting	Joints

components of phlegm, fire is of bile, and wind of wind. Space provides an environment for the activities and interactions of the elements and furnishes the openings and cavities of the body, but it is not a component of the humors. Accordingly, *phlegm* has the combined qualities of earth and water and is supported and increased by the presence of these elements. If we imagine what results from the combination of water and earth, we have a good idea of the characteristics of phlegm. It is moist, unctuous, and cold. In balance, phlegm contains nutrients, lubricates joints, and facilitates the smooth functioning of the body. Where present in excess, phlegm produces heaviness, dullness and sogginess. *Bile* has a hot nature and as such is responsible for heating and transformation within the body. Bile gives the body color and supports vision. When disturbed or present in excess, bile can cause pathological heat and disturbance in many organs. *Wind* is a mobile substance responsible for all aspects of movement in the body, from walking and respiration to the transport of vital substances and constituents. Wind is characterized in some contexts as essentially neutral and in others as cold.

Where wind is regarded as a cold humor, some consider *blood* as a fourth humor. Blood is also regarded as an important constituent of the body and is generally considered to be hot. Some scholars consider the schema that uses four substances as an indication of the incorporation of Persian and Arab traditions based on the four humors of Greco-Roman medicine into the Tibetan paradigm.

Thus, two common representations of these vital substances according to their hot and cold properties are as follows:

- *Hot:* bile
- *Neutral:* wind
- *Cold:* phlegm

or

- *Hot:* bile, blood
- *Cold:* phlegm, wind

Whether wind is to be regarded as cold or neutral depends on the context in which it is being discussed. In terms of wind's role as a vehicle of the other humors, it can be said to be neutral. Alone, wind is said to have a cold nature.

When discussing the faults or humors, it is important to recognize that, as with the elements, the faults are *tangible,* physically present substances in the body. In fact, the tantras specify not only their locations,

as we see later, but also the actual quantities of each that are expected to be present in the body. The amount of wind in the body is as much as could be contained in an inflated urinary bladder. The amount of bile is said to be that which would fill the scrotum, and the body contains three double handfuls of phlegm. Although we may question both the units of measure and the certainty with which they are presented, it is important to recognize that just as these vital substances are classified with other tangible constituents of the body, such as blood or brain tissue, they are themselves tangible. There is a contemporary tendency to gloss the problems presented by the equivocal anatomical status of the humors (especially in the popular presentations of Ayruveda in the West) by casting them as "energies." However, this is simply not the way they are understood within the tradition itself.

Each of the three humors is divided into five subcategories and described in terms of their proper functions and locations within the body.

> On the first branch [of the trunk of the body uncharacterized by disease] are fifteen leaves. The five winds are the life supporting, the upward moving, the pervasive, the fire accompanying and the downward moving. The five biles are the digesting, the radiance controlling, the accomplishing, the seeing and the color shining. The five phlegms are the supporting, the decomposing, the experiencing, the satisfying and the connecting.
> —The "Three Roots," from Padma Karpo's Commentary on the Four Tantras

By examining the subcategory of each of the three humors that pertains to the process of digestion, we can see how these express the nature of the three humors.

"Decomposing phlegm" is located in the upper portion of the stomach. This is "responsible for breaking down food into a semi liquid state" (Tsarong, 1981, p. 48).

"Digestive bile" (also referred to as "digestive heat") is located in the middle portion of the stomach, where it functions to transform the partially digested food into substances that can be used by the body. It is understood to support the separation of nutriment and waste during digestion and to be responsible for the growth and maintenance of the seven bodily constituents. Digestive heat is also responsible for the maintenance of bodily heat and for providing the essential warmth that supports the functions of vital substances, constituents, and organs. The disturbance or diminution of digestive heat can have numerous adverse consequences for health. It is said that if the three faults are balanced, the digestive heat will be balanced as well. Excess phlegm can weaken it, bile can cause it to become sharper, and wind can cause its intensity to vary.

The "fire equalizing wind" is firelike in nature and resides in the lower region of the stomach. Its pathway travels through the five solid organs and the six hollow organs, and it is responsible for digestion. This wind resides in the lower part of the stomach, where it is said to separate wastes from nutrients and to convey these nutrients through the body. Consequently, it is described as "ripening" the seven constituents of the body.

> First, mixing [decomposing] phlegm (in the upper region of the stomach) mixes together the food and drink of any of the six tastes that have been consumed. (During this process, the food and drink become) sweet and frothy, and (the power of) phlegm increases (throughout the body). During the middle period (of digestion), the digestive bile digests (the stomach contents and they become very hot and sour in taste, while the (power of) bile increases (throughout the body). Finally, the fire-accompanying wind [fire equalizing wind] (in the lower region of the stomach) separates the chyle [nutriment] from the wastes, and (the stomach contents) become bitter, causing the (power of) wind to increase (throughout the body). Due to the qualities of the food, which contains the five elements (earth, water, fire, air and space), elements of the body increase (Donden, 1977, p. 63).

As the five elements of the body increase, the seven constituents of the body are nourished by the nutriment (sometimes chyle or essence, Tib.dwangs) carried to them by the fire equalizing wind. The order of their presentation in the tree reflects the sequence of their nourishment and production in the body by increasingly refined portions of the nutriment or essence, as the process is described in the explanatory tantra. Thus (1) nutriment contributes to the formation of (2) blood, which develops (3) flesh. The essence of these tissues forms (4) fat, from which (5) bone is nourished. The essence of bone forms (6) marrow, whose essence forms the (7) regenerative fluid (Clark, 1995, p. 62; Tsarong, 1981, p. 49).

During this process the three *excretions* are also produced: feces, urine, and sweat. The excretions are composed of the wastes separated out of the digested food by the "fire equalizing wind" and expelled from the body by "the downward moving wind."

In this description of the healthy body, the three humors are shown to carry out actions that correspond to their qualities. Phlegm produces a moist, soft substance, which is transformed by the heat of bile, and the resultant products are moved through the body by the wind. Each stage in the process of digestion is shown to be accompanied by tastes that are associated with the currently dominant humor. Earlier, I related the humors to the five elements. The following discussion shows how these relationships provide a mechanism to describe the imbalance of the humors.

Other Features of Traditional Anatomy and Physiology

The amount of vital substances (the three faults) is described earlier in the discussion on the quantities of bodily constituents. This section of the *Explanatory Tantra* also enumerates the bones and other structures of the body. Tibetan anatomical concepts are similar to those described in the texts of Ayurveda and Chinese medicine but can differ in particulars. For example, the enumeration and description of the skeletal system may be inadequate from the perspective of systematic, bioscience-based anatomy. However, it is critical to recognize that the organization of these structures guides surgery and still is the basis for locating structures for the more aggressive methods of therapy in Tibetan medicine: venesection, cautery, and acupuncture.

The concept of *channels* (rtsa) is essential to the theory and practice of Tibetan medicine. Channels are differentiated in a variety of ways, and the term *rtsa* itself takes its meaning from context and qualifiers. It can have the sense of a distinguishable anatomical structure, such as vein, artery, nerve, or lymph vessel. A "white" channel (rtsa.dkar), for example, is typically nervous tissue. A channel can be "subtle" pathway, which conveys subtle winds and is accessed in meditation. In diagnostics, as shown later, *rtsa* can convey the sense of a pulse, and the palpated artery itself is a channel through which wind and blood flow.

Channels are extensively described and mapped. A clear conception of the channels permits an understanding of the movement of vital substances in the body, and the ability to locate channels permits the palpation and treatment of specific vessels.

BOX 24-1

Five Viscera and Six Bowels

Viscera	Bowels
Heart	Stomach
Liver	Large intestine
Lungs	Gallbladder
Spleen	Urinary bladder
Kidneys	Small intestine
	Reproductive organs

Although beyond the scope of this chapter, the progressive distinction among gross, subtle, and very subtle channels and the winds and substances that flow in them forms a progressive demarcation among the aspects of Tibetan anatomy and physiology that are critical to medicine, those that are primarily related to the practice of meditation in a religious context, and those that are shared by both.

The organs in Tibetan medicine are divided into the solid five organs, or *viscera* (don.lnga), and the hollow six organs, or *bowels* (snod.drug) (Box 24-1). These organs share certain similarities with the viscera and bowels (zang fu) of Chinese medicine, especially in being simultaneously real tissue structures and related to both physiological function and the surface of the body. At the same time, important differences exist between Chinese and Tibetan organ sets, since the "triple burner" and pericardium are omitted from the Tibetan model, and the reproductive organs are established in their own right as part of the bowels. The organs are also integrated into the Tibetan model of the three faults and the seven constituents in ways that are not the case in Chinese medicine.

The Two Flowers and Three Fruits

The metaphorical tree of Tibetan medicine (Figure 24-8) represents the benefits of a healthy body by describing the first trunk as bearing two flowers and three fruits. These are the flowers of *health* and *longevity* and the fruits of *spiritual practice, wealth,* and *happiness* (Figure 24-7). Health and longevity are considered the basis for all fundamental worldly and spiritual attainments.

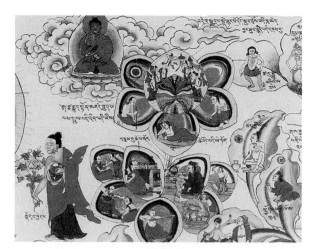

Figure 24-7 Three Fruits and Two Flowers. A detail from the upper left of The Root of Physiology and Pathology [the actual situation of the body] from plate 2, page 20, of Parfionovitch Y, Dorje G, Meyer F, eds. 1992, *Tibetan medical paintings: illustrations to the Blue Beryl treatise of Sangye Gamtso.* (Courtesy Harry N. Abrams, Inc., New York.)

THE BODY IN DISORDER

> The second trunk of the first root, the actual situation of the body, is the body characterized by disease, it has nine branches that cause illness to be produced: the substantive cause branch, the branch of coemergent conditions, the branch of entrances, the branch of locations, the branch of pathways, the branch of the time of arising, the branch of results, the branch of diverted flow (or changed causes), and the branch of epitomized meaning.
> —The "Three Roots," from Padma Karpo's Commentary on the Four Tantras

The discussion of the body marked by disease is comprehensive and organized around nine branches. The first two discuss causation. The next three discuss the way in which disease can progress through the body, the general location of diseases caused by the humors, and the movement of the humors through the bodily constituents. The sixth branch deals with the times and occasions that are conducive to diseases caused by the specific faults. The seventh pertains to factors leading to death in the course of disease, and the eighth addresses the way in which specific conditions of the humors can transform into each other. Finally, the humors are classified, as discussed earlier, according to the divisions of hot and cold.

This brief outline and the accompanying translation of the contents of the second trunk illustrate the complex understanding of the disease process in Tibetan medicine. These concepts are extensively elaborated in the *Explanatory Tantra*. Concepts of specific diseases presented within the tradition include an understanding of contagious diseases and disease caused by very small and difficult-to-see organisms.

However, the fundamental paradigm of the three faults guides the way in which the body is understood

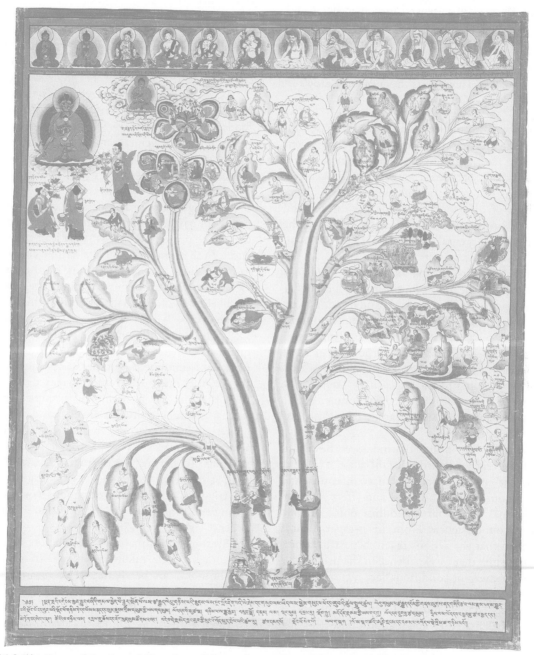

Figure 24-8 The Root of the Actual Situation of the Body as depicted in a scroll painting that includes the Three Fruits and the Two Flowers (top left). The Root of Physiology and Pathology [the actual situation of the body] from plate 2 page 20, of Parfionovitch Y, Dorje G, Meyer F, eds. 1992, *Tibetan medical paintings: illustrations to the Blue Beryl treatise of Sangye Gamtso.* (Courtesy Harry N. Abrams, Inc., New York.)

in health and sickness. The discussion that follows addresses the fundamental understanding of the disease process on this basis.

> The first branch, substantive causes, has three leaves. The cause of wind is desire. The cause of bile is hatred. The cause of phlegm is closed-mindedness.
> The second branch, coemergent conditions, has four leaves: the condition of time, the condition of harmful spirits, the condition of food, and the condition of behavior.
> —The "Three Roots" from Padma Karpo's Commentary on the Four Tantras

With regard to the fundamentals of disease causation, there are substantive causes and coemergent conditions. The three humors are said to be the "substantive causes" of disease and, when unbalanced, manifest the characteristics of disease. The substantive causes of disease are divided into distant and proximate, in that the faults have their roots in the ignorance and mental afflictions that cause all aspects of suffering.

Tibetan medicine is, after all, Buddhist medicine. This means that the roots of most manifest events lie in the past actions of body, speech, and mind. The *distant* aspect of substantive causes are the emotional afflictions familiar to students of Buddhism: desire, anger, and closed-mindedness. At the root of these lies the fundamental ignorance of the nature of reality. Thus, according to the *Explanatory Tantra*: "The sole cause of all disease is said to be ignorance due to lack of understanding of the meaning of selflessness" (Clark, 1995, p. 75).

Desire is the distant cause of wind, *anger* the distant cause of bile, and *ignorance* the distant cause of phlegm.

"Distant" means a span of many lifetimes and rebirths connected by the cause-and-effect relationships (karma) that, from a Buddhist point of view, conditions our existences. From this perspective, it is understood that the actions taken in past lives produce the results that we experience in the present.

The "coemergent conditions" are factors such as time or season; harmful influences such as spirits, inauspicious days, and unfortunate planetary aspects; unbalanced diet; and inappropriate behavior. Generally, the coemergent conditions, especially diet, behavior, and climate, act directly to imbalance the faults by furnishing conditions whose qualities or elemental character interact with them by *similarity*, exacerbating the tendency of a fault to imbalance, or

by *opposition*, diminishing the actions of the humors or faults to which they are opposed.

Diet, for example, is fundamental both to the cause and the cure of disease. Inappropriate foods are foods that are consumed to excess, in the wrong combination, at the wrong time, or by the wrong constitution. If an individual partakes of sweet foods to excess, this causes the phlegm to become unbalanced and also leads to a decrease in digestive heat. The elemental composition of the substances involved is crucial to an understanding of this process.

As explained earlier, the earth and water elements constitute phlegm. They are also the constituents of foods having a sweet taste. Digestive heat is produced through the fire element and is a healthy manifestation of the digestive bile. Fire is quenched and cooled by water, so an excess of the water element in the diet will damage the digestive fire.

Although current disorders are thought to originate with past actions, the behaviors associated with the three "poisonous minds" may lead to an imbalance of the humors and create karmic consequences in future lives. This suggests that, from the point of view of Buddhist medicine, avoiding anger can reduce the likelihood of bile disorder both in this life and in future lives.

Because the different emotional afflictions have qualities similar to the various humors, these afflictions can stimulate the humors and thus unbalance them. Other mental and emotional extremes can disturb the humors as well. For example, grief and intense mental activity can disturb wind.

Other behaviors that can disturb the humors are those that stress or alter the customary body rhythms. To suppress or restrain a natural function, such as suppressing and sneeze or an urge to urinate, can trigger wind disorders. Strenuous work under the wrong conditions can produce the heat of a bile disorder (Clark, 1995, p. 79).

Seasons and climates act to promote or suppress humors by their qualities as well. In some cases the humors can be disturbed in one season and the disorders emerge in another. An example is the disturbance of phlegm that occurs in the winter, only to emerge in the spring as the newly warm season reveals its character.

The status of spirits is problematic in a modern age. The Buddhist worldview is capable of simultaneously accepting a spirit as a reality and as the manifestation of a disturbed mind. Although some authors have expended great effort at establishing the spirit world of Tibetan medicine as form of psychiatry (Clifford 1984), it is important to note that the malign influence of spirits was a part of the Tibetan world. On this basis, the diagnosis of spirit-caused disease has been a relevant response to disease. Within the diagnostic tradition there are specific methods for determining the role of spirits in the disease process.

> The third branch, entrances, has six leaves: illness gets on the skin, spreads through flesh, circulates in the channels, gets attached to the body, settles in the solid organs, and falls into the hollow organs.
>
> The fourth, locations, has three leaves. Because phlegm depends on the brain, illness is located at the upper part of the body. Because bile rests on the seat of the liver, disease is located in the middle part of the body. As for wind, because it depends upon the hips and waist, illness is located in the lower part.
>
> The fifth branch, pathways, has fifteen leaves. Of the seven bodily constituents, wind moves through bone. Of the five senses, it moves through the ears. Of the impurities, it moves through the skin. Of the five viscera, it moves through the heart. Of the six bowels, it moves through the large intestine.
>
> Of the seven bodily constituents, bile moves through the blood. Of the five senses, it moves through the eyes. Of the impurities, it moves through sweat. Of the five viscera, it moves through the liver. Of the six bowels, it courses in the gallbladder and the small intestine.
>
> Of the seven bodily constituents, phlegm courses through the nutriment, flesh, fat, marrow, and regenerative fluid. Of the five sense organs, it moves through the nose and tongue. Of the impurities, it courses through the feces and urine. Of the five viscera, it courses through lungs, kidneys, and spleen. Of the six bowels, it courses through stomach, bladder and womb.
>
> —The "Three Roots," from Padma Karpo's Commentary on the Four Tantras

Disease is said to first affect the skin. Subsequently, the muscle tissue, channels, and then the bones are affected. After that, the disease passes into the five viscera and then the six bowels.

The general locations of the humoral disorders in the body are those associated with their characteristics and with the areas typically governed by the actions of the humor in health. Thus, wind disorders are often associated with the hips and waist. This pertains to the role of wind in activities such as movement, excretion, and reproduction. Bile disorders are associated with the middle of the body, because its seat is the liver. Phlegm is considered to have its seat in the brain, so its disorders frequently affect the upper body. Humoral imbalances also affect the specific areas and functions governed by the subcategories of the humors. The pathways of the humors, as described earlier, correspond roughly to the locations and roles of each of their five subcategories.

> The sixth branch, the time of arising, has nine leaves. There are three in the division of age. The elderly are wind people, the middle aged are bile people, and phlegm arises in youth. There are three in the division of place. Cold and breezy are the places of wind. Dry and tormented by heat are the places of bile. Very moist and oily are the places of phlegm. There are three in the division of the time of arising. Wind illness arises in the summer time, evening and dawn. Bile arises in the autumn, midday and midnight. Phlegm arises in the winter at dusk and in the morning.
>
> —The "Three Roots" from Padma Karpo's Commentary on the Four Tantras

The sixth branch, the conditions favorable to the development of a given fault, is especially interesting. Here, we can see clearly how a relationship continues to be created, between the qualities of an event and the nature of a given fault. There are three divisions, according to (1) age, (2) seasons and times, and (3) region; the division of seasons and times is addressed in the discussion of case histories. The division of regions is as follows (Tsarong, 1981, p. 53):

> Wind develops and accumulates in cold regions.
> Bile develops and accumulates in hot and dry regions.
> Phlegm develops and accumulates in wet and fertile regions.

Distinguishing the periods during which a fault will predominate permits the physician to anticipate occasions when specific diseases will flourish. This practice also permits the activities and diet of a patient to be guided according to seasonal and environmental influences and the nature of the disease. "The reason why wind accumulates in early summer is that early summer is characterized by lightness and roughness. Since these seasonal characteristics correspond to the characteristics of wind, accumulation of wind takes place during this period" (Donden, 1986, p. 61).

The Tibetan physician understands that phenomena such as the early summer and wind are produced by the five elements. That the wind and early summer have qualities in common is a sign of their common elemental constitution.

> The seventh, the branch of results, has nine leaves: the exhaustion of the three supports, life span, karma, and merit, the causes of disease become like enemies, therapeutic behavior and treatment are ineffective, damage to a vital point, a wind disease which interrupts the course of life, heat becomes excessive, cold deepens, the body cannot hold medicine, loss of life force.
>
> The eighth branch, diverted flow or changed causes, has twelve leaves. Wind having been pacified changes to bile and wind having been pacified changes to phlegm are two. Wind having not been pacified changes to bile and wind having not been pacified changes to phlegm are two. Bile having been pacified changes to wind and bile having been pacified changes to phlegm are two. Bile having not been pacified changes to wind and bile having not been pacified changes to phlegm are two. Phlegm having been pacified changes to wind and phlegm having been pacified changes to bile are two. Phlegm having not been pacified changes to wind and phlegm having not been pacified changes to bile are two.
>
> The ninth branch, epitomized meaning, has two leaves. Wind and phlegm are cold and have the nature of water. Blood and bile are hot and have the nature of fire. The temperature of worms and lymph is neutral. Because they enter they are not reckoned as leaves.
> —The "Three Roots," from Padma Karpo's
> Commentary on the Four Tantras

Branch seven deals with the result of disease (death) in all its manifestations. Branch eight discusses the possible transformation of the disorder through the suppression of one humor while another becomes unbalanced. The ninth branch has only two leaves, dividing the humors and blood into hot and cold. The concepts presented here are discussed earlier and reinforce the idea that understanding the predominant character of a condition, hot or cold, is critical.

More than one humor can become unbalanced at a time; in fact, any logically available combination is possible. Combinations of two and three humor disorders are described. In the case of three humors, a variety of relationships are described. A disorder may be one in which wind weakens, bile increases, and phlegm decreases. "Delicate" disorders, where one humor is diminished or dislocated by one or two oth-

ers, are also discussed. These and many more categories of illness are outlined in the twelfth chapter of the *Explanatory Tantra*, "The Classification of Illness."

This section has provided an overview of the way in which the body is conceptualized in health and sickness. We have examined the way in which the body is organized in Tibetan medicine and how the basis of disease, the humors, is understood in terms of the five elements.

The next problem confronting the Tibetan physician is forming a diagnosis.

THE ROOT OF RECOGNIZING SIGNS: DIAGNOSIS

> The root of the recognition of signs (diagnosis) has three trunks: the trunk of the science of observation, the trunk of the science of examination by feeling, and the trunk of communication skills, questioning and hearing.
> —The "Three Roots" from Padma Karpo's
> Commentary on the Four Tantras

Diagnosis is organized into the three trunks of observation, feeling the pulse, and questioning. *Observation* involves examination of the tongue and the urine, as well as observing the bearing and facial coloration of the patient. *Feeling the pulse* allows the practitioner to assess whether a disease has its origins in wind, bile, phlegm, or a combination of these and to understand which organs are affected. *Questioning* of the patient is used to evaluate prior behavior and current symptoms to determine the nature of the illness. All three of these diagnostic modes organize bodily information into signs that represent the state of the body to the physician and allow him or her to understand the nature of the patient's disease. These signs reveal the characteristics of disease, which then reveal the affected humors.

This section discusses the observation urine and the method of feeling the pulse in some detail. Both methods are considerably more complex than their representation on the trunk of diagnosis would suggest, since it presents only their basic principles. However, these two methods are the subject of extensive discussion in the *Final Tantra*. Tongue diagnosis is well summarized by Padma Karpo's description of the tree and is not discussed further here.

> The first trunk of the root of the recognition of signs has two branches: the branch of observing the tongue and the branch of examining the urine.

The first branch has three leaves. The wind tongue is red, dry and rough. The bile tongue is covered with thick, pale yellow phlegm. The phlegm tongue is pale, lusterless, soft and moist.

The second branch has three leaves. Wind urine is like water with big bubbles. Bile urine is red yellow with much steam and a strong smell. Phlegm urine is white having little vapor or smell.
— The "Three Roots" from Padma Karpo's Commentary on the Four Tantras

Observation of Urine

The texts describe preliminary compliances that are to be observed by the patient. Actions that are thought to alter the condition of the urine are forbidden. These include the consumption of tea, whey, and foods with a hot taste, which can affect the condition of wind, phlegm, and bile urines, respectively (Table 24-3). Strenuous activity is also forbidden (Rabgay, 1981, p. 52).

Other factors besides those traditionally presented may affect the color of urine. Tibetan physicians recognize the particular hue and qualities imparted to urine by vitamins or medicines. A physician may decide that a sample is not suitable for diagnosis because the patient had ingested medicines or vitamins the previous day, thereby distorting color or other factors.

Urine for observation is traditionally taken in the morning before eating. The medical scriptures state that the best time for examination is at dawn. In actual practice there are no stipulations concerning the length of time that may elapse before the urine itself is examined.

A small quantity of urine is placed in a white container (teacups are popular) and stirred vigorously with a stick (Figure 24-13). Tsarong (1981) describes the fundamental criteria applied as follows:

Wind urine is like water and big bubbles appear when stirred vigorously.

Bile urine is amber coloured, malodorous, steaming, and fast disappearing bubbles appear when stirred vigorously.

Phlegm urine is whitish, less odor and steam, saliva-like bubbles of medium size, appear when stirred vigorously (pp. 57-58).

The urine is inspected immediately after stirring (Figure 24-9) and then observed for changes (Figure 24-10).

The example provided is from a patient whose urine gave indication of a cold illness. The signs that helped make this determination were the comparative pale color of the urine, the small bubbles, and the bubbles persisting for a time after stirring. The second sample, depicted in Figures 24-11 and 24-12, supports a diagnosis of phlegm and wind. After stirring, the urine displays the large bubbles associated with wind (Figure 24-11), and for a time after stirring, the smaller bubbles persist, a sign of phlegm and cold (Figure 24-12).

The characteristics of urine indicating a blood disorder are similar to those of a bile disorder, except that the color approaches a dark red. Other factors to assess include the presence of sediment (ku.ya) and scum. If these are present in quantity, a hot disorder is indicated (bile or blood).

Some of these criteria are observable only in a fresh urine sample. Physicians will typically concentrate on the features that are not substantially affected by time. "There are nine stages in the analysis of urine, but among the nine, we mainly do the three types of analysis, color, odor, foam. The scum and sediment are also important" (Donden, 1980, p. 29).

The actual occurrence of a "pure" wind, bile, or phlegm disorder is a rarity. Combinations are said to occur more frequently. For example, a urine sample

TABLE 24-3

Two Medicines with Hot Taste

	Long pepper (pi.pi.ling)	Pomegranate (se.hbru)
Genus	*Piper longum*	*Punica granatum*
Treatment	Cold disorders	Cold wind and cold phlegm diseases
	Wind and spleen disorders	Increases digestive heat
Taste	Hot, salty, slightly sour	Sour, hot, slightly salty
Power	Sharp, rough, blunt	Hot, sharp, rough, oily, light
Quality	Warm, dry	Dry, mobile

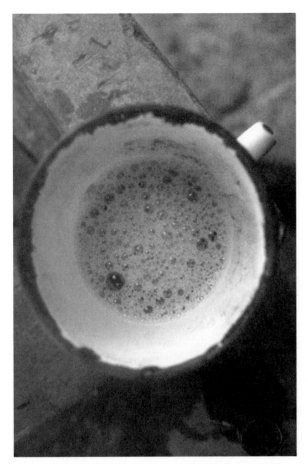

Figure 24-9 Cold illness urine immediately on stirring. (Courtesy Windhorse, © Kevin Ergil, 1982.)

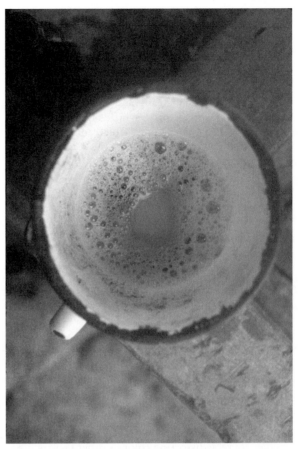

Figure 24-10 Cold illness urine shortly after stirring. (Courtesy Windhorse, © Kevin Ergil, 1982.)

indicating wind would be pale with many small viscous bubbles that remained for a long time after stirring and a few large bubbles scattered among them.

Urine may simply be distinguished in terms of hot and cold as well. "Hot disorder" urine, when fresh, is yellowish or reddish, hazy, and malodorous; steam is concentrated and stable; and it has minute bubbles that disappear quickly. "Cold disorder" urine is clear, white, and dilute; has little steam or color; and possesses large, stable bubbles (Rabgay, 1981, p. 58).

It is tempting to think of these diagnostic signs purely in terms of "contiguity," highlighting their indexical relationship with a given body state. It would be a mistake, however, to overlook the *qualitative* character of these signs. This is apparent in urine diagnosis, where the appearance of the urine is a sign not only because of its connection with the disorder, but also because of its similarity to the body state of which it partakes. Thus, phlegm urine has thick, vis-

cous bubbles and a dilute appearance; its appearance is not merely "indicative" but also *representative* of the cold, viscous quality of phlegm. Similarly, bile urine, which is steaming and reddish, both produces the appearance of heat and indicates its presence in the body. Wind urine embodies and indicates air with its large, rapidly disappearing bubbles.

Pulse diagnosis similarly reveals signs that express the state of the body in terms of quality.

Pulse Diagnosis

Pulse diagnosis is considered the most difficult medical skill to acquire within the Tibetan medical tradition. The pulse is taken at the radial artery on the wrist (Figure 24-14) to avoid the interference from the noise of lungs and heart and at the same time to be as close as possible to the internal organs. In this

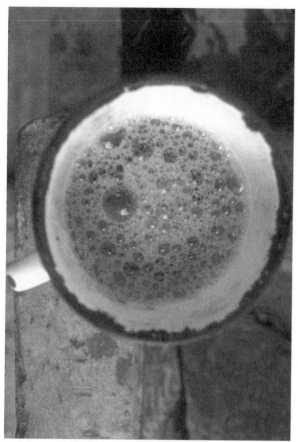

Figure 24-11 Phlegm and wind urine immediately on stirring. (Courtesy Windhorse, © Kevin Ergil, 1982.)

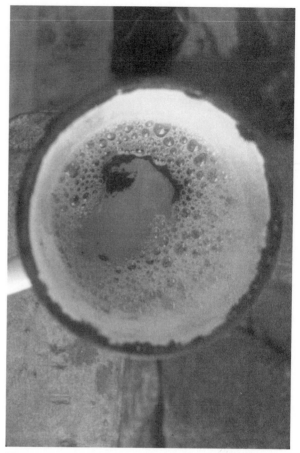

Figure 24-12 Phlegm and wind urine shortly after stirring. (Courtesy Windhorse, © Kevin Ergil, 1982.)

case, both the artery and the pulsation itself are understood through the Tibetan term *rtsa,* meaning "root" or "channel." To feel the channels is to palpate a pulse. Often the term *rtsa* has the sense of "pulse." As previously discussed, this term can also indicate many other types of channels in the body.

Wind produces movement in the body. Wind moves through certain channels by itself. In other channels, wind is responsible for the movement of the substances the channel carries, such as blood. In pulse diagnosis, although wind and blood flow together, the physician is more concerned with the quality of the wind. The channels (arteries in this case) are likened to messengers running between physician and patient. The distinction between the examination of the wind channels (assessing the quality of the motion displayed by a channel in which the wind flows), which indicate the condition of various internal organs, and the examination of the heart

rate is made. One physician admonishing his students made the following statement: "You don't feel the rlung [wind] pulse beat properly. I use a stethoscope to tell precisely the rate of the heart and arterial blood, but for rlung rtsa [wind pulse] this doesn't work" (Tsering, 1980).

Ideally, the pulse is taken in the morning before breakfast, when it gives the truest representation of the patient's condition. The patient and the physician should be calm. In practice, the pulse is taken throughout the day.

When the pulse is taken, three fingers of each hand are used. It is said that the index finger should rest lightly on the skin, the middle finger should feel flesh, and the ring finger should feel bone. The need for this variation of pressure derives from the shape of the channel, which is compared to a radish or carrot that tapers as it goes deeper into the ground.

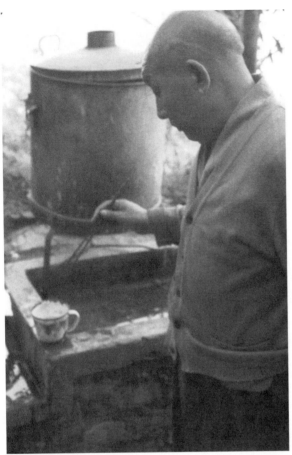

Figure 24-13 Dr. Yeshe Donden stirring urine. (Courtesy Windhorse, © Kevin Ergil, 1982.)

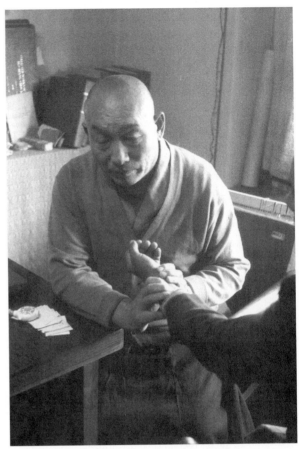

Figure 24-14 Dr. Yeshe Donden taking the pulse. (Courtesy Windhorse, © Kevin Ergil, 1982.)

An individual in normal health may be characterized by one of three pulse types: male, female, or neuter. Each of these has its own particular beat, as follows:

> A male constitutional pulse [is] the pulse of a person with a predominance of wind; consequently, his pulse beat is rough and thick. A female pulse is that [of] a person with a predominance of bile, and therefore has a rapid and thin beat. A neuter pulse beat is generally found in a phlegm-predominating person and the pulse beat is smooth and pliable (Rabgay, 1981, p. 48).

These pulses are "constitutional" in that they describe the dominant humor (as a trait) of an individual's body. A Tibetan physician is expected to recognize these and not confuse them with the pulses of wind, bile, and phlegm disorders.

The second trunk, the science of examination by feeling, has three branches: the branch of feeling the wind pulse, the branch of feeling the bile pulse, and the branch of feeling the phlegm pulse. There are three leaves. The first is the wind pulse; it is full and stalk like, it stops. The second is the bile pulse; it is quick, strong, hurried and forceful. The third is the phlegm pulse; it is sinking, thin and slow.

> —The "Three Roots," from Padma Karpo's Commentary on the Four Tantras

In its elaborated form, pulse diagnosis is used to asses the condition of the major organs in the body. As discussed, the internal organs are divided into the categories of the "solid" viscera and the "hollow" bowels. Specifically, the six bowels include the stomach, large intestines, gallbladder, small intestine, urinary bladder, and reproductive organs. The five viscera include the lungs, heart, liver, spleen, and kidneys.

Each of these organs is related to a point on the practitioner's fingers (Boxes 24-2 and 24-3). The

BOX 24-2

Pulse Diagnosis: Male Patient

Left Hand Touches	Right Hand Touches
Index finger	Index finger
Lung, large intestine	Heart, small intestine
Middle finger	Middle finger
Liver, gallbladder	Spleen, stomach
Ring finger	Ring finger
Right kidney, urinary bladder	Left kidney, reproductive organs

fingers are placed on the radial artery just on the proximal side of the styloid process of the radius. The right hand palpates the left radial artery. The lateral portion of the right index finger of the physician reads the heart pulse while the medial portion takes the pulse of the small intestine. The lateral portion of the middle finger reads the spleen while the stomach pulse is taken on the medial side. The lateral portion of the ring finger reads the left kidney while the medial side reads the reproductive organs.

The physician's left hand palpates the radial artery on the patient's right arm. The lateral index finger reads the lungs, medial index finger reads the large intestine; lateral middle finger reads the liver, medial middle finger reads the gallbladder; lateral ring finger reads the right kidney, and medial ring finger reads the urinary bladder. This configuration applies to male patients; when examining female patients, the pulses shown for the index fingers are interchanged.

Richard Selzer (1974) offers the following elegant description of a prolonged examination of the pulse,

BOX 24-3

Pulse Diagnosis: Female Patient

Left Hand Touches	Right Hand Touches
Index finger	Index finger
Heart	Lung
Small intestine	Large intestine
Middle finger	Middle finger
Liver	Spleen
Gallbladder	Stomach
Ring finger	Ring finger
Right kidney	Left kidney
Urinary bladder	Reproductive organs

carried out by Yeshe Donden at a hospital in the United States:

> At last he takes her hand, raising it in both of his own. Now he bends over the bed in a kind of crouching stance, his head drawn down into the collar of his robe. His eyes are closed as he feels for the pulse. In a moment he has found the spot, and for the next half hour he remains thus, suspended above the patient like some exotic golden bird with folded wings, holding the pulse of the woman beneath his fingers, cradling her hand in his. All the power of the man seems to have been drawn down into this one purpose. It is palpation of the pulse raised to the state of ritual. From the foot of the bed where I stand, it is as though he and the patient have entered a special place of isolation, of apartness, about which a vacancy hovers, and across which no violation is possible (p. 34).

In this instance, Donden correctly described the patient's condition as a congenital heart disorder. He also used metaphor to describe the state of the heart in a manner that was strikingly consistent with the biomedical diagnosis: interventricular septal defect with resultant heart failure.

This almost supernatural facility for knowing the body through the pulse is considered to be the mark of a master of Tibetan pulse diagnosis. The system itself builds on escalating levels of complexity. Pulse diagnosis in assessing a disorder can be considered to have three progressively more challenging levels: (1) the simple discrimination of the hot or cold quality of the condition; (2) the general quality of the pulse it self as a sign of the qualitative character of the disorder (the branch of feeling the pulse addresses this); and (3) the sensitive discrimination of the situation of areas of the body and the organs in relation to the characteristics of the disorders itself.

As with other diagnostic techniques, palpating the pulse may be used to determine something as basic as whether the patient's disorder is hot or cold or, as just shown, to derive extremely subtle information about the patient's condition.

To determine if a disorder is hot or cold, it is said that the pulse should beat five times in the period delimited by the physician's inhalation and exhalation. If it is much faster, the patient has a hot disease; if it is much slower, a cold disease is diagnosed.

The pulses for the several organs on each wrist will be about the same if the patient is in good health, except that the right hand pulse is stronger in women. If the individual is ill and there is an imbalance in an organ, the pulse location will manifest this by an irregularity of beat. In the case of bile disease, the beat is "fine, hard and strong." Phlegm disease is "slow and indistinct," and wind disease is characterized by a "hollowness" (Kunzang, 1973, p. 95). Many descriptive terms are available for the types of pulse, each signifying a specific sort of imbalance. Categories besides wind, bile, and phlegm are also represented. It is possible, for example, to feel a "lymph pulse."

The "organs" that are being assessed through palpation of the pulse have a slightly different status than those of biomedicine. The organs that a Tibetan physician is concerned with might best be viewed as "spheres of physiological function," the pathology of which has been described and organized in terms other than those of pathological change at a cellular level.

The accomplishments of a Tibetan physician lie in his or her ability to organize signs of quality clearly. This approach can be challenging to the biomedical perspective. A biomedical physician related the "problem of classifying his [the Tibetan physician's] system with ours." He cited such phrases as "the left hand is deep and weak" as ambiguous and difficult to interpret by Western physicians (Sarlson, 1981, p. 7). There is nothing necessarily ambiguous about this to the system's practitioner; we might suspect by now that a deep and weak pulse is a sign of a "cold" disease.

The pulse is regarded as a "messenger," and as such it must be understood as an index because this relationship expresses contiguity with its pertinent organ (Ergil, 1987, p 56.). This is the level of relation that is most common in biomedicine. A rapid pulse indicates the actual fact of a rapidly beating heart, and that fact must be placed in relation to others. When biomedicine attends to other features of the pulse, similar considerations arise; an indexical relation between tissue pathology and sign is specified. From the perspective of Tibetan medicine, however, the pulse is not simply a sign of a distant event to which it is related; it is also a sign regarded as being deeply infused with the character of what it represents, and as such the pulse has an iconic character. A pulse's qualities portray the actual state of an organ; they do not merely mark the presence of that state (Ergil, 1983, p 57).

Questioning

The third trunk of communication skills has three branches: the branch of questions about the customary state of illnesses conditioned by wind, the branch of questions about the customary states of illness conditioned by bile, and the branch of questions about the customary states of illness conditioned by phlegm.

The first branch has eleven leaves. Disease produced by light and rough food and behavior produces symptoms of yawning; stretching and sighing; shivering with cold; pain in all the hips, waist, bones, joints; vague pains; intermittent dry heaves; the sense organs become unclear; the mind is turbulent; there is pain at the time of being hungry. For those who tend to these symptoms, oily cures are of certain benefit.

The second branch has seven leaves. Disease produced by conditions of sharp and hot food and behavior produces such modes of illness as a bitter taste in the mouth; headache; great heat in the flesh; pain in the upper body; pain after digestion. For those who tend to these modes, coolness benefits.

The third has eleven leaves. Conditions of heavy, oily food and behavior produce symptoms of poor appetite; difficulty in digestion; vomiting; inability to taste; stomach cramps; belching; both mind and body are heavy; cold inside and out; feeling poorly after eating. If one tends to these, warmth restores health. Thus there are three trunks of sign modes with eight branches and thirty-eight leaves.

—The "Three Roots," from Padma Karpo's Commentary on the Four Tantras

A Tibetan physician's repertoire of diagnostic techniques includes the use of the "29 questions" just described. By determining what diet and behaviors the patient has engaged in, what symptoms the patient is experiencing, and the experiences that give relief, the physician can determine the nature of the patient's illness.

This last aspect of diagnosis clarifies how similarity in qualities pervades the causes, nature, and manifestation of disease. The rubric provided by the "29 questions" allow the physician to determine if the patient has engaged in activities or consumed a food that may have disturbed a humor. The cardinal signs of disturbances of the three faults are provided on each of the branches. Wind is characterized by the signs of windy motion: stretching and yawning. Vague, poorly defined pains signal the movement of wind, whereas pain in the joints signals the presence of wind in one of its customary seats. A turbulent or disturbed mind signals the unfettered stirring of the disturbed humor. The rising heat of bile produces headaches, with pain following digestion as the heat of digestion becomes disturbed by the bile imbalance. Phlegm shows signs of pervasive cold, impaired digestion from damage to the digestive heat, and a sense of heaviness caused by the thick, viscid humor. Physical states and symptoms maintain their qualitative relationship here as well. Heat produces bile disease, windy places engender wind, and cold, moist environments produce phlegm.

With these questions, a practitioner can validate the results that he or she has obtained by means of visual (tongue and urine) and pulse diagnosis. If the results of other methods are not clear, the process of interrogation can help the physician reach a diagnosis.

THERAPEUTICS: THE ROOT OF HEALING

The root of healing is the most prolific of the three roots. It produces four trunks whose order reveals the desirable sequence of their application.

The first trunk is the trunk of *diet* and has six branches pertaining to food and drink for diseases caused by each of the three humors. As discussed, diet is one of the factors that can easily cause an imbalance of the faults, and it can just as easily be used to correct the imbalance if applied in a timely manner.

Behavioral therapeutics follows diet. Just as *behaviors* can lead to a disturbance of the faults, the selection of appropriate behaviors can remedy an existing disturbance. This trunk has three branches describing behavior appropriate to the treatment of disease and to its engendering fault. Behavioral therapies in Tibetan medicine are not limited to the redressing of humoral imbalances; they also correct the ultimate cause of disease: the three "poisonous minds" of ignorance, desire, and anger.

The trunk of *medication,* examined in detail later, has 15 branches. Six of these describe the tastes and powers of medicines. These are important to consider because both dietary therapies and medications are selected and used according to the tastes and qualities that the five elements give to them. Six branches describe the forms of medications for pacifying disor-

ders, and three discuss cleansing medications. The fourth trunk discusses external therapies.

> The third, the root of the manner of healing, has four trunks: the trunk of food, the trunk of behavior, the trunk of medicine and the trunk of therapy.
> The first has six branches. The branch of foods that clear wind and the branch of beverages that clear wind are two. The branch of foods that clear bile and the branch of beverages that clear bile are two. The branch of foods that clear phlegm and the branch of beverages that clear phlegm are two.
> —The "Three Roots," from Padma Karpo's Commentary on the Four Tantras

Foods

Food as therapy is fundamental to Tibetan medicine. The principles of Tibetan dietetics are governed by the concepts that govern medicine, as discussed later. As mentioned, foods that contain tastes that promote a given humor, if taken to excess, may disturb it or suppress the actions of other humors. Thus the therapeutic foods discussed are those that will counteract the characteristics of a given humor. Although many of the chosen foods (e.g., donkey meat, treacle beer, marmot meat) represent dietary choices that are specific to Tibetan culture, the principles that govern the selection of foods and beverages can be applied broadly.

> The first branch of the root of healing describes the foods that clear wind and has ten leaves: horse meat, donkey meat, marmot meat, year old meat, human flesh, seed oil, year old butter, treacle, garlic, and onions. On the second branch of the root of healing, beverages that clear wind are described and it has four leaves: milk, grain beer containing angelica root and *Polygonatum cirrhifolium*, treacle beer, bone beer. In general there are fourteen wind foods in all.
> The third branch of the root of healing describes the foods that clear bile. It has nine leaves: yogurt, whey, fresh butter, deer and antelope meat, goat meat, ground grains, grey dandelion, dandelion stew. The fourth branch describes the beverages that clear bile. There are three leaves: spring water, cool water, and cool boiled water. Bile foods are twelve in all.
> The fifth branch describes the foods that clear phlegm. It has seven leaves: mutton, yak meat, the meat of wild carnivorous animals, fish, honey, warm porridge of meat and old grain, and yogurt

and whey. The sixth describes beverages that clear phlegm. It has two leaves: strong beer and boiled water. Phlegm foods are nine in all. In sum the leaves of food are thirty-five in number.

—The "Three Roots," from Padma Karpo's Commentary on the Four Tantras

Wind responds to heavy, oily foods and beverages, so seed oils, dense butters, garlic, and alcohol all have the ability to settle wind. Cooling foods such as dandelion (Figure 24-15), fresh butter, and cool water all counteract the hot characteristics of bile. The dense, heavy humor phlegm is addressed by means of warming foods such as mutton or foods such as honey, which is light and warm.

A taste calls to mind the elemental state of a substance. These principles are adaptable to newly encountered foods and substances. Just as the Four Tantras were revised and organized to reflect the dietary and environmental conditions of the Tibetan plateaus, the concepts of Tibetan medicine can be and are adapted to the prevailing diets and environments of South Asia and the West.

Behavior

Behavioral medicine is a striking aspect of the Tibetan tradition. Here we are shown that the wind humor, often implicated in nervous system disorders or psychological disorders, can be addressed by warmth and pleasant company. Phlegm disorders respond to activity and movement. A patient suffering from a phlegm condition might exhibit lethargy

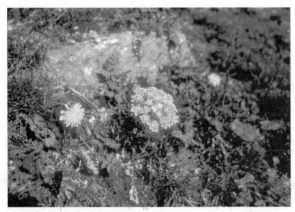

Figure 24-15 Tan kun and dandelion. (Courtesy Windhorse, © Kevin Ergil, 1982.)

and a preference for sleeping during the day. In these cases, warmth and activity are recommended.

The second trunk on the root of healing, behavior has three branches: wind behavior, bile behavior and phlegm behavior.

The first branch, behaviors that control wind, has two leaves: a warm place, and pleasing friends.

The second branch, behaviors that control bile, has two leaves: a cool place and behaving in a relaxed fashion.

The third branch, behaviors that control phlegm, has two leaves: staying in a warm place and strenuously walking. Altogether there are six leaves of behavior.

—The "Three Roots," from Padma Karpo's Commentary on the Four Tantras

Behavioral advice is provided extensively in the *Explanatory Tantra*. In addition to routine behavior for avoiding illness and adaptive seasonal behavior, suggestions are made with regard to behaviors for securing success in the world and for achieving the ultimate happiness and health associated with the practice of Buddhist doctrine.

Medicines

Tibetan medicine makes use of a wide variety of minerals, animal substances, and plant materials for therapeutic purposes. The Tibetan *materia medica* is substantial. It contains many plants and substances that are distinctive to the high-altitude meadows of Tibet and the Himalayas. Tibetan medicine also shares many medicinals with the Ayurvedic or Chinese *materia medica*. Although in general a standard nomenclature is used to reference the distinctive plants of the Tibetan tradition, many agents may be supplied by multiple plant species. Because of this, there can be problems with the precise identification of medicinals. This can be compounded where regional and historical substitutions have become well established. Standard references enumerate more than a thousand substances, and many of these may be supplied by multiple species, furnishing an extensive catalogue of medicinal agents.

The principles governing the selection and use of medicines are based on the systematic application of the relationship between tastes and the five elements.

The third trunk on the root of healing, medicine, has fifteen branches: the branch of wind clearing tastes, the powers that clear the wind, the tastes that clear bile, the powers that clear bile, the tastes that clear phlegm, the powers which clear phlegm, beverages that pacify wind, medicinal butters that pacify wind, decoctions which pacify bile, powders that pacify bile, pills that pacify phlegm, medicinal powders that pacify phlegm, enemas that cleanse wind, purgatives that cleanse bile, and emetics that cleanse phlegm.

—The "Three Roots," from Padma Karpo's
Commentary on the Four Tantras

The application of medicinal agents is based on a detailed theory that begins with simple principles based on tastes and is significantly elaborated with regard to more subtle principles. These principles, which are also applied to foods, provide the physician with a method of evaluating medicines from a perspective that is informed by the universal principle of the five elements or sources and their relation to the three faults. This means that once the physician has understood the body and assessed its condition in terms of the characteristics of the disease process embodied by the three faults, he or she is now prepared to use those same principles to treat the patient (Ergil, 1983, p 61, 1987, p 62).

Tastes, Powers, Potencies, and Qualities

In the first chapter of the *Root Tantra*, the tastes (ro), powers (nus.pa), and qualities (yon.tan) of medicines are mentioned in association with directions and medicinal substances. In the nineteenth and twentieth chapters of the *Explanatory Tantra*, these are explained, and their role in the treatment of illness is discussed in some detail.

The first branch of wind clearing tastes has three leaves: sweet, sour and salty. The second branch of wind clearing powers has three leaves: oily, heavy and soft.

The third branch, bile clearing tastes, has three leaves: sweet, bitter and astringent. The fourth branch, bile clearing powers, has three leaves: cool, liquefying and blunt.

The fifth branch, phlegm clearing tastes, has three leaves: hot, sour and astringent. The sixth branch, phlegm clearing powers, has three leaves: sharp, rough and light.

—The "Three Roots," from Padma Karpo's
Commentary on the Four Tantras

According to Tibetan medicine, there are six *tastes:* sweet, bitter, sour, salty, astringent, and hot. These include the four that are recognized by biomedical physiology and two extra "tastes," hot and astringent. Sweet, sour, and salty tastes are used for wind disorders. Sweet, bitter, and astringent tastes are given to persons with bile ailments. In case of phlegm, hot-, sour-, and astringent-tasting medicines are used (Box 24-4). Each taste has its elemental constituents, as follows:

- Sweet = earth and water
- Sour = earth and fire
- Salty = water and fire
- Bitter = water and air
- Hot = fire and air
- Astringent = earth and air

If this list is compared to the elemental components of the three faults, one sees that the faults are controlled by tastes that are not similarly constituted. For example, wind is composed of the air element and is pacified by tastes of substances containing earth, water, and fire elements. This reflects the essential or fundamental intention of Tibetan therapeutics: to remove a condition by opposing the factors (the faults and their elements) that have caused it to develop. The object is to restore bodily balance by the application of medicines, substances, or methods of opposing qualities. The "Science of Healing," therefore, is an allopathic system, in that it applies a therapy that is directly opposed to the character of the disease process.

The *powers,* of which there are eight, express the functions associated with a given taste. These powers reduce or oppose a given fault. The eight powers are heavy, oily, cool, blunt, light, rough, hot, and sharp (Box 24-5).

These powers also have a specific relationship with the five elements, as follows:

- Earth: heavy, blunt, oily
- Water: oily, cool, heavy
- Fire: sharp, rough, light, oily, hot
- Wind: light, rough

BOX 24-4

Tastes that Oppose Phlegm

- Sour = earth and fire
- Hot = fire and air
- Astringent = earth and air

For example, a phlegm condition can involve an overabundance of phlegm, which is made up of earth and water. In this case, it would be opposed by the four powers: light, rough, hot, and sharp and the use of hot-, sour-, and astringent-tasting medicines. While both the sour and astringent tastes contain earth, none of the tastes or their powers is associated with water, so the moist, muddy characteristics of phlegm are opposed.

The *potencies* are hot and cold. These are fundamental concepts, but it is essential that these principles be grasped correctly because failure to oppose a hot disease with a cold medicine, or vice versa, can lead to a significant worsening of the condition. Potencies reflect the general tendencies of a medication. Medicines having a hot potency are pomegranate and black pepper, while white sandalwood and camphor have cold potencies. The potencies are the most basic aspects of a medicine. Once a medicine's potencies, tastes, and powers are known, much of its therapeutic activity can be understood.

The concept of a medicine's qualities is a further elaboration of a given taste having specific powers. According to traditional sources, the powers may be viewed as "inherent forces due to having, in particular, special abilities that become the essence of all qualities" (bdud.rtsi, 1971, p. 192). In fact, the terms designating the powers are also included in the set of terms designating the qualities. The 20 characteristics of disease (mtsha.nyid) are said to be opposed by the 17 qualities. Although "qualities" and "characteristics" represent two intersecting sets of terms, different words are used because the term *quality* (yon.tan) has exclusively positive connotations, as follows:

> The qualities (are) soothing, heavy, warm, firm, cold, blunt, cool, flexible, liquefying, drying, oily, absorbent, hot, light, sharp, rough, and mobile. By the seventeen the twenty characteristics are subdued (bdud.rtsi, 1971, p. 192).

The powers and qualities are related to tastes in the following way:

> Salty, astringent and sweet in sequence (are) heavy. Similarly salty, sour and sweet (are) oily. Bitter, astringent and sweet are blunt. Sour, hot, bitter the three (are) light and rough. Hot, sour, and salty the three are hot and sharp (bdud.rtsi, 1971, p. 192).

In this way the link between the tastes and the powers that oppose the three faults is provided by their elemental constitution.

The elements are clearly understood as constituents of plants, contributing to their growth and development.

> Medicinal plants and herbs originate from the five elements of earth, water, fire and sky [space]. (a) The earth forms the base of the plants and herbs. (b) Water moistens them. (c) Fire generates heat and uses growth. (d) Air causes movement thus assisting growth. (e) The sky allows sufficient space for growth (Kunzang, 1973, p. 64).

According to the plant's own tendencies and their environments, a given element or elements will predominate. The medicinal effect of a plant lies in its elemental composition, which determines its powers and taste. Tastes can be determined directly, and qualities are said to be inferred from these tastes, as follows:

> Having determined the element composition of a drug by its taste, we can then infer the drug properties [qualities]. A drug with the predominant constituents of earth and water will have heavy, stable, blunt, smooth, oily and dry property [quality]. Consequently, the drug will produce an action of stabilization and physical and mental control and concentration. It is most efficacious for wind disorders (Topgay, 1980, p. 30).

Medicines are provided as beverages, medicinal butters, decoctions, powders, and pills, as well as in the form of suppositories. The nine branches dealing

---

BOX 24-5

Eight Powers and Effects on Three Faults

Powers removing *wind* and *bile:*
- Heavy
- Oily
- Cool
- Blunt

Powers removing *phlegm:*
- Light
- Rough
- Hot
- Sharp

Wind is increased by three powers:
- Light, rough, and cool

Bile is increased by three powers:
- Hot, sharp, and oily

Phlegm is increased by four powers:
- Heavy, oily, cool, and blunt

with specific medications present all aspects of medication in relation to the three faults.

The seventh branch, beverages that pacify wind, has three leaves: bone soup, the four essences and meat from a sheep's head.

The eighth branch, medicinal butters that pacify wind, has five leaves: medicinal butter of nutmeg, medicinal butter of pale garlic, medicinal butter of the three fruits, medicinal butter of the five roots and medicinal butter of Aconitum Ferrox.

The ninth branch, decoctions that pacify bile, has four leaves: decoction of camphor, decoction of mineral medicines, decoction of Tinasporia cordifolia, decoction of Swertia chirata, and decoction of the three fruits.

The tenth branch, powders that pacify bile, has four leaves: camphor powder, sandalwood powder, cardamom powder and bamboo manna powder.

The eleventh branch, pills that pacify phlegm, has two leaves: mineral pills and pills made from all sorts of salts.

The twelfth branch, medicinal powders that pacify phlegm, has five leaves: pomegranate, dwarf rhododendron, hot medicines, burned salt and ashes of burned calcite.

The thirteenth branch, enemas which cleanse wind, has three leaves: an enema followed by shaking legs upwards, an enema followed by clapping the soles of feet, enema followed by being shaken by feet.

The fourteenth branch, purgatives which cleanse bile, has four leaves: an ordinary purgative, a specific purgative, a strong purgative, a mild purgative.

The fifteenth branch, emetics which cleanse phlegm, has two leaves: a strong emetic and a mild emetic.

—The "Three Roots," from Padma Karpo's Commentary on the Four Tantras

Once we move from the therapeutic uses of single substances to the compounding of medicines, the matter becomes much more complex. Generally, texts such as the *Information Tantra* of the Four Tantras provide detailed instructions concerning the selection of medicinal compounds for specific conditions (Figure 24-16). The *compounding* of medicines is carried out in a variety of ways. The preparation of pills can be a simple matter of measuring and powdering medicinals and then mixing them with water before forming them into pills (Figures 24-17, 24-18, and 24-19), or it can be an exceptionally complex process involving the specific preparation of multiple ingredients accompanied by time-sensitive steps and religious ritual.

Most Tibetan medicines are named according to the principal ingredient and the total number of

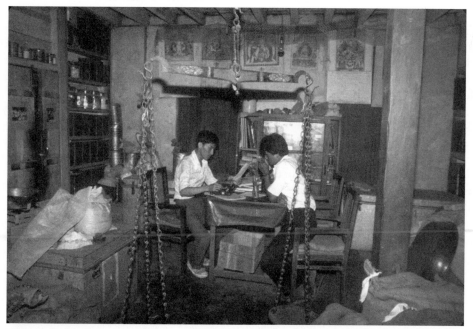

Figure 24-16 Tibetan physicians in the compounding room at the old Tibetan Medical Center in Upper Dharamsala, surrounded by processed medicinals, scales, and texts on the preparation of medicines. (Courtesy Windhorse, © Kevin Ergil, 1982.)

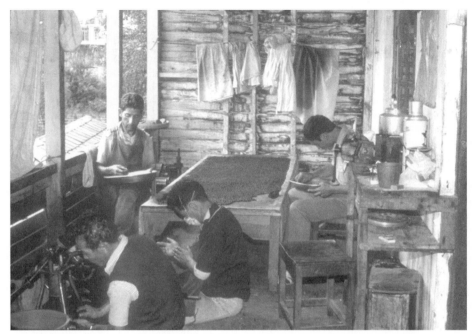

Figure 24-17 A team of workers preparing Tibetan medicinal pills. The powdered medicinals are mixed with water, extruded, cut into pill form, and shaped by hand. (Courtesy Windhorse, © Kevin Ergil, 1982.)

ingredients in the medicine. For example, one famous medicine, Aquilaria 31 (Agar So Chig), is made from *Aquilaria agallocha* and 30 other substances, including *Terminalia chebula, Terminalia belerica,* cardomum, saussurea, and sandalwood. Aloewood (a.ga.ru), *Aquilaria agallocha,* is its principal ingredient. The drug treats heart fevers, diseases of the life channel, and wind disease. Because of its slightly hot taste and its greasy power, as well as its warm, soft, dry qualities, it is considered an excellent medicinal for wind.

This medicine is used to treat a wide variety of disorders where an imbalance of the wind humor is indicated. These include emotional disorders, sleep disturbances, and symptoms such as dizziness. In these cases the powder prepared from the above ingredients is burned and inhaled. When mixed with melted butter, it may also be applied as an ointment to be massaged into related areas of the body. In this form it can be used for back pain.

Pomegranate Establish Essence, or "Say Dru Dwang Ma Nays" (se.'bru.dwangs.ma.gnas), is a useful illustration of an important formula with a limited number of ingredients. This medicine is used to strengthen the digestive processes in support of the "essence" or nutriment that is associated with the health of the body. It is indicated for conditions where phlegm and cold have impaired the digestive heat (digestive bile) and where phlegm and mucus are

said to have obstructed the channels. Some sources indicate its use in diabetes or leukemia with the appropriate presentation.

As discussed, pomegranate is considered a specific for stomach disorders, to support digestive heat and to treat cold and phlegm. Here again, the principal therapeutic agent gives the name to the formula. There are many variations of pomegranate formulas. Pomegranate Establish Essence has just five ingredients, which are blended proportionately (Box 24-6). The two major ingredients are pomegranate and safflower. Safflower (gur.gum), stigma crocus, or *Carthamus tinctorius,* treats liver disorders and is relevant here because the liver is the organ that converts food to blood and begins the process of establishing the essence of the body constituents. In addition, long pepper (pi.pi.ling) is a hot-tasting ingredient that treats cold disorders, and lesser cardamom (sug.smel) or *Elettaria cardamomum* is said to treat cold kidney. Cinnamon (shing.tsha) tastes hot, sweet, astringent, and salty. It also increases the heat of digestion and treats cold disorders of the stomach (see Table 24-3 p. 477).

The selection of an appropriate medicine for a disease according to its heat or coolness was and is a crucial aspect of therapy. It is said that if this is not done properly, the treatment has no hope of succeeding. Once the appropriate medicines are chosen, they are given to the patient at specific times of day according to the dominant humor. Thus a patient with a bile disease might receive a strong medicine to reduce bile at the time when it is most in the ascendant, noon.

Medicines are spiritual as well as material substances. Physicians will invite monks to come to their pharmacies and perform rituals and prayers to imbue the medicines with the healing power of the Medicine Buddha.

External Therapeutics

> The fourth trunk therapy has three branches: wind therapy, bile therapy and phlegm therapy.
> The first has two leaves, annointing with sesame oil and rubbing, and mongolian burning.
> The second has three leaves, sweating, venesection, and cold water bottle fomentation.
> The third has two leaves, burning and moxibustion.
>
> —The "Three Roots," from Padma Karpo's Commentary on the Four Tantras

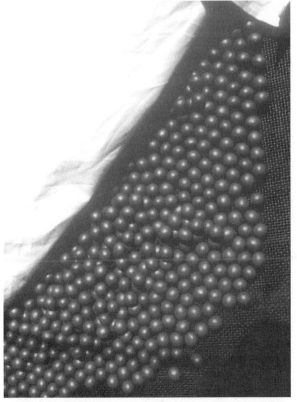

Figure 24-18 Finished Tibetan medicinal pills after drying and polishing. (Courtesy Windhorse, © Kevin Ergil, 1982.)

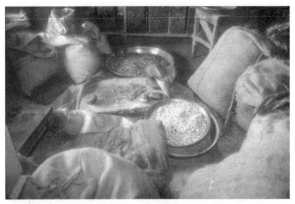

Figure 24-19 Fruit of the Chebulic myrobalan (a.ru.ra) that has had the seed removed from the dried flesh in preparation for grinding and mixing with other medicinals. Myrobalan fruit (a.ru.ra), *Terminalia chebula*, is said to treat diseases caused by wind, bile, and phlegm. (Courtesy Windhorse, © Kevin Ergil, 1982.)

The fourth trunk has three branches: wind therapy, bile therapy, and phlegm therapy. As with the other therapeutic methods, these are organized according to their qualitative effects on specific humors. Because wind has the characteristics of roughness and cold, therapies that are gentle, soothing, and warming are selected. The body is rubbed with oils and gentle heat applied to treat conditions that originate in a disturbance of the wind humor. Such a treatment might be appropriate for a wind condition where the skin feels tight, cracked, and rough and where any kind of physical contact is painful. Because bile conditions are characterized by heat, causing the body to sweat, bleeding and applying cold compresses are the methods chosen to release the heat of bile.

Phlegm, which is characterized by coldness and dampness, is treated with burning therapy and moxibustion. *Burning*, or cautery, involves the direct application of a heated instrument to a specific location on the body. Burning therapy can involve the use of a gemstone heated with friction or the application of a

---

BOX 24-6

Pomegranate Establish Essence

Se. 'bru.dwangs.ma.gnas	
Pomegranate	80 parts
Cinnamon bark	5 parts
Cardamom	5 parts
Long pepper	10 parts
Safflower flower	40 parts

heated iron. *Moxibustion* involves the burning of powdered herbs on the skin surface. A phlegm disorder that manifests in the bones might be treated with burning therapies of this type.

Three roots summarize a range of external or accessory therapies, which are presented in greater detail in the *Final Tantra*. Traditionally, therapies of this type are organized into two categories: gentle therapies and rough therapies. Rough therapies include techniques such as moxibustion, cautery (or burning), venesection, and the use of the golden needle (a distinctive form of acupuncture) (Figure 24-20). Gentle therapies include the use of oils and ointments, massage, soaking in herbal baths, and other types of bathing. Major and "petty" surgery has a history in Tibet as well. The practices described on this trunk are considered to be suitable when other therapies have been exhausted or have reached their maximum effect. These techniques are also used as preventive measures.

Surgery is said to have been practiced extensively in the Tibetan tradition at one time, but its practice has been limited to minor surgery. According to tradition, the mother of one of the ancient Tibetan kings lost her life during surgery that was intended to cure her. As a result, the son forbade the practice of surgery, and most surgery in Tibet was limited to minor surgical procedures. Based on the variety of medical practices in Tibet and the distances separating physicians, we have no way of knowing whether the king's ban was entirely honored. Also, other opinions existed. Some authorities believe that surgery was never extensively developed in the Tibetan tradition except for minor surgery, the treatment of wounds, the surgical treatment of hemorrhoids, bullet wounds, and infections, and that the allusions to more complex procedures are without basis in historical practice.

The status of acupuncture is somewhat contested in discussions of Tibetan medicine. Nothing closely resembling the developed acupuncture methodologies of China is specifically part of Tibetan tradition. However, there are techniques that bear points of similarity. Moxibustion and other types of burning therapy (including cautery), however, were widely used. Points suitable for acupuncture, for moxibustion and cautery, and for bleeding are vividly described in medical paintings (Figure 24-21).

There is a well-known method of external treatment in Tibetan medicine that is similar to the method of warming needles used in Chinese acupuncture. In Tibetan medicine this is known as the use of

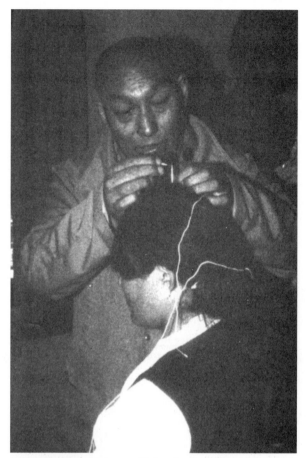

Figure 24-20 A patient suffering from severe headaches is treated with the golden needle and moxa. (Courtesy Windhorse, © Kevin Ergil, 1982.)

the "golden needle." A short, thick gold needle is shallowly inserted in the crown of the patient's head. Once this is in place, a dry herbal tinder is burnt on the head of the needle. The method is used to treat disturbed wind and can be used for severe headaches. Traditionally it is understood to cause the winds to move into the central channel. During this treatment the physician will invoke the Medicine Buddha and use his mantra to contribute to the healing process.

External Tibetan therapies include the following:

External Therapy for Wind
- *Anointing and rubbing:* The body is rubbed with sesame oil.
- *Mongolian burning:* A compress of hot oil and caraway seeds is prepared and applied to the skin.

External Therapy for Bile
- *Sweating:* The patient is wrapped in warm clothes to induce sweating.

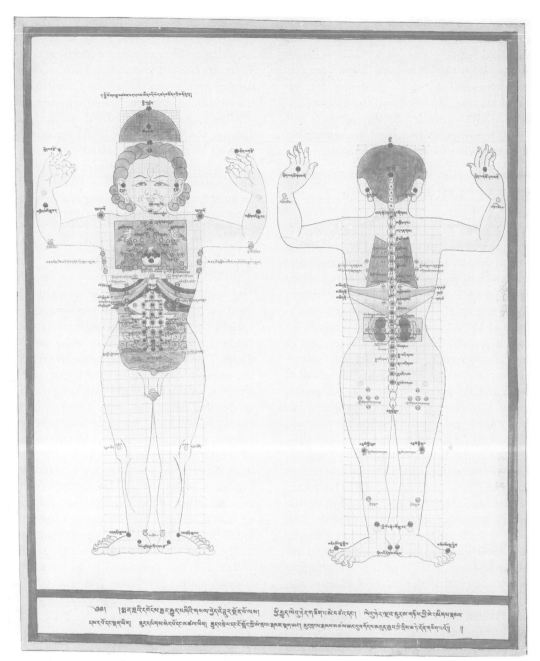

Figure 24-21 Bloodletting, surgical, and moxibustion locations on the body. (From Parfionovitch Y, Dorje G, Meyer F, editors: *Tibetan medical paintings: illustrations to the Blue Beryl treatise of Sangye Gamtso,* New York, 1992, Abrams.)

- *Venesection:* Small amounts of blood are taken from suitable veins.
- *Cold water application:* Cold water is applied to the patient.

External Therapy for Phlegm

- *Burning:* Instruments made of iron or other metals are heated and applied to selected points of the skin.

- *Moxibustion:* Powdered herbs are warmed or burned with powdered herbs.

Ultimately, all therapeutic methods in Tibetan medicine are linked directly to the physician's understanding of the patient's elemental and humoral situation. The method of treatment will be selected according to how these are understood. The goal of treatment is to bring the humors or faults into balance again and to remove the disease that their imbalance has engendered.

Additionally, the *Oral Instruction Tantra* contains extensive discussions of clinical strategies for the treatment of specific conditions and integrates the theoretical structure provided by the elements and humors with the empirically derived understanding of the best approaches for specific conditions.

CONTEMPORARY PRACTICE

Tibetan medicine is currently practiced in a surprising number of places. Its traditions, which embody the blending of practical therapy and compassion, are kept alive by Tibetan physicians in the Tibetan Autonomous Region (TAR), by Tibetan physicians in exile in India and Nepal, and by Tibetan physicians resident in many parts of the world. The government of H.H. Dalai Lama has made extensive efforts to preserve the traditions that were almost destroyed as a result of the invasion and the excesses of the cultural revolution. As mentioned earlier, in the TAR, where there has been relaxation of government restrictions on traditional Tibetan practices and a concerted effort since the late 1970s to provide greater support for the study and practice of Tibetan medicine, there are now centers for the study of Tibetan medicine as well as hospitals.

The Lhasa Mentsi Khang has increased in stature over the years. It came under the authority of the TAR government in 1980 and was established as a university around 1990. In addition, a 150-bed hospital was established in Lhasa in 1985. There now are a number of training facilities both within the TAR and in nearby areas such as Qing Hai Gansu, Yunan, and Sichuan. Industrial scale production of Tibetan herbal medicines is occurring. Research initiatives that focus on the tremendous knowledge of herbal medicine possessed by Tibetan physicians are beginning to emerge.

Organizations for the study and propagation of Tibetan medical traditions exist in England and the United States.

RESEARCH AND EVALUATION

Research in Tibetan medicine is not as extensively developed as the research activities that support the practices of acupuncture and herbal medicine in China, Japan, or Korea, or as those that support inquiry into the Ayurvedic materia medica in India. There are limited and isolated instances of preliminary inquiries into the use of Tibetan medicines in the treatment of cancers, and there have been minor studies in support of herbal products based on Tibetan medicines. There is some research on constituents of the Tibetan materia medica.

It is likely in the near term that the recently developed colleges and hospitals of Tibetan medicine will be the most promising source of studies exploring the clinical applications of these therapies in modern terms.

Acknowledgments

The contents of this chapter represent an engagement of longstanding with gso.rig and one that is entirely the result of the generosity of others. In particular Lama Thubten Yeshe, Geshe Jampel Thardo, Thepo Tulku, Dr. Yeshe Donden, Dr. Tenzin Trakpa, Dr. Pema Dorje, Dr. Lobsang Rabgyay, and Dr. Dawa Drolma, for their kindness in helping me to begin the study of Tibetan medicine. I owe a great deal of thanks to my very patient Tibetan teachers, especially Larry Epstein. I am, of course, dependent on the work of proper scholars in the field such as Barry Clark, Alan Wallace, Jeffrey Hopkins, Fernand Meyer, and Vincanne Adams, whose scholarship and enterprise in relationship to Tibetan medicine is of great benefit to many. My wife and colleague Marnae Ergil provided her invaluable skills as proofreader and editor, despite the demands of patients, students, and children. I owe especial thanks to my supremely patient editor, Dr. Marc Micozzi, who was kind enough to agree to this project and patient enough to wait for it to be completed.

References

Adams V: The sacred in the scientific: ambiguous practices of science in Tibetan medicine, *Cultur Anthropol* 16(4):542-575, 2001.

bdud.rtsi.snying.po.yan.lag. brgyud.pa.gsan.wa.men.nga. rgyud: *The Tibetan art of healing*, McLeod Ganj, India, 1971, Tibetan Medical Centre.

Clark B: *The quintessence tantras of Tibetan medicine*, Ithica, 1995, Snow Lion.

Dash B: Tibetan Medicine: with special reference to Yoga Sataka, 1976.

Dharamsala I: Library of Tibetan Works and Archives.

Donden Y, Tsering G: Methods of treatment in Tibetan medicine, *Tibet Med* 1:8-12, 1980.

Donden Y: *The ambrosia heart tantra*, Dharamsala, India, 1977, Library of Tibetan Works and Archives (Translated by J Kelsang).

Donden Y: *Health through balance: an introduction to Tibetan medicine*, Ithica, 1986, Snow Lion (Translated by J Hopkins, editor).

Ergil K: A discussion of the three roots of Tibetan medicine in the context of the treatment of rheumatism, Santa Cruz, CA, 1983, Semeiosis in Tibetan Medicine, University of Washington, 1987 (Unpublished MA thesis).

Finckh E: Tibetan medicine: theory and practice. In Aris M, Sun Kyi AS, editors: *Tibetan studies in honour of Hugh Richardson.* Proceedings of International Seminar on Tibetan Studies, Oxford, England, 1979, Aris & Phillips, pp 103-110.

Guenther HV: Early forms of Tibetan Buddhism, *Crystal Mirror* 3:80-92, 1974.

Hopkins J, Rinbochay L: *Death, intermediate state, and rebirth in Tibetan Buddhism*, Valois, New York, 1979, Gabriel.

Kunzang J, translator: *Tibetan medicine*, Berkeley, University of California Press.

Nor.Bu, mKHyen.Rab, et al: *Fundamentals of Tibetan medical practice*, Leh, 1974, sMan.Tsis.SHes.Rigs.sPen.dZod.

Padma dkarpo: rgyud bzhi'i 'grel-pa gzhan-la phan gteer. In *Collected works (gsun-'bum) of Kun-mkhyen Padma dKarpo* (Photo reproductions of 1920-1928 Gnam Brung se-ba byan-chub-glin-blocks) VI:325-476; Darjeeling, 1973, Kargyud Sangrab Nyamso.

Paul RA: *The Tibetan symbolic world*, Chicago, 1982, University of Chicago Press.

Rabgay L: The origin and growth of medicine in Tibet, *Tibet Med* 3:3-20, 1981.

Rabgay L: Urine analysis in Tibetan medicine, *Tibet Med* 3:53-60, 1981.

Sangs-rgyas-rgya-mtsho: Techniques of Lamaist medical practice being the text of man, ngag-yon-tan-rgyad-kyi-lhan-thabs-zug-rngai-tsha-gdang-sel-b'ai-kat-pu-ra-das-min-'chi-zhags-gcod-pa'i-ral-gri-sman-rtsis-shes-rig-spe-dzod. Vol 5, Leh, 1970, SW Tashigangpa.

Sarlson M: Herbal healing, *News Tibet* 3:6-7, 1981.

Selzer R: *Mortal lessons: notes of the art of surgery*, New York, 1974, Simon & Schuster.

Topgay S: Pharmacognosy in Tibetan medicine, *Tibet Med* 1:30-33, 1980.

Tsarong TJ, translator, editor: *Fundamentals of Tibetan medicine*, Dharamsala, India, 1981, Tibetan Medical Centre.

Tsering, N: Personal communication, 1980.

Suggested Readings

Avedon JF: *In exile from the land of snows*, New York, 1984, Knopf.

bdud.rtsi.snying.po.yan.lag.bryg.pa.gsan.men,nga.rgud: *The Tibetan art of healing*, London, 1979, Watkins.

Clark B: *The quintessence tantras of Tibetan medicine*, Ithica, 1995, Snow Lion.

Clifford T: *Tibetan Buddhist medicine and psychiatry*, York Beach, 1984, Samuel Weiser.

Donden Y: *Health through balance: an introduction to Tibetan medicine*, Ithica, 1986, Snow Lion (Translated by J Hopkins, editor).

Dorjee P, Richards E (editor): *150 Tibetan medicines*, McLeod Ganj, India, 1980, Tibetan Pharmaceutical Center.

Parfionovitch Y, Dorje G, Meyer F, editors: *Tibetan medical paintings: illustrations to the Bue Beryl treaeatis of Sangye Gamtso*, New York, 1992, Abrams.

Richardson HE: *A short history of Tibet*, New York, 1962, Dutton.

Website

Tibetan Medical and Astrological Institute: http://www.men-tsee-khang.org/

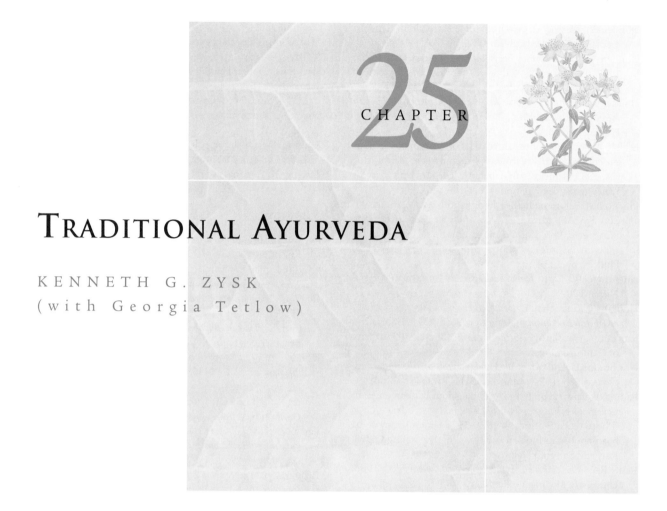

TRADITIONAL AYURVEDA

KENNETH G. ZYSK
(with Georgia Tetlow)

As health care professionals become better acquainted with the various forms of complementary, alternative, and integrative medical treatment, they often discover that India's traditional healing modality of Ayurveda is one of the world's oldest healing systems currently practiced. If only for this reason, health care practitioners who find themselves drawn to Ayurveda deserve the most reliable and up-to-date information about it. Therefore, the first part of this chapter discusses the fundamental principles and practices of traditional Ayurveda as understood from their original Sanskrit sources and traditional practitioners. The second part, devoted to the Ayurvedic clinical approach, offers specific maladies for which modern Ayurveda has shown effective results. The chapter concludes with a reading list of some of the most important sources on Ayurveda.

HISTORY

On the basis of available literary sources, the history of Indian medicine occurred in four main phases. The first, or "Vedic," phase dates from about 1200 to 800 BCE. Information about medicine during this period is obtained from numerous curative incantations and references to healing that are found in the *Atharvaveda* and the *Rigveda*, two religious scriptures that reveal a "magico-religious" approach to healing.

The second, or "classical," phase is marked by the advent of the first complete Sanskrit medical treatises, the *Caraka* and *Sushruta Samhitas*, which probably date from a few centuries before to several centuries after the start of the Common Era (CE). This period includes all subsequent medical treatises dating from before the Muslim invasions of India at the beginning of the eleventh century, since these works tend to follow the earlier classical compilations closely and provide the basis of traditional Ayurveda.

The third, or "syncretic," phase is marked by clear influences on the classical paradigm from Islamic or Unani, South Indian Siddha, and other nonclassical medical systems. *Bhavamishra's* sixteenth-century *Bhavaprakasha* is one text that reveals the results of these influences, which includes diagnosis by examination of pulse and urine. This phase extends from the Muslim incursions to the present era.

I would term the final or current phase as "New Age Ayurveda," wherein the classical paradigm is being adapted to the world of modern science and technology, including quantum physics, mind-body science, and advanced biomedical science. This recent manifestation of Ayurveda is most visible in the Western world, although much of New Age Ayurveda is filtering back to India.

These four phases of Indian medical history provide a chronological grid necessary to understanding the development of this traditional system of medicine.

THEORETICAL FOUNDATIONS

From its beginnings during the Vedic era, Indian medicine has always adhered closely to the principle of a fundamental connection between the microcosm and macrocosm. Humans are minute representations of the universe and contain within them everything that makes up the surrounding world. The interconnectedness of humans and their world makes it impossible to understand one completely without the other.

The Human Body

According to Ayurveda, the cosmos consists of five basic elements: earth, air, fire, water, and space or ether. Certain forces cause these to interact, giving rise to all that exists. In humans, these five elements combine in such a way as to produce the three *doshas*, psychophysical elements and forces that, along with the seven *dhatus* (tissues) and three *malas* (waste products), make up the human body.

The Three Doshas

The three doshas occur in varying amounts in every human body, and the proportion that is appropriate to an individual's body is called the person's innate, natural state, or *prakriti*, which is different for each person. When in equilibrium in the human body, the three doshas maintain health, but when an imbalance occurs among them, they defile the normal functioning of the body, leading to the manifestation of disease. An imbalance indicates an increase or decrease in one, two, or all three of the doshas. The three doshas are *Vata*, *Pitta*, and *Kapha*.

Vata, or *Vayu*, meaning "wind," is composed of the elements air and space. It is the principle of kinetic energy and is responsible for all bodily movement, evacuation, and nervous functions. It is located below the navel and in the bladder, large intestines, nervous system, pelvic region, thighs, bone marrow, and legs; its principal seat is the colon. When disrupted, its primary manifestation is gas and muscular or nervous energy, leading to pain.

Pitta, or bile, is made up of the elements fire and water. It governs enzymes and hormones and is responsible for digestion, pigmentation, body temperature, hunger, thirst, sight, courage, and mental activity. It is located between the navel and the chest and in the stomach, small intestines, liver, spleen, skin, and blood; its principal seat is the stomach. When disrupted, its primary manifestation is acid and bile, leading to inflammation.

Kapha, or *Shleshman*, meaning "phlegm," is made up of the elements of earth and water. It connotes the principle of cohesion and stability. It regulates Vata and Pitta and is responsible for keeping the body lubricated and maintaining its solid nature, tissues, sexual power, and strength. It also controls patience. Its normal locations are the upper part of the body, the thorax, head, neck, upper portion of the stomach, pleural cavity, fat tissues, and areas between joints; its principal seat is the lungs. When it is disrupted, its primary manifestation is fluids and mucus, leading to swelling, with or without discharge.

The attributes of each dosha help to determine the individual's basic bodily and mental makeup and to isolate which dosha or combination of doshas is responsible for a disease. The qualities of *Vata* are dryness, cold, light, irregularity, mobility, roughness, and abundance. Dryness occurs when Vata is disturbed and is a side effect of motion. Too much dryness produces irregularity in the body and mind. *Pitta* is hot, light, intense, fluid, liquid, putrid, pungent, and sour. Heat appears when Pitta is disturbed, resulting from change caused by Pitta. The intensity of excessive heat produces irritability in the body and mind. Kapha is heavy, unctuous, cold, stable, dense, soft, and smooth. Heaviness occurs when *Kapha* is disturbed and results from firmness caused by Kapha. The viscosity of excessive heaviness and stability produces slowness in body and mind.

The Seven Dhatus

The seven dhatus, or tissues, are responsible for sustaining the body. Each dhatu is responsible for the one that comes next in the following order:

1. *Rasa*, meaning "sap" or "juice," includes the tissue fluids, chyle, lymph, and plasma. It functions as nourishment and comes from digested food.
2. *Blood* includes the red blood cells and functions to invigorate the body.
3. *Flesh* includes muscle tissue and functions as stabilization.
4. *Fat* includes adipose tissue and functions as lubrication.
5. *Bone* includes bone and cartilage and functions as support.
6. *Marrow* includes red and yellow bone marrow and functions as filling for the bones.
7. *Shukra* includes male and female sexual fluids and functions in reproduction and immunity.

The Three Malas

The malas are the waste products of digested and processed food and drink. Ayurveda delineates three principal malas: *urine, feces,* and *sweat.* A fourth category of other waste products includes fatty excretions from the skin and intestines, ear wax, mucus of the nose, saliva, tears, hair, and nails. According to Ayurveda, an individual should evacuate the bowels once a day and eliminate urine six times a day.

Ayurveda considers digestion to be the most important function that takes place in the human body. It provides all that is required to sustain the organism and is the principal cause for all maladies from which an individual may suffer. The process of digestion and assimilation of nutrients is discussed under the topics of the *Agnis* (enzymes), *Ama* (improperly digested food and drink), and the *Srotas* (channels of circulation).

The Three Agnis

The Agnis, or enzymes, assist in the digestion and assimilation of food and are divided into three types, as follows:

- *Jatharagni* is active in the mouth, stomach, and gastrointestinal tract and helps break down food. The waste product of feces results from this activity.
- *Bhutagnis* are five enzymes located in the liver. They adapt the broken-down food into a homologous chyle according to the five elements and assist the chyle to assimilate with the corresponding five elements in the body. The homologous chyle circulates in the blood channels as rasa, nourishing the body and supplying the seven dhatus.
- *Dhatvagnis* are seven enzymes that synthesize the seven dhatus from the assimilated chyle homologized with the five elements. The remaining waste products result from this activity.

Ama

Ama, the chief cause of disease, is formed when there is a decrease in enzyme activity. A product of improperly digested food and drink, it takes the form of a liquid sludge that travels through the same channels as the chyle. Because of its density, however, it lodges in different parts of the body, blocking the channels. It often mixes with the doshas that circulate through the same pathways and usually gravitates to a weak or stressed organ or to a site of a disease manifestation. Because all diseases invariably come from Ama, the word *Amaya,* meaning "coming from Ama," is a synonym for disease. Internal diseases begin with Ama, and external diseases produce Ama. In general, Ama can be detected by a coating on the tongue; turbid urine with foul odor; and feces that is passed with undigested food, an offensive odor, or abundant gas. The principal course of treatment in Ayurveda involves the elimination of Ama and the restoration of the balance of the doshas.

The Thirteen Kinds of Srotas

The srotas are the vessels or channels of the body through which all substances circulate. They are either large, such as the large and small intestines, uterus, arteries, and veins, or small, such as the capillaries. A healthy body has open and free-flowing channels. Blockage of the channels, usually by Ama, results in disease. The 13 srotas are as follows:

1. Pranavahisrotas convey vitality and vital wind or breath *(prana)* and originate in the heart and alimentary tract.
2. Udakavahisrotas convey water and fluids and originate in the palate and pancreas.
3. Annavahisrotas convey food from the outside and originate in the stomach.
4. Rasavahisrotas convey chyle, lymph, and plasma and originate in the heart and in the 10 vessels connected with the heart. Ama primarily accumulates within them.
5. Raktavahisrotas convey red blood cells and originate in the liver and spleen.
6. Mamsavahisrotas convey ingredients for muscle tissue and originate in the tendons, ligaments, and skin.
7. Medovahisrotas convey ingredients for fat tissue and originate in the kidneys and fat tissues of the abdomen.
8. Asthavahisrotas convey ingredients for bone tissue and originate in hip bone.
9. Majjavahisrotas convey ingredients for marrow and originate in the bones and joints.
10. Shukravahisrotas convey ingredients for the male and female reproductive tissues and originate in the testicles and ovary, respectively.
11. Mutravahisrotas convey urine and originate in the kidney and bladder.
12. Purishavahisrotas convey feces and originate in the colon and rectum.
13. Svedavahisrotas convey sweat and originate in the fat tissues and hair follicles.

This broad outline shows Ayurveda understands that the human body's anatomical parts are composed of the five basic elements, which have undergone a process of metabolism and assimilation in the body. Humans differ, depending on their normal bodily constitution *(prakriti)*, which is determined at the moment of conception and remains until death. The four factors that influence constitutional type are (1) the father, (2) the mother (particularly her food intake), (3) the womb, and (4) the season of the year. A large imbalance of the doshas in the mother will affect the growth of the embryo and fetus, and a moderate excess of one or two of the doshas will affect the constitution of the child.

Prakriti

There are seven normal body constitutions based on the three doshas: *vata, pitta, kapha, vata-pitta, pitta-kapha, vata-kapha,* and *sama.* The last is a state in which all three occur in equal proportions. It is the best condition but is extremely rare. Most people are a combination of doshas, in which one dosha predominates. In general, vata-type people tend to be anxious and fearful, exhibit light and "airy" characteristics, and are prone to vata-diseases. Pitta-type people are aggressive and impatient, exhibit fiery and hot-headed characteristics, and are prone to pitta-diseases. Kapha-type people are stable and entrenched, if not sluggish at times; exhibit heavy, wet, and earthy characteristics; and are prone to kapha-diseases.

These are the principal factors that help the Ayurvedic physician determine the correct course of treatment to be administered to a patient for a particular ailment.

Three Mental States

In addition to physical constitution, Ayurveda understands that an individual is influenced by three mental states, which exhibit the three qualities *(gunas)* of balance *(sattva)*, energy *(rajas)*, and inertia *(tamas)*. In the state of balance the mind is in equilibrium and can discriminate correctly. In the state of energy the mind is excessively active, causing weakness in discrimination. In the state of inertia the mind is excessively inactive, also creating weak discrimination.

Ayurveda has always recognized that the body and the mind interact to create a healthy, normal (prakritic) or unhealthy, abnormal (vikritic) condition. An effective Ayurvedic physician will determine both the mental and the physical condition of the patient before proceeding with any form of diagnosis and treatment.

DISEASE

Aspects of the Ayurvedic understanding of disease are mentioned in the previous section. This section focuses specifically on the Ayurvedic classification of disease, the naming of disease, and the manifestations of disease.

Classification of Disease

Ayurveda identifies three broad categories of disease on the basis of causative factors.

Adhyatmika diseases originate within the body and may be subdivided into hereditary diseases, congenital disease, and diseases caused by one or a combination of the doshas.

Adhibhautika diseases originate outside the body and include injuries from accidents or mishaps and, in terms of modern science, from germs, viruses, and bacteria.

Adhidaivika diseases originate from supernatural sources, including diseases that are otherwise inexplicable, such as maladies stemming from providential causes, planetary influences, curses, and seasonal changes.

Disease Names

In Ayurveda, diseases receive their names in one of six ways. A disease is named for the misery it produces (fever, or *Jvara*), its chief symptom (diarrhea, or *Atisara*), its chief physical sign (jaundice, or *Pandu,* "yellowness"), its principal nature (piles, or *Arshas*), the chief dosha(s) involved (wind-disease, or *Vataroga*), or the chief organ involved (disease of the duodenum, or *Grahani*). Regardless of its given name, most diseases involve one or more of the doshas.

Manifestation of Disease

During the course of a disease, an Ayurvedic physician seeks to identify the malady's site of origin, its path of transportation, and its site of manifestation. The site of manifestation of a disease usually differs from its site of origin. Recognizing this distinction enables the physician to determine the correct course of treatment.

Ayurveda describes the manifestation of all diseases in the same fundamental way. Causative factors (e.g., food, drink, regimen, season, mental state) suppress enzyme activity in the body, leading to the formation of Ama. The circulating Ama blocks the channels. The site of the disease's origin is where the blockage occurs. The circulating Ama, often combining with one or more of the doshas, then takes a divergent course, referred to as the *path of transportation*. Finally, the mixture of dosha(s) and Ama comes to rest in and afflicts a certain body part, which is known as the site of *disease manifestation*. Treatment entails correction of all the steps in the process

leading to the disease's manifestation, thus restoring the entire person to his or her normal state (prakriti).

THERAPEUTICS

In Ayurveda, restoring a person to health is not viewed simply as the eradication of disease. It entails a complete process of diagnosis and therapeutics that takes into account both mental and physical components integrated with the social and physical worlds in which the patient lives, involving both immediate and long-term actions that often require changes in the patient's normal routine of life. Therefore this section briefly explains Ayurvedic diagnosis, examination of the disease, and types of therapeutics.

Ayurvedic Diagnosis

Ayurveda established a detailed system of diagnosis, involving examination of pulse, urine, and physical features.

After a preliminary examination by means of visual observation, touch, and questioning, the Ayurvedic physician may, if required, undertake a further eightfold method of detailed examination to determine more precisely the patient's abnormal condition.

Pulse Examination

Pulse examination is first mentioned in a medical treatise from the late thirteenth or early fourteenth century CE. It is a highly specialized art, often taking decades of practice finally to master. As a result, not every Ayurvedic physician uses pulse examination. The diagnostic process involves evenly placing the index, middle, and ring fingers of the right hand on the radial artery of the right hand of men and the left hand of women, just at the base of the thumb. A pulse resembling the movement of a snake at the index finger indicates a predominance of Vata; a pulse resembling the movement of a frog at the middle finger indicates a predominance of Pitta; a pulse resembling the movement of a swan or peacock at the ring finger indicates a predominance of Kapha; and a pulse resembling the movement of a woodpecker indicates a predominance of all three doshas. To obtain an accurate reading, the physician must keep in mind the times when each of the doshas is normally excited and should take the pulse at least three times early in the morning when the stomach is empty, or 3 hours after eating in the afternoon, making sure to wash his or her hands after each reading.

Urine Examination

As with pulse examination, urine examination probably was formalized in the syncretic phase of Indian medical history and may have come into Ayurveda from the Arabic Unani medical system. After collecting the morning's midstream evacuation in a clear glass container, the physician submits the urine to two kinds of examination after sunrise. First, the physician studies it in the container to determine its color and degree of transparency. Pale-yellow and unctuous urine indicates Vata; intense yellow, reddish, or blue urine indicates Pitta; white, foamy, and muddy urine indicates Kapha; urine with a blackish tinge indicates a combination of doshas; and urine resembling lime juice or vinegar indicates Ama. The physician also puts a few drops of sesame oil in the urine and examines it in sunlight. The shape, movement, and diffusion of the oil in the urine indicate the prognosis of the disease. The shape of the drops also reveals which dosha(s) is involved. A snakelike shape indicates Vata; umbrella shape, Pitta; and pearl shape, Kapha.

Examination of Bodily Parts

The physician concludes the diagnostic examination with careful scrutiny of the tongue, skin, nails, and physical features to determine which dosha(s) is affected. Using the basic characteristics of each of the doshas, the physician will examine the different parts of the body. Coldness, dryness, roughness, and cracking indicate Vata; hotness and redness indicate Pitta; and wetness, whiteness, and coldness indicate Kapha.

Having completed this phase of the diagnosis, the Ayurvedic physician proceeds to examine any malady present.

Examination of the Disease

A detailed examination of the disease involves a five-step process, leading to a complete understanding of the abnormality.

Etiology

A disease results from one or several of the following factors: mental imbalances resulting from the effects of past actions (*karman*); unbalanced contact between the senses and the objects of the senses affecting the body and the mind; effects of the seasons on the mental and doshic balance; and the immediate causes of diet, regimen, and microorganisms; doshas and Ama; and the combined interaction of individual components such as doshas and tissues or doshas and microorganisms.

Early Signs and Symptoms

Early signs and symptoms that appear before the onset of disease provide clues to the diagnosis. Proper diet and administration of medicine can avert disease if it is recognized early enough.

Manifest Signs and Symptoms

The most crucial step in the diagnostic process is manifest signs and symptoms. Their recognition involves determining the site of origin and of manifestation and of the path of transportation of the Ama and dosha(s). Most signs and symptoms are associated with the site of disease manifestation, from which the physician must work his or her way back to the site of the origin of disease to effect a proper diagnosis and complete cure. Although symptomatic treatment was largely absent in traditional Ayurveda, modern medicine in India has introduced Ayurvedic physicians to techniques of symptomatic treatment in cases of acute disease. This reflects a type of symbiotic relationship that has occurred between modern biomedical medicine and Ayurveda in India.

Exploratory Therapy

Exploratory therapy involves 18 different experiments that use drugs, diet, and regimens to determine the precise nature of the malady and suitable therapy by allopathic and homeopathic means.

Pathogenesis

Pathogenesis is a six-step process that determines the manner by which a dosha becomes aggravated and moves through the different channels to produce disease. An accumulation of a dosha leads to its aggravation, which causes it to spread through the channels until it lodges in a particular organ of the body, bringing about a manifestation of disease. Once a general form of the disease appears, it progressively splits into specific varieties. As in systems of medicine worldwide, many patients consult the

Ayurvedic physician only after their diseases have already appeared.

Ayurveda delineates seven basic varieties of disease on the basis of the doshas: diseases involving a single dosha, diseases involving two doshas, and diseases involving all three doshas together.

Prognosis is the final step in the Ayurvedic diagnostic process. Because Ayurvedic physicians traditionally did not treat persons with incurable diseases, it was important for the physician to know precisely the patient's chances of full recovery. Therefore, disease is one of three types. It is easily curable, palliative, or incurable or difficult to cure. In general, if the disease type (Vata, Pitta, Kapha) differs from the person's normal constitution, the disease is easy to cure. If the disease and constitution are the same, the disease is difficult to cure. If the disease, constitution, and season correspond in doshic type, the disease is almost impossible to cure through Ayurvedic means.

Having determined the patient's normal constitution (*prakriti*), diagnosed his or her illness, and established a prognosis for recovery, the Ayurvedic physician can begin a proper course of treatment.

Ayurvedic Treatment

Ayurveda recognizes two courses of treatment on the basis of the patient's condition. The first is *prophylaxis*, for the healthy person who wants to maintain a normal condition based on his or her physical constitution and to prevent disease. The second is *therapy*, for an ill person who requires health to be restored. Once the patient is healthy, Ayurveda recommends continuous prophylaxis based on diet, regimen, medicines, and regular therapeutic purification procedures, often requiring significant changes in the patient's lifestyle.

When a person is diagnosed with a doshic imbalance, purification therapy, alleviation therapy, or a combination of these is prescribed.

Purification Therapy

Purification therapy involves the fundamental *Pañchakarma*, or "Five Action" treatment. The fivefold process varies slightly in different traditions and regions of India, but a standard regimen generally is followed. All five procedures can be performed, or a selection of procedures can be chosen on the basis of different factors, such as the physical constitution of the patient, his or her condition, the season, and the nature of the disease. Before any therapeutic action is taken, the patient is given oil internally and externally (with massage) and is sweated to soften and loosen the dosha(s) and Ama. An appropriate diet of food and drink is prescribed. After this twofold preparatory treatment, called *Purvakarman*, the five therapies are administered in sequence over about a week.

Because of the profound effects on the mind and body, the patient is advised to set aside time for treatment. First, the patient might be given an emetic and vomits until bilious matter is produced, thus removing Kapha. Second, a purgative is given until mucous material appears, thus removing Pitta. Third, an enema, either of oil or decocted medicines, is administered to remove excess Vata. Fourth, head purgahon is given in the form of smoke inhalation or nasal drops to eradicate the dosha(s) that have accumulated in the head and sinuses. Fifth, leeches may be applied and bloodletting performed to purify the blood. Some physicians do not consider bloodletting in the five therapies of *Pañchakarma*, instead counting oily and dry enemas as two separate forms. The latter uses decocted medicines.

Alleviation Therapy

Alleviation therapy uses the basic condiments honey, butter or ghee, and sesame oil or castor oil to eliminate Kapha, Pitta, and Vata, respectively. This therapy and Pañchakarma often are used in conjunction with one another.

PHARMACEUTICS

Ayurveda prescribes a rich store of natural medicines that have been collected, tested, and recorded in medical treatises from ancient times. The tradition of collecting and preserving information about medicines in recipe books called *Nighantus* continues to the present. The most traditional source of Ayurvedic medicine is the kitchen. It is likely that, at an early stage of its development, Indian medical and culinary traditions worked hand in hand with each other.

Because of the close association between food and medicine, Ayurveda classifies foods and drugs (usually vegetal) by the tongue, potency, and taste after digestion and by special power.

Rasa, taste by the tongue, is categorized into six separate tastes, with their individual elemental composition and doshic effect as follows:

1. Sweet, composed of earth and water, increases Kapha and decreases Pitta and Vata.
2. Sour, composed of earth and fire, increases Kapha and Pitta and decreases Vata.
3. Saline, composed of water and fire, increases Kapha and Pitta and decreases Vata.
4. Pungent, composed of wind and fire, increases Pitta and Vata and decreases Kapha.
5. Bitter, composed of wind and space, increases Vata and decreases Pitta and Kapha.
6. Astringent, composed of wind and earth, increases Vata and decreases Pitta and Kapha.

Virya, potency, comprises eight types that are divided into four pairs: hot-cold, unctuous-dry, heavy-light, and dull-sharp.

Vipaka, postdigestive taste, identifies three kinds of aftertaste: sweet, sour, and pungent.

Prabhava, special power, is unique to the Ayurvedic pharmacopoeia. It refers to the drugs particular power or effect, which is known by means of a symbolic association rather that by rational and empirical means. For example, a certain type of cow's milk is effective as an aphrodisiac, when it has been fortified by a process which involves its warming by means of plunging heated golden rings into it, since it is believed that the milk and the rings symbolize respectively semen and the vagina, which in turn represent the Hindu deities Shiva and his female consort Parvati.

Contrary foods and drugs must always be avoided. For example, clarified butter and honey should not be taken in equal quantities, alkalies and salt must not be taken for a long period, milk and fish should not be consumed together, and honey should not be heated or be put in hot drinks.

Four important criteria are always considered when compounding plant substances and other ingredients into medical recipes. The substances that make up the recipe (1) should have many attributes that enable it to cure several diseases, (2) should be usable in many pharmaceutical preparations, (3) should be suitable for the recipe and not cause unwanted side effects, and (4) should be culturally appropriate to the patients and their customs. Every medicine should be able to treat the disease's site of origin, site of manifestation, and its spread simultaneously.

A brief survey of the different types of medical preparations indicates the depth and content of Ayurvedic pharmaceuticals. The botanically based medicines derive largely from the Ayurvedic medical tradition, whereas the mineral and inorganic-based drugs derive from the Indian Alchemical traditions, called Rasashastra, which became part of Ayurveda after about 800 CE.

1. *Juices* are cold-presses and extractions made from plants.
2. *Powders* are prepared from parts of plants that have been dried in the shade and other dried ingredients.
3. *Infusions* are parts of plants and herbs that have been steeped in water and strained.
4. *Cold infusions* are parts of plants and herbs that were soaked in water overnight and filtered the next morning.
5. *Decoctions* are vegetal products boiled in a quantity of water proportionate to the hardness of the plant part and then reduced by a fourth. It is then filtered and often used with butter, honey, or oils.
6. *Medicated pastes and oils.* Often the plant and herbal extracts are combined with other ingredients and formed into pastes, plasters, and oils. Used externally, pastes and plasters are applied for joint, muscular, and skin conditions, and oil is used for hair and head problems. Medicated oils also are used for massages and enemas.
7. *Large and small pills and suppositories.* Plant and herbal extracts are also formed into pills and suppositories to be used internally.
8. *Alcoholic preparations are made by fermentation or distillation.* Two preparations are delineated. One requires the drug to be boiled before it is fermented or distilled, and in the other, the drug, is simply added to the preparation. Fifteen percent is the maximum allowable amount of alcohol content in a drug. Several Ayurvedic medicines are prepared from minerals and metals and are derived ultimately from ancient traditions or later forms of medical alchemy.
9. *Sublimates* are prepared by an elaborate method leading to the sublimation of sulfur in a glass container. They are found in recipes (Rasayanas) used in rejuvenation therapies.
10. *Bhasmas* are ash residues produced from the calcination of metals, gems, plants, and animal

products. Most are metals and minerals that are first detoxified and then purified. An important bhasma is prepared from mercury, which undergoes an 18-stage detoxification and purification process. Ayurveda maintains that bhasmas are quickly absorbed in the blood and increase the red blood cells.

11. *Pishtis* are fine powders made by trituration of gems with juices and extracts.
12. *Collyrium* is made from antimony powder, lead oxide, or the soot from lamps burned with castor oil. Collyrium is used especially to improve vision.

Space does not allow a discussion of the individual plants used in Ayurvedic recipes. It is safe to say, however, that of the hundreds of plants and medical formulas mentioned in various Ayurvedic treatises, only a small portion are commonly used by most Ayurvedic physicians.

AYURVEDIC CLINICAL APPROACH

As mentioned, the first step undertaken in modern clinical Ayurveda is proper diagnosis of the patient and his or her condition. The general diagnostic procedure determines the individual's overall health and strength and the specific morbidity from which the person is suffering. The first step focuses on establishing the patient's normal doshic state, or prakriti, and assessing his or her mental and physical strength. The second step aims at identifying the illness from which the patient suffers in terms of the dosha(s) involved and the dhatus involved and srotas in which it is located. A specific name of a disease is not necessary if the twofold process of diagnosis is executed properly. The Ayurvedic doctor, Vaidya, now knows the patient's strength and weakness and the anatomical and physiological areas affected. Correct therapeutic treatment follows from this diagnosis.

Ayurvedic therapies are designed to rebalance and reintegrate the individual. They are classified as "toning" and "reducing" and are intended either to nourish deficiencies and tissue weakness or to detoxify and reduce aggravated doshas. Reduction usually comes first, followed by restoration therapies to rebuild the body's strength.

Reduction is often prescribed for Kapha disorders and toning for Vata disorders, whereas Pitta disorders normally require a mixture of both therapies. Reduction therapy itself is divided into two parts: palliation and purification. Palliation consists of strengthening the digestive fire, reducing Ama, and calming the excess doshas so that they can be removed during purification. Purification therapy involves five cleansing therapies, *Pañchakarma*.

An example of a specific disease illustrates the traditional Ayurvedic clinical approach. In Sanskrit terminology, the malady *Amavata* refers approximately to arthritic and rheumatic conditions.

Amavata (Arthritis)

As the word itself indicates, *Amavata* involves both Ama and the dosha Vata (wind). Traditional Ayurveda does not distinguish types of arthritis. This disease is caused by all factors that lead to the formation of Ama: unwholesome foods and regimens, bad digestive power, insufficient exercise, and excessive intake of unctuous foods and meat. The site of origin is principally the colon, but the entire alimentary canal is involved. Contrary foods and mental disturbance aggravate Vata and lead to the formation of Ama in the colon. Ama, forced by Vata, leaves the site of origin and affects the enzymes, causing Ama to form at every level. Ama then becomes lodged in the joints and the heart, the sites of manifestation. The path of transport is the *Rasavahasrotas*, the channels transporting chyle, lymph, and plasma.

Vata is the principal dosha affected. With the aggravation of Vata, symptoms include severe pain in the joints, rough skin, distention of the stomach, and indigestion. If Pitta is involved, a burning sensation spreads all over the body, especially in the joints. If Kapha is involved, the patient gradually becomes crippled. Little pain is experienced in the early morning because Ama is just beginning to move.

Both the ancient and the modern Ayurvedic treatments of Amavata involve therapeutic actions, medicines, and procedures to reduce Ama and alleviate Vata. The first course of action is to put the patient on a mild fast and to administer medicines that have a bitter taste, hot potency, and pungent postdigestive taste, all of which help to reestablish the digestive powers. Sweating might be recommended to aid the digestive process.

The second step of the treatment involves the purification therapy of *Pañchakarma*. The two preparatory actions, oleation and sweating, are administered first to soften and to dislodge the Ama. The remaining five procedures are performed over a week, during which time the patient maintains a strict diet. These actions will eradicate the dislodged Ama from the system and restore the balance of the doshas, especially Vata. One of two types of enema will be used, depending on the amount of Ama present. If Ama persists, an enema with decoctions is administered until Ama is removed, when an oily enema is given.

After the *Pañchakarma* therapy, the patient should assume a regimen that includes avoiding sleep during the day and after meals, as well as heavy foods that hinder digestion. Effective treatment of arthritic conditions, especially in children (childhood arthritis is an all too common disease in India), has included wet massage therapy in conjunction with the enemas of *Pañchakarma*. The affected areas are patted with a cloth bag filled with rice that has been cooked with milk and herbs. Massages with oils also are routinely prescribed.

Cancer (No Sanskrit equivalent in classic Ayurveda)

According to modern Ayurveda, under the influence of cancer, as defined by modern biomedical science, the three doshas destroy rather than preserve and nourish the body. Vata causes normal cells to proliferate and become cancerous. Pitta steals nutrients from other tissues *(dhatus)* to feed cancerous cells, and Kapha allows these cells to increase unchecked. Although cancer regulates the activities of all three doshas, it usually begins by domination in one. A doshic imbalance, accompanied by an overaccumulation of Ama and insufficient digestive fire, sets the stage for cancer. In addition, modern Ayurveda recognizes an intimate link between suppressed emotion and suppressed immunity. Other proposed factors include devitalized foods, a sedentary lifestyle, long-term exposure to radiation or chemical carcinogens, and a lack of spiritual purpose or effort in life.

Because Ama is one of the primacy causes and enablers of cancer, detoxification is the primary therapy. *Pañchakarma* rids the body of both Ama and any excessive accumulation of doshas. In modern Ayurveda, cancer is classified into Vata, Pitta, and Kapha varieties, according to the nature of the tumors themselves, the color of the patient's skin, the patient's demeanor, and other symptoms. Patients are put on powerful blood-cleansing herbs, strong circulatory stimulants, immune-strengthening tonics, and special Kapha-dispelling herbs. Specific anticancer herbs are administered differently for Vata, Pitta, or Kapha to obtain maximum assimilation. Vata patients are advised to imbibe fresh ginger tea with their herbs; Pitta patients should use aloe gel; and Kapha patients take honey and black pepper.

JVARA ROGA (FEVER)

Both traditional and modern Ayurveda views fever as both a disease and a symptom. Fever is also considered a positive sign when it indicates the loosening and release of Ama. Therefore, fever is often allowed to run its course unless one of the following is involved: fever that is both high and prolonged, a child who has had a febrile seizure in the past, or the individual who is rapidly becoming depleted. Causes other than infection include the wrong combination of foods (e.g., hot with cold, fruit with starch, bananas with milk), emotions such as excessive anger or fear, and overwork.

Vata fever is more likely to occur during the time of day when vata is most active (i.e., dawn or dusk) or during the fall. Pitta fever appears more often at midday and midnight and during the summer months. Kapha fever is noticed frequently in morning and evening and during late winter and spring.

In terms of pathogenesis, Vata fever begins in the colon, as is often the case in Vata disorders. An excess of Vata in the colon cools the digestive fire of the stomach and pushes it into the channels for transporting lymph, chyle, and plasma *(rasavahasrotas)*. Eventually this fire makes its way through the chyle into the blood and heats the blood.

Vata fever may be accompanied by shivering, tremors, extreme body ache, or headache. Constipation, insomnia, intense fatigue, and lower backache may also be present.

Pitta fever begins like a Vata fever, when the digestive fire in the stomach and small intestine are pushed out of their respective seats into the Rasavahasrotas. Symptoms include red eyes, diarrhea, nausea, vomiting, rash, nosebleeds, perspiration, and aversion to light. Pitta fever can cause severe dehydration and a significant reduction in blood pressure. It may be caused by alcohol abuse or consumption of very sour or fermented food. Aspirin is contraindicated in Pitta fever because it may damage the stomach lining.

Kapha fever occurs when the body produces excessive Kapha secretions in the stomach and dampens the digestive fire. With the fire diminished, undigested food accumulates in the stomach, and Ama increases; then, both Kapha and Ama are forced into the Rasavahasrotas. Precursor symptoms include runny nose, cold, and congestion. Causes may be overexposure to cold or improper combination of foods, especially when milk is involved. The fever itself is often low grade in nature; cough, breathlessness, or chest pain may be present. Laryngitis, hoarseness, sinus congestion, and sinus headache can be accompanying symptoms. Complete loss of appetite usually occurs during and for several days after the fever. The patient may feel heavy and dull and may have cold and clammy skin.

In addition to Vata, Pitta, and Kapha types of fevers, Ayurveda also recognizes and specifically treats fevers caused by intestinal parasites, continuous versus fluctuating fevers, and fevers that affect each of the seven tissues (dhatus).

Dhamani Pratichaya (Hypertension)

Because the heart regulates both the venous and the arterial systems, modern Ayurvedic practitioners believe that high venous blood pressure (sirabhinodhana) and arterial hypertension (dhamani pratichaya) are equally important in understanding blood pressure disorders. Arterial hypertension, the most common type, is examined here. Modern Ayurveda considers it a tridoshic disorder (i.e., one that can be caused by imbalances in any of the three doshas). With all types of hypertension, Ayurveda recommends that the patient follow a lifestyle and diet that reduce the primary aggravating dosha. In addition, caffeine, salt, sugar, and fatty or fried foods should be eliminated. Deep-breathing exercises, daily walk of at lease 3 miles, and meditation are recommended.

The disease pathway differs in each type of hypertension. In Vata-type hypertension, an excess of Vata dosha may lead to an accumulation of toxins in the colon. They are then absorbed into the blood, causing constriction of the blood vessels, especially the arteries. Blood pressure may rise and fall suddenly, the pulse may be erratic, and the diastolic pressure is often higher than the systolic pressure. The tongue may be dry, and the patient may experience insomnia. Puffiness under the eyes and constipation are also common. Colonic cleansing, often with a medicated enema, is the initial treatment, followed by a Vata-balancing diet that includes plenty of fish and the oily vitamins A, E, and D. Garlic is also recommended, especially with milk.

In Pitta-type hypertension, toxins from undigested foodstuffs in the small intestine can cause increased viscosity of the blood. Symptoms may include a violent headache, flushed face, red eyes, nosebleeds, sensitivity to light, anger, irritability, and a burning sensation. Both systolic and diastolic pressures tend to increase. Bitter herbs are prescribed, including aloe vera gel, bayberry, and Katuka, and purgation is recommended. The herb gotu kola is given to calm the mind, and other special herbal formulas act to pacify the Pitta dosha.

Kapha-type hypertension originates in the stomach. Kaphic mucosal secretions responsible for the production of triglycerides can overproduce the fatty molecules and cause increased blood viscosity and eventually arterial sclerosis. Symptoms often include obesity, tiredness, edema, hypothyroidism, and elevated cholesterol. Both systolic and diastolic pressures increase somewhat, but diastolic pressure may not rise as much as in Pitta hypertension. Dairy and high-fat foods should be aggressively eliminated, and appropriate herbs include cayenne, myrrh, garlic, motherwort, and hawthorn berries. Ayurveda recommends the use of diuretics only in Kapha hypertension.

Astmya (Allergies)

Modern Ayurveda understands allergies in terms of "changed reactivities," whose root cause is the body's weakened metabolism in one or more of the seven tissues (dhatus) of the body. Categories of allergic reactions are classified according to Vata, Pitta, and Kapha. All immediate, anaphylactic reactions are classified as Pitta-type, all intermittent allergies as Vata-Pitta–type or Vata-Kapha–type, and all delayed allergies, for example, seasonal sensitivities, as Kapha-type.

Vata-type allergic symptoms include headache, coughing, sneezing, gas, aches, and pains; sensitivity to dirt, dust, and pollens; heart palpitation; muscle spasms; nightmares; and wheezing. Patients having these allergies may be sensitive to nightshades (potato, tomato, eggplant), black beans, chick peas, and other beans. Emotionally, they are likely to experience anxiety, fear, insecurity, or hyperactivity. A Vata-pacifying diet is advised, along with appropriate Vata-reducing herbs.

Pitta-type symptoms include contact dermatitis, eczema, rash, acne, infections, heat and light sensitivity, insect bites, and sensitivity to foam mattresses, formaldehyde, and preservatives. Reactions to strawberries, bananas, grapefruit, eggs, carrots, onions, garlic, spicy food, pork, and some cheese products are considered Pitta allergies. A Pitta-pacifying diet and Pitta-pacifying herbs are recommended.

Kapha-type allergies include hay fever, bronchial asthma, laryngeal edema, colds, generalized edema, latent spring fever, allergic rhinitis, runny nose, teary eyes, and reactions to some forms of pollen. Individuals may be sensitive to avocado, bananas, lemons, watermelons, cucumbers, beef, lamb, pork, peanuts, and dairy products. A Kapha-reducing diet and teas are prescribed. The thymus gland and spleen play an important role in immunity and increased allergen reactivity. The warming (*agni*) factor of the thymus helps to maintain immunity, and its weakness may be one of the causes of Kapha-type allergies. The spleen is considered the root of the hematopoietic system and, according to modern Ayurvedic theory, not only acts as a blood reservoir but also contains components that destroy foreign particles and microorganisms. Any weakness in the spleen, detectable through Ayurvedic pulse diagnosis, is likely to be found in individuals prone to allergies.

Shira Shula (Headache)

According to both traditional and modern Ayurveda, headaches have many causes, including constipation, indigestion, colds and flu, poor posture, lack of sleep, overwork, stress, and muscle tension. Severe headaches or migraines specifically are thought to relate to congenital factors and are most often caused by Vata and Pitta imbalance.

Treatment for general headaches and migraines is similar. Diagnosis is based on identification of Vata,

Pitta, or Kapha symptoms. Vata headaches are characterized by extreme pain, anxiety, depression, constipation, and dry skin. The condition may worsen with lack of sleep, excessive activity, irregular lifestyle, and worry or stress. Pitta headaches involve burning sensation, red eyes and face, irritability, anger, light sensitivity, and sometimes nosebleeds. Often liver problems accompany the condition, or toxicity in the blood is detected. Kapha headaches, although usually not migraine in nature, bring feelings of tiredness, heaviness, and a dull ache. There may be nausea, phlegm, vomiting, or excess salivation. Often, Kapha headaches are caused by an accumulation of Kapha in the head and may be accompanied by pulmonary disorders.

Decongestant and expectorant herbs are selected for Kapha- or Vata-type sinus and congestive headaches, which are usually associated with common colds, coughs, or allergies. These herbs include calamus, ginger, bayberry, angelica, and wild ginger. Tulsi, holy basil, makes an excellent tea, and camphor, wintergreen, and eucalyptus provide effective soothing oils. If toxicity in the colon (Vata) is responsible for the headache, purgation is recommended. Herbal sedatives are also indicated to restore regular and restful sleep. If Pitta is to blame, the liver should be cleansed with aloe powder or rhubarb root. Sandalwood oil may be applied to the head for cooling purposes, and the herb gotu kola should be taken internally. Sun and heat should be avoided, and Pitta-pacifying fragrances, such as rose or lotus, should be inhaled. Application of medicated oils on the head and in the nose is prescribed in all forms of headaches, especially in migraines.

Meditation and yoga postures are extremely helpful for dealing with tension headaches and migraines. Another powerful tool is the Ayurvedic healing subsystem known as *Marman therapy*. Ayurveda had identified 107 specific points of the body, called *Marmans*, which, being the vulnerable points on the human body, are extremely sensitive to the touch. They are also effective for maintaining tridoshic balance. Known as "doors to the organs" and "gates of the doshas," marman points are accessible through the skin and intended to enhance immunity, raise serotonin levels, and increase other hormone secretions of the pineal gland. Five sets of marmam points are indicated for headache. They are located on the head and face, at the base of the eyebrows (above the tear ducts), on either side of the nose (a third way down), above the upper lip (evenly between the upper lip and base of the septum), and at the third eye (pineal) and at the top of the head.

Parinama Shula (Peptic Ulcer [Gastric and Duodenal])

In modern Ayurveda, peptic ulcers, often associated with excess stomach acid, involve painful inflammation of the mucous lining of the stomach. Unlikely factors such as shock, burns, and head injuries are thought to stimulate production of hydrochloric acid and create peptic ulcers, in addition to the more classic causative models involving the doshas. Each of the three doshas can cause stomach ulcers. For example, the nervousness and excessive mental activity characteristic of high-Vata can lead to stress, overwork, and potentially an ulcer. Aggression, frustration, and anger, classic high-Pitta symptoms, can lead to hyperacidity. A deficiency of the mucous secretions of the stomach (Kapha imbalance) can allow a normal or even low amount of stomach acid to burn through the lining of the stomach. The following prodromal symptoms are enumerated in Ayurveda: heartburn, belching of sour fluids, and perhaps nausea and vomiting. Those afflicted may have eaten an overabundance of sour or spicy food, greasy food, alcohol, or simply overate in general. *Amla Pitta* (hyperacidity), a common precursor to an ulcer, may be accompanied by migraine headache. Metabolism may become impaired, and vomiting may help the sufferer feel better. Pain between meals, but not during, may indicate a duodenal ulcer.

Ulcers can be classified into Vata-, Pitta-, and Kapha-type. In Vata-type ulcers there is more gas in the stomach, with radiating-like pain. In Pitta-type there is localized, sharp and penetrating pain that causes patients to waken in the middle of the night. Perforated ulcers are more likely in Pitta-type cases. Kapha-type ulcers are accompanied by dull, deep, and bearable pain.

For all types of ulcers, a Pitta-pacifying diet is given. It excludes all spicy and sour foods and citrus products, includes antacid foods such as milk or ghee, and prioritizes bland whole grains such as basmati rice. A milk fast may be recommended. An emphasis is placed on easy-to-digest foods. Alcohol and smoking should be avoided. The herbal compound *Avipattikara* is especially recommended for

ulcers and should be taken before meals. After meals, the herbal formula of Shatavari, Jatamamsi, and *Kamadudha* is recommended. A powerful remedy, Sat Isabgol, thought to seal a bleeding ulcer, may be taken with milk before sleep. Other specific herbal remedies are used if a duodenal ulcer causes blood to be passed in the stool.

CONCLUSION

Traditional Ayurveda is a sophisticated system of medicine that has been practiced in one form or another India for the last 2500 years. As with other forms of alternative, complementary, and integrative medicine, it focuses on the whole organism and its relation to the external world to reestablish and maintain the harmonious balance that exists within the body and between the body and its environment. Only a glimpse of this ancient form of medicine has been offered; there is much to be learned from a deeper exploration of Ayurveda. Studies of Ayurveda and related traditions in Tibetan medicine are being undertaken in India, Europe, and North America. Several Ayurvedic universities in India have designed special courses of Ayurvedic study for Westerners, ranging from 2 weeks to several years. Gujarat Ayurvedic University in Jamnagar and the faculty of Ayurvedic Medicine, Banaras Hindu University, Varanasi, India, are recommended.

Very few reliable sources for traditional Ayurveda are available in English. Most of the sound works are by and for specialists and are virtually inaccessible to the reader without knowledge of Sanskrit. To provide information on Ayurveda, the reputable Indian publisher with a worldwide distribution, Motilal Banarsidass, has undertaken the publication of a series of books devoted to Indian medicine, entitled *Indian Medical Tradition Series*, under the editorship of K.G. Zysk in Copenhagen and D. Wujastyk in London. It is specifically aimed at providing authoritative and reliable publications on the Indian medical traditions for the general public, health care professionals, and scholars. The series, whose currently available volumes are listed below by author, includes a selection of important classic studies, original works on specialized topics of Indian medicine and of Indian medical history, as well as rare and obscure texts and works on Indian medicine. A selective list of trustworthy and available books in English on traditional Ayurveda follows.

Suggested Readings

Das RP: *The origin of the life of a human being,* Indian Medical Tradition Series, vol 6, Delhi, 2003, Motilal Banarsidass.

Dash B: *Fundamentals of Ayurvedic medicine,* Delhi, 1980, Bansal.

Dash B, Kashyap L: *Basic principles of Ayurveda based on Ayurveda Saukhyam of Todarananda,* New Delhi, 1980, Concept Publishing.

Jolly J: *Indian medicine,* New Delhi, 1977, Munshiram Manoharlal (Translated by GC Kashikar).

Lad V: *Ayurveda: the science of self-healing,* Wilmot, Wis, 1990, Lotus Press.

Leslie C: *Asian medical systems,* Indian Medical Tradition Series, vol 3, New Delhi, 1998, Motilal Banarsidass.

Meulenbeld GJ: *A history of indian medical literature,* vols 1-3, Groningen, 1999-2002, Egbert Forsten.

Meulenbeld, GJ, Wujastyk D: *Studies on Indian medical history,* Indian Medical Tradition Series, vol 5, New Delhi, 2001, Motilal Banarsidass.

Nadkarni AK: *Dr. K.M. Nadkarni's Indian materia medica,* ed 3 (reprint), Bombay, 1908, Popular Prakashan.

Pitman V: *On the nature of the whole,* Indian Medical Tradition Series, vol 7, New Delhi, 2004, Motilal Banarsidass.

Sen Gupta KN: *The Ayurvedic system of medicine,* New Delhi, 1984 (1906, reprint), Logos Press.

Sharma PV, translator: *Caraka-Samhita: Agnivesha's treatise refined and annotated by Caraka and redacted by Dridhabala,* vols 1-4, Varanasi, India, 1981-1994, Chaukhamba Orientalia.

Sharma PV, translator: *Sushruta-Samhita with Dalhana's commentary and critical notes,* vols 1-3, Varanasi, India, 1999-2001, Chaukhamba Orientalia.

Singh RH: *Pañchakarma therapy,* Varanasi, 1992, Chowkhamba Sanskrit Series Office.

Singhal GD et al, translators: *Ancient Indian surgery [Sushruta Samhita],* vols 1-10, Varanasi, India, 1972-1993, Singhal Publications.

Srikanta Murthy KR, translator: *Sharngadharasamhita of Shrangadhara,* Varanasi, India, 1984, Chaukhamba Orientalia.

Srikanta Murthy KR, translator: *Vagbhata's AshtangaHridaya-Samhita,* vols 1-3, Varanasi, India, 1991-1995, Krishnadas Academy.

Srikanta Murthy KR, translator: *AshtangaSamgraha of Vagbhata,* vols 1-3, Varanasi, India, 1995-1997, Krishnadas Academy.

Srikanta Murthy KR, translator: *Bhavaprakasha of Bhavamishra,* vols 1 and 2, Varanasi, India, 1998-2000, Krishnadas Academy.

Svoboda RE: *Prakruti: your Ayurvedic constitution,* Albuquerque, NM, 1984, Geocom.

Upadhyay SD: *Nadivijana (ancient pulse science),* Delhi, 1986, Chaukhamba Sanskrit Pratisthan.

Zimmermann F: *The jungle and the aroma of meats,* Indian Medical Tradition Series, vol 4, New Delhi, 1999, Motilal Banarsidass.

Zysk KG: *Medicine in the Veda; Religious healing in the Veda,* Indian Medical Tradition Series, vol I, Delhi, 1996, Motilal Banarsidass.

Zysk KG: *Asceticism and healing in ancient India; Medicine in the Buddhist monastery,* Indian Medical Tradition Series, vol II, Delhi, 1998, Motilal Banarsidass.

Zysk KG: *Conjugal love in India,* Sir Henry Wellcome Asian Medical Series, vol 1, Leiden, Boston, Köln, 2002, EJ Brill.

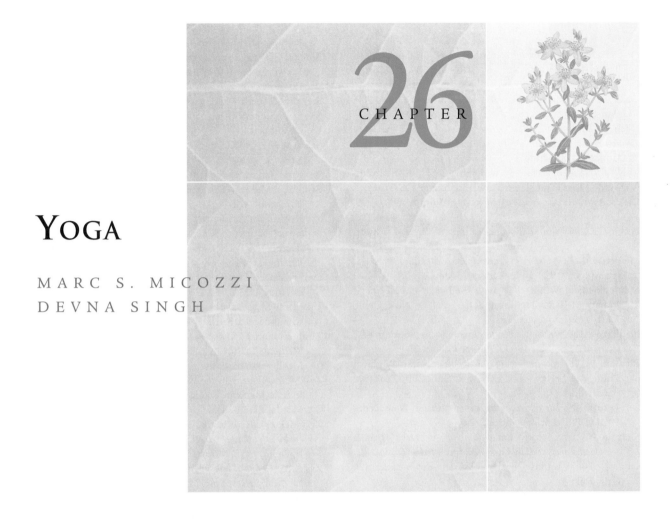

YOGA

MARC S. MICOZZI
DEVNA SINGH

Like Ayurveda, yoga is a textual and practical tradition that developed over time in India. Yoga is first a philosophical system with the purpose of spiritual development leading to the full realization of the soul. A wide range of modalities and techniques of yoga have developed to facilitate this journey on life's path. These techniques involve meditation (which may be likened to mind-body techniques), devotional practice, postural stretching and exercise, diet and nutrition, sound, and sexual exercises. Yoga may be seen in some ways as complementary medicine, but as with the practice of Ayurveda, it encompasses a philosophical system and lifestyle, as well as modalities that may be specifically therapeutic.

Traditional Ayurveda, until recently in "New Age Ayurveda," has remained separate from the tradition of yoga, which, on the other hand, has incorporated aspects of Ayurvedic medicine to help maintain the healthy bodily condition necessary for spiritual development.

In New Age Ayurveda, there is a special teacher-student relationship in which the yogi (one who knows yoga) acts as the mentor (or literally the guru) to impart knowledge of philosophy and technique to the pupil. Formulary versions in which the physical postures and techniques are taught without the philosophical basis would not be properly considered yoga but rather physical training and physical therapy, which nonetheless may be beneficial in its own right.

BACKGROUND AND HISTORY

Yoga is a common word in Sanskrit, an ancient Indo-European language. It has a range of meanings:

conjunction, constellation, team, or union. The term is related to words in other Indo-European languages, including the Latin *iugum,* German *joch,* and English *yoke,* all of which have the same meaning. According to the Advaita Vedanta, yoga is characteristic of philosophical teachings that subscribe to a nondualist metaphysical reality in which the self is the ultimate being underlying all phenomena. However, there is a dualist school, known as *Raja-Yoga,* or *Classical Yoga,* founded by the semimythical Patanjali. In this case, yoga represents not so much the union with an ultimate reality but disunion or separation from the ego. The ultimate outcome is the same because when the yoga practitioner succeeds in transcending the ego, he or she simultaneously realizes the true essence of the self or soul. Thus, yoga comprises schools that embrace total renunciation of the world *(samnyasa),* those that encourage proper performance of one's worldly obligations *(karman),* schools that regard dispassionate wisdom *(jnana)* as the means to spiritual enlightenment, and those that place love and devotion above all else *(bhakti).* One may observe these same ranges of expression within other spiritual traditions, such as Judaism, Islam, and Roman Catholicism. Although different versions of yoga are more or less religious and ritualistic, all are spiritual, and yoga may even be regarded perhaps as India's common brand of spiritualism.

Evidence of yoga beliefs and practices may be observed in the ancient *Rigveda* (or knowledge of praise), which serves as the source of the sacred heritage of Hinduism. It is the oldest of the four Vedas (knowledge), dating back to about 1200 BCE, the others being the Samaveda, the Yajurveda, and the Atharvaveda. The *Veda* is classic Sanskrit texts said to have been heard *(shruta)* by and thereby revealed to seers *(rshi)* in the form of poems or hymns based on their mystical visions, ecstasies, and insights and traditionally regarded as "revealed wisdom." All yogins within the Hindu tradition based themselves on this Vedic revelation *(shruti).* Those who do not, such as Gautama the Buddha and Mahavira, the founders of Buddhism and Jainism, respectively, deviated from the revealed teachings.

The *Bhagavad-Gita* (Lord's Song), the most popular and treasured of all yoga scriptures, dates to approximately 2500 years ago. Mahatma Gandhi referred to it as "my mother." It is embedded in the *Mahabharata,* one of two Hindu epics (the other being the *Ramayana*). It tells the story of a great war between two ancient Indian peoples: the Kurus and the Pandavas. Its mythical author Vyasa weaves spiritual teachings in the account of the events leading up to the war, the 18-day war itself, and the aftermath. The tale of the *Bhagavad-Gita* occurs on the morning of the first battle, when the Pandava prince Arjuna refuses to fight because he finds teachers and friends among the ranks of the enemy. Krishna, appearing in a divine incarnation as Arjuna's charioteer, encourages to him to do his duty because this is a "just war" to restore moral order. Yoga teachings are also given elsewhere in the *Mahabharata.*

During the period 500 BCE to about 100 CE, many *Upanishads* containing yoga teachings were composed. "Classical" yoga emerged in about 200 CE as codified by Patanjali in the famous *Yoga-Sutra,* or aphorisms of yoga. In Patanjala's text, yoga is defined as the stopping of the endless series of thoughts *(yogah cittavrittinirodhah).*

Later (post-Classical) sources of yogic knowledge are the *Tantras* (or webs), which belong to the tradition of Shiva-Shakti worship. *Shiva* manifests the universal male principle and is usually worshiped as a Hindu god; *Shakti,* meaning "power," refers to female principle or energy in the world, usually visualized as a goddess. Tantric yoga is concerned with enlisting this goddess energy in the yogic process.

Yoga is also an integral part of Shiva worship, as given in the *Agamas* (traditions).

Hatha-Yoga (or forceful yoga) is an important tradition that emerged in the eleventh century under the influence of Tantrism and has its own scriptures, including the *Geranda-Samhita* and the *Shiva-Samhita.*

The classic texts and history of yoga cover many traditions within Hinduism and can also be found within the tradition of Buddhism and Jainism. The Buddha's "noble eightfold path" presents an early form of non-Vedic yoga.

YOGA AS THE PATH OF WISDOM

The *Upanishads* are esoteric and philosophical scriptures describing the way to self-understanding, transcendence, and union with the universe. Wisdom is seen as the supreme means to this goal. Wisdom is seen as distinct from knowledge, which relies empirically on the senses and grasps the knowledge from the outside. Jnana-Yoga represents the spiritual discipline of wisdom.

In the words of Swami Vivekananda, a nineteenth-century yogin in the Hindu tradition of Advaita Vedanta, who represented Hinduism at the World Parliament of Religions in 1894:

> Every particle in the body is continually changing; no one has the same body for many minutes together, and yet we think of it as the same body. So with the mind: one moment it is happy, another moment unhappy; one moment strong, another weak—an ever changing whirlpool. That cannot be the Spirit which is infinite. . . . Any particle in this universe can change in relation to any other particle. But take the universe as one; then in relation to what can IT move? There is nothing besides IT. So this infinite unit is unchangeable, immovable, absolute, and this is the Real Man [sic].

The Real Man (or Woman) of Vivekananda is the eternal gender-transcending subject, the essential self of all beings and things. The insights of twentieth-century fundamental physics, as well as much of the knowledge of human physiology, biology, and pathology (see Chapter 1), came in large measure after Swami Vivekananda's insights of 1894.

Since the beginning, practitioners of yoga have cultivated the ideal of "renunciation" (samnyasa). Some interpret this to mean abandoning worldly life altogether. Others take renunciation primarily as an inner attitude. To the practitioner of Jnana-Yoga, renunciation comes naturally as a realization of the true pattern of life and nature of reality.

Yogic philosophy also holds that human suffering is caused by kleshas, which are:

1. Ignorance, or unawareness of reality
2. Ego
3. Attraction towards objects
4. Repulsion from objects
5. Fear of death

At the same time, it realizes that these kleshas are not independent but one leads to the next, the root cause being ignorance. Being unaware of the ultimate reality of connectedness gives rise to the a separate identity or ego; things or people who strengthen the ego are found attractive, whereas those that weaken the ego are considered repulsive or unattractive; and the ego or sense of identity leads to a deep aversion of death because it seems a loss of identity.

Reduction of the kleshas is also an aim of yoga as a predominance of kleshas is detrimental to meditation and progress on the spiritual path. As one progresses and evolves along the spiritual path, one realizes that one's view of life in the present state of consciousness is far inferior to the more subtle essence, which slowly reveals itself.

KARMA-YOGA

Traditional ancient Vedic spirituality was based on the ideal of outward sacrifice combined with inward meditation. The later Upanishads prescribed meditation as an inner sacrifice. This distinction was traditionally couched in terms of wisdom (jnana) versus action (karman). To the Jnana-yogin, the greater wisdom may be in non-action. The growth of the attractiveness of non-action as a path began to concern social leaders by the middle of the first millennium. They argued that a person should wait until his or her social duties were fulfilled to household and family before retiring to the mountaintop (an early and literal form of retirement). Indian lawgivers favored a lifestyle unfolding in four phases (ashrama): student, householder, forest-dweller (late maturity), and freely wandering ascetic (in old age).

The follower of Karman-Yoga acts in daily life so as to lessen lawlessness and restore virtue (dharma) or harmony. Like Mahatma Gandhi, the Karma-yogin works for the welfare of others. Devotionally, this practice may focus on the worship of God in personal form, notably Lord Krishna. Although love and devotion are central to Krishna's message, it is unthinkable without the corollaries of action and wisdom.

As a divine incarnation, Krishna is born whenever the moral order has collapsed and the world is enveloped in spiritual darkness. Krishna's Karman-Yoga is sometimes used to justify military action. It must be remembered that the war Krishna encouraged Arjuna to fight against the Kurus had the specific purpose of restoring moral order. The Karman-yogin may be seen as a "warrior" in this sense, whose good fight is manifest in the material world.

The link between Karman-Yoga and meditation is the loss of identification with the self while performing one's karma as the instrument of the supreme consciousness. When the individual no longer considers the self the doer but merely the instrument, the work becomes spiritualized. Desires and mental problems automatically disappear, as do likes and dislikes, which otherwise create obstacles to meditation. Also, Karman-Yoga further develops the faculty of concentration and the will. Briefly, the *will* can be defined as the ability to harmonize, motivate, and mobilize all one's abilities and actions to achieve a definite aim.

BHAKTI-YOGA: THE PATH OF DEVOTION

Bhakti means "devotion," generally devotion to God or the supreme consciousness in one of its manifestations. These manifestations may be one of numerous avatars or divine incarnations or may be one's guru or anyone or anything that evokes strong emotional feelings. Instead of directing the attention to an impersonal form of consciousness, as in Raja-Yoga and Jnana-Yoga, one's love is directed to something more tangible and concrete.

It is generally accepted that individuals are continually trying to find someone or something to which they can totally direct their emotion and devotion, and that this search carries on continually through life. In Bhakti-Yoga the state of meditation arises because a person who feels devotion automatically concentrates her or his mind, depending on the degree of devotion. This also results in the person losing awareness of "I-ness" or ego. Ideally, Bhakti-Yoga alone can be sufficient to bring about higher states of meditation, and no other practice is necessary. Important components of Bhakti-Yoga include the following:

1. Sravana, or hearing (glories of God)
2. Nama sankirtan, or repetition of God's name (s)
3. Smarana, or remembrance of God
4. Vandana, or prayers to God
5. Archana, or ritualistic worship

Although a devotional attitude in spiritual life is reflected in the writings of the seers of the Vedas, this independent path of Bhakti-Yoga emerged in the middle of the first millennium and centered on the theistic religions worshiping Krishna (a divine incarnation of Vishnu) and Shiva. Bhakti-Yoga draws from verses of the *Bhagavad-Gita*. Shiva worshipers in the same era created the *Shvetashvatara Upanishad* as a devotional text. The Bhakti-Yogin devotes himself or herself to the constant remembrance of the divine in all things, whether known as Krishna, Rama, Sita, Parvati, or other god or goddess. As mentioned, this worship takes the form of rituals, love-intoxicated chanting, singing, dancing, and meditation.

RAJA-YOGA

Raja-Yoga (or Classical Yoga) was formulated by Patanjali in the Yoga-Sutra around 200 BCE. This school is considered one of the six orthodox systems of Hindu philosophy. Raja-Yoga provides the most systematic access to the practical dimensions of Yoga. Patanjali enumerated eight principal limbs of yogic practice as follows:

1. Moral restraint: gentleness, truthfulness, honesty, chastity, and generosity (*Yama,* or social code)
2. Discipline: purity, contentment, asceticism, study, and devotion (*Niyamas,* or observances)
3. Posture (*asana*)
4. Breathing (*pranayama*)
5. Withdrawal of the senses (*pratyahara*)
6. Concentration (*dharana*)
7. Meditation (*dhyana*)
8. Ecstasy (*samadhi*)

These stages are progressive steps for attainment of successful meditation and indicate how obstacles on the spiritual path can be overcome. The first five stages have little direct connection with meditation but are extremely useful in preparation of the mind and body for the higher stages.

The social and personal codes of conduct (*Yama* and *Niyamas*) prepare the mind and body for the higher stages of meditation by reducing attachment and inducing tranquility. *Asanas,* or yogic postures, give a steady and comfortable position for the body to practice concentration and meditation without physical disturbance. Any position of the body even slightly uncomfortable will result in preoccupation of the mind with the body. At the same time, other asanas are more therapeutic than meditational. These therapeutic asanas are useful in removal and prevention of diseases of both body and mind, and they also induce tranquillity of mind, thereby encouraging successful meditation practice.

The word *prana* is often used in yoga and is often misunderstood to mean only "breath." *Prana* denotes "life force" or bioenergy. It is also the medium through which matter and mind are linked to consciousness. The aim of *pranayama* is control over the flow of prana, which is intimately linked to the breathing process. Pranayama results in redistribution of prana in the body, enabling the mind to go to the next stages of concentration.

Pratyahara is the method to withdraw the mind from association with the external world so that it can go to the stage of dharana and dhyana. This is done by reducing to zero the selection of sense impressions that are communicated to the mind. The mind is often likened to a naughty child, who does the opposite of what one wants the child to do. This idiosyncrasy of the mind is used for pratyahara, in which the mind is forced to think of external things with the eyes closed; in time, the mind tends to lose interest in the external sounds and does not associate with sense impressions. "Antarmouna" is a pratyahara technique that specifically exploits this behavior of the mind. Pratyahara also requires that the sitting position, or asana, be comfortable. Many techniques involve a systematic rotation of the awareness around different parts of the body, awareness of the breathing process, and awareness of sounds uttered either mentally or verbally. This satisfies the wandering tendency of the mind in a controlled manner.

Dharana, or concentration, is the method to eliminate memories of the past and projections of future events by concentrating totally on one object to the exclusion of all others. In yogic concentration the mind is not held completely rigid; the processes of the mind are not curtailed. The mind is held so that it is aware of one object, but it should move in the sense that it realizes deeper aspects of the object not perceivable earlier.

Dhayana is an extension of dharana and has been defined by Patanjali as the uninterrupted flow of concentration of mind on the object of meditation or concentration. The difference between dharana and dhyana is that the practitioner has to bring back the awareness to the object of concentration while in dhyana; the mind has been subjugated and is totally and continually absorbed in the object.

Samadhi is the fullest extension of dhyana and is the climax of meditation. Patanjali has defined Samadhi as that state in which there is only consciousness of the object and no concurrent consciousness of the mind.

The stages from dharana to samadhi are really different names for different degrees of attainment. One automatically and spontaneously leads to the next; these are not totally different practices as are the lower five stages. However, it is at these stages that the master or "Guru" becomes a necessity for guiding the aspirant safely.

KUNDALINI YOGA

In accordance with the ancient writings, kundalini yoga was designed to awaken the "serpent power" within the body. At present, kundalini awakenings are grouped under the medical rubric of "spiritual emergence," which is considered a psychological crisis. In *Kundalini Experience* (1976), American psychiatrist Lee Sannella argued that such "awakenings" should be considered spiritual rather than psychiatric in nature.

The Sanskrit word *kundalini* is the feminine form of *kundala,* meaning "ring" or "coil." It thus means "she who is coiled," like a serpent. This is an appropriate metaphor for the psychospiritual potential. Its power is conceived as the goddess counterpart of Shiva, which is pure consciousness.

Each level of the mind is associated with a psychic center, or chakra (see later discussion). The aim of kundalini yoga is to overcome he normal inactivity of the higher chakras so that they are stimulated and the individual is able to experience higher levels of the mind. The basic method of awakening these psychic centers in kundalini yoga is deep concentration on the centers and willing their arousal.

A fully awakened kundalini is said actually to restructure the body, leading to a reordering of control over vital functions, such as pulse, intestinal contractions, and brain activity. In Hatha-Yoga, various techniques are used to accomplish this by focusing the life breath or life force (*prana*) through mental concentration and controlled breathing. Because kundalini is thought to be dormant in the lowest chakra of the energetic body, effort is concentrated on that particular spot.

CHAKRAS: THE ENERGETIC BODY

The energetic body in yoga is thought to consist of five to seven energy centers, or *charkas* (literally, "wheels"). In Hatha-Yoga and many Tantric schools of yoga, the seven energy centers are, in ascending order, as follows:

1. *Muladhara:* "root-prop wheel," situated in the perineum (yoni), corresponding to the sacrococcygeal nerve plexus, associated with the earth element—the resting place of dormant kundalini.
2. *Svadhishthana:* "own-base wheel," located in the genitals, corresponding to the sacral plexus at the fourth lumbar vertebra, associated with the water element.
3. *Manipura:* "jewel-city wheel," located at the navel, corresponding to the solar plexus, associated with fire.
4. *Anahata:* "wheel of the unstruck," located at the heart, corresponding to the cardiac plexus, associated with the air element.
5. *Vishuddhi:* "wheel of purity," located at the throat, corresponding to the laryngeal plexus, associated with the ether element.
6. *Ajna:* "command wheel," located in the brain, corresponding to the vestigial third eye (known as the eye of Shiva, or the pineal gland in Western medicine), associated with the mind.
7. *Sahasrara:* "thousand-spoked wheel," located at the crown, associated with nonlocal consciousness.

These chakras as conceptualized here may be seen as illustrating two fundamental insights of yoga: matter is a low-velocity form of vibrational energy that exists in states of high velocity elsewhere, and consciousness is not inevitably bound in matter but is inherently free. Kundalini yoga is a method for finding that freedom of consciousness.

NADIS: THE PSYCHIC PATHWAYS

The word *nadi* means a "current," or "flow," connecting the different charkas and other psychic centers. There are said to be 72,000 such nadis; those of particular importance are the Sushumna, pingala, and ida nadis.

Sushumna is by far the most important nadi, with its base at the mooladhara chakra and traveling through the spinal column and terminating at the center of the Sahasrara chakra via the swadhishthana, manipura, anahata, and vishuddhi chakras. It is in this nadi that the kundalini flows when it is awakened.

The *pingala* and *ida* nadis start at the mooladhara and terminate at the ajna chakra, crossing the sushumna at the swadhishthana, manipura, anahata, and vishuddhi chakras in a serpent-like fashion, forming semicircular curves between two consecutive chakras. The pingala or "solar" nadi starts with a right curve from the mooladhara; the ida or "lunar" nadistarts with a left curve from the mooladhara.

HATHA-YOGA: THE PATH OF INNER POWER

Hatha means "force" or "forceful" and refers to the practice of yoga that uses physical purification and body strengthening as an arduous means of self-transformation and transcendence. A frail or diseased body may prove an obstacle on the path to enlightenment and therefore must be properly trained.

Physical and mental training and fitness are important because at the core of Hatha-Yoga is the potentially dangerous process of awakening the *kundalini-shakti*. This arousal of the power of consciousness at the lowest psychospiritual center (*chakra*) of the body and transmission to the highest center in the crown is tremendously powerful, physically and mentally. Historically, Hatha-Yoga is based on the development of Tantrism (Tantra-Yoga). The awakening of kundalini-shakti was central to Tantric esotericism, long before the emergence of Hatha-Yoga, as a practice for the preparation of the mind and body for this awakening.

In fact, another school of thought holds that in the word *hatha*, *ha* stands for the ida (lunar) nadi and *tha* stands for the pingala (solar) nadi. It is held that when the flow of prana in ida is equal to the flow of prana in pingala, kundalini automatically starts to rise. Therefore, Hatha-Yoga is concerned with the two nadis, ida and pingala, and its aim is balancing the flow of prana in each nadi. When the kundalini is activated in this way, it stimulates the chakras, and meditation automatically takes place.

Many of the Hatha-Yoga practices also attempt directly to stimulate the chakras and to clean and generally improve the condition of various physical organs that are linked to the chakras.

In preparation, Hatha-Yoga incorporates many techniques for cleansing and stabilization of body energy. It includes many postures or positions (*asanas*) to maintain or restore well-being, to improve vitality and flexibility, and to facilitate prolonged meditation. The basis is breathing and breath control (*pranayama),* and various techniques are used to modulate the body's vital winds (*prana)* through the breath. This is the form of yoga best known in the West, although its deeper philosophical foundations are rarely understood or practiced. It is widely reduced to another form of "fitness training."

The contemporary Hatha-Yoga master B.K.S. Iyengar, who has trained many American Hatha-Yoga teachers, said, "The original idea of Yoga is freedom and beatitude, and the by-products . . . including physical health, are secondary for the practitioner."

Physical Cleansing

Hatha-Yoga entails a complex program of physical cleansing (*shodhana).* The *Geranda-Samhita* describes six acts, as follows:

1. *Dhauti* (cleansing), consisting of four techniques: inner, dental, "heart" or chest, and "base" purification. "Inner cleansing" uses four exercises: swallowing the breath and expelling it through the anus, filling the stomach with water, stimulating the abdominal "fire" by repetitions of contracting the navel against the spine, and washing the prolapsed intestines (not medically recommended). "Dental cleansing" covers the teeth, tongue, ears, and frontal sinuses. "Heart cleansing" consists of induced or self-induced emesis. "Base cleansing" is manual cleansing of the anus with water or other solution.
2. *Vasti* or *Basti:* bladder cleansing by contracting the urinary sphincter, usually while standing in water.
3. *Neti:* threading a thin cloth through the nostril and out the mouth to remove mucus and "open up the third eye."
4. *Lauli* or *nauli:* rolling the abdominal muscles sideways to massage the inner organs.
5. *Trataka:* gazing steadily at a small, close object, such as a candle flame, until tears flow, to develop the powers of concentration.
6. *Kapala-bhati:* three practices involving breathing in through the right nostril and out through the left (and vice versa), drawing water through the nostrils and expelling it through the mouth, and sucking water up through the mouth and expelling it through the nose. This is done to purify the frontal portion of the brain.

Relaxation and Posture

Relaxation, as with purification, is another important preparatory aspect involving the postures (*asanas)* of Hatha-Yoga. Relaxation applies not only to the body but also to the mind. When posture is cultivated properly, it creates the sensation that the body is loosening up and widening out. Thus, posture is more than gymnastics or acrobatics; it is the art of relaxation to the point of meditation and beyond. Following are some *postures for meditation:*

- *Siddha-asana,* the "successful posture," is achieved by pressing the left heel against the perineum and placing the right foot above the genitals.
- *Padmasana,* the "lotus posture," is achieved by placing the right foot on the left thigh and the left foot on the right thigh. The classic texts also teach crossing the arms behind the back and grasping the left toe with the left hand and the right toe with the right hand, called the *bound lotus.* The lotus posture, in addition to promoting relaxation, is said to alleviate a number of diseases. It often is seen in depictions of the Buddha.
- *Sukhasana,* the "happy posture," favored by many Americans, is widely known as the *tailor's seat.*

Other well-known postures are the tree, triangle, hands-to-feet, adamantine, cow-face, back-stretching, serpent (cobra), all-limb, plow, and head postures. In addition to the postures, Hatha-Yoga has a series of *bandhas* (bonds or locks) and *mudras* (seals). There are three principal types of locks, in which the life force is forcibly retained in the body: The *root lock* is the contraction of the anal sphincter. The *upward lock* is executed by pulling the stomach up until there is a hollow below the rib cage, said to force the vital energy upward "like a great bird." The *throat contraction lock* is done by placing the chin down against the collarbone, stopping the downward flow of "ambrosial fluid" (possibly a reference to hormonal secretions). It prevents the life force (and the vital breath) from escaping through the nose or mouth.

The *Hatha-Yoga seals* consist of eight most important techniques, as follows:

1. *Space-seal:* turning the tongue back and inserting it in the nasopharynx (cavity at the back of the mouth leading to the nose), possible only if the frenulum underneath the tongue has been

deliberately cut. This mudra is said to satisfy hunger, quench thirst, cure disease, and postpone death.

2. *Power-stirring:* contracting the anus and forcing the vital energy into the central channel at the lowest chakra, the seat of the kundalini.

3. *Shambu:* a meditation technique more than a physical exercise, it requires a wide-eyed, unfocused gaze. Shambu, another name for Shiva, is regarded as the revealer of the secrets of Tantrism.

4. *Vajroli:* sucking the released semen back into the urethra. Females also learn this technique so as not to waste the valuable hormonal and chemical properties of semen.

5. *Sahajoli:* rubbing ejaculated semen into the skin.

6. *Amaroli:* drinking the midflow of the urine, thought to have certain healing properties.

7. *Womb:* while seated in the siddha-asana posture, with eyes, ears, and nostrils closed with the 10 fingers, the body's energy is forced through the six chakras by means of breath control, mantra, and visualization.

8. *Six-openings:* placing the thumbs on the two ears, the index and middle fingers on the two eyes, and the ring and the little fingers on the two nostrils.

Similarly, there are eight major breathing techniques (*pranayama*) for modulating the flow of vital energy into the body. Incorrect pranayama may cause hiccups, asthma, headache, and other ailments.

MEDITATION AND VISUALIZATION

Similar to mind-body interventions (see Chapter 16), yoga employs visualization as one of the traditional forms of meditation. Visualization has been practiced particularly in the Tantric Buddhism of Tibet. *Deity yoga* involves the visualization of deities and is the essential practice of what is called *Highest Yoga Tantra.* Deities are usually visualized together with their respective environments, known as *mandalas,* or "circles."

Physical Preparation

It is important to meditate in a secure environment where interruptions can be minimized. Having a usual location reserved for meditation and yoga is helpful. Repeated meditation in the same location may help develop an energetic environment (or *imprint*) that facilitates the meditative state.

Time of day is important. As with location, it is useful to meditate at a consistent time regardless of which time is chosen. Most traditions indicate that early morning is the best time to meditate. Yogins in India typically meditate at sunrise, known as the *hour of Brahma*. Meditation at noon, sunset, and midnight is also recommended.

It is advised at the outset to sit in meditation for no more than 15 minutes at a time. Initially the desire for sleep or mental indulgence in fantasies or daydreaming may tend to replace the meditative state. Being well rested is also important for meditation, as it is for general health, because tiredness merely invites sleep or daydreaming. Sexual activity should be avoided shortly before meditation because it may deplete the psychoenergetic centers (*chakras*).

MANTRA-YOGA: SACRED SOUNDS OF YOGA

The consciousness-altering effects of sound are well known and probably belong to the earliest expression of human culture (see Chapter 19). Sacred sounds preceded yoga and were most likely part of the early Vedic rituals and religion.

Some of the mystical insights and writings of the ancient Vedic sages have been reinterpreted in light of modern understanding of fundamental physics, namely, that the universe is "an ocean of vibrations." According to the schools of Siddha-Yoga, also known as *Mantra-Yoga,* all perceptible sounds ultimately derive from a universal matrix of sound. This expression has been translated as "sonic absolute," which is typically articulated as the monosyllabic sound "OM (A-U-M)." Classic physics states that sounds are waves of consecutive compressions and rarefactions of air or other fluid.

Mantra-Yoga uses the vehicle of sonic vibration to unify consciousness through recitation and contemplation of special numinous sounds such as OM. In addition, the monosyllables HAM, YAM, RAM, VAM, LAM, AH, HUM, and PHAT are also used

Few mantras have a denotative meaning but rather are used to produce specific states of energy and consciousness. After continuous and dedicated practice, the mantra is repeated automatically without strain or effort. The mantra spontaneously manifests itself and becomes an integral part of the mind. The mind vibrates with the sound of the mantra. This is a powerful way of approaching meditational states, since the mind is rendered calm and concentrated. The mantra acts as a pathway between normal states of consciousness and superconsciousness.

SEXUAL ENERGY: TANTRISM AND YOGA

Tantric yoga posits that sexual energy is an important reservoir of energy that should be used wisely to facilitate the spiritual process rather than block it through orgasmic release.

There are right-handed and left-handed practices of Tantric yoga. In left-handed Tantra, sexual union is a central ritual. In many countries throughout the Middle East and South Asia, the left hand is the taboo hand used for private bodily functions, not for eating or greeting. (The Latin term *sinister* also means "left.") In left-handed Tantra, things that are taboo are charged with energy because of the negative attention they receive, and this yoga makes a point of breaking with established norms by using taboo functions such as sexuality in the service of spiritual transformation.

At the center of left-handed Tantra are the five prohibitions: sex, wine, meat, fish, and parched grain. In the West, a tantric ritual involving all five taboos includes random coupling. The sexual union itself is accomplished according to strict ritual and with great dignity and meditative visualization. Generally, the purpose of sexual union is the healthy circulation of vital energy between the male and female partners.

Tantrism is neither orgiastic nor hedonistic in principle on the one hand, nor is it ascetic. Discipline is essential to Tantric practice. For example, semen is equated with the impulse toward enlightenment and should not be discharged. Orgasm does not lead to bliss but merely to pleasurable sensations. Thus the earnest practitioner must forgo orgasm. Men are advised to apply pressure to the perineum to prevent ejaculation. Some practitioners learn to control their genital functions to the point where they can suck the ejaculated semen back through the penis.

The same consideration applies to women, although in Chinese Taoism, for example, orgasm is not seen to have the same depleting effect as in men. The female equivalent of semen is called *rajas,* which may refer to the hormone-rich vaginal secretions released during sexual arousal. In some schools, men are urged to absorb the female rajas into their own bodies.

In Tantrism and yoga, sexual activity is not a moral matter, and sexual drive is considered inherently divine. The only reason for suggesting chastity is purely a matter of economics: conservation of energy.

THE HEART OF THE MATTER

In yoga, individual consciousness is thought to be connected with the physical body at the heart. This consciousness in an unenlightened individual is labeled "self-contraction." This contraction, felt at the level of the heart, is a sense of separation, isolation, loneliness, fear, and uncertainty. At the level of the mind, this contraction manifests itself as doubt. Yoga endeavors to expand this contraction.

In the West, yoga often is reduced to fitness training bereft of the consciousness that can be brought to heart and mind. Although reductionist yoga practice helps many people maintain and restore physical health, it does not provide the full potential benefits of yoga. Many practitioners of yoga, in India as well as the West, know only this reductionist form of yoga.

Yoga was never intended for quick fixes or as a cheap service to the ego. Promises of enlightenment over a weekend or a week are blatant misconceptions. Like anything in life, the benefits from yoga are commensurate with the attention, discipline, and effort put into it. Yoga must be learned from a knowledgeable master. A mature student will have no difficulty in learning from a master in any given field. We must, however, examine our teachers carefully. As proven constantly in our daily experience, neither education nor age is any guarantee of wisdom.

The mass media have profitably manipulated public opinion by confusing the guru tradition with the vexing issues of cult leadership and brainwashing. As more flamboyant and questionable gurus are replaced through experience with true spiritual masters, the practice of yoga should gain in strength.

RESEARCH ON YOGA

As age-old traditions of yoga and meditation enter contemporary health care, they represent ways to help manage stress and chronic diseases and to promote good health.

Yoga has also become a fertile field for scientific research. There is much research on hypnotherapy, biofeedback, and relaxation techniques independent of yoga (covered in other chapters), as well as research specifically associated with yoga. The biofeedback technique in particular has great promise for beginners and for those who are not making discernible progress in meditation, even after constant practice.

The practice of yoga produces physiological changes in the body, as scientifically proven. The monitoring and understanding of these changes have led to a greater understanding of the human body, particularly with regard to the bioenergetic aspects (see Chapter 17). Basic research has also been done on the psychological aspects of yoga practice. Personal psychology has methods for assessing states of consciousness, and alterations in consciousness through yoga practice have also been shown scientifically. *Psychosynthesis,* for example, has the same aims as yoga: integration of the whole being of an individual and eventual self-realization. Both modern psychology and yoga emphasize the importance of evolution and growth from "less wholeness" to "more wholeness."

Although yoga has been studied as part of traditional scientific research in physiology and psychology to gain a better understanding of the human body and mind, it is also now forming a part of research specifically on complementary medicine as an aid to good health.

Clinical studies have shown that yoga is effective therapy for several chronic conditions, as well as for stress management. Yoga has been found helpful in the treatment of heart disease and high blood pressure.

As with many other complementary therapies using mechanisms of action not fully understood, yoga is helpful in the management of asthma and other breathing disorders. It also helps improve mood and counter mild depression.

Yoga is helpful in the management of a number of musculoskeletal disorders, such as carpal tunnel syndrome and osteoarthritis, and of common occupational health problems, such as low back pain. Preliminary evidence indicates that yoga may be helpful in disorders of the immune system, such as rheumatoid arthritis and lupus. Yoga has also been seen to improve physical performance in schoolchildren, potentially contributing to healthy growth and development.

Yoga is a practice that involves the total body and total mind. Yoga and meditation act as a holistic treatment concerning the whole mind-body complex. They are a powerful way of controlling physiological processes and also of controlling physiological reactions to psychological events.

One of the most important changes that take place in the body during meditation is the slowing down of the metabolism, resulting in a sharp reduction in oxygen consumption and carbon dioxide output by up to 20%. Although blood pressure and heart rate decrease overall, blood flow increases during meditation; activities of the sympathetic nervous system are reduced, and constriction of the blood vessels is decreased. This in turn ensures the oxygen is more efficiently delivered to the muscles and that lactate is more quickly and effectively removed. Reduction of lactate level has a direct effect on reduction of blood pressure and anxiety levels.

The quality of relaxation produced by yoga and meditation is superior to that produced by sleep. This allows recuperation of the body from the damaging effects of overproduction of adrenaline and activity of the sympathetic nervous system.

Through meditation, the septal region of the limbic system becomes operational for the predominant part of our life. This leads to a life of relaxation, which at the same time is more efficient and disease-free.

Scientific studies continue to prove the beneficial health effects of yoga.

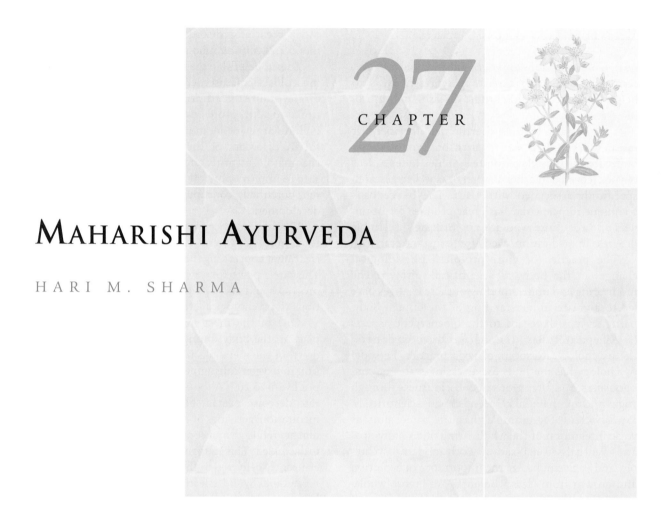

CHAPTER 27

MAHARISHI AYURVEDA

HARI M. SHARMA

HISTORY

Ayurveda is a holistic system of natural health care that originated in the ancient Vedic civilization of India. During the centuries of foreign rule in India, which began in the fifteenth century, Ayurvedic institutions declined or were suppressed, and much of the Ayurvedic knowledge was fragmented, misunderstood, and not used in its totality. Recently, Ayurveda has been revived in its completeness in accordance with the classical texts by Maharishi Mahesh Yogi and in collaboration with leading Ayurvedic scholars and physicians, known as *vaidyas*. This specific reformulation of Ayurveda is known as *Maharishi Ayurveda* (MAV).

The Sanskrit name "Ayurveda" is a compound of two words: *Ayus,* which means "life" or "life span,"

and *Veda,* which means "knowledge," with a connotation of completeness or wholeness of knowledge. The element of "wholeness" in Ayurvedic knowledge has profound clinical significance: the MAV clinician uses more than 20 treatment approaches that deal with the full range of the patient's life: the body, mind, behavior, environment, and most importantly, the patient's consciousness, his or her "innermost life." MAV considers consciousness to be of primary importance in maintaining optimal health and emphasizes meditation techniques to develop integrated holistic functioning of the nervous system.

MAV includes a sophisticated theoretical framework that provides clinical insight into the functioning of both mind and body. Understanding of the patient's mind-body type is essential to diagnosis and

518

treatment, and special emphasis is placed on the therapeutic effects of diet and healthy digestion, as well as techniques to balance behavior and emotions. An extensive materia medica describes the therapeutic use of medicinal plants, and there is a detailed understanding of biological rhythms, which form the basis for daily and seasonal behavioral routines to strengthen the immune system and homeostatic mechanisms.

Ancient Ayurvedic texts[*] typically begin with a thorough description of strategies of prevention before discussing modalities for treatment. In addition to preventive techniques, MAV offers a holistic theory of prevention. Western medical attempts to develop preventive medical strategies, although laudable, conspicuously lack such a theory. As for the fields of diagnosis and treatment, MAV offers a large body of procedures and protocols, including a set of noninvasive diagnostic techniques, and addresses certain deficiencies of Western allopathic medicine. For example, functional diseases, such as irritable bowel syndrome and poor digestion, account for approximately one third of patient visits to family practitioners: Western medicine, however, lacks well-developed theories or methods of treatment for these disorders.

Another example is iatrogenic (physician-caused) diseases, which one study found afflicted 36% of hospitalized patients (Steel et al., 1981). Another study found that 17.7% of hospital patients had at least one serious "adverse event" (another term for iatrogenic occurrence) resulting from inappropriate care, which lengthened their hospital stay (Andrews et al., 1997). A different study on adverse events found that almost 14% of the adverse events led to death (Berwick and Leape, 1999). A large percentage of iatrogenic illnesses are the result of side effects from drugs. Incredibly, adverse drug reactions have now become the fourth leading cause of death in the United States (Lazarou et al., 1998). To consider one example of this scenario, Western approaches to cancer treatment have severe side effects, and some antitumor drugs even contribute to the development of new cancers. MAV modalities have been effective in reducing the side effects of several of these treatments (Misra et al., 1994; Sharma et al., 1994; Srivastava et al., 2000), and laboratory research has shown that some MAV herbal preparations reduce cancer growth directly (Mazzoleni et al., 2002; Patel et al., 1992; Prasad et al., 1992, 1993; Sharma et al., 1990, 1991).

MAV is being practiced in clinics worldwide in India, Europe, Japan, Africa, Russia, Australia, and South and North America by specially trained physicians, many of whom also practice privately. In various ways, MAV directs its objectives not only to individual patients, but also to the life of society as a whole.

THEORETICAL BASIS: A "CONSCIOUSNESS MODEL" OF MEDICINE

Maharishi Ayurveda's contribution to patient care and clinical practice results from the model of health and disease on which it is based. Whereas Western medicine bases its model for understanding health and disease on the *material* of the body, Maharishi Ayurveda is based on the body's *non*material substrate, which is conceived as a field of pure intelligence. Western medicine's paradigm may seem to be seen as more scientific, but in certain respects, Ayurveda's may be seen to presage today's advanced theories of physics.

From the time of Newton until the early twentieth century, the field of physics was based on a materialist approach to the natural world (see Chapter 1). The allopathic medical paradigm, developed in the nineteenth century, is based on this theory of materialism; it views the body as a complex machine. However, discoveries by twentieth-century physicists have undermined this materialist worldview and uncovered a fundamental role for consciousness in the physical world. Because the nature and importance of consciousness are not usually considered in allopathic medicine, twentieth-century physics provides a useful background for understanding Maharishi Ayurveda.

---

[*] These include three major texts (*Brihat Trayi*), the *Charaka Samhita*, *Sushruta Samhita*, and *Ashtanga Hridaya* of Vagbhata, and three minor texts (*Laghu Trayi*), the *Sarngadhara Samhita*, *Bhavaprakash Samhita*, and *Madhava Nidanam*. Most of these texts have been translated into English (Charaka Samhita, 1977; Madhavakava, 1986; Sarngadhara, 1984; Sushruta Samhita, 1963; Vagbhata, 1982). These texts address eight main sections of Ayur-Veda: *Shalya*, surgery in general; *Shalakya*, surgery for supraclavicular diseases; *Kaya chikitsa*, treatment, diagnosis, and internal medicine; *Kaumarya Birtya*, pediatrics, obstetrics, and gynecology; *Agad Tantra*, toxicology and medical jurisprudence; *Bhut Vidya*, psychosomatic medicine; *Rasayana*, materia medica to promote vitality, stamina, resistance to disease, and longevity; and *Vajikarana*, fertility and potency.

According to the materialist theory that dominated physics until the 1900s, the universe is made up of solid, discrete bits of matter. These particles affect each other only through direct interactions. Four basic principles support this "common sense" view of reality, as follows:

1. *Solid matter*. The world is fundamentally made up of solid material objects, the building blocks of nature.
2. *Strict causality*. Change in motion of one object can be caused only by direct interaction with another object.
3. *Locality*. Interactions between particles can occur only through collisions or through influences radiated through the electromagnetic or gravitational fields at the speed of light, or less. No nonlocal interaction can occur.
4. *Reductionism*. Large systems in nature—including, in principle, the human body and even the entire universe—can be understood completely by understanding the properties and local, causal interactions of their smallest discrete components.

In the materialist theory the consciousness of the scientist is considered separate from the material objects being studied. The knower (consciousness) and the known (object) are thought to exist in completely distinct domains. This separation is thought to be the basis of "objective" science. Throughout the history of science, however, the separation of consciousness from the apparently material world has led to theoretical difficulties. For example, if consciousness is completely separate from matter, it is difficult to explain how consciousness could arise from the purely mechanical interactions of solid matter within the brain.

In the twentieth century the terms of this discussion were changed by the fundamental discoveries of quantum physics. Experiments performed in the first quarter of the twentieth century indicated that subatomic particles, the supposed building blocks of nature, did not appear to be composed of solid matter. In some of these experiments, particles behaved as if they were waves. In others, electrons took instantaneous, discontinuous quantum jumps from one atomic orbit to another, with no intervening time and no journey through space—an impossible act for a classic particle. It also was shown that an individual subatomic particle cannot have both a precise position and a precise momentum simultaneously (the

"uncertainty" principle), another situation that would not apply to a solid material particle. Finally, it was found that electrons can, with predictable regularity, tunnel through a solid barrier that, classically, would be impenetrable.

On the basis of these findings, the basic principles of quantum mechanics (often known as the *Copenhagen interpretation*) challenge the materialist worldview, as follows:

1. *No solid matter*. This interpretation accepted the scientific findings (wave/particle, quantum jumps, uncertainty, tunneling) that contradict the notion of solid matter.
2. *No strict causality*. Precise predictions for individual subatomic particles are impossible. Quantum mechanics thus loses the ability to trace causal relations among individual particles.
3. *No locality*. Quantum mechanical equations indicate that two particles, once they have interacted, are instantaneously connected, even across astronomical distances. This defies the strictly local connections allowed in classic materialism.
4. *No reductionism*. If apparently separate particles actually are connected nonlocally, a reductionist view based on isolated particles is untenable.

The Copenhagen interpretation was not put to experimental test for decades, leaving some physicists unconvinced that solidity, causality, locality, and reductionism had to be abandoned. In the 1980s, however, a number of different experiments produced results that consistently contradicted the theories of materialism (often called *local realism*) and consistently confirmed the predictions of quantum mechanics (Aspect et al., 1981; Rarity and Tapster, 1990). These studies found that once two particles have interacted, they are instantaneously correlated nonlocally, over arbitrarily vast distances—an impossibility in materialism.

These results do not invalidate materialism altogether. In the everyday world of "large" objects, the mechanistic causation of Newtonian physics is approximately correct, which is why much of medicine has been able to rely on it without apparently ill consequences. However, at the fundamental, subatomic level, materialism conflicts both with theory and with frequently replicated experimental evidence. This gives rise to a fundamentally different worldview. Many physicists now argue that nature is composed of *probability waves* that are a function of *intelligence alone,* not of discrete physical particles. The equations of quantum mechanics thus describe a world made of abstract patterns of intelligence.

> In view of these uniformly idea-like characteristics of the quantum-physical world, the proper answer to our question, "What sort of world do we live in?" would seem to be this: "We live in an idea-like world, not a matter-like world." There is, in fact, in the quantum universe no natural place for matter. This conclusion, curiously, is the exact reverse of the circumstance that in the classic physical universe there was not a natural place for mind (Stapp, 1994).

Quantum field theory, the most accurate version of quantum mechanics, can be related to the core tenet of Maharishi Ayurveda's paradigm. In quantum field theory the probability wave for a particle is described as a fluctuation in an underlying, nonmaterial field (known as a *force field* or *matter field*). Furthermore, in the most recent superunified theories, physicists have described all the force and matter fields that make up the universe as modes of vibration of one underlying, unified field, sometimes called the *superfield* or *superstring field*. All the order and intelligence of the laws of nature arise from this one fundamental, nonmaterial field, as does all matter. Not only are particles really just waves, but those waves ultimately are made of an underlying field, as ocean waves are made of ocean water. This field is one of pure intelligence, having the attributes that we associate with consciousness. This lends support to the statement of the quantum mechanical pioneer Max Planck, who said, "I regard consciousness as primary. I regard matter as derivative from consciousness," and to Sir Arthur Eddington, the physicist who first provided evidence in support of Einstein's general theory of relativity, who said, "The stuff of the world is mind-stuff" (Eddington, 1974).

Unified field theory may seem worlds away from the concerns of a clinician. The current allopathic approach assumes that the body can be explained by material reductionism, analogous to machinery. Maharishi Ayurveda, by contrast, has viewed it as an abstract pattern of intelligence. Because this latter view appears to be consistent with fundamental science, it is not unreasonable to consider that it might contribute to the clinician's capacity to promote health. Let us examine how Maharishi Ayurveda's "consciousness model" is applied in clinical practice.

APPLYING THE CONSCIOUSNESS MODEL IN MAHARISHI AYURVEDA

Transcendental Meditation

To understand the most basic application of the consciousness model, we must briefly touch on physics again. Vedic thought discusses a unified field of pure, nonmaterial intelligence and consciousness whose modes of vibration manifest as the material universe. These modes of vibration are called *Veda.** The Vedic description is strikingly similar to that of physics but emphasizes an idea less often discussed in physics: that the unified field is the field of pure consciousness. The differentiation between consciousness and matter, between knower and known, loses its significance at the level of the unified field.

In Maharishi Ayurveda the ultimate basis of disease is losing one's connection to (or, to use a central Vedic description, one's memory of) the unified field, which is the innermost core of one's own being and experience. This loss is known technically as *pragya-aparadh.* The ultimate basis of prevention and cure is restoring one's conscious connection to (or memory of) this innermost core of one's being and experience. This reconnection is the basis of an integrated approach to health care; integration of the different layers of life begins with reconnecting one's life to the substrate on which all its layers are based. The innermost core of one's experience is considered identical to the home of all the laws of nature that operate throughout the universe. The body contains, at its basis, the total potential of natural law, and all of Maharishi Ayurveda's modalities aim to enable the full expression of the body's inner intelligence.

The foremost means for accomplishing this are the Vedic techniques for developing consciousness, the most important of which is Transcendental Meditation (TM). The term *transcendental* indicates that the mind *transcends* even the subtlest impulses of thought and settles down to the simplest state of awareness (in MAV terms, identical to the unified

---

* These various modes of vibration known as *Veda* are described and written down in the voluminous Vedic literature. Recently the different aspects of Vedic literature have been found to correspond with different areas of the human physiology (Nader, 1993).

field). This state of awareness is known technically as *Transcendental Consciousness* (TC).

Interestingly, a large body of published research has demonstrated that, during the subjective experience of TC, the body's metabolism and electroencephalogram (EEG) take on a unique pattern of profound physiological rest and balance, with a metabolic reduction significantly deeper than that experienced during sleep or eyes-closed rest (Gallois, 1984; Wallace, 1970). Periods of clear experience of TC have been characterized by suspension of respiration without oxygen deprivation (Badawi et al., 1984; Farrow and Hebert, 1982), stabilization of the autonomic nervous system (Orme-Johnson, 1973), and a decrease in plasma lactate, a chemical marker of metabolic activity (Jevning et al., 1983) and cortisol levels (Jevning et al., 1978). Simultaneous with this metabolic rest, the brain displays "restful alertness," characterized by greatly increased coherence between the EEG patterns of different areas of the brain (i.e., stable phase relations between two EEG signals, as measured by Fourier analyses that attain correlations of more than 0.95) (Badawi et al., 1984; Levine, 1976). Also, blood flow to the brain increases markedly (Jevning et al., 1978).

The state of TC can thus be defined physiologically and experientially. This corroborates Maharishi Ayurveda's view of TC as the fourth major state of human consciousness, in the sense that the three common states of waking, sleeping, and dreaming can be defined physiologically as well. MAV also discusses three higher states of consciousness (as yet untested in the laboratory) in which the full potential of consciousness progressively unfolds.

Maharishi Ayurveda views unfolding consciousness as the most important strategy of both prevention and cure. Consistent with this theory, data suggest that regular experience of TC has significant health benefits. Such research supports the MAV concept that "remembering" the unified field enlivens the orderly patterns that prevail in a healthy body. For example, TM has been found in several studies to retard biological aging (Glaser et al., 1992; Wallace et al., 1982). In a Harvard study of elderly nursing home residents that compared TM with two other types of meditation and relaxation techniques over 3 years, the TM group had the lowest mortality rate and the greatest reductions in stress and blood pressure (Alexander et al., 1989). Several subsequent studies found that TM significantly reduces high blood pressure (Cooper and Aygen, 1978; Schneider et al., 1992;

Wallace et al., 1983). Schneider and colleagues (1995) found TM to be approximately twice as effective as progressive muscle relaxation in reducing hypertension in older African Americans. Barnes and associates (2004) studied the effect of TM on African American adolescents with high normal blood pressure and found that the TM group had greater decreases in daytime systolic and diastolic blood pressure compared with a control group who received health education. A previous study by Barnes and colleagues (2001) on adolescents found that TM had a beneficial effect on cardiovascular functioning, as measured by blood pressure, heart rate, and cardiac output. Studies on TM have also shown that it significantly reduces cholesterol (Cooper and Aygen 1978, 1979) and lipid peroxide, fat that has been damaged by free radicals and can in turn cause damage of its own (Schneider et al., 1998). In addition, a study on catecholamine levels in TM practitioners showed that epinephrine and norepinephrine levels were significantly lower in the TM group compared with the control group, and anxiety levels were similar in both groups (Infante et al., 2001). This indicates that the regular practice of TM results in a low hormonal response to daily stress.

High blood pressure, high levels of cholesterol and lipid peroxide, and stress are risk factors for heart disease. Since TM has been shown to reduce high blood pressure, cholesterol, and lipid peroxide and modulate the body's response to stress, TM should be helpful in the treatment of heart disease. Research has borne this out: patients with heart disease were challenged by exercising on a bicycle and those who practiced TM showed better performance in several heart-related parameters (Zamarra et al., 1996). Also, a randomized controlled clinical trial showed that TM is associated with a reduction in atherosclerosis—hardening of the blood vessels that can lead to heart attack or stroke (Castillo-Richmond et al., 2000).

A meta-analysis of research on meditation and trait anxiety conducted at the Stanford Research Institute found that TM is approximately twice as effective as other meditation techniques in reducing trait anxiety (Eppley et al., 1989). Orme-Johnson and Walton (1998) conducted an analysis of meditation and relaxation techniques that showed TM to be more effective than other approaches in reducing anxiety, improving psychological health and reducing tobacco, alcohol, and drug use. These and similar studies and meta-analyses (Alexander et al., 1991, 1994a, 1994b) seem to corroborate Maharishi Ayurveda's theory, in that relaxing or meditating appeared to be not as significant a variable as experiencing the fourth state of consciousness: Transcendental Consciousness. Hundreds of other published studies on TM have documented a wide range of benefits in such areas as intellectual development and rehabilitation, but these are not of immediate relevance here. (Many of these studies are reprinted in Chalmers et al., 1989a, 1989b, 1989c; Orme-Johnson and Farrow, 1977; and Wallace et al., 1989.)

Regular practice of TM also has been found to reduce health care costs significantly, as measured by insurance statistics; TM practitioners needed hospitalization for illness or surgery 80% less often than a matched control group (Orme-Johnson, 1987). A more recent study of Canadian citizens enrolled in the government health insurance program showed that over a 6-year period, practice of the TM technique reduced government payments to physicians by 13% each year (Herron and Hillis, 2000). This translates into significant savings for health insurance companies struggling with the soaring cost of today's health care.

Prevention, Pathogenesis, and Balance

Seeing the body as a pattern of intelligence is the basis of a central tenet of MAV: for optimal health, it is necessary to maintain the body's natural state of internal balance. This tenet has applications for strengthening immunity, as well as for prevention, diagnosis, and treatment. The natural state of balance is understood in terms of another important Ayurvedic concept: three principles known as *doshas,* which govern the functioning of the body. The three doshas are Vata, Pitta, and Kapha; each has specific qualities and governs certain physiological activities. The doshas are not thought of as specifically physiological but as subtle principles that emerge early in the manifestation of the unified field. Therefore they are understood to operate throughout nature.[*]

[*]The doshas are considered to derive from combinations of still subtler expressions, the five *mahabhutas,* or "great elements." The physicist John Hagelin, a major contributor to grand unification theory, has pointed out that physics too now identifies five basic "elements," known as *spin types*. All the force and particle fields of physics belong to one of these five categories, and the characteristics of the five spin types correspond closely to those of the five mahabhutas.

In terms of the body, *Vata,* which governs flow and motion, is said to be at the basis of the activity of the locomotor system. It controls functions such as blood circulation and the expansion and contraction of the lungs and heart, intestinal peristalsis and elimination, activities of the nervous system, the contractile process in muscle, ionic transport across membranes (e.g., the sodium pump), cell division, and unwinding of deoxyribonucleic acid (DNA) during the process of transcription or replication. Vata is of prime importance in all homeostatic mechanisms and controls the other two principles, Pitta and Kapha.

Pitta governs bodily functions concerned with heat and metabolism and directs all biochemical reactions and the process of energy exchange. For example, it regulates digestion, functions of the exocrine glands and endocrine hormones, and intracellular metabolic pathways such as glycolysis, the tricarboxylic acid cycle, and the respiratory chain.

Kapha governs the structure and cohesion of the organism. It is responsible for biological strength, natural tissue resistance, and proper body structure. Microscopically, it is related to anatomical connections in the cell, such as the intracellular matrix, cell membrane, membranes of organelles, and synapses. On a biochemical level, Kapha structures receptors and the various forms of chemical binding.

When the doshas are balanced in their natural states and bodily locations, they produce health; when aggravated or imbalanced, they produce disease. A balanced Pitta dosha, for example, ensures healthy digestion, but an aggravated Pitta can cause ulcers and acid indigestion. MAV holds that all disease results from disruption of the natural balance of the doshas, and immune strength results from maintaining balance of the doshas. As Table 27-1 shows, the natural dosha balance can be thrown off by a wide variety of factors, such as unhealthy diet, poor digestion, unnatural daily routine, pollutants, and certain behaviors. The balance is restored by a variety of dietary and behavioral modalities, as well as other modalities discussed in this chapter, such as TM and herbal mixtures.

Each dosha has five subdivisions that govern different aspects of the body. For example, one subdivision of Pitta, *Bhrajaka Pitta,* relates to the skin. When balanced, it gives luster to the skin; when aggravated, Bhrajaka Pitta results in acne, boils, and rashes.

TABLE 27-1

The Three Doshas

Dosha	Effect of Balanced Dosha	Effect of Imbalanced Dosha	Factors Aggravating Dosha
Vata	Exhilaration Clear and alert mind Perfect functioning of bowels and urinary tract Proper formation of all bodily tissues Sound sleep Excellent vitality and immunity	Rough skin Weight loss Anxiety, worry Restlessness Constipation Decreased strength Arthritis Hypertension Rheumatic disorder Cardiac arrhythmia Insomnia	Excessive exercise Wakefulness Falling Bone fractures Tuberculosis Suppression of natural urges Cold Fear or grief Agitation or anger Fasting Pungent, astringent, or bitter foods Late autumn and winter (November-February)
Pitta	Lustrous complexion Contentment Perfect digestion Softness of body Perfectly balanced heat and thirst mechanisms Balanced intellect	Yellowish complexion Excessive body heat Insufficient sleep Weak digestion Inflammation Inflammatory bowel diseases Skin diseases Heartburn Peptic ulcer	Anger Strong sunshine Burning sensations Fasting Sesame products Linseed Yogurt Wine, vinegar Pungent, sour, or salty foods Midsummer and early autumn (July-October)
Kapha	Strength Normal joints Stability of mind Dignity Affectionate, forgiving nature Strong and properly proportioned body Courage Vitality	Pale complexion Coldness Lethargy Excessive sleep Sinusitis Respiratory diseases Asthma Excessive weight gain Loose joints Depression	Sleeping during daytime Heavy food Sweet, sour, or salty food Milk products Sugar Spring and early summer (March-June)

The concept of doshas—underlying metabolic principles—simplifies the practitioner's tasks and increases his or her effectiveness. The tridosha concept can help in clarifying the possible side effects of any treatment, customizing treatments for a specific patient, predicting risk factors and tendencies toward specific diseases, and noticing clusters of apparently unrelated syndromes that may have a similar underlying cause.

Some of these aspects result from the doshas' ability to provide the basis for a more precise description of the individual's natural state of balance. An individual may have a natural predominance of one or more doshas. These doshas need not be present in equal proportion to ensure physiological balance, but they need to be functioning in harmony with each other. This state is called *prakriti*. When the doshas are out of balance, they create *vikriti*, resulting in disorder and disease. Box 27-1 describes the classic characteristics of Vata, Pitta, and Kapha prakritis. More common than these are mixed prakritis, which involve various combinations of the three classic types, such as Vata-Pitta, or Pitta-Kapha, also describing the normal state of balance for individuals who possess them. Treatment in MAV is tailored to the individual patient through careful evaluation of both prakriti and vikriti.

Because Maharishi Ayurveda views disease as resulting from disruption of the natural balance of the doshas, the doshas play a key role in MAV's approach to understanding pathogenesis. In Western medicine a disease is detected as a result of its symptoms. The emergence of symptoms, however, must be preceded by earlier stages of imbalance. MAV locates six stages of pathogenesis, the first three of which have highly subtle symptoms with which allopathic medicine is not familiar. These first three stages involve aggravation of the normal functioning of the doshas. A skilled MAV diagnostician can detect these early pathogenic stages before overt symptoms emerge, using the techniques discussed in the next section.

BOX 27-1

Classic Characteristics of Vata, Pitta, and Kapha Prakritis

Vata Prakriti
Light, thin build
Performs activity quickly
Tendency to dry skin
Aversion to cold weather
Irregular hunger and digestion
Quick to grasp new information, also quick to forget
Tendency toward worry
Tendency toward constipation
Tendency toward light and interrupted sleep

Pitta Prakriti
Moderate build
Performs activity with medium speed
Aversion to hot weather
Sharp hunger and digestion
Medium time to grasp new information
Medium memory
Tendency toward irritability and temper
Enterprising and sharp in character
Prefers cold food and drink
Cannot skip meals
Good speakers
Tendency toward reddish complexion and hair, moles, and freckles

Kapha Prakriti
Solid, heavier build
Greater strength and endurance
Slow, methodical in activity
Oily, smooth skin
Tranquil, steady personality
Slow to grasp new information, slow to forget
Slow to become excited or irritated
Sleep is heavy and for long periods
Hair is plentiful, tends to be dark color
Slow digestion, mild hunger

Diagnosis

Maharishi Ayurveda adds a number of diagnostic techniques to the clinician's repertoire. All of them are noninvasive and reveal much information both about specific illnesses and about underlying imbalances. Chief among these techniques is *nadi vigyan* (pulse diagnosis), which allows one to retrieve detailed information about the internal functioning of the body and its organs through signals present in the radial pulse. This information involves not only the cardiovascular system but other bodily systems as well. From the pulse, the diagnostician gains information about the functioning of the bodily tissues, the state of the doshas, and much more. Pulse diagnosis reveals early stages of imbalance that precede full-blown symptoms. In this and other MAV diagnostic modalities, perceiving the body as a pattern of intelligence enables physicians to retrieve enormous amounts of information in a noninvasive manner.

Pharmacology

This paradigm in which the body is understood in terms of patterns of intelligence also is demonstrated in Maharishi Ayurveda's approach to pharmacology, which makes sophisticated use of thousands of herbs and other plants.

Western pharmacology, applying the mechanistic model of the body, isolates and then synthesizes single active ingredients from herbs and plants. For example, the Ayurvedic remedy willow bark was the source of acetylsalicylic acid, and the Ayurvedic remedy rauwolfia was the source of reserpine. The active-ingredient model reflects a weakness of the scientific method: its inability to deal with complex systems and its requirement that the researcher radically simplify a process to evaluate it (Sharma, 1997). By contrast, Ayurvedic pharmacology, called *dravyaguna,* uses the synergistic cooperation of substances as they *co*exist in natural sources. It uses either single plants or, more often, mixtures of plants whose effects are complementary. Such synergistic effects are gaining consideration in Western medical research, which is finding, for example, that *combinations* of antioxidants may stop oxidation damage and cancer cell growth more effectively than these substances acting alone.

In terms of MAV's consciousness model, the effectiveness of herbal mixtures relative to active ingredients can be explained by the idea that plants, especially herbs, are concentrated repositories of nature's intelligence, which, when used properly, can increase the expression of that intelligence in the body. Research and experience with Maharishi Ayurveda herbal mixtures, known as *rasayanas,* show that synergism enhances the free radical–scavenging properties of herbs and mitigates the harmful side effects that often accompany Western drugs (Sharma, 2002).

According to Maharishi Ayurveda, rasayanas promote longevity, stamina, immunity, and overall well-being (Sharma, 1993). Research has shown several rasayanas to have significant antioxidant properties (Bondy et al., 1994; Cullen et al., 1997; Dwivedi et al., 1991; Engineer et al., 1992; Hanna et al., 1994; Niwa, 1991; Sharma et al., 1995). The rasayana known as *Maharishi Amrit Kalash* (MAK) is approximately 1000 times more effective at scavenging free radicals than vitamin C, vitamin E, and a pharmaceutical antioxidant (Sharma et al., 1992).

MAK has been researched extensively in laboratory, animal, and clinical settings, and found to have a wide range of significant beneficial properties. MAK prevented and treated breast cancer (Sharma et al., 1990; Sharma et al., 1991); prevented metastasis of lung cancer (Patel et al., 1992); caused nervous system tumor cells (neuroblastoma) to regain normal cell functioning (Prasad et al., 1992); enhanced the effect of nerve growth factor in causing morphological dif-

ferentiation of nervous system tumor cells (pheochromocytoma) (Rodella et al., 2004); inhibited the growth of skin cancer cells (melanoma) (Prasad et al., 1993); and prevented liver cancer (Mazzoleni et al., 2002). In clinical studies, MAK has been shown to reduce the side effects of chemotherapy, without reducing the efficacy of the cancer treatment (Misra et al., 1994; Srivastava et al., 2000).

MAK also reduces several risk factors for heart disease. It prevented human platelet aggregation (Sharma et al., 1989) and reduced atherosclerosis in laboratory animals by 53% (Lee et al., 1996). In clinical studies on patients with heart disease, MAK reduced the frequency of angina, improved exercise tolerance, and lowered systolic blood pressure and lipid peroxide levels (Dogra et al., 1994; Dogra and Bhargava, 2000). A study on hyperlipidemic patients showed that MAK increases the resistance of low-density lipoprotein to oxidation, which is important for the prevention of atherosclerosis (Sundaram et al., 1997).

A strong immune system is vital to the maintenance of health. Several studies have shown that MAK significantly enhances immune functioning (Dileepan et al., 1990, 1993; Inaba et al., 1995, 1996, 1997). MAK has also demonstrated antiaging effects. It improved age-related visual discrimination in older men (Gelderloos et al., 1990) and has been shown to rejuvenate the antioxidant defense system and protect against mitochondrial deterioration in the aging central nervous system (Vohra et al., 1999, 2001a). In the aging brain, MAK reduced lipid peroxidation and lipofuscin pigment accumulation, restored normal oxygen consumption, and enhanced cholinergic enzymes (Vohra et al., 2001b, 2001c). It has also been shown to decrease the number of dark neurons in the brain, which indicates that MAK protects the neurons from injury (Vohra et al., 2002).

Diet and Digestion

Western medical research is accumulating more and more evidence that diet plays a critical role in the development of heart disease and cancer. The American Cancer Society reports that about one third of the cancer deaths in the United States each year have diet as a significant risk factor (*Cancer Facts and Figures,* 2004). Scientists estimate that 60% to 70% of cancers can be prevented by simple changes in diet and lifestyle (Sharma et al., 2002). It is also known that a diet rich in the wrong types of fat creates a higher risk of heart disease, the number-one killer in the United States today (Sharma and Clark, 1998). Ayurveda has long considered problems of diet and digestion to be among the central causes of all disease and has considered improvement of diet and digestion to be crucial to almost any therapeutic regimen. Ayurveda views faulty diet as not only contributing to specific degenerative diseases, but also throwing off the body's natural balance, thus weakening immunity.

MAV's approach to diet rests on the "consciousness model"; food is viewed as providing not only matter and energy to the body but also intelligence, order, and balance. This brings to mind the observations of the Nobel Laureate physicist Erwin Schrödinger that food helps the body resist the second law of thermodynamics, which normally leads any complex system into chaos (Schrödinger, 1967). By this view, when we eat, we are eating not only nutrients but also "orderliness." MAV dietetics considers not only the nutritional value and caloric content of food but also the food's impact on the body's underlying state of balance; food affects the doshas, and diet must be suited to the individual vikriti and prakriti. It also must reflect the climate and season, as well as specific health conditions.

The influence of food on the doshas is specific to the food but usually can be determined by knowing in which generic categories of tastes and qualities the food belongs. According to MAV, the six categories of taste are sweet, sour, salty, pungent, astringent, and bitter. The six major categories of quality are heavy, light, cold, hot, oily, and dry. Box 27-2 summarizes how taste and food qualities affect the doshas, and Box 27-3 gives examples of foods that possess these various qualities and tastes.

To give an example of how this information would be applied clinically, a patient with Kapha syndromes (e.g., sinusitis, certain types of obesity) would be told to minimize eating cold, oily, and heavy foods, as well as foods with sweet, sour, and salty tastes. The patient would be advised instead to give predominance to foods exhibiting the remaining qualities and tastes.

Maharishi Ayurveda recommends a lactovegetarian diet for optimal health. Meat is more difficult to digest and has been linked to numerous diseases, including heart disease and cancer. MAV also recom-

BOX 27-2

Taste and Food Quality Effects on the Doshas

Tastes	
Decrease Vata	*Increase Vata*
Sweet	Pungent
Sour	Bitter
Salty	Astringent
Decrease Pitta	*Increase Pitta*
Sweet	Pungent
Bitter	Sour
Astringent	Salty
Decrease Kapha	*Increase Kapha*
Pungent	Sweet
Bitter	Sour
Astringent	Salty

Major Food Qualities	
Decrease Vata	*Increase Vata*
Heavy	Light
Oily	Dry
Hot	Cold
Decrease Pitta	*Increase Pitta*
Cold	Hot
Heavy	Light
Oily	Dry
Decrease Kapha	*Increase Kapha*
Light	Heavy
Dry	Oily
Hot	Cold

mends the use of fresh produce. These emphases map well with emerging Western findings on diet, which have shown significant health benefits from a meatless diet and from increasing consumption of fruits and vegetables (*Harvard Health Letter*, 2004). A long-term study on vegetarians revealed that eating fresh fruit daily results in a significant reduction in mortality from ischemic heart disease, cerebrovascular disease, and all causes combined (Key et al., 1996). A separate study showed that vegetarians have a 25% lower mortality from ischemic heart disease compared with nonvegetarians (Key et al., 1999). Another study on ischemic heart disease showed that the risk of developing this illness is significantly lower in older vegetarian women compared with older nonvegetarian women (Kwok et al., 2000).

BOX 27-3

Common Examples of the Six Tastes and Major Food Qualities

Six Tastes and Common Examples

Sweet: sugar, milk, butter, rice, breads, honey
Sour: yogurt, lemon, cheese
Salty: salt
Pungent: spicy foods, peppers, ginger, cumin
Bitter: spinach, other green leafy vegetables
Astringent: beans

Six Major Food Qualities and Common Examples

Heavy: cheese, yogurt, wheat products
Light: barley, corn, spinach, apples
Oily: dairy products, fatty foods, oils
Dry: barley, corn, potato, beans
Hot: hot (temperature) food and drink
Cold: cold food and drink

Other studies also indicate that vegetarians have a significantly lower incidence of coronary heart disease (Claude-Chang et al., 1992; Dwyer, 1988; Slattery et al., 1991). Patients on a vegetarian diet have reduced frequency, duration, and severity of angina; regression of atherosclerosis; and improvement in coronary perfusion (Segasothy and Phillips, 1999). Research has also found that long-term vegetarians have a reduced risk of lipid peroxidation (Krajcovicova-Kudlackova et al., 1995a, 1995b) and lower levels of cholesterol (Key et al., 1999; Kwok et al., 2000).

A vegetarian diet has proven beneficial in other chronic diseases as well. A study showed that women who eat red meat daily are at twice the risk of developing colon cancer compared with women who eat red meat less than once a month (Willett et al., 1990). A study on Seventh-Day Adventists showed that the prevalence of diabetes and hypertension was lower among long-term vegetarians compared with non-vegetarians (Brathwaite et al., 2003). Considering all the benefits of a vegetarian diet, it is not surprising that studies have shown vegetarians have a longer life span. A long-term study found that vegetarians have a mortality rate that is half that of the general population (Key et al., 1996). A separate long-term study of male Seventh-Day Adventists found that meat eating correlated with all forms of mortality measured (Snowdon, 1988).

Maharishi Ayurveda focuses not only on what one eats but also on how one digests it. The emphasis on digestion contrasts with Western allopathic medicine, which deals with digestion only when it is significantly disrupted. In MAV, excellent digestion is critical to robust health. MAV contains a number of techniques for improving digestion and treating digestive disorders. They center on the concept of *agni,* which literally means "fire," and refers to metabolic and digestive activities that convert foodstuff into bodily substances. Ayurveda describes 13 types of agni in the body. Their importance in Ayurvedic health care is suggested by the fact that one of the eight branches of Ayurveda, *Kaya Chikitsa* (internal medicine), focuses on the strength or weakness of the agnis.

This becomes clearer when we consider the end product of poor digestion, which Ayurveda calls *Ama.* Ama plays a key role in pathogenesis, interacting with aggravated doshas and causing them to "stick" to areas where they do not belong. Healthy digestion reduces the amount of Ama produced.

To rid the body of accumulated Ama, pollutants, and other pathogenic impurities that disrupt or block the natural expression of the body's inner intelligence, Maharishi Ayurveda emphasizes the importance of purification therapies that rid the body of these substances. Foremost among these purification therapies is *Panchakarma* (or Pañchakarma; see Chapter 25), which literally means "five activities," because it includes five main treatment modalities, as follows:

1. Whole-body massage with herbalized oil *(abhyanga)*
2. Continuous flow of warm herbalized oil on the forehead *(shirodhara)*
3. Fomentation of the body with herbalized heat *(swedana)*
4. Special herbalized oil head massage and nasal administration of herbs *(nasya)*
5. Sesame oil retention or herbalized eliminative enemas *(basti)*

Daily treatments, administered for 2 to 14 days or longer, are recommended with each change of the seasons. Certain aspects of Panchakarma can fit easily into a patient's daily preventive regimen. Preliminary research has shown that regular Panchakarma reduces several cardiovascular risk factors, including cholesterol (Sharma et al., 1993; Waldschutz, 1988).

Sesame oil, which is used topically and for colonic irrigation in Panchakarma, has been shown to inhibit in vitro malignant melanoma growth (Smith and Salerno, 1992) and human colon adenocarcinoma cell line growth (Salerno and Smith, 1991). Preliminary research on Panchakarma has also shown that it reduces fat-soluble toxicants in humans. Levels of polychlorinated biphenyls (PCBs) and agrochemicals were reduced by 50% in subjects who received Panchakarma. PCBs have been banned for years, but previous exposure can result in a lingering accumulation of the toxicant in fat tissue. Lipophilic toxicants have been associated with hormonal disorders, suppression of the immune system, reproductive disorders, cancer, and other diseases (Herron and Fagan, 2002).

The central role of food and digestion is demonstrated particularly well by consideration of another central MAV concept: the importance of a substance called *ojas*. Ojas is said to be the finest manifestation of the unified field, which serves as a sort of glue to link consciousness and matter. Ojas maintains the integrity of the seven bodily tissues *(dhatus)*: plasma *(rasa)*, blood *(rakta)*, muscle *(mamsa)*, fat *(meda)*, bone *(asthi)*, bone marrow and nervous system *(majja)*, and sperm/ovum *(sukra)*. Most MAV therapies and behavioral advice are designed to maximize the presence of ojas, and almost all MAV proscriptions are designed to minimize the depletion of ojas. The end product of truly healthy diet and digestion is said to contain significant amounts of ojas. According to an MAV expression, "Like a bee which gets honey from the flowers, we get ojas from our food." MAV also asserts that positive, loving emotions increase the abundance of ojas; food should be eaten in a warm, congenial, and uplifting atmosphere. Arguing or any other negativity at meals interferes with digestion, producing a harmful end product (Ama) instead of ojas.

Behavior, Emotions, and the Senses

The recommendation for a positive emotional tone during meals reflects a general concept of MAV regarding behavior, speech, and emotions, and their effect on health. This concept springs naturally from the model that places consciousness at the basis of the body. Emotions can be understood as fine fluctuations of consciousness (or the unified field); as such, their impact on the more expressed physical levels of the body are immense. Recently, Western medicine has begun to investigate the effect of emotions on health, with interesting findings; Ayurveda has discussed this field for millennia. Ayurvedic texts include detailed discussions of lifestyle and behavior, and their impact on health. Interestingly, traditional virtues—such as respect for elders, teachers, loved ones, and family members; pardoning those who wrong you; practicing nonviolence; and not speaking ill of others—are understood to promote health for the individual's mind and body, as well as for the community and society.

In addition to emotion, sensory input is understood to have an impact on health. This idea is applied clinically, not only in terms of behavioral advice but also in the form of sensory therapies, such as aromatherapy and sound therapy involving both music (called *Gandharva-Veda*) and primordial sounds that are used for their healing qualities. A study on Maharishi Ayurveda primordial sound therapy (specifically, Vedic sounds known as *Sama Veda*) found it to reduce in vitro human tumor cell growth significantly, whereas hard rock music tended to increase growth significantly (Sharma et al, 1996) (see Chapter 25).

Biological Rhythms

In Maharishi Ayurveda, attuning the patient's lifestyle to natural biorhythms is considered a crucial element of prevention and treatment. MAV gives a detailed analysis of circadian and circannual rhythms, with recommendations for daily and seasonal routines. These include such advice as rising and retiring early and eating one's main meal at lunchtime, when the digestive "fires" are strongest. Many other recommendations are also given; as always, this advice must be tailored to the individual. Emerging Western data on biorhythms correlate well with the ancient Ayurvedic knowledge. Again, the idea of a connection between patterns of order in nature and in the human body was obvious to Ayurveda millennia ago.

The three-dosha concept plays a key role in understanding these connections. Different times of the day are associated with different doshas, as are different seasons and the different stages of the human life cycle (Box 27-4). For example, the summer is dominated by Pitta (the dosha that governs heat and

BOX 27-4

Seasons and Times of Day Classified
According to the Doshas

- Kapha season: Spring-early summer (approximately March to June)
- Kapha time: Approximately 6 AM (sunrise) to 10 AM and 6 PM to 10 PM
- Kapha period in life cycle: Childhood
- Pitta season: Midsummer-early autumn (approximately July to October)
- Pitta time: Approximately 10 AM to 2 PM and 10 PM to 2 AM
- Pitta period in life cycle: Adulthood
- Vata season: Late autumn-winter (approximately November to February)
- Vata time: Approximately 2 AM to 6 AM (sunrise) and 2 PM to 6 PM
- Vata period in life cycle: Old age

metabolism), whereas the spring is dominated by Kapha (which has qualities of coolness and moisture). Childhood is dominated by Kapha (which governs structure, substance, and growth) and old age by Vata. In fact, physicians see a preponderance of Kapha-based disorders in children, such as colds and respiratory illnesses, and an ever-increasing number of Vata disorders in elderly patients, such as constipation and lighter, shorter, and more frequently interrupted sleep. They also see more Kapha-type disorders in spring and Pitta disorders in summer. Understanding the concept of doshas is helpful in treating these ailments.

COLLECTIVE HEALTH AND THE ENVIRONMENT

Maharishi Ayurveda holds great promise in several areas of collective health. In terms of infectious disease and epidemics, the Western approach of using antibiotics has an inherent limitation and risk caused by the process of natural selection that produces new, resistant strains of microbes. As a result, overreliance on antibiotics can foster the growth of serious new infectious diseases. MAV's focus on strengthening immunity and its techniques for dealing directly with epidemics offer a more effective and safer means of ensuring collective health.

In terms of chronic disease, Western medicine has long recognized that preventing and treating these disorders requires changes in lifestyle, diet, and behavior. However, allopathic medicine has been at a loss as to how to effect these changes in patients for a prolonged time. Research has shown that those who practice TM are better able to give up harmful habits, such as cigarette smoking, alcohol consumption, and illegal drug use, and to incorporate healthy dietary and lifestyle changes (Alexander et al., 1994b; Gelderloos et al., 1991; Monahan, 1977). MAV also offers other time-tested modalities that benefit individual patients, such as daily routine and purification procedures, which could be useful in large-scale applications. Finally, MAV offers an overall theory of prevention, involving such elements as the three-dosha concept, that could have value for future research on preventive medicine.

The most significant public health approach of Maharishi Ayurveda deals with larger social disorders and the dangers they pose. War, crime, and violence rarely are considered subjects of public health policy, but their implications for health are obvious. As with individual disease, Maharishi Ayurveda understands these as originating not in material factors but ultimately in consciousness: in this case, both individual and collective consciousness. Just as an abstract field of consciousness underlies the individual's mind and body, so such a field underlies societal trends. Society reflects the influence of its members not only in a linear, additive way—in the sense that a green forest is made of green trees—but also through a field effect—in the sense that a gravitational field's influences are not localized. If the individual consciousness of a sufficient number of members of a society is coherent, harmonious, and life supporting, those influences spread through the "field" of the collective consciousness of the society, influencing the whole society.

This idea has been tested by a number of studies. One study found that when a sufficiently large group of practitioners of the TM and advanced TM-Sidhi techniques meditated together as a group in Israel, war deaths in Lebanon were significantly reduced compared with casualty rates on days when the number of practitioners meditating together decreased below a certain threshold (Orme-Johnson et al., 1988). Similar findings have emerged in studies of other localities, usually involving reductions in the rate of violent crime (Dillbeck et al., 1981, 1988; Orme-Johnson and Gelderloos, 1988). For example, a

1993 study in Washington, DC, showed that when a large group of practitioners of the TM and TM-Sidhi programs assembled to meditate during the summer, it produced an 18% reduction in violent crime compared with levels that had been predicted on the basis of previous years' crime and weather trends (Hagelin et al., 1999). There has been much discussion and debate regarding these observations and the validity of what has been called the *Maharishi effect*.

FUTURE DIRECTIONS

Many central elements of Ayurveda, such as the ideas that diet and emotions play a crucial role in disease and prevention, were not taken seriously by Western medicine a generation ago but are now major themes of research. Other areas of Ayurveda might prove to be of value both in clinical work and in research. Already, the Transcendental Meditation technique and herbal preparations have produced bodies of significant research findings whose implications have yet to be fully explored. Other areas, such as prakriti and vikriti, will likely prove equally interesting to researchers.

The clinical use of Ayurveda appears to be most dramatic when applied to diseases that Western medicine finds difficult to treat, such as poor digestion, heart disease, cancer, and other chronic diseases (Janssen, 1989; Orme-Johnson, 1987). Its clinical value extends to other areas not discussed previously, such as pediatrics, where it has been found to reduce significantly the incidence of childhood ailments such as frequent colds, and gynecology, where it reduces the severity of menstrual and premenstrual disorders.

Several medical institutions have incorporated Ayurveda into their teaching curricula. In the future it is likely that Ayurveda will gain further recognition as a valuable system of natural health care. Its comprehensive modalities can be used to create health and well-being in the individual and in society as a whole.

References

Alexander CN, Langer EJ, Davies JL, et al: Transcendental Meditation, mindfulness and longevity: an experimental study with the elderly, *J Pers Soc Psychol* 57:950-964, 1989.

Alexander CN, Rainforth MV, Gelderloos P: Transcendental Meditation, self-actualization, and psychological health: a conceptual overview and statistical meta-analysis, *J Soc Behav Pers* 6:189-247. 1991.

Alexander CN, Robinson P, Orme-Johnson DW, et al: The effects of Transcendental Meditation compared to other methods of relaxation and meditation in reducing risk factors, morbidity and mortality, *Homeostasis* 35:243-264, 1994a.

Alexander CN, Robinson P, Rainforth M: Treating alcohol, nicotine, and drug abuse through Transcendental Meditation: a review and statistical meta-analysis, *Alcoholism Treatment Q* 11:13-87, 1994b.

Andrews LB, Stocking C, Krizek T, et al: An alternative strategy for studying adverse events in medical care, *Lancet* 349:309-313, 1997.

Aspect A, Grangier P, Roger G: Experimental tests of realistic local theories via Bell's theorem, *Phys Rev Lett* 47:460, 1981.

Badawi K, Wallace RK, Orme-Johnson DW, Rouzere AM: Electrophysiologic characteristics of respiratory suspension periods occurring during the practice of the Transcendental Meditation program, *Psychosom Med* 46:267-276, 1984.

Barnes VA, Treiber FA, Davis H. Impact of Transcendental Meditation on cardiovascular function at rest and during acute stress in adolescents with high normal blood pressure, *J Psychosom Res* 51(4):597-605, 2001.

Barnes VA, Treiber FA, Johnson MH: Impact of Transcendental Meditation on ambulatory blood pressure in African-American adolescents, *Am J Hypertens* 17:366-369, 2004.

Berwick DM, Leape LL: Reducing errors in medicine, *BMJ* 319:136-137, 1999.

Bondy SC, Hernandez TM, Mattia C: Antioxidant properties of two Ayurvedic herbal preparations, *Biochem Arch* 10:25-31, 1994.

Brathwaite N, Fraser HS, Modeste N, et al: Obesity, diabetes, hypertension, and vegetarian status among Seventh-Day Adventists in Barbados: preliminary results, *Ethn Dis* 13(1):34-39, 2003.

Cancer facts and figures, Atlanta, 2004, American Cancer Society, p 43.

Castillo-Richmond A, Schneider RH, Alexander CN, et al: Effects of stress reduction on carotid atherosclerosis in hypertensive African Americans, *Stroke* 31:568-573, 2000.

Chalmers RA, Clements G, Schenkluhn H, Weinless M, editors: *Scientific research on Maharishi's Transcendental Meditation and TM-Sidhi program: collected papers,* vol 2, Vlodrop, The Netherlands, 1989a, MVU Press.

Chalmers RA, Clements G, Schenkluhn H, Weinless M, editors: Scientific research on Maharishi's Transcendental Meditation and TM-Sidhi program: collected papers, vol 3, Vlodrop, The Netherlands, 1989b, MVU Press.

Chalmers RA, Clements G, Schenkluhn H, Weinless M, editors: *Scientific research on Maharishi's Transcendental Meditation and TM-Sidhi program: collected papers,* vol 4, Vlodrop, The Netherlands, 1989c, MVU Press.

Charaka Samhita, Varanasi, India, 1977, Chowkhamba Sanskrit Series Office (Translated by RK Sharma and B Dash).

Claude-Chang J, Frentzel-Beyme R, Eilber U: Mortality pattern of German vegetarians after 11 years of follow-up, *Epidemiology* 3(5):395-401, 1992.

Cooper MJ, Aygen MM: Effect of Transcendental Meditation on serum cholesterol and blood pressure, *Harefuah J Israel Med Assoc* 95(1):1-2, 1978.

Cooper MJ, Aygen MM: A relaxation technique in the management of hypercholesterolemia, *J Hum Stress* 5:24-27, 1979.

Cullen WJ, Dulchavsky SA, Devasagayam TPA, et al: Effect of Maharishi AK-4 on H_2O_2-induced oxidative stress in isolated rat hearts, *J Ethnopharmacol* 56:215-222, 1997.

Dileepan KN, Patel V, Sharma HM, Stechschulte DJ: Priming of splenic lymphocytes after ingestion of an Ayurvedic herbal food supplement: evidence for an immunomodulatory effect, *Biochem Arch* 6:267-274, 1990.

Dileepan KN, Varghese ST, Page JC, Stechschulte DJ: Enhanced lymphoproliferative response, macrophage mediated tumor cell killing and nitric oxide production after ingestion of an Ayurvedic drug, *Biochem Arch* 9:365-374, 1993.

Dillbeck MC, Banus CB, Polanzi C, Landrith G III: Text of a field model of consciousness and social change: the Transcendental Meditation and TM-Sidhi program and decreased urban crime, *Mind Behav* 9(4):457-486, 1988.

Dillbeck MC, Landrith G III, Orme-Johnson DW: The Transcendental Meditation program and crime rate change in a sample of 48 cities, *J Crime Justice* 4:24-45, 1981.

Dogra J, Bhargava A (SPON: Sharma H): Lipid peroxide in ischemic heart disease (IHD): Inhibition by Maharishi Amrit Kalash (MAK-4 and MAK-5) herbal mixtures, *FASEB J* 14(4):A121, 2000 (abstract).

Dogra J, Grover N, Kumar P, Aneja N: Indigenous free radical scavenger MAK4 and 5 in angina pectoris: is it only a placebo? *J Assoc Physicians India* 42(6):466-467, 1994.

Dwivedi C, Sharma HM, Dobrowki S, Engineer F: Inhibitory effects of Maharishi Amrit Kalash (M-4) and Maharishi Amrit Kalash (M-5) on microsomal lipid peroxidation, *Pharmacol Biochem Behav* 39:649-652, 1991.

Dwyer JT: Health aspects of vegetarian diets, *Am J Clin Nutr* 48:712-738, 1988.

Eddington A: *The nature of the physical world,* Ann Arbor, 1974, University of Michigan Press, p 276.

Engineer FN, Sharma HM, Dwivedi C: Protective effects of M-4 and M-5 on Adriamycin-induced microsomal lipid peroxidation and mortality, *Biochem Arch* 8:267-272, 1992.

Eppley KR, Abrams A, Shear J: Differential effects of relaxation techniques on trait anxiety: a meta-analysis, *J Clin Psychol* 45:957-974, 1989.

Farrow JT, Hebert JR: Breath suspension during the Transcendental Meditation technique, *Psychosom Med* 44(2):133-153, 1982.

Gallois P: Modifications neurophysiologiques et respiratoires lors de la practique des techniques de relaxation, *Encephale* 10:139-144, 1984.

Gelderloos P, Ahlstrom HHB, Orme-Johnson DW, et al: Influence of a Maharishi Ayur-Vedic herbal preparation on age-related visual discrimination, *Int J Psychosom* 37:25-29, 1990.

Gelderloos P, Walton KG, Orme-Johnson DW, Alexander CN: Effectiveness of the Transcendental Meditation program in preventing and treating substance misuse: a review, *Int J Addict* 26:293-325, 1991.

Glaser J, Brind J, Vogelman J, et al: Elevated serum dehydroepiandrosterone sulfate levels in practitioners of the Transcendental Meditation (TM) and TM-Sidhi programs, *J Behav Med* 15(4):327-341, 1992.

Hagelin JS, Orme-Johnson DW, Rainforth M, et al: Results of the National Demonstration Project to Reduce Violent Crime and Improve Governmental Effectiveness in Washington, DC, *Soc Indic Res* 47:153-201, 1999.

Hanna AN, Sharma HM, Kauffman EM, Newman HAI: In vitro and in vivo inhibition of microsomal lipid peroxidation by MA-631, *Pharmacol Biochem Behav* 48:505-510, 1994.

Harvard Health Letter: Vegetarianism: addition by subtraction, *Harv Health Lett* 29(4):6, 2004.

Herron RE, Fagan JB: Lipophil-mediated reduction of toxicants in humans: an evaluation of an Ayurvedic detoxification procedure, *Altern Ther Health Med* 8(5):40-51, 2002.

Herron RE, Hillis SL: The impact of the Transcendental Meditation program on government payments to physicians in Quebec: an update, *Am J Health Promot* 14(5):284-291, 2000.

Inaba R, Sugiura H, Iwata H: Immunomodulatory effects of Maharishi Amrit Kalash 4 and 5 in mice, *Jpn J Hygiene* 50(4):901-905, 1995.

Inaba R, Sugiura H, Iwata H, et al: Immunomodulation by Maharishi Amrit Kalash 4 in mice, *J Appl Nutr* 48(1-2):10-21, 1996.

Inaba R, Sugiura H, Iwata H, Tanaka T: Dose-dependent activation of immune function in mice by ingestion of Maharishi Amrit Kalash 5, *Environ Health Prev Med* 2(1):35-39, 1997.

Infante JR, Torres-Avisbal M, Pinel P, et al: Catecholamine levels in practitioners of the Transcendental Meditation technique, *Physiol Behav* 72(1-2):141-146, 2001.

Janssen GW: The application of Maharishi Ayur-Ved in the treatment of ten chronic diseases: a pilot study, *Ned Tijdschr Geneeskd* 5(35):586-594, 1989.

Jevning JR, Wilson AF, Davison JM: Adrenocortical activity during meditation, *Horm Behav* 10:54-60, 1978.

Jevning JR, Wilson AF, O'Halloran JP, Walsh RN: Forearm blood flow and metabolism during stylized and unstylized states of decreased activation, *Am J Physiol* 245 (*Regul Integr Comp Physiol* 14):R100-R116, 1983.

Key TJ, Davey GK, Appleby PN: Health benefits of a vegetarian diet, *Proc Nutr Soc* 58(2):271-275, 1999.

Key TJ, Thorogood M, Appleby PN, Burr ML: Dietary habits and mortality in 11,000 vegetarians and health-conscious people: results of a 17-year follow-up, *BMJ* 313(7060):775-779, 1996.

Krajcovicova-Kudlackova M, Simoncic R, Babinska K, Bederova A: Levels of lipid peroxidation and anti-oxidants in vegetarians, *Eur J Epidemiol* 11(2):207-211, 1995a.

Krajcovicova-Kudlackova M, Simoncic R, Bederova A, et al: Plasma fatty acid profile and prooxidative-antioxidative parameters in vegetarians, *Nahrung* 39(5-6):452-457, 1995b.

Kwok TK, Woo J, Ho S, Sham A: Vegetarianism and ischemic heart disease in older Chinese women, *J Am Coll Nutr* 19(5):622-627, 2000.

Lazarou J, Pomeranz BH, Corey PN: Incidence of adverse drug reactions in hospitalized patients, *JAMA* 279:1200-1205, 1998.

Lee JY, Hanna AN, Lott JA, Sharma HM: The antioxidant and antiatherogenic effects of MAK-4 in WHHL rabbits, *J Altern Complementary Med* 2(4):463-478, 1996.

Levine JP: The Coherence Spectral Array (COSPAR) and its application to the study of spatial ordering in the EEG, *Proc San Diego Biomed Symp* 15:237-247, 1976.

Madhavakava: *Madhava Nidanam,* Delhi, 1986, Chaukambha Orientalia (Translated by KR Srikanta Murthy).

Mazzoleni G, Hsiao WLW, Statuto M, et al: Anti-tumor effects of the antioxidant natural products Maharishi Amrit Kalash-4 and -5 (MAK) on cell transformation in vitro and in liver carcinogenesis in mice, *J Appl Nutr* 52(2/3):45-63, 2002.

Misra NC, Sharma HM, Chaturvedi A, et al: Antioxidant adjuvant therapy using a natural herbal mixture (MAK) during intensive chemotherapy: reduction in toxicity—a prospective study of 62 patients. In Rao RS, Deo MG, Sanghvi LD, editors: *Proceedings of the XVI International Cancer Congress,* Bologna, Italy, 1994, Monduzzi Editore, pp 3099-3102.

Monahan RJ: Secondary prevention of drug dependence through the Transcendental Meditation program in metropolitan Philadelphia, *Int J Addict* 12:729-754, 1977.

Nader T: *Human physiology: expression of Veda and the Vedic literature,* Vlodrop, The Netherlands, 1993, MVU Press.

Niwa Y: Effect of Maharishi-4 and Maharishi-5 on inflammatory mediators—with special reference to their free radical scavenging effect, *Indian J Clin Pract* 1:23-27 1991.

Orme-Johnson DW: Autonomic stability and Transcendental Meditation, *Psychosom Med* 35:341-349, 1973.

Orme-Johnson DW: Medical care utilization and the Transcendental Meditation program, *Psychosom Med* 49:493-507, 1987.

Orme-Johnson DW, Alexander CN, Davies JL, et al: International peace project in the Middle East: the effects of the Maharishi Technology of the Unified Field, *J Conflict Resolut* 32(4):776-812, 1988.

Orme-Johnson DW, Farrow JT, editors: Scientific research on the Transcendental Meditation program: collected papers, vol 1, Rheinweiler, W Germany, 1977, MERU Press.

Orme-Johnson DW, Gelderloos P: The long term effects of the Maharishi Technology of the Unified Field on the quality of life in the United States (1960-1983), *Soc Sci Pers J* 2(4):127-146, 1988.

Orme-Johnson DW, Walton KG: All approaches to preventing or reversing effects of stress are not the same, *Am J Health Promot* 12(5):297-299, 1998.

Patel VK, Wang J, Shen RN, et al: Reduction of metastases of Lewis lung carcinoma by an Ayurvedic food supplement in mice, *Nutr Res* 12:667-676, 1992.

Prasad KN, Edwards-Prasad J, Kentroti S, et al: Ayurvedic (science of life) agents induce differentiation in murine neuroblastoma cells in culture, *Neuropharmacology* 31:599-607, 1992.

Prasad ML, Parry P, Chan C: Ayurvedic agents produce differential effects on murine and human melanoma cells in vitro, *Nutr Cancer* 20:79-86, 1993.

Rarity JG, Tapster PR: Experimental violation of Bell's inequality based on phase and momentum, *Phys Rev Lett* 64:2495, 1990.

Rodella L, Borsani E, Rezzani R, et al: MAK-5 treatment enhances the nerve growth factor–mediated neurite outgrowth in PC12 cells, *J Ethnopharmacol* 93:161-166, 2004.

Salerno JW, Smith DE: The use of sesame oil and other vegetable oils in the inhibition of human colon cancer growth in vitro, *Anticancer Res* 11:209-216, 1991.

Sarngadhara: *Sarngadhara Samhita,* Delhi, 1984, Chaukhambha Orientalia (Translated by KR Srikanta Murthy).

Schneider RH, Alexander CN, Wallace RK: In search of an optimal behavioral treatment for hypertension: a review and focus on Transcendental Meditation. In Johnson EH, Gentry WD, Julius S, editors: *Personality, elevated blood pressure, and essential hypertension,* Washington, DC, 1992, Hemisphere, pp 123-131.

Schneider RH, Nidich SI, Salerno JW, et al: Lower lipid peroxide levels in practitioners of the Transcendental Meditation program, *Psychosom Med* 60:38-41, 1998.

Schneider RH, Staggers F, Alexander CN, et al: A randomized controlled trial of stress reduction for hypertension in older African Americans, *Hypertension* 26:820-827, 1995.

Schrödinger E: *What is life?* Cambridge, Mass, 1967. Cambridge University Press.

Segasothy M, Phillips PA: Vegetarian diet: panacea for modern lifestyle diseases? *QJM* 92(9):531-544, 1999.

Sharma H: *Freedom from disease: how to control free radicals, a major cause of aging and disease,* Toronto, 1993, Veda Publishing.

Sharma H, Clark C: *Contemporary Ayurveda: medicine and research in Maharishi Ayur-Veda,* London, 1998, Churchill Livingstone.

Sharma H, Mishra RK, with Meade JG: *The answer to cancer,* New York, 2002, SelectBooks.

Sharma H, Guenther J, Abu-Ghazaleh A, Dwivedi C: Effects of Ayurvedic food supplement M-4 on cisplatin-induced changes in glutathione and glutathione-S-transferase activity. In Rao RS, Deo MG, Sanghvi LD, editors: *Proceedings of the XVI International Cancer Congress,* vol 1, Bologna, Italy, 1994, Monduzzi Editore, pp 589-592.

Sharma HM: Phytochemical synergism: beyond the active ingredient model, *Altern Ther Clin Pract* 4(3):91-96, 1997.

Sharma HM: Free radicals and natural antioxidants in health and disease, *J Appl Nutr* 52(2-3):26-44, 2002.

Sharma HM, Feng Y, Panganamala RV: Maharishi Amrit Kalash (MAK) prevents human platelet aggregation, *Clin Ter Cardiovasc* 8:227-230, 1989.

Sharma HM, Kauffman EM, Stephens RE: Effect of different sounds on growth of human cancer cell lines in vitro, *Altern Ther Clin Pract* 3(4):25-32, 1996.

Sharma HM, Dwivedi C, Satter BC, Abou-Issa H: Antineoplastic properties of Maharishi Amrit Kalash, an Ayurvedic food supplement, against 7,12-dimethylbenz(a)anthracene-induced mammary tumors in rats, *J Res Educ Indian Med* 10(3):1-8, 1991.

Sharma HM, Hanna AN, Kauffman EM, Newman HAI: Inhibition of human LDL oxidation in vitro by Maharishi Ayur-Veda herbal mixtures, *Pharmacol Biochem Behav* 43:1175-1182, 1992.

Sharma HM, Hanna AN, Kauffman EM, Newman HAI: Effect of herbal mixture Student Rasayana on lipoxygenase activity and lipid peroxidation, *Free Radic Biol Med* 18:687-697, 1995.

Sharma HM, Nidich SI, Sands D, Smith DE: Improvement in cardiovascular risk factors through Panchakarma purification procedures, *J Res Educ Indian Med* 12(4):2-13, 1993.

Sharma HM, Dwivedi C, Satter BC, et al: Antineoplastic properties of Maharishi-4 against DMBA-induced mammary tumors in rats, *Pharmacol Biochem Behav* 35:767-773, 1990.

Slattery ML, Jacobs DR Jr, Hilner JE, et al: Meat consumption and its associations with other diet and health factors in young adults: the CARDIA study, *Am J Clin Nutr* 54(5):930-935, 1991 (erratum 55(1):iv, 1992).

Smith DE, Salerno JW: Selective growth inhibition of a human malignant melanoma cell line by sesame oil in vitro, *Prostaglandins Leukot Essent Fatty Acids* 46:145-150, 1992.

Snowdon DA: Animal product consumption and mortality because of all causes combined, coronary heart disease, stroke, diabetes, and cancer in Seventh-Day Adventists, *Am J Clin Nutr* 58:739-748, 1988.

Srivastava A, Samaiya A, Taranikanti V, et al: Maharishi Amrit Kalash (MAK) reduces chemotherapy toxicity in breast cancer patients, *FASEB J* 14(4):A720, 2000 (abstract).

Stapp HP: *Mind, matter and quantum mechanics,* New York, 1994, Springer-Verlag, pp 220-221.

Steel K, Gertman PM, Crescenzi C, Anderson J: Iatrogenic illness on a general medical service at a university hospital, *N Engl J Med* 304:638-642, 1981.

Sundaram V, Hanna AN, Lubow GP, et al: Inhibition of low-density lipoprotein oxidation by oral herbal mixtures Maharishi Amrit Kalash-4 and Maharishi Amrit Kalash-5 in hyperlipidemic patients, *Am J Med Sci* 314(5):303-310, 1997.

Sushruta Samhita, Varanasi, India, 1963, Chowkhamba Sanskrit Series Office (Translated by KL Ghisagrantne).

Vagbhata (Upaohyaya VY, editor): *Ashtanga Hridayam,* Varanasi, India, 1982, Chaukambha Sanskrit Sansthan.

Vohra BPS, James TJ, Sharma SP, et al: Dark neurons in the ageing cerebellum: their mode of formation and effect of Maharishi Amrit Kalash, *Biogerontology* 3:347-354, 2002.

Vohra BPS, Sharma SP, Kansal VK: Maharishi Amrit Kalash rejuvenates ageing central nervous system's antioxidant defence system: an in vivo study, *Pharmacol Res* 40(6):497-502, 1999.

Vohra BP, Sharma SP, Kansal VK: Effect of Maharishi Amrit Kalash on age-dependent variations in mitochondrial antioxidant enzymes, lipid peroxidation and mitochondrial population in different regions of the central nervous system of guinea pigs, *Drug Metab Drug Interact* 18(1):57-68, 2001a.

Vohra BPS, Sharma SP, Kansal VK: Maharishi Amrit Kalash, an Ayurvedic medicinal preparation, enhances cholinergic enzymes in aged guinea pig brain, *Indian J Exp Biol* 39:1258-1262, 2001b.

Vohra BPS, Sharma SP, Kansal VK, Gupta SK: Effect of Maharishi Amrit Kalash, an Ayurvedic herbal mixture, on lipid peroxidation and neuronal lipofuscin accumulation in ageing guinea pig brain, *Indian J Exp Biol* 39:355-359, 2001c.

Waldschütz R: Influence of Maharishi Ayur-Veda purification treatment on physiological and psychological health [translation], Erfahrungsheilkunde *Acta Medica Empirica* 11:720-729, 1988.

Wallace RK: Physiological effects of Transcendental Meditation, *Science* 167:1751-1754, 1970.

Wallace RK, Dillbeck MC, Jacobe E, Harrington B: The effects of the Transcendental Meditation and TM-Sidhi program on the aging process, *Int J Neurosci* 16:53-58, 1982.

Wallace RK, Orme-Johnson DW, Dillbeck MC, editors: *Scientific research on Maharishi's Transcendental Meditation and TM-Sidhi program: collected papers,* vol 5, Fairfield, Iowa, 1989, MIU Press.

Wallace RK, Silver J, Mills P, et al: Systolic blood pressure and long-term practice of the Transcendental Meditation and TM-Sidhi program: effects of TM on blood pressure, *Psychosom Med* 45:41-46, 1983.

Willett WC, Stampfer MJ, Colditz GA, et al: Relation of meat, fat and fiber intake to the risk of colon cancer in a prospective study among women, *N Engl J Med* 323:1664-1672, 1990.

Zamarra JW, Schneider RH, Besseghini I, et al: Usefulness of the Transcendental Meditation program in the treatment of patients with coronary artery disease, *Am J Cardiol* 77:867-870, 1996.

Suggested Reading

Sharma H: *Freedom from disease: how to control free radicals, a major cause of aging and disease,* Toronto, 1993, Veda Publishing.

Sharma H: *Awakening nature's healing intelligence: expanding Ayurveda through the Maharishi Vedic approach to health,* Twin Lakes, Wis, 1997, Lotus Press.

Sharma H, Clark C: *Contemporary Ayurveda: medicine and research in Maharishi Ayur-Veda,* London, 1998, Churchill Livingstone.

Sharma H, Mishra RK, with Meade JG. *The answer to cancer,* New York, 2002, SelectBooks.

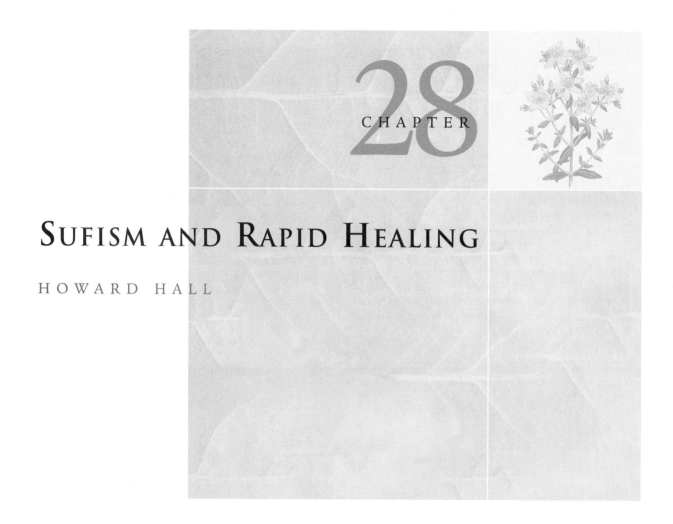

SUFISM AND RAPID HEALING

HOWARD HALL

HISTORICAL BACKGROUND

The history of Sufism is rooted back about 15 centuries, or around 600 years after Jesus, to the time of the Prophet Muhammad (may the blessings and peace of Allah be on him) (P) and the birth of Islam. The Prophet Muhammad (P) lived from 570 CE (Common Era) to 632 CE and was born in the city of Mecca, which is today in Saudi Arabia. He was an orphan by age 6 years and was taken in by his uncle Abu Talib. At age 25, he worked as a merchant for a widow, Khadija, transporting goods to Syria. Khadija was 15 years older than Muhammad (P) but was so impressed with his character that she later proposed marriage to him. They were married for about a quar-

ter of a century until her death, during which time he never took any other wives, even though polygamy was common practice (Fatoohi, 2002).

Muhammad (P) would frequently retire for meditation to a cave, later known as "Hira," on top of a mountain north of Mecca called "Nur," or light. At age 40 in the year 610 CE, while meditating in that cave, the Prophet Muhammad (P) received the first of a series of revelations from God though angel Gabriel. These revelations continued over about 23 years through this "unlettered" prophet and were memorized and written down by his followers and became the *Quran*, or the holy text of Islam. The Quran (or Qur'an) consists of 114 chapters and has not been modified since it was written down; thus it is the same text today as was revealed to the Prophet during his lifetime (Fatoohi, 2002). Tradition also holds that the Quran is divinely protected from being corrupted (verse 15:9). The Quran is also remarkable for its internal consistency, its external agreement with historical and archaeological evidence, as well as providing new information and scientific findings that did not come to light until the nineteenth and twentieth centuries (Fatoohi and Al-Dargazelli, 1999). For example, human fetal development was vividly described well before the dawn of scientific knowledge of embryology (Quranic verses 22:5, 23:12-14, and 40:67). Furthermore, unlike other religious traditions, Muhammad (P) is not worshiped or seen as divine, but rather is credited with the revelation of a literary masterpiece, along with the founding of a major religion and a new world power (Armstrong, 1993).

The terms "Islam" and "Muslim" were never meant to represent an elusive religion, but the universal concept of peace through "surrendering oneself to the will of **Allah**" (the Arabic word for *the God*). Likewise, a Muslim is one who surrenders his or her whole self to the one God. Thus, all living creatures, including animals and insects, are natural Muslims following God's divine design by their instinctual behaviors (Armstrong, 1993). However, it is only humans who can choose to surrender to the will of Allah or rebel and follow selfish desires. This struggle between surrender and rebellion represents the history of human spiritual evolution, with Allah sending prophets to lead people back to the creator. Also, Islam is the religion of peace, as expressed in the letters that form the word "Islam" from "Salam," which means "peace." In addition, one of the beautiful names of Allah as described in the Quran is "Al-Salam." Further, the greeting of the believers is peace, or "Asalamualaikum." Finally, believers are ordered by the Prophet of Islam, Muhammad (P), to spread "Salam."

The Quran teaches that Allah sent the same basic religion and revelation to humans, without holding one of the earlier religions above the later ones, including Judaism, Christianity, and Islam. This universal religion was revealed to the first human, Adam, and all the earlier prophets: Noah, Abraham, Ishmael, Isaac, Jacob, Joseph, Moses, Aaron, David, Solomon, Zachariah, John, and Jesus. As stated in the Quran: "The same religion has He established for you as that which He enjoined on Noah—that which We have sent by inspiration to thee—and that which We

enjoined on Abraham, Moses, and Jesus; Namely, that ye should remain steadfast in Religion, and make no divisions therein" (42:13).

Contrary to popular belief, Islam is not anti-Judaism or anti-Christian but commands that all Muslims respect and revere all the previous messengers, books, and messages that Allah revealed to them. Because Jews and Christians received earlier revelations from Allah, they are referred to as "People or family of the Book" in the Quran. (Fatoohi, 2002). Thus the Quran holds that Allah's universal message has come to people across the ages through appointed messengers as a type of "progressive revelation" (2:106). The form of this message may change according to the needs of the people and their circumstances, but it is the same basic message of surrender. Thus, true Islamic view is acceptance of these other religions as noted in the Quran: "The Messenger believeth in what hath been revealed to him from his Lord, as do the men of faith. Each one (of them) believeth in Allah, His angels, His books, and His Messengers. 'We make no distinction between one and another of His Messengers'" (2:285).

Islam also sees people as equals, only distinguished by their righteousness: "O mankind! We created you from a single (pair) of a male and a female, and made you into nations and tribes, that ye may know each other (Not that ye may despise each other). Veril the most honoured of you in the sight of Allah is (he who is) the most righteous of you" (49:13).

In addition to the believing in prior messengers and scriptures, the central belief of Islam is in the Oneness of God (Allah). Not only is there just one God, but God (Allah) is in control of everything in the universe, regardless of whether we humans judge outcomes in the world as positive or negative. Islam also accepts the existence of angels and the Day of Judgment and that Muhammad (P) is the last prophet and the Quran is the last of Allah's holy books (Fatoohi, 2002).

Sufism is the mystical spiritual tradition within Islam, which directs humans toward a "nearness" to the God (Allah) so that they can become agents for Allah. As noted in the introduction of the Quran (C:1):

> Glory to Allah Most High, full of Grace and Mercy; He created All, including Man. To Man He gave a special place in His Creation. He honoured man to be His Agent, and to that end, endued him with understanding, purified his affections, and gave

him spiritual insight; so that man should understand Nature, understand himself, and know Allah through His wondrous Signs, and glorify Him in Truth, reverence, and unity.

The Quran then discusses how humans were given a "will" so that they may choose to follow the will of Allah (i.e., submission or Islam) (C:2) and how humans became distant from Allah when their lower self rebelled against Allah's will (C:3):

> For the fulfillment of this great trust man was further given a Will, so that his acts should reflect Allah's universal will and Law, and his mind, freely choosing, should experience the sublime joy of being in harmony with the Infinite, and with the great drama of the world around him, and with his own spiritual growth.
>
> But, created though he was in the best of moulds, man fell from Unity when his Will was warped, and he chose the crooked path of Discord. And sorrow and pain, selfishness and degradation, ignorance and hatred, despair and unbelief poisoned his life, and he saw shapes of evil in the physical, moral, and spiritual world, and in himself.

Thus the spiritual tradition of Sufism represents the direct path back to Allah or, as noted in the Quran's "Opening" Surah 1:6, "the straight way."

The Sufi musician Hazrat Inayat Khan (1983) provides the following description of spiritual development: "The word 'spiritual' does not apply to goodness or to wonder-working, the power of producing miracles, or to great intellectual power. The whole of life in all its aspects is one single music; and the real spiritual attainment is to tune oneself to the harmony of this perfect music" (p. 129).

The foundation of Sufism is based on belief in the mystical aspects of the spirituality of the Prophet (P) (Hussein et al., 1997). During his lifetime, pious individuals from different nations learned under his guidance the Spiritual Laws of Islam, because these laws led toward direct experience of the Divine or nearness to Allah (Ansha, 1991).

The spiritual leader of a Sufi school is known as a *Shaikh*. The spiritual knowledge of the Shaikh can be traced back to the Prophet Muhammad (P), who later converted his cousin and son-in-law "Ali bin abi Talib." Ali is considered a spiritual heir to the Prophet and the one who inherited his spiritual knowledge and power. Thus, all Sufi Masters are his students, directly or indirectly, and this is the origin of the title

"Shaikh of the Shaikhs." Through a line of succession, each Shaikh would initiate a successor based on revelations from Allah, maintaining a direct spiritual link or attachment with the Prophet Muhammad (P) to the present spiritual leader (Chishti, 1991). This chain from the Prophet Muhammad (P) down to the present Master of a Sufi school is known as a *silsila* (Hussein et al., 1997). At present, there are more than 150 orders or schools of Sufism.

A Shaikh is a *mediator* or guide to Allah in Sufism to help the student draw near to Allah, battle their lower self (jihad), and help channel the spiritual power from Allah to perform paranormal events (discussed under the metapsychology of Sufism). As noted by the teaching of Shaikh Gaylani:

> The mediator is essential. Ask your Lord for a physician who can treat the diseases of your hearts, a healer who can heal you, a guide who can guide you and take you by the hand. Draw near to those whom He has brought near to him, His elite, the ushers of His nearness, the keepers of His door. You have consented to serving your lower selves and pursuing your passions and natural inclinations. You work hard to satisfy and satiate your lower selves in this world, although this is something that you will never achieve. You keep to this state hour after hour, day after day, month after month and year after year, until you find that death has suddenly come to you and you cannot release yourselves from its grip (Al-Casnaszani al-Husseini, 1999, p. 15).

If Allah did not reveal someone with the attributes that qualify the person to be a Shaikh, the Shaikh would not name a successor, and the silsila of that particular *tariqa* (way) would discontinue. In this case the dervishes would have to join another tariqa after the departure of their Shaikh to maintain the spiritual link necessary for the attainment.

The unifying factor and ultimate aim of the Sufi way is the attainment of "nearness" to Allah by following a chain of masters who have already attained nearness to Allah and by following the path of the Prophet (P). This process of drawing near also is related to purifying one's lower self through personal internal struggle, or *Jihad*. The process of drawing near to Allah may include the acquisition of paranormal powers, such as rapid wound healing and paranormal knowledge, including Quranic knowledge. One of the great Sufi masters, Shaikh "Abd al-Qadir al-Gaylani," used to describe what the dervish would obtain as being "something that no eye has ever seen, no ear has ever heard, and has never occurred to any human heart." In Sufi terms, the attainment to Allah means the transformation into light by becoming absorbed or extinct in the Light (i.e., Allah). Allah describes Himself in the Holy Qur'an as being "nur" (light): "Allah is the Light of the heavens and the earth" (24:35). The nearer the dervish draws to Allah, the more Allah attributes he acquires. When the dervish achieves the ultimate goal of total "extinc-tion" (Arabic *fana*) in Allah, he will lose his own will and become an instrument in the hands of Allah, thus experiencing the ultimate submission of one's will to Allah. With this nearness to Allah, one can reach the high stage of being an agent (vicegerent) for Allah, with spiritual guidance, vision, and power to help transform the world and people. The broad implication for society is having an *umma*, or com-munity, united by following the will of Allah versus the traditional tribal, blood, and kinship allegiances with accompanying blood feuds that were so preva-lent during the time of the Prophet (P) and today (Armstrong, 1993).

Sufism is not associated with terrorism or funda-mentalism. The Sufi spiritual viewpoint may not be generally accepted by some traditional Muslims; it has even been met with hostility from other Muslim schools of thought (Hussein et al., 1997).

THE WAY

An integral part of Sufism is the notion of a "path" or "way" toward Allah through self-understanding, cer-tain practices, and discipline (Ansha, 1991). Thus, Sufism is the straight path, or one of the shortest paths, to God. Many great spiritual traditions use the concept of a path or way toward the experience of the divine. For example, Buddhism is known as a path toward Nirvana or enlightenment (Clarke, 1993). In the Bible, Psalm 25:4 states, "Show me thy ways, O Lord; teach me thy paths." Continuing with verses 9-10, "The meek will he guide in judgment: and the meek will he teach his way. All the paths of the Lord are mercy and truth unto such as keep his covenant and his testimonies." In the New Testament, Jesus said, "I am the way, the truth, and the life; no man cometh unto the Father, but by me" (John 14:6). Similarly, in the beginning chapter of the Holy Qur'an, *Al Fatihah* ("The Opening") 1:6-7, Allah teaches the people how to pray to Him in these verses:

"Show us the straight way, The way of those on whom Thou hast bestowed Thy Grace, Those whose portion is not wrath, and who go not astray."

The idea of a spiritual path has a corollary within the Western philosophy concept of "means" versus an "end." As John Dewey (1922) noted when discussing means and end concerning an activity:

> The distinction of means and end arise in survey-ing the course of a proposed line of action, a con-nected series in time. The "end" is the last act thought of; the means are the acts to be performed prior to it in time. To reach an end we must take our mind off from it and attend to the act that is next to be performed. We must make that the end.

Dewey's concept of means and end were greatly influenced by the mind-body movement therapy work of F. Matthias Alexander (1910). Alexander observed that many postural problems people encountered were caused by unconscious movements to gain some end, such as sitting or standing, without much thought as to the means, way, or path of accomplish-ing this goal. Alexander taught individuals to focus on the "means whereby" of doing a simple act such as the process of moving from sitting to standing versus focusing on the end results or "end gaining," as he termed it. The process of attending to the "means" or "way" resulted in increased conscious guidance and control of the self. As Alexander (1910) noted:

> This triumph is not to be won in sleep, in trance, in submission, in paralysis, or in anaesthesia, but in a clear, open-eyed, reasoning, deliberate conscious-ness and apprehension of the wonderful potential-ities possessed by mankind, the transcendent inheritance of a conscious mind.

From this perspective, following a path or way or attending to a means may be associated with increased awareness or consciousness or perhaps even a higher consciousness. This is comparable to the increased consciousness or awareness found in one's body movements following instructions with the Alexander method (Alexander, 1910) (see Chapter 9).

ISLAMIC TRADITIONS AND HEALTH

As a spiritual tradition within Islam, Sufism follows the five pillars of Islam: the statement of belief or

Shahada ("There is no God, but The God [Allah] and Muhammad [P] is the messenger of Allah"), prayer, fasting, charity; and *hajj* (pilgrimage). Traditional Islam includes spiritually based and healthy practices, such as prayer five times a day (early morning, noon, midafternoon, sunset, and evening), fasting, and prohibition against the consumption of pork products and intoxicating liquors. There are also prohibitions against gambling, sexual relations outside of marriage, and behavior or dress that is indecent (Abdalati, 1996).

There are obvious health benefits for avoiding such high-risk behaviors as prescribed by Islamic tradition. Avoiding alcohol intoxication also helps prevent the disinhibition effects and the accompanying social problems. "It has been said that the super-ego is the alcohol-soluble portion of the personality" (Friend, 1957, p. 84). Avoiding pork would also provide protection against swine-related foodborne diseases, such as *Salmonella typhimurium* gastroenteritis (Gessner anad Beller, 1994); *Yersinia* enterocolitis (Tauxe, 1997); and viral illnesses from pork or pork products, including foot-and-mouth disease, classic swine fever (hog cholera), African swine fever, and swine vesicular viral disease (Farez and Morley, 1997; McKercher et al., 1978). Even the use of modern microwave ovens may fail to protect against pork-related illness such as salmonellosis (Gessner and Beller, 1994). Pork is not the only source of foodborne diseases, and such pathogens in general are emerging as a major public health challenge (Tauxe, 1997).

FASTING

Being hungry is better than the maladies that come with satiety. Subtlety and lightness and being true to your devotion are some of the advantages of fasting.

—RUMI (1991)

During the lunar holy month of Ramadan, Muslims all over the world fast from sunrise to sunset. This fasting means abstaining completely from foods, drinks, and sexual intercourse from dawn to sunset (Abdalati, 1996). Fasting is done for spiritual purposes in Islam. As stated in the Qur'an (2:183): "O ye who believe! Fasting is prescribed to you as it was prescribed to those before you, so that ye may learn self-restraint." As Woodward (1985) stated, "Fasting is thought to purge the body of passion and sin and reduce the risk of disease. Once passion has been con-

trolled, it is possible to clear the mind (an element of the spiritual body) of conscious thought. This allows the mystic to establish contact with saints, spirits, sources of magical power and ultimately with Allah." Fasting also teaches patience and unselfishness, for when a person fasts, he or she can identify with the pains and deprivations of others less fortunate (Abdalati, 1996).

In naturopathic medicine, fasting is used as a method of detoxifying the body (see Chapter 13). It is a rapid way to increase the elimination of wastes within the body to facilitate healing. Also, a number of medical conditions have been treated with fasting, ranging from obesity, allergies, and chemical poisoning to irritable bowel syndrome (Murray and Pizzorno, 1991). Obesity is becoming epidemic within the United States. Further, intermittent fasting, caloric restriction, and undernutrition (but not malnutrition) have been associated with increased life span for both animals and humans (Walford, 1983). As suggested by Rumi, one of the maladies that come with overeating may be a shorter life.

MEDITATION

When you neglect your meditation, you contract with pain. This is God's way of telling you that your inner pain can become visible. Don't ignore it.

—RUMI (1991)

Meditation is one of the most important Sufi tools for drawing nearer to Allah by "remembering" God and thus treating one's inner heart that has become distant, diseased, and hardened. Worshipful meditation is an integral part of Sufism and is also known as "Divine Remembrance," *Dhikr*, or *Zekr* (Chishti, 1991). As noted in the Qur'an: "Then do ye remember Me, I will remember you" (2:152). The place of worship or the Takiya is also known as the "House of Remembrance." These Sufi meditation practices are above and beyond the traditional prayers.

Such meditation practices involve a prescribed number of recitations of verses from the Qur'an using prayer beads (i.e., a rosary to keep count), such as "la illaha illa Allah," or "there is no god but Allah (The God)" (Ansha, 1991), or other remembrances, such as "The Beautiful Names" of Allah. For some tariqas (e.g., Tariqa Casnazaniyyah), this recitation is done aloud with accompanying head movements symbolizing a hammer slamming the heart that has become "hardened like a stone." The remoteness from Allah causes this hardness and the remembrance is the remedy. As noted in the Qur'anic verse 2:74, "Thenceforth were your hearts hardened: they became like a rock and even worse in hardness." Other tariqas use silent remembrances or use different movements altogether. Meditation has been suggested to help treat diseases (see Chapter 16). It has been suggested that the number of recitations to treat diseases end with a zero (e.g., 100, 300) (Chishti, 1991). Again, from the Sufi perspective, worshipful meditation is a means of drawing near to Allah, and with that connection may come transcendent events.

Research has documented the many health and physiological benefits of meditation, including decreasing blood pressure, rate of breathing, heart rate, and oxygen consumption. The positive effects of meditation are associated with the production of a physiological "relaxation response" that is opposite to the "fight-or-flight response" (Benson, 1975). Thus the regular worshipful meditative practice of Sufism may also contribute to increased health.

PRAYER

The healing benefits of prayer are now becoming recognized within the disciplines of science and medicine (Dossey, 1996, 2001). "Prayer works. More than 130 controlled laboratory studies show, in general, that prayer or a prayer like state of compassion, empathy, and love can bring about healthful changes in many types of living things, from humans to bacteria. This does not mean prayer always works, any more than drugs and surgery always work, but that, statistically speaking, prayer is effective" (Dossey, 1996).

THE PSYCHOLOGY OF SUFISM

The notion of the heart and the ego or lower self (Arabic *nafs*) has played a prominent role in Sufi psychology (Ansha, 1991; Chishti, 1991). The spiritual path of Sufism is geared toward inner spiritual development by helping the follower in the purification or extinction (*fana'*) of the ego/lower self (*nafs*) or more basic appetitive aspects of the body and selfish and mean-spirited desires. The health benefits of a system

that helps manage the excessive appetitive motives would have positive implications for a number of disorders of overindulgence, such as weight problems and addictions. Disorders of excesses provide significant causes of morbidity within the West, with obesity one of the most serious threats.

The heart, in Sufism, is related to one's spiritual self. As mentioned earlier, the head movement that accompanies the recitation meditation, Dhikr practice, symbolizes a hammer slamming the heart that has become a stone so that its true luster can shine through. The Prophet (P) stated, "There is a polish for everything that taketh away rust; and the polish of the Heart is the invocation of Allah" (Ling, 1977). It is within the heart or inner being where spiritual development and battles occur. This internal battleground is the true concept of jihad.

Jihad

One of the most misunderstood concepts in Islam is the term "Jihad," usually associated with the notion of "holy war" and terrorism. The definition of Jihad from the Quran means "exerting the best efforts," or some type of "struggle" and "resistance," to achieve some goal (Fatoohi, 2002). The Quran discusses two types of Jihad, "peaceful jihad" and "armed jihad." Armed jihad was permitted as a temporary response for Muslims against armed aggression. The early Muslim community lived 14 years under the guidance of the Prophet's revelations before they were given permission from Allah to fight back to defend themselves. The Quran uses a different term, *qital*, when referring to fighting an enemy. It is also forbidden in Islam to take an innocent life because killing one innocent person is like killing the whole group, and conversely, saving one person is like saving the whole community (Quran 5:32).

Peaceful jihad, however, is the permanent struggle in which every Muslim must continuously exert efforts against evil desires within the lower self. Shaikh Muhammad al-Casnazani refers to this perpetual internal holy war or jihad as "Spiritual sport." Such an ongoing inner struggle uses such facilities as intuition to allow oneself to overcome lower drives and draw nearer to Allah, with all the spiritual, material, and metaphysical benefits. This struggle often comes down to a choice. As mathematics professor Jeffrey Lang pointed out:

The Qur'an presents human history as a perennial struggle between two opposing choices: to resist or to surrender oneself to God. It is in this conflict that the scripture immerses itself and the reader; it could be said to be the very crux of its calling. This choice must be completely voluntary, for the Qur'an demands, 'Let there be no compulsion in religion—the right way is henceforth clearly distinct from error' (2:256) (Lang, 2000, p. 27).

Afflictions

One of the greatest challenges people currently face in the world is trying to understand and endure personal crises, illness, and afflictions. The Islamic and Sufi perspective holds that whatever happens to an individual occurs only by the will of Allah. However, one might ask, "Why would Allah allow bad things to happen to people?" Sufi Shaikh Gaylani notes that given the Oneness of Allah, afflictions bring people closer to God:

> The people of Allah accustom themselves to afflictions and do not get annoyed like your annoyance. . . . Afflictions are of various kinds; some affect the body, while some affect the heart. Some of them are suffered in relation to creatures, while others in relation to the Creator. There is no good in someone who has not been subjected to suffering. Afflictions are the hooks of the True One (i.e. Allah) (Al-Casnaszani al-Husseini, 1999, p. 183).

Shaikh Gaylani goes on to point out the Oneness of Allah in terms of afflictions and the lessons learned from such adversities:

> Obey and do not disobey. Believe in the oneness of Allah and do not attribute partners to Him. Your reliance on creatures is a form of polytheistic idolatry. Woe unto you! You are mad! Dissatisfaction and protestation do not give you something or take away another. Your anger cannot delay something or bring forward another. Affliction and the removal of affliction are both in the hand of Allah. It is He who has sent down the disease and the remedy. It is He who has created the disease and has created the remedy. He afflicts you with tribulations to make you come to know Him through affliction, to show you His signs and His power in sending down the affliction and in removing it and to show you the removal and the putting down

of His plate (of grace). Afflictions show the way to the door of Allah ('Azza wa Jall) and knock on it. They bring the heart and the True One ('Azza wa Jall) together. They promote the status. Do not hate afflictions for you have many benefits in these things that you hate. Set aside asking "why" and "how." If you endure the afflictions with patience, they will purify you of outward and inward sins. The Prophet (Salla Allah ta'ala alayhi wa sallam) is reported to have said: "Afflictions will continue to come the believer's way until he comes to walk on the earth carrying no sin." His sins will be erased from his scrolls and the angels who recorded them will forget them (Al-Casnaszani al-Husseini, 1999, p. 186).

Thus, affliction teaches humility, patience, and thankfulness from Allah, when relief and blessing come. It is our lower self that rebels against Allah during afflictions and distances one from the source of needed help. The psychology of human behavior is keenly noted in the Quran (C:4) where people tend to "boast in prosperity, and curse in adversity." Faith in the oneness of Allah and enduring these struggles is the heart of peaceful Jihad and brings one closer to The God.

FAITH

Faith has also been suggested as an important factor in the psychology of healing from a Sufi perspective as in other healing traditions. As noted by a contemporary Sufi, M.R. Bawa Muhaiyaddeen (1991):

> Illnesses can be treated in many ways, but no matter how many different treatments are used, they may still fail to heal the patient. In order for a treatment to work, first of all, even if the patient does not have faith in God, he must have faith in the doctor and in whatever treatment he suggests. Secondly, the doctor who is performing the treatment must have faith in God; he must have God's qualities, His love, and His patience. The doctor must give all responsibility to God, instead of thinking that he is the one who is responsible for curing the patient.
>
> When these conditions exist, when the patient has faith in the doctor and the doctor has faith in God, then treatment becomes very easy and the illness will be cured, at least to a certain extent (p. 253).

PAN ISLAMIC SUFISM AND HEALING TRADITIONS

Although the primary focus of Sufism is on attainment to Allah, some Sufis have developed a particular focus on healing. Often there is a blend of Sufi philosophy with other healing traditions, as well as incorporating the use of herbs, food, and other practices (Chishti, 1991).

The Sufi Healing Order, currently under the guidance of Himayat Inayati, offers both training and services in spiritual healing. Some healing services are conducted within a group prayer circle, where Divine help is requested for healing. Members also visit ill persons, offering spiritual support. Himayat Inayati incorporates a number of different traditions within his Sufi healing approach (website: www.sufihealingorder.org).

Sufi philosophy has played a major role in influencing traditional medical practices in the Indonesian island of Java. As Woodward (1985) noted:

> The Javanese medical system draws on a wide variety of symbols, roles and interactional patterns, none of which may be understood as uniquely medical. Concepts of personhood, cosmology, power and knowledge are melded into a corpus of closely related theories explaining the origins of disease and motivating highly diverse treatment strategies. Medical pluralism is, therefore, an inherent feature of Javanese traditional medicine. There are two primary modes of medical practice. One practiced by Sufi saints *(wali)* is based on Islamic mystical concepts of miracles and gnosis. The other, practiced by *dukun* (curers), involves the use of morally suspect forms of magical power.

It is interesting to note that Sufism fits well in the current complementary and integrative (CIM) and alternative (CAM) medical movement.

Integrative and Alternative Medicine

The 1990s were the era of a "silent revolution" in health care for some of the wealthiest, most highly educated mainstream citizens of major industrialized countries of the world, from the United States to Europe. A U.S. survey revealed that Americans with chronic non–life-threatening conditions made about 427 million visits to alternative medicine practitioners, compared with 388 million visits to all primary care physicians (Einsenber et al., 1993). By 1997, the number of visits to "alternative medicine practitioners" continued to increase (629 million visits), eclipsing the number of visits to all U.S. primary care physicians (386 million) (Einsenber et al., 1998). When these data were examined in terms of percentage of people using "unconventional medicine," for the 1990 survey about 34% of individuals interviewed had used at least 1 of 16 alternative therapies in the previous year. By 1997 this number increased to 42%, and it continues to increase. The nature of these alternative therapies ranged from relaxation techniques, hypnosis, biofeedback, imagery, herbal medicines, and chiropractic manipulations to such healing practices as acupuncture, homeopathy, and folk remedies (Einsenber et al., 1993). In 1990, Americans spent about $15 billion on services for alternative medicine practitioners, and by 1997 this figure had increased to more than $21 billion.

This growing use of alternative medical practices by highly educated Americans with chronic non–life-threatening health conditions may not represent irrational behavior when one considers the finding that a combined total of about 225,000 deaths occur each year in the United States from medication errors and adverse effects, hospital mistakes, unnecessary surgeries, and nosocomial infections. This places our "high-tech" medical interventions as the third leading cause of death in the United States, after heart disease and cancer (Starfield, 2000). Medical interventions for emergency situations are critical, but interventions for chronic non–life-threatening conditions could prove lethal.

There is a paradigm shift within mechanistic medicine best described by Dossey's three eras. Larry Dossey (1993) described medicine moving through three distinct eras. *Era I* was mechanical, material, or physical medicine; this was the Newtonian view of the world where the human body was seen as operating like a machine. At present this is our reductionistic, high-tech medicine. *Era II* was the mind-body medicine movement; in the United States, one can place relaxation, meditation, and many Sufi approaches within the alternative medicine movement. *Era III* is "spiritual healing" or "energy healing"; Dossey also called this "nonlocal" or "transpersonal" medicine. The metaphysical aspects of Sufism can be viewed within this context.

ERA III: Energy Medicine or Spiritual Healing (Nonlocal, Transpersonal Medicine or Vitalism)

The "silent revolution" or paradigm shift of the 1990s incorporated global healing traditions from other cultures that were thousands of years old. These non-Western practices involved nonmechanistic and whole-person approaches to healing. Such global healing traditions included Ayurveda medicine of India with its various yogas (Zysk, 1996), Chinese medicine with acupuncture (Ergil, 1996), and Qigong (McGee et al., 1996). Western religious traditions provided intercessory prayer and distant healing intention research (Dossey, 1993).

Daniel Benor, a practicing holistic psychiatrist, addressed the evidence-based question of spiritual healing:

> "Does spiritual healing work? Does research confirm that healing is an effective therapy?" An impressive number of studies with excellent design and execution answer this question with a "Yes." If we take a broad view, out of 191 controlled experiments of healing, . . . close to two thirds (64.9 percent) of all the experiments demonstrate significant effects (Benor, 2001, p. 371).

Spiritual healing effects can be demonstrated on animals, plants, single-celled organisms, bacteria, yeasts, and DNA. Similarly, cellular biologist and physiologist James Oschman states the following:

> Medical research is demonstrating that devices producing pulsing magnetic fields of particular frequencies can stimulate the healing of a variety of tissues. Therapists from various schools of energy medicine can project, from their hands, fields with similar frequencies and intensities. Research documenting that these different approaches are efficacious is mutually validating. Medical research and hands-on therapies are confirming each other. The common denominator is the pulsating magnetic field, which is called a biomagnetic field when it emanates from the hands of a therapist (Oschman, 2000, p. XIV).

With the "silent revolution," people are moving toward whole-person health and global healing traditions (Weil, 1983). One global healing tradition from the Middle East that has received little attention from the West (probably for geographical and political reasons) is the spiritual practice of rapid wound healing from "deliberately caused bodily damage" at a major Sufi school in Iraq. This has been the focus of my research for the past several years.

THE METAPSYCHOLOGY OF SUFISM AND RAPID WOUND HEALING

The extraordinary phenomenon of instantaneous wound healing from "deliberately caused bodily damage" (DCBD) has been reported by the Tariqa Casnazaniyyah School of Sufism in Baghdad, one of the largest Sufi schools in the Middle East (Hussein et al., 1994a, 1994b, 1994c, 1997). Followers (dervishes) of this Sufi school have been observed to demonstrate instantaneous healing of DCBD. For example, dervishes have inserted a variety of sharp instruments (e.g., spikes, skewers) into their body, hammered daggers into the skull bone and clavicle, and chewed and swallowed glass and sharp razor blades without harm to the body and with complete control over pain, bleeding, and infection, as well as rapid wound healing within 4 to 10 seconds (Figure 28-1). This Sufi school's name, *Tariqa Casnazaniyyah*, is an Arabic-Kurdish word meaning "the way of the secret that is known to no one" (Hussein et al., 1997). Researchers report that such extraordinary abilities are accessible to anyone and not restricted to only a few talented individuals who have spent years in special training. These unusual healing phenomena have also been reproduced under controlled laboratory conditions and are not similar to hypnosis (Hall et al., 2001).

Similar observations of DCBD phenomena have been observed in various parts of the world in a variety of religious and nonreligious contexts (Don and Moura, 2000; Hussein et al., 1997). For example, trance surgeons in Brazil have employed sharp instruments to cut, pierce, or inject substances into a patient's body for therapeutic purposes. Laboratory electroencephalogram (EEG) investigation of trance surgeons has shown that this "state of spirit possession" for the healers was associated with a hyper-aroused brain state (waves in the 30- to 50-Hz band) (Don and Moura, 2000). Unfortunately, besides little scientific attention being given to the investigation of these rapid healing claims in the United States, such claims for extraordinary healing abilities have been met with scorn and have even been challenged by so-called skeptic groups, such as the Committee for the Scientific Investigation of Claims of the Paranormal (CSCIOP). These groups offer monetary incentives to discredit such claims in unscientific and dangerous settings (Mulacz, 1998; Posner, 1998). (See Dossey, 1999, and Fatoohi, 1999, for a response.)

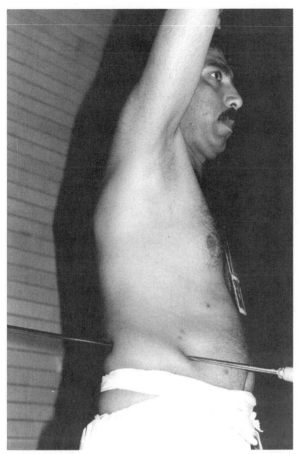

Figure 28-1 A dervish at the major school in Baghdad demonstrating Sufi wound healing.

From a spiritual perspective, this type of healing is described in terms of healing energies (Husseinet al., 1994a, 1994b, 1994c). This "higher energy" is alleged to be instantly transferable mediated through a spiritual link from the current shaikh of the Tariqa Casnazaniyyah Sufi School and through the chain of masters to Muhammad (P) and ultimately from Allah (Husseinet al., 1997). As noted in the Quran: "The Prophet is closer to the Believers than their own selves" (33:6). Followers of this Sufi school describe the ability to accomplish DCBD as an "others-healing phenomenon," which goes beyond traditional mechanistic and psychological factors that influence healing. It is also argued that hypnosis and altered states of consciousness as explanations for DCBD have little logical, theoretical, or empirical support (Hall, 2000).

How might Western scientists empirically investigate such claims of usual wound healing from the Middle East? First, it would entail travel to Baghdad to observe and document such claims directly through video recording. Second, one might also want to experience such rapid wound healing in that setting. Third, one might desire to see if such a Middle Eastern demonstration can be transported to the United States within a traditional medical setting. In 1998, with an invitation from the Shaikh of the Tariqa Casnazaniyyah School of Sufism in Baghdad and support from the Kairos Foundation in Illinois, I traveled alone to Baghdad to meet with the spiritual leader of this group, Shaikh Muhammad al-Casnazani, and witnessed a group demonstration of DCBD at their major school (Hall, 2000). At this meeting, which was professionally videotaped, I had the opportunity to examine firsthand the objects that were employed during the DCBD demonstrations, such as the knives, razor blades, and glass, and observe them being inserted into various parts of the body. What I witnessed and recorded was consistent with the extraordinary claims made by this group about rapid wound healing and no apparent pain.

Although I saw no evidence of a ruse, I imagined that some skeptics might question if I had somehow been deluded, even with video footage. Thus, while at this demonstration, I had requested permission to experience DCBD by having my cheek pierced (Hall, 2000). After witnessing several demonstrations of DCBD, an assistant asked if I was ready. I said, "Yes," and he asked me to face the Shaikh to ask permission to allow the healing energy for rapid wound healing. The Shaikh nodded, indicating that I had his permission. What was most striking was that I did not feel any different or in an altered state, and my cheek was not numb. The assistant then inserted a metal ice pick through the inside of my left cheek to the outside. It felt like a poke, but with no pain (Figure 28-2). I walked around the group circle with the ice pick in my cheek, introspecting on how it was not hurting, bleeding, or numb. I could feel the weight of the object and notice the metal taste in my mouth, but I felt no discomfort. Again, consistent with their reports, my cheek healed rapidly in minutes with only a couple of drops of blood. This personal experience was very compelling to me despite much doubt that I had, as well as not being particularly fond of pain. Nonetheless, I still imagined that skeptics would question if such practices could be demonstrated outside this religious context and exported to the West. A demonstration of such rapid wound healing was clearly needed within a Western medical setting, given

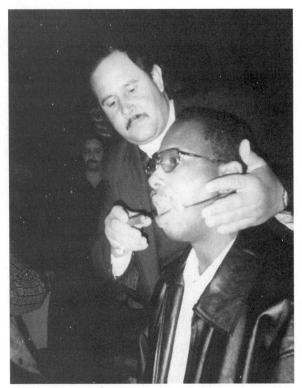

Figure 28-2 The author, Howard Hall, having his cheek pierced at the major school in Baghdad.

the scientific implications for such healing. If such spiritually based healing approaches are genuine, they hold much promise for addressing some of today's most serious medical issues.

The investigation of such unusual healing phenomena in the West raises many questions. What should be measured within a scientific context? Would standard measures of brain and immune activity be associated with changes in rapid wound healing, or should standard measures, such as EEG activity, be used in less standard ways? Would high-frequency EEG activity need to be examined for hyperaroused brain states? Would new approaches be needed to detect "fields of consciousness," such as the examination of changes in the output from a "random event generator"?

Case Report

With the support of the Kairos Foundation of Wilmette, Illinois, a Sufi practitioner (J.H.) was invited from the Middle East to a local radiology

facility in Cleveland, Ohio on July 1, 1999. He had permission from the Shaikh of the Casnazaniyyah Sufi school to perform a demonstration of rapid wound healing after insertion of an unsterilized metal skewer, 0.38 cm thick and approximately 13 cm long, while being videotaped by a film crew in the presence of scientists and health care professionals (Hallet al., 2001). This was apparently the first demonstration from this Sufi School in the United States. The practitioner consented to sign a release of liability for the medical facility and personnel against claims from possible injuries. Emergency medical technicians were present. The major goal of this demonstration was to observe the authenticity of rapid wound healing following a deliberately caused injury within a medical setting.

The demonstration was also conducted with radiological, immunological, and EEG evaluations, as well as a "zener noise diode random event generator," similar to the one employed at Princeton University by Dr. Robert Jahn and colleagues. Based on previous studies in Brazil with healer-mediums engaged in quasisurgical practices, it was hypothesized that DCBD would be accompanied by alterations in brain waves and effects on random event generators (REGs). The alterations in brain waves found with the Brazilian healer-mediums showed statistically significant enhancement of broadband 40-Hz brain rhythms (Don and Moura, 2000). A statistically significant deviation from random behavior in REGs was found, run covertly while the Brazilian healer-mediums were in trance. This methodology was developed by Robert Jahn and Associates at the Princeton Engineering Anomalies Research Laboratory (PEAR) (Nelson et al, 1996, 1998). Such energy fields have been considered as theoretically associated with rapid wound healing (Don and Moura, 2000).

Nineteen-channel EEGs were recorded during baseline resting conditions, while the dervish inserted the skewer through his cheek, and immediately after removing the instrument.

An REG, plugged into the serial port of a computer, was run in the background without informing the dervish. The distribution of binary digits was tested for possible significant deviations from random behavior. Data were acquired before and after the self-insertion, as well as during the skewer insertion condition. Before insertion of the skewer and about 1 hour after the piercing, blood was collected from the practitioner and three volunteers for an immunological analysis of the percent change in CD4, CD8, and total T cell counts.

Results

Radiological images were done while the skewer was inserted. Axial computed tomography (CT) images through the lower mandibular region showed artifact from dental metal. In addition, a horizontally oriented metallic bar elevated the left lateral soft tissues just anterior to the muscles of mastication. There was no associated underlying mass. A single frontal fluoroscopic image showed a presence of EEG leads over the maxilla and mandibular regions. A transverse metal was superimposed extending from the soft tissues on the right through to the left without interval break.

Because of movement and scalp muscle artifacts throughout the experimental self-insertion condition, it was impossible to assess the EEG for the hypothesized 40-Hz brain rhythms. The frequency spectrum of scalp muscle discharge overlaps the 40-Hz EEG frequency band of interest.

The REG during baseline periods did not differ significantly from random behavior. However, during the self-insertion condition, there was a trend toward significant nonrandomness. The chi-square test result was 3.052, df = 1, and p was approximately .07.

Discussion

The behavior of the REG was in the predicted direction of nonrandomness. This has been interpreted by our laboratory and the PEAR laboratory as being associated with states of heightened attention and emotion. Further, PEAR has proposed that a "field of consciousness" is associated with such nonrandomness. Unfortunately, the 40-Hz brain wave hypothesis was not testable because of the excessive amount of scalp artifact and thus awaits further exploration. The presence of increased theta rhythms after the insertion condition (and a slight decrease in average alpha power) suggests a mild hypoaroused altered state of consciousness. The Sufi performing this feat was doing so for the first time. With further practice or by testing more experienced subjects, it may be feasible to obtain EEG data without large amounts of scalp artifact. Because the subject reported no perceived pain during the self-insertion, preliminary relaxation exercises might eliminate all or most of the artifact. This would enable us to test the 40-Hz hypothesis definitively. Clearly, further work is indicated.

The immunology did not reveal any major difference between the Sufi practitioner and the controls. These data suggest that the variation found in the practitioner was not different from normal controls.

The radiological film documented that the skewer had actually penetrated both cheeks, thus addressing skeptic groups that such practices are the result of fakery. After the removal of the skewer, there was a slight trickle of blood, which stopped with compression of clean gauze to the cheek. The physicians and scientists present documented that the wound healed rapidly within a few moments. The practitioner also reported that there was no pain associated with the insertion or removal of the metal skewer. This demonstration was conducted outside the traditional religious context, where chanting, drumming, and head movements are generally part of the ceremony when done in the Middle East. Thus, our case study argues against the necessity of a religious context, with its accompanying state of consciousness being important for the successful outcome of such a demonstration. This case study also demonstrated that DCBD could be done at such a large distance separating the dervish from the Master (Baghdad and Cleveland). This would suggest that this is a robust phenomenon independent of the distance separating its source and the scene where the DCBD phenomenon occurs.

It should also be noted that the skewer stayed in the dervish's cheeks for more than 35 minutes, longer than the few minutes I had observed during my field observations at the Major School of Tariqa. Thus, this case study argues against the necessity of a brief piercing for a successful outcome of DCBD. Further, the dervish of this demonstration reported that there was no pain associated with this piercing, minimal bleeding, and no postprocedural infection. Finally, about a half-hour after the completion of the demonstration, the dervish, along with seven other people who witnessed the DCBD event, had dinner together.

Personal Rapid Wound Healing

After witnessing rapid wound healing in the Middle East and experiencing it myself there, I was initiated into the Sufi Order with the ritualistic handshake taking about 2 to 3 minutes. After a subsequent visit with the Shaikh in the United Kingdom in June 2000, I was given a license to perform DCBD.

I first requested permission from the Shaikh in Baghdad to perform a cheek piercing on myself in May at the 2001 World Congress on Complementary Therapies in Medicine in Washington, DC. After lecturing on DCBD, I informed the audience that I needed to take an earlier flight home because of a family medical emergency in Cleveland. Skipping a break, I went right into the cheek piercing for the first time on my own. My state of mind was on the family medical crisis back home, but I was instructed to focus on connecting with the Shaikh, asking mentally for spiritual energy for rapid wound healing before the piercing. This took about a minute. One physician in the audience was particularly skeptical, so I invited him to stand next to me when I did the piercing. Please note that this was about 4 months before September 11, so I took a skewer from my kitchen drawer to be used for the demonstration.

After the 1-minute mental connection with the energy from the Shaikh and much nervousness, I pushed a very dull skewer through my left cheek. Yes, I was quite worried about the medical situation at home. The most difficult aspect of this experience was getting this dull object through my cheek. Eventually it went through with no pain. My skeptical medical colleague was very quiet after that. I pulled it out and there were a couple of drops of blood, which I blotted with a tissue until the bleeding stopped. From there, I had a friend take me directly to the airport.

The second time I demonstrated DCBD on myself was at the Fifth World Congress on Qigong in November 2002. Since this was after 9-11-2001, I had to shop for a better piercing instrument. This demonstration was preceded by a video interview by some of the leading scientists in the field of energy healing attending the conference. The video camera was then set on a stand on the side of my left cheek. I again focused on connecting with the energy of the Shaikh for rapid wound healing. I did not feel different, but I had faith that the connection was there, despite the distance in space. Again, I found that pushing the metal pick through my cheek was very difficult. After some effort (Jihad), both physical and mental, it went through. I also spoke on camera about how I was feeling with the object through my cheek. After the interview, I pulled the pick out and padded a tissue against my cheek with a few drops of blood. The wound closing was also documented on film for the first time. I had cut myself shaving early in the morning flying to

California, and the piercing was the next day. The shaving cut was more noticeable than the piercing after the demonstration. I went out for a late dinner after this demonstration.

How does Sufism explain how this can occur?

Sufism can form a unified theory for mechanistic, mind-body, and spiritual healing. Traditional Islamic theology recognizes that Allah (God) created a world that can apparently operate under mechanistic and Newtonian principles. As noted in the Holy Qur'an (Surah 6:95-99), Allah (God) created order in this world, causing seed to sprout, the rising and setting of the sun, and the rain to fall. "Such is the judgment and ordering of (Him) the exalted in Power, the Omniscient" (6:96).

This is consistent with the mechanistic Newtonian view of the world and humans. Thus, there is no rejection of mechanistic views from traditional Islamic philosophy. Sufi philosophy goes further, noting that mechanistic views can also be explained within a vitalistic perspective. From this point of view, Sufism can predict both mechanistic and energy-based DCBD healing phenomena in ways that Newtonian models cannot explain.

As explained by Sufi Shaikh Gaylani:

> The belief of the followers of the Book and the Sunna of the Messenger of Allah (Salla Allah ta'ala 'alayhi wa sallam) is that the sword does not cut because of its nature, but it is rather Allah ('Azza wa Jall) who cuts with it, that the fire does not burn because of its nature, but it is rather Allah ('Azza wa Jall) who burns with it, that food does not satisfy hunger because of its nature, but it is rather Allah ('Azza wa Jall) who satisfies hunger with it and that water does not quench thirst because of its nature, but it is rather Allah ('Azza wa Jall) who quenches thirst with it. The same applies to things of all kinds; it is Allah ('Azza wa Jall) who uses them to produce their effects and they are only instruments in His hand with which He does whatever He wills (Al-Casnazani al-Husseini, 1998, p. 42).

Thus, most of the time the world operates by mechanical laws allowed by Allah, but mediation by a Sufi Shaikh based on the Shaikh's nearness to Allah and through Allah would allow for fire not to burn or a knife not to cut, thus suspending mechanistic laws. The Quran is clear in several verses that so-called natural laws can be suspended by Allah. For example, in Surah 2:117, "when He (Allah) decreeth a matter, he saith to it: 'Be,' and it is."

The goal of the Sufi and all spiritual paths is nearness to God. In Sufism, this is done by following the Sufi path and practices and Jihad or struggling against the lower self or *nafs*. It is the lower self that keeps humans distant from God. Islam and Sufism are about surrendering to the will of God through following this path. Once near God, alterations of mechanistic laws may occur. This nearness to Allah is the explanation for "miracles" performed within religious contexts of ancient times and today.

Rapid wound healing is a very impressive phenomenon to observe and experience, but Islam and Sufism teaches that one's heart is the center of one's being that becomes diseased (Surah 5:52) and hardened (6:43) from wrong acts (sins). Sufism, however, offers healing for the heart, as noted in the Quran: "O mankind! There hath come to you a direction from your Lord and a healing for the (diseases) in your hearts—and for those who believe a guidance and a Mercy" (10:57). Thus, when the heart has been purified through jihad, the nearness and true healing will occur.

CONCLUSION

Sufism is a mystical tradition within Islam and is based on drawing nearer to Allah, through the spirituality of the Prophet Muhammad (P). Masters of present Sufi schools trace their origins back to the Prophet (P) through a chain of Masters. Sufism can be described as a path or way of attainment to Allah with its possible paranormal powers, knowledge, and healing. The psychology of Sufism is geared toward this attainment. The Sufi way involves following orthodox Islamic practices such as daily prayer, fasting, and some dietary prohibition, as well as frequent worshipful meditation. These practices may have not only spiritual purposes, but also many positive health implications.

Although Sufism generally is focused on spiritual development, some Sufi schools have focused on healing. This healing is a blend of Sufi philosophy with other Islamic healing traditions. Paranormal Sufi healing abilities have been observed and explained on the basis of a spiritual link mediated through the Sufi Master back to the Prophet (P) and Allah. Such phenomena from the Sufi way do not appear to result from meditative or altered states of consciousness but may be caused by a higher consciousness.

The implications of Sufism for integrative health is that Western high-tech medicine can be helpful for medical and surgical emergencies but may not be as helpful for chronic non–life-threatening conditions. What is needed today is a blending of "high tech" with "high touch." Sufism is one of the least studied approaches that offered an integration of Eras I, II, and III of medicine.

The Sufi way is the universal path for spiritual traditions, including prayer, fasting, and meditation; avoiding intoxicants, pork, sex outside marriage, and jihad (or battle against the lower self); and ultimate attainment of nearness to The God (Allah). Dossey (2001) anticipated the "respiritualization of medicine" when he noted the following:

> Modern medicine has become one of the most spiritually malnourished professions in our society. Because we have thoroughly disowned the spiritual component of healing, most healers throughout history would view our profession today as inherently perverse. They would be aghast at how we have squeezed the life juices and the heart out of our calling. Physicians have spiritual needs like anyone else, and we have paid a painful price for ignoring them. It simply does not feel good to practice medicine as if the only thing that matters were the physical; something feels left out and incomplete (p. 242).

Acknowledgments

Thanks go to Jeanie Hall, PhD, Lillian Hawkins, and Hadele Banna for their comments on earlier drafts of this manuscript.

References

Abdalati H: *Islam in focus*, Plainfield, 1996, American Trust Publications.

Al-Casnazani al-Hussesini M: *Jila'al-khatir: purification of the mind*, Philadelphia, 1999, Alminar Books.

Alexander FM: *Man's supreme inheritance: conscious guidance and control in relation to human evolution in civilization*, London, 1910, Chaaterson.

Ansha N: *Principles of Sufism*, Fremont, Calif, 1991, Asian Humanities Press.

Armstrong K: *Muhammad: a biography of the prophet*, San Francisco, 1993, HarperCollins.

Benor D: *Spiritual healing: scientific validation of a healing revolution*, 2001.

Benson H: *The relaxation response*, New York, 1975, Avon.

Chishti HM: *The book of Sufi healing*, Rochester, NY, 1991, Inner Traditions International.

Clarke PB, editor: *The world's religions: understanding the living faiths*, Pleasantville, NY, 1993, Reader's Digest Books.

Dewey J: *Human nature and conduct*, New York, 1922, Henry Holt.

Don NS, Moura G: Trance surgery in Brazil, *Altern Ther Health Med* 6(4):39-48, 2000.

Dossey L: Healing words, New York 1993, HarperSan-Francisco.

Dossey L: *Prayer is good medicine*, New York, 1996, HarperSanFrancisco.

Dossey L: Response to Peter Mulacz, *J Soc Psychical Res* 63(856):246-250, 1999 (letter to the editor).

Dossey L: *Healing beyond the body: medicine and the infinite reach of the mind*, Boston, 2001, Shambhala.

Ergil KV: Chinese medicine in M Micozzi: Fundamentals of complementary and alternative medicine second edition, New York, Churchill Livingstone, 303-344, 1996.

Eisenberg D, Kessler R, Foster C, et al: Unconventioal medicine in the united states: Prevalence, costs, and patterns of use, *N Engl J Med* 328(4): 246-252, 1993.

Eisenberg D, Davis RB, Ettner SL, et al: Trends in alternative medicine use in the united states, 1990-1997, *JAMA* 280(18): 1569-1575, 1998.

Farez S, Morley RS: Potential animal health hazards of pork and pork products, *Revue Scientifique Technique* 16(1):65-78, 1997.

Fatoohi L: Response to Peter Mulacz, *J Soc Psychical Res* 63(855):179-181, 1999 (letter to the editor).

Fatoohi L: *Jihad in the Qur'an*, Kuala Lumpur, Malaysia, 2002, AS Noordem.

Fatoohi L, Al-Dargazelli S: *History testifies to the infallibility of the Qur'an*, Kuala Lumpur, Malaysia, 1999, AS Noordem.

Friend MB: Group hypnotherapy treatment. Hospital treatment of alcoholism: a comparative, experimental study, *Menninger Clin Monogr Series* 11:77-120, 1957.

Gessner BD, Beller M: Protective effect of conventional cooking versus use of microwave ovens in an outbreak of salmonellosis, *Am J Epidemiol* 139(9):903-909, 1994.

Hall H: Deliberately caused bodily damage: metahypnotic phenomena? *J Soc Psychical Res* 64(861):211-223, 2000.

Hall H, Don NS, Hussein JN, et al: The scientific study of unusual rapid wound healing: a case report, *Adv Mind-Body Med* 17:203-213, 2001.

Hussein JN, Almukhtar N, Fatoohi LJ, Al-Dargazelli SS: The role of ambiguous terminology of consciousness in misunderstanding healing phenomena, *Frontier Perspect* 6(1):27-32, 1996.

Hussein JN, Fatoohi LJ, Al-Dargazelli SS, Almuchtar N: Deliberately caused bodily damage phenomena: mind, body, energy or what? Part 1, *Int J Altern Complementary Med* 12(9):9-11, 1994a.

Hussein JN, Fatoohi LJ, Al-Dargazelli SS, Almuchtar N: Deliberately caused bodily damage phenomena: mind, body, energy or what? Part 2, *Int J Altern Complementary Med* 12(10):21-24, 1994b.

Hussein JN, Fatoohi LJ, Al-Dargazelli SS, Almuchtar N: Deliberately caused bodily damage phenomena: mind, body, energy or what? Part 3, *Int J Altern Complementary Med* 12(11):25-28, 1994c.

Hussein JN, Fatoohi LJ, Hall H, Al-Dargazelli SS: Deliberately caused bodily damage phenomena, *J Soc Psychical Res* 62:97-113, 1997.

Khan HI: *The music of life*, New Lebanon, NY, 1983, Omega Publications.

Lang J: *Even angels ask: a journey to Islam in America*, Beltsville, Md, 2000, Amana Publications.

Lings M: *What is Sufism?* Berkeley, 1977, University of California Press.

McGee CT, Sancier K, Chow EPY: Qigong in Traditional Chinese Medicine, in M Micozzi: *Fundamentals of complementary and alternative medicine*, New York, Churchill Livingstone, 225-230, 1996.

McKercher PD, Hess WR, Hamdy F: Residual viruses in pork products, *Appl Environ Microbiol* 16(1):65-78, 1978.

Muhaiyaddeen MRB: *Questions of life, answers of wisdom by the contemporary Sufi M.R. Bawa Muhaiyaddeen*, vol 1, Philadelphia, 1991, Fellowship Press.

Mulacz WP: Deliberately caused bodily damage (DCBD) phenomena: a different perspective, *J Soc Psychical Res* 62:434-444, 1998.

Murray M, Pizzorno J: *Encyclopedia of natural medicine*, Rocklin, Calif, 1991, Prima Publishing.

Nelson RD, Bradish GJ, Dobyns YH, et al: Field REG anomalies in group situations, *J Sci Explor* 10(1):111-141, 1996.

Nelson RD, Bradish GJ, Dobyns YH, et al: FieldREG II: consciousness field effects—replications and explorations, *J Sci Explor* 12(3):425-454, 1998.

Oschman J: *Energy medicine: the scientific basis*, 2000.

Posner G: Taking a stab at a paranormal claim (http://www.csicop.org/sb/9509/posner.html), 1998.

Rumi J: *Feeling the shoulder of the lion*, Putney, Vt, 1991, Threshold Books.

Starfield B: Is US health really the best in the world? *JAMA* 284(4):483-485, 2000.

Tauxe RV: Emerging foodborne diseases: an evolving public health challenge, *Emerg Infect Dis* 3(4):425-434, 1997.

Walford RL: *Maximum life span*, New York, 1983, Avon Books.

Woodward MR: Healing and morality: a Javanese example, *Soc Sci Med* 21:1007-1021, 1985.

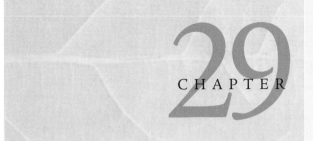
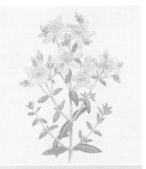

CHAPTER 29

NATIVE AMERICAN HEALING

R I C H A R D   W .   V O S S
V I C T O R   D O U V I L L E
E .   D A N   E D W A R D S
(w i t h   G a y l a   T w i s s)

Opening Cautionary Note

Indian people are understandably wary of the written word. Some may criticize the inclusion of this chapter in this edition. This criticism is understandable, because often the written word objectifies understandings and can be manipulated outside the relationship in which the understanding was shared. This is a concern and a risk in contributing this chapter to the third edition of *Fundamentals of Complementary and Integrative Medicine*. However, not to include a chapter on American Indian views about medicine and health care is also a concern, because it helps perpetuate the invisibility of Indian people amidst the dominant social, political, and religious factions. The untold history of Native American people is a sobering context through which one must view contemporary concerns. The purpose of this chapter is to honor the continuing journey of understanding between medical science practitioners and traditional Indian medicine practitioners to see how these two medicine paths can help restore health to the people and to bring about increased understanding—*wo'wa'bleza*—among peoples. This chapter is not intended to encourage "mixing" Indian medicine with allopathic or "alternative" medicines, but rather to emphasize the importance of respecting the integrity of each of these paths in bringing health and help to people in need.

> It is this loss of faith that has left a void in Indian life—a void that civilization cannot fill. The old life was attuned to nature's rhythm—bound by mystical ties to the sun, moon, stars; to the waving grasses,

flowing streams and whispering winds. It is not a question (as so many white writers like to state it) of the white man "bringing the Indian up to his plane of thought and action." It is rather a case where the white man had better grasp some of the Indian's spiritual strength. I protest against calling my people savages. How can the Indian, sharing all the virtues of the white man, be justly called a savage? The white race today is but half civilized and unable to order his life into ways of peace and righteousness (Luther Standing Bear, 1931).

These words of Luther Standing Bear provide a sobering orientation toward understanding a pan-Indian perspective of medicine and health. Long before Columbus landed in what he thought was Hindustan, the indigenous peoples of the Americas practiced a highly advanced medicine that was effective in combating diseases then common in the Americas (Iron Shell, 1997; Little Soldier, 1997; Looking Horse, 1997; Red Dog, 1997; Standing Bear, 1933). These medicine ways emphasized the "right order of things" and viewed humans not as some higher intellectual being above lower animal and inanimate beings but as a kindred partner in the universe (creation), reliant on the other beings in creation for life itself.

However, the worldview of the new European visitors to the Americas prompted misunderstandings and exploitation of the peoples they called *Indios,* a corruption of the Spanish, derived from Columbus' perception of the people he encountered in the New World. He described them as *"una gente en Dios,"* which literally means "a people in with God" (Means, 1995).

Tragically, this early perception of the natural peacefulness, harmony, and ease of temperament of these "Indians" prompted Columbus to conclude that "they would make excellent slaves" (Means, 1995). This set the stage for the subsequent historical events that led to the degradation of the indigenous, or natural, people of the Americas who were called *Indians.* The "natural" style of these people was to be perceived as "brutish" and "savage"; their attentiveness to primal experience would be perceived as "primitive"; their understanding of the creation (all of the universe) as infused with life and spirit would be seen as "animistic." In all these assessments, what was "Indian" was evaluated as inferior to the European cultural standards, including advanced technology and "higher" (theistic) religion(s).

The term *Indian* was imposed on the indigenous peoples of the Americas erroneously, because they were not a homogeneous group but rather distinct "nations" or "peoples" with different languages, beliefs, customs, social and political structures, and historical rivalries. The term *American Indian* is used today to talk about common values and a certain shared identity among many Native American people, and it is also used as the legal title of federally recognized tribes holding jurisdiction on reservation lands in the United States. The indigenous people of Canada and the Six Nations' People (Iroquois) preferred the term *Natives,* which is the official term used by the Canadian government to identify indigenous people. The terms *American Indian, Native American,* and *Indian people* are used interchangeably throughout this chapter, with an awareness of the historical and political complexity associated with these terms (Means, 1995).

HISTORY

To understand American Indian health care and approaches to medicine, one needs to "get the history right" and take a critical look at the "other" American history that most Americans were never taught, that was never included in their textbooks, and that continues to be glossed in mainstream American classrooms—the largely invisible history of Native Americans in the United States. Non-Indian people need to learn both sides of American history, to understand the "bad medicine" that has infected relations between Indians and non-Indian people. Recall the interaction between Tosawi, chief of the Comanches and General Sheridan after Tosawi brought in the first band of Comanches to surrender. Addressing

---

*These include three major texts *(Brihat Trayi),* the *Charaka Samhita, Sushruta Samhita,* and *Ashtanga Hridaya* of Vagbhata, and three minor texts *(Laghu Trayi),* the *Sarngadhara Samhita, Bhavaprakash Samhita,* and *Madhava Nidanam.* Most of these texts have been translated into English (Charaka Samhita, 1977; Madhavakava, 1986; Sarngadhara, 1984; Sushruta Samhita, 1963; Vagbhata, 1982). These texts address eight main sections of Ayur-Veda: *Shalya,* surgery in general; *Shalakya,* surgery for supraclavicular diseases; *Kaya chikitsa,* treatment, diagnosis, and internal medicine; *Kaumarya Birtya,* pediatrics, obstetrics, and gynecology; *Agad Tantra,* toxicology and medical jurisprudence; *Bhut Vidya,* psychosomatic medicine; *Rasayana,* materia medica to promote vitality, stamina, resistance to disease, and longevity; and *Vajikarana,* fertility and potency.

Sheridan, Tosawi spoke his own name and two words in English: "Tosawi, good Indian." Sheridan responded with the now-infamous words: "The only good Indians I ever saw were dead" (Ellis, 1900) cited in Brown, 1970, p. 170.

Beyond the larger cultural-historical context, one also needs to consider the distinctive Indian tribal culture. It is important to know how each tribe dealt with its own survival in the wake of U.S. expansionism, policies of extermination, and the extent to which each tribe was exposed to racial and cultural genocide. It is also important to understand how its tribal leadership related with the U.S. government and to assess the degree of broken trusts and treaties. With this background information, one can then develop an awareness of, and sensitivity to, the issues that have an impact on the consciousness and sense of well-being or disease and distrust of government and other social institutions by many Native American people today. One needs to be informed about the issues of loss of land and culture, repeated broken trusts, and unenforced treaties. One must be sensitive about the forced assimilation policies, programs, and depersonalizing attitudes directed toward Indian people, both formally and informally, by the U.S. government, missionaries, and other social institutions that were embedded in the "progressive American consciousness" and committed to civilizing and incorporating the Indian into this larger consciousness.

Although some Indian people claim to have benefited from their boarding school experience, the greater number of Indian people are beginning to speak out about the cultural trauma of the boarding school systems. Through assimilation programs, what was "natural" and basic to Indian self-identity was suppressed, discouraged, and literally "beaten out" of them through systematic resocialization. Indian children were separated from their families and their traditional ceremonial practices, which were intimately linked to the extended family and reinforced by social, moral, political, and spiritual life, and introduced to what was perceived as a more civilized (materialistic) view of life, which devastated Indian society (Clark, 1997; Clifford M, 1997; Douville, 1997a; Little Soldier, 1997; Mestheth, 1993; White Hat Sr, 1997). For Indian people, all aspects of life were intimately connected to good health and well-being. The interconnections among family, tribe or clan, moral, political, and ceremonial life all con-tributed to a sense of harmony and balance that was called *wicozani* (good total health) by the Lakota and *hozhon* (harmony, beauty, happiness, and health) by the Navajo.

Traditional Navajo healing practices revolve around the notion of *Hozho*, a term that embodies the concepts of balance, harmony, and spirituality. When people achieve a life of *Hozho*, they walk the "Beauty Way," and their lives are filled with peace, contentment, and positive health—physically, mentally, emotionally, and spiritually. Positive interconnections among family, clan, tribe, nature, all living things, and ceremonial life all contribute to a sense of harmony and balance, which is the achievement of *Hozho*. When a Navajo medicine man performs a healing ceremony, a circle of healing is formed by the interconnection among the sick person, family, relatives, the spirits, and singers who help with ceremonial songs. For traditional Navajo, the world is a dangerous place requiring due caution and respect; there is an emphasis on preventing harm from occurring through prevention-type ceremonies (*hozonji*) to better meet this dangerous world. Navajo healers (*Hatalie*) use sand painting to cure the sick person. A very stylized sand painting is drawn using various colors of sand; on its completion, the patient is instructed to sit on the painting while the healing ceremony is performed. Healing takes place as the sick person absorbs the power or spirits that exist in the sand painting (Figure 29-1) (Edwards, 2004).

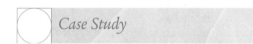

Case Study

Robert, a full-blood American Indian, has lived most of his life in a large metropolitan area. He was hospitalized in a residential treatment facility for depression, anxiety, weight loss, verbal and social regression, agitated moods, hysterical behaviors, and night terrors. During his hospitalization, these behaviors worsened, and he was noncompliant with the treatment plan, which included group and individual psychotherapy. Additional background included the following: Robert lived with his mother and two half-siblings; his mother was recently divorced from his stepfather; and Robert's father died 6 years earlier.

An urban American Indian social worker from Robert's tribe was called in as a clinical consultant with the hospital staff regarding Robert's deteriorating mental and physical health status. The clinical consultant first met with staff and then with Robert. In their initial meeting, Robert and the American Indian clinical consultant

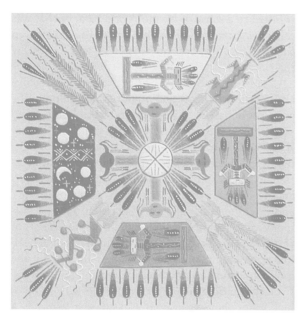

Figure 29-1 Traditional sand painting (Artist: Frank Martin). (Courtesy Penfield Gallery of Indian Arts, Albuquerque, NM, http://www.penfieldgallery.com/.)

conversed in their Native language regarding their parents, siblings, clans, home reservation areas, and cultural activities in which they both participated. They then talked about Robert's current situation, including his hospitalization, his separation from his family, and his fears. Robert believed that his father had been hexed (someone had placed an evil spell over him) and died as a result of evil forces associated with this hex. Robert also believed that these evil forces could be unleashed on him, and that he, too, might die.

The clinical consultant talked with Robert about the spiritual ceremonies that could be arranged for him on his home reservation to restore balance and harmony in his life. Robert knew and understood the significance of these healing ceremonies and was willing to participate with the clinical consultant in arranging the ceremony for him. The clinical consultant, an enrolled member of a recognized American Indian tribe, gave Robert an eagle feather and talked to Robert about the power and protective nature of the eagle feather, the value of his cultural healing traditions, and the importance of his Native culture in restoring balance and harmony in his life. A healing ceremony was arranged for Robert on his home reservation, where the Indian medicine people were able to provide information and healing to Robert, effectively allaying much of his anxiety, to the point where he was amenable to participate in the recommended clinical treatment available at the hospital. The combined therapies contributed to a positive treatment outcome. ∾

This case example illustrates a number of important components of the relationship between traditional healing methods and Western medicine practices relevant to this discussion. First, the clinical consultant was able to speak the Native language of the patient and could comprehend the cultural significance of the problems Robert was facing, as well as the corresponding cultural resources available to address these problems in a culturally compatible manner. Second, the consultant was able to explain to the non-Indian hospital staff Robert's perceptions of his problems and desire to participate in a traditional healing ceremony. Third, the clinical consultant, as an enrolled member of a recognized tribe, was able to give Robert, also an enrolled member, an eagle feather (which is illegal for non-Indians to possess), which requires considerable generosity from the giver and is a sign of utmost respect for the person to whom the gift is given. Fourth, it is important to note that regardless of the current residence or length of time Native people have lived off the reservation, identification with Native traditions and cultural practices may play a very important role in their construction of meaning in life events, as well as in their understanding of health and well-being. Finally, the case study illustrates well how Western medicine and traditional Indian medicine may complement each other in promoting good health and wellness among traditional American Indians, both living on the reservation and off the reservation. (A version of this case study appears in *Social Work: a Profession of Many Faces* [Edwards and Edwards, 1998, pp. 477-478].)

For Indian people, life is like a circle, continuous, harmonious, and cyclical, with no distinctions. Medicine was a coming together of all the elements in this circular pattern of life. The circle of healing was formed by the interconnections among the sick person, his or her extended family or relatives, the spirits, the singers who helped with the ceremonial songs, and the medicine practitioner (Figures 29-2 and 29-3).

Therefore, as ceremonial practices were suppressed and as government policies undermined the integrity of traditional Indian practices, the cultural fabric of Indian peoples was also torn. Official U.S. government assimilation policies forced many traditional Indian medicine practitioners "underground" for risk of being cited for committing actions prohibited by government regulation or being accused of "devil worship" and held up to public ridicule. Archie

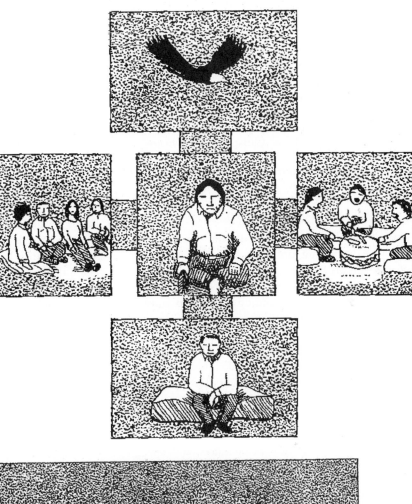

Figure 29-2 Spirits, relatives, singers, and sick person in the shape of two intersecting lines. (Courtesy Sinte Gleska University.)

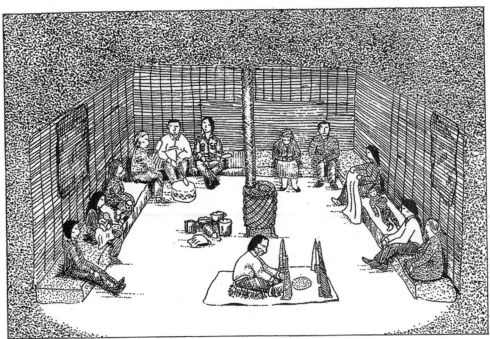

Figure 29-3 All of the elements from Figure 29-2 are depicted in this ceremony of the extended family in the healing process. The drawing shows a quiet gathering of people in a darkened room. (Courtesy Sinte Gleska University.)

Fire Lame Deer and Richard Erdoes note, "Between 1890 and 1940, the Sundance, as well as all other native ceremonies, were forbidden under the Indian Offenses Act." They continue, recalling the following:

> One could be jailed for just having an Inipi [a sweatlodge ceremony] or praying in the Lakota way, as the government and the missionaries tried to stamp out our old beliefs in order to make us into slightly darker, "civilized" Christians. Many historians believe that during those fifty years no Sundances were performed, but they are wrong. The Sundance was held every year . . . but it had to be done in secret, in lonely places where no white man could spy on us (1992, p. 230).

Clyde Holler notes the official ban of the Sundance beginning on April 10, 1883, with the enforcement of "Rules for Indian Courts," which were in effect up until 1934, with the ban on piercing up until 1952 or later, depending on interpretation (Holler, 1995; see also Commissioner of Indian Affairs, 1883).

Luther Standing Bear reflected on the profound shift that was occurring as he recalled his experience traveling to the Carlisle Indian School as a boy. He wrote:

> It was only about three years after the Custer battle, and the general opinion was that the Plains people merely infested the earth as nuisances, and our being there simply evidenced misjudgment on the part of Wakan Tanka. Whenever our train stopped at the railway stations, it was met by great numbers of white people who came to gaze upon the little Indian "savages." The shy little ones sat quietly at the car windows looking at the people who swarmed on the platform. Some of the children wrapped themselves in their blankets, covering all but their eyes. At one place we were taken off the train and marched a distance down the street to a restaurant. We walked down the street between two rows of uniformed men whom we called soldiers, though I suppose they were policemen. This must have been done to protect us, for it was surely known that we boys and girls could do no harm. Back of the rows of uniformed men stood the white people craning their necks, talking, laughing, and making a great noise. They yelled and tried to mimic us by giving what they thought were war-whoops. We did not like this (Standing Bear, 1933).

To this day many older Indian people are reluctant to talk about the older traditional ways, and many middle-age Indian people who were educated in the boarding school system were literally removed from their tribes and forced to assimilate white man's ways. Resocialized in often-abusive environments, many never learned the older traditions and their native languages. Often, students from western tribes were sent east to the Carlisle Indian School at Carlisle, Pennsylvania, and students from eastern tribes were sent west (e.g., the Nanticokes of Delaware were sent to the Haskell Indian School in Kansas) (Clark, 1997).

Other Indians whose behavior seemed odd or troublesome were sent to the infamous Hiawatha Insane Asylum for Indians, also known as the *Canton Insane Asylum,* which was the only segregated asylum built exclusively for American Indians in the United States, located in Canton, South Dakota (Hoover, 1997; Iron Shield, 1992; Putney, 1984). This institution was opened in 1902 as the second federal institution for the insane (predated by St. Elizabeth's Hospital in Washington, DC) to provide psychiatric care exclusively to Indian people by an act of Congress, despite opposition from the Department of the Interior and the Superintendent of St. Elizabeth's Hospital when the bill was first passed by Congress in 1898 (Iron Shield, 1988, 1992). Under the abusive administration of Dr. Harry Hummer, the institution would become the subject of a 150-page report filed by Dr. Samuel Silk in 1929 detailing the abhorrent conditions endured by the patient-residents there.

As a result of Dr. Silk's report, Dr. Hummer was dismissed, and in December 1933, after further study, the Hiawatha Asylum for Indians was closed, its remaining 71 Indian patients transferred to St. Elizabeth's Hospital. Over the 31 years of operation, the asylum housed 370 Indians. There are 121 Indians buried on the grounds of the former asylum; the causes of these deaths are unknown. Although the asylum was founded "as a place to alleviate the suffering of mentally ill tribesmen from the Indian reservations, it ended as an institution that itself caused genuine human misery" (Putney, 1984). The asylum was turned into a community hospital in the 1950s and is now the Canton-Inwood Memorial Hospital. The Indian burial ground is now located next to the Hiawatha Golf Course, which sits adjacent to the grounds of the asylum in Canton (Iron Shield, 1991, 1994, 1997). Harold Iron Shield is currently leading a movement to identify relatives of those buried at the Canton (Hiawatha) Asylum and is seeking to repatriate their remains to their respective tribes, where possible, and preserve the cemetery as a National Historic Site.

Medical treatment and health care for American Indians was historically grossly inadequate and often seen as antagonistic with traditional Indian medicine ways. There was no supervision of agency doctors, and "not until 1891 were physicians placed in a classified service and required to pass examinations in addition to having a medical degree" (DeMallie and Jahner, 1991). Charles Alexander Eastman, a Lakota Sioux Indian who served as an agency physician at Pine Ridge from 1890 to 1892, observed the practice of government-sponsored medical care. He wrote:

> The doctors who were in the service in those days had an easy time of it. They scarcely ever went outside of the agency enclosure, and issued their pills and compounds after the most casual inquiry. As late as 1890, when the Government sent me out as a physician to ten thousand Ogallalla Sioux and Northern Cheyennes at Pine Ridge Agency, I found my predecessor still practicing his profession through a small hole in the wall between his office and the general assembly room of the Indians. One of the first things I did was to close that hole; and I allowed no man to diagnose his own trouble or choose his pills (DeMallie and Jahner, 1991).

Physicians in the Indian Service had to use their own funds and gifts of money from friends to buy medicines and supplies. Drugs supplied to the Indians were "often obsolete in kind, and either stale or of the poorest quality" (DeMallie and Jahner, 1991). In 1893, Dr. Z.T. Daniel recommended that the procedures for Indian Service doctors be reappraised, modernized, and compiled in serviceable form. He also recommended that an agency physician be sent annually as a representative of the American Medical Association, and he urged that Indian Service doctors be supplied with medical textbooks and medical journals.

In light of the inadequate health care provided to Indian people, it is important to keep in mind the decimation Indian people faced by the exposure to Old World diseases. Henry Dobyns (1983) estimated that Native people faced serious contagious diseases that caused significant mortality at approximately 4-year intervals from 1520 to 1900. The pandemics affecting Indian people are often treated by white historians and others as types of "natural disasters," never intended by Europeans (Jaimes, 1992). How-

ever, Indian people are cognizant of their history and remember their oral history in which forms of germ warfare were conducted by military operations against them. One example often cited was the distribution of smallpox-infected blankets by the U.S. Army to Mandan (Indians) at Fort Clark on June 19, 1837, thought to be the causative factor in the smallpox pandemic of 1836-1840 (Chardon, 1932; Jaimes, 1992).

The shame nurtured by decades and centuries of efforts to "civilize the heathen Indian" has taken its toll on our American consciousness. One cannot begin to appreciate traditional Indian medicine ways without a profound awareness at a "gut level" of how much effort went into the eradication of what is now being perceived as "alternative medicine." This is the uneasy starting point of understanding traditional Indian medicine. Within this historical context, one can better perceive the basis for many Indian peoples' objections to the growing "popularity" of their traditional spirituality and healing practices among non-Indians—by the *wasicun*. This Lakota word described the early white hunter's propensity to take the fatty, choice portion of the buffalo, and leave the rest to rot; Buechel translates it as, "One who takes things." This term is still used today to express their perception of the narrow, materialistic, and destructive worldview of mainstream white culture. Interest among whites in seeking out "Indian medicine men and shamans" and the resultant exploitation of Indian ceremonies (e.g., buying Indian spirituality in weekend or half-day workshops, seminars, paying fees for sweatlodge ceremonies) have prompted some Lakota leaders to issue a "declaration of war" against such exploitation (Mestheth et al., 1993). There are strong feelings about the contemporary curiosity of whites about Indian medicine ways.

WILLIAM PENN'S ACCOUNT OF TENOUGHAN'S SWEATBATH

One of the earliest accounts of a European observing an American Indian healing ceremony is in *William Penn's Own Account of the Lenni Lenape or Delaware Indians* (Meyers, 1970). The account portrays many factors relevant to understanding Indian medicine ways and the quality of interaction of Indian people with Europeans. The account cited here is Penn's observation of a Lenape man named Tenoughan involved in a healing sweatbath (Figure 29-4).

> I called upon an Indian of Note, whose Name was Tenoughan, the Captain General of the Clan of Indians of those Parts. I found him ill of a Fever, his Head and Limbs much affected with Pain, and at the same time his Wife preparing a Bagnio for him: The Bagnio resembled a large Oven, into which he crept, by a Door on the one side, while she put several red hot Stones in a small Door on the other side thereof, and fastened the Doors as closely from the Air as she could. Now while he was Sweating in this Bagnio, his Wife (for they disdain no Service) was, with an Ax, cutting her Husband a passage into the River, (being the Winter of 83 the great Frost, and the Ice very thick) in order to the Immersing himself, after he should come out of his Bath. In less than half an Hour, he was in so great a Sweat, that when he came out he was as wet, as if he had come out of a River, and the Reak or Steam of his Body so thick, that it was hard to discern any bodies Face that stood near him. In this condition, stark naked (his Breech-Clout only excepted) he ran into the River, which was about twenty Paces, and duck'd himself twice or thrice therein, and so return'd (passing only through his Bagnio to mitigate the immediate stroak of the Cold) to his own House, perhaps 20 Paces further, and wrapping himself in his woolen Mantle, lay down as his length near a long (but gentle) Fire in the midst of his Wigwam, or House, turning himself several times, till he was dry, and then he rose, and fell to getting us Dinner, seeming to be as easie, and well in Health, as at any other time (Surveyor General Thomas Holme's letter, dated 5th Month [May] 7, 1688, concerning the running of a survey line) (Meyers, 1970).

Penn made this observation when he was on a surveying expedition of the "farthest northern region of his Provence," which was actually near Monocacy, Berks County, Pennsylvania, today about a 45-minute commute from Philadelphia. The river would be the Schuylkill River, now polluted by a century of industrial contaminants and washoff from coal mines and agriculture farther north. This old account provides a powerful illustration of the cultural chasm that separated Penn from Tenoughan's world of medicine and health care. This story conveys the tremendous gap in appreciating what was happening during the observation. Penn was intent on buying land from the Lenape people, so it was on an economic venture that he stumbled on a healing bath taken by Tenoughan, a Lenape leader of some stature.

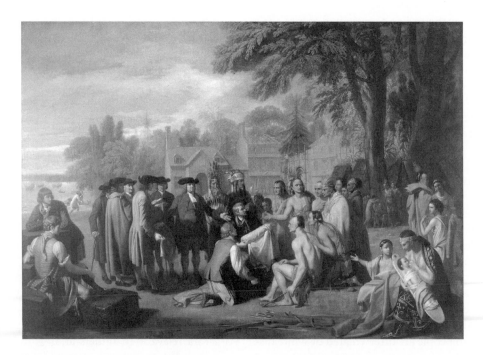

Figure 29-4 Benjamin West's painting of William Penn's Treaty with the Indians (1771-2). (Courtesy Pennsylvania Academy of the Fine Arts, Philadelphia.)

The story provides a model for understanding the complexity and the obstacles that confront non-Indian people, embedded in Eurocentrism, in not comprehending Indian medicine ways. Penn was struck by the exotic and the unusual nature of the event he witnessed, as well as the apparent efficacy of the sweatbath on Tenoughan, but the observation lacks any real personal encounter between Penn and Tenoughan, although we read that *Tenough* served dinner for his guests after the sweatbath. As old and as minimally detailed as this account is, it illustrates a number of important insights into American Indian medicine and health care.

First, the sweatbath was located near Tenoughan's home. It was familiar, literally, in his backyard. Second, the practice included the assistance by a family member, Tenoughan's wife, who actually prepared the sweatbath for him, carried the red hot stones into the Bagnio, and assisted in closing the door securely. Much of Indian medicine is family oriented; it is not something that is done by strangers. Medicine is a family matter; family is intimately involved and plays a significant role in the healing process. Later, Tenoughan's wife assisted in the arduous task of cutting a path through the ice for the "patient" to plunge into the river. Indian medicine often brings the patient into close interaction with the natural world and the elements. After the sweatbath, Tenoughan rests by the fire in his wigwam, and he then serves dinner to his guests. For many Indian people, stone, fire, air, water, food, spirits, and social and familial relationships are seen as medicine.

CULTURE

Sutton and Broken Nose cite a powerful clinical vignette about how the cultural differences can create real tension between expectations of clinical practitioners from the dominant culture and Indian sensibilities and practices. Although they cite the experience of a social worker sent to run an alternative school program on a Montana Indian reservation, the setting could be any health care or service-oriented setting. The vignette is quoted in the following:

> One day I came into work and no one was there. There were no teachers, students, or counselors. At first I thought it was Saturday or some holiday I had forgot about. I checked my calendar and the one the tribe printed to see if it was some special kind of Indian holiday, but it was not. Finally, I went riding around in my car. I saw one of the counselors and asked where everyone was. He said Albert Running Horse had died. I found out later that Albert was one of the oldest men in the tribe and was somehow related to almost everyone at school. When I tried to find out when everyone would be back at work, I couldn't get a definite answer because they weren't sure when some of Albert's relatives would come in from out of state. I was upset because I felt we had been making progress with some particularly difficult cases. I was concerned about the continuity of therapy and the careful schedule we had all worked out. When I expressed my frustration to one of my counselors she just shrugged her shoulders and said we all have to grieve. All I could think of is how am I going to explain this to my superiors (McGoldrick et al., 1996).

This example illustrates the fundamental difference in worldview between Indian and non-Indian Americans and presents a common "clinical dilemma" that is likely to occur between mainstream approaches to health care and the "natural" approach to healing and human relationships typical among Indian people. Which is the better medicine, following the prescribed treatment plan or attending to the sense of community loss and grief on the death of an esteemed elder? Health care practitioners need to look for ways to affirm and support the values, beliefs, and needs of Indian people. Conversely, these values, beliefs, and needs may well be the same for non-Indian people as well, but denied in the face of economic expediency. Appreciating the impact of diverse cultures on medical and health care practice is essential and is perhaps the most important thing the health care practitioner needs to address in developing cultural competence with Indian people or with any group not often credited or valued by the larger, dominant culture.

First, the concept of "professional helper/healer" is foreign to traditional Indian peoples and has no precedent in prereservation Lakota society. The idea of "paid professionals" conflicts with the tradition that "helping other people" is a social responsibility for everyone, not just for a few. Professional/paid health care practitioners are often viewed with suspicion by some traditionalists as governmental "agents of forced assimilation." Along with government-sanctioned missionary activity, the legacy of Indian boarding schools, and psychiatric hospitalization, health care professionals were associated with oppressive social structures that were intended to "civilize the Indian." Thus, a Lakota-centric view of health care starts with the awareness of the power of the institutionalized systems (e.g., social, health care, educational systems) to influence and assert social control, which although aimed at "improved health care" or social well-being, may also reflect and enact the larger, more pervasive oppression of racist attitudes, policies, and procedures of "civilizing the Indian."

Although no permanent or paid professional "health care providers" were among the Lakota bands or tribes in prereservation days, various individuals, groups, and societies within Lakota bands provided health care functions to the people. In effect, every tribal member was expected to follow the "natural law of creation," or the *Wo-ope*, the unwritten natural law that guides Lakota life, which emphasizes unselfishness and generosity. The *Wo'ope* embodies the philosophy of *mitakuye oyas'in*, which, according to White Hat "is what keeps us together." It is the knowledge "that we come from one source, and we are all related." However, to make this work, "we must identify the good and evil in us, and practice what is good" (White Hat Sr, 1997). Lakota philosophy does not separate good and evil, sickness and health, or right and wrong as distinct realities, they coexist in each person, in every creation; even in the most sacred thing there is good and evil. The important thing is to understand that there is the negative and the positive within everyone and everything, and to be responsible in one's life to live in a good, moral, healthy way, in balance with all creation.

The natural law is the way nature acts. Understanding Lakota philosophy begins with understanding the natural law or the seven laws of the Creator (Iron Shell, 1997; Looking Horse, 1997; Lunderman, 1997). The "natural law" or the *Wo'ope* required each person to exercise shared values, which, if acted on in one's life, gave the person and the extended family *(tios'paye)* and the tribe *wicozani*, which was understood as total or perfect health, balance and harmony, good social health, and well being (Iron Shell, 1997); it implies physical and spiritual health (White Hat Sr, 1997).

Another orienting value of helpers and healers among the Lakota is *Nagi'ksapa*, or self-wisdom is the awareness of your aura/spirit (Iron Shell, 1997). White Hat, Sr., translates and explains the *nagi'ksapa* as "one's spirit, the wise spirit in a person." White Hat, Sr., notes that "The Lakota are very much aware of the spirit within [us]—we talk to our spirit—we ask our spirit to be strong and to help us in our deci-

sions" and life (1997). *Iha'kicikta* is the ability to look out for one another. If you move camp, you should be concerned that everyone is going to move together. You want to make sure there is enough water and food for everyone (Iron Shell, 1997). *Wo'onsila* is the ability to have pity on each other (Iron Shell, 1997). Albert White Hat, Sr., explains the word as "recognizing a specific need of someone or something, and you address that (specific) need." According to White Hat, Lakota philosophy does not encourage people to "stay stuck" or dependent. *Iyus'kiniya* is the ability to go do things with a happy attitude (Iron Shell, 1997). *Wi'ikt ceya* is the measure of wealth by how little one has; it is the capacity to give to others; it is one's capacity for self-sacrifice (Iron Shell, 1997). *Teki'ci' hilapi* is the ability to cherish, esteem, and treasure each other (Iron Shell, 1997). Practicing these social values ensured good social functioning.

The primary orientation of traditional Indian medicine was universalistic. Health and welfare resources were made available to everyone through their family and community. Prereservation Lakota society emphasized tribalism over individualism, social harmony over self-interest, and a commitment or loyalty to the people or the larger extended family relations over individual success. Health care functions were accomplished by one's extended family *(tios'paye)*; it was the extended family that provided for the social support and material assistance of all its members. Wealth was distributed through the practice of the giveaway ceremony *(wopila)*, which is still practiced by traditional Lakotas. This practice ensured that no one person's or one family's wealth or resources dominated.

Mental health and physical health are viewed as inseparable from spiritual and moral health. The good balance of the one's life in harmony with the *Wo'ope*, or natural law of creation, brings about *wicozani*, or good health, which was both individual and communal. Rather than viewing the individual as a mind-body split, which has influenced much of Western psychiatric thinking, traditional Lakota philosophy viewed the individual person as an unexplainable creation with four constituent dimensions of self. The *nagi* is one's individual soul; Buechel (1983) translates the word as, "The soul, spirit; the shadow of anything, as of a man *(wicanagi)* or of a house *(tinagi)*." The *nagi la* is the divine spirit immanent in each human being. The *niya*, or "the vital breath," gives life to the body and is responsible for the circulation of the blood and the breathing process. The fourth element of the person is the *sicun,* or "intellect" (Goodman, 1992, p. 41). Albert White Hat, Sr., however, describes the *sicun* as "your (spirit's) presence [that] is felt on something or somebody." Beuchel (1983) translated the word as, "That in a man or thing which is spirit or spiritlike and guards him from birth against evil spirits." Often a person appeals to his *nagi la* for assistance. This is a power within each person that can help him or her overcome obstacles. When one goes on the *hanbleceya,* or pipe fast, one leaves the physical world as a *nagi.*

According to Gene Thin Elk, "We are not humans on a soul journey. We are nagi, 'souls,' who are making a journey through the material world" (Goodman, 1992). The *nagi la* has been described as the "little spirit," which is the "divine spirit immanent in each being" (Goodman, 1992). Existence in the material world is tenuous for the newborn, according to Lakota philosophy: Ms. Edna Little Elk commented: "The most important things for infants and little children are to eat good, sleep good and play good," and by doing so, the *nagi* of the child is persuaded to become more and more attached to its own body (Goodman, 1992). Traditional Lakota philosophy sees abuse, rejection, or neglect affecting the child's *nagi,* where it may detach from the child's body and not come back. In this case, ceremonies are conducted by a medicine man to find the child's *nagi* and bring it back (Goodman, 1992). Such a condition has been called *soul loss.* Thus, good mental or emotional health is intimately related to good spiritual, moral, and physical health; these cannot be separated out.

(See Appendix 29 for a discussion of Native American herbs and medicinal plants.)

CONTRIBUTIONS OF INDIAN PEOPLE TO MEDICINE AND HEALTH CARE

Despite that Native American people have ancient oral traditions of healing and helping tribal members in need during reservation times, prereservation times, and the traumatic transition periods in between (Douville, 1997a; Lunderman, 1997; Red Dog, 1997), much of the health care literature reviewed focused on practice issues concerning Native American people where they were viewed primarily as a special client or health care risk group in need of a specialized approach to treatment (DuBray, 1985, 1992; Garrett and Garrett, 1994; Good Tracks, 1973; Williams and Ellison, 1996). This literature generally treats "Native Americans" as a generic, homogeneous group and does not examine specific tribal traditions or practices of help and healing indigenous to specific tribal traditions.

DuBray calls for a more holistic approach to treatment intervention based on Native American (Lakota) practices. DuBray (1992) discusses the use of the vision quest, the importance of food as a symbol of love and respect, the role of cultural healing ceremonies, and the importance of the collective unconscious in Indian experience of reality. The contributions of Native American practices, philosophies, and traditions of help and healing have also been discussed in anthropological studies (Wallace, 1958), rehabilitation medicine (Braswell and Wong, 1994; Hodge, 1989), nursing (Reynolds, 1993; Turton, 1995), and psychiatric literature (Garro, 1990; Hammerschlag, 1988, 1992; Lewis, 1982, 1990). There is a growing use of traditional medicine ways in alcohol treatment programs for American Indians, both on and off the reservation (Hall, 1985, 1986; Red Dog, 1997; Thin Elk, 1995), as well as in health programs for Indian children and youth (e.g., Healthy Nations Program at the Cheyenne River Sioux Tribe) (Red Dog, 1997).

The timing is ripe for health care and medical educators to look carefully at how Native practices, traditions, and values can shape theory, practice, and policy at a foundational level. This is particularly important as tribal governments develop strategies and responses to welfare reform with the implementation of the Temporary Assistance to Needy Families (TANF) program, which is being met with great concern by many Native American tribal leaders and health care providers (Goldsmith, 1996).

ORIENTING CONCEPTS TO INDIAN MEDICINE

In a report to the National Institutes of Health, *Alternative Medicine: Expanding Medical Horizons* (1992), the Lakota (Sioux Tribe) were cited for the use of healing ceremonies by specialists who are essentially shamanic in their approach to treatment. Although the report cites key ceremonies and practices used by healers and helpers, the report reflects a number of important inaccuracies. To understand Indian medicine ways, one cannot rely solely on written accounts. Although written ethnographical studies may provide a wealth of descriptive data, it is best to talk to authoritative sources personally.

Although the sweatlodge, Sundance, and vision quest are all used by Lakotas for health, help, and healing, not all were always conducted by "medicine women" or "medicine men." The report tends to project an exclusivity of these ceremonies, when in fact there is considerable variation and scope for these practices, most of which were family oriented (Douville, 1997b).

The sweatlodge or "purification ceremony," for example, is very common and may be conducted by anyone who has "been on the hill" or completed the *hanbleceya,* often called the "vision quest" (Figure 29-5). Although the English name emphasizes the physiological reaction of the "sweat," this ceremony of the common man (Lakota *ikce wicasa*), it is really an encounter with one's spiritual self and one's spirit relatives. This is a purification that "gives life" (*inip-i'kogapi,* that which gives life) to the participants and represents a form of rebirth. This is a family-oriented ceremony and is an integral part of all other Lakota ceremonies. Participants enter a small lodge made of willow saplings (for support) and covered with heavy, darkening canvas. Between 7 and 16 or more red-hot stones are brought into this little lodge, which can be 10 to 15 feet in diameter. The stones represent the "first creation" and have deep spiritual meaning in this ceremony. Water is poured over the stones by someone who is permitted to conduct this ceremony, and the steam from this generates intense heat. There is deep spiritual significance to this.

Family members usually participate in this ceremony on a regular basis. Often, sweatlodges are located behind one's home. There is a prohibition that excludes menstruating women from ceremonies out of respect for the ceremony the woman's body is undergoing (i.e., menstruation, which is seen by Lakota people as a purification with its own proper spiritual power). This is often viewed by white culture as "discriminatory," but the tradition is not intended to be discriminatory. It is an affirmation of the natural feminine power, which white culture tends to minimize, often viewing menstruation as a handicap or a problem (e.g., PMS).

There are also different types of "medicine" people among the Lakota. It is difficult to generalize about the diverse functions using the English term

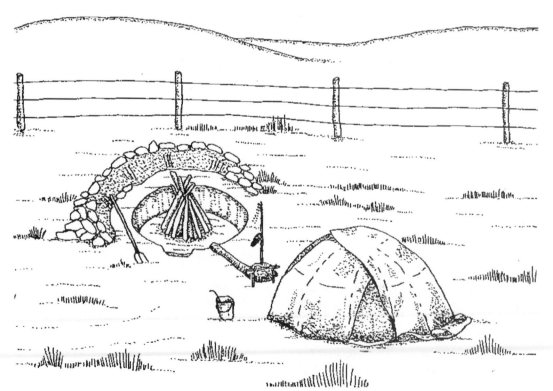

Figure 29-5 Sweatlodge. (Courtesy Sinte Gleska University.)

"medicine man/woman." The Lakota practiced common medicines that included herbal remedies known to families whose primary medical care was prevention and geared to building up the immune system (Douville, 1997b). The various common medicines included teas, ointments, and smudging (smoke from burning certain herbs, e.g., prairie sage or "flat cedar"). This first line of medical care was performed by knowledgeable family members or friends. When required, more spiritual consultations were sought from a shaman medicine man or an interpreter for the *Wakantanka* (the great mystery in all creation), which represents sacred medicine.

A "ceremony" may be requested by the patient and is usually held at night with family members, close friends, and singers (see Figure 29-3). Usually the patient presents a sacred pipe to the medicine man, who will smoke it if he accepts the request. The ceremony (which usually describes a *Lowanpi* or a spirit ceremony) takes place in a darkened room in the home. All furniture is removed, and the windows are covered. Certain ceremonial objects are used (e.g., various-colored flags, tobacco offerings, earth). During the ceremony, the Spirits instruct the medicine man or interpreter on what remedies would be provided by *Unci Maka* ("Grandmother Earth") to heal the patient. This process is done with the support of the *tios'paye*, or the extended family, for the *wicozani* (good health) of the patient.

Along with these practices, family members actively participated in a ceremonial life, which revolved around the *wo'ope*, or "natural law of creation," which included the behaviors and attitudes for right living. The *wo'ope* is embodied in the philosophy of *mitakuye oyas'in*, which recognizes that all things, persons, and creations (both animate and inanimate, seen and unseen) are related (White Hat Sr, 1997). These laws are not written down; they are learned through observing the creation. These behaviors for "right living" were reinforced by the ceremonial life of the extended family system, or *tios'paye*.

Health care was primarily an extended family matter. Medical care was common and free to everyone who needed it, because the herbs or materials for ceremonies used natural elements that could be harvested from nature's bounty. Although medical care was "free," it was not provided without cost, because in Lakota philosophy, when someone gives you something, you are expected to return it fourfold the value. When treated by healers, the people who received help gave something back. The concept of receiving "something for nothing" is not part of Indian philosophy (White Hat Sr, 1997). The Lakota philosophy encourages self-reliance *and* mutual relations. Something changed when white man's medicine became institutionalized in the United States, emphasizing intervention over prevention, the individual over the tribe or extended family, materialism over spirituality, and the physical body-self over the spirit-body-self.

TRENDS IN CONTEMPORARY INDIAN MEDICINE AND HEALTH CARE

Today, many of the old Indian healing traditions are experiencing a renaissance and are beginning to be viewed with a renewed sense of respect and credibility as an alternative and complement to more invasive or secular Western medical models of treatment (*Alternative medicine*, 1992; Hall, 1985, 1986; Thin Elk, 1995a, 1995b, 1995c). For example, on the Cheyenne River Indian Reservation at Eagle Butte, the tribal council approved alcohol treatment programs and delinquency prevention programs based on traditional methods and approaches to helping people with alcoholism, viewed as a problem with social, emotional, physical, and spiritual dimensions (Red Dog, 1997). These traditional methods include the *inipi*, or purification ceremony (popularly called the sweatlodge); the *hanbleceya*, or pipe fast (often called the vision quest), and the *wiwang wacipi*, or the gazing-at-the-sun dance. The infusion of these ceremonies within the treatment process, collectively, has been called the *Red Road Approach* (Thin Elk, 1995a, 1995b, 1995c).

A number of medical facilities on various reservations include medicine men as consultants on a formal and informal basis (Clifford, 1997; Douville, 1997a; Erickson, 1997; Twiss, 1997) and the use of traditional ceremonies in health care settings is encouraged and respected (Erickson, Rosebud Indian Health Services Hospital, 1997; Richards, Rapid City Regional Hospital, 1997). Where the ceremonial burning of sage (a common medicinal herb burned for purification) had been discouraged in the past, hospital staff report increased acceptance of this practice and now arrange appropriate space for traditional ceremonial practices both within the health care facility and outside on hospital grounds

(Erickson, 1997; Richards, 1997). One Lakota friend commented on his recent hospitalization at an allopathic hospital. He was visited by a medicine man, who placed a bundle of sage under his pillow. This made him feel better and showed how simple cooperation can be between allopathic medicine and alternative health care practices.

Rapid City Regional Hospital has initiated a Diversity Committee to discuss cultural sensitivity in both employee-administration and staff-patient relationships and credits this committee for improved retention rates of Indian staff (Montgomery, 1997). The Diversity Committee, which meets monthly, provides an opportunity to express areas of cultural awareness, tension, and misperception, whereby understanding across culture can take place. Conflicts in cultural views and values are inevitable, but there are growing opportunities for understanding and joint efforts.

Mike Richards, Discharge Planner and Liaison with the tribes at Rapid City Regional Hospital, noted one situation in which a Lakota client was discharged to his extended family. The plan was for the child to live in a tent in the backyard. This plan was challenged by State Social Services, failing to recognize that it is not uncommon for Lakota children to share close space in the family home or relative home. During my visits and stays with Lakota friends, I might see many children from an extended family share a small space in the family dwelling or occupy outbuildings or tents on the family compound or community (tios'paye) during the summer months. Although this practice might be considered "inappropriate" based on middle-class white standards, it affirms the Lakota value of close kinship bonds and enjoyment of children and illustrates the "bifurcating-merging family structure," a traditional Lakota kinship structure that considered parallel family relationships (e.g., one's aunts and uncles as "mothers" and "fathers"). Close kinship among all family members was reinforced by this family structure, whereby households and family resources were shared generously (Douville, 1997a; Driver, 1969).

The mental health liaison to the tribe advocated the child's return to his extended family, and the plan was eventually approved. The case illustrates how simple cultural misunderstanding can occur when service delivery is not centered on the values, family system organization, and beliefs of the traditional Indian perspective. Further illustrating this cultural insensitivity at a structural level is the fact that reser-

vation housing financed by U.S. Housing and Urban Development (HUD) grants are on a lottery basis and "invent" communities that are not based on natural, extended family relationships. This social invention (i.e., building housing developments and populating them on the basis of governmental criteria) often conflicts with the natural, familial basis of the tios'paye, or extended family system, of Lakota people (Lunderman, 1997). Such practices undermine the natural sense of community among Indian people and unwittingly create community tensions.

There is active cooperation between medical practitioners and traditional medicine men on Lakota reservations. Referrals are made both ways; medicine men will refer patients to medical doctors when they have exhausted their repertoire of remedies, and medical doctors will refer to medicine men when they have exhausted their treatment repertoire. The relations between traditional and medical health care providers appear cooperative and fluid. Antagonism between these distinct and complementary approaches to health care has subsided somewhat, although suspicions toward Western approaches to medicine remain among some traditional Indian people, which is understandable.

While traditional Western psychiatric thought has emphasized the mechanics of the mind, traditional American Indian philosophy looks at the "natural" flow of the individual's spirit-body-mind-self in relation to "everything that is." The Lakota term *mitakuye oyas'in* is often heard during ceremonies, reminding and reaffirming the participants of their relationships to ancestral spirits, powers, and energies of creation and to their kinship relatives, or *tios'paye*, the extended family and community. All these elements are considered essential for *wicozani*, or good health. The notion of *mitakuye oyas'in* is consistent with family systems theory that examines the impact of intergenerational family dynamics on the present functioning of family members.

Shamanic traditions and healing practices are very active among traditional American Indians today and seem to be gaining ground after generations of official and unofficial prohibitions and sanctions. There is diversity among traditional Indian tribal practices. The Lakotas have been open and receptive to sharing knowledge and technology with other nations. Lakota medicine people rely on their spirit helpers to "give them permission" to treat people and conduct ceremonies (Holler, 1995; Little Soldier, 1997; Running, 1987; Smith, 1987; Twiss, 1997). This permission is very specific; for example, a medicine man may be instructed to use certain herbal medicines for men only, women only, or people in general. The spirits work through the healer. The medicine man is only as effective as the spirits "working through him." He is responsible and accountable to the spirits for everything. This is a serious responsibility that these people accept.

Although many similarities exist in approaches to health and healing practices among American Indian healers (e.g., emphasis on prevention, involvement of family and community in healing ceremonies), important differences must be taken into consideration as well when treating American Indians. The best advice is for the health care practitioner to ask patients about their traditional practices, assuring them that the practitioner may not understand all their cultural traditions, but that he or she is interested in learning about these practices and, perhaps most importantly, is willing to work in a collaborative way that incorporates traditional healing practices without dismissing them. Individuals who use traditional methods of help and healing need to sense that their traditions will be respected when they seek medical care in mainstream medical facilities, or they may not accurately inform their physician about what traditional measures and remedies they are taking to restore health, balance, and healing in their lives (Lunderman, 2004).

One of the most important trends in Indian health care today may be the concern about the impact of welfare reform on Indian peoples, along with the national trend of individual states to reduce welfare rolls and move Medicaid services under managed care providers. An article in the *Journal of the American Medical Association* noted that American Indians know a lot about government program reforms. "If some people had had their way, Native American tribes would have been reformed out of existence a century ago. So it's not surprising that members of some 500 federally recognized tribes that remain are wary when talk in their locality turns to 'health care reform'" (Goldsmith, 1996, p. 1786).

At present, the Indian Health Service (IHS), a federally administered Indian health care program that is accredited by the Joint Commission on Accreditation of Healthcare Organizations (JCAHO), is facing severe budget deficits, overall receiving only 50% to 75% of what it needs to operate (Goldsmith, 1996, p. 1787). At the same time, IHS Director Michael H. Trujillo, MD, MPH, reported that the

service population has increased by more than 2% per year. It is safe to say that although there have been increasing federal appropriations for IHS over the years, the actual amount of "real money" has gone down. For many Indian people, the IHS is the only medical provider in their often-remote areas, serving a population with disproportionately higher incidence rates of diabetes and cervical cancer, for example, than the general American population. In the wake of anticipated health care reform, Dr. Gerald Hill, the Director of the Center for American Indian and Minority Health in the Institute for Health Services Research at the University of Minnesota, reminds health care planners of the statistic that in the American Indian population, 31% of the people die before their forty-fifth birthday (Goldsmith, 1996). The present situation of Indian health care is at another critical crossroad. Trends in Indian Health 2000-2001 (2004) reports that the age-specific death rate for American Indians/Alaskan Natives between 1996 and 1998 was more than double the U.S. rate during 1997 for whites aged 1-4 years and 15-54 years. It is interesting to note that the only age group with a lower death rate than U.S. whites, was those 85 and older (p. 70). Recent evidence provides some reason for optimism since the overall death rate for American Indians/Alaskan Natives was 28% between 1996 and 1998 for individuals under 45 years of age (Trends, 2004, p. 72).

Questions for Further Discussion

In light of the growing interest and expanding practice of traditional healing methods across American Indian communities, a number of questions deserve further study. It is first important to note that in raising these questions, the authors recognize the complex cultural divide in which these questions are framed as they straddle Western diagnostic categories that relate to empirical facts and traditional methods of healing that relate to the subject's belief system and spiritual practices. Thus, what is being questioned here is not traditional spirituality, but the specific medical implications of certain physical activities, often part of the spiritual healing practices. These questions are raised for both Western health care practitioners and traditional healing practitioners to consider as both seek continuing understanding in promoting good health among all people.

Since diabetes is a leading cause of death among American Indian people, 291% greater than the U.S. mortality rate for all races (Trends in Indian Health, 2000-2001, p. 7), the question is raised as to the efficacy of moderate, sustained, or prolonged fasting from food and water on the renal system. Because some traditional healing practices, such as the *hanble-ceya* (pipe fast, vision quest) and the *wi'wang wacipi* (Sundance), involve fasting from food and water from 1 to 4 days, we still do not know the long-term effect of such practices on renal functioning. Traditional Indian people differentiate physical healing and spiritual healing; sometimes both occur during a ceremony, and at other times a spiritual healing may take place without a physical cure. A powerful example of this is reflected in the sobering account reported by Archie Fire Lame Deer (1992, pp. 186-188), in which a man with diabetes died while on a "vision quest," having fasted without food or water for 4 days. Lame Deer noted, "Ron's autopsy showed that, besides diabetes, he had been suffering from three other deadly conditions. He had already been in the process of dying when he went to the mountain to leave this world in prayer" (p. 186). In this case, the individual faster was advised to take his insulin during the vision quest, but as Lame Deer later reports, "He had not touched his insulin."

Although this case may represent a rare occurrence, researchable questions can be asked, such as, "What are the physiological effects of such prolonged fasts on individuals with early, middle, and advanced stages of diabetes?" Because practices vary among traditional healers in the use of fasting, other questions could explore the effects of complete or absolute fasts, partial fasts from sundown to sundown, and partial fasts that include some liquid nourishment (e.g., herbal teas, medicines) on the individual faster. It would be interesting to know which of these practices offers the best opportunity for physiological healing or cure. Some might argue that such inquiry is not appropriate or perhaps even disrespectful to traditional healing practices. However, the authors also note the long tradition of holding so-called medicine men (women) accountable to demonstrate their power in public ways before the extended *tios'paye*, or extended family or community. For example, the test of a true *Heyoka* (Medicine Man) has been the demonstration of plunging his hand into the boiling hot kettle and pulling out the medicine for the people. This ceremony was (and is) conducted publicly and in full daylight. The witnessing community attests to the power and truth of the *Heyoka*, so there are precedents for such demonstrations of efficacy among traditional healers.

Another aspect of these questions is to challenge any romanticized notion or exploitation of traditional healing, particularly among or by non-Indians, who may attempt to engage in such healing practices without the appropriate guidance or understanding. This is an extremely serious concern among genuine traditional practitioners and healers, and it has been repeatedly raised as a concern by the elders, traditional spiritual leaders, and others.

CONCLUSION

A pan-Indian perspective of health care and medicine challenges the intervention model and offers a prevention model as the starting place for social health and assistance. A Lakota-centric view of health and wellness prioritizes a universal approach to health care opposed to an exceptional approach typical of most Western medicine currently in the United States. Traditional Lakota values emphasize the participation of the family in the healing process, including the extended family as well as the larger kinship of community to bring about *wicozani,* or good health. The help and healing process is not impersonal, but rather is highly personalized and individualized around specific needs. This personal dimension touches on all of reality (creation) as fundamentally relational and ecological, challenging the mechanism of Cartesian dualism. For the Lakotas and other Indian peoples, there is no split or dualism in reality or creation. Health and sickness, good and evil, and mind and body are intrinsic, interrelated, and unified. The roles of medicine practitioners include that of healer, counselor, politician, and priest (Figure 29-6).

Another important contribution of a pan-Indian perspective of health is that it provides a rich topology of spirit. The human creation, like all creations, is a spirit-being composed of multilayered aspects of spirit. "Spirit" here is not some "supernatural" reality outside the human being, but rather an intrinsic dimension of everything that is, including the human creation (person). To speak of humans is to speak about spiritual reality. Medical treatment or any form of social or human/mental health service is

WHAT IS A MEDICINE MAN?

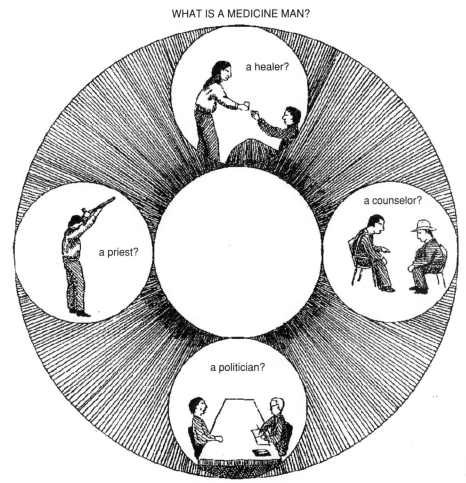

Figure 29-6 Illustration of the multiple roles of the medicine man: healer, priest, counselor, and politician. (Courtesy Sinte Gleska University.)

first and foremost a spiritual endeavor. A pan-Indian view of medicine and health care forces us to look at a broader, more encompassing view of the human person. Rather than taking a narrow biomedical approach, a pan-Indian view of health and well-being looks at the human as part of a lively and interacting bio-psycho-social-spiritual creation, in which the human person is viewed as a peer to other beings in a highly personalized universe and is intimately related to all creation (i.e., the natural world of plants, animals, insects, fish, stone, earth, fire, air, water, wind, and spirit entities).

The human being, or to use the Lakota term, the *ikce wicasa,* is the common (wo)man—a peer to all other beings. He or she is not above creation and as a peer depends on good relations with all the other creations for survival and good health. If anything,

the human creation is the most needy of all the created beings and depends on the medicine of other beings (e.g., plant nations and various animal nations) to overcome sickness. The Lakota view of life is based on a radical mutuality, interrelationships, and respect among all the members or peoples of creations. They have no word for "animal"; the birds belong to a nation and have status, as everything does (Smith, 1987; White Hat Sr, personal communication, 1997).

The most obvious implication of a pan-Indian perspective of health care and medicine is that it compels health care educators and practitioners to begin "indigenizing" our own consciousness, not only about the "missing chapter" in our introductory textbooks, but also about the fundamental influence of Western materialism and Eurocentrism on our thinking.

As we begin to take multicultural perspectives seriously, the Eurocentrism of our epistemologies, pedagogies, and professional practice of medical and health services will come under greater scrutiny, and we may even question some long-held beliefs about how to provide medical and health services. There will be a greater awareness of the role and importance of spirituality, shamanic practices, and common or herbal remedies as a complement to clinical practice. Finally, there will be a reaffirmation of the importance of grassroots community development in health care delivery services, an expanding awareness of the prescribed limitations of our dominant Eurocentric models of help and healing in the United States, and the increasing need, as well as opportunities, to incorporate integrative, alternative, and complementary models of health care in our mainstream health care services (see Chapter 1).

The increasing cooperative relations between medical and health care service personnel and traditional Indian medicine practitioners provides ground for encouragement that a multicultural approach is not only possible but is also actually taking root in Indian country. It is time for the diverse medical and health care disciplines to learn more about Native American and pan-Indian ways of healing and health. The benefits of this cross-cultural collaboration not only affect Indian people but everyone in the larger culture who will benefit from greater access to a more holistic health care model, recognizing both the physiological and the spiritual causes of disease and sickness, as well as the efficacy of both biological and spiritual remedies.

Hecetu'yelo! (Lakota: "the way it is")

References

Alternative medicine: expanding medical horizons. A report to the National Institutes of Health on alternative medical systems and practices in the United States, Washington, DC, 1992, US Government Printing Office.

Braswell ME, Wong HD: Perceptions of rehabilitation counselors regarding Native American healing practices, *J Rehabil* 60(2):33-43, 1994.

Brown D: *Bury my heart at Wounded Knee: an Indian history of the American West,* New York, 1970, Henry Holt.

Buechel E: 1983. Dictionary-Oie Wowapi Wan of Teton Sioux. Manhart, P. (Editor), published in cooperation with the Institute of Indian Studies, University of South Dakota and the Red Cloud Indian School, Inc., Pine Ridge, South Dakota.

Chardon FA: *Journal at Fort Clark: 1834-39,* Pierre, 1932, State Historical Society of South Dakota.

Clark C Jr: Personal communication, 1997 (Member and Tribal Historian of Nanticoke Tribe, Millsboro, Del).

Clifford B: Personal communication, June 21, 1997 (Dean, Human Services Department, Sinte Gleska University, Mission, SD).

Clifford M: Personal communication, June 10, 1997 (Member of Pine Ridge Sioux Tribe, Rapid City, SD).

Commissioner of Indian Affairs: Annual Report of the Commissioner of Indian Affairs to the Secretary of the Interior, Washington, DC, 1872-1892, US Government Printing Office.

Deloria EC: *Waterlily,* Lincoln, 1988, University of Nebraska Press (Afterword by RJ DeMallie).

DeMallie R, Jahner EA, editors: *Lakota belief and ritual: James R. Walker,* Lincoln, 1991, University of Nebraska Press.

Dobyns HF: *Their numbers become thinned: Native American population dynamics in Eastern North America,* Knoxville, 1983, University of Tennessee Press, p 24.

Douville V: Personal communication, June 12, 1997a (Member of Rosebud Sioux Tribe, Sinte Gleska University, Mission, SD).

Douville V: Personal communication, Sept 5, 1997b.

Driver HE: *Indians of North America,* ed 2 (revised), Chicago, 1969, University of Chicago Press.

DuBray WH: American Indian values: critical factor in casework, *Soc Casework* 66(1):30-37, 1985.

DuBray WH: *Human services and American Indians,* Minneapolis/St. Paul, 1992, West Publishing.

Edwards: Personal communication, 2004.

Edwards ED, Edwards ME: Social work practice with American Indians and Alaskan Natives. In Morales AT, Sheafor BW, editors: *Social work: a profession of many faces,* ed 9, Boston, 1998, Allyn & Bacon, pp 463-489.

Erikson J: Personal communication, 1997 (Intake social worker, Indian Health Services Hospital, Rosebud, SD).

Garrett JT, Garrett MW: The path of good medicine: understanding and counseling Native American Indians, *J Multicultur Counsel Dev* 22:134-144, 1994.

Garro LD: Continuity and change: the interpretation of illness in Anishnaabe (Ojibway) community, *Cult Med Psychiatry* 14:417-454, 1990.

Goldsmith MF: First Americans face their latest challenge: Indian health care meets state Medicaid reform, *JAMA* 275(23):1786, 1996.

Good Tracks JG: Native American non-interference, *Soc Work* 18(6):30-34, 1973.

Goodman R: *Lakota star knowledge: studies in Lakota stellar theology,* ed 2, Rosebud, SD, 1992, Sinte Gleska University.

Hall R: Distribution of the sweat lodge in alcohol treatment programs, *Curr Anthropol* 26(1):134-135, 1985.

Hall R: Alcohol treatment in American Indian populations: an indigenous treatment modality compared with traditional approaches (*Ann NY Acad Sci* 472). In Babor TF, editor: *Alcohol and culture: comparative perspectives from Europe and America,* New York, 1986, New York Academy of Sciences, pp 168-178.

Hammerschlag CA: *The dancing healers: a doctor's journey of healing with Native Americans,* New York, 1988, Harper San Francisco.

Hammerschlag CA: *The theft of the spirit: a journey to spiritual healing,* New York, 1992, Fireside, Simon & Schuster.

Hodge F.: Disabled American Indians: A Special Population Requiring Special Considerations, *American Indian Culture and Research Journal,* 13(3-4), 83-104,1989.

Holler C: *Black Elk's religion: the sun dance and Lakota Catholicism,* Syracuse, NY, 1995, Syracuse University Press.

Hoover H: Personal communication about the Canton File, Sept 26, 1997 (University of South Dakota, Vermillion).

Iron Shell JT: Personal communication, June 19, 1997 (Member of Rosebud Sioux Tribe, Public Relations and Cultural Resource Coordinator, Mission, SD).

Iron Shield H: Research indicates asylum wasn't in Indians' best interest, *Argus Leader* (Different Voices), Sioux Falls, SD, Aug 8, 1988.

Iron Shield H: Indian activist wants 119 bodies reburied, *Sioux City Journal,* Nov 11, 1991.

Iron Shield H: The legacy of an infamous institution: Hiawatha Insane Asylum for American Indians, *Native American Press,* Vermillion, SD, Nov 13, 1992, p 3.

Iron Shield H: Journalist talks about Indian asylum, *Minnesota Daily,* May 20, 1994.

Iron Shield H: Personal communication, 1997 (Coordinator of Native American Reburial Restoration Committee, 116 12th St, Moorhead, MN 56560, phone: 218-236-5434).

Jaimes MA, editor: *The state of Native America: genocide, colonization, and resistance,* Race and Resistance Series, Boston, 1992, South End Press.

Lame Deer, Fire A, Erdoes R: *Gift of power: the life and teachings of a Lakota medicine man,* Santa Fe, NM, 1992, Bear & Co (Introduced by AM Josephy Jr).

Lewis T: Group therapy techniques in shamanistic medicine, *Group Psychother Psychodrama Sociometry* 35(1)24-30, 1982.

Lewis T: *The medicine men: Oglala Sioux ceremony and healing,* Lincoln, 1990, University of Nebraska Press.

Little Soldier A (Lunderman A Sr): Federal policy and social disparity on Indian reservations: problems and solutions for the 1990s (a study of the Rosebud Sioux Tribe social structure), 1992 (unpublished paper).

Little Soldier A: Personal communication, June 12, 15, 1997 (Elder of Rosebud Sioux Tribe, Ring Thunder, SD).

Looking Horse M: Personal communication, June 24, 1997 (Member of Cheyenne River Sioux Tribe, Green Grass, SD).

Lunderman A Jr: Personal communication, 1997 (Rosebud Sioux tribal member and Lakota student, Mission, SD).

Lunderman M: Personal communication, 2004.

McGoldrick M, Giordano J, Pearce JK, editors: *Ethnicity and family therapy,* ed 2, New York, 1996, Guildford Press.

Means R: *Where white men fear to tread: the autobiography of Russell Means,* New York, 1995, St Martin's Press (with MJ Wolf).

Mestheth W, Standing Elk D, Swift Hawk P: Declaration of war against exploiters of Lakota spirituality, 1993 (http://maple.lemoyne.edu/ ~ bucko/war.htm).

Meyers AC: *William Penn's own account of the Lenni Lenape or Delaware Indians,* tercentenary edition, Wilmington, Del, 1970, Middle Atlantic Press (Foreword by JE Pomfret).

Montgomery J: Personal communication, June 16, 1997 (Licensed practical nurse and member of Cultural Diversity Committee at Rapid City Regional Hospital, Rapid City, SD).

Putney D: Canton Insane Asylum for Indians, *South Dakota History* 14(1):1-30, 1984.

Red Dog G: Personal communication, June 25, 1997 (Member of Cheyenne River Sioux Tribe and Tribal Council, Eagle Butte, SD).

Red Dog L: Personal communication, June 24, 1997 (Member of Cheyenne River Sioux Tribe, On the Tree, SD).

Reynolds C: The nature of health promotion with Ojibwe culture, Detroit, 1993, Wayne State University (dissertation).

Richards M: Personal communication, June 16, 1997 (Social Worker and Discharge Planner, also clinical tribal liaison at Psychiatric Unit, Rapid City Regional Hospital, SD).

Smith H (Program Director): *Wokiksuye: live and remember,* New York, 1987, Solaris Lakota (videotape; includes interview with traditional medicine man and elders).

Standing Bear L: *Land of the spotted eagle,* Lincoln, 1933, University of Nebraska Press (Foreword by RN Ellis).

Thin Elk G: Wounded warriors: a time for healing (as told to Doyle Arbogast). In *The Red Road approach,* Minneapolis/St. Paul, 1995a, Little Turtle Publications, pp 319-320.

Thin Elk G: *The Red Road to sobriety,* San Francisco, 1995b, Kifaru Productions (videotape; written and directed by C Pierce).

Thin Elk G: *The Red Road to sobriety video talking circle,* San Francisco, 1995c, Kifaru Productions (videotape; written and directed by C Pierce).

Trends in Indian health (2000-2001), Indian Health Service, US Department of Health and Human Services, Washington, DC, February 2004, US Government Printing Office.

Turton CLR: Spiritual needs of hospitalized Ojibwe people, *Mich Nurse* 68(5):11, 1995.

Twiss GJ: Personal communication, 1997 (Administrator, Rosebud Public Health Services Indian Hospital).

Wallace AC: Dreams and the wishes of the soul: a type of psychoanalytic theory among the seventeenth century Iroquois, *Am Anthropologist* 60:234-248, 1958.

White Hat A Sr: Personal communication, June 11, 1997 (Member of Rosebud Sioux Tribe, Sinte Gleska University, Mission, SD).

Williams EE, Ellison F: 1996. Culturally informed social work practice with American Indian clients: Guidelines for non-Indian social workers, *Social Work* 41:147-151, 1996.

Suggested Readings

Attneave CL: American Indians and Alaska Native families: emigrants in their own homeland. In McGoldrick M, Pearce J, Giorando J, editors: *Ethnicity and family therapy,* New York, 1982, Guilford Press, pp 55-83.

Black Elk: *The sacred pipe: Black Elk's account of the seven rites of the Oglala Sioux,* Norman, 1953, University of Oklahoma Press (Recorded and edited by JE Brown).

Brown Wolf O: Personal communication, 1997 (Elder of Cheyenne River Sioux Tribe).

Canda ER, Sun-in Shin, Hwi-Ja Canda: Traditional philosophies of human service in Korea and contemporary social work implications, *Soc Dev Iss* 15(3):84-104, 1993.

Catches P, Catches P: *Oceti Wakan: sacred fireplace,* Pine Ridge, SD, 1997, Oceti Wakan Press.

D'Andrea M: The concerns of Native American youth, *J Multicultur Counsel Dev* 22:173-181, 1994.

Dauphinais P, Dauphinais L, Rowe W: Effects of race and communication style on Indian perceptions of counselor effectiveness, *Counselor Educ Supervision* 21:72-80, 1981.

DeMallie R, editor: *The sixth grandfather: Black Elk's teachings given to John G. Neihardt,* Lincoln, 1984, University of Nebraska Press (Foreword by H Neihardt Petri).

Erikson EH: Observations on Sioux education, *J Psychol* 7:101-156, 1937.

Gross ER: Deconstructing politically correct practice literature: the American Indian case, *Soc Work* 40(2):206-213, 1995.

Gross G: Postmodern social work: no truths outside the gates of Eden? *J Baccalaur Soc Work* 2(1):63-77, 1996.

Hartman A: In search of subjugated knowledge, *Soc Work* 37:483-484, 1992 (editorial).

Herring RD: The clown or contrary figure as a counseling intervention strategy with Native American Indian clients, *J Multicultur Counsel Dev* 22:153-164, 1994.

Keith S: Personal communication, June 16, 1997 (Elder of Cheyenne River Sioux Tribe, Rapid City, SD).

Kelley ML, McKay S, Nelson CH: Indian agency development: an ecological practice approach, *Soc Casework* 66(10):594-602, 1985.

Lakota Cultural Center and Manual Productions: *Lakota: land of survivors,* Eagle Butte, SD, 1997, HVJ Lakota Cultural Center (videotape).

Looking Horse S: Personal communication, June 24, 1997 (Elder of Cheyenne River Sioux Tribe, Green Grass, SD).

Mehl-Madrona L: Call me Coyote: Stanford-trained Cherokee physician talks of coyote medicine and other Native American healing techniques, *Nat Health* 27(3):96, 1997.

Morales et al: *Social work: a profession of many faces,* ed 7, Needham Heights, Mass, 1995, Simon & Schuster.

Neihardt JG: *Black Elk speaks: being the life story of a holy man of the Ogalala Sioux,* New York, 1932, William Morrow (reprints, Lincoln, University of Nebraska Press, 1961, 1979, with new preface, introduction, illustrations, appendixes).

Niess R: Personal communication, June 14, 1997 (Member of Rosebud Sioux Tribe, Ring Thunder Wacipi, Mission, SD, Alliance of Tribal Tourism Advocates).

Porterfield KM: Sitting Bull Pipe returns, *Indian Country Today,* Nov 10-17, 1997, pp B1, B3.

Powers WK: *Yuwipi: vision and experience in Oglala ritual,* Lincoln, 1982, University of Nebraska Press.

Red Bird S: Personal communication, June 19, 1997 (Member of Rosebud Sioux Tribe, Rosebud, SD).

Red Dog L: *Leon speaks: wounded warriors: a time for healing,* as told to D Arbogast, editor, Omaha, 1995, Little Turtle Publications, pp 146-170.

Smith WC: *Faith and belief,* Princeton, New Jersey, 1979, Princeton University Press.

St Pierre M: *Madonna Swan: a Lakota woman's story as told through Mark St. Pierre,* Norman, 1991, University of Oklahoma Press.

St Pierre M: Personal Communication, June 17, 1997 (Author and educator, Cheyenne River Sioux Cultural Center, Eagle Butte, SD).

St Pierre M, Long Soldier T: *Walking in the sacred manner: healers, dreamers, and pipe carriers—medicine women of the Plains Indians,* New York, 1995, Touchstone.

Schacht AJ, Tafoya N, Mirabla K: Home-based therapy with American Indian families, *Am Indian Alaska Native Mental Health Res* 3(2):27-42, 1989.

Simms TE: *Otokahekagapi (first beginnings): Sioux creation story,* Chamberlain, SD, 1987, Tipi Press (Lakota translations by B Black Bear Jr).

Standing Bear L: The tragedy of the Sioux, *American Mercury* 24(95), 1931.

Sutton CharlesEtta T, Broken Nose MA: American Indian families: an overview. In McGoldrick M, Giordano J, Pearce JK, editors: *Ethnicity and family therapy,* ed 2, New York, 1996, Guilford Press.

Thomason TC: Counseling Native Americans: an introduction for non-Native American counselors, *J Counsel Dev* 69:321-327, 1991.

Walker JR (DeMallie RJ, Jahner EA, editors): *Lakota belief and ritual,* Lincoln, 1980, University of Nebraska Press.

Native American Medicinal Plants

DANIEL E. MOERMAN

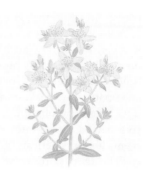

ative American peoples developed a sophisticated plant-based medical system in the millennia before the European arrival in America. Many of the plants that these people used are familiar medicinal species and have taken a role in contemporary medicine.

Echinacea is well known in Europe and increasingly in North America as a treatment for colds and particularly as an "immune system stimulant." The cone flowers, Native American species, were used more than 100 ways by a dozen Midwestern tribes (e.g., Blackfoot, Cheyenne, Dakota, Omaha, Pawnee, Paiute) to treat a variety of diseases and conditions, including headaches, burns, and toothaches. The Winnebago used *Echinacea* in an interesting way: fire handlers used the plant to make themselves insensitive to hot coals that they put in their mouths.

Another very interesting plant—*Podophyllum peltatum,* the mayapple—is less well known to the public but is probably more important medically than *Echinacea.* American Indians used the plant in many ways, but the most common use was as a laxative or purgative, which was a common use of the plant in early American medicine as well. For many years, podophyllum resin has been a standard treatment for venereal warts. Also, etoposide (VePesid), a semisynthetic derivative of podophyllotoxin, another may apple constituent, is an effective treatment for refractory testicular tumors and for small cell lung cancer.

Plants used by Native Americans as medicinal species can also be dangerous. This is apparent with toxic species such as *Datura meteloides* (jimsonweed) and *Heracleum maximum* (cow parsnip), but others are less obviously dangerous. A classic case is ephedrine, derived from several species of the genus *Ephedra,*

notably *E. sinica.* The American species, *E. viridis,* contains less ephedrine than the Asian species. It was used by many Native American groups for internal illnesses. It has a long use in the American Southwest as a stimulating drink known as "teamster's tea" or "Mormon tea," and the drug and various synthetic variations (particularly pseudoephedrine) is a useful decongestant. In the past few years, herbal drug companies have made capsules containing from 7 to more than 40 mg of ephedrine, along with other *Ephedra* alkaloids, and sold them under such names as "Herbal Ecstacy," "Ultimate Xphoria," and "Cloud 9." These drugs presumably mimic the action of the street drug MDMA (4-methyl-2, dimethoxyamphetamine)—illegal in the United States—which produces euphoria; the street name of the drug is "Ecstacy." A number of people taking six to eight of these "herbal highs" have died of heart attack, stroke, and various types of seizures.[1] Just because a drug is "natural" does not mean it is safe.

There are many such interesting stories about Native American drug plants and their modern uses, and these accounts are readily found. However, there are other approaches to the medicinal plants of native North America, as I describe here. Although significant differences existed between the systems developed by the many native groups,[2] there were also many broad similarities. There are approximately 21,000 species of plants in North America. Native Americans used more than 2800 of them medicinally.[3]

Over the past 25 years, I have built a database with 44,775 entries listing uses of plants by Native American peoples as drugs, foods, dyes, fibers, and so on. The database contains 25,025 entries on uses of drugs, representing a total of 2865 different species of plants. An additional 11,079 entries describe the uses of 3896 species that were used as food. The database was constructed by gathering together several hundred published works on the ethnobotany of Native American peoples and coding all the information in a systematic way. Because many of these publications were originally obscure and often difficult to find, this database facilitates making such global statements about American Indian plant use.

The used portion of the flora (the "medicinal flora") is a distinctly nonrandom assortment of the plants available. The richest sources of medicines are the sunflower family (Asteraceae), the rose family (Rosaceae), and the mint family (Lamiaceae). By contrast, the grass family (Poaceae) and the rush family (Juncaeae) produce practically no medicinal species. This remarkable volume and extraordinary selectivity demonstrate the falseness of demeaning claims that suggest that Native American medicines were chosen at random, that they "just used everything and stumbled on something useful (like *Echinacea* or *Podophyllum*) once in a while."

HEALTH AND DISEASE

To understand the character and effectiveness of a medical system, one must understand the health status of the people who use it. Native American peoples were typically very healthy. They generally did not have the degenerative diseases of the heart and circulatory systems so common today; their diets were rich in fiber and carbohydrates and low in fats. They lived vigorous lives that provided hearty exercise on a daily basis. They experienced little cancer. Cancer is largely a modern disease of civilization; although the situation is complex, an apparently necessary condition for cancer is carcinogens, which are largely products manufactured by industrial societies (e.g., organic chemicals and dyes, nuclear radiation). Even current evidence indicates that the traditional Navajo have lower rates of cancer than surrounding people (Csordas, 1989).

In addition, Indian people had fewer classic infectious diseases, which have ravaged European society over the past two millennia. In large part, this seems to be because many such diseases (e.g., plague, typhoid, smallpox, cholera) are *zoonoses,* diseases of animals that, under conditions of domestication, underwent evolutionary change and subsequently affected the human keepers of these animals. Native Americans

never domesticated animals to any significant degree (the guinea pig and llama of Peru were apparently only coming under domestication in the few hundred years before European contact). Once these diseases were introduced into North America, they devastated native populations, which had no natural immunity to them.[4] Until the sixteenth century, when Europeans underwent successive epidemics that regularly killed a quarter or half of the population, Native Americans were spared this devastation.

What medical problems *did* Native Americans face? In the Southeast and Southwest, evidence suggests a decline in health status after the invention of agriculture as the diet became simpler (less varied), which apparently led to some deficiency diseases. Hunting and gathering peoples avoided that problem, but they, like Europeans, may have experienced some zoonotic infections, particularly from beaver, and some trichinosis from bears. However, these would have been "direct" zoonoses that individuals contracted directly from the infected animal, not "remote" zoonoses, which, once passed to one human, were subsequently passed from person to person. As with rabies, a terrible disease for the individual who contracts it, these direct zoonoses are not serious threats to a whole society because they are not "contagious" in the ordinary sense of the term: from human to human.

Native Americans probably paid a price for the vigorous life they led. Accidents, sprains, broken bones, cuts, lacerations, and other trauma were common. There was a range of arthritic conditions, with some probably the result of injury and some similar to rheumatoid arthritis. Ample evidence indicates that native peoples engaged in warfare, which would have been a source of serious medical problems. There was a range of occasional problems associated with menstruation, pregnancy, childbirth, and lactation that required attention. Living in smoky houses, it is not surprising that they had a wide range of treatments for irritated eyes and skin; they also treated colds, headaches, cold sores, and bruises, the normal insults of daily life everywhere.

HERBAL MEDICINES

To address this range of problems, Native Americans inevitably resorted to medicines based on various plants.[5] Although a good deal of research has been done on this ethnobotany, much is difficult to find and use. Most of the research has been done on a "tribe-by-tribe" basis. This means that if you are interested in what plants the Iroquois used for medicines and how they used them, you could look in James Herrick's doctoral dissertation, *Iroquois Medical Botany,* and find out (Herrick, 1977). However, if you were interested in how different cultural groups used the same plant, it was a much more challenging proposition. My database, described earlier, makes this work much more practical.

Every Native American group for which we have any information had a botanical pharmacopeia. Although some were quite small (the Inuit had few plant resources on which to rely), most were quite elaborate, with hundreds of plant drugs used for a broad range of conditions. This straightforward proposition raises a number of much more challenging questions. Native American healers, even into the early twentieth century, regularly knew the identity of 200 or 300 medicinal plants, which they could readily distinguish from the 3000 to 5000 species that grow in any particular area. Among 100 sophisticated and well-educated modern Americans or Europeans, few could identify 200 species of plants of any kind unless they were professional botanists. How did nonliterate people, without reference to botanical keys or floras compiled by professionals, maintain this extraordinary amount of knowledge?[6]

If a Native American discovered, by whatever means, a marvelous medicinal plant that cured a child of a terrible rash, and if the plant were very rare and unusual, an annual of uncertain provenience, she might be hard pressed to find it a second time, and harder pressed yet to teach her daughter or niece or neighbor where to find it. Such a plant would be unlikely to become part of the common knowledge of the community. If the situation were compounded by the fact that the plant were drab, with no particularly visible flowers or leaves—an undistinguished, rare, annual forb, for example—it is even less likely that it would become part of common knowledge. Such a proposal can lead to some testable propositions. For example, I would predict that, compared with other species, medicinal plants will *tend* to be the following:

- Abundant
- Perennial
- Large (e.g., trees rather than forbs)

- Widespread
- Distinctive, that is showy and visible

This does not mean that a tiny, drab, undistinguished, rare annual occurring in one forest in Tennessee could not be part of the Native American medicinal flora. It means it is *more likely* that a large, common, perennial tree found in 20 states will be used medicinally than the rare one.

Abundance

I cannot directly test the proposition that "medicinal plants tend to be relatively abundant" because I have no data set listing the relative abundance of North American plants. However, I can test a variation on that proposition, which states that "medicinal plants tend *not* to be rare and endangered."

The United States has a law called the Endangered Species Act, which seeks to protect endangered and threatened species of plants and animals. To administer the act, the U.S. Department of Agriculture (USDA) maintains a list of such species (many of which are actually varieties or subspecies). Currently there are 389 species (or subspecies or varieties) on the list in four categories: proposed threatened, threatened, proposed endangered, and endangered. These are all taxa that, by definition, are found in limited areas, which are infrequent in their ranges. Two of 2572 medicinal species (0.08%) are on the list, whereas 387 of the remaining 28,543 taxa (species, subspecies, varieties, quads) in North America (1.3%) are on the list. This difference is highly statistically significant. By this admittedly flawed test, medicinal plants tend *not* to be rare and unusual. If it were possible to measure directly the abundance of a good sample of American species, a much better test of this proposition could be performed.

Distribution[7]

In addition, evidence accumulated by the USDA is available for the distribution of North American plant species. There is information on the presence or absence of species in 60 states and territories and 12 Canadian provinces. Species used as drugs are found in an average of 15.6 states or provinces, whereas species not used as drugs are found in an average of only 5.2 states. Drug plants are much more widespread than nondrug plants.

Growth Habit

Evidence indicates, first, that among native North Americans, a disproportionate share of medicinal plants have a *perennial* rather than annual growth habit. There are many more perennials (12,284) than annuals (3060); 16% of the perennials are used medicinally, whereas only 8.7% of the annuals are used medicinally.

Growth Form

The most commonly used growth form is trees and shrubs, followed by forbs, vines, and grasses. Table 29-1 shows the numbers and percentages of each type. Although these differences may not seem large, they are, again, highly statistically significant; a given tree or shrub is 30% more likely to be used as a medicine than a given forb.

Flavor

Circumstantial evidence from a number of cases indicates that medicinal plants often have a distinctive and in particular a bitter taste. This cannot be easily tested because no evidence is available on the flavors of plants *not* used as medicines (because botanists do not consider a plant's flavor to be an important characteristic).

Showiness

Finally, there is evidence that plants used for medicine by Native American peoples are more showy or visible than other plants. The test for this is an indirect one. As I became more interested in flower gardening, I had a sense that most of the garden plants I was learning about were also in my database of medicinal plants. Why do we put this plant in a flower garden, and not that one? Generally it is because the garden species has beautiful, or unusual, or colorful flowers, or leaves, or scent, or growth habits or the like; garden plants are typically recognizable and distinctive. Many of our garden varieties are much different from their wild ancestors, but the hybridizers rarely began with nothing. I reasoned that medicinal plants would be more likely to show up in gardens than plants not used as medicinals.

I looked among my garden books and found *Ortho's Complete Guide to Successful Gardening*. The book has a 122-page encyclopedic chart of plants of value in a garden, alphabetically arranged from *Abelia* to *Zoysia*. I checked genera in the gardening book, which also appeared in a standard list of the flora of North America (Kartesz, 1994). There are 3138 genera in this list, of which 852 appear in my database of medicinal plants. In addition, there were 423 genera of plants listed in the garden book that appear on the Kartesz checklist (a few items in the book were not in the checklist because they do not appear outside of gardens). If all were distributed randomly, and if medicinal plants were not favored for use in the garden, we would predict that 115 of the garden plants would have appeared on the list of 852 medicinal species. However, there are actually almost twice that many, 213, again a highly statistically significant difference. Medicinal plants tend to be visible, recognizable, and showy (Box 29-4).

CONCLUSION

The medicinal knowledge of native North American peoples is extraordinary. Just how this knowledge was developed remains a mystery. Native American peoples are thought to have come from Asia; the flora of Asia is similar to that of North America in many ways. It is likely that the first migrants to the New World brought detailed knowledge of medical botany, much of which was applicable to this new flora.

TABLE 29-1

Growth Forms for Native American Medicinal Plants

Growth Form	Drug Plants	Total Plants	Percentage
Trees	340	2213	13.32
Shrubs	598	4002	13.00
Forbs	1386	11,753	10.55
Vines	103	1037	9.04
Grasses	75	2039	3.55

BOX 29-4

Four Native American Medicinal Plants

Echinacea angustifolia

There are a total of 123 records for *Echinacea*, the coneflowers, in my database. They represent 26 distinctly different use categories, such as "analgesic," "antirheumatic," and "cold remedy." There are 18 different tribes represented in those data, and 93 combinations of tribe and use (e.g., "Pawnee analgesic," "Crow cold remedy"). Nine different tribes are reported to have used echinacea as an analgesic. Some tribes used it several different ways: The Winnebago used it in a wash for pain from burns and also put it in a smoke treatment for headaches. The Ponca used it the same two ways.

Toxicodendron radicans

Poison ivy is a common North American plant that causes serious, itchy rashes on many people. Children are taught "leaflets three; let it be." The toxic chemical urishol is found throughout the plant: in the soft woody stem, the leaves, and the berries. It is particularly dangerous when burned with dead leaves in the fall; contact with the smoke can also cause serious allergic reactions. Several other members of this genus have similarly noxious properties, including *T. diversilobum* (Pacific poison oak), *T. pubescens* (Atlantic poison oak), and *T. vernix* (poison sumac).

It may be somewhat surprising, therefore, to discover that Native American people found this genus to be useful as a medicine. There are 57 listings of *Toxicodendron* in the database. Although some of these listings indicate simply that the people recognized the plant as being poisonous, others found medicinal uses for the plants. The Yuki Indians of California, for example, used Pacific poison oak to treat warts, whereas the Cherokee used a decoction of the bark of Atlantic poison oak as an emetic. The Kiowa Apache rubbed poison ivy leaves over boils or other skin eruptions, and the Houma of Louisiana took a decoction of the leaves as a tonic and "rejuvenator." In homeopathic preparations, *Toxicodendron* is a leading remedy for several common symptoms.

Continued

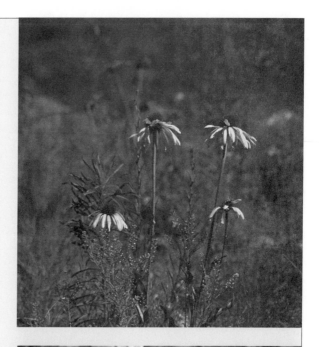

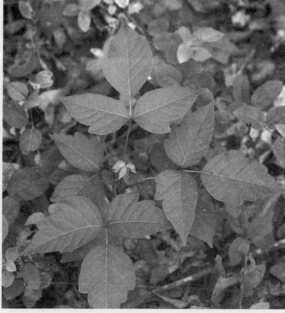

Four Native American Medicinal Plants—cont'd

Geranium maculatum

Eight species of wild geraniums were used medicinally by Native American peoples (note that these are not the same as the common ornamental plants often called *geraniums,* which are actually Pelargoniums). The most widely used is *Geranium maculatum,* the wild cranesbill. This plant produces a long, pointed seed that has a series of small but distinct hooks on the end, which probably serve to catch the seeds in the fur of passing animals to aid in their dispersal. However, these hooks also provide the Iroquois with a rationale for using a poultice of the roots of this plant on chancre sores; the "hooklike and ensnaring qualities" of the plant (implied by its hooked seeds) are precisely what to use on a "loose, running, everted" sore. The plant is therefore a "meaningful" medicine for the Iroquois. The roots also contain substantial quantities of tannin, which would probably be an effective treatment for sores. Medicines typically have this double quality of "meaning and chemistry" in all medical systems.

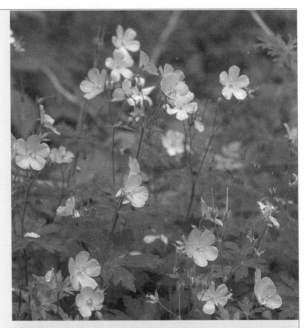

Daucus carota

The wild European carrot, or Queen Anne's Lace, is a common medicine for American Indian people. This is true of a number of introduced species; other common European plants that became widely used are mullein *(Verbascum thapsus),* curly dock *(Rumex crispus),* catnip *(Nepeta cataria),* and the common tansy *(Tanacetum vulgare).* The Delaware and Mohegan Indians used wild carrot to treat diabetes; the Iroquois used it as a diuretic; and the Cherokee used an infusion of the plant as a wash for swellings.

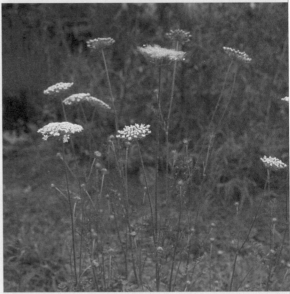

Most remarkable, however, may be this: I am unaware of any significant medicinal use of any indigenous American plant species that was *not* used medicinally by one or another Native American group. An interesting example involves recent research on taxol, a substance of great potential medical value found in the common yew, *Taxus brevifolia,* and the Canadian yew, *Taxus canadensis.* Taxol has shown substantial effect in the destruction of tumors in several forms of cancer, particularly ovarian cancer, a highly refractory form. Native Americans did not use yew to treat cancer (see previous discussion), but they did use it for a variety of other conditions, including skin problems, wounds, rheumatism, and colds.

In general, if one is interested in finding potentially useful botanical chemicals from the North American flora, it would be wise to focus first on that portion of the flora that has been used by Native

Americans. Their experience and knowledge can yet guide our scientific efforts to enhance human health.

Acknowledgments

The work reported here has been generously supported by the National Science Foundation (SBR-9200674). I also wish to thank Claudine Farrand for helpful discussions about gardening, and Michael Heinrich for his wise counsel on this appendix.

Notes

1. For a review of this situation, see the detailed article by Blumenthal and King (1996).
2. Many fine works on the medical systems of particular groups are available, although sometimes difficult to find. Perhaps the finest is by James Herrick on the Iroquois (1977). For a superb overview of the range of forms of treatment and understanding of illness, see Vogel's classic work, *American Indian Medicine* (1970).
3. The most comprehensive available listing of Native American medicinal plants is Moerman's *Medicinal Plants of Native America* (1986). For a more recent and much larger database, see Moerman's *Native American Ethnobotany* (1997). Also available at www.umd.umich.edu/cgi-bin/herb.
4. For a fascinating and controversial review of the impact of European diseases on Native Americans, see Calvin Martin's *Keepers of the Game* (1978). The classic work on the zoonotic origins of modern diseases is R.N. Fiennes' *Zoonoses and the Origins and Ecology of Human Diseases* (1978).
5. There were some nonplant substances used medicinally. Castoreum from beaver was used for various conditions, and some minerals and clays were used as well. The preponderance of medicinal substances came from plants.
6. The definitive treatment of non-Western botanical knowledge is Brent Berlin's *Ethnobiological Classification* (1992); the best modern treatment of the problems of the origins of knowledge of food and drug plants is Timothy Johns' *With Bitter Herbs They Shall Eat It* (1990).
7. The next three sections on distribution, habit, and form are based on data from the USDA National Plants Database (http://trident.ftc.nrcs.usda. gov/plants/plntmenu.html).
8. A detailed comparison of the ethnobotany of North America and China awaits scholarly attention. A preliminary account by James Duke (in Duke and Ayensu, *Medicinal Plants of China*, 1985) is provocative.

References

Berlin B: *Ethnobiological classification: principles of categorization of plants and animals in traditional societies,* Princeton, NJ, 1992, Princeton University Press.

Blumenthal M, King P: The agony of the ecstasy: herbal high products get media attention, *HerbalGram J Am Botanical Council Herb Res Foundation* 37, 1996.

Csordas T: The sore that does not heal: cause and concept in the Navajo experience of cancer, *J Anthropol Res* 45(4): 457-485, 1989.

Duke JA, Ayensu ES: *Medicinal plants of China,* Algonac, Mich, 1985, Reference Publications.

Fiennes RN: *Zoonoses and the origins and ecology of human diseases,* New York, 1978, Academic Press.

Herrick JW: Iroquois medical botany, Ann Arbor, 1977, University Microfilms International (Dissertation).

Johns T: *With bitter herbs they shall eat it: chemical ecology and the origins of human diet and medicine,* Tucson, 1990, University of Arizona Press.

Kartesz J: *Synonymized checklist of the flora of North America,* Portland, Ore, 1994, Timber Press.

Martin C: *Keepers of the game: Indian-animal relationships and the fur trade,* Berkeley, 1978, University of California Press.

Moerman DE: *Native American ethnobotany,* Portland, Ore, 11997, Timber Press.

Vogel VJ: *American Indian medicine,* Norman, 1970, University of Oklahoma Press.

Suggested Readings

Brower LP, Nelson CJ, Seiber JN, et al: Exaptation as an alternative to coevolution in the cardinolide-based chemical defense of monarch butterflies *(Danaus plexippus L.)* against avian predators. In Spencer KC, editor: *Chemical mediation of coevolution,* San Diego, 1988, Academic Press, pp 447-476.

Moerman DE: The medicinal flora of native North America: an analysis, *J Ethnopharmacol* 31:1-42, 1991.

Wrangham RW, Goodall J: Chimpanzee use of medicinal leaves. In Heltne PG, Marquardt L, editors: *Understanding chimpanzees,* Chicago, 1987, University of Chicago Press.

LATIN AMERICAN CURANDERISMO

ROBERT T. TROTTER II

HISTORY

Curanderismo, from the Spanish verb *curar* (to heal), is a broad healing tradition found in Mexican American communities throughout the United States. It has many historical roots in common with traditional healing practices in Puerto Rican and Cuban American communities, as well as traditional practices found throughout Latin America. At the same time, curanderismo has a history and a set of traditional medical practices that are unique to Mexican cultural history and to the Mexican American experience in the United States.

Seven historical roots are embedded in modern curanderismo. Its theoretical beliefs partly trace their origins to Greek humoral medicine, especially the emphasis on balance, and the influence of hot and cold properties of food and medicines on the body.

Many of the rituals that provide both a framework and a meaningful cultural healing experience in curanderismo date to healing practices contemporary to the beginning of the Christian tradition and even into earlier Judeo-Christian writings. Other healing practices derive from the European Middle Ages, including the use of traditional medicinal plants and magical healing practices in wide use at that time.

The Moorish conquest of Southern Europe is visible in the cultural expression of curanderismo. Some common Mexican American folk illnesses originated in the Near East and then were transmitted throughout the Mediterranean, such as belief in *mal de ojo,* or the evil eye (the magical influence of staring at someone). Homeopathic remedies for common health conditions such as earaches, constipation, anemia, cuts and bruises, and burns were brought from Europe to the New World to be passed down to the present time within curanderismo. There also is significant sharing of beliefs with Aztec and other Native American cultural traditions in Mexico. Some of the folk illnesses treated in pre-Columbian times, such as a fallen fontanelle *(caida de la mollera)* and perhaps the blockage of the intestines *(empacho)* are parts of this tradition. The pharmacopeia of the New World also is important in curanderismo (and added significantly to the plants available for treatment of diseases in Europe from the 1600s to the present). Some healers *(curanderos)* keep track of developments in parapsychology and New Age spirituality, as well as acupuncture and Eastern healing traditions, and have incorporated these global perspectives into their own practices.

Finally, curanderismo is clearly a deeply rooted traditional healing system, but it also actively exists within the modern world. Biomedical beliefs, treatments, and practices are very much a part of curanderismo and are supported by curanderos. On the border between the United States and Mexico, it is not unusual for healers to recommend the use of prescription medications (which can often be purchased in Mexico over the counter) for infections and other illnesses. These healers also use information obtained from television and other sources to provide the best advice on preventive efforts such as nutrition and exercise and on explanations for biomedical illnesses.

Individual healers vary greatly in their knowledge of the practices that stem from each of these seven historical sources. The overall system of curanderismo is complex and not only maintains its cultural link to the past but evolves toward accommodation with the future as well.

Cultural Context

This chapter is based partly on research that was conducted in the Lower Rio Grande Valley of Texas for more than 15 years. That information is enhanced by data from other regions near the U.S.-Mexican border, and from Mexican American communities in Colorado, Nebraska, Chicago, and Florida. Multiple research environments, both rural and urban, have affected the practice of curanderismo. Alger (1974) described one possible outcome of urbanized curanderismo, in which the folk healing system mimics the modern medical system, but this mimicry does not exist to any significant extent in southern Texas,

where both curanderos and their patients have extensive knowledge of the medical system in urban and rural areas. However, unlike attitudes reported in earlier studies of the area (Madsen, 1961; Rubel, 1966), curanderos and their patients accept the use of modern medicine. These multiple environments of curanderismo practice create a complex healing system with core elements that are common to each place and modifications that respond to local cultural, political, and legal circumstances.

The earliest systematic research was done on curanderismo in the late 1950s, when modern medicine was inaccessible, or only recently available to significant segments of the Mexican American population. Since that time, the efficacy of modern medicine has been demonstrated empirically numerous times, so it is an integrated part of the cultural system, although many access barriers still exist to prevent its full use by everyone. These barriers reflect the same reasons that the holistic health movement and the charismatic healing movements are becoming increasingly popular. Although traditional healers in Mexican American communities believe that modern medicine is as capable in certain types of healing, their experience shows that their own practices are not recognized in hospitals and clinics and that they can accomplish those same tasks better than modern medicine. Thus, curanderismo and modern medicine often assume complementary roles in the minds of the curanderos and their patients, although not necessarily in the minds of the medical professionals of the area.

Intellectual Tradition

Traditional Mexican American healers perceive health and illness to contain a duality of "natural" and "supernatural" illnesses. This duality forms the theoretical base on which curanderismo is constructed. The natural source of illness is essentially a biomedical model of illness that includes lay interpretations of some diseases inspired by Mexican American culture. Biomedical aspects such as the germ theory of disease, genetic disorders, psychological conditions, and dietary causes for medical conditions are accepted. These natural illnesses are treated by physicians with herbal remedies. A parallel supernatural source of illness also is recognized by this healing tradition. These illnesses are not considered amenable to treatment by the medical establishment. They can be repaired only by the supernatural manipulations of curanderos. The curanderos fault the scientific medical system for its failure to recognize the existence of magic or of supernatural causation. One curandero commented that as many as 10% of patients in mental institutions were really *embrujados* (hexed or bewitched), and because physicians could not recognize this condition, it went untreated. This curandero was willing to test his theory scientifically in any way that the mental health professionals set up as a research project. However, the mental health professionals were not willing to allow the tests to be conducted because of their attitudes toward curanderismo. In this case, it appeared to the anthropologists that the curanderos had a stronger belief and trust in science, even when it was directed at the supernatural, than the physicians and other health professionals.

Supernaturally induced illnesses are most often said to be initiated by either evil spirits *(espiritos malos)* or by *brujos* (individuals practicing antisocial magic). They form a significant part of the curanderos' work; these healers explain that any particular illness experienced by a patient could be caused theoretically by either natural or supernatural processes. For example, they believe there is a natural form of diabetes and a form that is caused by a supernatural agent, such as a *brujo*. The same is true for alcoholism, cancer, and other diseases. Identifying the nature of the causal agent for a particular illness is a key problem for the curandero. Some identify more supernatural causes for illnesses, and others take a more biomedically balanced approach. In either case, there is much less dichotomizing of physical and social problems within curanderismo than within the medical care system (Holland, 1963; Kiev, 1968).

Curanderos routinely deal with problems of a social, psychological, and spiritual nature, as well as physical ailments. Many cases overlap into two or more categories. Bad luck in business is a common problem presented to curanderos. Other problems include marital disruptions, alcoholism or alcohol abuse, infidelity, supernatural manifestations, cancer, diabetes, and infertility. One healer distinguishes between the problems presented by women and men. The central focus of the problems brought by women is the husband; the husband drinks too much, does not work, does not give them money, or

is seeing other women. Men bring problems of a more physical nature, such as stomach pain, headaches, weakness, and bladder dysfunction. Men also bring problems that deal directly with work; they need to find a job, cannot get along with people at work, or are having trouble setting up a business. The wife rarely is the focal point of their problems. The total list of problems presented to curanderos includes almost every situation that can be thought of as an uncomfortable human condition. Curanderismo seems to play an important, culturally appropriate psychotherapeutic role in Mexican American communities (Galvin and Ludwig, 1961; Klineman, 1969; Torrey, 1972).

Another element of curanderismo that forms an important intellectual foundation for its practices is the concept that healers work by virtue of "a gift of healing" *(el don)* (Hudson, 1951; Madsen, 1965; Romano, 1964; Rubel, 1966). This inherent ability allows the healer to practice his or her work, especially in the supernatural area. In the past this was believed to be a gift from God. However, a secular interpretation of the *don* is competing with the more traditional explanation. Many healers still refer to the *don* as a gift from God and support this premise with Biblical passages (Corinthians 12:7 and James 5:14), but other healers explain the *don* as an inborn trait that is present in all humans, just like the ability to sing, run, or talk. Almost any person can do these things, but some do them better than others, and a few people can do them extremely well. Curanderos, according to this theory, are the individuals with a better ability to heal than is normative for the population as a whole. Healers refer to this concept as "developed abilities."

Another element common to Hispanic-based folk medicine is the hot-cold syndrome (Currier, 1966; Foster, 1953; Ingham, 1940). This belief system is not common in southern Texas (Madsen, 1961), where the only indications of a hot-cold syndrome found among the patients were scattered folk beliefs, such as not eating citrus during menses, not ironing barefoot on a cement floor, or taking a cold shower after prolonged exposure to the sun. None of these beliefs was organized systematically or shared extensively within the Mexican American population. In other areas, there is extensive knowledge and use of this system of classifying foods, treatments, and elements of illnesses to provide the basis for deciding which remedies apply to specific illnesses.

THEORETICAL BASIS

The community-based theoretical structure for curanderismo has three primary areas of concentration, called *levels (niveles)* by the healers: the material level *(nivel material),* the spiritual level *(nivel espiritual),* and the mental level *(nivel mental).* More curanderos have the *don* for working at the material level, which is organized around the use of physical objects to heal or to change the patient's environment. This theoretical area can be subdivided into physical and supernatural manipulations. Physical treatments are those that do not require supernatural intervention to ensure a successful outcome. *Parteras* (midwives), *hueseros* (bone setters), *yerberos* (herbalists), and *sobadores* (people who treat sprains and tense muscles) are healers who work on the *nivel material* and effect cures without any need for supernatural knowledge or practices. All the *remedios caseros* (home remedies) used in Mexican American communities are part of this healing tradition.

The supernatural aspect of this level is involved in cures for common folk illnesses found in Mexican American communities, such as *susto, empacho, caida de mollera, espanto,* and *mal de ojo.* These illnesses are unique to Hispanic cultural models of health and illness. This area of healing also includes the spells and incantations that are derived out of medieval European witchcraft and earlier forms of magic, such as the cabala, that have been maintained as supernatural healing elements of curanderismo. Supernatural manipulations involve prayers and incantations in conjunction with such objects as candies, ribbons, water, fire, crucifixes, tree branches, herbs, oils, eggs, and live animals. These treatments use a combination of common objects and rituals to cure health problems.

The spiritual level *(nivel espiritual)* is an area of healing that is parallel to the channeling found in New Age groups and in shamanistic healing rituals around the world (Macklin, 1967, 1974a, 1974b, 1974c; Macklin and Crumrine, 1973). Individuals enter an altered state of consciousness and, according to the curanderos, make contact with the spirit world by one or all of the following methods: opening their minds to spirit voices, sending their spirits out of the body to gain knowledge at a distance, and allowing spirits the use of the body to communicate with this world.

The mental level *(nivel mental)* is the least often encountered of the three levels. One healer described working with the mental level as the ability to transmit, channel, and focus mental vibrations *(vibraciones mentales)* in a way that would affect the patient's mental or physical condition directly. Both patients and healers are confident that the curanderos can effect a cure from a distance using this technique.

The three levels are discrete areas of knowledge and behavior, each necessitating the presence of a separate gift for healing. They involve different types of training and different methods of dealing with both the natural and the supernatural world. The material level involves the manipulations of traditional magical forces found in literature on Western witchcraft. Spiritualism involves the manipulation of a complex spirit world that exists parallel to our own and the manipulation of *corrientes espirituales,* spiritual currents that can both heal and provide information or diagnosis from a distance. The mental level necessitates the control and use of the previously mentioned *vibraciones mentales.* Thus the levels are separate methods of diagnosing and treating human problems that are embedded into a single cultural tradition.

Not all problems can be dealt with successfully using each level. An example of this is serious alcohol abuse (Trotter, 1979; Trotter and Chavira, 1978). Alcohol abuse and alcoholism are treated by curanderos using techniques of both the material and the mental level. The techniques of the spiritual level, however, were considered ineffective in dealing with alcohol-related problems. Therefore, if one has the *don* for working with the spiritual level alone, he or she is excluded from the process of curing alcohol problems.

One theme that is common to the practices of all three levels is the use of energy to change the patient's health status. On the material level, this energy often is discussed in relation to the major ritual of that level, known as the *barrida* or *limpia* (a "sweeping" or "cleansing"). In this ritual a person is "swept" from head to foot with an object that is thought to be able either to remove bad vibrations *(vibraciones malos)* or to give positive energy *(vibraciones positives)* to the patient. The type of object used (e.g., egg, lemon, garlic, crucifix, broom) depends on the nature of the patient's problem and whether it is necessary to remove or to replace energy. On the spiritual level, the energy used for both diagnosis and healing is the previously mentioned *corrieiites espirituales.* The mental level is almost totally oriented around generating and channeling *vibraciones mentales.* The following sections provide more detail on the actual practices of the curandero's work on each level.

The Material Level (*Nivel Material*)

The material level is the easiest of the three levels to describe; it is the most extensively practiced and the most widely reported. At this level the curandero manipulates physical objects and performs rituals (or *trabajas,* spells). The combination of objects and rituals is widely recognized by Mexican Americans as having curative powers. Practitioners of the material level use common herbs, fruits, nuts, flowers, animals and animal products (chickens, doves, and eggs), and spices. Religious symbols, such as the crucifix, pictures of saints, incense, candles, holy water, oils, and sweet fragrances, are widely used, as are secular items, such as cards, alum, and ribbons. The curandero allows the patients to rely extensively on their own resources by prescribing items that either are familiar or have strong cultural significance. Thus a significant characteristic of the objects used at the material level is that they are common items used for daily activities such as cooking and worship.

Natural Illnesses and Herbal Cures

Curanderos recognize that illnesses can be brought about by natural causes, such as dysfunction of the body, carelessness or the inability of a person to perform proper self-care, and infection. Curanderos at the material level use large amounts of medicinal herbs *(plantas medicinales)* to treat these natural ailments. Some traditional curanderos classify herbs as having the dichotomous properties considered essential for humoral medicine, based on a hot-cold classification system common throughout Latin America (Foster, 1953). They use these dual properties to prescribe an herb or combination of herbs, depending on the characteristics of the illness. If a person's illness supposedly is caused by excessive "heat," an herb with "cold" properties is given. Conversely, if a person's illness is believed to be caused by excessive "coldness and dryness," a combination of herbs having "hot and wet" properties is administered.

Other curanderos recognize herbs for their chemical properties, such as poisons *(yerba del coyote, Karwinskia humboldtuna Roem. et Sch.),* hallucinogens *(peyote, Lophaphora williams Lem.),* sedatives *(flor de tila, Talia mexicana Schl.),* stimulants *(yerba del trueno),* and purgatives *(cascara sagrada).* These individuals refer to the beneficial chemical properties of the herbs that allow them to treat natural illnesses.

Curanderos prescribe herbs most frequently as teas, baths, or poultices. The teas act as a sort of formative chemotherapy. *Borraja* (borage, *Borajo officialis* L.), for example, is taken to cut a fever; *flor de tila,* a mild sedative, is taken for insomnia; *yerba de la golondrina* (*Euphorbia prostrate* Ait.) is used as a douche for vaginal discharges; and *peilos de elote* are used for kidney problems. Herbal baths usually are prescribed to deal with skin diseases; *fresno* (ash tree, *Fraxinus* species) is used to treat scalp problems such as eczema, dandruff, and psoriasis; and *linaza* is prescribed for body sores. For specific sores such as boils, *malva* (probably a *Malvastrum*) leaves are boiled until soft and then applied to the sores as a poultice. Other herbs are used as decongestants. A handful of *oregano* (oregano, *Oregenum vulgare* L.) is placed in a humidifier to treat someone with a bad cold.

Some herbal lore is passed on as an oral tradition, and other information is available in Spanish-language books for Mexico that are widely circulated among both curanderos and the public (Arias; Wagner). These works describe and classify numerous herbs. Herbal remedies are so important to Mexican American folk medicine that their use often is confused with the art of curanderismo itself by the mass culture. Indeed, some curanderos known as *yerberos* or *yerberas,* specialize in herbs, but their knowledge and skills go beyond the mere connection of one disease to one herbal formula. For curanderos to be genuine, even at the material level, an element of mysticism must be involved in their practice. Herbs are typically used for their spiritual or supernatural properties. Spiritual cleansings *(barridas)* often are given with *ruda (Ruta graveolens L.), romero* (rosemary, *Rosmarinus officianalis* L.), and *albacar* (sweet basil, *Ocimum basiticum* L.), among others. Herbs are used as amulets; *verbena* (verbena, *Verbena officinalis* L.), worn as an amulet, is used to help open a person's mind to learn and retain knowledge.

Some curanderos have successful practices on the material level without resorting to the use of herbs. Some nonherbal treatments are described in the following section.

Supernaturally Caused Illnesses and Ritual Cures

Supernatural illnesses, which occur when supernatural negative forces damage a person's health, sometimes can be confused with natural illnesses. One healer stated that these supernatural illnesses may manifest as ulcers, tuberculosis, rheumatism, or migraine headaches, but in reality, they are believed to be hexes that have been placed on the person by an enemy. Supernatural influences also disrupt a person's mental health and his or her living environment. Physicians cannot cure a supernatural illness. The curandero usually deals with social disruption, personality complexes, and sometimes, serious psychological disturbances. One healer gave the following description of a case that contained several of these elements:

> This patient worked for the street maintenance department of (a small city in south Texas). Every day after work a voice would lead him out into the brush and sometimes keep him there until 2:00 am. This activity was wearing out the man and his family and he was going crazy. A bad spirit was following this man and would not leave him alone. The man was cured, but it took three people to cure him: myself, a friend, and a master *(maestro)* from Mexico. This man was given three *barridas* each day for seven days, one by each of us. The tools used were eggs, lemons, herbs, garlic, and black chickens. The man was also prescribed herbal baths and some teas to drink. He was also given a charm made from the *haba mijrina* designed to ward off any more negative influences which might be directed at him. This patient regained his sanity.

Also, a number of illnesses are both supernaturally caused and of a supernatural nature and can be treated on the material level. The following account is an example of such an illness and cure:

> My brother-in-law was working at a motel . . . in Weslaco. When he started working they laid off this other guy who had been working there for several years. This guy didn't like it, and he's been known to be messing around with black magic. I don't know what he did to my brother-in-law, but every other day he'd have to be taken home because he was sick. He started throwing up, had shaky knees, and weak joints. So my mother and I went over to see this lady in Reynosa, and she told my mother just what to do. My sister rubbed her husband with a lemon every night for three days. She also gave him some kind of tea. . . . On the third day, a big black spot appeared on the lemon, so we threw it away, and he's been fine ever since.

Rituals and the Material Level

Curanderos use several types of rituals for supernatural cures. The *barrida* is one of the most common

rituals. These cleansings are designed to remove the negative forces that are harming the patient, while simultaneously giving the patient the spiritual strength necessary to enhance recovery. Patients are always "swept" from head to toe, with the curandero making sweeping or brushing motions with an egg, lemon, herb, or whatever object is deemed spiritually appropriate. Special emphasis is given to areas in pain. While sweeping the patient, the curandero recites specific prayers or invocations that appeal to God, saints, or other supernatural beings to restore health to the patient. The curandero may recite these prayers and invocations out loud or silently. Standard prayers include the Lord's Prayer, the Apostles' Creed, and *Las Doce Verdades de Mundo* (The Twelve Truths of the World).

The following description of a *barrida* illustrates how the material objects, the mystical power of these objects, the invocations, the curandero, and the patient come together to form a healing ritual designed for a specific patient and a specific illness: In this case, five eggs, four lemons, some branches of *albacar* (sweet basil), and oil were used. To begin the healing process, the lemons and eggs were washed with alcohol and water to cleanse them spiritually. Before beginning the ritual, the participants were instructed to take off their rings, watches, and other jewelry; high-frequency spiritual and mental vibrations can produce electrical discharges on the metal, which might disturb the healing process. The sweeping itself is done by interchanging an egg and a lemon successively. Sweeping with the egg is intended to transfer the problem from the patient to the egg by means of conjures *(conjures)* and invocations *(rechasos)*. The lemon is used to eliminate the *trabajo* (magical harm) that has been placed on the patient. The patient is swept once with *albacar* (sweet basil) that has been rinsed in *agua preparada* (prepared water). This sweeping purifies the patient, giving strength and comfort to his spiritual being. The ritual ends by making crosses with *aceite preparado* (specifically prepared oil) on the principal joints of the patients, such as the neck, under the knees, and above the elbow. This oil serves to cut the negative currents and vibrations that surround the patient, which have been placed there by whoever is provoking the harm. The crosses protect against the continued effect of these negative vibrations. *Agua preparada* is then rubbed on the patient's forehead and occiput *(cerebro)* to tranquilize and to give mental strength. All the objects used in the *barrida* are then burned to destroy the negative influences or harm transferred from the patient.

Another common ritual is called a *sahumerio,* or "incensing." The *sahumerio* is a purification rite used primarily for treating businesses, households, farms, and other places of work or habitation. This ritual is performed by treating hot coals with an appropriate incense. The curandero may prepare his or her own incense or may prescribe some commercially prepared incense, such as *el sahumerio maravilloso* (miraculous incense). A pan with the smoking incense is carried throughout the building, making sure that all corners, closets, and hidden spaces, such as under the beds, are properly filled with smoke. While incensing, the healer or someone else recites an appropriate prayer. If the *sahumerio maravilioso* is used, the prayer often is one to Santa Marta, requesting that peace and harmony be restored to the household. After the *sahumerio,* the healer may sprinkle holy water on the floor of every room in the house and light a white candle that stays lit for 7 days. The *sahumerio* is an example of the curandero treating the general social environment, seeking to change the conditions of the persons who live or work there. Incensing of a house removes negative influences such as bad luck *(salaciones),* marital disruptions, illness, or disharmony. For business and farms, incensing helps ensure success and growth and protects against jealous competitors. These rituals are designed to affect everyone in the environment that has been treated.

Another type of ritual, called a *sortilegio* (conjure), uses material objects such as ribbons to tie up the negative influences that harm the curandero's patients. These negative influences are often personal shortcomings, such as excessive drinking, infidelity, rebellious children, unemployment, or any other problem believed to be imposed by antisocial magic *(un trabajo).* One *sortilegio* that I observed required four ribbons in red, green, white, and black, each approximately 1 yard in length. The color of each ribbon represents a type of magic, which the curanderos can activate to deal with specific problems. Red magic involves domination, green deals with healing, white with general positive forces, and black with negative or debilitating forces.

When working with a specific area of magic, one uses material objects that are the appropriate color naturally or that have been made that color artificially. The color-based division of magic also is carried over into another type of ritual system used on the material level, *velacione,* or burning candles to produce supernatural results. The *velaciones* and the colored material objects used in the *sortilegios* tie into the energy theme that runs throughout curanderismo, because the colors and objects are believed to have specific vibratory power or energy that can affect the patient when activated by the incantations used in conjunction with the objects. For example, blue candles are burned for serenity or tranquility; red candles are burned for health, power, or domination; pink candles are burned for good will; green candles are burned to remove a harmful or negative influence; and purple candles are burned to repel and attack bad spirits *(espiritus obscuros)* or strong magic. Once the proper color of candle has been chosen to produce the proper mental atmosphere, the candles are arranged in the correct physical formation and activated by the *conjuros y rechasos.* If a patient asks for protection, the candles might be burned in a triangle, which is considered to be the strongest formation, one whose influence cannot be broken easily. If they want to dominate someone—a spouse, a lover, or an adversary—the candles might be burned in circles. Other formations include crosses, rectangles, and squares, depending on the results desired (Buckland, 1970).

Another relatively common use of candles is to diagnose problems by studying the flame or the ridges that appear on the melted wax. A patient may be swept with a candle while the healer recites an invocation asking the spirit of the patient to allow its material being to be investigated for any physical or spiritual problems that may be affecting the person. This ritual also can be performed by burning objects used in a *barrida.* Lighting the candle or burning the object after the *barrida* helps the curandero reveal the cause and extent of the patient's problems. Similarly, if a petitioner asks for candling, the wax of the candles burned for the *velacione* may be examined for figures or other messages that point to the source of a patient's problems.

One of the organizing principles of the material level of curanderismo is synchronicity with Christianity in general and the Catholic Church in particular. Special invocations often are directed at saints or spirits to bring about desired results. For example, San Martin de Porres is asked to relieve poverty, San Martin Caballero to ensure success in business, San Judas Tadeo to help in impossible situations, and Santa Marta to bring harmony to a household. Ritual materials used by the Church, such as water, incense, oils, and candles, are extensively used by folk healers. The ways in which these religious objects are used and the theories for their efficacy closely mirror the concepts found within the healing ministry of the Church, which are not incompatible with European witchcraft, from which curanderismo partly derives.

The Spiritual Level *(Nivel Espiritual)*

Curanderos who have the *don* for working on the spiritual level *(nivel espiritual)* of curanderismo are less numerous than those who work on the material level. These practitioners also must go through a developmental period *(desarrollo)* that can be somewhat traumatic. Spiritual practices in communities revolve around a belief in spiritual beings who inhabit another plane of existence but who are interested in making contact with the physical world periodically. Healers become a direct link between this plane of existence and that other world. In some cases the curanderos claim to control these spirit beings, and in other cases they merely act as a channel through which messages pass. Some of these practices are carried out by individual healers, whereas other activities occur in conjunction with spiritual centers *(centros espiritistas)* that are staffed by trance mediums and other individuals with occult abilities. These centers often work through two prominent folk saints: El Niño Fidencio from Northern Mexico and Don Pedrito Jaramillo from southern Texas (Macklin, 1974a, 1974b, 1974c). This trend in visiting spiritualist centers appears to be relatively recent, not having been reported during the 1950s and 1960s by those doing research on Mexican American folk medicine (Clark, 1959; Madsen, 1964; Rubel, 1960, 1966).

The practice of spiritualism rests on "soul concept," a belief in the existence of spirit entities derived from once-living humans. The soul is thought to be the immortal component, the life and personality force of humans, an entity that continues to exist after physical death on a plane of reality separate from the physical world. This concept is important not only to curanderismo but also to the religions and mystical beliefs found in all Western cultures.

The soul is alternatively described by curanderos as a force field, ectoplasm, concentrated vibrations, or group of electrical charges that exist separate from the physical body. It is thought to retain the personality, knowledge, and motivations of the individual even after the death of the body. Under proper conditions the soul is ascribed the ability to contact and affect persons living in the physical world. Although souls occasionally can be seen as ghosts or apparitions by ordinary humans, they exist more often in the spiritual realm previously mentioned. Some people view this realm as having various divisions that have positive or negative connotations associated with them (e.g., heaven, limbo, purgatory, hell). Other people see the spiritual realm as parallel to the physical world. They state that the spiritual is a more pleasant plane on which to live, but few attempt any suicidal test of this belief. One healer commented that "spirits" *(espiritos)* and "souls" *(almas)* are the same thing. These spirits' activities closely parallel their former activities in this world. Because the personality, knowledge, and motivation of the spirits are much the same as they were for the living being, there are both good and evil spirits, spirits who heal and spirits who harm, and wise spirits and fools.

These spirits might communicate with or act on the physical plane. Some have left tasks undone in their physical lives that they want to complete; others want to help or cause harm; and many want to communicate messages to friends and relatives, telling them of their happiness or discontent with their new existence. Therefore, curanderos with the ability to work on the spiritual realm become the link between these two worlds. Some curanderos believe that there are multitudes of spirits who want to communicate with the physical world, and they tend to hover around those who have the *don* to become a medium, waiting for an opportunity to enter their bodies and possess them. This explains the cases of spirit possession in Western cultures. Individuals who become possessed are people with a strong potential to be trance mediums who have not had the opportunity to learn how to control this condition.

The ability to become a medium is thought to be centered in the *cerebro*, that portion of the brain found at the posterior base of the skull. Those with the gift are said to have a more fully developed cerebro, whereas those who do not are said to have a weak cerebro *(un cerebro debil)*. This weakness has no relationship either to the intelligence or to the moral nature of the individual, only to his or her ability to communicate with the spiritual realm. Weak cerebros represent a danger for anyone who wants to become a medium. Only rare individuals demonstrate mediumistic potential spontaneously and can practice as mediums without further training. Therefore, curanderos often test their patients and friends for this gift of healing, and those with the gift are encouraged to develop their ability.

The development of this ability is called *desarrollo* and is a fairly lengthy process that might last from 2 months to more than 6 months initially, with periodic refresher encounters often available from the *maestro* (teacher). *Desarrollo* is a gradual process of increasing an apprentice's contact with the spirit world, giving the apprentice more and more experiences in controlled trances and possessions, as well as the knowledge necessary to develop and protect the apprentice as a spiritualist. The teacher also is responsible for giving the apprentice knowledge at a safe pace. The curandero does not always explain what each sensation means; each person, as he or she develops, becomes more sensitive to the environment. The apprentice must expect to encounter odd sensations, such as bright lights, noises, changes in pressure, and other sensations associated with developing powers. At the end of these *desarrollo* sessions, the conversation reverts to social chatting for some time before the apprentice leaves. This developmental process continues, with variations, until the apprentice is a fully developed medium.

Fully developed mediums control how, where, and when they work, and several options are available to them. Some mediums work alone and treat only family problems (Box 30-1); others might use their abilities only for their own knowledge and gratification. Some mediums work in groups with other mediums or with other persons whom they believe have complementary spiritual or psychic powers. Some mediums work in elaborate spiritual centers (*centros espiritistas*) that are formal churches, often dedicated to a particular spirit (e.g., Fidencio, Francisco Rojas, Don Pedrito Jaramillo). The spiritual centers and the activities surrounding them take on the major aspects of a formalized religion.

Sometimes a trance session is open to more than one person at the same time. This group session can be carried out by a lone curandero but more often is found at spiritual centers. The process of the development of these centers is described elsewhere (Trotter and Chavira, 1975a). Once a temple has been established, it may house from 1 to 20 mediums. The more mediums, the better; otherwise, a medium may have to let his or her body be used by too many different spirits, exhausting them and laying them open to supernatural harm. Larger temples might have four or five *videnntes* (clairvoyants), as well as the mediums, and might be putting several apprentices through *desarrollo* at the same time. Many of the accounts provided to these authors about spiritual healing were from individuals who had had experiences with spiritual temples in Mexico. Some temples were located in *Espinaso,* the home of El Niño Fidencio and a center of pilgrimage for mediums practicing in his name, and others were in urban centers such as Tampico and Mexico City. Large numbers of people make pilgrimages to these healing centers in Mexico to deal with health care problems that they have not resolved in the United States.

One healing center is called *Roca Blanca,* after the spirit that speaks most often in that place. The owner, Lupita, founded it about 30 years ago, after discovering her ability to cure. She was granted permission to practice by a spiritual association. The following report is from a visitor to Lupita's healing center:

> I went to this place simply because I was curious. I was swept with *albacar* and the medium was at my side. While I was being swept, the medium went into trance. The sister who was sweeping me asked the spirit who he wanted to talk to. He said, "with the one you are sweeping." Then, the sister finished sweeping me and directed me to talk with the person who was addressing me. When she (the medium in trance) talked to me, she sounded like a man. He asked me, "Do you know who I am?" I have a cousin who got killed in a place in Tampico. "You must be my cousin," I said. "Yes, exactly, I am your cousin." "Look," he said, "You have come here with your husband." On other occasions I really had been there with my husband, mother and different relatives. "You have come here with your husband because you think he is hexed and that is why he is sick. But that's not true. He has a physical illness that the doctor can cure. Don't believe it's anything bad."
>
> He said, "I'm going to prove who I am by coming to your house. Tell my cousin I'm going to see her." You see, I have a sister who's not nervous at all and who isn't afraid of anything. On Tuesday, as my sister was leaning by the window watching a television show, she felt someone embrace her. She turned and saw no one.

BOX 30-1

Curanderos

Many curanderos able to work on the spiritual level prefer to work at home, alone. Their practices tend to be less uniform than the practices of mediums working at spiritual centers, because they do not have to conform to the calendric and ritual structure found in more formalized temples. However, there is enough commonality to their actions to provide an accurate description of a lone medium. This healer is described by a student in his early 20s who was one of her patients; she had been handling problems for him and his family for several years.

R: Can you describe how this *curandera* works, in as great detail as you can?

S: We drive up into the driveway of a fairly decent-looking place. She walks out and greets us, shakes our hands, asks how we are doing and how we have been. Then we go inside. She's got a small room perhaps 8 by 10 feet. She has an altar with saints and candles and flowers on it. She has a small vase shaped like a crystal ball sitting on a table. Sometimes it has water on it and sometimes turned upside down.

You walk in there and sit down and she's talking with you. She's not in her trance; it's just social talk. Then she sits and puts her hand on that crystal-deal. She taps it, closes her eyes, and she starts asking you what kind of problem you have or whatever you want to ask her.

R: Her voice changes?

S: Yes, it does. It's a lot lower. All of a sudden her voice becomes soft, sort of like whispering. Really mild.

R: Does she keep her hands on the glass all of this time?

S: No. Sometimes she grabs a folder with papers in it and starts writing down things on it, using her finger.

R: Can she read what she has written?

S: I'm pretty sure she can.

R: How does she cure people?

S: She does it in a number of ways. Some time ago my mother had pains on both of her heels. She went to the doctor and the doctor didn't find anything wrong. So she went over to this lady again who said it was something (a *trabajo* or hex) that [a woman across the alley from his house] had put in the yard. When my mother's out hanging up clothes she's barefooted and she stepped on it. And that's what was hurting her. So the *curandera* gave her a "shot" on her arm like a regular shot. And that cured her.

R: How did she give her the shot?

S: (Simulated the action of giving an injection without a syringe or hypodermic.)

R: Could your mother feel it?

S: She told me she didn't. But it cured her.

The informant went on to tell of several other cures that this curandera had performed for his family. She had prescribed herbs, suggested the use of perfumes to ward off the *envidia* (envy) of their neighbors, and suggested that the mother perform a series of *barridas* on her son-in-law to remove a hex against him that was making him ill and keeping him from work. Each of these cures could just as easily have been suggested or performed by a curandero working on the material level of curanderismo, but this curandera did it from a trance state. Therefore, what sets this curandera apart from those working strictly on the material level is not the tools she uses or the rituals she suggests to her clients, but the source of her diagnosis and cure—her contact with a spirit world.

These spiritual centers vary according to their size, their owners, and the spirits who are associated with them, but there is considerable regularity in the services they perform. Sometimes mediums prescribe simple herbal remedies for physical problems. These recipes are virtually identical to the ones presented in the previous section on the material level, although, occasionally, it is said that a spirit will recommend a new use for an herb. The mediums might suggest that the patient perform the already familiar rituals of curanderismo, such as the *barrida*. The spirits are thought to be able to influence people's lives directly, in addition to imparting knowledge about remedies. The curanderos state that spirits control spiritual currents (*Corrientes espirituales*) and mental vibrations (*vibraciones mentales*); they can manipulate the patient's health by directing positive or negative forces at them from the spiritual realm.

During spiritual sessions observed at a developing spiritual center in southern Texas, a spirit repeatedly presented himself over the course of several weeks to treat several patients. One of these patients was a man with lower back pain. One week the spirit told him to buy a bandage and bring it to the next session. The man did so, but then the spirit chided him for not following instructions correctly. The bandage was too narrow and not long enough. The man was instructed to buy a new bandage and place it on the window ledge to catch the morning dew, which is thought to have healing properties. He then was to place a glass of water under the head of his bed and a jar of alcohol at the side of the bed. He was to wrap himself in the bandage according to given instructions and lie quietly on his bed for no less than 2 hours, during which time the spirit promised to visit him and complete the cure. The man followed these instructions and stated that he did gain relief from his back pain. The same spirit treated a young college girl who periodically had asthma attacks. The girl's mother, a regular member of the group, brought her to the session. The spirit, in the person of the medium, stood and clasped the girl's head with one hand on her *cerebro* and the other on her forehead, sending *Corrientes espirituales* through her brain. The spirit then told her to take a sip of *agua preparada* and sit back down in the circle. The treatment was successful in overcoming this particular attack, and the mother mentioned after the session that these cures relieved her own asthma for several months.

Another patient requested a social and emotional treatment. Her husband recently had begun to practice witchcraft *(btujeria),* and she was worried that he or his friends might attack her or members of her family. A considerable amount of tension existed between the couple's families. She felt under continual stress and had gone to a doctor for help. The physician prescribed a mild sedative, which she had taken for 3 weeks without relief. The medium's spirit probed her mind and told her to take three sips of *agua preparada* to break any spells that had been cast on her. The spirit promised to provide her with protection and help from the spiritual realm to counteract anything that her husband might do. She appeared to be content with the spirit's activities on her behalf and was greatly relieved.

Several aspects of the spiritual level have not been covered in this brief description but are described in more detail elsewhere (Trotter, 1975). These aspects include the actual techniques of testing for *el don,* the physical and supernatural dangers of trance mediumship, the acquisition of spiritual protectors to overcome those dangers, detailed descriptions of the trance state from the subjective perspective of the developing medium and the objective perspective of an observer, and finally, the existence and purpose of mediums' associations.

The Mental Level *(Nivel Mental)*

Conducting observational, descriptive, and experimental research on the practices of the mental level has proved to be the most difficult task in exploring all the aspects of curanderismo. The mental level has the fewest rituals and the least outward complex behavior associated with it. To date, it has the fewest practitioners, which severely limits the number of people who could be approached for an opportunity to investigate the phenomenon. All the cases the author observed followed a similar pattern. For example:

> After the curandero chatted with the patient and asked them about the basic problem, he asked the patient to state her complete name *(el nombre completo).* The curandero wrote the name on a piece of paper. Sitting behind the desk he used for consultations, he leaned his arms on the desk, bent forward slightly, closed his eyes, and concentrated on the piece of paper. After a few minutes, he opened his eyes, told the patient more about his or her problem, and stated that it was being resolved.
>
> The curandero stated that he had learned to use his mind as a transmitter through *desarrollo.* He could channel, focus, and direct *vibraciones mentales* at the patient. These mental vibrations worked in two ways—one physical, one behavioral. If he was working with a physical illness, such as cancer, he channeled the vibrations to the afflicted area, which he already had pinpointed, and used the vibrations to retard the growth of damaged cells and accelerate the growth of normal cells. In a case of desired behavioral changes, he sent the vibrations into the person's mind and manipulated them in a way that modified the person's behavior. The curandero gave an example of one such case in which a husband had begun drinking excessively, was seeing other women, was being a poor father to his children, and was in danger of losing his job. The curandero stated that he dominated the man's thought processes and shifted them so that the husband stopped drinking to excess, and became a model husband and father (Trotter, 1981, p. 473).

There also are a number of syncretic beliefs drawn from other alternative healing traditions—such as New Age practices, the "psychic sciences," and Eastern philosophy—that have been incorporated into this area of curanderismo. For example, some healers state that they are able to perceive "auras" around people and that they can use these auras to diagnose problems that patients are encountering. They conduct the diagnosis on the basis of the color or shape of the patient's aura. Some state that they learned these practices from other healers, whereas others indicate that they learned them from books on parapsychology.

The mental level is practiced most often by individual healers working with individual patients, rather than in groups. It appears to be a new addition to this healing system and does not have, as yet, a codified body of ritual associated with it. It therefore constitutes an area in which additional descriptive work will be necessary to unify healers' behavior.

Theoretical Unification

The three levels of curanderismo unify the theories of disease and illness found in the Mexican American folk medical model. They create a framework for determining the therapeutic approaches of curanderos in southern Texas. The system emphasizes a holistic approach to treatment and relies heavily on the intimate nature of the referral system and the extensive personal knowledge of the patient's social environment that is normally held by the curandero. Christian symbols and theology provide both tools (candles, incense, water) and organization models (rituals, prayers, animistic concepts) for the material and the spiritual levels, but not to a similar degree for the mental level. An *energy* concept is the central idea that integrates the three levels and forms a systematic interrelationship among them. This energy concept derives from belief in forces, vibration, and currents that center in the mind of those who have the gift for healing and that can be transmitted to cause healing from a distance, by affecting the patient's social, physical, spiritual, or psychological environment.

All three levels of healing are still evolving. The variations in the practices of curanderismo can be explained partly by differences in the curanderos' personality, differences in their treatment preferences or abilities, and differences in their emphasis on theoretical or experiential approaches. There also are variations produced by individual interpretations of an underlying body of theory. A study of these variations would be useful, now that the underlying theoretical

system provides a common starting point and common objectives.

SETTINGS FOR CURANDERISMO HEALING SYSTEM

Curanderismo is a community-based healing system. It is complex and widespread. At one level, it may be practiced in any area where Mexican Americans know about it. Part of this healing tradition is the information that is spread throughout the Mexican American culture on home treatments for common physical ailments (colds, flu, arthritis, asthma, diabetes) and for common spiritual or "folk illnesses" (*susto, mal de ojo,* and *empacho*). This is analogous to the biomedical information that is spread throughout all European cultures, including the Mexican American culture, where the home is the first line of defense for the diagnosis of illnesses that eventually might necessitate a physician or hospital. On the other hand, some aspects of curanderismo require the use of special locations, preparations, and tools. This is especially true of spiritual practices on the spiritual level and for the effective treatment of supernatural harm on the material level.

The first setting where this knowledge is used is at home. When people become ill, they use their existing cultural model of health and illness to come up with solutions. One type of solution is home diagnosis and home treatment. Therefore, both biomedical concepts and folk medical concepts are applied immediately, and home treatments are attempted. In the case of curanderismo, this often results in the use of home remedies (*remedio caseros*) that have been part of the culture for generations, especially herbal cures. When the diagnosis identifies a magical or supernaturally caused illness, the illness results in a home-based ritual. These interventions are done by mothers, grandmothers, cousins, friends, or knowledgeable acquaintances.

Illnesses that appear to be too serious to handle at home, both natural and supernatural, are taken to professional healers who have a locally widespread reputation for being able to treat both biomedical and traditional health care problems. Most of these healers work in a silent, but positive, partnership with physicians, although the physicians often are unaware of the link. The curanderos interviewed in various studies of Mexican American folk medicine are consistent in their positive regard for modern medicine. They consistently refer patients to modern health care services, where they see the efficacy of that approach to be equal to or greater than their own. At the same time, they note significant differences in the models of health and illness between their own practices and modern medicine, especially in the areas of supernatural illnesses, in addressing social (marital, business, interpersonal) problems and in dealing with psychological problems. In these cases the treatments take place either in the patient's home or work environment or in special workrooms established by the curanderos as part of their practices. The cure might call for working directly in the environment that is affected. In other cases the venue of choice is the curandero's area because the cure depends on careful preparation and protection from outside influences. These work areas contain altars, medicinal plants, tools for supernatural rituals, and other items, and the atmosphere is considered most beneficial for the healing process, particularly in the case of supernatural problems and treatments (Trotter and Chavira, 1981).

RESEARCH AND EVALUATION APPROACHES

The research that is available on curanderismo is broad in interest and historical depth. Unlike specific healing techniques, such as acupuncture, which can be studied in relation to specific illnesses with relative ease, curanderismo is a complex brew of both theoretical approaches to healing and an interrelated set of healing techniques. The techniques range from herbal cures, which must be approached from an ethnopharmacological perspective; to rituals, which can be studied symbolically as projective psychiatric techniques; to methods such as massages, natural birth, nutritional prescriptions, and dietary practices. Some studies have investigated the scientific efficacy of the practices of curanderismo, whereas others have approached it from a sociopolitical or symbolic viewpoint. Some practices have not been studied at all. Therefore, although the efficacy of some parts of the system is clearly defined, other parts remain to be explored.

Early research on curanderismo can be found in the classic anthropological works on Mexican American folk medicine, published primarily in the 1960s (Clark, 1959a; Currier, 1966; Kiev, 1968; Madsen, 1961, 1964; Romano, 1965; Rubel, 1960, 1964, 1966). These authors produced descriptive baseline data on the prominent folk medical practices of Hispanic communities in the United States. They provide an initial view of curanderismo that is rich in descriptions of Mexican American folk illnesses, such as *susto, empacho, mal de ojo, caida de mollera, bilis,* and *espanto* (Nail and Speilberg, 1967). These works generally treat traditional healing in Mexican American communities as a body of knowledge that is widely distributed throughout the culture, rather than as a theoretical healing system. Therefore the works consider the consensual data on what is available to a significant segment of the existing Mexican American population but spend less time describing the professional actions of curanderos, because these mass cultural phenomena are generally thought of as having themes or unifying elements rather than a theoretical structure. This viewpoint is well represented in articles about curanderismo and its form and function within Mexican American communities (Clark, 1959b; Edgerton, et al., 1970; Foster, 1953; Martinez and Martin, 1966; Torrey, 1969).

Later research maintains the strengths of this approach but adds folk theoretical concepts. Early epidemiological approaches to folk illnesses give an idea of the geographical spread and variation in beliefs, illnesses, and healing rituals, whereas later studies identify or discuss the common denominators that unify curanderos: their underlying perception of illness. Traditional anthropological research techniques were used to gather the data for these studies, primarily participant observation and interviewing over prolonged periods. Most of the authors used personal networks to identify individuals who were known locally as healers. Emphasis often was placed on finding individuals who were full-time healers rather than talking to those who treated only family members and neighbors. Therefore a curandero can be defined as an individual who is recognized in his community as having the ability to heal, who sees an average of five or more patients a day, and who has knowledge of and uses the theoretical structure described in this chapter. These people can be viewed as both specialists and professionals. Several areas of curanderismo have received a considerable amount of research attention.

Home Remedies

Herbal and chemical treatments for both natural and supernatural illnesses are common in Mexican American communities. More than 800 *remedios caseros* have been identified on the U.S.-Mexican border alone (Trotter, 1981a, 1981b). Many of the remedies have been tested for biochemical and therapeutic activities (Etkin, 1986; Trotter, 1981, 1983; Trotter and Logan, 1986). Overall, the remedies are not only biochemically active; more than 90% have demonstrated therapeutic actions that matched the folk medical model for their uses. At the same time, only a small proportion of the herbs have been tested. This lack of information is being overcome by an ongoing project to study the efficacy of the complete range of herbal cures available in Mexican American communities (Graham, 1994), by use of combined ethnographic and biomedical methods (Browner et al., 1988; Croom, 1983; Ortiz de Montellano and Browner, 1985; Trotter, 1985).

The exceptions to the general rule of efficacy are the use of remedies for illnesses such as the common cold, where the remedies relieve symptoms but do not directly treat the illness. The actions of these remedies, some of which are described earlier, include diuretics, treatments for constipation, abortifacients, analgesics, sedatives, stimulants, cough suppressants, antibacterial agents, coagulants and anticoagulants, vitamin and mineral supplements, and plants with antiparasitic actions. Most have proved safe and effective when used in the manner described and recommended by the curanderos. This area and the therapeutic, culturally competent counseling practices of the healers are the most clearly acceptable and useful approaches for articulation with modern medicine.

Additional Information on Epidemiology of Folk Illnesses

Of all the complex areas of Mexican American traditional healing, the one that has received the most research attention has been the study of common folk illnesses that are experienced and treated in Mexican American communities. The most frequently reported are *susto,* an illness caused by a frightening event; *mal de ojo,* an illness that can be traced to the Near East, which involves a magically powerful glance taking away some of the vital essence of a susceptible person; *empacho,* a blockage of the intestines caused by eating the wrong type of food at the wrong time or by being forced to eat unwanted food; and *caida de la mollera,* a condition of fallen fontanelle in infants. A number of others also are well defined, if not as commonly studied, but these four receive most of the research attention.

The epidemiology and the cognitive models of these illnesses have been well documented (Rubel, 1964; Trotter, 1982, 1985; Weller et al., 1993). These illnesses have been studied both singly and in combination (Baer et al., 1989; Logan and Morrill, 1979; Rubel et al., 1984; Weller et al., 1993), in terms of their cognitive structure within and between Hispanic cultural groups, their frequency of treatment, belief and mention in various communities, and their relationships to medical conditions and to the treatment of medical conditions (Collado-Ardon et al., 1983; Trotter, 1991; Trotter et al., 1989). In the case of *susto,* clear evidence indicates that it is linked directly to serious morbidity patterns in Latin American communities and acts as an excellent indicator that biomedical personnel should investigate multiple conditions and problems among patients complaining of its symptoms. *Caida de la mollera,* on investigation, is a folk medicine label that corresponds to severe dehydration in infants caused by gastrointestinal problems. It is life threatening and, when identified by parents, is an excellent indicator that the child should be brought in immediately for medical care. *Empacho* is a severe form of constipation based on its description and is treated with numerous remedies that cause diarrhea. Because it is thought to be a blockage of the intestines, the purgative effect of these remedies signals that treatment has been effective. To date, no studies have linked *mal de ojo* to any biomedical condition; however, because the symptoms include irritability, lethargy, and crying, some connection may be made in the future.

Healing and Psychiatry

Another area of significant endeavor in curanderismo is the identification of parallels and areas of compatibility between the processes and rituals of curanderismo and the use of psychiatry in cross-cultural settings (Kiev, 1968; Klineman, 1969; Torrey, 1969; Trotter, 1979; Velimirovic, 1978). The parallels are clear, especially when healers concentrate on psychological conditions that they recognize from their knowledge of psychology and psychiatry. A number of successful collaborations have been conducted in this area between traditional healers and individuals from modern medical establishments in several states.

Unexpected Consequences

It is clear that Mexican American folk medicine contains a very high ratio of useful, insightful, and culturally competent healing strategies that work well in Hispanic communities. As seen previously, these range from proven herbal cures to therapeutic models to culturally important labeling systems that can help physicians identify the cultural labels for certain types of biomedical problems. The complexity of curanderismo ensures that these findings will increase.

At the same time, no health care system exists that does not have side effects and unexpected results. With allopathic medicine, these range from the birth defects of thalidomide to dreadful side effects of chemotherapy and the limited ability of psychology to deal with chronic mental health conditions such as alcohol and drug abuse. In curanderismo, allopathic conditions are not the bulk of its use, and a few unexpected consequences have been discovered in treating *empacho* (Baer and Ackerman, 1988; Baer et al., 1989; Trotter, 1983b). These occurrences are rare but must be taken into account and understood within the overall cultural context of curanderismo and within the context of the much more pervasive positive benefits that the communities derive from having these alternative health care practices available.

With the complexity and the diversity of practices within this traditional healing system, there remains a great deal of useful and insightful research that can be conducted beneficially in relation to curanderismo.

Acknowledgments

The initial phase of the research findings reported by the author was supported by a grant from the Regional Medical Program of Texas (RMPT Grant No. 75-108G). Further efforts at data collection were supported by the Texas Commission on Alcoholism, Pan American University, and the author himself.

References

Alger N, editor: The Curandero-Supremo. In *Many answers,* New York, 1974. West Publishing.

Arias HyF, Costas: *Plantas medicinales,* Biblioteca Practica, Mexico.

Baer R, Ackerman A: Toxic Mexican folk remedies for the treatment of empacho: the case of azarcon, greta and albayalde, *Ethnopharmacology* 24:31-39, 1988.

Baer R, Garcia de Alba DJ, Cueto LM, et al: Lead based remedies for empacho: patterns and consequences, *Soc Sci Med* 29(12):1373-1379, 1989.

Browner CH, Ortiz de Montellano BR, Rubel AJ: A new methodology for ethnomedicine, *Curr Anthropol* 29(5):681-701, 1988.

Buckland R: *Practical candle burning,* St Paul, Minn, 1970, Llewellyn Publications.

Clark M: *Health in the Mexican American culture,* Berkeley, 1959a, University of California Press.

Clark M: Social functions of Mexican-American medical beliefs, *Calif Health* 16:153-155, 1959b.

Collado-Ardon R, Rubel AJ, O'Nell CW: A folk illness (susto) as indicator of real illness, *Lancet* 2:1362, 1983.

Croom EM: Documenting and evaluating herbal remedies, *Econ Botany* 37(1):13-27, 1983.

Currier RL: The hot-cold syndrome and symbolic balance in Mexican and Spanish American folk medicine, *Ethnology* 4:251-263, 1966.

Edgerton RB, Karno M, Fernandez I: Curanderismo in the metropolis: the diminished role of folk psychiatry among Los Angeles Mexican-Americans, *Am J Psychiatry* 24:124-134, 1970.

Etkin N, editor: *Plants used in indigenous medicine: biocultural approaches,* New York, 1986, Redgrave Publications.

Foster GM: Relationships between Spanish and Spanish-American folk medicine, *J Am Folklore* 66:201-247, 1953.

Galvin JAV, Ludwig AM: A case of witchcraft, *J Nerv Ment Dis,* 1961, pp 161-168.

Graham JS: Mexican American herbal remedies: an evaluation, *Herbalgram* 31:34-35, 1994.

Holland WR: Mexican-American medical beliefs: science or magic? *Arizona Med* 20:89-102, 1963.

Hudson WM: The healer of Los Olmos and other Mexican lore, *Texas Folklore Soc* XXIV, 1951.

Ingham IM: On Mexican folk medicine, *Am Anthropol* 42:76-87, 1940.

Jaco EG: Social factors in mental disorders in Texas, *Soc Probl* 4(4):322-328, 1957.

Kiev A: *Curanderismo: Mexican American folk psychiatry,* New York, 1968, Free Press.

Klineman A: Some factors in the psychiatric treatment of Spanish-Americans, *Am J Psychiatry* 124:1674-1681, 1969.

Macklin J: *El Niño Fidencio: un estudio del Curanderismo en Nuevo Leon,* 1967, Anuario Huminitas, Centro de Estudios Humanisticos, Universidad de Nuevo Leon.

Macklin J: Santos folk, curanderismo y cullos espiritistas en Mexico: eleccion divina y seleccion social, *Anuario Indigenista* 34:195-214, 1974a.

Macklin J: Folk saints, healers and spirit cults in northern Mexico, *Rev Interamericana* 3(141):351-367, 1974b.

Macklin J: Belief, ritual and healing: New England spiritualism and Mexican American spiritism compared. In Zaretsky IT, Leone MP, editors: *Religious movements in contemporary America,* Princeton, NJ, 1974c, Princeton University Press.

Macklin J, Crumrine NR: Three north Mexican folk saint movements, *Comp Studies Soc History* 15(1):89-105, 1973.

Madsen C: A study of change in Mexican folk medicine, *Mid Am Res Inst* 25:93-134, 1965.

Madsen W: Shamanism in Mexico, *Southwest J Anthropol* 11:48-57, 1955.

Madsen W: Society and health in the Lower Rio Grande Valley, Austin, Texas, 1961, Foundation for Mental Health, Hogg.

Madsen W: *The Mexican Americans of South Texas,* New York, 1964a, Holt, Rinehart & Winston.

Madsen W: Value conflicts and folk psychotherapy in South Texas. In Kiev A, editor: *Magic, faith and healing,* New York, 1964b, Free Press, pp 420-440

Martinez C, Martin HW: Folk diseases among urban Mexican-Americans, *JAMA* 196:161-164, 1966.

Nall FC, Speilberg J: Social and cultural factors in the responses of Mexican-Americans to medical treatment, *J Health Soc Behav* 7(1):299-308, 1967.

Ortiz de Montellano BR, Browner CH: Chemical basis for medicinal plant use in Oaxaca, Mexico, *J Ethnopharmacol* 13:57-88, 1985.

Romano O: *Don Pedrito Jaramillo: the emergence of a Mexican-American folk saint,* Berkeley, 1964, University of California (PhD dissertation).

Romano O: Charismatic medicine, folk-healing, and folk sainthood, *Am Anthropol* 67:1151-1173, 1965.

Rubel AJ: Concepts of disease in a Mexican-American community in Texas, *Am Anthropol* 62:795-814, 1960.

Rubel AJ: The epidemiology of a folk illness: Susto in Hispanic America, *Ethnology* 3:268-283, 1964.

Rubel A: *Across the tracks: Mexican-Americans in a Texas City,* Austin, 1966, University of Texas Press.

Torrey FE: The case for the indigenous therapist, *Arch Gen Psychiatry* 20(3):365-373, 1969.

Torrey FE: *The mind game: witch doctors and psychiatrists,* New York, 1972, Bantam Books, Emerson Hall.

Trotter RT II: Evidence of an ethnomedical form of aversion therapy on the United States-Mexico border, *J Ethnopharmacol* 1(3):279-284, 1979a.

Trotter RT II: *Las yerbas de mi abuela (grandmother's tea),* San Antonio, 1979b, Institute of Texas Cultures (slide series, filmstrip).

Trotter RT II: *Don Pedrito Jaramillo,* San Antonio, 1981a, Institute of Texas Cultures (slide series, filmstrip).

Trotter RT II: Folk remedies as indicators of common illnesses, *J Ethnopharmacol* 4(2):207-221, 1981b.

Trotter RT II: Remedios caseros: Mexican American home remedies and community health problems, *Soc Sci Med* 15B:107-114, 1981c.

Trotter RT II: Contrasting models of the healer's role: South Texas case examples, *Hispanic J Behav Sci* 4(3):315-327, 1982a.

Trotter RT II: Susto: within the context of community morbidity patterns, *Ethnology* 21:215-226, 1982b.

Trotter RT II: Azarcon and Greta: ethnomedical solution to an epidemiological mystery, *Med Anthropol Q* 14(3):3-18, 1983a.

Trotter RT II: Community morbidity patterns and Mexican American folk illness: a comparative approach, *Med Anthropol* 7(1):33-44, 1983b.

Trotter RT II: Ethnography and bioassay: combined methods for a preliminary screen of home remedies for potential pharmacologic activity, *J Ethnopharmacol* 8(1):113-119, 1983c.

Trotter RT II: Greta and Azarcon: unusual sources of lead poisoning from Mexican American folk medicine, *Texas Rural Health J,* May-June, 1983d, pp 1-5.

Trotter RT II: Letter to the editor: Greta and Azarcon: two sources of lead poisoning on the United States-Mexico border. *J Ethnopharmac* 8(1):105-106, 1983e.

Trotter RT II: Greta and Azarcon: a survey of episodic lead poisoning from a folk remedy, *Health Care Hum Organization* 44(1):64-71, 1985.

Trotter RT II: A survey of four illnesses and their relationship to intracultural variation in a Mexican American community, *Am Anthropol* 93:115-125, 1991.

Trotter RT II, Chavira JA: *The gift of healing.* A monograph on Mexican American folk healing, Edinburg, Texas, 1975a, Pan American University.

Trotter RT II, Chavira JA: *Los Que Curan* (South Texas Curanderismo), 1975b (43-minute color 16-mm film).

Trotter RT II, Chavira JA: Alcohol abuse, 1978.

Trotter RT II, Chavira JA: *Curanderismo: Mexican American folk healing system,* Athens, 1981, University of Georgia Press.

Trotter RT II, Logan M: Informant consensus: a new approach for identifying potentially effective medicinal plants. In Etkin N, editor: *Plants used in indigenous medicine: biocultural approaches,* 1986, Redgrave Publications, pp 91-112.

Trotter RT II, Ortiz de Montellano B, Logan M: Fallen fontanelle in the American Southwest: its origin, epidemiology, and possible organic causes, *Med Anthropol* 10(4):201-217, 1989.

Velimirovic B, editor: Modern medicine and medical anthropology in the United States-Mexico border population, Scientific Publication No 359, Washington, DC, 1978, Pan American Health Organization.

Wagner F: *Remedios caseros con plantas medicinales,* Hermanos, SA, DF Medicina, Mexico.

Weller SC, Pachter LM, Trotter RT II, Baer RM: Empacho in four Latino groups: a study of intra- and inter-cultural variation in beliefs, *Med Anthropol* 15(2):109-136, 1993.

Suggested Readings

Baca J: Some health beliefs of the Spanish speaking, *Am J Nurs* 69:2171-2176, 1969.

Bard CL: Medicine and surgery among the first Californians, *Touring Topics,* 1930.

Bourke IH: Popular medicine customs and superstitions of the Rio Grande, *J Am Folklore* 7:119-146, 1894.

Capo N: *Mis observaciones clinicas sobre el limon, el ajo, y la cebolla,* Ediciones Natura.

Cartou LSM: Healing herbs of the Upper Rio Grande, Santa Fe, 1947, Laboratory of Anthropology.

Chavez LR: Doctors, curanderos and brujos: health care delivery and Mexican immigration in San Diego, *Med Anthropol Q* 15(2):31-36, 1984.

Comas J: Influencia indigena en la Medicina Hipocratica, en la Nueva Espana del Sigio XVI, *America Indigena* XIV(4):327-361, 1954.

Creson DL, McKinley C, Evans R: Folk medicine in Mexican American subculture, *Dis Nerv Syst* 30:264-266, 1969.

Davis J: Witchcraft and superstitions of Torrance County, *NM Histor Rev* 54:53-58, 1979.

Dodson R: Folk curing among the Mexicans. In *Toll the bell easy,* Texas Folklore Society, 1932, Southern Methodist University Press.

Esteyneffer J de SJ: Florilegio medicina vide todos las enfermedades, acadodevarios, y clasicos autores, para bien de los pobres y de los que tienen falia de medicos, en particular para las provincial remotas en donde administran los RRPP, Mexico, 1711, Misioneros de la Compania de Jesus.

Esteyneffer J de SJ: Florilegio medicinal o oreve epidomede las medicinas y cirujia: la primera obra sobre esta ciencia impresa en Mexico en 1713, Mexico, 1887.

Fabrega H Jr: On the specificity of folk illness, *Southwest J Anthropol* 26:305-315, 1970.

Farfan A: *Tratado breve de medicina: obra impresa en Mexico por Pedro Orcharte en 1592 y ahora editada en facimil,* Coleccion le Incinables Americanos, vol X, Madrid, 1944, Ediciones Cultura Hispanica.

Gillin J: Witch doctor? A hexing case of dermatitis, *Cutis* 19(1):103-105, 1977.

Gobeil O: El susto: a descriptive analysis, *Int J Soc Psychiatry* 19:38-43, 1973.

Gudeman S: Saints, symbols and ceremonies, *Am Ethnol* 3(4):709-730, 1976.

Guerra Fmonardes: Diologo de Hierro. Compania Fundido de Fierro y Acero de Monterrey, SA, Mexico. Los Cronistas-Hispanoamericanos de la Materia Medicina Colonial al Professor Dr Teofilo Hernando por sus amigos y in Homenaje o discipulos, SA, Madrid, 1961, Libreria y Casa Editorial Hernando.

Hamburger S: Profile of Curanderos: a study of Mexican folk practitioners, *Int J Soc Psychiatry* 24:19-25, 1978.

Jaco EG: Mental health of the Spanish-American in Texas. In Upler MK, editor: *Culture and mental health,* New York, 1959, Macmillan.

Johnson CA: Nursing and Mexican-American folk medicine, *Nurs Forum* 4:100-112, 1964.

Karno M: The enigma of ethnicity in a psychiatric clinic. A paper presented at the Southwestern Anthropological Association Annual Meeting, UCLA, April 16, 1965.

Karno M: Mental health roles of physicians in a Mexican-American community, *Community Ment Health J* 5(1), 1969.

Karno M, Edgerton RB: Perception of mental illness in a Mexican-American community, *Arch Gen Psychiatry* 20:233-238, 1969.

Kay M: Health and illness in the barrio: women's point of view, Tucson, 1972, University of Arizona (PhD dissertation).

Kay M: The fusion of Utoaztecan and European ethnogynecology in the florilegio medicinal. Paper presented at Medical Anthropology Symposium, XLI International Congress of Americanists, Mexico City, Mexico, 1974a.

Kay M: Florilegio medicinal: source of southwestern ethnomedicine. Paper presented at Society for Applied Anthropology, Boston, 1978; Parallel, Alternative, or Collaborative: Curanderismo in Tucson. In Velimirovic B, editor: *Modern medicine and medical anthropology in the United States-Mexico border population,* Scientific Publication No 359, Washington, DC, 1974b, Pan American Health Organization.

Klein J: Susto: the anthropological study of diseases of adaptation, *Soc Sci Med* 12:23-28, 1978.

Kleinman A: Culture, illness, and care: clinical lessons from anthropological cross-cultural research, *Ann Intern Med* 88:251-258, 1978.

Kreisman JJ: Curandero's apprentice: a therapeutic integration of folk and medical healing, *Am J Psychol* 132:81-83, 1975.

Langner TS: *Psychophysiological symptoms and the status of women in two Mexican communities: approaches to cross-cul-*

tural psychiatry, Ithaca, NY, 1965, Cornell University Press, pp 360-392.

Macklin J: Current research projects: Curanderismo among Mexicans and Mexican-Americans, New London, Conn, 1965, Connecticut College.

Madsen N: Anxiety and witchcraft in Mexican-American acculturation, *Anthropol Q,* 1966, pp 110-127.

Maduro R: Curanderismo and Latino views of disease and curing, *West J Med* 139:868-874, 1983.

Marcos LR, Alpert M: Strategies and risks in psychotherapy with bilingual patients, *Am J Psychiatry* 113(11):1275-1278, 1976.

Marin BV, Marin G, Padilla AM: Utilization of traditional and nontraditional sources of health care among Hispanics, *Hispanic J Behav Sci* 5(1):65-80, 1983.

Martinez C Jr, Alegria D, Guerra E: El Hospital Invisible: a study of Curanderos, Department of Psychiatry, University of Texas Health Science Center at San Antonio.

Montiel M: The social science myth of the Mexican-American family, *El Grito* 3:111, 1970.

Morales A: Mental health and public health issues: the case of the Mexican Americans in Los Angeles, *El Grito* 3:111(2), 1970.

Moustafa A, Weiss G: *Health status and practices of Mexican-Americans,* Berkeley, 1968, University of California Graduate School of Business.

Moya B. Superstitions and beliefs among the Spanish-speaking people of New Mexico, Albuquerque, 1940, University of New Mexico (master's thesis).

Padilla AM: *Latino mental health: bibliography and abstracts,* Washington, DC, 1973, US Government Printing Office.

Paredes A: *Folk medicine and the intercultural jest in Spanish-speaking people in the U.S.,* Seattle, 1968, University of Washington Press, pp 104-119.

Pattison M: Faith healing: a study of personality and function, *J Nerv Ment Dis* 157:397-409, 1973.

Press I: The urban Curandero, *Am Anthropol* 73:741-756, 1971.

Press I: Urban folk medicine, *Am Anthropol* 78(1):71-84, 1978.

Romano O: Donship in a Mexican-American community in Texas, *Am Anthropol* 62:966-976, 1960.

Romano O: The anthropology and sociology of the Mexican-American history, *El Grito* 2, 1969.

Rubel AJ: Ethnomedicine. In Johnson TM, Sargent CF, editors: *Medical anthropology: contemporary theory and methods,* New York, 1990, Praeger, pp 120-122.

Rubel AJ, O'Neil CW: Difficulties of presenting complaints to physicians: Susto illness as an example. In Velimirovic B, editor: *Modern medicine and medical anthropology in the United States-Mexico border population,*

Scientific Publication No 359, Washington, DC, 1978, Pan American Health Organization.

Ruiz P, Langrod J: Psychiatry and folk healing: a dichotomy? *Am J Psychiatry* 133:95-97, 1976.

Samora J: Conceptions of disease among Spanish Americans, *Am Cath Soc Rev* 22:314-323, 1961.

Sanchez A: *Cultural differences and medical care: the case of the Spanish-speaking people of the Southwest,* New York, 1954, Russell Sage Foundation.

Sanchez A: The defined and the definers: a mental health issue, *El Sol* 4:10-32, 1971.

Saunders L, Hewes GW: Folk medicine and medical practice, *J Med Educ* 28:43-46, 1953.

Smithers WD: Nature's pharmacy and the Curanderos, Alpine, Texas, 1961, Sul Ross State College Bulletin.

Snow LF: Folk medical beliefs and their implications for care of patients, *Ann Intern Med* 81:82-96, 1974.

Speilberg J: Social and cultural configurations and medical cure: a study of Mexican-American's response to proposed hospitalization for the treatment of tuberculosis, 1959, University of Texas (master's dissertation).

Trotter RT II: A case of lead poisoning from folk remedies in Mexican American communities. In Fiske S, Wulff R, editors: *Anthropological Praxis,* Boulder, Colo, 1978a, Westview Press.

Trotter RT II: Discovering new models for alcohol counseling in minority groups. In Velimirovic B, editor: *Modern medicine and medical anthropology in the United States-Mexico border population,* Scientific Publication No 359, Washington, DC, 1978b, Pan American Health Organization, pp 164-171.

Trotter RT II: Folk medicines and drug interactions, *Migrant Health Newsline* 3(171):3-5, 1986.

Trotter RT II: Folk medicine in the Southwest: myths and medical facts, *Postgrad Med* 78(8):167-179, 1986.

Trotter RT II: Caida de mollera: a newborn and early infancy health risk, *Migrant Health Newsline,* 1988.

Trotter RT II: The cultural parameters of lead poisoning: a medical anthropologist's view of intervention in environmental lead exposure, *Environ Health Perspect* 89:79-84, 1990.

Trotter RT II, Chavira JA: Curanderismo: an emic theoretical perspective of Mexican American folk medicine, *Med Anthropol* 4(4):423-487, 1980.

Unknown Jesuit: *Rudo Ensayo,* Tucson, 1951, Arizona Silhouettes Publication (Original 1763 by J Nentuig).

Uzzell D: Susto Revisited: illness as a strategic role, *Am Ethnol* 1(2):369-378, 1974.

Weclew RV: The nature, prevalence and levels of awareness of "Curanderismo" and some of its implications for community mental health, *Community Ment Health J* 11:145-154, 1975.

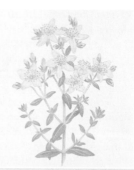

CHAPTER

31

SOUTHERN AFRICAN HEALING AND PROFESSIONALIZATION

M A R I A N A   H E W S O N

We waited patiently for the healer to call us for the interview. The waiting room was small, containing only six chairs and a dresser. Prepared with the specified money and gift, we reviewed our questions, the way in which the interpretation would be handled, and how our notes would be taken. Eventually, the traditional healer appeared in full regalia: copious strands of white beads around her neck, wrists, and ankles; decorative strands of animal skins hanging from her waist; her legs clad in animal skins decorated with beads, shells, and beer bottle tops; and an impressive headdress (much like a bishop's miter) made of cowhide. She had several ceremonial tools, highly decorated with intricate beadwork: a fly whisk (made of a cow tail) to signify the healer's status, a long-handled spear for slaughtering animals, and a smoking pipe and drum that she used to contact ancestral spirits. Two younger apprentices in more modest dress stayed close at her side and ministered to her needs. To initiate my interview, I put the required fee (about $20) plus a gift on the floor of the waiting room. One of the apprentices burned a local dried plant, *bepo*, in an open dish, and the master healer ceremonially smoked her long pipe to invoke the spirits to be present in our conversation. She tipped a little ash onto the money and gifts to bless them, a necessary part of developing our relationship (Hewson, 1998).[*]

---

[*]This interview was one of eight similar interviews with female traditional healers in southern Africa.

In this chapter, I outline the professional components of traditional African healing based on interviews with traditional healers (Hewson, 1998). The value of studying a phenomenon outside of one's own culture is to identify aspects of one's own culture that are not readily apparent to those who practice within that culture.

PROFESSIONALISM AND THE HEALING ARTS

Is traditional African healing a profession? In the Western view the medical profession consists of specialists who diagnose and prescribe in areas that draw on comprehensive knowledge and skills that transcend those available to non-specialists. Education for the professions involves questions about legitimate knowledge, license to practice, arrangements for providing services, entry to education and training, the curriculum offered, standards of achievements, and assessment (Goodlad, 1984). Similarly, Cassidy describes professional considerations of a health care system in Chapter 4 of this volume. Following Cassidy's categories, I discuss (1) the explanatory model of illness that underlies traditional healing in southern Africa, (2) the educational process of healers, (3) the professional accreditation of the practitioners, (4) the professional organization of practitioners who monitor and maintain standards of care, and (5) the social mandate through which the community influences the provision of care. Finally, I highlight unique aspects of traditional healing that can transcend both the traditional and the allopathic system of healing.

EXPLANATORY MODEL UNDERLYING TRADITIONAL HEALING IN SOUTHERN AFRICA

Concepts of Health, Illness, and Healing

Traditional healing in southern Africa existed long before the arrival of modern medicine, and it remains an intact system of caregiving among many African people. This system of healing is shamanic in nature.

The term *shaman* refers to medicine men and women, and *shamanism* is a methodology (not a religion) used to describe the practices of healers in the regions of central and north Asia. Shamanism represents "the most widespread and ancient methodological system of healing known to humanity" (Harner, 1990, p. 40). This practice, including assumptions and methods, occurs all over the world, in areas as diverse as Australia, New Zealand, North and South America, Siberia, Central Asia, eastern and northern Europe, and Africa. In all these regions, the shaman is seen as "the great specialist of the human soul: he alone 'sees' it, for he knows its 'form' and its destiny" (Eliade, 1964, p. 8). Shamanic practitioners generally make use of "non-ordinary reality" or controlled entrancement, to access the information they seek on behalf of their patients.

Africa, in particular southern Africa, is thought to be the "cradle of mankind," but little has been written about the traditional healers of southern Africa. Traditional healers in southern Africa are not called "shamans," yet their practices are similar to those described by Eliade (1964) and Harner (1990). At present, their ancient practices coexist in a modern society that subscribes to and practices allopathic medicine. Despite regional differences throughout southern Africa, there appears to be a common system aimed to relieve illness and disease (feelings of being "out of sorts," or ill at ease socially and spiritually).

In the southern African view, illness is thought to be caused by psychological conflicts or disturbed social relationships with persons living or dead. The accompanying disequilibrium is expressed as physical or mental problems (Frank, 1973). Traditional healers believe that psycho-social-spiritual imbalances must be rectified before a patient can recover physically. Traditional healing thus focuses on psychological and spiritual suffering, as well as on physical suffering, and aims to correct the disequilibrium. Traditional healers view healing as the removal of impurities from the body or disequilibrium from the patient's mind, with the hope of reducing the anxieties it has produced. For example, a common concept of healing involves purification by draining the body of harmful substances, resulting in wide use of purgatives and emetics. Healing also involves appeasing the patients' spirits (in particular the recently departed members of the family), who might be angry with the patient for some reason. Warding off bad spirits, such as the *tokoloshe* (a mischievous or evil spirit responsible for life's misadventures and accidents), the curses from living people, or the ill will of angry ancestral spirits constitutes a version of preventive medicine. Furthermore, in several southern African groups, such as the Basotho of Lesotho, the state of disequilibrium manifests in the form of being "hot" (not feverish) (Hewson and Hamlyn, 1985), and treating people who are "hot" involves cooling with appropriate agents such as ash, water plants, or aquatic animals. These views are quite distinct from modern allopathic medical concepts of disease as the malfunctioning of physiological systems.

Traditional Healing Processes

Traditional healers hold an esteemed and powerful position in modern African societies, and their role is a combination of physician, counselor, psychotherapist, and priest. Traditional healers prevent and treat illnesses mainly with plant and some animal products in combination with divination. There are two types of traditional healers: those who are mainly herbalists and those who use divination. However, the distinction between the two is becoming increasingly blurred, and most traditional healers appear to practice both types of medicine. Sorcery (evil or malevolent doctoring) is practiced by some healers in southern Africa but is not considered further in this chapter.

Traditional healers appear to work most successfully with illnesses that have a high psychological or emotional content related to envy, frustration, or guilt (Frank, 1973). In allopathic medicine, these might be called *somatic illnesses*. Currently, healers also appear to concentrate on illnesses for which allopathic medicine has little effective curative power, such as stroke, tuberculosis, cancer, and human immunodeficiency virus and acquired immunodeficiency syndrome (HIV/AIDS). Traditional healers claim to be effective in helping to treat pregnancy, malaise, arthritis, and social problems, especially those involving interpersonal disputes. All the healers seemed to be able to distinguish between those illnesses that need to be helped by Western medicine (e.g., broken bones, hernias) and those that respond to traditional healing. The claims to heal illnesses such as stroke, cancer, and HIV/AIDS appear to relate to the psychosocial and emotional components of the illness rather than the pathological or pathophysio-

logical conditions. For example, traditional healers make no claims to be able to deal directly with bacterial or viral impurities, but rather with the patient's ability to cope with and eliminate them. This view of healing suggests that if one takes care of the psychodynamics of illness, the body will heal. This is in contrast to the modern view that if one takes care of the body, the mind will heal itself (Hewson, 1998).

As part of the diagnostic process, traditional healers "throw the bones." The "bones" consist of a set of 10 to 15 items, such as bones and shells and various collectibles (e.g., dice, coins, bullets, domino pieces). These are usually "thrown" (like dice) in the belief that clues to the problem can be read in the configuration of the items. The "bones" are made up of an idiosyncratic collection of items that have attributed meanings, depending on the context and the meaning attributed by particular healers. Each item signifies an important aspect of a person's life (e.g., happiness, children, bad luck, ancestral spirits). The consistencies among these items are in the attributions of the items rather than in the items themselves. For example, a traditional healer from Mozambique had a red die signifying war (the country had experienced a civil war for many years), and a healer from South Africa had a bullet signifying death or misfortune (South Africa was, at that time, engulfed in violence).

Traditional healers use drumming and dance to augment the diagnostic and therapeutic processes. Drumming helps the healer enter non-ordinary reality. Similarly, frenzied dance has the same effect. In non-ordinary reality, healers use their dreams as manifestations of the higher wisdom of the spirits, especially their ancestors. The healers use their own spiritual powers, as well as those of the patient, to discern causes of the patient's spiritual, psychological, or social disequilibrium that cause physical ailments and bad luck To encourage their own dreams, healers wash with herbal solutions, drink herbal potions, smoke a pipe, or use snuff (all of which appear to have psychotropic effects).

Healers prepare and prescribe therapeutic herbal remedies for their patients. A traditional healer must know the symptoms of a disorder and the conditions of the patient's life before prescribing a treatment. There is a lack of uniformity, however, about the prescribed remedies for particular illnesses. A medicine may be used for multiple problems. The actual prescription depends on the spiritual advice received by the healer through normal dreams and through the dreams of non-ordinary reality or entrancement. Each prescription is driven by the particulars of the patient and the details of the situation in which the patient became ill. The lack of a systematic, generalized approach to healing promotes individualistic practices that often seem idiosyncratic to Westerners. This phenomenon is one of the reasons African traditional healing remains so baffling and inscrutable to Western scientists.

Traditional healers seek causes for illness from a variety of areas. The common areas concern relationships with family, friends, and people at work. Healers are especially concerned about disturbed relationships involving jealousy, anger, loss, grief, and resentment. They seek to identify possible causes of illness from the following situations: someone wishes the patient ill; the patient wants something he or she does not or cannot have; the patient has known or unknown enemies; the patient experiences unrequited love or loss of a loved one; the patient has an unfaithful spouse or partner; the patient longs for progeny; and the patient's ancestors (the "recently departed") may be displeased with the patient for some reason, known or unknown. The healer inquires into every aspect of a patient's present and past activities, focusing on behaviors that would be most likely to provoke conflict with others in the community or even internal psychological conflict (e.g., in personal values). This is a process of divination commonly referred to as "seeing." A healer must "see" forward into the future as well as backward into the past. The process is similar to that used by shamans around the world (Harner, 1990). Although southern African healers do make some use of totemic animal spirits, their emphasis is mainly focused on the spiritual forces of the "recently departed" family members. These ancestors are the source of key information and are powerful forces in the lives of their living family members.

If the divination process does not provide immediate answers, the process may take longer. In this situation the healer may say, "The bones are not talking today," and request subsequent visits. When healers cannot find an answer to the patient's problems, they will refer the patient to another traditional healer or to a Western physician. All healers are concerned with truth and trust in their relationship with a patient. If the healer discerns a lack of either, he or she will ask the patient to leave.

EDUCATIONAL PROCESS

Selection: the Call to Be a Healer

Traditional healers are "called" to become healers and need to be verified by the group's elders, who check whether the call is real or not. First, the future healer experiences an unusual, mysterious illness that does not respond to usual herbal or allopathic treatment. Some examples recounted by my respondents included heart problems, lung problems, abdominal pain, swollen abdomen unrelated to pregnancy, amenorrhea, problems with feet, dizziness, headaches, mental problems (e.g., forgetfulness), pains throughout the body, and "fevers that are not real fevers" (which may relate to the cultural metaphor of being "hot"; see Hewson and Hamlyn, 1985).

The illness is often followed by dreams with significant, recognizable components. The future healer then asks his or her elders (e.g., parents, aunts, uncles, grandparents) about the dreams. If an elder recognizes the special components of the dream, the elder advises the future healer to consult a traditional healer. At the discretion of the traditional healer, the patient is then both treated and taken as an apprentice for several years. A traditional healer named Emily tells how she was called by her ancestral spirits to be a healer (Hewson, in preparation):

> First I was sick for a whole year, like I didn't know where I was, like becoming mad, my mind wasn't working properly. I felt pains everywhere and I didn't know what to do. I was forgetful. I forgot what I did the day before, like washing dishes, and I felt like sitting alone and no one should come near me. I went to the doctors and they could not see what the problem was with me. Then I had a dream. In my sleep I saw three grand people, old people, sitting next to me. One was holding a bible. My father's mother was holding beads in a dish and some bones—little bones—with two hands. And my mother's father was holding a bible. They said to me I must wear a white dress. And I dreamed I was in this big hall and on the other side was a church. The people were dancing and preaching. And in the hall the *sangomas* and *nyangas* [widely used terms for traditional healers in southern Africa] were dancing and beating drums. And I said "What kind of a dream is this?"
>
> Then I told my aunty that I had this kind of funny dream. I described the old people and she said they really were my grand people who I had

never seen before in life. And she called another woman [a healer], and I told her this same dream. Then she took me to the river and prayed and talked to my old people [ancestral spirits] who are called *amanyangas*. And then she prayed there for me and I took the water. She made beads for me and put them round my neck, and then I was alright. I never got sick again.

A second healer, Elizabeth, described her sickness (headaches and fevers that were not really fevers) followed by a dream in which her ancestor came to her and told her to go to the forest to find herbs. This she did and encountered a man, sitting in the light, who instructed her. This dream was interpreted as being a call to be a healer. A third healer described her mysterious sickness and said that she went to consult a healer, who made a mixture of stringy roots mixed with a grated rhizome-like substance in water. Using a twig as a mixer, this solution created a profusion of bubbles. The future healer was asked to drink the bubbles by her trainer, which induced dreams that "helped me see what I should do to help people." She used the same techniques for inducing the spirits in her apprentices.

To refuse the calling by the ancestors is to invite worse sickness, madness, and possible death. One healer recounted the story of a woman who had denied the call and had become "mad." A man in Cape Town, a renowned drunkard, believed he was being called to be a healer, but the elders of his family disabused him of this idea, saying that his dreams and sickness were the consequence of alcohol.

Training

Training involves an apprenticeship, usually with a well-known master healer. If the master healer lives far away, the apprentices live in his or her master healer's compound (many small dwellings inhabited by extended family members) for the duration of the training. The art of the healer is thought to be transmitted through the ancestral spirits who speak to healers through dreams. Apprentices are encouraged to have dreams and to learn how to interpret them on behalf of their patients. Dreams can be induced by herbal potions, inhaled smoke, or snuff. As one traditional healer put it, "Through the dreams, your ancestors open your eyes to signs. I trust the dreams every time." Another said that anyone can learn about the practice of traditional healing, but "unless you have contact with the spirits through dreams, you cannot be a healer."

The master healer first demonstrates the use of herbs and animal parts and then teaches the apprentices how to administer them. Then, in a progressive weaning process, the master healer withdraws and expects the apprentices to perform independently. One healer described being taken into the bush by her teacher to find *muti* (medicinal substances, such as herbs, roots, and barks, and animal parts, such as hooves, bones, and horns) that are used for healing. She had to rise at 4:30 AM "because the spirits only come early in the morning." She had to prepare herself to obtain the *muti* by bringing on the ancestral spirits. This she did by taking a herbal bath, drinking herbal concoctions, beating the drums, and dressing with a special outfit.

The training process is strenuous and challenges the mental and physical strength of the apprentices. One healer said, "I went to the bush for many days with my teacher to seek *muti*, with only *putu* [cornmeal porridge] and black tea. It was hard to live like that, but it is necessary for *nyangas* to suffer because this kind of work is *swarig*" (Afrikaans word for "heavy" or "burdensome"). Because this process is so exacting, not every apprentice completes the training.

Apprentices help their master healers with patient consultations, seemingly acting as a team for the duration of the training program. On one occasion I observed an apprentice and master healer in a Lesotho mountain village who entered a trancelike state in which both danced with extremely rapid movements to the accompaniment of drums. In a trancelike state, they called on the ancestors and revealed spiritual insights to the assembled small crowd (Hewson, 1993).

PROFESSIONAL ACCREDITATION OF PRACTITIONERS

Tests and Standards

Throughout training, apprentices are tested on their ability to find things, to identify and administer herbs, and to contact the ancestors through dreams to discern people's physical, psychological, or spiritual problems. Some of the objects to be found become part of the divining "bones," and others are used as medicines. The items that are needed are often given to the apprentice by patients, friends, or family members in recognition of the demonstrated healing skills and power of the apprentice. The master healer may also help the apprentices find things they need. For example, one healer described how, on occasions, the very item she had been instructed to find would be given to her by someone, apparently in a serendipitous manner (McCallum, 1992). Another described how she went to the beach with her teacher and collected the perfect shells for her set of "bones." Other objects must be gleaned from the countryside, found in the bush, or purchased from stores that specialize in the healers' equipment and accoutrements.

Several levels of tests must be passed by the apprentice healers. Tests of competence may involve oral examinations. For example, one healer described how her master healer asked all the apprentices in her cohort "to stand like a choir" and to answer numerous questions. Then, each apprentice was asked to declare whether he or she was able to cure.

The final test often involves finding a hidden object. For her final test, one healer had to find an unknown object that had been hidden somewhere in the vicinity of a village (McCallum, 1992). The final test also involves "finding" the animal(s) that will be slaughtered as part of the graduation ceremony, such as a chicken, goat, or cow. The procurement of these animals may involve gifting the apprentice's family, friends, or satisfied patients and is an additional social accreditation that represents faith and trust in the apprentice as a healer.

An apprentice graduates when the master healer is satisfied that he or she has passed all the tests; that, through dreams, the ancestral spirits have confirmed the apprentice's readiness; and that the apprentice has paid the stipulated fees, including procuring the necessary animal(s) for slaughter. The master healer consults his or her own ancestral spirits concerning the sufficiency of each apprentice's knowledge. When all the criteria have been satisfied, the master healer may give each apprentice a gift, such as a set of bones or a braided bracelet. Thus, both the teacher and the apprentice, and indirectly the community, assess the readiness for graduation. Patients also play a part in this judgment through their gifts.

More importantly, the ancestral spirits indicate, through dreams, when a trainee is ready. One healer explained that she knew that she was ready to graduate when she had a dream in which her ancestor (grandfather) "sent me to a *rondavel* [Afrikaans for 'small round dwelling'] that had a half door made of glass. There was a man standing behind the door who asked, 'What do you want here? I don't know what you are doing here any more.'" Then she heard the words coming from behind her: "Go and help people." At this point, she went through the final graduation ceremony, collected all her medicines and divining tools, and traveled back to her home, some 300 miles away.

Graduation often involves a final test of slaughtering an animal with the ceremonial spears. The apprentice drinks the animal's blood and selects various body parts, such as pieces of hoof or bone, to become part of his or her healer's tools *(bones)* or as *muti*. For example, the skin of the slaughtered goat may be used as the mat for throwing bones, the animal's stomach may be used as a pouch for carrying other medicine, or a vertebra may become part of the divining tools. The rest of the animal is then consumed by the community to celebrate the occasion.

PROFESSIONAL ORGANIZATION: MONITORING STANDARDS OF CARE

Continuing Education

Traditional healers engage in meetings with other healers. One group described meetings that occurred on weekends, in which they would assemble, fully dressed in their ceremonial costumes (clothing, wigs, necklaces, anklets), to discuss healing matters, to share their latest healing stories, and to compare notes. The group may collectively criticize certain healers for dangerous or unwise practices. The regular meetings also include singing, dancing, drumming, drinking herbal potions, and engaging the ancestral spirits. The meetings appear to be important social events in the lives of traditional healers.

The business of traditional healers includes their formal organization (South African healers are now organized and provide their healers with certificates), their practice in the context of new diseases (e.g., HIV/AIDS), and their relationship with Western medicine. The World Health Organization (WHO) has recognized traditional healers in Mozambique and elsewhere, and traditional healers are being increasingly recognized and incorporated into the general medical system.

Ongoing Relationships with Teachers

Traditional healers typically maintain a lifelong relationship with their master healers, who serve as mentors. These relationships appear to be deep and profound. One healer from Maputo in southern Mozambique returned approximately once a year to visit her teacher in northern Mozambique. These visits were casual in nature, and the master healer might teach "depending on his mood. If he is not happy he doesn't teach anything!" This particular healer had trained five of her own apprentices, and she used the same methods as those used by her own teacher. She liked to teach, but reflected that to be a teacher, "You have to be happy all the time," suggesting the essential relationship between teacher and learner involves enthusiasm and effort.

Mutual Caring

Mutual caring among healers becomes necessary under stressful or strained conditions, especially death. According to one healer, when a patient dies, the traditional healer becomes spiritually contaminated and loses his or her healing powers because the relationship with the patient has been broken and the healer, of necessity, grieves. In this situation the healer removes his or her necklaces, ceremonial clothes, and artifacts and does not practice as a healer. This afflicted healer must be treated by another healer in a purification ceremony that restores the healing powers.

The role of being a traditional healer does have dangers. Healers may practice in a team context, which provides them with a measure of protection in terms of the accuracy of their diagnoses and treatments. Team practice also protects a healer against the malevolent practices of other healers or sorcerers in this competitive field.

SOCIAL MANDATE: COMMUNITY INFLUENCE ON PROVISION OF CARE

Community control is exerted through remuneration and accreditation systems. Traditional healers are paid according to the type of service they provide. For straightforward dispensing of *muti,* patients pay over-the-counter fees for the medicines they receive. For diagnosis of physical, psychological, social, or spiritual problems, the patient must first "open his or her pockets" and pay a flat fee at the beginning of the process. This amount is prorated on the approximate cost of one head of cattle and appears to be approximately one sixth of the total cost. When cured, the patients must pay an additional fee that appears to be independent of time spent or for medicines but is measured in proportion to the patient's satisfaction with the care, the cure, or both. Thus a moderately satisfied patient might provide a modest offering, such as food bought from a store (sugar, flour, or vegetables) or picked from a vegetable garden, whereas a highly satisfied patient might offer a live animal, such as a chicken or a goat. This offering would be ceremonially slaughtered at a later date. In urban areas, money is the usual mode of payment. The amount of money is often a loose translation of the worth of a cow, goat, sheep, chicken, pumpkin, and so on.

For training services, an apprentice needs to pay a relatively large fee, equivalent to at least one head of cattle, and must also provide the animal(s) for the graduation ceremony. Apprentices are helped in paying the required fees by other people (patients, friends, family members) who pay or provide necessary items in proportion to their belief in the healing powers of the apprentice. This linking of the payment, patient satisfaction, and the accreditation process provides a complex system of checks and balances in an otherwise unregulated training system.

The healers referred to their own satisfaction in terms of "happiness." For example, one healer said that "to heal someone is to give life to that person," and when the person is healed, "both the traditional healer and the patient become happy." This happiness is manifest at a celebration in which the food offered is consumed in thanksgiving for the healing and for the continued goodwill of the spiritual beings whose power over the living is great.

UNIQUE ASPECTS OF TRADITIONAL HEALING

Differences between traditional and allopathic professionalism are summarized in Tables 31-1 and 31-2. Despite these differences, interesting phenomena characterize traditional healing and the professional training of the healers that are important to the fundamental, perhaps archetypal, contract between healer and patient.

Spiritual Context of Healing

Spiritual powers are loosely defined within African cosmology as those spiritual powers that derive ultimately from God (within the African worldview) and that are present in decreasing amounts through the various levels of spirits of the ancestors (the forefathers) and the "recently departed" family members, living people, animals, vegetation (e.g., trees), and the earth itself (Mbiti, 1969).

Traditional healing deals with spiritual powers that are manifest through an integrated conception of body and mind at all levels. For example, in the call to be a healer, the person experiences a mysterious physical illness and has dreams that reveal a connection with ancestral spirits. In the training process the apprentice learns both the physical skills of an herbalist and the spiritual skills of interpreting problems through dreams that involve the ancestral spirits. When traditional healers graduate, the tests involve knowledge and skills in both herbal medicine and spiritual healing.

Truth and Trust in the Healer-Patient Relationship

The traditional system of healing in southern Africa is consistent with the worldview of the people indigenous to this region. This worldview constitutes a paradigm that emphasizes some ways of thinking (e.g., the body-mind connection) and deemphasizes others (e.g., the objective, rational scientific approach). To be effective, traditional healing requires that patients who seek healing within this paradigm must subscribe to it. Thus, traditional healers are cautious in

TABLE 31-1

Steps to Becoming a Professional in Traditional Healing and in Western Medicine

Step	Traditional Healing	Western Medicine
Call to healing	Mysterious illness, significant dreams, interpreted and sanctioned by elders in community	Individual, personal "call" to become a clinician, family suggestion, augmented by academic counseling
Selection of trainees	Based on mysterious illness and recognizable evidence of healing capability and spiritual power	Based on standardized test scores, essay(s), and interviews with medical school personnel
Training	Rigorous, prolonged, relatively expensive; emphasis on subjective witness of healing powers by patients and/or trainers	Rigorous, prolonged, expensive; emphasis on objective measures of competence designed by professional boards
Accreditation	Approval by master healer, community members, and guidance from ancestral spirits	Approval on basis of national test scores in certifying/licensing examinations
Continuing education	Regular and frequent meetings and celebrations with other healers, and regular ongoing communication with trainer	Regular and frequent conferences, with regulated continuing medical education (CME) accreditation
Professional relationships	Lifelong relationship with trainer and ongoing relationships with colleagues	Occasional mentors, ongoing relationships with professional colleagues, especially focused on research

TABLE 31-2

Characteristics of the Practice of Traditional Healing and Western Medicine

Step	Traditional Healing	Western Medicine
Concepts of curing the patient	Take care of the mind and the body will take care of itself.	Take care of the body and the mind will take care of itself.
Diagnosis	Use spiritual powers and psychological techniques involving non-ordinary reality to "see" causes of spiritual, psychological, or social disequilibrium.	Use technological and scientific tools to recognize directly or indirectly the pathology or pathophysiology. Use clinical reasoning and evidence-based medicine.
Prevention	Very important to ward off negative spirits and harmful circumstances.	Increasing importance of preventive medicine.
Treatment	Resolve disequilibrium and return person to harmonious state.	Treat the biological causes of disease.
Relationship to patient	Subjective, interpersonal involvement, counselor, confessor.	Objective, scientific, rational, clinical relationship.
Relationship to community and individual patients	Paternalistic relationship based on healers' spiritual and social status and reputation.	Paternalistic relationship based on clinicians' accreditation level, social status, and reputation.
Professional satisfaction and rewards for healing	Directly linked with patient satisfaction and monetary payment or "in kind" gifts.	Indirectly linked with patient satisfaction; salary negotiated with health care organization.

checking the adherence of patients to their traditional African way of thinking. In addition, there is the "dark side" to this practice: malevolent sorcery. For similar reasons that benevolent traditional medicine is effective, sorcery is powerful and greatly feared. Traditional healers need to discern the intentions of their patients, and they are alert to desires for "dirty witch doctoring." If a patient is thought to be untruthful or distrustful, the healer will send the patient away.

Psychosocial Medical Model and Interpersonal Communications

Based on the central premises concerning the connection between body and mind and between the earthly and spiritual realms, traditional healing is a form of integrated bio-psycho-social healing. The role of the healer is to "see" the cause of the problem that afflicts the patient, and this "seeing" includes spiritual dimensions. The healers pay close attention to the ways in which their patients describe their illnesses and to the contexts within which the illnesses occur. Healers concentrate on looking for signs that indicate the reasons for the disequilibrium that causes sickness. The holistic approach allows traditional healers to integrate body-mind phenomena and to provide healing, despite being extremely limited in terms of modern medical science.

Patients Contribute to Accreditation of Professionals

In the training of traditional healers, patients have the opportunity to play a role in certifying the apprentice through the voluntary gifts they make. To the extent that patients believe they are healed by a particular healer, they gift that healer. These gifts are often in the form of materials needed in the practice, for example, a special necklace or a medicine pouch. These gifts may be worn to signify the healing power of the particular healer.

Establishment of Lifelong, Mentoring Relationship

Traditional healers in southern Africa appear to engage in lengthy apprenticeships with one master healer. Although the length of training may last from one to many years, the relationship with the master healer does not end at graduation. Instead, these relationships are treasured and maintained for life, which suggests that trainees benefit from the deeper, more sustained relationships, similar to those in traditional apprenticeships. The cross-fertilization of styles and standards of practice takes place at regular meetings of traditional healers. These gatherings can be seen as analogous to Grand Rounds and national and regional conferences.

Apprenticeship Methods

The apprenticeships of traditional healers initially involve being shown how to do things (e.g., to recognize herbs, to interpret dreams) through role modeling and coaching. As the apprentices become more competent, the master healer allows them more independence and takes on a role more akin to that of an evaluator, in which the apprentice is tested for knowledge and skills and for evidence of the power of healing. At the same time the teacher personally rewards the apprentice with small, highly desired gifts that are needed as part of the prescribed collection of accoutrements (e.g., divining "bones," various medications). In addition, the apprentice might wear some of the gifts from the master healer as a visible testament to the healer's skills.

This apprenticeship style of teaching is effective in developing professional competence. It makes use of several teaching approaches, such as role modeling (performing so that the learner can see what the teacher does) and coaching (helping the learner by providing assistance as well as feedback). The strategies also include experiential learning throughout the training process, such as collecting and preparing herbs and animals for medicines and helping with all patients seen by the master healer. The apprentices are expected to do much of the work around the master healer's practice, which includes helping the master healer to dress in ceremonial clothes, often involving an elaborate ensemble of beads, skins, necklaces, anklets, and headdresses, as well as gathering and carrying the items needed for healing processes.

Hardship as a Necessary Part of Professional Training

The training of traditional healers is strenuous because the practice of medicine is difficult. Healers are expected to lead a lifestyle characterized by a high level of personal and social responsibility, and their training is thus a test of physical and mental endurance. The requirement for this type of physical and mental testing is also present in the cultural initiation rites that take place at puberty for boys and girls in southern African cultures. Indeed, in Xhosa, the word for a healer-in-training is *mkweta,* which is the same word used for young boys and girls who undergo initiation.

CONCLUSION

In the practice of traditional medicine in southern Africa and the training of these traditional healers, there are substantial differences between this tradition and Western practice and healers. However, although traditional healers lack the science and power of modern medicine, they are highly effective in a way that has stood the test of time for 20,000 to 30,000 years. As in modern medicine, the knowledge and skills of traditional healers are based on empirical experiences, and interesting similarities exist in the professional training of the practitioners. These similarities may reduce the negative perceptions of traditional healers and offer possibilities for a synergism between the two traditions, with potential mutual benefits for both types of healers, for the training of these healers, and for the ultimate benefit to patients.

Acknowledgments

The author thanks Thomas Lang for his earlier suggestions concerning this topic.

References

Eliade M: *Shamanism: archaic techniques of ecstasy,* Bollingen Series LXXVI, Princeton, NJ, 1964, Princeton University Press.

Frank JD: *Persuasion and healing: a comparative study of psychotherapy,* Baltimore, 1973, Johns Hopkins University Press, pp 46-77.

Goodlad S, editor: *Education for the professions: quis custodiet . . . ?* Guildford, UK, 1984, Society for Research in Higher Education, NFER-Nelson.

Harner M: *The way of the shaman,* San Francisco, 1990, Harper & Row.

Hewson MG: Training in the traditional arts: some thoughts, *Medical Encounter* 9(3):3-4, 1993.

Hewson MG: Traditional healers in southern Africa, *Annals of Internal Medicine* 128:1029-1034, 1998.

Hewson MG, Hamlyn D: Cultural metaphors: some implications for science education, *Anthropol Educ Q* 16:31-46, 1985.

Mbiti JS: *African religions and philosophy,* ed 2, London, 1969, Heinemann Educational Books.

McCallum TG: *White woman witchdoctor: tales from the African life of Rae Graham,* as told by Rae Graham, Miami, 1992, Fielden Books.

Suggested Readings

Cassel EJ: *The nature of suffering and the goals of medicine,* New York, 1991, Oxford University Press.

Ngubane H: Clinical practice and organization of indigenous healers in South Africa. In Feierman S, Janzen JM, editors: *The social basis of health and healing in Africa,* Los Angeles, 1992, University of California Press.

INDEX

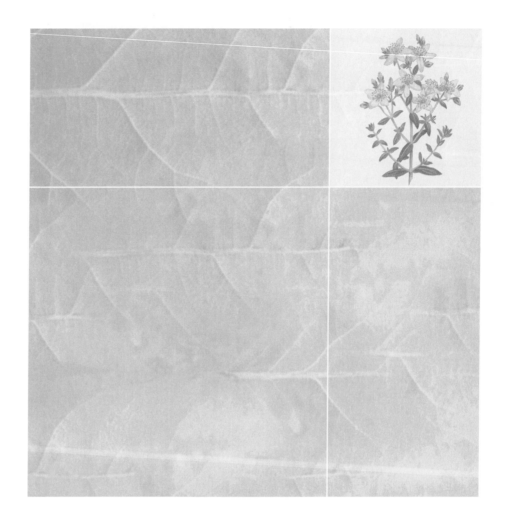

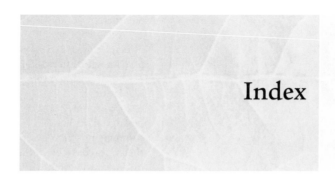

Index

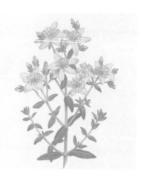

Page numbers with "t" denote tables; those with "f" denote figures; and those with "b" denote boxes